D1582287

HAM'S HISTOLOGY

NINTH EDITION

HAM'S HISTOLOGY

David H. Cormack, Ph.D.

Associate Professor of Anatomy
Department of Anatomy
Faculty of Medicine
University of Toronto
Toronto, Canada

J. B. Lippincott Company

Philadelphia

London•Mexico City•New York•St. Louis•São Paulo•Sydney

Acquisitions Editor: David Barnes
Sponsoring Editor: Richard Winters
Manuscript Editor: Margaret E. Maxwell
Indexer: David H. Cormack
Art Director: Tracy Baldwin
Design Coordinator: Susan Hess Blaker
Production Supervisor: J. Corey Gray
Production Coordinator: Kathleen R. Diamond
Compositor: TAPSCO, Inc.
Printer/Binder: R. R. Donnelley & Sons Company

1 3 5 6 4 2

Library of Congress Cataloging-in-Publication Data
Ham, Arthur W. (Arthur Worth), DATE
   Ham's histology.
   Rev. ed. of: Histology/Arthur W. Ham,
David H. Cormack. 8th ed. c1979.
   Includes bibliographies and index.
   1. Histology.   I. Cormack, David H.   II. Title.
III. Title: Histology.   [DNLM: 1. Histology.
QS 504.3 H198h]
QM551.H147   1987   611′.018   86-30535
ISBN 0-397-50681-3

HARPER INTERNATIONAL EDITION
ISBN 0-06-320159-3

The authors and publisher have exerted every effort to ensure that
drug selection and dosage set forth in this text are in accord with
current recommendations and practice at the time of publication.
However, in view of ongoing research, changes in government
regulations, and the constant flow of information relating to drug
therapy and drug reactions, the reader is urged to check the package
insert for each drug for any change in indications and dosage and
for added warnings and precautions. This is particularly important
when the recommended agent is a new or infrequently employed
drug.

Marking the centennial of the incorporation of the Department of
Anatomy into the Faculty of Medicine at the University of Toronto.
                                                              —*D.H.C.*

PREFACE

The major role of a histology course in the medical curriculum is to provide an initial basic understanding of many different aspects of the internal structure and function of the body. This textbook therefore presents a comprehensive survey of many of the complex interrelationships that exist between the structure and the function of cells and tissues. Other aspects of histology explore the respective origins, proliferative behavior, and various interactions of the 200 or so cell types that, together with their respective cell products, make up the human body. The medical relevance of a detailed study of the body tissues will probably become more apparent as the medical student approaches his clinical training, because in many ways histology sets the stage for subsequent studies of abnormal structure and function.

A number of outstanding advances in biomedical research have had a major impact on the subject matter and teaching of histology since the eighth edition of *Ham's Histology* was published. Remarkable progress was made in the 1970s and 1980s when revolutionary new techniques of molecular biology were added to innovative applications of established histological techniques such as radioautography and immunocytochemistry. Also, when monospecific monoclonal antibodies became commercially available, the reliability of immunocytochemical staining methods was greatly increased.

This accelerating progress was foreseen almost 60 years ago when Alexis Carrel, who won the Nobel prize for physiology and medicine in 1912, subsequently wrote

Modern cytology is endowed with new and powerful methods of investigation and is ready for the attack of fundamental problems. A more profound and scientific knowledge of the cell itself and of its relations with the humors of the organism will be the starting point of great progress in physiology and pathology.

Another result of such progress is that it has substantially broadened the scope of histology. Formerly concerned only with describing the details of body structure, histology now addresses such matters as how cell and tissue components carry out specific functions, how cells communicate and interact, and how the body regulates and coordinates its manifold cellular activities.

Major textbooks are a helpful asset, especially when they require no previous familiarity with the subject. This ninth edition of *Ham's Histology* is tailored to meet the requirements of students entering medicine at the end of the 1980s. Its text incorporates a substantial amount of recent information, and to facilitate learning, its contents have been appropriately compacted and restructured. Many scanning electron micrographs and other useful new illustrations have been added. In an effort to keep the book from becoming too daunting and cumbersome, and in recognition of the time constraints imposed by most medical curricula, the total length of this edition has been decreased by 25%.

If there were ever any question about whether a medical curriculum required a comprehensive survey course dealing with body structure and function at the cellular and tissue levels, this ninth edition should help in answering that question. Medical students and their teachers will recognize the same functionally and clinically oriented, widely integrated approach that characterizes the preceding editions. Considerable emphasis is again placed on medically important aspects of histology and their clinical implications, and more illustrations of human material are included. Also, significant shortening of the text will help to reduce the number of unnecessary details. Although there is likely to be some diversity of opinion about what should have been included, few would disagree that overall comprehension of the subject is more valuable than presentation of every minute detail. Certain details are accordingly either relegated to condensed type or omitted to allow important facts, concepts, and generalizations to emerge with greater emphasis. This does not mean that students can afford to ignore the condensed passages entirely, but they would be well advised to inquire whether they are required, for examination purposes, to know the very detailed contents of such passages.

Some of the principal changes that will be found in this largely rewritten edition, which is now made up of 25 chapters instead of 28, are as follows. The section on cell biology has been revised extensively, with increased emphasis on the structure of chromatin and certain other aspects of the cell nucleus. The cell nucleus is now described in two chapters (Chaps. 2 and 3) instead of three. The details of meiosis are given in the context of the female reproductive system (Chap. 23) instead of being included in the section that deals with cell biology. In the chapter on the cytoplasm (Chap. 4), new sections have been added that describe receptor-mediated endocytosis, endosomes, and peroxisomes.

Chapter 5, which is a fairly detailed consideration of cellular differentiation and proliferation, now includes a section on oncogenes and should have something to offer to readers interested in neoplasia. It also incorporates a brief new account of human embryonic development that sets the stage for subsequent study of the body tissues.

A single chapter, Chapter 7, now describes the various intercellular substances and cells of connective tissue, whereas in earlier editions these topics were spread over two chapters. The sections dealing with collagen and basement membranes are both expanded and present new information and terminology. Blood cells are likewise described in a single chapter (Chap. 8) instead of two, and new color plates of blood cells and bone marrow cells can be found in Chapters 8 and 9.

The chapters dealing with myeloid tissue (Chap. 9) and lymphatic tissue (Chap. 10) have been thoroughly revised and contain a substantial amount of new information about blood cell formation, lymphocytes, and the cellular basis of immunity. Chapter 10 also contains a new section describing gut-associated lymphoid tissue and mucosal immunity.

In the chapters that deal with bone (Chap. 12) and joints (Chap. 13), some recent information is provided on the process of calcification and on the coupling that occurs between the processes of bone formation and bone resorption. Readers with an interest in orthopedics will find that the sections relating to the repair of articular cartilage and fracture healing have been revised and refer to new work.

The recently recognized peptide hormone atrial natriuretic factor is discussed in Chapter 15, and additional emphasis is placed on atherosclerosis in Chapter 16. Also, the section dealing with the lymphatic system in Chapter 16 has been revised.

A new section on cutaneous immune responses has been added to the chapter on the integumentary system (Chap. 17), and more information is provided about normal pigmentation of the skin. In Chapter 19, increased emphasis has been given to the acinar concept of liver structure in recognition of the fact that it is fast gaining almost universal acceptance. Chapter 20 has a revised section on lung development and a new section on bronchus-associated lymphoid tissue.

The most significant change in the chapters dealing with the endocrine system (Chap. 22) and the reproductive system (Chaps. 23 and 24) is the increased emphasis now placed on the hypothalamic control of endocrine secretion. In addition, many of the former micrographs of endocrine organs have been replaced by fine new illustrations of human biopsy specimens. In Chapter 23, the endocrine regulation of ovarian function receives attention commensurate with its clinical importance, and in Chapter 24, more details are supplied about spermiogenesis and spermatozoa. Chapter 25 incorporates a new section on photoreceptor disks. Finally, of the 600 illustrations in this edition, 206 are new.

Although this textbook now appears somewhat shorter, neither its coverage nor the clinical relevance of its contents are diminished, so it retains its suitability for medical curricula. Students who understandably might be horrified at seeing everything they could be expected to know may be reassured that very few histology courses would require them to commit all of this material to memory. This textbook will nevertheless continue to serve them well as a valuable reference source as they progress through medicine and consider, in ever-increasing detail, the many internal workings of the human body.

David H. Cormack, Ph.D.

ACKNOWLEDGMENTS

A substantial number of people offered me advice and help while I was preparing this edition. Their kindness and enthusiasm are greatly appreciated and have made the task of revising such a large book more enjoyable than it otherwise might have been. First, it would be remiss of me not to acknowledge the encouragement, sound advice, and helpful suggestions offered by Arthur Ham, other colleagues in the Department of Anatomy, and several members of other departments in the Faculty of Medicine, University of Toronto. Three other individuals who deserve special mention for their help are Dr. L. Arsenault, who supplied numerous excellent micrographs of skeletal and other tissues and provided me with new information on calcification obtained through electron spectroscopic imaging; Dr. R. B. Salter who, along with his research associates, supplied me with recently obtained information about the regeneration of articular cartilage; and D. J. McComb, who assisted me greatly in obtaining many excellent new micrographs of biopsied human tissues. I would also like to express my sincere gratitude to Dorothy Irwin for executing the new drawings in this edition and to Bruce Smith for the substantial number of new photomicrographs he prepared. The quality of the artwork and photography in this edition will be appreciated by all who see it.

Among the many contributors of outstanding new illustrations for this edition, I would particularly like to thank Dr. L. Arsenault of the University of British Columbia, Dr. S. L. Erlandsen and J. Magney of the University of Minnesota, Dr. J. Sturgess of the Department of Pathology, Hospital for Sick Children, Toronto, and the several staff members of the Department of Pathology, St. Michael's Hospital, Toronto, who contributed micrographs of human material.

I am also indebted to the following individuals for their kind assistance. Dr. M. W. Thompson reviewed the revised manuscript on chromosomes and cytogenetics. Dr. F. P. Ottensmeyer provided some recent information on nucleosomes that was derived from his newly perfected technique of electron spectroscopic imaging. Dr. K. L. Moore reviewed the newly written outline of human embryonic development. Dr. R. L. Van was of assistance in revision of the section on adipose tissue. Dr. A. O. Anderson provided a number of useful illustrations on the lymphatic tissues. Drs. R. B. Salter, S. W. O'Driscoll, and J. Schatzker made a number of helpful suggestions regarding the sections describing the healing of articular cartilage and fracture healing, and I am particularly indebted to Drs. S. C. Marks and J. N. M. Heersche for their advice on revision of the sections on bone resorption, parathyroid hormone, calcitonin, and the regulation of blood calcium levels. Dr. P. Lea supplied a number of micrographs of the skin. Dr. R. L. Owen provided relevant information and illustrations of the antigen-sampling M cells of the digestive tract. Dr. E. R. Weibel provided a number of superb micrographs illustrating the fine structure of the lungs. Dr. S. W. Carmichael read the revised section on the adrenal medulla and provided a micrograph of the two kinds of chromaffin cells. Dr. J. Sturgess supplied me with several excellent illustrations of spermatozoa and cilia of the respiratory tract. Dr. B. Borwein provided several new illustrations and relevant information on the retina.

I am deeply grateful to all the others who also contributed valuable illustrations for this edition. Each person is individually acknowledged in the captions, so I shall refrain from trying to mention everyone here.

Lastly, it is a pleasure to acknowledge the valuable advice and assistance provided by the editorial staff of the J. B. Lippincott Company, for which thanks are due to Richard Winters, David Barnes, and Peggy Maxwell.

CONTENTS

HAM'S HISTOLOGY

PART ONE

INTRODUCTION

The first part of this textbook will prepare those who have no experience at all in histology with the background necessary to understand this subject. As well as outlining the scope of histology and the principal methods employed in the microscopic study of cells, tissues, and organs, it will set the stage for the subsequent detailed study of the cells and tissues of the body. Its main aims are to provide the perspective necessary for an in-depth study of cellular and subcellular detail and to make clear to the student what is entailed in studying this subject.

1

Histology and the Methods Used for Its Study

This chapter, which is addressed specifically to those who are not yet acquainted with the subject of histology, should provide students with an initial overview of the range of subject matter involved in learning the subject, and should also familiarize them with the basic procedures used for the preparation and study of slides and electron micrographs that they will see in the laboratory. In addition, it will serve to introduce some of the basic terms used in the subject. Students will soon find that learning histology is not just a question of mastering a new subject. It is also necessary to become familiar with a new and somewhat technical vocabulary of biological and medical terms. Most early contributors to science were also very well versed in the classics, and the terms they introduced for their discoveries and concepts were generally derived from Greek or Latin roots. The rewards of exploring the derivations of the various technical terms used in subjects such as histology are that medical terminology becomes increasingly meaningful and its usage eventually becomes second nature. It is therefore advisable to take note of the various derivations of the new terms being introduced and, on occasion, to reinforce the learning of such terms through the use of an illustrated medical dictionary or similar reference source.

THE SUBJECT MATTER OF HISTOLOGY

Histology (Gr. *histos*, tissue; *logia*, a branch of learning) means the *science of the tissues.* What then is a tissue? Derived from the French *tissu*, meaning weave or texture, the word *tissue* was first used in a biological sense by Bichat, a French anatomist and physiologist who was impressed by the different textures of the various layers and structures that came to his attention as he dissected the body. Microscopic observations confirmed that the body is made up of different tissues and revealed that *cells* are the ultimate living units from which animals and plants are constructed.

Another important discovery was that living cells possess a number of *functional attributes* that set them apart from inanimate objects. Furthermore, it became evident that such attributes were expressed to varying extents in the different tissues, suggesting that each tissue performed its own specific functions. For example, it was discovered that cells could react to particular kinds of chemical or electrical stimuli, a fundamental property known as *irritability*. In response to such a stimulus, the covering membrane of the cell could develop a wave of altered ionic permeability that spread over the cell surface as a wave of excitation. The term used for such a spread is *conductivity*. This, in turn, could cause the cell to shorten, a property referred to as *contractility*. All cells need to absorb and to utilize essential nutrients and also the chemical building blocks required to synthesize more of their own cell substance and their respective cell products; this is referred to as *absorption* and subsequent *assimilation*. Oxygen, too, must be available to the cell so that it can derive essential energy through the oxidation of foodstuffs, which is described as *cell respiration*. Certain cell products may perform useful functions outside the cell, requiring regulated release to its exterior; such a release is known as *secretion*. The cell also has to rid itself of potentially toxic by-products of metabolism that it allows to diffuse through its covering membrane. This process is known as *excretion*. Finally, the cell increases in size by synthesizing additional amounts of its own cell substance, the process of cell *growth*. Because a very large size would not be compatible with many of these physiological processes, the cell avoids becoming too large by dividing into two daughter cells, which is referred to as cell *reproduction*. However, the ability to divide is sacrificed in certain types of cells (*e.g.*, heart muscle cells) that attain an extreme level of functional specialization.

Fundamental Physiological Properties of Cells Are Expressed in Four Basic Tissues.   Though Bichat envisioned the existence of more than twenty different body tissues, subsequent microscopic studies indicated that there were really only *four basic tissues*, the others being variants of these. The four basic tissues are (1) *epithelial tissue*, (2) *connective tissue*, (3) *nervous tissue*, and (4) *muscle tissue*. It requires ten chapters to deal with the specialized structure and functions of these tissues. All that needs to be said about them at this point is that the cells of each tissue are structurally specialized to express one or more of the physiological properties described above. For example, we shall find that although the cells of *epithelial tissue* (Gr. *epi*, upon) generally serve a protective function (because membranes made of epithelial cells cover external and line internal body surfaces), there is another division of this tissue consisting of groups of cells that are situated more deeply in the body and that function to provide external or internal secretions important to the body.

Connective tissue plays many roles; one in particular will be mentioned here. When we say that the body is composed of cells, we are not telling the whole truth, because if the body consisted only of cells, it would be as soft as cells and hence would amount to no more than a big mound of jellylike material. In the body the function of producing nonliving supportive materials is allotted almost entirely to certain cells of connective tissue that are specialized for this purpose. Such materials are called *intercellular substances* (L. *inter*, between). They sometimes lie between individual cells and sometimes between groups of cells. Some intercellular substances are delicate whereas others have great tensile strength or are weight-bearing. The intercellular substance lying between the cells of bone, for instance, is much like reinforced concrete. It is because of intercellular substances that man is able to stand erect and that his body tissues remain intact. We shall find that connective tissue permeates the other body tissues and thereby serves two main purposes. First, its intercellular substances support cells of other tissues. Secondly, it supports the walls of blood vessels because these all develop within connective tissue and remain ensheathed by it. Thus connective tissue keeps the cells of other tissues in place, and its blood vessels provide for their nourishment. However, not all the cells in connective tissue are involved in producing intercellular substances. Other types of tissues with varying functions, such as dense ordinary connective tissue, adipose (fat) tissue, blood cells and the blood cell-forming tissues, cartilage, and bone, are also classified as connective tissues.

Nervous tissue is highly specialized with respect to irritability and conductivity. Long nerve fibers extend from nerve cells in the brain or spinal cord to all parts of the body and provide a means of extremely rapid communication. However, nerve cells are so highly specialized that they have relinquished all capacity for cell division.

Finally, *muscle tissue* is highly specialized for contractility. It is, of course, our skeletal muscles that allow us to move our bones relative to one another, facilitating locomotion. Again, in two of the three different types of muscle, the cells are too highly specialized to be able to divide.

Cells and Tissues Represent Building Blocks of Two Different Orders.   An analogy might be helpful here. There are two different orders of building blocks from which chemical compounds are assembled. The specific atoms are arranged together to form molecules. In studying the composition of these compounds, it is often easier to visualize how they are built up from molecules than from atoms. Likewise, in studying the organs (L. *organum*, a part of the body that serves a special function), it is often easier to visualize how these are assembled from the four basic tissues than from individual cells. For example, once it is appreciated why connective tissue, with its intercellular substances and blood vessels, needs to be present in an epithelial organ whose function is secretion, it is easy to understand why such an organ would be constructed of both epithelial and connective tissue.

Histology Is Essentially a Study of Cell Societies. The body was likened to a *cell state* more than a century ago by the eminent pathologist Virchow. There is a truly remarkable parallelism in how cell societies and industrialized states operate. The main basis of similarity is the profound division of labor (function) that exists in cell societies. However, the cell's capacity to perform all the functions necessary for its survival is sacrificed so that it can do a few specialized tasks well. In other words, specialization is only achieved at the expense of independence. Hence a second similarity is that just as the individuals in an industrialized state are obliged to exchange their own specialized services or products of their work for those of their fellows, a continuous exchange of function and products is necessary among the specialized cells of the body, without which none of the cells can survive. Rapid exchanges between specialized cells are made possible by the bloodstream, which serves as a highly efficient mode of transportation. In addition, two body-wide communications systems regulate functional activities in specialized cells. First, impulses traveling by way of the nervous system can elicit or suppress cellular activities. Secondly, chemical messages called *hormones* (Gr. *hormaein*, to set in motion) traveling by way of the bloodstream can regulate the activities of cells distant from those cells sending the hormones.

The cell population within a cell state undergoes continual turnover. Cells that die are generally replaced by new ones of the same kind, except that certain types of specialized cells are not replaced. This leaves a deficit that in certain cases (*e.g.,* that of heart muscle cells) can have clinical repercussions. Once enough cells of a given kind have been produced to do their type of work, production of that kind of cell ceases until a further need arises. Several different kinds of cells can arise from a common ancestor within a cell society, yet the cells in a specific family generally breed true to their own kind.

Finally, the cell state, like a state made up of people, is vulnerable to attack by various outside enemies, including viruses, bacteria, and other microorganisms and parasites. Hence certain cells, specialized to fend off invaders, can reach them by way of the bloodstream and destroy them.

Histology Bears a Close Relationship to Several Other Biological and Medical Sciences. Although some distinction was initially made between histology and microscopic anatomy, histology soon came to include microscopic anatomy as well. Then the development of the electron microscope ushered in a whole new era of exploration of subcellular detail that resulted in a very significant increase in knowledge about cell structure and its relation to function. Mean-while, innovative methods were evolving whereby the various kinds of structures present inside cells could be separated from one another, enabling their respective functions to be investigated at the biochemical level. The knowledge gained soon became incorporated into histology, greatly expanding the valuable contribution that cell biology made to medical histology. Histology eventually became a truly interdisciplinary subject. In other words, it embodied relevant information gained from all possible sources instead of relying on one particular discipline. This, of course, now makes the subject rather hard to define. However, few would dispute that an important purpose of learning histology is to gain some understanding of the *relation between normal body structure and function at the cellular level.* Indeed, many now perceive the subject as having more to do with exploration of the cellular basis of bodily function than with an attempt to satisfy the obsessive desire to describe everything in the body in the greatest possible detail. Of course, physiology is likewise concerned with the functions of the body, but in far greater detail and depth, involving itself, for example, with the measurement of bodily functions. The relation between physiology and histology is nevertheless so close that in some countries the teaching of histology is considered the responsibility of physiology departments. Furthermore, it is primarily the functional aspects of histology that make it relevant to medicine. Certainly, histology can be a useful subject in the medical curriculum if it provides insight into the internal workings of the body and the various ways in which these matters become perturbed by disease (*i.e.,* pathology and pathophysiology). In fact, students often seem quite surprised by how much they can perceive about the functions of a tissue or about the nature of its involvement in a disease process by observing it under a microscope. Students also will find histology a helpful preparation for applied subjects such as pathology, immunology, and hematology because of its integrated approach to tissue structure and function.

Terms Used in Describing Cells

Microscopic observation has revealed that almost all human cells have a central part with a refractive index that is noticeably different from that of the remainder of the cell. This central part came to be known as the *nucleus* (L. *nux*, nut) because of its similarity to a nut lying in the midst of a shell. For the same reason, the Greek prefix *karyo-* (Gr. *karyon*, nut) was often used in words that refer to the nucleus (*e.g., karyolysis,* the term used for dissolution of the nucleus when a cell dies). The membrane that encloses the nucleus was called the *nuclear membrane.* When the electron microscope (EM) subsequently revealed that this was, in fact, a double-membrane system, it became known as the *nuclear envelope* instead, but either term remains acceptable (Fig. 1-1). One or more rounded, darkly staining bodies in the interior of the nucleus (Fig. 1-1) were each called a *nucleolus* (diminutive form of L. *nux*). Tiny granules or irregular clumps of darkly staining material scattered in the nucleus were called *chromatin* (Gr. *chroma,* color) to indicate their affinity for certain dyes. The unstained component in which the nucleoli and chromatin granules appeared to be suspended became known as the *nuclear sap* (Fig. 1-1).

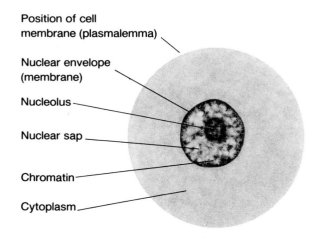

Position of cell membrane (plasmalemma)

Nuclear envelope (membrane)

Nucleolus

Nuclear sap

Chromatin

Cytoplasm

Fig. 1-1. Diagrammatic representation of the cell, showing the main parts seen under the light microscope.

The outer part of the cell was called the *cytoplasm* (Gr. *kytos*, a covering or something hollow; *plasma*, something molded) because it seemed to be molded around the nucleus. Particular functions are performed by specialized components of the cytoplasm referred to as *cytoplasmic organelles* (*dim.* of organ) that lie in a *cytoplasmic matrix* (*cytosol*). The term *inclusion* is used to denote such features as pigment granules or droplets of stored fat and is applied to cytoplasmic accumulations of *exogenous* (external) as well as *endogenous* (internal) origin. Such materials were classified as *inclusions* because they were considered nonessential components of the cytoplasm. The *cell membrane* covering the surface of the cell is so thin that cross sections of it cannot be distinguished in the light microscope (LM). Although its existence was certainly known, the cell membrane was never actually seen until it became possible to observe it directly in the EM. By way of analogy with the bark of a tree, the cell membrane is also sometimes referred to as the *plasmalemma* (Gr. *lemma*, bark). However, it is now customary to use the unqualified term *cell membrane* to mean the *external membrane* of the cell, and it is in this sense that we shall be using the term throughout this book.

Finally, it should be mentioned that two different kinds of cells are recognized in cell biology: those with a nucleus and those without. The former are known as *eukaryotic* cells. From its derivation (Gr. *eu*, good + *karyon*), this term indicates the possession of a true nucleus confined by a nuclear membrane (envelope). All animals and plants, including microorganisms other than bacteria and the blue-green algae, are *eukaryotes*. Bacteria and the blue-green algae are classified as *prokaryotes* because they are believed to have evolved before eukaryotes. They differ from eukaryotes in that their nuclear material is *not* confined within a nuclear envelope. Our present-day understanding of how eukaryotic cells function at the molecular level depends in no small measure on what has been learned from research on prokaryotic cells.

THE COMPOSITION OF BODY COMPONENTS

The body is composed of three basic components. One of these, *cells*, has already been described and is the main component of three of the four basic tissues (epithelium, nervous tissue, and muscle). In addition to cells, the connective tissues contain very substantial amounts of nonliving *intercellular substances*. Cells, the living component of the body, obtain their nutrients and oxygen from *tissue fluid* (known also as *intercellular* or *extracellular fluid*). The three basic components of the body are therefore its *cells*, *intercellular substances*, and various *body fluids*.

The Composition of Cells

Four major classes of organic compounds enter into the composition of cells: *proteins, nucleic acids, carbohydrates,* and *fats* (*lipids*). For our present purposes, we need only deal with the proteins; carbohydrates and lipids will be considered later in this chapter, and nucleic acids will be dealt with in Chapters 2 and 3.

Proteins Represent the Main Constituent of Cells. Proteins can be present by themselves or in combination with (1) carbohydrates either as *glycoproteins* or as *proteoglycans* (Gr. *glykys*, sweet), (2) lipids (Gr. *lipos*, fat) as *lipoproteins*, or (3) nucleic acids as *nucleoproteins*. The functional and structural importance of proteins is manifested in the diversity seen between different cell types, which is caused by specific differences in the sets of proteins that different types of cells synthesize. Because each individual type of cell makes its own distinctive set of proteins, it expresses specific distinguishing features, described as the cell's *phenotype* (Gr. *phainein*, to show; *typos*, type), that enable the histologist to characterize it as a particular kind of cell.

Proteins are macromolecules that are made up of one or more component polypeptide chains linearly assembled from 20 different amino acids and their derivatives. Each amino acid possesses an amino ($-NH_2$) group as well as a carboxyl ($-COOH$) group. Whereas plants are able to synthesize amino acids (and therefore proteins) from inorganic nitrogen, carbon dioxide, and water, animals lack the facility to do this. They must therefore obtain building blocks for protein synthesis from organic foods that include vegetable and animal products. Proteins in the food are broken down in the intestine, from which their constituent amino acids are absorbed into the bloodstream and are carried to all parts of the body. Each cell of the body is then responsible for synthesizing its own particular proteins from the pool of amino acids.

Once synthesized, cellular proteins are occasionally sacrificed as fuel even though the amount of energy obtainable from proteins is not very great compared with that liberated from carbohydrates and lipids. The principal functions of cellular proteins, however, are that they constitute much of the *structural* material of the cell and that they are instrumental in *regulating* its very large number of internal biochemical reactions.

Proteins Play a Key Role in the Regulation of Metabolism. The sum total of all the chemical reactions that proceed in a cell, conferring on it the properties of life, constitute its *metabolism* (Gr. *metaballein*, to throw into a different position, change). Some of these metabolic reactions involve either destruction or production of cell substance. Those concerned with the breakdown of cell substance are termed *catabolic* (Gr. *kata*, down; *ballein*, to throw). Those concerned with the synthesis of new cell substance are termed *anabolic* (Gr. *anaballein*, to throw up). In some cells anabolic and catabolic activity remain in balance; such cells are said to be in a metabolically *steady state*. Growth is dependent on anabolic reactions exceeding catabolic reactions.

The chemical reactions involved in metabolism are catalyzed by *enzymes* (Gr. *en*, in; *zyme*, leaven), all of which are proteins. However, not all proteins are enzymes, because some provide structural material for cellular components. For example, many of the cytoplasmic organelles are composed of *membranes*, which are made of lipids in association with proteins. Membranes also subdivide the cytoplasm into different compartments, each with different functions. Such membranes can serve to separate particular constituents, thereby preventing them from interacting. Moreover, enzymatic proteins are commonly incorporated into membranes, and enzymatic reactions commonly occur on the surface of membranes. However, neither enzymatic nor structural proteins last forever; they are always being catabolized and replaced. Hence life depends on the continuous synthesis of proteins.

Intercellular Substances

Two different sorts of intercellular substances are necessary for the adequate support and nourishment of cells. These two kinds of intercellular substances are described as *fibrous* and *amorphous* (Gr. *a*, without; *morphē*, form) respectively. The most abundant fibrous intercellular component is called *collagen* (Gr. *kolla*, glue; *gennan*, to produce) because boiling it down produces glue. The protein collagen constitutes fibers of great tensile strength and is found, for example, in tendons, which must resist stretching as they transmit the pull of muscles on bones.

Another protein that can exist in the form of fibers is *elastin*. As well as forming fibers, this protein also forms layers called *laminae* (L. *lamina*, flat layer) in the walls of arteries. Unlike collagen, elastin can be stretched. It is because elastin stretches that the pulse can be felt every time the heart pumps blood into an artery; its elastic recoil restores the artery's former diameter between heartbeats. Elastin is a particularly long-lasting product, some persisting to the present day in arteries of Egyptian mummies. Most of the elastin in arteries is produced by muscle cells, but

elsewhere it is produced, like collagen, by connective tissue cells.

Amorphous intercellular substances, sometimes referred to as the *ground substance,* contain carbohydrate bound to protein. The carbohydrate is in the form of polysaccharides in which hexuronic acids and amino sugars are alternately linked together to form long-chained molecules called *glycosaminoglycans,* a name that reflects how such molecules are made up of repeating disaccharide units. When glycosaminoglycans are covalently bound to proteins, the molecules are called *proteoglycans.*

As anyone knows who has thickened a sauce by adding cornstarch (which is a polysaccharide) and heating it, polysaccharides can exist in the form of viscous solutions, and this is the form they take in amorphous intercellular substances. As well as forming viscous solutions, often referred to as *sols,* polysaccharides can also exist in the form of semisolid (or virtually solid) *gels.* The sols in most parts of the body act as fillers between blood vessels and cells. Gels such as that in cartilage are solid enough to bear weight. Yet, whether they take the form of sols or gels, it is important to realize that amorphous intercellular substances hold enough water to permit the ready diffusion of dissolved substances (*e.g.,* oxygen and nutrients) from sites of higher to sites of lower concentration.

Body Fluids

The main body fluids are (1) *blood,* (2) *tissue fluid,* and (3) *lymph.* The *blood* consists of two components: *blood cells* and a slightly viscous fluid called *plasma* in which they are suspended. The blood circulates throughout the body in *blood vessels,* the narrowest of which are called *capillaries* (L. *capillaris,* hair). Capillaries pervade the intercellular substance so extensively that few cells are far from a capillary (Fig. 1-2).

Through minute openings in their walls, capillaries exude a clear watery fluid called *tissue fluid* that is more or less a dialysate of blood plasma. This fluid permeates the amorphous intercellular substances lying between capillaries and cells (Fig. 1-2) and is held there by their carbohydrate-containing macromolecules. The blood plasma within the capillaries contains both nutrients and oxygen (released from red blood cells) in simple solution. Because both of these necessities are in greater concentration in the plasma than in tissue fluid, they diffuse out through the thin walls of the capillaries into the tissue fluid, and by this means they reach the tissue cells (Fig. 1-2). The cells in turn release waste products that, being more concentrated in tissue fluid than blood, diffuse in the opposite direction and are carried away by the blood (Fig. 1-2).

More tissue fluid can be produced than can be absorbed back into the capillaries; any excess is carried away by a series of vessels called *lymphatics.* The fluid they absorb (which is really tissue fluid) is called *lymph* (L. *lympha,* wa-

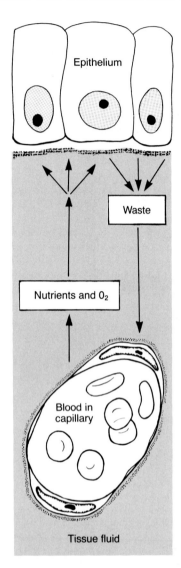

Fig. 1-2. Schematic diagram of the route by which the cells in a tissue obtain their nutrients and oxygen from underlying capillaries. Metabolic waste products pass in the reverse direction and are carried away in the bloodstream. In each case, diffusion occurs through the tissue fluid that permeates the amorphous intercellular substances lying between the capillaries and the tissue cells.

ter) as soon as it lies within a lymphatic. The lymphatics eventually empty into the bloodstream.

THE MICROSCOPIC STUDY OF CELLS AND TISSUES

Cells Can Be Observed Directly in the Living State. Valuable information can generally be obtained by encouraging cells to grow in culture systems amenable to study by microscopy and related methods. This is known

as growth *in vitro* (L. *vitrum*, glass) even though the cells are now generally grown in plastic containers. Under *in vitro* conditions, many kinds of cells continue to perform functions that they carried out in the body. If provided with the appropriate culture conditions, they can even undergo further specialization and express new features and functions. However, the artificial *in vitro* environment in which the cells now find themselves seldom supports their preexisting pattern of intercellular organization and may even affect the way they behave, leaving some room for doubt as to whether *in vitro* findings invariably reflect the behavior of cells in the body. By means of *microsurgical techniques*, it is also possible to operate on cells *in vitro;* for example, it is possible to transplant the nucleus from one cell into another. Moreover, cells from two different tissues or two different species can be induced to fuse with one another *in vitro*.

In many cases, cell cultures can be prepared by dissociating tissues with a proteolytic enzyme such as trypsin. If the cells obtained in this manner are incubated at body temperature in a suitable serum-containing medium, they will grow in suspension or as a monolayer on the floor of the culture vessel. Normal cells rarely proliferate for more than a few months in culture. However, some of them may acquire the potential to proliferate more or less indefinitely as a result of some alteration in their genetic constitution. Such cells will go on to produce *continuous cell lines* that can be frozen and restarted as needed.

One of the many purposes for which cell cultures are well suited is to ascertain the chromosomal sex of an individual. *In vitro* methods are also widely used to establish whether a particular substance is toxic to living cells and to study cell specialization and malignant changes in cells. Furthermore, *in vitro* methods represent the only ethical way of experimenting with human tissues.

The Preparation of Histological Sections

In vitro methods involving the isolation of cells from their former surroundings reveal very little about the cell's respective living arrangements under normal conditions and in disease. To preserve the structural relationship between cells in tissues, it is necessary to cut very thin slices of tissue, called *sections*, that are suitable for light or electron microscopy. Tracer methods exist by which cells in a living animal can be labeled, so that their life histories can be followed in tissue sections obtained at various time intervals after labeling. It is even possible to follow what happens to labeled molecules by such a procedure. Thus sections fulfill much the same purpose as snapshots do in capturing and indicating to an observer what is going on in a tissue at any given moment. Sections cut for light microscopy must be thin enough to transmit sufficient light and to avoid visual superimposition of their various components. Thinner than the diameter of most cells, an LM section is extremely fragile and must be attached to a glass slide to be

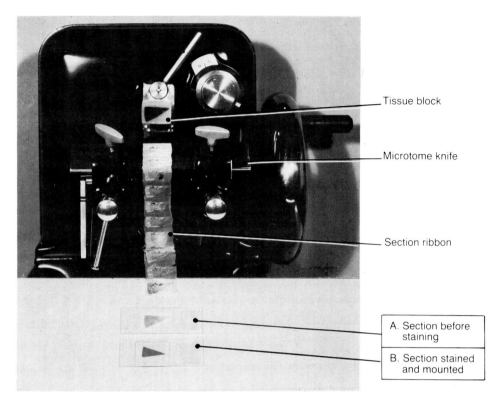

Tissue block

Microtome knife

Section ribbon

A. Section before staining

B. Section stained and mounted

Fig. 1-3.   Paraffin sections for light microscopy are cut on a microtome.

handled with ease (Fig. 1-3). The final product (*i.e.,* a stained and mounted preparation) is also referred to as a *section.* For light microscopy, sections are generally prepared by the *paraffin technique,* which is described in the following discussion. Other ways of preparing tissues will be described in the context of the tissues to which they apply.

The Paraffin Technique Is Routinely Used for Preparing Tissue Sections.   The standard procedure used includes the following stages:

1. *The Tissue Sample.* A small sample of tissue called the *tissue block* is obtained by *biopsy* (diagnostic sampling) or surgical excision, or postmortem. If the sample is taken from a cadaver, it is essential to remove it promptly after death to avoid postmortem degeneration. The tissue has to be dissected out with care, using sharp instruments to avoid distorting its microscopic appearance. For adequate fixation, its size must not exceed 1 cm in any dimension. As soon as it has been removed, it must be immersed in a fixative.

2. *Fixation. Fixatives* prevent postmortem degeneration and other misleading structural changes in cells and tissues, and they harden soft tissues. Much of this action is attributable to the fact that they coagulate proteins, which are present in great abundance in cells and tissues. Certain chemical fixatives are more effective than others in preserving specific tissue components. *Formaldehyde,* 4% in an aqueous solution buffered to neutral *p*H (*formalin*), is routinely employed for LM fixation in the laboratory. Chemical fixatives either crosslink protein molecules or denature and precipitate them by replacing the

water associated with them. As a result, tissues become harder. A further important action is that the fixative prevents cellular hydrolytic enzymes, which are released when cells die, from degrading tissue components and thereby spoiling tissues for microscopy. *Prompt fixation is essential* to avoid such postmortem degeneration. Coagulation due to fixation also locks into place certain kinds of carbohydrate- and fat-containing macromolecules that would otherwise be lost during tissue processing. Most fixatives are also strong antiseptics, killing pathogenic microorganisms, such as bacteria present in infected tissues, with the result that these no longer constitute a health hazard to those who handle them. Fixation can also enhance subsequent staining of the tissue.

3. *Dehydration.* The principle of the paraffin technique is to substitute paraffin wax for the water initially present in the tissue so that the tissue block can be sectioned easily. This is achieved in two stages. The first stage is a process of gradual *dehydration,* which is accomplished by passing the block of fixed tissue through increasing strengths of alcohol to absolute alcohol. However, alcohol does not act as a paraffin solvent, so it is necessary to replace the alcohol with xylol or some other paraffin solvent that is also miscible with alcohol. This second stage is termed *clearing.*

4. *Clearing.* The solvent routinely used for clearing is xylol. The alcohol-dehydrated block of tissue is passed through successive changes of xylol until all the alcohol has been replaced by xylol in preparation for embedding.

5. *Embedding.* The xylol-permeated tissue block is passed through several changes of warm paraffin, which dissolves

readily in the xylol. The melted wax fills in all the spaces formerly occupied by water, and when it hardens on cooling, it renders the tissue block ready for sectioning.

6. *Sectioning.* Once the excess wax has been trimmed away, sections can be cut from the tissue block by means of a cutting instrument called a *microtome* (Fig. 1-3). Equipped with a dreadfully sharp knife that is evidently a direct descendant of the cut-throat razor, this instrument can be adjusted to deliver any required thickness of section. At the cutting edge of the knife, the wax shavings accumulate in the form of a continuous ribbon (Fig. 1-3) from which individual sections can readily be separated with forceps once the ribbon has been floated on water.

Section Thickness. For routine purposes, sections are generally cut to a thickness of 5 to 8 micrometers. A *micrometer* is 0.001 mm (1×10^{-6} m) and is represented by the symbol μm. (In the older literature, it was referred to as a *micron* and it was given the symbol μ.) If a thinner section is required, the tissue is embedded in plastic or epoxy resin instead of paraffin wax. *Semithin* sections for light microscopy are usually cut to a thickness of 1 μm to 2 μm. Frozen sections, described below, are not always cut quite as thinly as paraffin sections and are commonly 6 μm to 10 μm thick. However, with enough expertise, it is possible to cut them to a thickness of 5 μm.

7. *Staining and Mounting.* Most staining is done in aqueous solution, so the wax that permeates the section needs to be replaced by water. This is achieved by attaching the section to a slide and passing it through xylol to remove the paraffin, through absolute alcohol to remove the xylol, through alcohol rinses of decreasing strength, and then through water. The section is now ready for staining, after which it appears as in Figure 1-3A. Once stained, it is passed through a series of increasing strengths of alcohol to absolute alcohol and then xylol. Finally, it is *mounted* in a drop or two of mounting medium dissolved in xylol. Mounting eliminates unwanted diffraction of the light passing through the section. A protective glass coverslip is carefully positioned over the section so that when the xylol in the mounting medium evaporates, the coverslip becomes tightly bonded to the slide (Fig. 1-3B).

Frozen Sections.   Whenever there is some urgency about obtaining tissue sections, as for example during surgery when rapid confirmation of the nature or spread of a diseased tissue is required, they can be prepared in great haste by another procedure. This rapid procedure can also furnish the experimental investigator with sections of fresh tissue that have not been submitted to the relatively harsh processing required to prepare paraffin sections. Moreover, virtually everything present in the living tissue is still present in the same place in *frozen sections,* but it is necessary to examine these sections promptly to avoid fixation. Supplemental fixation is essential for a permanent preparation. To cut frozen sections, the block of fresh tissue is frozen very rapidly using liquid nitrogen. It is then sectioned inside the refrigerated cabinet of a *cryostat,* an apparatus designed to maintain the microtome knife and tissue at a subzero temperature throughut the entire cutting operation. Frozen sections are most easily obtained if they are cut slightly thicker than paraffin sections and if they are prepared in small batches.

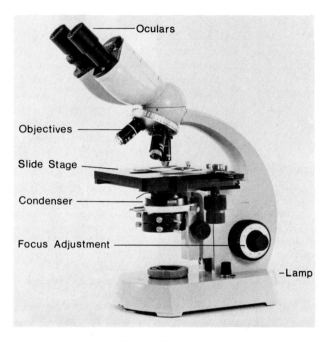

Fig. 1-4.   The essential parts of a light microscope. (Courtesy of C. Zeiss Company)

Light Microscopy and Its Applications

The intelligent use of the light microscope is so important in histology that it is essential at the outset to have some idea of what the microscope can and cannot do. First, of course, it can make things appear larger. The compound microscope is, in effect, a two-stage magnifying system in which the specimen is magnified first by an elaborate lens system in the *objective* and then again by a second lens in the *ocular (eyepiece).* The position of these two optical parts on the microscope is shown in Figure 1-4. The total magnification of the instrument is simply the product of the magnifications resulting from the objective and ocular, respectively.

The second feature of the compound microscope is that it enables its user to see more detail. The importance of this property can hardly be overemphasized, because unless clarity of detail stays hand in hand with an increase in size, the image becomes increasingly blurred and indistinct. Hence we must distinguish between the extent to which the size of an object appears increased in the image, which is called *magnification,* and the extent to which the details in the object are faithfully reproduced in the image, which is termed *resolution.* Resolution is the degree of separation that can be seen between adjacent points (details) in the specimen. The smaller the distance that can be distinguished between such points, the more detail there is in the image. At close range, points appear as different entities to the unaided eye only if they are separated by a distance of 0.2 mm (200 μm) or more; but if a good light microscope is used, points as close as 0.25 μm can be distinguished from one another. This distance is the smallest that can be detected between any two details in an object using a light microscope and represents its *limit of resolution*. The fidelity with which a microscope can reproduce in its image the details present in a specimen is limited, because resolution is a function of the wavelength of the energy (light) employed for illumination. The only way around this particular limitation is to employ energy of shorter wavelength, which, as we shall see, can be achieved if an electron beam is employed instead of light rays.

The other optical parameter that determines how detailed the image will be is the proportion of the potential visual detail in the specimen that is able to enter the objective lens. Optically dense details in the specimen reduce the amplitude of all the light waves extending from them in every direction. However, not all this potential visual information can be used to form the image, because only the light rays entering the optical pathway of the microscope are used to build the image. The proportion of light rays put to good use in forming image details is determined by the aperture size of the objective lens, which depends on the angle of the cone of light rays accepted by the objective from the condenser. The wider the angle of this cone, the greater the proportion of potential detail reproduced in the image. The aperture size (fraction of wavefront admitted) is expressed as the *numerical aperture (NA)* of the lens,* and its value is engraved on each objective, beside the magnification. Not only detail, but also the brightness of the image depends on NA. For maximum resolution and adequate illumination at any given magnification, it is important that the NA of the condenser lens be matched as closely as possible with the NA of the objective. In practice it turns out that no further detail can be seen if the total magnification exceeds 1000 times the NA of the objective. The maximum useful magnification of the LM is about ×1400.

Phase-Contrast Microscopy Permits the Direct Observation of Living Cells. Almost all parts of the cell have similar optical densities, which means that they all decrease the amplitude of light rays to approximately the same extent. Unless stained, they have so little effect on the *amplitude* of the light waves passing through them that most of them cannot be distinguished by means of an ordinary light microscope. However, individual cell components can differentially alter the *phase* of the light waves they transmit. Although the eye is insensitive to phase differences, light waves that are in or out of phase interfere with each other, with the result that the amplitude of the resultant waves increases or decreases. The *phase-contrast microscope* is designed to convert invisible phase differences into visible amplitude differences. Light waves incident to the specimen are recombined with those leaving the specimen, with the result that these two sets of waves interfere with each

---

* The *numerical aperture (NA)* of a lens is calculated from its *half angle of aperture,* that is, the angle between its optical axis and the most inclined rays of light it can accept. The angle is expressed as its sine value (to make it numerical) and is multiplied by the refractive index of the medium (air or oil) between the specimen and the objective. The product gives the NA of the lens. The resolution that can be attained with an objective is directly proportional to the wavelength of the light used for illumination and inversely proportional to the NA of the objective lens. The brightness of the field is directly proportional to the square of the NA.

other to different extents. Because this enables the various components present in cells and tissues to be distinguished from one another under the light microscope without any staining, cells can be observed in the living state (see Fig. 4-6).

Fluorescence Microscopy Reveals Sites of Specific Localization. The light microscope has been adapted in yet another way that permits constituents of cells and tissues to be localized in a highly specific manner. Certain substances absorb light energy of short wavelength and emit it as visible light of longer wavelength. This property is known as *fluorescence*, and it can be observed directly by means of the *fluorescence microscope*. Basically similar to an ordinary light microscope, the fluorescence microscope is equipped with a high-pressure mercury vapor or quartz–iodine lamp capable of emitting light of high intensity, some of which is in the *ultraviolet* range. This light is transmitted through an exciter filter that screens out all the unnecessary wavelengths, leaving only those that are required to elicit fluorescence. To avoid injury to the eyes from the ultraviolet light, a barrier filter that excludes short wavelengths but permits the passage of longer wavelengths in the visible range is inserted below the level of the eyepieces. A similar filter is necessary to prevent the ultraviolet light from fogging the film when a fluorescent preparation is being photographed.

Immunofluorescent Staining. The fluorescence microscope is used often in histological investigations because the fluorescent dyes fluorescein (which emits green light) and lissamine rhodamine (which emits red light) are both suitable for *tagging proteins*. Such fluorescent-labeled proteins are readily detectable under the fluorescence microscope. Moreover, specific antibodies can be labeled with either of these fluorescent dyes without losing their antigenic specificity. Thus it is possible to produce a *fluorescent-labeled antibody* that will recognize a particular cellular or intercellular protein with a remarkable degree of specificity. The basis of its specificity is that a complementary lock-and-key configuration enables a region of the antibody molecule to recognize an antigenic site on the protein molecule. Fluorescent staining methods based on such specific immunological recognition are known as *immunofluorescence* techniques. (A good example is shown in Fig. 4-29.) Immunofluorescent staining may be direct or indirect as explained in the following section.

If the protein being studied is of high molecular weight, it may elicit the production of an antibody when injected into another species. To raise an antibody, the protein is freed of contaminants and is then injected on a repeated basis into a laboratory animal such as a rabbit. The immunoglobulin (antibody) fraction of serum obtained from the immunized animal can then be conjugated to a fluorescent dye, whereupon the antibody retains its immunological specificity. If the antibody itself is labeled and is employed for localizing the antigen, the method is known as *direct* immunofluorescent staining. However, *indirect* immunofluorescent staining may be more appropriate in certain situations. The indirect method takes advantage of the fact that once an immunoglobulin has been raised in a given species, the immunoglobulin itself is recognized as a foreign protein when it is injected into another species. Hence it is possible to raise a secondary or *anti-immunoglobulin* antibody directed against the initial antibody. Furthermore, if the antigenic site against which the secondary antibody is directed happens to lie in the constant region of the initial antibody molecule, the secondary antibody will have the capacity to interact with immunoglobulins of every conceivable specificity made by the first species. (This will be easier to understand when we consider antibodies in Chap. 10.) Thus it is possible to prepare a single fluorescent-labeled antibody that will recognize all immunoglobulins of any given species regardless of antigenic specificity. The general procedure for indirect immunofluorescent staining is as follows. The microscopic preparation is first overlaid with *unlabeled* specific antibody raised in a certain species. The excess is washed away, and any antibody that has become specifically bound to the tissue is then visualized microscopically by applying a *fluorescent-labeled antibody* raised in a different species and directed against immunoglobulins of the first species. This indirect method is more sensitive than the direct one because of the number of antibody molecules bound at each stage of the procedure. It is also more economical because only a single fluorescent-labeled antibody is involved in localizing a large number of different antigens.

Immunogold Staining. A similarly direct or indirect approach can be used for the immunocytochemical localization of specific tissue proteins using an antibody labeled with *colloidal gold* instead of a fluorescent dye. The advantage of *immunogold staining* with antibody-coated gold particles is that they constitute an excellent marker in the EM as well as in the LM. Such particles are ideal for immuno-electron microscopy because of their tiny size and high electron density. At the LM level, they appear reddish-brown when seen in large numbers under an ordinary light microscope.

Use of the Light Microscope

Before a section is observed under a microscope, it should always be held up to the light and examined with no magnification. This will show which side of the slide has the section on it, and will reveal whether there is dirt or immersion oil on the coverslip, which should be cleaned off. Also, in cases in which the source of the section is unknown, this cursory inspection sometimes provides helpful hints about the identity of the section. On occasion, it is advantageous to utilize an inverted eyepiece as a simple magnifying glass.

The Low-Power Objective. It is a great mistake to be too eager to use the highest possible magnification at the earliest possible opportunity. Beginning with a low magnification, preferably a *scanning objective,* has a real advantage in that it allows a fairly large area of the section to be seen at any given time, and by racking the slide back and forth under the scanning or low power, every part of the section can be examined. This is important to do because sometimes the best clues about the nature of the section can be found only in a part of it, and these clues might be missed unless the entire section is thoroughly examined under low power. This preliminary survey of the whole section will also disclose suitable areas for further observation under higher magnification.

The High-Power Objective. There should be no problem in swinging the high-power objective into position to examine the preselected area. However, if this area cannot be focused properly, the slide may be upside down, in which case the section remains too far away from the objective to be brought into sharp focus.

The Oil-Immersion Objective. Because the oil-immersion objective has to be brought very close to the coverslip, it is possible to break the coverslip or damage the objective when trying to focus the microscope. To do this correctly, the coarse adjustment should first be used to lower the stage before the oil-immersion objective is swung into place. A small drop of immersion oil is then applied to the coverslip and, while watching the objective from one side, the stage is raised until the objective makes contact with the oil. The section is then brought into focus using the fine adjustment. If this takes more than a couple of turns, the problem may be that no part of the section is under the objective, or the objective lens may already be *below* the level required for focus. If some color can be seen, the first possibility can be ruled out; if the image sharpens with further focusing, the objective lens may still be too high. It is advisable for the beginner to proceed with caution until he has gained some experience.

Lenses Should Be Kept Clean. The field of view may appear irregularly clouded, distorted, or even covered with specks. This can indicate (1) dirt on the coverslip, (2) oil on an objective lens (especially the ×40 objective), (3) dirt on an eyepiece, or (4) dirt on the top lens of the condenser. If the distortion or specks rotate when an eyepiece is turned, the problem is a dirty eyepiece lens. Dirty lenses should be cleaned off *very gently* with lens paper. Specks of dirt should be blown off, preferably with a puff of air from a rubber bulb kept for this purpose. Oil should be gently wiped from coverslips or objective lenses with lens paper and, if necessary, the barest trace of xylol.

Field of View

The Field of View Is Inversely Related to the Magnification Used. A thorough initial scan of a section is essential because only a small area of it comes into view at any given moment. Under low power, for example, the diameter of the field of view is only 1.5 mm across, which happens to be the area within a letter "o" as printed on this page. The unit used to record length in light microscopy, the *micrometer* (μm), is equal to 0.001 mm; hence the area seen under low power has a diameter of 1500 μm. The diameter of the field of view bears an inverse relation to the magnification used, as may be seen in Table 1-1.

Plate 1-1 provides an example of what can be observed at these different magnifications. Under low power, it is just possible to discern that a liver section is basically made up of radiating rows of cells (called hepatocytes) separated by long slitlike spaces (Plate 1-1*A*). Under high power, the blue-stained nuclei of hepatocytes can be readily distinguished from the pink-stained cytoplasm (Plate 1-1*B*), and under oil immersion, some of the finer details can be observed (Plate 1-1*C*). Cell boundaries are difficult to discern because the cell membrane is too thin to be seen in the LM. However, an indistinct pink line sometimes marks the border between two cells (the arrows in Plate 1-1*C* indicate the positions of such borders).

Table 1.1   Magnification and Field of View

	Eyepiece	Objective	Magnification	Diameter of Field of View
Low-power	10×	10×	100×	1,500 μm
High-power	10×	40×	400×	375 μm
Oil immersion	10×	100×	1,000×	150 μm

Line drawings can be a great help in interpreting what is seen in sections because they incorporate a substantial amount of information garnered from many different sources, including different kinds of preparations and even observations made on the living tissue. They can also illustrate microscopic structure in three dimensions. Learning to visualize structures in three dimensions from what is seen in sections is such an essential part of histology that we shall now consider it in some detail.

Three-Dimensional Interpretation

Some idea of the difficulties involved in visualizing three-dimensional structure from the appearance of single sec-
tions can be gained by mentally reconstructing a hard-boiled egg. Some of the misconceptions that can arise are illustrated in Figure 1-5. Only slice *D* in this figure contains enough information to reveal the true structure of an egg. In some cases, the internal microscopic structure of parts of the body is so complicated that it can only be understood by mounting photographic enlargements of *serial* (consecutive) sections on material of appropriate thickness and assembling them in the proper order to constitute a large *reconstruction.*

It is very important to "think" in three dimensions when trying to match the shapes of areas seen in histological sections to the shapes of structures encountered in gross anatomy. We will therefore review the various *planes* in which histological sections can be cut.

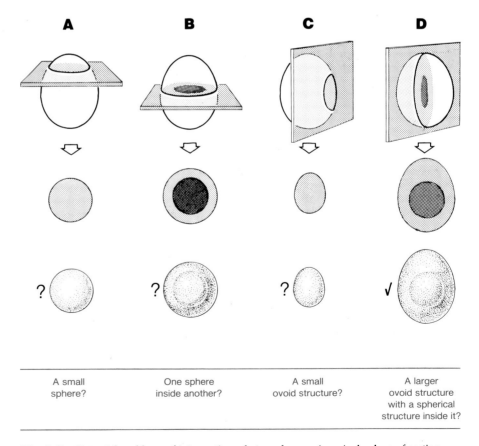

| A small sphere? | One sphere inside another? | A small ovoid structure? | A larger ovoid structure with a spherical structure inside it? |

Fig. 1-5.   Potential problems of interpreting what can be seen in a single plane of section.

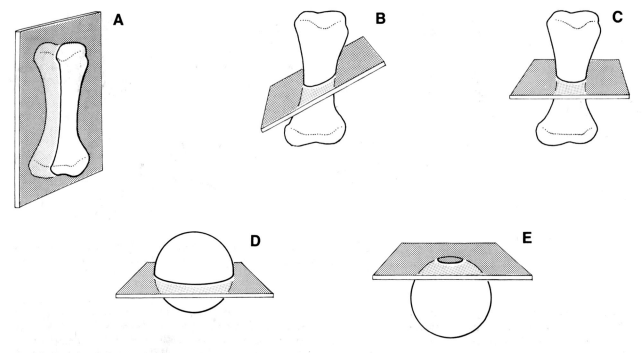

Fig. 1-6. Diagrams showing the various planes of histological section. A long structure may be cut in (A) longitudinal, (B) oblique, or (C) transverse or cross section. A rounded structure may be cut in (D) transverse or cross section, or (E) grazing or tangential section.

Planes of Histological Section. Any cut parallel to the longest dimension of a structure produces a *longitudinal section* (Fig. 1-6A), and any cut that is perpendicular to it produces a *cross section* (Fig. 1-6C). A cut at any angle between these two planes results in an *oblique section* (Fig. 1-6B). However, most cells and many body parts are round. A cut through the middle of a spherical structure produces a *cross section* (Fig. 1-6D), and one that only grazes the surface produces a *grazing section* (Fig. 1-6E), otherwise known as a *tangential section* (L. *tangere*, to touch).

We shall now consider the various appearances encountered when parts of the body with familiar shapes are cut in different planes.

Tubes. The body abounds with tubes of various diameters; those most frequently seen in histological sections are blood vessels and lymphatics. Also, many glands are equipped with tubular *ducts* that convey their secretions. It so happens that blood vessels, lymphatics, and ducts all can be conveniently observed at the same time in the small patches of connective tissue scattered throughout sections of the liver, particularly if this organ is taken from the pig, because in this species the supporting connective tissue is extremely prominent (see Fig. 1-9). Thus the representative area seen in Figure 1-9C contains a vein (*v*), a small artery (*a*), a lymphatic (*l*), and a duct (*d*), all of which have been cut in cross section. The tube labeled *o*, however, is sectioned obliquely and is less easy to recognize as a lymphatic

than the one labeled *l*. Hence tubes are most easily recognized if they have been cut in cross section, as depicted in Figure 1-7D. When they have been cut longitudinally (Fig. 1-7A, B, and C) or obliquely (Fig. 1-7E), or have been sectioned in places where they are curved (Fig. 1-8A, B, and C), it is necessary to visualize them in three dimensions in order to recognize them as tubes.

Partitions. Most glandular organs are subdivided internally by connective tissue partitions made up primarily of fibrous intercellular substances. Such partitions are termed *septa* (L. *saeptum*, wall). Pig liver is an excellent example of an organ that is subdivided into discrete compartments by septa (labeled *s* in Fig. 1-9), but human liver is not subdivided in this manner. Even though the individual compartments of a subdivided organ may be comparable in size and shape, some will appear larger and others smaller (Fig. 1-9A), depending on the level of section. This is readily verifiable by cutting an orange in different planes and observing the size of its segments (Fig. 1-10). By the same token, apparent differences in the size of nuclei or even whole cells can be due to differences in the level at which they were cut.

Rows of Cells. One possible interpretation of what can be seen in Plate 1-1C is that hepatocytes are arranged in single rows. However, by comparing this photomicrograph with the three-dimensional drawing in Figure 1-11, it will

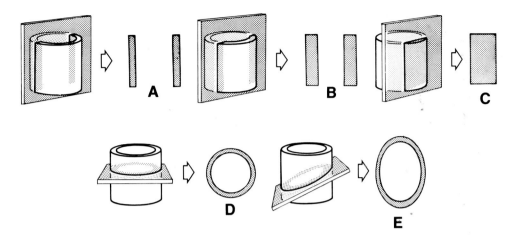

Fig. 1-7. Series of diagrams illustrating the appearance of sections of a straight tube cut in various planes. (*A, B,* and *C*) Longitudinal sections cut at different levels relative to the center of the lumen. Section *C* does not disclose the presence of a lumen. (*D*) Transverse or cross section. (*E*) Oblique section.

be appreciated that such an appearance is not inconsistent with an arrangement that is more than one cell deep. It is always necessary to think of what might have been present above or below the plane of section before arriving at a conclusion. Some histological terms take three-dimensional reconstruction into account, but a few disregard it entirely.

Histological Staining

Until tissue components have been suitably stained, they are all of fairly uniform optical density; hence most of what is present in a section appears indistinct and fails to stand out in sufficient contrast to the remainder (in this respect, phase-contrast microscopy is an exception). Staining is essential if all the components of a section are to be distinguished under the ordinary LM. The fact that different tissue components absorb these stains on a selective basis is a great asset that facilitates their recognition. Used in appropriate combinations, histological stains can act in two different ways. First, they enable the observer to recognize

certain tissue components by *differentially coloring* them. Secondly, they can impart their colors to different extents, which results in *graded depth of staining.* Such gradation becomes very important in EM staining, which is entirely dependent on it.

The two stains routinely used for histological sections are *hematoxylin* and *eosin;* the finished product is known as an *H & E section. Hematoxylin* is derived from the brownish-red wood of the logwood tree. In H & E staining, a weak dye called *hematein* is used in combination with Al^{3+} ions; *alum hematoxylin,* the dye complex formed, has a deep purple color. The second stain is *eosin,* which imparts a pink-to-red color to most of the tissue components that are not stained bluish-purple by hematoxylin. However, several factors can influence the final outcome of H & E staining, and considerable variation in these colors should be expected.

Basophilic and Acidophilic Staining. *Basophilic* substances are so called because they have an affinity for *basic*

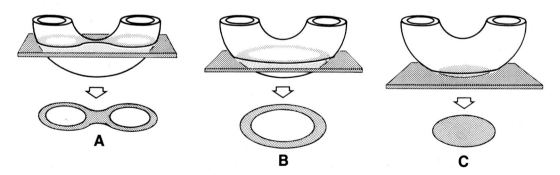

Fig. 1-8. Series of diagrams illustrating the appearance of sections of a curved tube cut at different levels relative to the center of its lumen. Sections *A* and *B* include the lumen. Section *C* does not disclose the presence of a lumen.

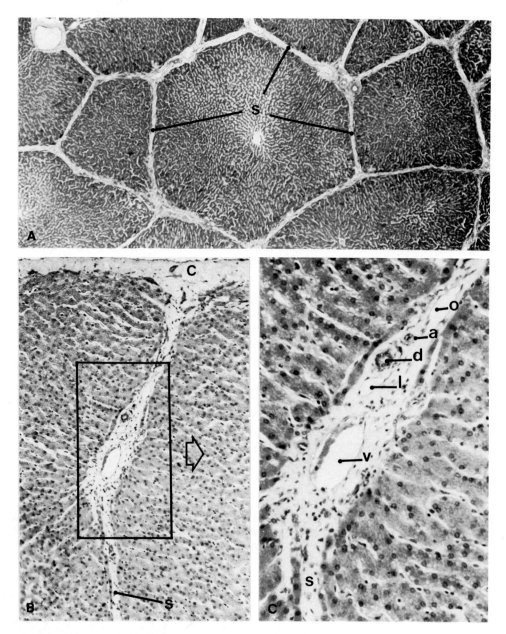

Fig. 1-9. Photomicrograph of a section of pig liver, illustrating how fibrous septa and tubular structures such as vessels and ducts appear when cut in cross or oblique section. (*A*) Pig liver differs from undiseased human liver in that it is subdivided into discrete lobules by fibrous septa (*s*). (*B*) These supporting septa (*s*) are made up of connective tissue that is continuous with the fibrous capsule (*c*) of the liver. (*C*) The following tubular structures can be distinguished within the septum (*s*): *v,* vein; *l* and *o,* lymphatics; *d,* duct; and *a,* arteriole.

stains, whereas *acidophilic* substances exhibit an affinity for *acid stains.*

The basic and acid stains we are talking about here are, in fact, neutral salts, each with an acid radical and a basic radical. In *basic* stains, the color resides in the *basic radical,* whereas in *acid* stains it resides in the *acid radical.* Hematoxylin acts as a basic stain; its

color-imparting component is the complex [hematein + Al^{3+}]. Substances stained by hematoxylin are accordingly described as *basophilic.* Substances that stain with eosin, an acid stain, are described as *acidophilic* (*eosinophilic*). These stains are now more often considered in terms of whether their color-imparting moiety is positively or negatively charged. If the color resides in their acid radical, which in ionic form is negatively charged, the stain is an

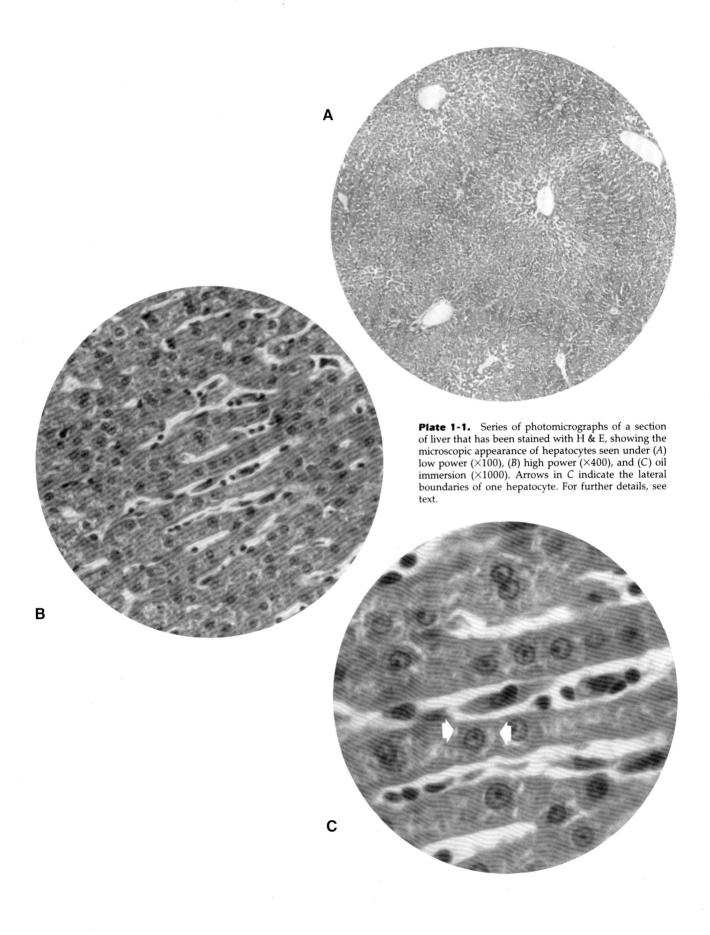

Plate 1-1. Series of photomicrographs of a section of liver that has been stained with H & E, showing the microscopic appearance of hepatocytes seen under (*A*) low power (×100), (*B*) high power (×400), and (*C*) oil immersion (×1000). Arrows in *C* indicate the lateral boundaries of one hepatocyte. For further details, see text.

providing a different color. Such *neutral stains* are widely employed for staining blood cells.

The Colors Seen in H & E Sections Reflect General Charge Distributions. The color-containing radicals of hematoxylin and eosin bind to tissue components of opposite charge. Thus the [hematein + Al^{3+}] complex in hematoxylin binds to negatively charged (anionic) sites on basophilic components, and the colored anion of eosin binds to positively charged (cationic) sites on acidophilic components. However, there is nothing specific about such binding. Apart from indicating general charge distributions, the colors seen after H & E staining tell the observer very little about the chemical composition of tissue components. Furthermore, factors such as the *p*H at which the sections were stained can affect the final colors, making them difficult to interpret. From Plate 1-1C it can be seen that the chromatin granules scattered about in the nucleus and associated with the nuclear envelope and nucleolus are intensely basophilic because of their content of nucleic acids, which are rich in PO_4^{3-} groups. Cytoplasmic proteins, on the other hand, are mostly acidophilic; hence the cytoplasm generally stains some shade of pink in contrast to the bluish-purple color of hematoxylin (Plate 1-1C). However, in cells that are synthesizing proteins very actively, there is sufficient nucleic acid (RNA) in the cytoplasm for this also to stain blue. Furthermore, the depth of cytoplasmic acidophilia seen is very dependent on the *p*H used during staining (generally in the range *p*H 5 to 6). At acid *p*H, a larger number of positively charged ionized groups (*e.g.*, NH_3^+) become available on cytoplasmic protein molecules to adsorb the eosin. Depending on the kind of tissue being

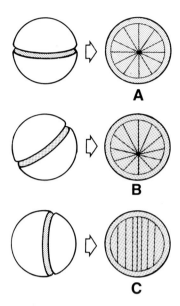

Fig. 1-10. Series of diagrams showing the appearance of the segments of an orange that has been cut in various planes of section. (*A*) Transverse or cross section. (*B*) Oblique section. (*C*) Nonmedial longitudinal section. Although the segments are septum-bounded compartments with similar dimensions, noticeable inequalities in size are seen in certain planes of section (*B* and *C*).

anionic stain. Conversely, if the color resides in their basic radical, which is positively charged, the stain is a *cationic stain*. Hence eosin, an acid stain, is also an anionic stain; hematoxylin, a basic stain, is also a cationic stain. Certain other stains are able to impart two different colors at the same time, their anion and cation each

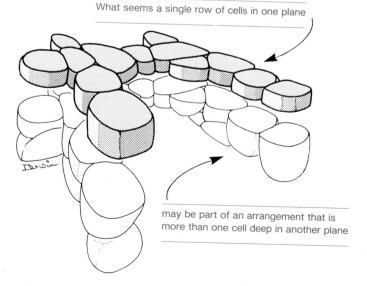

What seems a single row of cells in one plane

Fig. 1-11. When interpreting what is seen in a single plane of section, it is necessary to think about what could have been present above or below the plane of section.

may be part of an arrangement that is more than one cell deep in another plane

stained, it may be necessary to adjust the *p*H to achieve the desired depth of staining. Hence any temptation to try to attach too much importance to color should be resisted, and it is a good idea to learn to rely on black and white illustrations instead of colored ones, which may manifest excessive variability in color. This is also good training for the interpretation of electron micrographs, which are never in color because there is no color spectrum in an electron beam. In black and white photomicrographs, blue-to-purple staining is seen as black tones and pink-to-red staining appears in shades of gray, but the amount of contrast seen between blues and reds may have been artificially enhanced for photographic purposes through the use of appropriate color filters. Basically, however, the darker tones are due to staining with hematoxylin and the lighter tones are due to staining with eosin.

In addition to H & E staining, special methods exist for demonstrating tissue components that do not stain well with routine stains. Some of these methods will be described subsequently in connection with the particular tissues for which they are used. Also, certain staining procedures generate colors that do indicate the chemical nature of the component being stained, but these represent a special case. Thus in *histochemical* staining, known color reactions specific to particular chemical groups in tissue components are employed for their detection. An example of such a reaction is described in the following section.

The Periodic Acid–Schiff (PAS) Reaction for Staining Polysaccharides.   The liver plays an important role in maintaining a constant level of blood sugar. Glucose absorbed from the intestine after meals is absorbed by hepatocytes and is converted into *glycogen,* a polysaccharide storage product. Neither eosin nor hematoxylin stain glycogen, translucent deposits of which are recognized in the cytoplasm as empty-looking *spaces* with *ragged edges* (Fig. 1-12A; Plate 1-1C). A widely used histochemical reaction employed to demonstrate glycogen in cells is the *PAS reaction.* In this two-step histochemical procedure, *periodic acid* (HIO$_4$) is employed first to oxidize hexose and hexosamine residues in polysaccharide chains to aldehyde groups. The *Schiff reagent,* which is decolorized basic fuchsin, is then used to detect the aldehyde groups, with which it combines to produce a magenta- or purple-colored complex. In Figure 1-12, the appearance of glycogen-storing hepatocytes stained by the PAS procedure is compared with their appearance in an H & E section.

However, glycogen is not the only polysaccharide-containing constituent of tissues; hence a further step is necessary to determine whether a given PAS-positive constituent is glycogen. It so happens that glycogen is readily degraded by an enzyme present in saliva (α-*amylase,* also known as *diastase*), so it is standard procedure to incubate a control section with amylase (or saliva) before staining it by the PAS procedure and to ascertain whether this di-

gests the reactive substance from the section. If unextractable by amylase, the stained material is usually *glycoprotein* or *proteoglycan,* although *glycolipid* is also PAS positive.

Fat Stains.   Another kind of seemingly empty space can be seen in the cytoplasm of the cells of some livers. Such spaces differ from those of glycogen in that they are round and have sharp edges (Fig. 1-13A) instead of irregular shapes and fuzzy edges. Round empty spaces are left by the dissolution of stored droplets of fat by the reagents employed in making paraffin sections. If the cells of liver contain a great many of these round holes or a single large one, as in Figure 1-13, the person is said to have a *fatty liver.* Commonly, this condition is seen in individuals who have, for a lengthy period, omitted nourishing food from their diets in favor of considerable amounts of alcohol.

Because the fat in liver cells dissolves during preparation of a paraffin section, frozen sections are used to demonstrate fat with such special stains as scharlach R or Sudan III (Fig. 1-13B).

Artifacts

An *artifact* (L. *ars,* art; *factum,* made) is something artificial. In histology, this term is used for unwanted features in sections that are the result of accident or poor technique. Because artifacts are sometimes seen in sections studied in the laboratory, it is helpful to learn how to recognize common ones now in order to disregard them later. The inexperienced student sometimes spends a lot of time worrying about a feature in a slide about which he has received no instruction, only to find out later that this feature does not exist in living tissue at all. We shall mention here a few common artifacts.

Postmortem Degeneration.   Although this is the most common cause of poor quality in sections, postmortem degeneration is, strictly speaking, not a true artifact. This is because instead of being something inflicted on the tissue by human hands, it is the result of something that is not being done properly. The importance of rapid and thorough fixation has already been emphasized. Unless tissues are fixed as soon as they are obtained, they suffer a prolonged period of *anoxia* (Gr. *an,* without; meaning without oxygen) and this causes hydrolytic enzymes to be released from cytoplasmic organelles known as lysosomes. The hydrolytic enzymes commence to digest the cells, so that details are lacking when seen under the microscope.

Shrinkage.   The various reagents used in preparing sections, including hot paraffin, often cause shrinkage of tissues. As a result, tissues that are attached in life may become pulled away from each other, leaving empty spaces, as indicated by the arrows in Figure 1-14A. This is a very common artifact, and the student should be forewarned

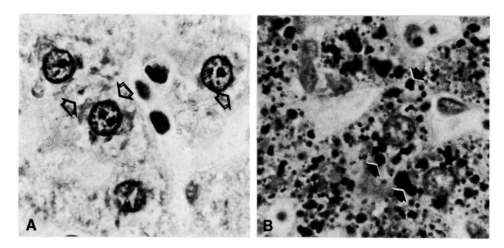

Fig. 1-12. Photomicrographs of hepatocytes that are storing glycogen in their cytoplasm. (*A*) In H & E sections, glycogen deposits (*arrows*) appear as clear spaces with ragged edges. (*B*) In PAS-stained sections, glycogen deposits (*arrows*) are stained a bright magenta color.

that with the exception of true anatomical spaces filled with tissue fluid or other special fluids, there are no such seemingly "empty" spaces in the living body.

Precipitate.   Numerous particles of precipitate are frequently seen (Fig. 1-14*B*) in tissues fixed in formaldehyde solutions that are poorly buffered and therefore acidic. When acidic formalin reacts with the red pigment *hemoglobin* of erythrocytes (or *myoglobin* in muscle cells), a brown granular pigment is also formed, called *formalin pigment.*

This artifact increases with the length of time the tissue is left in formaldehyde. Other fixatives, too, will form precipitates unless properly removed.

Precipitation can also occur during certain staining procedures, especially in connection with the use of blood stains. It can be avoided by not allowing the stain to become too concentrated or dried out during staining.

Folds and Wrinkles.   Paraffin sections are so thin that it is not unusual for them to become wrinkled or folded when

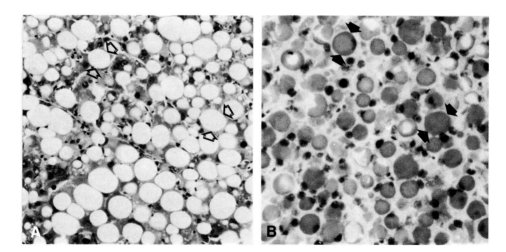

Fig. 1-13. Photomicrographs of hepatocytes that are storing excess fat in their cytoplasm (fatty liver). (*A*) In H & E sections, the sites where fat droplets were present (*arrows*) appear as round empty spaces with distinct edges. (*B*) In frozen sections stained with a Sudan dye, fat droplets (*arrows*) persist and stain positively for fat.

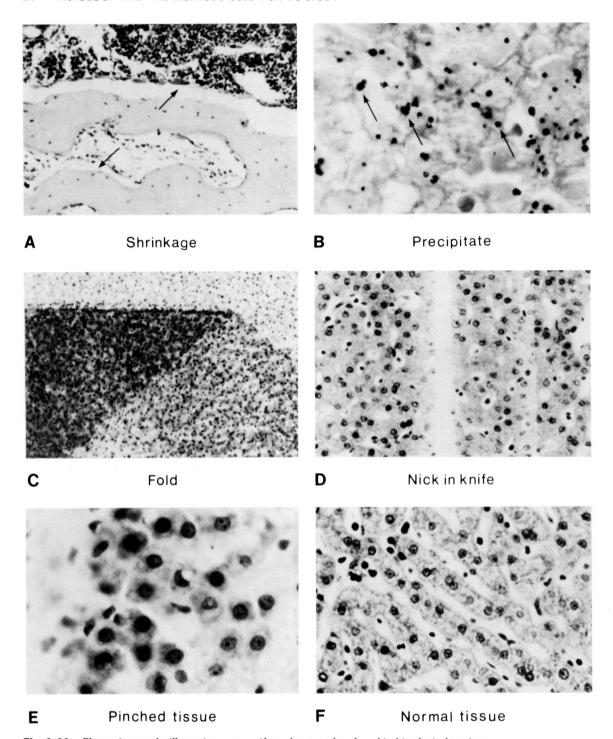

A   Shrinkage

B   Precipitate

C   Fold

D   Nick in knife

E   Pinched tissue

F   Normal tissue

Fig. 1-14. Photomicrographs illustrating some artifacts that are often found in histological sections.

the section is being mounted on a slide. They then appear as shown in Figure 1-14C.

Knife Nicks.   Any little nicks in the cutting edge of the microtome knife will cause straight lines to appear across the sections as the knife cuts through the embedded block (Fig. 1-14D).

Rough Handling of the Tissue.   An artifact that can create the impression of some pathological change is produced by rough handling of the tissue while it is being obtained (*e.g.,* pinching it with forceps or cutting it with dull scissors). This appearance, illustrated in Figure 1-14E, may be compared with Figure 1-14F, which shows how this tissue appears when it is not mistreated.

Electron Microscopy

From physics it was established that the *limit of resolution* (*i.e.,* maximal resolution) of the LM, about *0.2 μm,* is imposed by the wavelength of visible light. However, the discovery that electromagnetic lenses could be employed to shape and focus an electron beam then led to an enormous advance in microscopy because it was realized that the wavelength of a voltage-accelerated electron beam is very short indeed, giving it the potential for much greater resolution than formerly obtainable using light rays. This led to the design of an *electron microscope* (EM) based on the principle of using of an electron beam in place of light rays. This is an instrument that is now capable of *resolving about 1 nm* in biological specimens (1 nm is equal to 0.001 μm). Although the first electron microscopes were built in the 1930s, it was not until the mid-1950s that the preparation of biological materials became advanced enough to permit the effective study of cells and tissues (see Pease and Porter). This achievement opened up a whole new world of knowledge about the detailed structure of the body.

Transmission Electron Microscopy. The optical path of the EM is easily understood if it is compared with that of the LM. In the type of EM most commonly employed for the study of tissues, the electron beam is used much like a beam of light and passes right through many parts of the specimen. This particular kind of EM is therefore called a *transmission electron microscope* (TEM), and we shall describe the design and operation of this type of EM first. However, to compare its optical path with the LM, it is necessary first to consider how an image is produced in the LM.

The optics of the LM are shown on the left side of Figure 1-15, but, to compare them readily with those of the EM, the optical path of the LM is drawn upside down.

In the LM, light is focused with a *condenser lens* onto the object—for example, a stained specimen. The light passing through the object enters the *objective lens,* which brings an image of the object into focus somewhere between the objective lens and the *ocular lens;* the latter then further magnifies this image. Alternatively, the ocular lens can be used to bring the enlarged image into focus on *photographic film* placed at the site indicated by the bottom arrow (Fig. 1-15, *left*), to produce a *photomicrograph.*

The optics of the *transmission EM* are illustrated in the middle of Figure 1-15. The electrons are deflected by the variable electromagnetic fields of the electromagnetic lenses (stippled in Fig. 1-15). The whole instrument (Fig. 1-16) is, in essence, a cathode-ray tube in which a vacuum must be maintained by continuous pumping, because electrons can travel only for very short distances in air. From the electrically heated *cathode,* which is a V-shaped tungsten filament, electrons are emitted and accelerated toward the *anode* (usually by a potential difference of 50 to 100 kilovolts). The anode has an aperture through which the electron beam passes before being focused by the *condenser lens* onto the specimen.

As the electrons pass through the specimen, some are scattered out of the beam by the electron-dense parts of the specimen. The scattered electrons are removed from the beam by the blocking action of a very fine *aperture* (not shown in the diagram) positioned just above the objective lens. The role of this aperture is to provide more contrast in the image. The electrons not scattered by electron-dense parts of the specimen are focused by the *objective lens* to produce an enlarged image of the specimen. This image is then enlarged further, first by a lens known as an *intermediate lens* (not shown) and then by a *projection lens;* the latter projects the image either onto a *fluorescent screen* or onto *photographic film* for taking *electron micrographs.* EM sections are prepared as follows.

1. *Fixation. Glutaraldehyde* fixation followed by *osmic acid* postfixation is routinely used for electron microscopy. The addition of *tannic acid* to the glutaraldehyde sometimes reveals more details (see Fig. 3-10, *left*). If it is necessary to preserve enzymatic activity, *formaldehyde* is used in place of glutaraldehyde, and any histochemical staining is done prior to osmic acid postfixation.
2. *Embedding.* Following dehydration, the specimen is infiltrated with unpolymerized embedding medium. The medium has to be harder than wax to permit the cutting of EM sections, which must be extremely thin because electrons cannot penetrate very far into tissues. Epoxy resins are used most often. The specimen is kept at 60°C for several days to allow the resin to harden by polymerization.
3. *Sectioning.* EM sections are cut on an *ultramicrotome* using the broken edge of fractured plate glass or a diamond knife. The sections are then floated onto water and picked up on a small copper grid coated with a supporting film of carbon or plastic. Electrons pass through the supporting grid by way of its perforations.
   Section Thickness. EM sections, sometimes referred to as *thin sections,* are routinely cut to a thickness of 60 to 80 nanometers. A *nanometer* (*nm,* from the Gr. *nanos,* dwarf) is 0.001 micrometer; a *micrometer* (*μm*) is 0.001 *millimeter* (*mm*). The *Angström unit* (Å), previously used very extensively for EM measurements, is 0.1 nm; hence 1 nm equals 10 Å.
4. *Staining.* Salts of *heavy metals* combine with tissue components to various extents, rendering some of them more electron dense than others. This increases the amount of contrast obtained. *Osmic acid* acts both as a fixative and as a stain, scattering electrons very effectively. Other electron stains, which are generally applied to sections already placed on grids, include soluble salts of *uranium* and *lead.*

Electron Micrographs. Electrons cannot be seen, so the EM image is formed on a fluorescent screen that converts the energy of electrons into light. This energy can also produce *silver grains* in a photographic emulsion, enabling film to be used to obtain the negative of an *electron micrograph.* Electron-dense regions in the specimen scatter electrons and thereby produce white areas on the negative. Because photographic printing reverses black and white, such white areas on the negative appear black on the print. Accordingly, the electron-dense regions of transmission electron micrographs appear *black.* In the course of learning about the fine structure (*ultrastructure*) of cells and tissues, histology students have to become familiar with a great many types of electron micrographs. The conventional electron micrographs seen in histology textbooks are taken with a *transmission* EM that requires electrons to pass through the section in order to produce an image. Because more detail can be recorded by photography than can be seen by direct observation of the fluorescent screen, enlarged prints of EM negatives are used to take fullest advantage of the resolving power of the instrument.

In interpreting transmission electron micrographs, it is

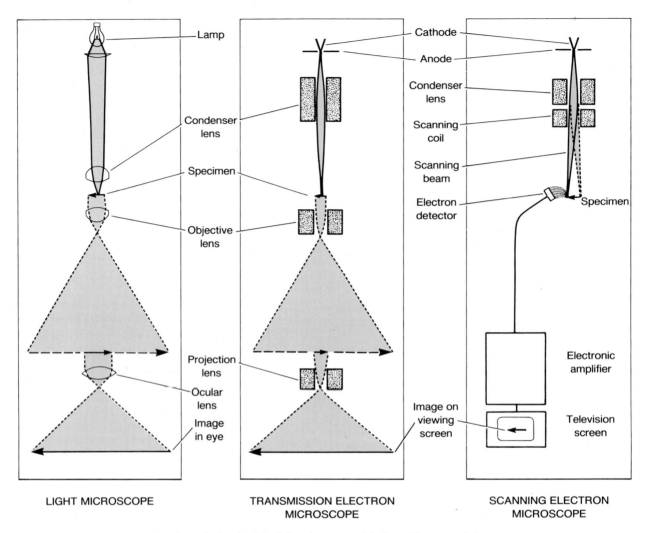

Fig. 1-15. Diagram comparing the optical path of the light microscope with that of the transmission electron microscope and scanning electron microscope. The optical path of the light microscope has been inverted to facilitate comparison.

always necessary to remember that EM sections are generally very much thinner (60 nm to 80 nm) than LM sections (5 μm to 8μm). Whereas two or three LM sections are sufficient to disclose the entire contents of most cells, about 400 routine EM sections would be required to achieve the same purpose. Hence, the amount of representative information gained about cells from the usual kind of EM section is somewhat limited. Also, everything present in such a section is seen in the *same plane of focus*. Unlike an LM section, it is not possible to tell by focusing up and down whether a given component of the section lies above or below another; they will both appear to lie in the same plane.

High-Voltage Electron Microscopy.   If an EM section is not representative of the entire cell, the problem can be circumvented by using a *high-voltage electron microscope*. In this special kind of TEM, increased acceleration of the electrons by a much greater potential difference (1000 to 3000 kilovolts) substantially increases their ability to penetrate the tissue, enabling thicker sections to be used and even making it possible to observe the full thickness of tissue culture cells up to 3 μm thick. This type of EM can provide better resolution (0.2 nm) and can also give an impression of section depth, as may be seen in Figure 11-3*B*. If the specimen is too thick to be viewed under a high-voltage EM, it is still possible to study its surface features by means of another type of EM designed on an altogether different principle, as described in the following section.

Scanning Electron Microscopy.   In the *scanning electron microscope* (SEM), the electron beam *scans* the surface of the specimen instead of passing through it. Electrons reflected and emitted as secondary electrons from a thin, heavy-metal coating on its surface are converted into electrical signals that build up an image of the surface on a television screen (Fig. 1-15). The photographic record of

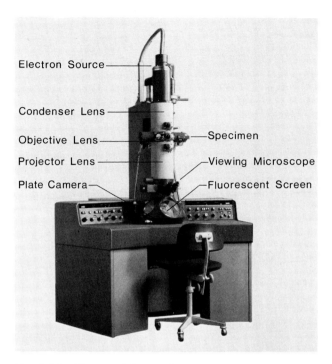

Electron Source

Condenser Lens

Objective Lens

Projector Lens

Plate Camera

Specimen

Viewing Microscope

Fluorescent Screen

Fig. 1-16. The essential parts of a transmission electron microscope. (Courtesy of Phillips Electronics)

the image on the screen is termed a *scanning electron micrograph*. The great advantage of such a micrograph is that it reveals surface contours *in three dimensions*. (A good example may be seen in Fig. 4-30.)

The basic design of the SEM is depicted in the right-hand panel of Figure 1-15. The *condenser lens* is used to produce a narrow pencil-like beam of electrons; this passes through a *scanning coil* that moves it back and forth over the surface of the specimen in a rapid scanning motion corresponding to the scanning pattern on a television screen. At each place that the scanning beam strikes the specimen, secondary electrons are emitted from its surface coating. These secondary electrons are collected by *electron detectors* and their energy is converted into an electrical signal, the intensity of which is displayed at the corresponding position on a *television screen*. The scanning beam follows the same path as the image-producing spot on the television screen and travels in synchrony with it so as to build up the image. Micrographs are obtained by photographing the image on the television screen.

A specimen has to be specially prepared for its surface features to be examined in the SEM; it does not need to be cut into sections. Following suitable fixation, the specimen is first *dehydrated* as gently as possible to avoid distortion. After it has been mounted, it is coated with a thin layer of heavy metal, such as gold or platinum, that scatters electrons and thereby enables the surface features of the specimen to be observed.

Scanning electron micrographs are generally easier to interpret than transmission electron micrographs because they disclose structure in three dimensions. However, the resolving power of the SEM is not quite as great as that of the TEM (3 nm to 5 nm in the SEM compared with 1 nm in the TEM).

SELECTED REFERENCES

Light Microscopy

BARER R: Lecture Notes on the Use of the Microscope. Oxford, Blackwell, 1968

DIXON K: Principles of some tinctorial and cytochemical methods. In Champion RH, Gilman T, Rook AJ, Sims RT (eds.): An Introduction to the Biology of the Skin, chap. 4. Oxford, Blackwell, 1970

GAUNT PN, GAUNT WA: Three Dimensional Reconstruction in Biology. Baltimore, University Park Press, 1978

JAMES J: Light Microscopic Techniques in Biology and Medicine. The Hague, Martinus Nijhoff, 1976

KAWAMURA A, JR (ed): Fluorescent Antibody Techniques and Their Application, 2nd ed. Baltimore, University Park Press, 1977

KRSTIĆ RV: Illustrated Encyclopedia of Human Histology. Berlin, Springer-Verlag, 1984

PEARSE AGE: Histochemistry—Theoretical and Applied, 3rd ed, Vols 1 and 2. Boston, Little, Brown, 1968

WILLMER EN (ed): Cells and Tissues in Culture. Methods, Biology and Physiology, Vols 1 to 3. London, Academic Press, 1965

Electron Microscopy

AGAR AW, ALDERSON RH, CHESCOE D:Principles and practice of electron microscope operations. In Glauert AM (ed): Practical Methods in Electron Microscopy, Vol 2. Amsterdam, North Holland, 1974

ALLEN DJ, MOTTA PM, DIDIO JA (eds): Three Dimensional Microanatomy of Cells and Tissue Surfaces. New York, Elsevier North-Holland, 1981

DEMEY J: Colloidal gold probes in immunocytochemistry. In Polak J, van Noorden S (eds): Immunocytochemistry: Applications in Pathology and Biology. London, John Wright & Sons, 1983

EVERHART TE, HAYES TL: The scanning electron microscope. Sci Am 226:54, Jan. 1972

GLAUERT AM: Fixation, dehydration and embedding of biological specimens. In Glauert AM (ed): Practical Methods in Electron Microscopy, Vol 3, Part 1. Amsterdam, North Holland, 1975

GOODMAN SL, HODGES GM, TREJDOSIEWICZ I, LIVINGSTON DC: Colloidal gold markers and probes for routine application in microscopy. J Microsc 123:201, 1981

HAYAT MA: Basic Electron Microscopy Technics. New York, Van Nostrand Reinhold, 1972

HAYAT MA: Principles and Techniques of Electron Microscopy. New York, Van Nostrand Reinhold, 1972

HAYAT MA: Introduction to Biological Scanning Electron Microscopy. Baltimore, University Park Press, 1978

KOEHLERED JK: Advanced Techniques in Biological Electron Microscopy, New York, Springer-Verlag, 1973

LEWIS PR, KNIGHT DP: Staining methods for sectioned material. In Glauert AM (ed): Practical Methods in Electron Microscopy, vol 5. Amsterdam, North Holland, 1977

PEASE DC, PORTER KR: Electron microscopy and ultramicrotomy. J Cell Biol 91:287s, 1981

REID N: Ultramicrotomy. In Glauert AM (ed): Practical Methods in Electron Microscopy, Vol 3, Part 2. Amsterdam, North Holland, 1975

WISCHNITZER S: Introduction to Electron Microscopy, 2nd ed. New York, Pergamon Press, 1970

PART TWO

CELL BIOLOGY

Cell biology is the keystone around which histology is built. A thorough understanding of the nature of the cell and its component parts is therefore an important step toward mastering histology. Cell biology now incorporates a wealth of information derived from many different disciplines, including biochemistry, molecular biology, and genetics. Students with some background in modern cell biology will find Part Two to be a broad-based review of certain relevant facets of the subject. Those lacking such a background will find that Part Two constitutes an essential preparation for studying the tissues in Part Three and the systems in Part Four.

2

The Interphase Nucleus

NUCLEAR ENVELOPE

NUCLEAR PORES

NUCLEAR MATRIX

NUCLEAR DNA AND OTHER COMPONENTS OF CHROMATIN
Chromatin

PROTEIN SYNTHESIS: ROLE OF NUCLEIC ACIDS

NUCLEOLUS

NUCLEAR CHANGES INDICATING CELL DEATH

Eukaryotic cells (cells with a true nucleus) have a more complex level of organization than prokaryotic cells (cells that lack a true nucleus). They are characterized by a *nuclear envelope* that segregates a discrete central compartment, the cell *nucleus*, from the remainder of the cell, which is known as its *cytoplasm*. The nucleus is essentially a storage compartment for DNA, the very important self-perpetuating nucleic acid that codes for the various kinds of proteins synthesized in the cytoplasm of the cell. It is also the part of the cell that begins the process of putting genetic instructions into effect. Unlike the cytoplasm, which in many instances shows evidence of specialization for specific tasks, the nucleus performs fundamentally similar functions in all kinds of cells and, with relatively few exceptions, exhibits the same kind of internal structure. Its characteristic appearance at the light microscopic and electron microscopic levels and its main functions during the lifetime of the cell will be considered in this chapter; the radical changes that it undergoes when the cell divides will be dealt with in Chapter 3.

The nondividing phase in which the body cells perform their various specialized functions is described as *interphase*, a term that came into being as a result of studies of continuously dividing cells growing *in vitro*. Cells that were not engaged in the process of cell division were viewed as being between phases of division, hence the term *interphase*. As we shall see, in most instances, it is more applicable to use the term *nondividing cell* for *interphase cell*, but it has nevertheless become customary to refer to the nucleus of a nondividing cell as the *interphase nucleus*.

Whereas the various stages of cell division were already known from light microscopic studies completed before the turn of the century, the nature of the interphase nucleus, particularly the structure and functions of its chromatin, have only recently begun to be elucidated through the use of applied electron microscopy, sophisticated biochemical methods, molecular genetics, and other newly emerging investigative techniques of molecular cell biology.

General Features of the Interphase Nucleus.   Interphase nuclei of all cells are made up of the same basic components. Yet they do not look exactly the same in all kinds of cells, and this can be helpful in cell recognition. For example, the nuclei of some cells have such tightly packed contents that their individual components cannot be distinguished with the light microscope (LM). The cells lining liver sinusoids exemplify this type of cell (Fig. 2-1). There are also cells with nuclei of unusual shape (*e.g.*, elongated instead of round to ovoid, or pinched into a segmented shape as in the neutrophil; see Fig. 8-11).

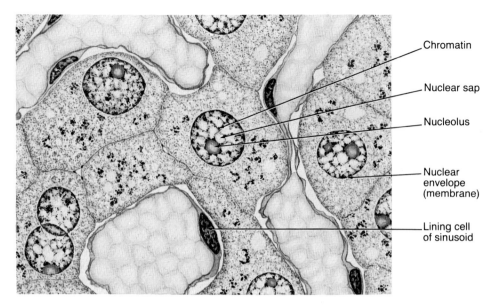

Chromatin

Nuclear sap

Nucleolus

Nuclear envelope (membrane)

Lining cell of sinusoid

Fig. 2-1.   The appearance of the interphase nucleus in a liver section stained with H & E. The nucleus in hepatocytes contains extended chromatin and chromatin granules, whereas that in the lining cells of sinusoids contains tightly packed condensed chromatin.

Figure 2-1 illustrates the characteristic features of the interphase nucleus as seen in hepatocytes in hematoxylin and eosin (H & E) sections. The boundary of the nucleus is marked by a blue-purple line that indicates the position of its *nuclear envelope* (sometimes referred to as the *nuclear membrane*). Within the nucleus, there are one or more fairly large and heavily stained masses called *nucleoli,* as well as many smaller and less rounded aggregates of *chromatin* (Fig. 2-1). The intense staining of these components is due to a high concentration of nucleic acids. Between them is a nonstaining colloidal sol still sometimes referred to as the *nuclear sap.* As we shall see, the presence of *chromatin granules* in the nucleus is a reflection of the fact that interphase chromosomes exist in a partly condensed and partly extended condition that gives them the collective appearance of granules. The type of chromatin that constitutes chromatin granules is described as *condensed chromatin,* and that representing the extended regions of chromosomes, not visible in the LM, is referred to as *extended chromatin.*

Chromosomes and the Nucleic Acids: Historical Perspective.   Early light microscopic studies revealed that dividing cells contained dark-staining, thread-shaped *chromosomes* (Gr. *chroma,* color; *soma,* body) in place of *chromatin granules,* and cell division thereupon came to be known as *mitosis* (Gr. *mitos,* thread; *osis,* condition). It was then observed that each mitotic chromosome divided longitudinally, with the result that the two daughter cells received an identical set of chromosomes. Because it was known that the daughter cells also inherited identical genes, it became evident that *genes are carried on chromosomes.*

The next key development was discovery of the nucleic acids and elucidation of their chemical structure. *Nucleic acids* were found to be long linear macromolecules made up of alternating sugar

and phosphate groups with nitrogenous bases extending as side chains from the sugars (see Fig. 2-6). There are two different nucleic acids, *deoxyribonucleic acid (DNA)* and *ribonucleic acid (RNA),* each with its own constituent sugar: 2-deoxy-D-ribose in DNA and D-ribose in RNA. Moreover, there is one difference between their respective nitrogenous bases that we shall consider later in this chapter. DNA can be distinguished histochemically from RNA by means of the *Feulgen reaction.* A section of fixed material is first subjected to a mild acid hydrolysis capable of removing the purine groups from the deoxyribose residues of DNA. This treatment yields an aldehyde group on each deoxyribose residue. The aldehyde groups are then detected by means of the Schiff reaction, which is described in Chapter 1 in connection with PAS staining. Any DNA present in the section is thereby colored magenta. The specificity of the Feulgen reaction is due to the fact that the initial hydrolysis employed is too mild to generate aldehyde groups from the ribose residues that characterize RNA. With Feulgen staining, it was conclusively demonstrated that the predominant constituent of chromatin granules and mitotic chromosomes is DNA.

Then came the important discovery that DNA extracted from a specific strain of bacteria possessed the remarkable potential of conferring inheritable characteristics on another strain. Since then a wealth of additional evidence has been obtained in support of the conclusion that *DNA represents the chemical basis of genes.*

With this introductory account of the microscopic structure and chemical nature of the cell nucleus as general background, we shall now go on to describe the parts of the interphase nucleus in more detail.

NUCLEAR ENVELOPE

In H & E sections, the *nuclear envelope (membrane)* appears as a substantial, darkly stained line (Fig. 2-1). Its apparent

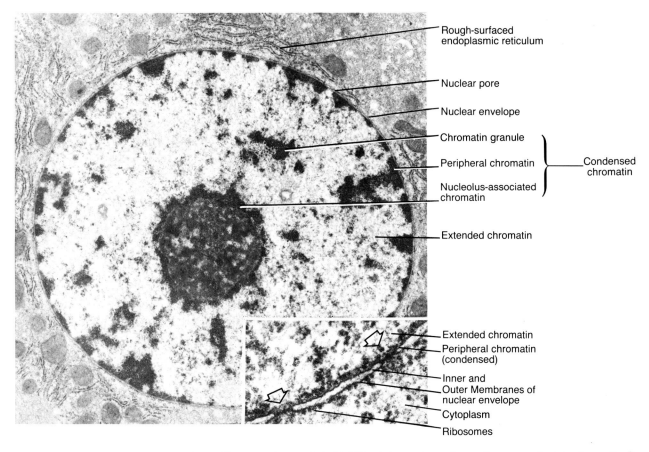

Rough-surfaced endoplasmic reticulum

Nuclear pore

Nuclear envelope

Chromatin granule

Peripheral chromatin } Condensed chromatin

Nucleolus-associated chromatin

Extended chromatin

Extended chromatin
Peripheral chromatin (condensed)
Inner and Outer Membranes of nuclear envelope
Cytoplasm
Ribosomes

Fig. 2-2. Electron micrograph (×14,000) of the nucleus of a rat hepatocyte in interphase. (*Inset*) Higher magnification micrograph of the nuclear envelope. The *arrows* indicate nuclear pores. (*Large micrograph,* Miyai K, Steiner JW: Exp Mol Pathol 4:525, 1965; *inset,* courtesy of V.I. Kalnins)

thickness and depth of staining are due to the condensed chromatin adherent to its inner surface, as becomes evident if a section treated with DNAase (which hydrolyzes DNA) is compared with one that has not been treated with this enzyme. The adherent *peripheral chromatin* is more readily distinguished in electron micrographs (Fig. 2-2). It will also be seen from Figures 2-2 to 2-4 that the nuclear envelope is made up of *two membranes* about 8 nm thick, separated by a space of approximately 25 nm. These membranes, which are below the limit of resolution of the LM, are seen clearly in the electron microscope (EM) only where they have been cut in a perpendicular plane. They are like the other membranes in the cell in that they have a *unit membrane* structure. This means that although at low magnification each membrane appears as a single electron-dense line (Fig. 2-2), under high magnification with good staining and resolution it has a trilaminar appearance (see Fig. 2-4A). The general basis of this more complex staining pattern will be considered at the molecular level when we deal with the cell membrane in Chapter 4. Thus the constituent membranes of the nuclear envelope are both typical unit membranes with a molecular structure that is basically

similar to the other membranes of the cell. The lumen of the nuclear envelope lies *between* these two unit membranes (Fig. 2-3).

The *outer membrane* of the nuclear envelope (*i.e.,* the membrane next to the cytoplasm) is continuous with that of a cytoplasmic membrane system known as the *rough-surfaced endoplasmic reticulum,* which will be described in Chapter 4. Hence the outer membrane of the nuclear envelope and the membrane of the rough-surfaced endoplasmic reticulum have one feature in common: both are *studded with ribosomes,* which are electron-dense organelles involved in the synthesis of proteins (Fig. 2-2, *inset,* and Fig. 2-3).

NUCLEAR PORES

An exchange of macromolecules between the nuclear and cytoplasmic compartments occurs by way of the *nuclear pores,* which are specialized apertures in the nuclear envelope (Fig. 2-2, *inset,* indicated by arrows, and Fig. 2-4). Almost circular in face view (Fig. 2-4B and C), these pores

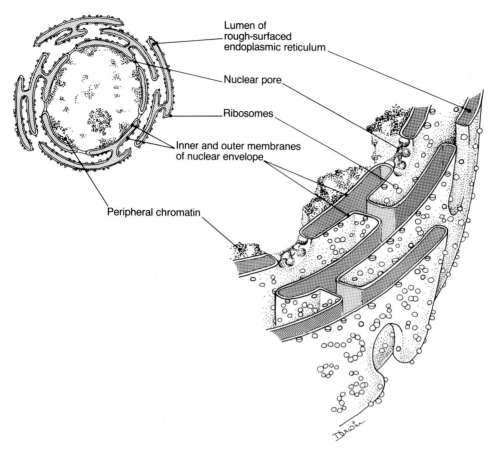

Lumen of
rough-surfaced
endoplasmic reticulum

Nuclear pore

Ribosomes

Inner and outer membranes
of nuclear envelope

Peripheral chromatin

Fig. 2-3. Schematic diagram of the interconnections between the nuclear envelope and cisternae of the rough-surfaced endoplasmic reticulum. The inner and outer membranes of the nuclear envelope are continuous with each other at the periphery of the nuclear pores.

actually exhibit an octagonal substructure. Most cells have several thousand nuclear pores, spaced roughly 100 nm to 200 nm apart. At the periphery of each pore, there is direct continuity between the inner and outer membranes of the nuclear envelope (Figs. 2-2, 2-3, and 2-4B). Nuclear pores range in diameter from 30 nm to 100 nm, depending on the cell type. Detailed studies show that they contain intricate structures that can be isolated as distinct entities from the nuclear envelope. From each pore a cylindrical channel extends for a short distance into the nucleus on the one side and into the cytoplasm on the other. Within the nucleus, condensed chromatin encircles the periphery of the pore but is absent from the inner surface of the pore (Figs. 2-3 and 2-4A). On the cytoplasmic side, a short channel encircled by a ring of slightly increased electron density extends from the pore region (Fig. 2-4A). The entire arrangement is known as a *nuclear pore complex.*

Macromolecular exchanges occur *in both directions* across the nuclear pores, which evidently regulate which molecules pass from the nucleus to the cytoplasm and vice versa. In this connection, there are indications that the nuclear

pore aperture is covered by a shelflike partition composed of some kind of fibrillar material (Fig. 2-2, *inset,* and Fig. 2-4A and B). Nuclear pores also sometimes exhibit a central electron-dense granule (Fig. 2-4C), which is currently believed to be a tiny mass of ribonucleoprotein, possibly a ribosomal subunit, that is in the process of passing through the pore complex toward the cytoplasm. There is evidence to suggest that macromolecules and macromolecular aggregates with diameters approaching 10 nm to 15 nm can traverse some kind of selective central channel that seems to exist or open up in the middle of each nuclear pore. However, entire ribosomes exceed the width of this channel and remain in the cytoplasm where they are assembled. Accordingly, proteins are synthesized in the cytoplasm but not in the nucleus.

NUCLEAR MATRIX

The interphase nucleus also possesses a protein-containing skeletal framework called the *nuclear matrix.* The main

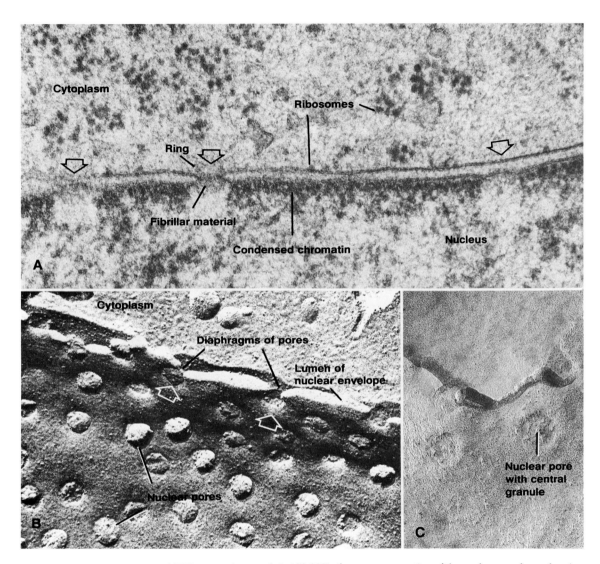

Fig. 2-4. (*A*) Electron micrograph (×120,000) of a transverse section of the nuclear envelope, showing sites of three nuclear pore complexes (*arrows*). In the pore situated left of center, fibrillar material is visible in the pore aperture, and the external ring that extends from the periphery of the pore into the cytoplasm can just be discerned, along with the closing diaphragm. Peripheral chromatin is not seen at the aperture site. A few ribosomes are attached to the outer membrane of the nuclear envelope. (*B*) Freeze-fracture replica (×76,000) of the nuclear envelope, showing its nuclear pore complexes. Diaphragms can be seen closing over the pore apertures of the fractured pores (*arrows*). Continuity between the inner and outer membranes of the nuclear envelope can be seen at the pore periphery. (C) Freeze-fracture replica of the outer surface of the nuclear envelope (×120,000). In the pore complex seen in face view at right, a central ribonucleoprotein granule is in the process of escaping through the pore aperture. (For details of the procedure used to prepare the replicas shown in *B* and *C*, see Fig. 4-3, discussed in Chap. 4 in connection with the cell membrane.) (Courtesy of L. Arsenault)

component of this matrix is a thin, uniform layer of tightly intermeshed fibrillar material that adheres to the internal surface of the nuclear envelope. Known as the *fibrous (nuclear) lamina,* this layer can just be discerned in Figure 2-5, but in most other cell types, its thinness and lack of distinctive staining make it very difficult to distinguish. The nuclear pore complexes remain attached to this layer if it

is isolated. The second component of the nuclear matrix is a fibrogranular network that extends from the fibrous lamina into the interior of the nucleus. The third component is a similar framework supporting the nucleolus.

The role of the fibrous lamina is to shape and reinforce the inner membrane of the nuclear envelope, to strengthen and secure the nuclear pore complexes, and to anchor

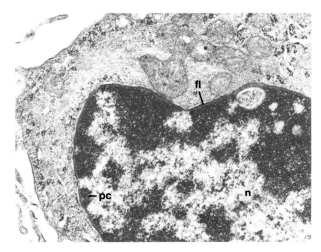

Fig. 2-5. Electron micrograph showing the fibrous lamina (*fl*) in the nucleus (*n*) of an epidermal keratinocyte (biopsy of human skin). This component of the nuclear matrix is generally difficult to distinguish from the peripheral chromatin (*pc*). (Courtesy of P. Lea)

chromatin to the inner aspect of the nuclear envelope. This crucial role in maintaining the general organization of the interphase nucleus is only briefly interrupted when the nuclear envelope fragments during mitosis. After undergoing transitory disassembly, the fibrous lamina already appears fully reconstructed by the end of mitosis. Hence the state of assembly of the nuclear lamina and the special binding properties of its three constituent proteins are believed to play a key role in determining the overall structure and organization of the interphase nucleus. The nuclear matrix also seems to be involved in gene transcription, the process whereby genetic information is copied from DNA into RNA. An intimate association is found between active steroid-induced transcription and the nuclear matrix of chicken cells, for example. Moreover, this close association is lost when the inducing hormone is withdrawn and there is an accompanying cessation of active transcription, and other genes that are not expressed at all show no evidence of being closely bound to the nuclear matrix. There are also indications that the nuclear matrix provides replication sites for the duplication of chromosomal DNA, which is discussed below.

NUCLEAR DNA AND OTHER COMPONENTS OF CHROMATIN

Genetic Information Is Encoded in Nuclear DNA.   Each DNA molecule consists of two long strands (*polynucleotide chains*) wound together in the form of a double helix (Fig. 2-6). Both strands have a backbone of alternating phosphate and deoxyribose groups. A side chain representing one of the four nitrogenous bases, *adenine, thymine, cytosine,*

or *guanine* (represented in Figs. 2-6 and 2-7 by the letters *A, T, C,* and *G,* respectively), extends laterally from each sugar group. The apposed bases of the two strands are attached to each other as depicted in Figure 2-6. However, there is obligatory base pairing between *adenine* and *thy-*

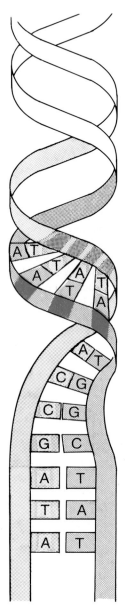

Fig. 2-6. Diagram representing the DNA molecule according to the model of Watson and Crick. This consists of two polynucleotide chains arranged in the form of a double helix. The nitrogenous bases adenine (*A*), thymine (*T*), cytosine (*C*), and guanine (*G*) extend as side chains from each strand, the backbone of which is made up of alternating deoxyribose and phosphate groups. There is obligatory base pairing between A and T and also between G and C. In the bottom half of the diagram, the two component strands of the molecule are beginning to separate in preparation for DNA replication.

mine and also between *cytosine* and *guanine*. Such *complementary base pairing* ensures error-free replication during DNA synthesis. There can be several million of these *base pairs* along a single DNA molecule. The individual pieces of information coded on DNA molecules are called genes; the most familiar kind (the *structural gene*) specifies the amino acid sequence of a polypeptide chain. However, because there are also other types of genes, a broader definition of a *gene* is a *stretch of DNA coding for a particular RNA molecule.*

Genetic information is carried in the DNA molecule much as information is carried in a string of words. Any three letters selected from four possible options can be combined in a number of ways to form three-letter words that constitute a meaningful sentence. Similarly, different combinations of any three of the four kinds of nitrogenous bases along a polynucleotide chain can be arranged so that they encode the amino acid sequence of a specific polypeptide. Chemical "code words" constructed of three nitrogenous bases designate which particular amino acids are to be incorporated. The code word sequence prescribes the specific order in which these building blocks are to be assembled. In the synthesis of a polypeptide chain, the genetic information in DNA is first *transcribed* into RNA. The intermediate message encoded in RNA then enters the cytoplasm, where its instructions become *translated* into a polypeptide chain. Thus in eukaryotic cells, the processes of transcription and translation take place in *two different compartments* separated by the nuclear envelope.

Duplication of DNA. Not all the genetic information embodied in nuclear DNA is utilized by the cell. In any given cell type, a great many genes are not expressed. Yet DNA does have to disclose all its information when the cell replicates its nuclear DNA in preparation for its next cell division. In the same way as a book has to be opened to copy the information on its pages, the DNA molecule has to be opened a short distance at a time to duplicate its genetic information. At the numerous sites where its two strands (polynucleotide chains) come apart, each original strand acts as the template for the new strand synthesized beside it (Fig. 2-7). Complementary base pairing determines the base sequence of the newly synthesized strand, ensuring that it is complementary to the preexisting strand. Hence in the two double-stranded molecules of DNA that are formed, only one strand in each molecule is synthesized anew and the other strand persists from the original molecule (Fig. 2-7). This arrangement is termed *semiconservative* replication. As we shall see, nuclear DNA replicates during interphase, several hours in advance of mitosis.

Replication complexes for duplicating chromosomal DNA do not seem to be randomly intermixed with the extended chromatin of interphase chromosomes, as once assumed. Studies of DNA synthesis in hepatocytes and fibroblasts suggest that DNA replication sites are closely associated with the nuclear matrix. The general picture emerging from such studies is that during DNA replication,

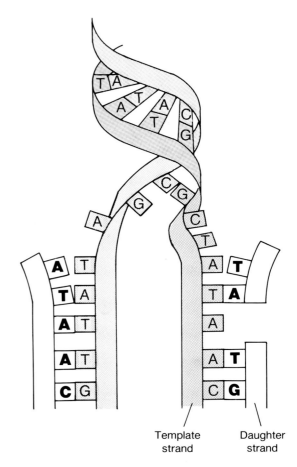

Template strand   Daughter strand

Fig. 2-7. Diagrammatic representation of the next stage in DNA replication. Each separated strand now serves as a template for the synthesis of a daughter strand, the base sequence of which is complementary to the template strand. As a result, two identical daughter molecules are produced from the parent molecule and each incorporates one strand of the original molecule.

loops of interphase chromatin may be reeled through replication complexes attached to the nuclear matrix. The merit of such an arrangement is that it would preserve the orderly looped arrangment of interphase DNA, which will be described in the following section.

Chromatin

The term *chromatin* is used for the somewhat complex basophilic material of which chromosomes are composed. In addition to its genetic component (*DNA*), chromatin contains a small number of highly conserved, strongly basic DNA-associated proteins called *histones,* together with a variable number of less basic *nonhistone proteins* and a certain amount of *RNA* transcribed from DNA. One role of such proteins seems to be to confer various orders of structural and functional organization on the chromatin. Due to the relatively high content of positively charged amino acids in the five types of histones, these proteins possess a marked affinity for the negatively charged phosphate groups of DNA. A striking consequence of their interaction with the DNA double helix is that they cause it to assume a characteristic configuration made up of a linear series of roughly spherical structural subunits called *nucleosomes,* which are described below. Some nonhistone chromosomal proteins may also be required to maintain additional orders of chromatin organization within the chromosome. However, one of the main reasons for recent interest in this class of proteins lies in the possibility that it would include the functionally important proteins responsible for regulating gene expression.

Nucleosomes.   Biochemical studies and detailed analysis of chromatin structure by x-ray crystallography and electron spectroscopic imaging have done much to unravel the complexities of how each DNA molecule, the extended length of which would be several centimeters, becomes compacted into a chromosome that is thousands of times shorter. The manner in which this is thought to be achieved is depicted in Figure 2-8. A first order of compaction is achieved by winding of the DNA double helix around a repetitive series of spool-like cores composed of certain histones. The histone-associated regions of DNA lie evenly spaced along the molecule, interconnected by short stretches of *linker DNA* (Figs. 2-8 and 2-9A). This arrangement has the EM appearance of a string of beads; each beadlike particle is known as a *nucleosome.* The same general pattern of elementary subunits with histone cores seems to be common to both heterochromatin and euchromatin. Moreover, nucleosomes are present even while DNA is undergoing transcription or replication. The core of each nucleosome consists of two molecules of each of four of the five histones (H2A, H2B, H3, and H4) that combine to form an octamer around which the double helix takes almost two-and-one-half turns (Figs. 2-9B and C) before extending on to the next nucleosome (Harauz and Ottensmeyer). Single molecules of the remaining histone (H1) interconnect neighboring nucleosomes and the intervening stretches of linker DNA in such a way as to lock the nucleosomes into a linear array.

Further orders of supercoiling, looping, and winding achieve an almost 10,000-fold reduction in the overall length of the single DNA molecule in each half of a mitotic chromosome. In electron micrographs of chromosomes that have been isolated at the metaphase stage of mitosis and have been prepared as whole mounts (Fig. 2-10), it can be seen that each half of the chromosome seems to be made up of a continuous nucleoprotein thread extending as multiple radial loops from some kind of axial scaffold, as depicted at the top of Figure 2-8. The 20-nm to 30-nm diameter of the looping *chromatin fiber* seen in mitotic and meiotic chromosomes is consistent with the basic configuration depicted in Figure 2-8, which shows the fiber as a continuous supercoiled nucleoprotein thread composed of approximately six nucleosomes per helical turn. Although much less is known about chromatin organization during interphase, there are reports that looped nucleosome-containing fibers of comparable diameter are present in interphase chromatin as well. It now seems likely that a close correspondence will be found between the looped domains of chromatin fibers and individual functional units of gene expression.

Chromatin Classification.   Gene transcription occurs from extended chromatin but not from the condensed type of chromatin that can be seen in the LM. To emphasize the functional disparity between *condensed chromatin,* which is *genetically inactive,* and *euchromatin* (chromatin in the extended state necessary for gene transcription), *heterochromatin* (Gr. *heteros,* other) is often used as an alternative name for condensed chromatin. Except during DNA synthesis, over 90% of the interphase chromatin remains in a condensed state. Some of it, termed *constitutive heterochromatin,* is permanently condensed and devoid of usable genetic information. Never transcribed, such chromatin is thought to have some sort of conformational role; it characterizes the centromere region and certain other regions of chromosomes and hence is the same in all types of cells. The remainder of the condensed chromatin, classified as *facultative heterochromatin,* is also transcriptionally inactive during interphase. Here, however, *genes have been inactivated* on a selective basis. The precise pattern of inactivation is distinctive for specific cell lineages and developmental stages. As a result, there is considerable variation in the gene content and relative abundance of facultative heterochromatin from one cell type to the next. The total amount present accounts for much of the difference in microscopic detail seen between the nuclei of different kinds of interphase cells.

Any *changes in gene expression* require the selective unlocking of genes formerly secluded in condensed chromatin, and presumably they involve reversal of the processes that led to chromatin condensation and gene suppression in the first place. Such changes enable the same gene complement to be expressed in a variety of ways. Diversification of cells through the acquisition of characteristic structural features and specialized functions (overt signs of *altered gene expression*) is termed *cell differentiation.*

Fine Structure of Chromatin.   The granular masses of electron-dense chromatin seen in EM sections (Fig. 2-11) are made up of both kinds of *condensed chromatin.* This form of chromatin is associated with the nuclear envelope (*peripheral chromatin,* Figs. 2-2 and 2-3) and nucleolus (*nucleolus-associated chromatin,* Fig. 2-2). It also constitutes the *chromatin granules* scattered about with extended chromatin in the nuclear sap (Fig. 2-2). *Extended chromatin,* which is more widely dispersed, is not as electron dense. Where it is extended, chromatin occasionally manifests short lengths of chromatin fibers (Fig. 2-11), the diameters of which are consistent with the several orders of coiling of the DNA double helix illustrated in Figure 2-8. However, occasional

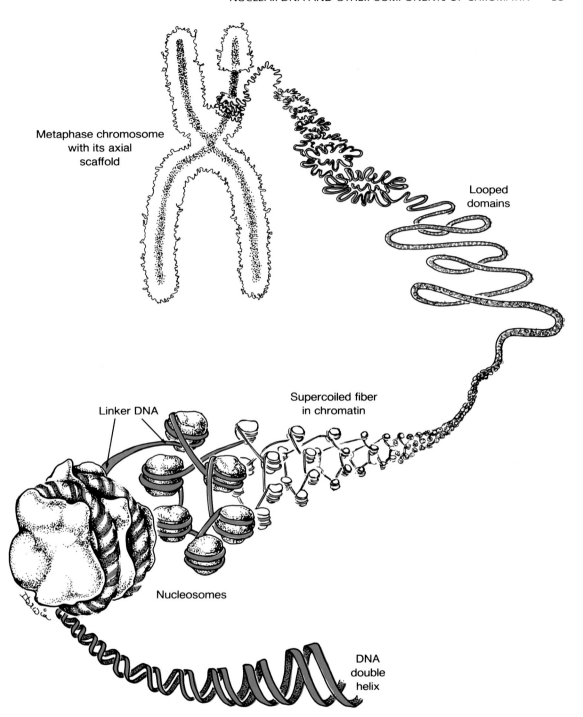

Metaphase chromosome
with its axial
scaffold

Looped
domains

Linker DNA

Supercoiled fiber
in chromatin

Nucleosomes

DNA
double
helix

Fig. 2-8. Diagrammatic representation of the increasing orders of compaction of DNA in chromatin and mitotic chromosomes. For details, see text.

short lengths of these fibers are all that can be discerned in the plane of an EM section because they are highly convoluted, looping around in every conceivable direction. A further limitation of using EM sections to observe chromatin is that there are usually gentle gradations between areas of condensed and extended chromatin, with remarkably few clear-cut delineating borders (Fig. 2-11). It was not until other more informative ways of preparing chromatin could be devised that our present-day understanding of the elaborate structure of chromatin began to emerge.

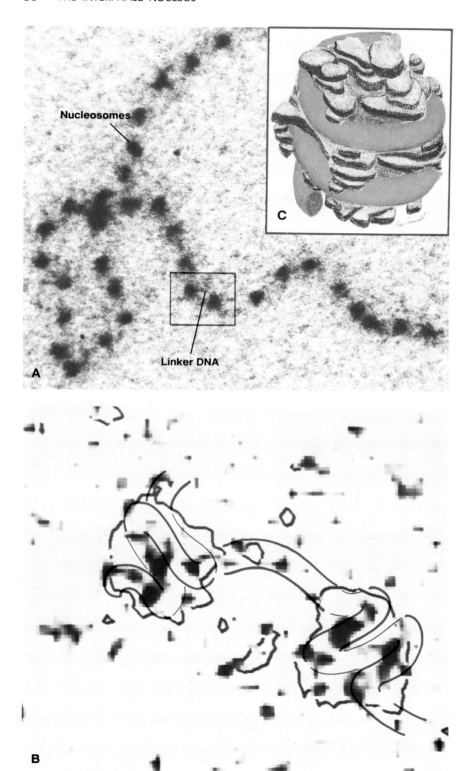

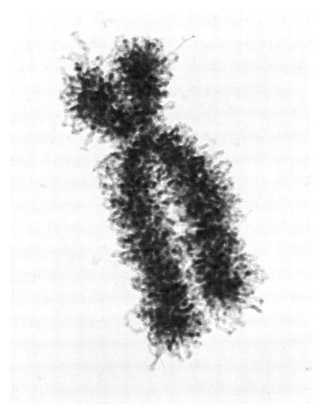

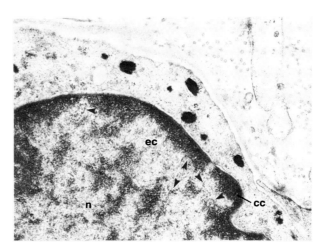

Fig. 2-11. Electron micrograph of part of the nucleus (*n*) of a melanocyte (biopsy of human skin). Electron-dense condensed chromatin (*cc*) can easily be distinguished from extended chromatin (*ec*), but there are intermediate gradations. In this section, short lengths of chromatin fibers (*arrowheads*) can be recognized in the extended chromatin. (Courtesy of P. Lea)

Fig. 2-10. Electron micrograph (×60,400) of a chromosome 12 at metaphase (whole mount preparation). A continuous chromatin fiber 20 nm to 30 nm across can be seen extending from the axial scaffold of each half of the chromosome (chromatid) in the form of radial loops. (DuPraw EJ: DNA and Chromosomes. New York, Holt, Rinehart & Winston, 1970)

PROTEIN SYNTHESIS: ROLE OF NUCLEIC ACIDS

The essential differences between *ribonucleic acid* (RNA) and DNA are that in RNA (1) the sugar groups are *D-ribose*

instead of 2-deoxy-D-ribose, and (2) *uracil* replaces the nitrogenous base thymine. Hence thymine is unique to DNA, and uracil is unique to RNA. Moreover, there are three different forms of RNA, termed *messenger RNA, ribosomal RNA,* and *transfer RNA,* each with a specific role to play in protein synthesis. The genetic information specified in the three-letter code words (*codons*) of nuclear DNA is *transcribed* into molecules of *messenger RNA* (mRNA). Ribosomal and transfer RNA are then required for the genetic instructions, now copied into mRNA molecules, to be put into effect in the cytoplasm.

Complementary base pairing, which was described above in connection with DNA synthesis, also provides the basis for *transcription* from extended chromatin. However, the genetic information embodied in any given gene is confined to one strand of the DNA double helix; the other strand

Fig. 2-9. (*A*) Electron micrograph of a string of nucleosomes in chromatin isolated from calf thymus. (*B*) Computer-generated video image of the phosphorus distribution of the two nucleosomes and linker DNA enclosed by the box in *A*. This phosphorus map was obtained by electron spectroscopic imaging (see Harauz G, Ottensmeyer FP: Nucleosome reconstruction via phosphorus mapping. Science 226:936, 1984; some information about this technique will also be found in the section on calcification in Chap. 12). The outer border of the histone core of each nucleosome is traced in black outline. The corresponding net phosphorus distribution is shown superimposed on this outline in shades of gray; sites of highest phosphorus concentration are represented in the darkest shade of gray. By assuming that this phosphorus distribution represents the spatial distribution of DNA, it is possible to follow the helical path of DNA around each nucleosome core. A three-dimensional interpretation of its path is indicated in blue outline. The DNA double helix, which is 2 nm wide, makes 2.4 turns around the histone core. The length of this supercoiled part of the double helix is 146 base pairs. The outer diameter of the supercoil is 8.5 nm and its pitch is 4 nm (data from Harauz and Ottensmeyer). (*C*) Diagrammatic representation of a nucleosome with its histone core and, in blue, the helical path of the part of the DNA double helix that is wound around it. (*A* and *B* courtesy of F. P. Ottensmeyer; *C*, courtesy of L. Arsenault)

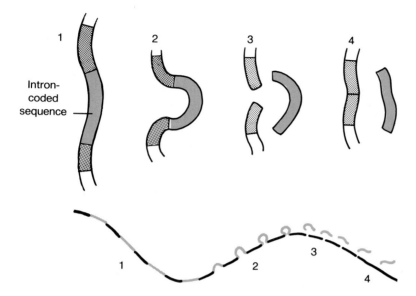

Intron-coded sequence

Fig. 2-12. Schematic diagram of the steps involved in the removal of an intron-coded sequence from a precursor RNA molecule, which is the processing of a primary RNA transcript. (*1*) A gene-coded sequence (the two parts of which are shown in *gray*) is interrupted by an intron-coded sequence (indicated in *blue*). (*2*) The nonadjacent parts of the gene-coded sequence are brought into juxtaposition by looping of the intron-coded portion. (*3*) The intron-coded sequence is excised. (*4*) The previously nonadjacent parts of the gene-coded sequence are spliced together. Once its intron-coded sequences have been removed, the resealed transcript is known as mature RNA.

conveys only complementary information. Furthermore, in this case, the obligatory base pairing results in RNA molecules that incorporate *uracil* (U) in place of thymine (T). The four-letter alphabet of RNA is therefore made up of A, C, G, and U, with a U being incorporated wherever an A is present in the DNA molecule from which it is being transcribed (see Fig. 2-14, *top*).

Transcribed RNA Undergoes Processing. Gene transcription initially results in the formation of *precursor RNA* molecules that are relatively long. Besides embodying transcribed genetic instructions, such molecules commonly include transcripts of genetically meaningless spacer DNA, which is interposed between genes. Moreover, even though each structural gene is a stretch of DNA that gives rise to a single polypeptide chain, the length of DNA involved may exceed that of the encoding base sequence. In such cases, the protein-coding sequences, called *exons* because they are the ones that are *expressed,* are separated from one another by *introns,* the term used for *interpolated* base sequences that do not code for proteins. Where introns interrupt the specific base sequence of a gene and make it discontinuous, or where a gene is flanked by irrelevant base sequences, the extraneous sequences are transcribed along with the gene. However, all the spurious sequences are then excised from this primary transcript, purging the mature RNA molecules of nonsensical sequences encoded by introns or spacer DNA (Fig. 2-12). Following the excision of intron transcripts, the formerly nonadjacent regions encoded by the exons are *spliced* together to constitute the mature RNA molecule (Fig. 2-12). This production of mature RNA molecules from primary transcripts is known as *RNA processing,* and it is thought to occur exclusively within the nucleus. Hence an important advantage conferred by the bicompartmental organization that characterizes eukaryotic cells is the unique opportunity it furnishes for the intranuclear processing of RNA molecules before they are translated in the cytoplasm.

Ribosomes and Transfer RNA Are Also Required for Translation. From the nuclear compartment, mRNA molecules pass by way of the nuclear pores into the cytoplasm. Such mRNA molecules can be isolated and specially prepared for electron microscopy, whereupon they are seen as long thin strands (Fig. 2-13). The sum total of their transcribed genetic information collectively specifies the amino acid sequences of every kind of protein molecule synthesized by the cell. In the cytoplasmic compartment, such information is *translated* into protein molecules. This process involves consecutive linking of the specified amino acids on *ribosomes,* which are cytoplasmic organelles made up of proteins and *ribosomal RNA.*

Each *ribosome* is a more or less round, electron-dense particle that is 20 nm to 30 nm in diameter (Fig. 2-13) and is made up of a *large* and a *small subunit,* both of which contain *ribosomal RNA* (rRNA) complexed with protein as ribonucleoprotein. As we shall see, the precursor of rRNA is transcribed from the *nucleolar genes* situated in the nucleolus. Because rRNA is a structural constituent of ribosomes, it does not show variation in base sequence as mRNA does. Ribosomes provide the requisite sites for linking amino acids together according to the codon sequence on mRNA molecules. For this assembly to proceed, however, *transfer RNA* is also necessary.

The *transfer RNA* (tRNA) molecule possesses a specific attachment site for one of the twenty amino acids (Fig. 2-14). It also embodies a three-letter code word (*anticodon*) that, by complementary base pairing, specifically matches its complementary codon on an mRNA molecule.

Mechanism of Translation. Genetic instructions inscribed on mRNA must reach the cytoplasm to be translated. Here

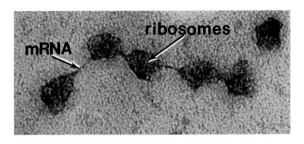

Fig. 2-13. Electron micrograph (×400,000) of a polysome consisting of five ribosomes attached to an mRNA molecule that codes for a globin chain of hemoglobin. (Courtesy of H. Slater and A. Rich)

the mRNA molecule passes between the large and small subunits of a ribosome and extends out on the far side (Fig. 2-14). As the mRNA molecule works its way through the ribosome, like thread passing through the eye of a needle, the ribosome implements the encoded instructions. The leading end of the molecule soon extends far enough to reach other ribosomes, with the result that several of these structures may become attached to the same mRNA molecule at fairly regular intervals (Fig. 2-13). Such an arrangement is termed a *polysome* (*polyribosome*).

The tRNA-mediated recognition mechanism outlined above enables ribosomes to assemble amino acids in the order specified by each mRNA molecule (Fig. 2-14). Gen-

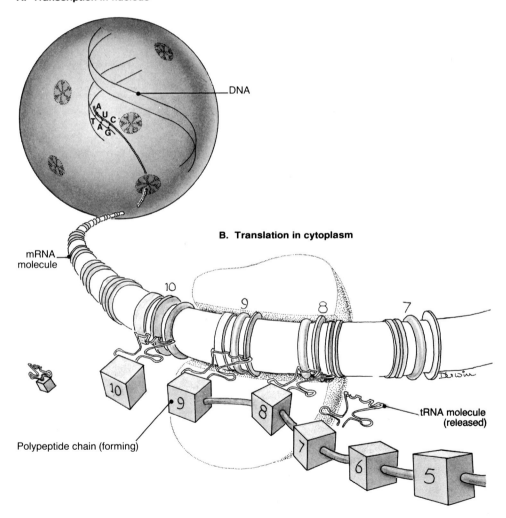

Fig. 2-14. Schematic representation of protein synthesis, depicting the consecutive processes of (*A*) transcription and (*B*) translation. Amino acid molecules (represented as numbered blocks) are being incorporated into a forming polypeptide chain according to the genetic instructions transcribed into the mRNA molecule. Only one of the ribosomes translating these instructions is shown.

erally speaking, several polypeptide chains are assembled concurrently, one by each of the several ribosomes through which the mRNA molecule is passing. As soon as an amino acid has been incorporated, its tRNA molecule is released (Fig. 2-14) and then reutilized for adding another molecule of the same amino acid. Ribosomes are recycled, too, because they are used repeatedly for synthesizing different protein molecules.

Once a particular mRNA molecule reaches the cytoplasm, protein synthesis proceeds automatically. This is true even if it is an inappropriate protein that is being artificially produced as a result of the introduction of exogenous mRNA molecules. Molecules of mRNA continue to direct protein synthesis until they become degraded. Most species of mRNA are short-lived, but a few are known to persist for several days in cells that dispense with their nucleus.

Regulation of Protein Synthesis.   Whenever more of a particular protein is needed, the gene directing its synthesis becomes active and remains active for the appropriate length of time. There must therefore be some molecular mechanism that turns the gene "on" or "off" according to specific requirements. Yet, in most cases, the demand for such a protein arises elsewhere in the body and not in the cells that are synthesizing it. For example, the quantities of pancreatic enzymes needed for the digestive process have no direct relation to the needs of the enzyme-secreting cells themselves. Any increase in demand for such proteins would have to be signaled to the cells that produce them, whereupon the message would have to be relayed by way of the cytoplasm to the nucleus, in order to augment transcription of the genes coding for these proteins.

However, the transcriptional level does not represent the only level at which protein synthesis can be regulated. Once a gene has been turned "on," the pattern in which its corresponding primary RNA transcript becomes processed, the accessibility of its specific mRNA to ribosomes in the cytoplasm, the effective lifespan of these specific mRNA molecules, and any post-translational modification of the gene product all will affect the nature and quantity of the protein being produced. Transcriptional control is nevertheless regarded as one of the most important regulatory mechanisms determining the spectrum of proteins produced in each cell type, and recently there has been considerable interest in trying to establish the molecular mechanisms involved.

NUCLEOLUS

Within the *nucleolus*, rRNA is transcribed from multiple copies of *nucleolar genes* that lie along five different pairs of chromosomes. Accordingly, there can be more than one nucleolus in the same nucleus. However, multiple nucleoli generally fuse into one or two larger structures as a result of association between the so-called *nucleolar organizer re-*

gions of these chromosomes. The nucleolar gene product, mRNA, thereupon aggregates into one or two confluent masses. Although easily seen in the LM in large nuclei that contain well-dispersed chromatin (see Fig. 3-24), nucleoli are commonly obscured by the large quantity of condensed chromatin present in smaller nuclei. Their intense basophilia in H & E sections is reduced following treatment with DNAase but is not much affected by pretreatment with RNAase. This indicates that their intense basophilia is primarily due to nucleolus-associated chromatin (Fig. 2-2). Nucleoli are prominent in cells actively engaged in protein synthesis, and they are particularly large in cells of rapidly growing tumors (see Fig. 2-17, *upper left corner*).

Nucleolar Genes.   In the case of rRNA and also tRNA, transcription occurs from multiple copies of genes. However, the nucleolus is the only part of the nucleus where rRNA is transcribed. The genes that code for rRNA are known as *nucleolar genes;* they are present on the satellited chromosomes 13, 14, 15, 21, and 22 (see Chromosome Identification in Chap. 3). When the *nucleolar organizer regions* containing these genes are transcriptionally active, they stain selectively with reducible silver salts, probably reflecting their content of acidic proteins.

An innovative procedure whereby nucleolar gene-bearing DNA is isolated in its transcriptionally active state from amphibian oocytes and then is suitably prepared for study in the EM has revealed, in remarkable detail, the electron microscopic appearance of newly synthesized molecules of precursor rRNA (Miller and Beatty). Figure 2-15 shows a number of these rRNA precursor molecules in the process of being transcribed by RNA polymerase I from four of the multiple nucleolar genes that occur repetitively along such DNA. Each nucleolar gene, separated from its neighboring nucleolar genes by stretches of spacer DNA, resembles the trunk of a *Christmas tree*, the branches of which represent primary transcripts of precursor rRNA. The shortest branches are rRNA transcripts that are still in the early stages of synthesis, and the longest ones are transcripts that are nearing completion. Before these primary transcripts are incorporated into ribosomal subunits, they are submitted to RNA processing, which yields mature rRNA molecules that rapidly complex with protein as ribonucleoprotein.

Maturation of rRNA.   The primary rRNA transcript has a sedimentation coefficient of 45S (Svedberg units), corresponding to about 13,000 base pairs. From this large molecule, a 28S (5000 base pair) rRNA molecule is formed and incorporated into a large (60S) ribosomal subunit, and an 18S (2000 base pair) rRNA molecule is formed and incorporated into a small (40S) ribosomal subunit. Two much smaller rRNA molecules are also produced and incorporated into each large subunit. These four mature rRNA molecules are all formed from the same primary transcript, ensuring that they are produced in the requisite equimolecular proportions.

The newly synthesized rRNA transcripts rapidly associate with ribosomal proteins that reach the nucleus from the

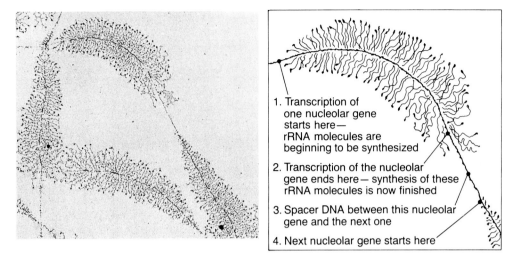

Fig. 2-15. Electron micrograph (×25,000) and interpretive diagram of nucleolar genes isolated from newt oocytes. These genes are in the process of being transcribed into rRNA. (*Micrograph,* Miller OL, Beatty BR: Science 164:955, 1969)

The labeled callouts in the diagram read:

1. Transcription of one nucleolar gene starts here— rRNA molecules are beginning to be synthesized
2. Transcription of the nucleolar gene ends here— synthesis of these rRNA molecules is now finished
3. Spacer DNA between this nucleolar gene and the next one
4. Next nucleolar gene starts here

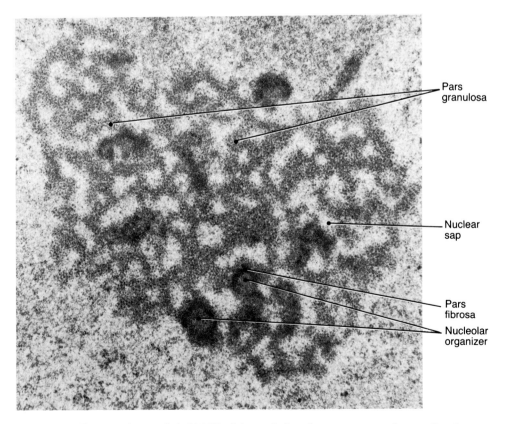

Fig. 2-16. Electron micrograph (×26,000) of the nucleolus of a mouse oocyte. Surrounding the nucleolar-organizer regions of the five pairs of chromosomes that possess nucleolar genes, there are lighter-staining regions called fibrillar centers. Electron-dense filamentous material surrounds the fibrillar centers and constitutes the pars fibrosa. (Courtesy of L. Chouinard)

cytoplasm, which is the only part of the cell that can synthesize proteins. Complexed with protein, the cleavage products of these transcripts accumulate in the nucleolus in the form of *ribonucleoprotein particles.* Final assembly of ribosomes occurs only when ribosomal subunits reach the cytoplasm; the ribosomal nucleoprotein escapes by way of the nuclear pores.

Fine Structure of the Nucleolus. The direct electron microscopic visualization of nucleolar genes undergoing transcription, as described above, has been a great help in interpreting the internal organization of the nucleolus. This relatively diffuse structure has the EM appearance of an irregular spongy network that is not limited by any membrane of its own (Fig. 2-16). Its light-staining interstices are filled with nuclear sap. Most of its electron-dense material, referred to as the *pars granulosa* because of its granular appearance, represents an accumulation of 15-nm ribonucleoprotein particles, which correspond to ribosomal subunits in various stages of formation. The remainder of the nucleolus is known as the *pars fibrosa* because it is composed of a fine filamentous material (Fig. 2-16). The tightly packed filaments characterizing this part of the nucleolus probably represent newly transcribed precursor rRNA that is only just beginning to become complexed with protein. There is no sharp border between the pars fibrosa and the pars granulosa. Surrounded by the electron-dense filamentous material that characterizes the pars fibrosa, there are less electron-dense *fibrillar centers* containing the *nucleolar organizer regions* of the five pairs of chromosomes that bear nucleolar genes (Fig. 2-16). As described above, these regions of the chromosomes bear repetitive nucleolar genes, each resembling a Christmas tree, the lateral branches of which correspond to growing precursor rRNA molecules that collectively comprise the pars fibrosa. Thus it is likely that rRNA transcription occurs toward the periphery of the fibrillar centers.

When the cell begins mitosis, its nucleolus disappears late in prophase and re-forms in the daughter cells at telophase. The tiny new nucleoli that then form in association with the nucleolar organizer regions of the five pairs of chromosomes subsequently coalesce into one or two large nucleoli.

NUCLEAR CHANGES INDICATING CELL DEATH

When histologists and pathologists use the term *dead cells,* they mean cells that died when the individual was still alive. Such cells may be encountered in sections under two different kinds of circumstances. First, it is normal for the cells of certain tissues to die and to be replaced by new cells; this occurs, for example, in the outer layers of the skin. Secondly, there are situations in which the presence of dead cells is indicative of disease. Thus occlusion of an

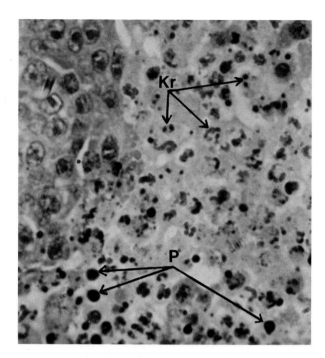

Fig. 2-17. Photomicrograph of part of a malignant tumor (high power). The cells shown at upper left are still viable; the remainder show nuclear changes indicative of necrosis. Nuclei that have shriveled up and condensed into a homogeneous hyperchromatic mass have undergone pyknosis (*P*). Nuclei that have broken up into fragments have undergone karyorrhexis (*Kr*).

artery supplying a particular region of the body can lead to local cell death as a result of deprivation of oxygen and nutrients. There is a similar tendency for rapidly growing tumors to acquire a central *necrotic* zone (Gr. *nekros,* dead) as they outgrow their blood supply; such necrotic cells can be seen in Figure 2-17.

Although there are also cytoplasmic changes in dead cells, the most positive indication that cells are dead is given by the appearance of their nuclei. The nuclear changes indicating cell death are of three general kinds. The most common is called *pyknosis* (Gr. for condensation) and entails shrinkage of the nuclear material into a homogeneous and darkly staining (*hyperchromatic*) mass (Fig. 2-17, *P*). It is important not to confuse a nucleus showing pyknosis with a nucleus containing much condensed chromatin or with a mitotic figure. When difficulty is encountered in this respect, it is advisable also to examine the cytoplasm of the cell in question, because if the cell is dead, the cytoplasm, too, will commonly present an abnormal appearance, as may be seen in Figure 2-17. Often it will lack detail and present a generally "muddy" appearance; moreover, it may be harder to distinguish cells as separate entities, as is the case in the middle of Figure 2-17.

In other instances, cell death is indicated by the nucleus breaking up into fragments, a type of nuclear change called *karyorrhexis* (Gr. *karyon + rhexis,* breaking). Thus instead

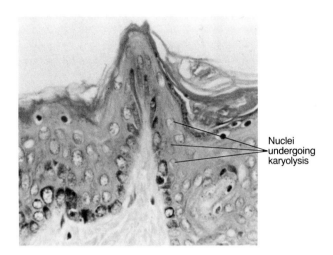

Nuclei
undergoing
karyolysis

Fig. 2-18. Photomicrograph of thin skin, showing epidermal cell nuclei undergoing karyolysis as they approach the body surface.

of shrinking, nuclei may completely disintegrate (Fig. 2-17, *Kr*), with the ultimate formation of such tiny fragments of nuclear material that these are sometimes referred to as nuclear "dust."

The third appearance presented by nuclei in dead or dying cells is that of dissolving away. This type of nuclear change, which is illustrated in Figure 2-18, is termed *karyolysis* (Gr. *lysis*, dissolution).

SELECTED REFERENCES

Structure of the Interphase Nucleus

ALBERTS B, BRAY D, LEWIS J et al: The cell nucleus. In Molecular Biology of the Cell, p 385. New York, Garland Publishing, 1983

BEREZNEY R, BUCHHOLTZ LA: Dynamic association of replicating DNA fragments with the nuclear matrix of regenerating liver. Exp Cell Res 132:1, 1981

CIEJEK EM, TSAI M-J, O'MALLEY BW: Actively transcribed genes are associated with the nuclear matrix. Nature 306:607, 1984

FAWCETT DW: The Cell, 2nd ed. Philadelphia, WB Saunders, 1981

FELDHERR C: Structure and function of the nuclear envelope. In DuPraw EJ (ed): Adv Cell Molecular Biology, Vol 2. New York, Academic Press, 1972

FRANKE WW: Structure, biochemistry and functions of the nuclear envelope. Int Rev Cytol (Suppl) 4:72, 1974

GALL JG: Octagonal nuclear pores. J Cell Biol 32:391, 1967

HOPKINS CR: Structure and Function of Cells. London, WB Saunders, 1978

KESSEL RG: Structure and function of the nuclear envelope and related cytomembranes. In Progress in Surface and Membrane Science, Vol 6, p 243. 1973

PARDOLL DM, VOGELSTEIN B, COFFEY DS: A fixed site of DNA replication in eukaryotic cells. Cell 19:527, 1980

Chromatin and Chromosome Structure and Protein Synthesis

DARNELL JE: The processing of RNA. Sci Am 249(4):90, 1983

DARNELL JE: RNA. Sci Am 253 No. 4:68, 1985

DUPRAW EJ: The Biosciences: Cell and Molecular Biology. Cell and Molecular Biology Council, Stanford, CA, 1972

DUPRAW EJ: DNA and Chromosomes. New York, Holt, Rinehart and Winston, 1970

FELSENFELD G: DNA. Sci Am 253 No 4:58, 1985

FRANKE WW, SCHEER U: Morphology of transcriptional units at different states of activity. Philos Trans R Soc Lond [Biol Sci] 283:333, 1978

GURDON JB, WYLLIE AH, DEROBERTIS EM: The transcription and translation of DNA injected into oocytes. Philos Trans R Soc Lond [Biol Sci] 283:375, 1978

HARAUZ G, OTTENSMEYER FP: Nucleosome reconstruction via phosphorus mapping. Science 226:936, 1984

KORNBERG RD, KLUG A: The nucleosome. Sci Am 244(2):52, 1981

LANE C: Rabbit hemoglobin from frog eggs. Sci Am 235:60, August, 1976

LEWIN B: Gene Expression, Vol 2: Eucaryotic Chromosomes, 2nd ed. New York, John Wiley & Sons, 1980

LEWIN B: Genes. New York, John Wiley & Sons, 1983

MARSDEN M, LAEMMLI UK: Metaphase chromosome structure: Evidence for a radial loop model. Cell 17:849, 1979

PAULSON JM, LAEMMLI UK: The structure of histone-depleted metaphase chromosomes. Cell 12:817, 1977

RICH A, KIM SH: The three-dimensional structure of transfer RNA. Sci Am 238:52, January, 1978

RIS H, KORENBERG JR: Chromosome structure and levels of chromosome organization. In Goldstein L, Prestcott DM (eds): Cell Biology, p 268. New York, Academic Press, 1979

STEIN GS, STEIN JS, KLEINSMITH LJ: Chromosomal proteins and gene regulation. Sci Am 232:46, February, 1975

WATSON JD: Molecular Biology of the Gene, 2nd ed. New York, WA Benjamin, 1970

Nucleolus

BLOOM SE, GOODPASTURE C: An improved technic for selective silver staining of nucleolar organizer regions in human chromosomes. Hum Genet 34:199, 1976

BUSCH H, SMETANA K: The Nucleolus. New York, Academic Press, 1970

DENTON TE, HOWELL WM: The use of AgNO$_3$ and ammoniacal silver to study nucleolar organizer and satellite regions of chromosomes. Mammalian Chromosomes Newsletter 16:178, 1975

GHOSH S: The nucleolar structure. Int Rev Cytol 44:1, 1976

JORDAN EG: The Nucleolus, 2nd ed. Oxford, Oxford University Press, 1978

MILLER OL, JR: The visualization of genes in action. Sci Am 228:34, March, 1973

MILLER OL, JR, BEATTY BR, HAMKALO BA, THOMAS CA, JR: Electron microscopic visualization of transcription. Cold Spring Harbor Symp Quant Biol 35:505, 1970

3

The Dividing Nucleus

Before the cell divides it replicates its full complement of nuclear DNA, so that by the time mitosis starts, each threadlike chromosome already contains two complete DNA molecules. To see how the timing of nuclear DNA synthesis relates to the onset of mitosis, we shall now consider the *cell cycle,* a valuable conceptualization of the cell's life history that has a number of broad implications in histology.

THE CELL CYCLE

A *cycle* (Gr. *kylos,* circle) is a sequence of events that is repeated over and over again in the same sequence. The concept of the *cell cycle* arose from the study of cells that divided at regular intervals (*cycling* cells) when they grew under *in vitro* conditions. Basically, this cycle consists of (1) *mitosis* and (2) *interphase,* the term for the interval between consecutive phases of mitosis (Fig. 3-1A). At any given moment most body cells are not in mitosis but in *interphase,* the stage *between* divisions during which the cells carry out their specialized work. Such cells are accordingly referred to as *interphase cells.* At first it was thought that there were only these two basic parts to the cell cycle. However, it soon became obvious that the nuclear DNA would have to be duplicated at some time during interphase, before chromosomes became visible as threadlike structures. So the period of interphase during which the new DNA was synthesized

Fig. 3-1. Diagrammatic representation of the cell cycle in cycling cells, showing (*A*) the two major divisions of the cycle and (*B*) the three subdivisions of interphase with the relative durations of each phase drawn to scale. Although there are variations in the length of each phase between different cell types and between different species, representative durations measured for cycling mouse cells growing in suspension culture are as follows: G_1: 8 hr, *S*: 7 or 8 hr, G_2: 4 hr, *M*: 1 hr.

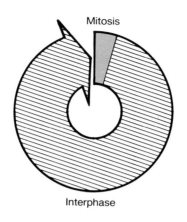

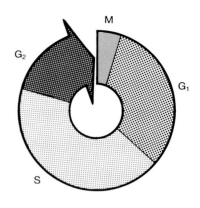

A   **B**

was termed the *S phase* (*S* for *synthesis*), indicated in Figure 3-1*B*. In cycling mammalian cells growing *in vitro*, it was found that this stage begins approximately 8 to 12 hours after the end of mitosis (*mitosis* is denoted by *M*) and takes approximately 7 or 8 hours to complete. The intervening *gap* between the end of mitosis and the beginning of S is called G_1 (*G* for *gap*), and the *gap* between the end of S and the beginning of mitosis is termed G_2. So it is now accepted that the cell cycle is made up of four stages: M, G_1, S, and G_2. For cycling mouse cells maintained under *in vitro* conditions, these stages have the durations specified in Figure 3-1*B*. The cell cycle is significantly longer in total duration in most types of human cells.

The finding that nuclear DNA replicates during one portion of interphase made it necessary to modify the earlier view that interphase is entirely occupied with the performance of special functions. It now seems logical to assume that during the S phase, the cell would be more involved with replicating its DNA than with discharging its special duties. Any specialized work would therefore have to be carried out during G_1 or G_2. Yet from *in vitro* studies it soon became evident that continuously cycling cells rarely spend enough time in either of these stages to perform much specialized work, and as a result, they show little evidence of extensive specialization. Most of their G_1 stage is, in fact, occupied with the cell growth necessary to produce two daughter cells at the end of the cycle.

To assume a highly specialized role, interphase cells either leave the cell cycle permanently, generally making an exit in G_1 (Fig. 3-2*A*), or they enter an extension of this cycle, in most cases a prolonged G_1 phase (Fig. 3-2*B*). Very few cell types escape from the cycle during G_2 in order to specialize. Hence most specialized functions are carried out by cells that have either entered an *extended G_1 phase* or have *left the cell cycle* during G_1, never to cycle again.

The Concept of a G_0 State

Certain kinds of interphase cells seem to be able to withdraw from the cycling state during G_1 for an indefinite

period without going on to specialize. Many believe that such cells enter a special sort of standby noncycling state called G_0. The term G_0 is reserved for quiescent (nonproliferating) cells that for the time being are *out of cycle*. However, appropriate stimuli are able to *trigger their reentry* into G_1. Hence unlike the second type of cell just mentioned, these cells have not left the cell cycle permanently. There are a few subtle quantitative biochemical indications that the hypothetical and still virtually immeasurable G_0 state may be distinct from an extremely prolonged but uninterrupted cell cycle. However, this issue remains unresolved and opinion is divided as to whether such cells are in a *reversibly arrested* G_1 (*i.e.*, G_0) phase or an *indefinitely extended* G_1 phase.

CELL RENEWAL

We have seen that almost all types of specialized functional cells exist in a prolonged G_1 phase, or have made a final exit from the cell cycle and in so doing have become what are termed *end cells*. Yet there are many instances in which highly specialized end cells are either rapidly wearing out or are frequently becoming lost from a body surface. In certain of these cases, compensatory cell replacement is essential to maintain function. New cells are also needed for the regeneration of damaged tissues. Hence mitosis is an absolute requirement in certain kinds of cell populations. The body is nevertheless made up of three different kinds of populations of cells that differ in their capacity to progress through the cell cycle, as we shall explain in the following sections. Furthermore, as a general rule, the greater the level of specialization of a cell, the less likely it is to retain the capacity for mitosis.

Nonrenewing Populations

Certain types of very highly differentiated cells have *no proliferative capacity whatsoever*. Moreover, there is no pro-

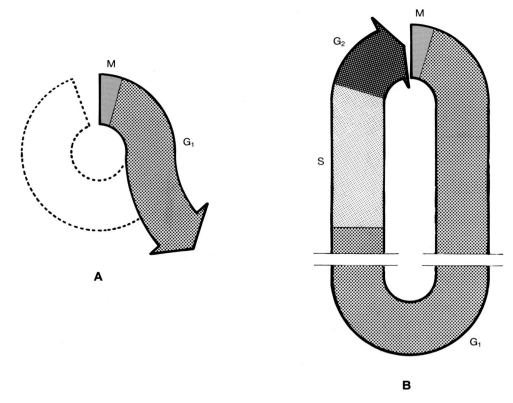

Fig. 3-2. Diagrammatic representation of the cell cycle in specialized cells. (*A*) Certain highly specialized cell types (*e.g.,* neurons and cardiac muscle cells) exit the cell cycle in G_1. (*B*) Most other specialized cell types pass into an extended G_1 phase (the breaks are used to emphasize that this phase can be very prolonged).

vision for the replacement of such end cells when they wear out or are destroyed, and they are characterized by a lifelong decline in absolute numbers. The nerve cells of the brain and heart muscle cells are both classic examples of this type of cell population.

Continuously Renewing Populations

In continuously renewing populations, the highly specialized end cells are similarly unable to reproduce themselves, but there is an alternative mechanism for their replacement. In this case, cell renewal is brought about by less highly differentiated cells of the same cell lineage or family that have not yet specialized to the extent of losing their capacity for mitosis. From this pool of less differentiated cycling cells, new cells emerge that will go on to specialize and provide replacements for the nonproliferating end cells that are lost. This mechanism produces a continual and, in some cases, rapid turnover of the cell population. Because a balance exists between cell production and cell loss, a *steady state* is maintained by continuously renewing populations.

A good example of a continuously renewing population is the epithelial lining of the intestine, cells of which are continually sloughing off into the intestinal lumen. The replacements for these cells arise from less specialized cells of the same family type situated deeper in the wall of the gut in invaginations known as *crypts*. When the new lining cells exit the cell cycle in G_1 in order to specialize, they migrate from the crypts into the lining layer and keep this lining intact. Through this mechanism the intestinal lining is able to renew itself completely approximately every 3 to 5 days. For a second example, we can cite certain types of circulating blood cells that survive for only a few days, after which they have to be replaced by new cells arising from less highly differentiated cycling cells of the same family type. The task of these cycling progenitors is to keep up the production of specialized blood cells in adequate numbers to maintain normal blood cell counts.

Role of Stem Cells. Two important terms used in describing continuously renewing populations are *progenitor cells* and *stem cells*. The main characteristics of *progenitor* (L. for parent or ancestor) *cells* may be summarized as follows. They are sufficiently differentiated that their daughter cells are not restricted to the same level of differentiation as the parent cell, but they are insufficiently differentiated to preclude the potential for active proliferation. As a result, progenitor cells can *proliferate very rapidly* and provide large numbers of end cells, but they generally have a somewhat limited capacity or virtually no detectable capacity for *self-renewal* (*self-replacement*). In addition to being in cycle, progenitor cells eventually become restricted to *specific lines* *of differentiation* and are finally committed to producing a single type of end cell.

In contrast, the term *stem cell* is reserved for quiescent ancestral cells that remain *incompletely differentiated* throughout life. Although most of these cells are *not in active cycle,* they can be triggered back into cycle, out of G_o (arrested G_1, which is virtually indistinguishable from an indefinitely prolonged G_1), by exceptional demands or by end cell depletion brought on by some emergency situation. An important characteristic of stem cells is their latent but not necessarily freely expressed potential for *very extensive proliferation.* Indeed, they seem to have been given the name *stem cells* because of their remarkable potential for producing progenitor cells when these are needed in increased numbers. Under steady-state conditions, the two daughter cells resulting from a stem cell division are believed to manifest a roughly equal likelihood of (1) *differentiating further* and becoming committed progenitor cells, or (2) *not differentiating further* and remaining stem cells. Both daughter cells commonly make the same choice, producing either two progenitor cells or two stem cells. Furthermore, under most circumstances, the numbers of daughter cells settling for each option stay in roughly equal balance. The second option is called *self-renewal* because it leads to the creation of a subsequent generation of identical stem cells. Hence, a unique feature of all stem cells is their *extensive capacity for self-renewal,* a characteristic that guarantees that there will not be total exhaustion of the stem cell supply. We shall come across several examples of tissues and organs in which the continuing renewal of highly differentiated functional cells with no proliferative potential ultimately depends on the maintenance of adequate pools of stem cells.

In certain instances, a single type of stem cell can give rise to several different kinds of specialized end cells. Because the progeny of these stem cells have the potential to differentiate in more than one direction, such stem cells are often described as *pluripotential* (L. *plus,* more; *potentia,* power). However, if the number of different kinds of end cells is relatively large, such stem cells are sometimes referred to as *multipotential* stem cells. Stem cells that are restricted to producing only one type of end cell are described as *unipotential.* Blood cells and the epithelial cells that line the intestine are examples of continuously renewing populations derived from multipotential and pluripotential stem cells, respectively. Spermatozoa and the keratin-producing cells of skin represent populations that are continuously renewed from unipotential stem cells.

Hence the important role of stem cells is to provide the basis for lifelong renewal of highly specialized cells that have lost all capacity for proliferation.

Potentially Renewable Populations

There are few exceptions to the general rule that very highly differentiated cells cannot divide. Nevertheless, in one or two instances, long-lived specialized cells maintain the ca-

pacity to assume an actively cycling state in response to critical cell depletion. Even so, this latent capacity for cell renewal is not very evident unless cell replacement has become a virtual necessity. The best example of such a population is seen in the fully grown liver when portions of this organ are removed or destroyed. The hepatocyte population thereupon goes into active cycle and continues to proliferate until the liver is restored to its original mass. Certain kinds of hormone-secreting cells, which are also comparatively specialized, behave in a similar manner.

Following from this discussion of cell renewal, we shall next consider how the cell prepares itself for mitosis. Our first task will be to explain how DNA duplication can be recognized microscopically.

RADIOAUTOGRAPHY (AUTORADIOGRAPHY)

Known also as *autoradiography,* the technique of *radioautography* is an extremely versatile histological procedure that, over the years, has substantially broadened the scope of what can be learned about cells at the light microscope (LM) and electron microscope (EM) levels. Besides serving as a specific means of identification of cells in the S phase, this procedure has proved useful for following and timing a number of other important cellular processes. It also furnishes a reliable means of estimating rates of cell turnover and enables undetermined cell lineages to be traced.

Advantage is taken of the fact that the cell handles low levels of radioisotopes, or of compounds into which radioactive isotopes have been introduced, in the same manner as it handles their unlabeled counterparts. Detection of the isotope is relatively easy because the radiation it emits affects photographic emulsion in the same way that light does. Indeed, hospital or laboratory personnel that work in places where x-ray machines and radioisotopes are often being used wear individual badges containing special photographic film that is shielded from light. Pieces of film are issued and then developed on a regular basis to monitor total body exposure to ionizing radiation. Radioisotopes can be localized in tissues at the LM or EM level in much the same manner. All that is necessary to localize such isotopes is to coat suitable tissue preparations with a nuclear emulsion in a darkroom, after which they are stored in the dark for several weeks and then are photographically developed and fixed. Discrete *silver grains* can then be seen over the sites that emit radiation; their position indicates sites of incorporation of the radioisotope (Fig. 3-3). Such a preparation is termed a *radioautograph* or *autoradiograph* (Gr. *radio,* raylike; *autos,* self; *graphō,* to write). Tissue constituents containing labeled precursors are referred to as *products.* Although the precursors are soluble, the macromolecular products that incorporate them are generally insoluble. Hence although residual precursors are lost in processing the tissue, the products are retained. Radioautography can therefore be used to locate labeled product that

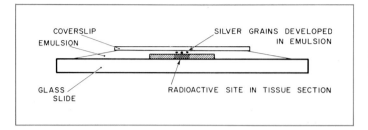

Fig. 3-3.   Diagram showing how the sites of incorporation of a radioactive precursor in a tissue section are detected by radioautography.

is locked into position through fixation. The details of the procedure are as follows.

Once the labeled precursor has become incorporated, sections or whole-cell preparations are made from the tissue and are fixed and processed for the LM or EM, depending on the level of resolution required. Supplementary histological staining can be carried out before or after radioautography, but prestaining must be used with caution because certain staining methods can extract radioactivity or interfere with emulsion responsiveness to radioactivity. In some cases post-staining is preferable, but even this is not without its share of attendant difficulties. The tissue preparation is coated with emulsion for radioautography, dried, and stored in a lightproof box. Nuclear emulsions used to record the tracks of subatomic particles are basically similar to photographic emulsions in that they are suspensions of silver bromide crystals in gelatin. Each site of radioactivity in the preparation is a source of radiation that is capable of causing the conversion of silver ions to silver atoms in silver bromide crystals. When the emulsion has been photographically developed and fixed, the latent image that forms in each critically affected silver bromide crystal becomes expressed as a characteristic *grain* of metallic silver. Thus the presence of grains in the developed emulsion indicates that a radioactive product lies beneath them (Fig. 3-3).

Where present in a tissue preparation, a radioactive isotope acts as a point source from which subatomic particles emanate in all directions. Yet isotopes such as ^{32}P that emit β particles (electrons of nuclear origin) endowed with high energy do not provide satisfactory localization within the tissue. In addition to electrons that traverse the preparation perpendicularly and affect the emulsion directly above the label, electrons given off at other angles are also able to reach the emulsion, although they travel farther to do so. The emitter can thereby affect the emulsion for some distance on all sides, and the site of radioactivity cannot be pinpointed with precision. For precise localization, it is essential to use a *low-energy* β emitter. Such isotopes give off electrons with short tracks that ideally are only long enough to affect the emulsion directly above the isotope and are too short to reach the emulsion obliquely. This is one of the main reasons why *tritium* (^3H, with a track length in water of about 1 μm) is widely used for radioautography. Other requirements for optimal resolution are that the coating of emulsion should lie as close as possible to the tissue and that the section should be sufficiently thin to ensure that all perpendicularly tracking particles reach the emulsion. Provided that the section and emulsion layer are thin enough and that the radioisotope is a short-tracking β emitter, the radioactive sites can be assumed to be located directly under the grains in the developed emulsion. Under optimal conditions, radioautography enables sites of precursor incorporation to be localized to within 80 nm or so.

Radioactive isotopes can be used in a direct manner to explore the cellular processing of inorganic constituents. Examples include the use of radioisotopes of calcium or phosphorus to investigate the process of calcification (*i.e.,* calcium phosphate deposition) in cartilage or bone. Once radioactive iron has been incorporated into the red pigment hemoglobin, it can be used to investigate clinical conditions affecting red blood cells. Thyroid hormone contains iodine; hence its formation can be followed by administering radioactive iodine.

Detecting Macromolecular Synthesis

Tritiated Thymidine Is Used to Detect DNA Synthesis.   During the replication of DNA molecules in the S phase, each new strand (polynucleotide strand) must be constructed from nucleotides. If conditions are arranged so that one of these nucleotides (consisting of a nitrogenous base, deoxyribose, and a phosphate group) becomes *radioactive,* any cells that are undergoing DNA synthesis can be identified by radioautography. The base *thymine* is incorporated solely into DNA and is therefore the ideal marker for DNA synthesis. However, to be incorporated, thymine must be made available as the nucleoside *thymidine,* which contains deoxyribose as well as thymine. *Tritiated thymidine* (*i.e.,* thymidine labeled with *tritium,* a readily available radioisotope of hydrogen) is therefore universally employed as a specific marker for the radioautographic recognition of cells that are replicating their nuclear DNA in the S phase.

Both strands of the DNA molecule serve as templates for the synthesis of a corresponding new strand (see Fig. 2-7), so each of the resulting double-stranded molecules is made up of an old strand and a new strand. This *semiconservative* pattern of replication is depicted in Figure 2-7. Thus if tritiated thymidine is made available during the S phase, the thymine incorporated into the new strand will be radioactive (Fig. 3-4). However, because the preexisting thymine in the old strand is devoid of any radioactive label, only the newly synthesized strand of each new DNA molecule will become labeled. Accordingly, in a cell that enters mitosis after replicating its DNA in the presence of tritiated thymidine, all the chromosomes passing into the two daughter cells will carry the label in one of their two strands.

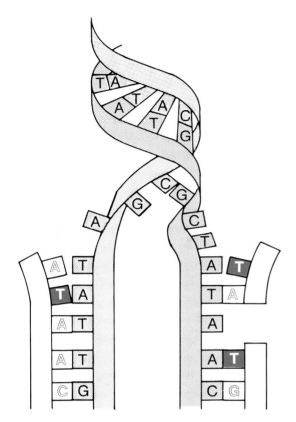

Fig. 3-4. Diagram showing the incorporation of radioactively labeled thymine (represented as the blue squares labeled *T* on each daughter strand) into a replicating DNA molecule. Such incorporation occurs when tritiated thymidine (a radioactive thymine precursor) is made available during the S phase of the cell cycle. Only the daughter strand of each new molecule becomes labeled; the template strand remains unlabeled.

Even though tritiated thymidine is confined to the newly formed strand of each new DNA molecule, it labels DNA very satisfactorily for radioautographic studies of DNA synthesis. It is, for example, possible to see the label over chromosomes of cells that took up labeled thymidine during the S phase and then entered mitosis. Figure 3-5*A* shows the way silver grains appear over and immediately beside chromosomes in a radioautograph of a spread of a mitotic cell, in which DNA synthesis took place during the preceding S phase in the presence of labeled thymidine. More commonly, the label is seen over interphase cells. If the interval between giving labeled thymidine and obtaining the cells is short, label is found over cells that have not yet entered mitosis and so are still in G_2 (Figs. 3-5*B* and 3-6). If, however, the cells are taken some time after giving labeled thymidine, labeled cells may have already passed through mitosis and entered G_1. Figure 3-5*B* is an LM radioautograph showing two interphase cells of bone marrow obtained shortly after injecting labeled thymidine into an animal. Here silver grains indicate incorporation of labeled

thymidine into the DNA of one of the cells, which was in S phase at the time of labeling. Although some grains lie outside the limits of its nucleus (a result of the track length of the β particles), the label is clearly confined to one cell and is lacking from the other.

The tritium label can be localized much more precisely by carrying out radioautography at the EM level. Silver grains, which are composed of metallic silver, have the EM appearance of irregularly convoluted ribbons. Figure 3-6 shows many of them lying over peripheral chromatin following the incorporation of labeled thymidine during the S phase.

Detecting RNA Synthesis.   RNA synthesis can be investigated by allowing cells to take up *tritiated uridine*, which is a specific precursor for RNA. Indeed, the radioautographic tracing of RNA synthesis to diffusely distributed chromatin, but not to condensed chromatin, became the first major piece of evidence that gene transcription occurs only from extended chromatin.

Detecting Protein Synthesis.   A suitable precursor for most newly synthesized proteins is the amino acid leucine into which ³H has been incorporated. For collagen, which is rich in proline and glycine, tritiated proline is often used because it provides more specificity.

Detecting Carbohydrate Synthesis.   Glucose labeled with ³H is satisfactory for following the synthesis of glycogen. Any radioactivity that persists following treatment with α-amylase, an enzyme that breaks down glycogen, would suggest that the labeled glucose was incorporated into glycoprotein, proteoglycan, or glycosaminoglycan. (These are complex carbohydrate–containing macromolecular compounds that will be described in later chapters.)

We shall next go on to consider some other important ways in which the use of tritiated thymidine has resulted in noteworthy advances in histological knowledge.

Estimating Mitotic Index

The *mitotic index* of a cell population or tissue is a measure of the proportion of its cells that are undergoing mitosis at any given time. Until tritiated thymidine became available, this parameter was generally determined by counting the number of mitotic cells present in sections of tissue obtained after the injection of colchicine, a drug that allows mitotic cells to accumulate because it blocks cellular proliferation. However, for mitotic cells to be recognized they must be cut in some plane that discloses that they are dividing. A more accurate estimate of the mitotic index of a tissue can be obtained by radioautography after the injection of tritiated thymidine, which is described below.

Administration of the labeled thymidine should be restricted to a 1-hour period to keep exposure to the labeled precursor brief. After an appropriate interval, the tissue is fixed, sectioned, and

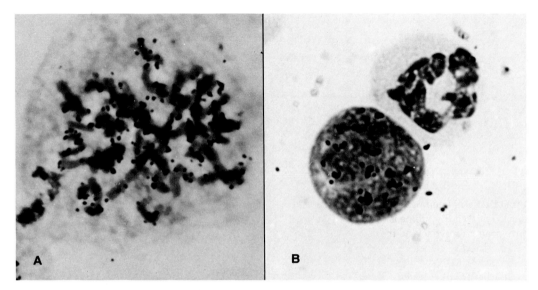

Fig. 3-5.   LM radioautographs prepared following the incorporation of tritiated thymidine. Rounded black grains of silver are seen lying over (*A*) metaphase chromosomes and (*B*) an interphase nucleus. Due to the track length of the β particles from the tritium, some of the grains lie outside the limits of the rounded nucleus, which is situated somewhat eccentrically in the upper left part of the cell. The nucleus of the other cell in *B* (a neutrophil) is not labeled with the isotope. (*A*, Stanners CP, Till JE: Acta Biochim Biophys 37:406, 1960; *B*, Courtesy of D. Osmond and S. Miller)

prepared for radioautography. However, the time allowed before taking the tissue should be short enough to prevent any labeled cells from going through mitosis, because otherwise there would be two labeled cells to count when there should have been only one. Provided these requirements are met, every cell showing radioactive label in the radioautograph represents a cell destined to undergo mitosis during the next few hours. Generally speaking, this radioautographic procedure provides the same sort of infor-

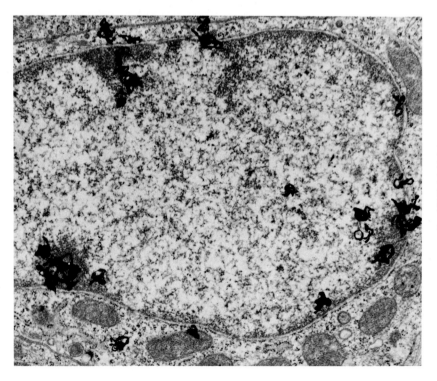

Fig. 3-6.   EM radioautograph (×9500) prepared following the incorporation of tritiated thymidine. Silver grains, seen here lying primarily over the peripheral chromatin of an interphase nucleus, appear as irregularly convoluted, electron-dense ribbons. These are seen to advantage at right. (Cheng H, Leblond CP: Am J Anat 141:537, 1974)

mation as a direct count of mitotic cells. However, although the reasoning is complex, estimates obtained using the two different methods will not be exactly the same if the total duration of mitosis in the cell type concerned differs significantly from the 1-hour period allowed for thymidine uptake.

Tracing Cell Origins and Lineages

Thymidine labeling has also been used with a certain amount of success in investigating the origins of the cells responsible for growth, regeneration, and the daily maintenance of tissues. Because all cells except red blood cells possess a nucleus, the ideal marker for tracing cell lineages is a nuclear label that will keep passing from one cell generation to the next. Tritiated thymidine is invaluable in this respect; the only major drawback at this stage is that its initial uptake is restricted to cells that are in cycle. Once incorporated into the nuclear DNA of a cell, however, it serves as an excellent marker for the progeny of that cell and is therefore well suited to exploring parent–progeny relationships between cells.

Cells that multiply and serve as ancestral or progenitor cells to more specialized cells can be identified (and traced to the nondividing specialized cells) by administering tritiated thymidine to several animals at the same time. In radioautographs of tissues taken a short time after the thymidine was injected, the label will be present only in cycling unspecialized cells that were in S phase at the time of labeling. However, radioautographs of tissues taken at later times will then begin to show labeled specialized cells, and in due course, the label will be found only in specialized cells. Such findings reflect the fact that it is only the unspecialized cells in the family that are capable of dividing. Because label does not appear in the specialized cells until after the labeled thymidine has been cleared from the animal's circulation, the labeled specialized cells must have originated from previously labeled unspecialized cells.

A further potentially frustrating limitation that has to be taken into consideration when using tritiated thymidine to establish cell lineages is that every time a labeled cell divides, its content of radioactive DNA diminishes by a factor of two. Indeed, if the labeled cells continue to proliferate in the absence of further label, the amount of label persisting in future generations eventually becomes undetectable. The reason for this is described below.

By the time the first mitosis after labeling is under way, all the DNA molecules will have replicated in the presence of label during the preceding S phase and so will carry label in one of their two strands (Fig. 3-4). Hence, when the daughter chromosomes separate from each other, each contains a DNA molecule with label in one of its two strands. As a result, all the chromosomes entering both daughter cells are labeled. In the S phase of the next cell cycle, however, the DNA of the daughter cells replicates in the *absence* of further label. Both strands of each DNA molecule now serve as templates for the formation of new strands (Fig. 3-7). The labeled strand gains an unlabeled strand beside it (Fig. 3-7, *lower right*), but the DNA molecule is still labeled. The unlabeled strand

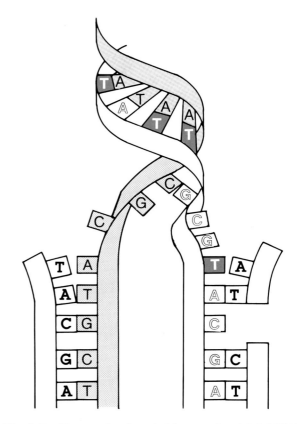

Fig. 3-7. Diagram showing what happens to a labeled DNA molecule when it replicates during the next S phase in the absence of further label (labeled thymine is represented as blue squares labeled *T*). The new DNA molecule shown at lower left has had no opportunity to incorporate any label. The new DNA molecule seen at lower right retains the label that was incorporated into its template strand, but its new daughter strand acquires no further label. The net result is that one of the new DNA molecules formed remains labeled but the other molecule is totally unlabeled.

also gains an unlabeled strand (Fig. 3-7, *lower left*), but in this case, it becomes part of a DNA molecule that carries no label. The two newly formed DNA molecules, one labeled and the other unlabeled, then segregate to different daughter cells. Furthermore, it is a matter of chance as to whether a daughter cell will receive the labeled or the unlabeled chromosome. On average, 50% of the labeled chromosomes finish up in one daughter cell and 50% go to the other cell. As a result, only one half of the chromosome complement carries the label in second-generation daughter cells. The drastic reduction in total amount of label that occurs over the course of several successive divisions unfortunately makes it an unrealistic endeavor to try to follow cell lineages over more than a few generations. However, if the labeled cells go on to specialize instead of continuing to divide, the label persists, and it can be detected by radioautography until its radioactivity decays.

Timing the Cell Cycle

Without the adoption of special measures for inducing synchronous cell division, cells growing in culture manifest a random distribution with respect to their stage in the cell cycle. The durations of these stages can nevertheless be readily estimated by labeling such cells with tritiated thymidine and by preparing radioautographs. Mitosis (M) can even be timed without the use of labeled thymidine by observing the process directly in living cells under a phase-contrast microscope. In most cases, the duration of mitosis is approximately 1 hour, but it takes up to 1.5 hours in certain cell types. The other stages can be timed as described in the following section.

Estimating the Duration of G_2.   The duration of G_2 is estimated by *pulse labeling* cells, that is, by adding labeled thymidine for up to 1 hour and then changing the medium to prevent further uptake of the labeled precursor. Under these conditions, only the small proportion of cells that are in S phase during the exposure to labeled thymidine become labeled. The cells taking up the label range from those just commencing an S phase to those just finishing S during the exposure period. As might be expected, in cells sampled immediately following the removal of labeled thymidine, label is found only in interphase nuclei; mitotic cells are devoid of label. However, if samples continue to be taken at subsequent intervals, there comes a time when label begins to appear in the chromosomes of the mitotic cells as well. Because the label is taken up by cells that include some that are just beginning and others that are just finishing an S phase at the time of labeling, those cells close to the termination of S are the first to undergo mitosis and reveal labeled mitotic chromosomes. The interval between (1) removal of labeled thymidine from the culture and (2) the first appearance of labeled mitotic cells is therefore a minimal estimate of the duration of the G_2 stage of the cell cycle.

Estimating the Duration of the S Phase.   Cells just ending an S phase during labeling are the first cells to enter M and, conversely, those just commencing an S phase a short time before removal of the label are the last to go into M and to manifest labeled mitotic chromosomes. In consecutive samples taken at regular intervals and examined radioautographically, the proportion of mitotic cells showing label in their chromosomes increases until virtually all the mitotic cells are labeled. The first labeled cells to finish M are, of course, the first to have entered it, and the last labeled cells to leave M are the last to have entered it. Accordingly, the interval between the times at which (1) the label is *first* seen in 50% of the mitotic cells and (2) the label is *last* seen in the same proportion of mitotic cells provides a mean estimate of the duration of the S phase. To stay consistent with this convention, the endpoint adopted for measuring G_2 is also sometimes taken as the time at which 50% of the mitotic cells first show label, even though this endpoint provides a *mean* estimate of G_2 and not a *minimal* estimate as described above.

Estimating the Total Length of the Cell Cycle.   If samples continue to be taken after the proportion of labeled mitotic cells drops to zero, labeled mitotic cells reappear. These represent the daughter cells of cells that took up the label when they were in S phase. In other words, the mother cells have now passed through an entire cell cycle. The time taken to complete a cell cycle is known as the *generation time* of the cell, T_G. The total length of the cell cycle, represented by the period between successive labeling peaks, is generally measured as the interval between consecutive times at which the proportion of labeled mitotic cells reaches a level of 50%.

Estimating the Duration of G_1.   Because the durations of the other three stages of the cell cycle can all be estimated or timed directly and the generation time can be determined as outlined above, the duration of G_1 can be calculated by subtracting the combined duration of G_2, S, and M from the generation time, T_G. Though fairly constant for any given cell line, the length of G_1 differs a great deal from one kind of cell to another and is the most variable stage of the cell cycle. As noted earlier, it can be very prolonged in cells that are specialized.

It should be noted that the use of tritiated thymidine provides *average values* for the lengths of stages of the cell cycle. Within the same population, there can be considerable variation from one cell to another, both in the relative duration of the individual phases and also in the total length of the cell cycle.

MITOSIS

By the time the cell enters mitosis, the nuclear DNA that was present in G_1 has been replicated during the S phase, with the result that two DNA molecules are present in each chromosome. Each chromosome now condenses along its entire length, with the result that the formerly partly extended, single chromatin threads that characterized G_1 have now become double threads composed entirely of condensed chromatin. The two constituent chromatin threads of each mitotic chromosome lie side by side, joined at a single site termed the *centromere* (Gr. *kentron*, center; *meros*, part).

A Note on Terminology.   Certain terms used to describe cell division were devised in the last century and now need clarification. These include the terms *chromatid*, *chromosome*, and *daughter chromosome*. The two threads of a mitotic chromosome were called *chromatids* (Gr. *idio*, small or young) long before it was known that each chromatid continued to exist throughout interphase as an intact chromatin thread, namely, a *chromosome*. Indeed, the chromatids entering the daughter cells were thought to break up into chromatin granules that, in turn, reassembled into chromosomes for the next division. Furthermore, chromatids that had parted company were described as *daughter chromosomes* even though they were still essentially the same structures split from each other at the centromere. Finally, the word *chromosome* is used both for the single threads present in G_1 and also for the double-threaded structures present during G_2 and the first two stages of mitosis. Medical students tend to think of chromosomes as double structures because these are what they see when chromosomes are prepared for cytogenetic analysis. However, the chromatin granules seen in interphase cells represent amassed condensed regions of *single-threaded* chromosomes in G_1 and are distinct from *double-threaded* chromosomes in G_2. To aid in comprehension, when it becomes necessary to draw a distinction between single- and double-threaded chromosomes, we shall refer to the former as *s-chromosomes* (s for single) and the latter as *d-chromosomes* (d for double). Nevertheless, it should be understood that our only justification in introducing these two terms here is that they reduce the number of words needed, and we should stress that neither term belongs to the classical language of cytogenetics.

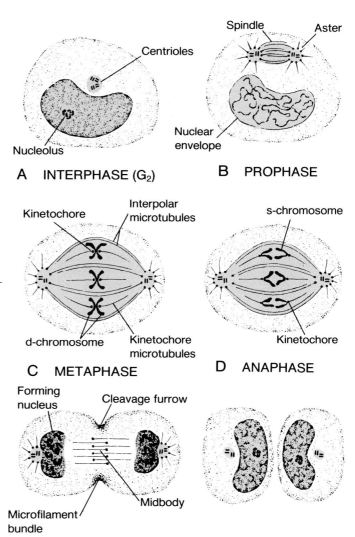

Fig. 3-8. Diagrammatic representation of the stages of mitosis. For details, see text. (Courtesy of V. I. Kalnins)

Although mitosis is one continuous process, it is classically subdivided into four sequential phases called *prophase* (Gr. *pro*, before), *metaphase* (Gr. *meta*, beyond), *anaphase* (Gr. *ana*, again), and *telophase* (Gr. *telos*, end). These stages are illustrated schematically in Figure 3-8, and their appearance in the LM is shown in Figure 3-9. As already stated, the whole process takes from 1 to 1.5 hours to complete, depending on the cell type. When a typical human cell starts to divide, it contains 46 d-chromosomes. During the course of mitosis, the two chromatids of each d-chromosome separate from each other, producing 92 daughter chromosomes (s-chromosomes). Half the complement of s-chromosomes then moves toward each pole of the spindle, where it later becomes incorporated into a daughter cell nucleus. At this time the cell pinches itself in half, producing two daughter cells with identical chromosome complements. A further distinctive feature of mitosis is the assembly of a transitory structure known as the *mitotic spindle*, which also plays a role in the alignment and segregation of mitotic chromosomes.

In addition to nuclear components, we also have to consider paired cytoplasmic organelles known as *centrioles*, which are present at the poles of the mitotic spindle.

Centrioles Replicate in Preparation for Mitosis. A cell in G_1 contains a pair of small, closely associated structures that are called *centrioles* (Gr. *kentron*, center) because they have a tendency to be situated beside the nucleus, somewhere near the middle of the cell and commonly in a nuclear indentation (Fig. 3-8*A*). In special kinds of LM preparations, the centrioles are just detectable as two tiny dots. In the EM it can be seen that they are cylindrical structures that are 0.5 μm in length and 0.2 μm in diameter. The walls of each centriole are made up of nine longitudinal bundles of microtubules (Fig. 3-10). *Microtubules* are long tubular

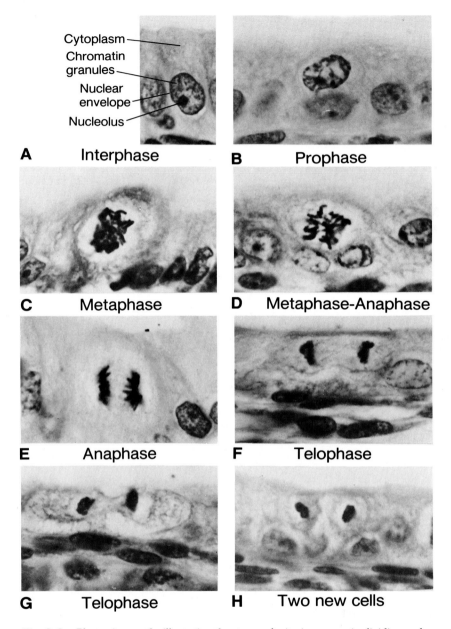

Cytoplasm
Chromatin granules
Nuclear envelope
Nucleolus

A   Interphase

B   Prophase

C   Metaphase

D   Metaphase-Anaphase

E   Anaphase

F   Telophase

G   Telophase

H   Two new cells

Fig. 3-9.   Photomicrographs illustrating the stages of mitosis, as seen in dividing endometrial cells of a rat (oil immersion).

structures with a distinct central channel that is relatively electron lucent. (They will be considered again in more detail in Chapter 4.) Although variable in length, they have a constant external diameter of 25 nm. Individual microtubules cut in longitudinal section may be seen by turning to Figure 3-13; their appearance in cross section can be seen in Figure 3-12, in the region marked *K*. Microtubules are polymerized from dimeric subunits made up of two slightly different forms of the protein *tubulin.* By referring

to the cross section of a centriole shown in Figure 3-10, it can be seen that (1) the microtubules of centrioles are arranged as bundles of three, and (2) these so-called *triplet microtubules* lie embedded in finely fibrillar material.

In the G_1 phase, there are two centrioles lying at right angles to each other (Fig. 3-8*F*). By the time a cell reaches G_2, a daughter centriole has assembled beside and at right angles to each preexisting centriole (Fig. 3-8*A*). As a result, a cell in G_2 contains *two pairs* of centrioles.

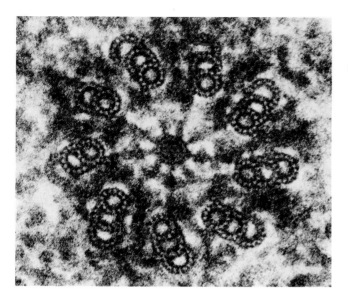
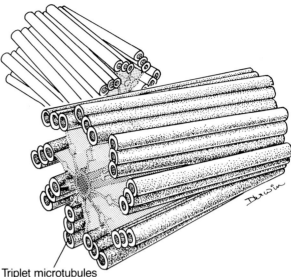

Triplet microtubules

Fig. 3-10. Electron micrograph (×330,000) of a centriole in a chick tracheal epithelial cell, showing its appearance in transverse section, and an interpretive diagram of a centriole pair. Staining has been enhanced with tannic acid to show the subunit structure of its constituent microtubules (discussed in Chap. 4). Nine triplet microtubules, embedded in a fine fibrillar material, are arranged in a characteristic radiating pattern around an axial structure. This axial component is present at one end of the centriole and is frequently described as a cartwheel because in cross section it appears as a central hub with nine radiating spokes. (Courtesy of M. Wassmann and V. I. Kalnins)

Prophase

At the beginning of prophase, the two pairs of centrioles start migrating toward opposite ends (*poles*) of the cell (Fig. 3-8*B*). At the same time, microtubules grow out in a radiating pattern from the fuzzy, electron-dense material surrounding each centriole pair. This shell of fuzzy material contains multiple sites (represented as black dots in Fig. 3-8*B*) from which microtubules grow out in all directions away from the centrioles. Such sites are therefore known as *microtubule organizing centers*. At first, the two radiating groups of microtubules, termed *asters* (Gr. *astron*, star), are hardly noticeable in mammalian cells. However, the interdigitating microtubules situated in the region where both of these radiating arrangements overlap then begin to lengthen, pushing the two centriole pairs apart (Fig. 3-8*B*). These progressively elongating microtubules, termed *interpolar*, *polar*, or *continuous microtubules* (continuous in

the sense of extending from one pole to the other), soon constitute a spindle-shaped mass called the *mitotic spindle* (Figs. 3-8*B* and 3-11). In early prophase the nuclear envelope is still intact, so the spindle starts to develop outside the nucleus (Fig. 3-8*B*). As prophase proceeds, however, the nuclear envelope fragments and the nucleolus disappears. There is now no structural barrier to prevent the developing spindle from assuming a central position in the cell, and the chromosomes are able to associate with the lengthening spindle microtubules. Prophase chromosomes first appear as double threads and then become more rod-shaped (Fig. 3-8*B*).

Thus in prophase, the nucleus and nucleolus both disappear as visible entities, and the cell assumes an ovoid shape with a centriole pair at each pole. The d-chromosomes associate with the lengthening interpolar microtubules of the mitotic spindle, which now lies where the nucleus was located.

Fig. 3-11. Photomicrographs of the mitotic spindle of cells in metaphase (*A*) stained with iron hematoxylin and (*B*) following immunofluorescent staining for tubulin, the protein from which microtubules are assembled (see Chap. 1 for the basis of such staining). All of the chromosomes are arranged in the equatorial plane. (*A,* courtesy of Y. Clermont and C. P. Leblond; *B,* Connolly JA, Kalnins VI: In DeBrabander M, DeMay J [eds]: Microtubules and Microtubule Inhibitors, p 175. Amsterdam, Elsevier/North Holland Biomedical Press, 1980)

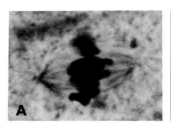
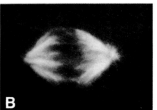

Metaphase

Chromosome condensation (shortening and thickening) continues into metaphase. When metaphase chromosomes are appropriately spread out and stained, they are suitable for study under the LM (see Fig. 3-16). The structural characteristics by which they are classified for cytogenetic analysis will be considered later in this chapter.

The most striking feature of metaphase is that all the chromosomes become aligned with their centromeres in a single transverse plane (Figs. 3-8C and 3-11). This plane lies perpendicular to the long axis of the spindle and is known as the *equatorial plane* of the cell because of its equivalence to the plane of the world's equator. Easy to recognize in the LM, this highly characteristic chromosome arrangement is often described as a *metaphase plate.*

To understand why all chromosomes become arranged in the equatorial plane, we must next consider a second set of microtubules that are now added to the spindle. These

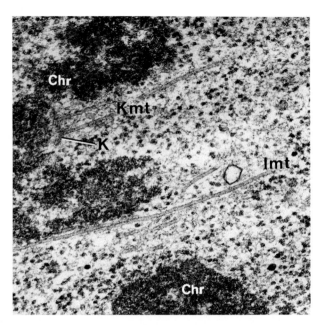

Fig. 3-13. Electron micrograph (×50,000) of metaphase chromosomes (*Chr*), showing kinetochore microtubules (*KMt*) attached to a kinetochore (*K*). The microtubule labeled IMt is probably an interpolar microtubule. (Courtesy of V. I. Kalnins)

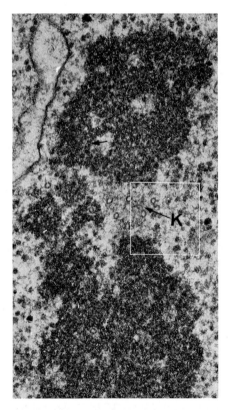

Fig. 3-12. Electron micrograph (×50,000) of the centromere region of a mitotic chromosome, showing a kinetochore region (labeled *K*). The two electron-dense masses represent parts of the same chromosome, bent around so that both arms of the chromosome lie in the plane of section. In the kinetochore region, which lies at the junction of the two arms, chromosomal microtubules may be seen cut in cross section. The granular appearance of the chromosome is due to its chromatin thread (visible at the *arrow* as a curving thread) being sectioned innumerable times. (Courtesy of V. I. Kalnins)

additional microtubules become attached to the chromosomes in their centromere region, at which site each chromatid possesses a layered, platelike attachment plaque for microtubules called a *kinetochore* (Fig. 3-12, labeled *K*). It should be noted that the term *kinetochore* (Gr. *kinetos*, movable; *chora*, space; movable in the sense of varying in position on different chromosomes) refers to the tiny disk-shaped structure seen at this site with the EM and not to the entire centromere. Kinetochores persist throughout interphase and replicate during the S phase along with the s-chromosomes to which they belong. Because the second set of microtubules contributing to the spindle become anchored to kinetochores, they are called *kinetochore* or *chromosomal microtubules.* Such microtubules are shown cut in transverse section in Figure 3-12 and in longitudinal section in Figure 3-13. They appear within the spindle when tubulin from the cytoplasm becomes freely available in the previously nuclear area as a result of fragmentation of the nuclear envelope. Recent evidence does not favor the earlier contention that their assembly is initiated by kinetochore-associated microtubule organizing centers. Instead, it seems likely that the kinetochores have the capacity to latch onto microtubules that grow out from the centriole pairs. There is also evidence that kinetochore microtubules can exert pull on chromosomes, but opinion is divided about whether this action depends on interaction of kinetochore microtubules with (1) interpolar microtubules or (2) some other as yet unidentified component of the spindle. Every metaphase chromosome acquires two groups of kinetochore microtubules (a group for the kinetochore on each of its chromatids). The opposing poleward forces exerted on the component chromatids of the chromosome keep it in a state of *dynamic equilibrium.* From the behavior of metaphase chromosomes, it can be inferred that they are submitted to pole-directed forces that are proportional to the length of the kinetochore microtubules attached to either side of the chromosome. Once a balance is achieved between these opposing forces, metaphase chromosomes all become aligned, with their centromeres in a plane that is equidistant from either pole, namely, the equatorial plane. Moreover, their two chromatids are now facing opposite poles of the spindle in the appropriate orientation for their impending separation at anaphase.

Anaphase

Early in *anaphase,* each d-chromosome splits at its centromere, allowing its two component s-chromosomes to separate from each other (Fig. 3-8D). Half the total number of s-chromosomes then approaches each pole of the cell. Yet the source of the motive forces that bring about such pole-directed movements remains a contentious issue. Nevertheless, as the daughter chromosomes progress toward the poles, the kinetochore microtubules attached to them shorten by undergoing net disassembly at their polar end. Hence as well as pulling on the chromosomes, this set of microtubules is believed to be rate-limiting for the speed of poleward migration of the chromosomes, ensuring that the two sets of daughter chromosomes segregate in a precise and orderly manner.

Mechanisms invoking the intracellular redistribution of calcium ions and the participation of actin and other contractile proteins (a general term for cytoplasmic proteins that are involved in contractile arrangements) have also been proposed to explain how spindle forces are generated. Nevertheless, several of the models currently favored continue to be based on the hypothesis that the microtubules in each half of the spindle are somehow involved in generating the forces responsible for separating and drawing daughter chromosomes toward opposite poles during anaphase.

Also contributing to separation of the daughter chromosomes at anaphase is further elongation of the spindle, which can double in length before the cell reaches telophase. Such elongation, a continuation of the process whereby lengthening of the interpolar microtubules pushes the two ends of the spindle farther apart, is believed to involve an active sliding movement of the two half-spindles away from each other.

Telophase

At the end of anaphase or at the beginning of telophase, a constriction develops around the middle of the elongated cell (Fig. 3-8E). This constriction is called the *cleavage furrow* because by deepening it eventually cleaves the cell into two (Fig. 3-8F). Under the cleavage furrow, a ring-shaped bundle of actin-containing microfilaments can generally be found near the cell membrane (Fig. 3-8E). By interacting with other contractile proteins, the actin in these filaments produces a force that tightens the ring and deepens the cleavage furrow. The bundle of spindle microtubules that still connects the daughter cells while this furrow is deepening is termed the *midbody* (Fig. 3-8E). When the daughter cells separate at the end of cleavage, a remnant of the midbody may remain attached to one of the daughter cells and persist well into interphase. In the meantime, the chromosomes of each daughter cell become partly extended and chromatin granules reappear. The nucleoli re-form and a new nuclear envelope is assembled, restoring interphase organization to each daughter nucleus.

Recognition of Mitotic Figures

The various chromosome arrangements in mitotic cells are referred to as *mitotic figures,* and their presence in a section indicates that cell division was occurring when the tissue was obtained. Mitotic figures are encountered in most body tissues until growth is over, after which they are seen at sites where cells are (1) dividing to maintain cell populations or (2) increasing in number in response to hormonal stimulation or increased functional demands. In addition, they appear at sites where tissue repair is in progress and also in abnormal cellular growths such as tumors, where their prevalence is an important clue in diagnosing cancer. The spotting of mitotic figures in a section is important, and all students of histology and pathology should learn how to recognize them.

In LM sections only sizable, well-stained structures are obvious. Also, the cells are cut in every conceivable plane, so it takes much searching to find mitotic figures cut in a plane in which they can be recognized. Chromosomes are seldom as well fixed in sections as in spreads, and they have an unfortunate tendency to aggregate. Mitotic figures must be carefully distinguished from the nuclei of dead cells in which the chromatin has aggregated into a solid mass. They can generally be spotted by looking for clusters of deeply stained chromosomes that are not confined within a nuclear envelope (Fig. 3-9C to F). A spiky appearance, due to chromosomes sticking out at angles (Fig. 3-9C to E), is indicative of a mitotic figure, as distinct from the rounded contours of the nucleus of a dead cell.

Metaphase, anaphase, and telophase mitotic figures are easy to spot if the cell has been sectioned perpendicular to its equatorial plane (Fig. 3-9C to F). Special fixation and staining also make it possible to see the spindle, at least during metaphase (Fig. 3-11). However, it takes patience and the use of several sections to find representative examples of all stages of mitosis. Also, it is necessary to visualize the appearance of mitotic figures sectioned in other planes. Prophase is the hardest stage to find, particularly during its early stages when the nuclear envelope is still intact. Beginners sometimes mistake two interphase nuclei

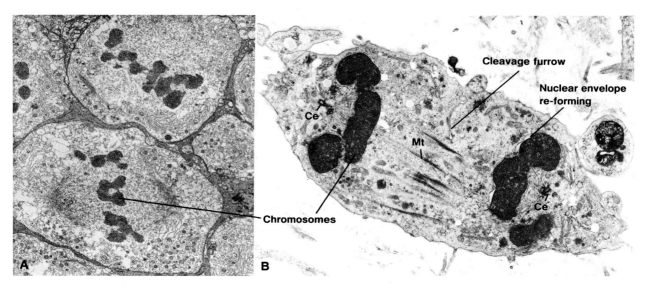

Fig. 3-14. (*A*) Electron micrograph (×1400) of two spermatocytes in metaphase. Note the characteristic shape of mitotic chromosomes in the bottom cell. Metaphase mitotic figures are readily recognizable at the EM level by the orientation of the centromeres within the equatorial plane of the cell. (*B*) Electron micrograph (×2800) of a human dermal cell in telophase. This section includes both poles of the spindle as well as the cleavage furrow. Note the two groups of electron-dense daughter chromosomes, the re-forming nuclear envelope around each group, the two pairs of centrioles (*Ce*), and the residual microtubules (*Mt*) that will persist as the midbody. (*A*, courtesy of L. Arsenault, *B*, courtesy of S. Marie)

lying close together for a telophase mitotic figure. Unless the nuclei belong to two noticeably small daughter cells, they are not likely to represent telophase.

Mitotic figures are fairly easy to recognize at the EM level under low magnification, provided the nuclear envelope has fragmented and large masses of condensed chromatin are in evidence (Fig. 3-14). Such areas of coarsely granular chromatin are irregular in outline because of variable orientation of the chromosomes. However, their general pattern of distribution in the cell can indicate the stage of mitosis, as may be seen by comparing parts A and B of Figure 3-14. EM sections disclose very little about the internal structural organization of mitotic chromosomes. Most of our current understanding of the arrangement of chromatin in mitotic chromosomes comes from specially prepared whole mounts of entire isolated chromosomes (Fig. 2-10). The complex coiling and looping of the chromatin fiber that can be seen in such preparations was discussed under Chromatin in Chapter 2 and is depicted in Figure 2-8.

Radiation and Drug Effects on Mitosis

Radiation Interferes with Cellular Proliferation. The damage done to cells by ionizing radiation is unlike that inflicted by other kinds of damaging physical agents such as heat. Thus injury due to heat is greatest at the body surface, diminishing in relation to depth, and it soon becomes evident. The damage caused by ionizing radiation, on the other hand, is more insidious because it does not necessarily diminish in relation to depth and it may not be manifested for a relatively long time.

High-energy radiation can be more damaging below the body surface. The high-energy photons of x or γ radiation set energetic electrons in motion in the living cells that lie in their path. These electrons then knock out other electrons from atoms in cell constituents, with the result that such atoms become intensely reactive and enter into new and sometimes inappropriate chemical combinations, changing the chemical composition of the constituent involved. Some of this damage may be of little immediate consequence to an interphase cell, affecting only unexpressed or repetitive genes, or molecules that can be synthesized anew or replaced through metabolism. However, any such lesion that damages nuclear DNA can then present an insurmountable problem if the cell attempts to undergo mitosis. Indeed, this remarkable capacity of ionizing radiation to interfere with cellular proliferation constitutes the basic rationale for utilizing radiotherapy in the treatment of cancer.

When irradiated cells begin mitosis, their chromosomes may appear altered in form, fragmented, or joined together in anomalous ways, and portions of them may become lost. The spindle, too, may show abnormalities. Instead of having two poles, for example, it may have three, with the result that the chromosomes attempt to separate into three groups rather than two. The mitotic chromosomes may also act as if they were sticky, and at anaphase they may pull apart unevenly. Some may lag behind, forming bridges between groups of chromosomes. The daughter chromosomes may also dissociate without the nucleus itself dividing, resulting in an extra large nucleus that contains more than the normal number of chromosomes.

The reason why radiation damage becomes evident as soon as cells attempt to undergo mitosis is because this represents the first occasion on which the total effect of all the damage done to their nuclear DNA becomes manifest. Every molecule of DNA, not all of which is expressed in G_1, has to be replicated in the S phase before a cell can divide. Critical damage to DNA can interfere with this essential replication process. Manifested as broken chromosomes or abnormal mitotic figures, such damage can interfere with all further attempts at mitosis, halting cell division. A single chromosome break can be sufficient to stop a cell from dividing. Hence the purpose of employing radiation for the treatment of cancer is to damage nuclear DNA so that the cancer cells will never be able to divide again. This radiation has to be delivered in a way that ensures that the cancer cells receive more radiation than the nearby normal tissues because radiation damage is nonspecific.

Radiosensitivity. A factor known to influence the amount of damage inflicted by radiation is the local *oxygen tension;* damage to DNA is greatest at sites of higher oxygen tension. Broadly speaking, cells are no more sensitive to radiation during mitosis than during interphase. However, cells that divide at frequent intervals are more radiosensitive than cells that remain in interphase for a prolonged period. This is because they continue to enter mitosis, the stage at which the effects of radiation damage become manifest. Nevertheless, when rates of cell turnover are similar, all types of body cells exhibit a *roughly equal sensitivity* to radiation at all stages of the cell cycle.

It should always be borne in mind that tissues with a rapid cell turnover are more radiosensitive than tissues in which cell turnover is slow. Thus with total body radiation, greater damage can be expected in cells of the intestinal lining and blood cell-forming tissues than in those of the brain or heart. Yet this has nothing to do with the fact that many cells are in mitosis during irradiation. It is more a reflection of the fact that short-lived specialized cells need to be replaced on a continuous basis through rapid cellular proliferation. By retarding the necessary production of new cells, substantial doses of total body radiation can interfere with cell renewal in the intestinal lining and can cause a precipitous drop in the numbers of white cells in the blood. Thus when tissues with a rapid turnover of cells are described as more susceptible (sensitive) to radiation than tissues with a slow turnover, it is not because their cells are intrinsically more sensitive to radiation. What it really means is that the tissue concerned is very sensitive to anything (including radiation) that interferes with proliferation and the production of new cells.

Ionizing Radiation Is Mutagenic. The damage done to DNA by ionizing radiation is sometimes a comparatively minor alteration that is manifested as an altered gene product. When genes are duplicated in preparation for mitosis, the altered gene is also duplicated. Accordingly, all

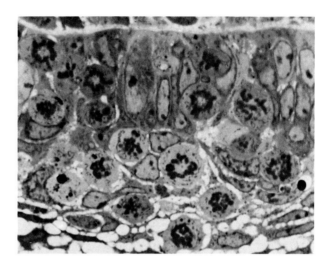

Fig. 3-15. Photomicrograph showing C-metaphases in preameloblasts and preodontoblasts of a tooth (stained with toluidine blue). This tissue was obtained from an animal 8 hours after the injection of colchicine and shows a high proportion of dividing cells trapped in a typical metaphaselike configuration. A good example is seen below center. (Courtesy of C. Smith)

progeny of the affected cell inherit any new qualities conferred by the altered gene. In this case the radiation, in a dose that was not lethal to the cell, has induced a cell *mutation* (L. *mutare,* to change). If a mutation occurs in a germ cell, it can be inherited by an offspring that is then known as a *mutant.*

Drugs That Block Mitosis. *Colchicine,* an alkaloid isolated from *Colchicum autumnale* (the meadow saffron), can also arrest mitosis. In the presence of this drug, no mitotic spindle is formed, hence chromatids fail to separate from one another even though they continue to condense. Mitotic chromosomes prepared using colchicine may therefore appear somewhat shorter and thicker than they usually do (Fig. 3-15).

Colchicine acts by *inhibiting formation of the spindle microtubules.* It becomes attached to a high-affinity binding site on the tubulin subunit, thereby forming a colchicine–tubulin complex. Once such complexes have been incorporated into a microtubule, they block the further addition of tubulin subunits, halting the process of microtubule assembly. This action of colchicine will be considered further in Chapter 4 when we deal with cytoplasmic microtubules.

Because colchicine inhibits the formation of spindle microtubules, no microtubules develop to push the two pairs of centrioles toward opposite poles of the cell. As a result, both pairs of centrioles stay in the middle of the cell and the double chromosomes assume a spherical distribution around them. Seen in sections, this chromosome arrangement can be suggestive of a metaphase mitotic figure (Fig. 3-15), so it is referred to as a *C-metaphase* (C for colchicine). An advantage of using colchicine to arrest mitosis is that its action can be reversed. When colchicine is removed, a mitotic spindle develops and a true metaphase follows in which the double chromosomes become aligned in the equatorial plane. The daughter chromosomes then segregate in the normal manner.

Vinblastine and a derivative called *vincristine* are drugs of lower toxicity that are obtained from *Vinca* (the periwinkle plant). Both of these alkaloids also block spindle formation by preventing microtubule assembly and cause the tubulin subunits with which they complex to aggregate into crystal-like arrays. These two drugs are unsurpassed for putting tubulin out of commission and are used clinically as antimitotic drugs in cancer chemotherapy.

Because these drugs block mitosis by inhibiting microtubule assembly, they arrest cellular proliferation in a different manner from ionizing radiation.

Cell Turnover Can Be Estimated Using Colchicine. Once colchicine is administered *in vivo* or is added to cells that are growing *in vitro*, mitotic figures (C-metaphases) begin to accumulate because the cells that enter mitosis are unable to complete it. It is therefore possible to use this drug to estimate the number of cells entering mitosis over a given period. In situations in which cell proliferation is compensating for cell loss, this estimate also provides a rough measure of the *turnover rate* of the total cell population. However, the information gained through the use of colchicine is not as reliable as that obtained using radioautography following the uptake of tritiated thymidine, as outlined earlier in this chapter.

Chromosomes for Cytogenetic Analysis Can Be Obtained Using Colchicine. Pairs of chromosomes can be readily identified at the C-metaphase stage obtained when mitosis is arrested with colchicine. This alkaloid (or its synthetic analogue, colcemid) is therefore much used in preparing chromosomes for the cytogenetic investigation of chromosomal abnormalities. For example, certain blood cells can be induced to proliferate *in vitro* and colchicine can then be added to block cell division. This method of preparing chromosomes, which will be described in the following section, greatly facilitates the diagnosis of genetic disorders and is standard procedure in most cytogenetics laboratories.

CHROMOSOME IDENTIFICATION

The fertilized human ovum contains 46 chromosomes, and typical *somatic cells* (Gr. *soma*, body) arising from it have the same chromosome number. Half this chromosome complement (made up of single representatives of each chromosome pair) comes from an *ovum*, and the other half is derived from a *spermatozoon* (the *female* and *male germ cells*, respectively). *Meiosis* (Gr. for diminution), the complex process by which these germ cells are produced, will be described in connection with the female and male reproductive systems in Chapter 23 and 24. One of the 23 chromosomes in the nucleus of each germ cell is a *sex chro-*

mosome; the other 22 are known as *autosomes* (Gr. *autos,* self). In every ovum the sex chromosome is an X chromosome, whereas in a spermatozoon it can be either an X (the female sex chromosome) or a Y (the male sex chromosome). Maleness is absolutely dependent on inheritance of a Y chromosome. Accordingly, when an ovum (which always has an X chromosome) is fertilized by a spermatozoon carrying an X chromosome, it will develop into a female with 44 autosomes and 2 X chromosomes in each somatic cell. In cases where the spermatozoon carries a Y chromosome, the fertilized ovum will develop into a male with 44 autosomes and the XY combination in each somatic cell.

The *chromosome number* of typical somatic cells (22 pairs of autosomes + one pair of sex chromosomes = 46 pairs) is referred to as the *diploid* chromosome number (Gr. *diplous,* double), twice the *haploid* (Gr. *haplous,* single) chromosome number (23) that characterizes germ cells. However, it is not abnormal for certain types of somatic cells to acquire a chromosome number that is more than twice the haploid number. Such cells are described as *polyploid* (Gr. *polys,* many).

Karyotyping for Cytogenetic Analysis. The chromosome constitution of an individual is established by investigating the chromosome complement of a representative sample of somatic cells. It is a relatively easy matter to induce lymphocytes to enter mitosis, after which they can be stopped at the C-metaphase stage by adding colchicine. Spreads can then be made of the so-called metaphase chromosomes obtained from such cells. From a photomicrograph of these chromosomes, it is possible to assemble a map or *karyotype* (Gr. *typos,* mark or prevailing character) portraying the individual's chromosome constitution. A close scrutiny of the karyotype will generally indicate any abnormality thay may exist in (1) the chromosome number or (2) the morphology of individual chromosomes. The significance of such an anomaly is that it can indicate a specific disorder of the individual concerned.

Chromosomal anomalies in somatic cells that are representative of the body as a whole originate at the germ cell level. However, it is also possible for chromosomal aberrations to arise at the somatic cell level in individuals with an otherwise normal karyotype. To investigate this type of anomaly, it is, of course, essential to obtain the karyotype of cells that are representative of the affected cell population.

Laboratory Procedure. First, the white blood cells are separated from a blood sample provided by the patient. These cells are then grown *in vitro* in a medium containing the plant-derived lectin *phytohemagglutinin*, which acts as a *mitogen* (Gr. *gennan,* to produce), stimulating lymphocytes to divide. Colchicine or colcemid is later added to accumulate C-metaphases. Next, the cells are suspended in a very dilute (hypotonic) medium that makes them swell up osmotically, and this causes their chromosomes to spread apart. The cells are then fixed and are made to spread out

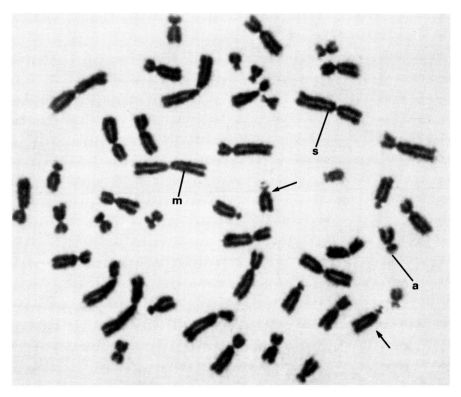

Fig. 3-16. Photomicrograph of metaphase chromosomes of a normal human male. Preparation made from a blood cell culture. Metacentrics (*m*), submetacentrics (*s*), and acrocentrics (*a*) can be distinguished. The arrows indicate satellited acrocentrics. (Courtesy of C. E. Ford)

flat on a slide. After staining, the chromosome complement of single cells selected on the basis of representative morphology and chromosome number are photographed under the LM (Fig. 3-16). Photographic representations of each individual chromosome are then cut out from such a photomicrograph and are arranged so as to construct a *karyotype.* The first step is to match them together in pairs, as described in the following section.

Chromosomes Are Assembled as Homologous Pairs. For every maternally derived autosome in a somatic cell, there is a paternally derived counterpart or *homologue.* Alternate forms of the same genes, termed *alleles,* are present on the two homologues. Females possess 23 pairs of homologues because the two X chromosomes in every somatic cell constitute a homologous pair. Males have only 22 pairs of homologues together with the XY sex chromosome constitution. The X chromosome and the Y chromosome are not considered homologues because almost all the genes they bear are different.

Because there are two chromatids in a metaphase chromosome, each of the two so-called arms extending from its centromere is actually a double structure. For assembly into a karyotype, the chromosome is oriented with its shorter arm (if it has one) uppermost. By referring to Figure 3-17, it can be seen that a chromosome whose centromere is situated near its middle is described as *metacentric.* If its

centromere lies closer to one end, the chromosome is described as *submetacentric.* A chromosome whose centromere lies close to one end is classified as *acrocentric* (Gr. *akron,* extremity). In man, there are no chromosomes that have their centromere situated at one end.

Satellites are small terminal regions of chromosomes attached by a narrow, nonstaining region, called a *secondary constriction,* to the ends of the short arms of certain acrocentric chromosomes (Fig. 3-17). Satellites are present on chromosomes 13, 14, 15, 21, and 22. The secondary constrictions associated with satellites become more obvious if silver salts are used for staining. Their functional significance is that they represent the sites where *nucleolar genes* coding for rRNA are distributed repetitively along the chromosome.

To prepare a karyotype, the 23 chromosome pairs are assembled in order of decreasing length and are numbered 1 to 22. As shown in Figure 3-18, they are assigned to 7 groups designated A to G. Group A, for example, consists of chromosome pairs 1 to 3, which are the longest metacentric chromosomes, and Group G includes pairs 21 and 22, which are the shortest acrocentric chromosomes. In males, group G also contains the Y chromosome (Fig. 3-18), which is an acrocentric chromosome like the others, but is usually the longest in the group, and its long arms

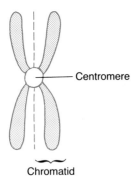

Centromere

Chromatid

Metacentric

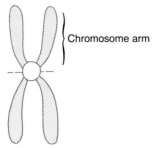

Chromosome arm

Submetacentric

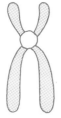

Acrocentric

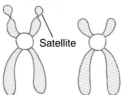

Satellite

Fig. 3-17.   Diagram showing the three shapes and the component parts of human chromosomes. This classification is based on the relative position of the centromere.

are usually parallel to one another, rather than divergent as in the other members of the G group. The X chromosome is very similar to certain members of the 6 to 12 (C) group (Fig. 3-18).

Each Chromosome Pair Is Recognized by Its Characteristic Banding Pattern. More recently developed methods of staining have made it possible to identify every pair of chromosomes in each group. These innovative

staining techniques disclose that each pair of chromosomes possesses a unique *pattern of bands* formerly unobtainable using conventional staining. Because such patterns are specific for each homologous pair, it is possible to recognize all the chromosome pairs unequivocally. We shall now go on to consider some of the banding techniques currently used to facilitate cytogenetic investigation and genetic counseling.

Virtually all major centers for antenatal detection and diagnosis of chromosomal defects have the laboratory facilities for staining chromosomes of prenatally sampled fetal cells for either *G-bands* or *Q-bands*, which are described below. The structural basis for such banding is not yet clear, but it seems to be due to localized condensation of configurationally uniform chromatin, possibly reflecting a measure of structural compatibility between looped domains of the chromatin fiber or some other kind of conformational uniformity. Although the bands revealed by Giemsa and quinacrine staining are virtually identical, there seem to be certain differences in their basis of staining, as we shall now go on to explain.

Q-Bands. The chromosome bands revealed by *quinacrine*, a derivative of the dye acridine, are termed *Q-bands* (the Q denoting quinacrine). This drug was first introduced as an antimalarial agent, but its use for this purpose has since been discontinued. Nevertheless, it became apparent that quinacrine and its closely related derivatives, like other acridine dyes, have an affinity for chromatin and are intensely *fluorescent,* meaning that when exposed to ultraviolet radiation they emit light of a visible wavelength. When observed under the fluorescence microscope (which was described in Chap. 1 under Light Microscopy and Its Applications), quinacrine was found to fluoresce a bright greenish-yellow color. Then came the important discovery by Caspersson and his coworkers that *discrete bands* along the length of mitotic chromosomes stained with quinacrine mustard. Moreover, between different chromosomes there were differences in band thickness and interband spacing, providing a specific pattern that now allowed the pairs of chromosomes to be individually identified with certainty. For example, a particularly large and brightly fluorescent Q-band is evident on the distal region of the long arm of the Y chromosome. In human cells this band is even quite prominent in interphase, appearing as an intensely fluorescent little spot approximately 0.2 μm in diameter.

Not much is known about how quinacrine and its derivatives stain chromosome bands, except that, in general, the brightly fluorescing stretches of DNA present in Q-bands are richer in the bases adenine and thymine than they are in guanine and cytosine. However, this pattern of staining probably reflects some enhancement or quenching of fluorescence rather than differential binding of the dye, and it remains unclear whether Q-bands are a direct result of underlying regional base specificity or mirror an uneven distribution of associated chromosomal protein. Q-banding nevertheless seems to reflect a certain amount of gross qualitative variation in base-pair composition along the length of the mitotic chromosome.

G-Bands. Following the discovery of Q-bands, alternative banding methods were developed that made the use of a fluorescence microscope unnecessary. These techniques utilize *Giemsa stain,* which is also widely used to stain blood cells. However, they

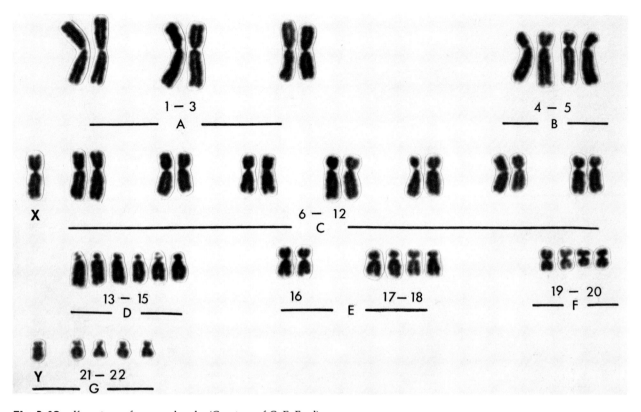

Fig. 3-18.   Karyotype of a normal male. (Courtesy of C. E. Ford)

also require *denaturation treatment* of the chromosomes before staining. This entails mild treatment of the fixed chromosomes with proteolytic enzymes, salts, heat, detergents, or urea, all of which are agents capable of denaturing chromosomal proteins. When the chromosomes are stained with Giemsa after such treatment, *G-bands* can be seen under an ordinary light microscope. The banding pattern is similar to that obtained using quinacrine. Figure 3-19 shows a karyotype assembled from chromosomes stained by this procedure. Like the DNA of Q-bands, that of G-bands is comparatively rich in adenine and thymine. It also replicates late in the S phase and has been reported to have fewer active genes than does the DNA of negative G-bands. These observations are consistent with the fact that it is present as heterochromatin during most of the cell cycle.

The mechanism of G-banding has not yet been clearly elucidated. However, it appears to depend on uneven removal of chromosomal proteins as a result of denaturation, perhaps in relation to some local gross variation in the underlying base-pair composition of the DNA with which such proteins are associated.

It is nevertheless fairly well established that positively charged thiazin dyes in Giemsa stain side-stack on the negatively charged phosphate groups of DNA molecules, whereupon a thiazin-eosin complex becomes preferentially deposited in the dark-staining G-band regions of the pretreated chromosomes. Moreover, there are indications that (1) this dye complex forms in regions where the phosphate groups lie a certain critical distance apart, and (2) such regions may be rich in hydrophobic proteins. Thus regional differences in the kinds of proteins present along the length of a chromosome could well determine the staining affinity of any given

region of its DNA, and its negative G-bands could fail to stain because of extraction or some configurational change in these hydrophobic proteins. Another hypothesis is that protein extraction might cause the chromatin fiber or its loops to become rearranged and thereby increase the chromatin content of the G-bands. A third possibility is that in the negative G-band regions, the phosphate groups may be blocked by denatured nonhistone proteins.

The negative G-band regions of chromosomes can also be demonstrated by a modification of the Giemsa procedure that discloses them as bands of a third type known as *R-bands.*

C-Bands.   Yet another modification of the Giemsa procedure provides a totally different pattern of staining. Prior to staining, most of the DNA is extracted from the fixed chromosomes by relatively harsh treatment with alkali, acid, salts, or heat. In this case, it is the constitutive heterochromatin in the centromere region that stains darkly as a *C-band* (C for *centromere*). The DNA in this region seems to be able to survive the harsh extraction procedure that precedes staining, and the thiazin dye molecules in Giemsa stain then side-stack on the phosphate groups of the unextracted DNA. The Y chromosome shows more general staining, reflecting broader distribution of constitutive heterochromatin in this particular chromosome. The fact that only the Y chromosome shows this unusual staining can facilitate the recognition of cells bearing a Y chromosome.

From a pool of collected data, the bands found on each chromosome pair have now been standardized. Figure 3-20 shows the positions of the principal bands on human

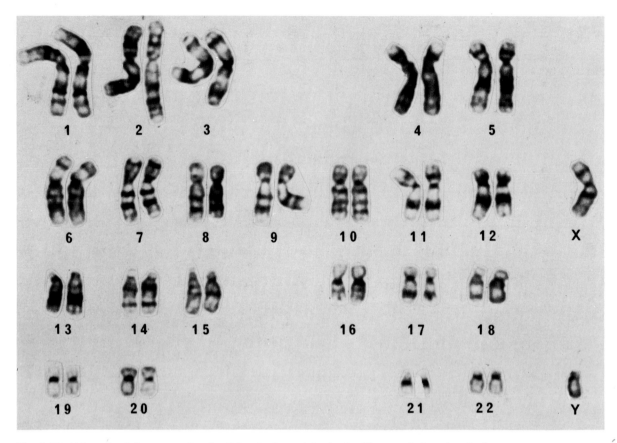

Fig. 3-19. Normal male karyotype, showing G-bands after staining by the Giemsa technique described in the text. The characteristic banding pattern permits each chromosome pair to be identified. (Courtesy of M. Seabright)

chromosome 12. This diagram may be compared with Figure 2-10, which shows an entire chromosome 12 prepared for the EM as a whole mount. Similar chromosomes stained for G-bands can also be seen in the karyotype shown in Figure 3-19. Here we might also add that in karyotypes prepared from such banded chromosomes, it is seldom easy to see that each chromosome in a homologous pair is actually double, that is, it consists of two chromatids joined by a centromere.

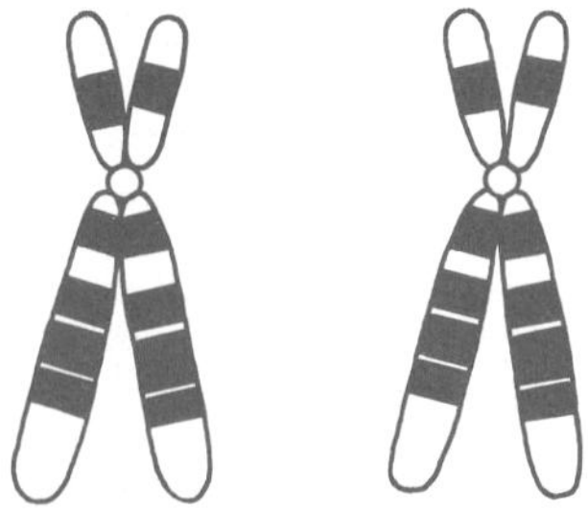

Besides assisting greatly in the preparation of karyotypes, chromosome banding techniques made it possible to visualize hitherto undetected chromosomal anomalies such as deletions of small portions of chromosomes and translocations of tiny parts of chromosomes from one chromosome to another. Because such procedures also enabled each pair of chromosomes to be distinguished individually, it finally became possible, for example, to recognize chromosome 21 from chromosome 22, helping to further our understanding of the chromosomal basis of certain important genetic disorders.

CHROMOSOMAL ANOMALIES

A *chromosomal anomaly* is some kind of deviation from (1) the normal diploid chromosome number of 46 or (2) normal chromosomal morphology. It may involve either the sex chromosomes or the autosomes. As noted, chromosomal

Fig. 3-20. Diagram of a pair of human chromosomes (chromosome 12), depicting their principal bands. (Based on an illustration in Paris Conference [1971], Supplement [1975]: Standardization in Human Cytogenetics. In Bergsma D [ed]: Birth Defects: Original Article Series, XI, 9, 1975. White Plains, the National Foundation)

anomalies originating at the germ cell level characterize all body cells and are therefore generally disclosed by karyotyping. Anomalies arising at the somatic cell level, because they are *not* typical of the body as a whole, are generally discovered by other means.

Anomalies Arising at the Germ Cell Level

Chromosomal aberrations inconsistent with full-term development *in utero* cause spontaneous abortions or miscarriages. Thus karyotypic investigations have disclosed that roughly 50% of all spontaneous abortions involve some sort of chromosomal abnormality of the conceptus. Yet there is a wide variety of chromosomal aberrations that do not preclude full-term fetal development, and about 1 out of every 160 newborn babies inherits some kind of cytogenetic abnormality.

The Sex Chromosome Constitution Is Responsible for Primary Sex Determination. The *sex chromosome* constitution, which is different in males and females, determines the *gonadal sex* of an individual. Certain genes on the Y chromosome have the effect of steering differentiation of the previously indifferent embryonic gonads in the direction of *testicular* development. A long-established hallmark of testicular development is that it is accompanied by the expression of a distinctive cell-surface constituent called the *H-Y antigen*. However, the significance of this particular marker is somewhat obscure and requires further elucidation. During the course of normal development, the fetal testes produce sufficient quantities of male sex hormone to bring about the differentiation of male genital ducts and male external genitalia. However, if the primary testis-organizing determinants carried by the Y chromosome are absent, and at least one X chromosome is present, the indifferent gonads undergo ovarian development instead. The X chromosome is also of general importance to the body as a whole because it bears a significant number of other genes.

Normal Sexual Development in Males Also Requires Responsiveness to Androgen. The nature of a male's external genitalia, as well as his secondary sexual characteristics, are profoundly influenced by expression of the *testicular feminization* locus on the X chromosome. Wherever the dominant form (allele) of this gene is expressed, an individual's cells can produce receptor protein for male sex hormone (androgen); this receptor is just as necessary as the hormone for normal sexual development of the male. However, the small number of individuals who inherit the recessive allele at this locus are only able to produce a *defective receptor protein* that will not bind androgen or that has insufficient androgen-binding capacity, with the result that their androgen-dependent cells fail to respond adequately to the hormone. These individuals possess an X and a Y chromosome and hence develop testes but may then fail to manifest any male external characteristics. Individuals with this rare X-linked condition, which is known as the *testicular feminization syndrome*, can develop genitalia that are typically female in external appearance, undergo breast enlargement at puberty, and except for being unable to menstruate or bear children can be physically and psychologically similar to fe-

males. The testes are nonfunctional and generally remain intra-abdominal and hence undetected. Pubic and axillary hair may also be missing since hair growth in these regions is androgen-dependent in both sexes.

Characteristic Anomalies of the Sex Chromosomes. One of the most common anomalies of the sex chromosomes is the presence of an extra X chromosome in a male, who therefore has the XXY sex chromosome constitution. Males with this anomalous combination have unusually small testes and are infertile. Later in life they may also show evidence of being intellectually impaired. This condition, called *Klinefelter syndrome*, can be due to failure of the two X chromosomes in a maternal diploid germ cell precursor to separate and segregate to different cells at meiosis; instead, both chromosomes go to an ovum that becomes fertilized by a spermatozoon carrying a Y chromosome. Less frequently, the XXY constitution arises when an XY-bearing spermatozoon (resulting from a corresponding failure of the paternal X and Y chromosomes to segregate at meiosis) fertilizes a normal X-bearing ovum. The sex chromosomes of a parent's cells can even fail to segregate at both divisions of meiosis (described in Chap. 23), and this can result in XXXY or XXXXY chromosome constitutions. Such variants of Klinefelter syndrome are characterized by fairly severe mental retardation.

Another anomaly in males is the XYY constitution. Men with this particular combination tend to be tall, and there are indications that some of them can be predisposed to aggressive or antisocial behavior (a claim that may have received more than its due share of publicity). The intelligence of such individuals can also be subnormal, but their fertility is generally unimpaired. In this case, erroneous segregation of the paternal sex chromosomes at the second meiotic division of spermatogenesis produces a YY spermatozoon that, at fertilization, contributes two Y chromosomes instead of one.

Females born with an extra X chromosome (in other words, females with an XXX constitution) can also be mentally retarded and some of them are infertile. The inheritance of further supernumerary X chromosomes (XXXX and XXXXX, for example) only serves to compound these problems.

Females born with only one X chromosome instead of two manifest a rarer condition called *Turner syndrome*. The general term for denoting that one of a pair of homologous chromosomes is missing from diploid cells is *monosomy* (Gr. *monos*, single). Apart from the few surviving babies manifesting monosomy of the X chromosome and occasional reports of monosomy 21, monosomies are incompatible with survival; embryos with the YO constitution, for example, are totally nonviable. Two X chromosomes are nonetheless required for the ovaries to undergo full development. Females born with the XO constitution (the O denoting that the homologue of this X chromosome is absent) possess only poorly developed ovaries and, in addition, are short in stature and exhibit certain other typical physical characteristics. The breasts fail to enlarge and other female secondary sexual characteristics may not appear when expected at the age of puberty. Such individuals possess a normal level of intelligence but rarely menstruate and are almost all infertile.

Theoretically, the XO condition could be due to failure of the mother's two X chromosomes to segregate at meiosis, because if both of these chromosomes were to segregate to a polar body, the ovum would not receive either of them. Fertilization of such an ovum by an X-bearing spermatozoon could then result in the offspring receiving only the paternal X chromosome. Yet a virtual absence of maternal-age dependence in this syndrome suggests that such an occurrence is a less common cause of the XO condition than the loss of an X or a Y chromosome either during spermatogenesis or following zygote formation. In the former case, the condition would be the result of fertilization of a normal X-bearing ovum by a spermatozoon that had no sex chromosome. It is probably significant that a substantial proportion of surviving cases of Turner syndrome show various kinds of *mosaicism* with respect to monosomy of the X chromosome, with the result that at least some of their cells possess more than one X chromosome.

Example of an Anomaly of an Autosome.   Approximately 1 out of every 800 babies is born with *trisomy 21,* another name for which is *Down syndrome.* This disorder is the most common chromosomal aberration of newborn babies. Moreover, the risk of a mother having a baby with Down syndrome increases considerably with her age, representing more of a hazard if she becomes pregnant in the latter part of her reproductive life. Individuals with Down syndrome are short in stature and are readily recognizable by their characteristic facial features and certain other typical but less striking physical characteristics. Although generally happy and affectionate in disposition, they are all mentally retarded.

In most cases, individuals with Down syndrome have an entire extra chromosome in their cells. When it was established that this chromosome belongs to the G group, it was agreed to classify it as an extra chromosome 21. Banding techniques subsequently confirmed that it was indeed another chromosome 21. The name *trisomy 21* is now widely adopted because it indicates that in classic cases of Down syndrome, there are three representatives of chromosome 21 in each cell. These three chromosomes are marked with arrows in Figure 3-21, which is a photomicrograph of chromosomes prepared from a fetal cell obtained during the course of a pregnancy.

Cells such as these can be collected from *amniotic fluid* tapped from the mother by *amniocentesis* (Gr. *kentesis,* puncture). This is a fairly straightforward procedure in which a sample of amniotic fluid is withdrawn by way of a needle carefully inserted through the anterior abdominal and uterine walls of the mother into the amniotic cavity surrounding the fetus. Such samples of aspirated amniotic fluid yield viable fetal cells (mostly desquamated from the fetal skin and respiratory tract) that are suitable for antenatal chromosomal analysis.

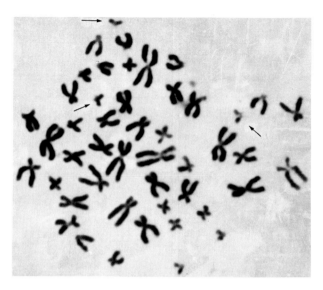

Fig. 3-21.   Chromosome preparation of a cell obtained by amniocentesis (for details, see text). The fact that there is one extra chromosome 21 (chromosome 21 is indicated by *arrows*) shows that the fetus had the chromosome constitution of Down syndrome, thus allowing a diagnosis to be made prenatally. (Courtesy of H. Nadler)

The chromosomal basis of trisomy 21 will be discussed in further detail when we deal with the process of meiosis as it occurs in the female (see Chap. 23).

Symbols Used in Specifying Karyotypes and Chromosomal Anomalies.   To denote a person's chromosome constitution, the total number of chromosomes is recorded first, followed by the sex chromosome complement. No specific mention is made of individual autosomes unless there is some detectable abnormality in them. Thus the normal male karyotype is designated 46,XY. The chromosome constitution of a female with Down syndrome who has an extra chromosome 21 would be specified as 47,XX,+21 (the + denoting that an extra autosome is present). The karyotype of a male having Klinefelter syndrome with two X chromosomes would be recorded as 47,XXY. A female with Turner syndrome would be designated 45,X or 45,XO (either of these conventions is acceptable).

The symbol *p* (Fr. *petit,* small) denotes the shorter arm of a chromosome; the longer arm is designated *q,* the next letter in the alphabet. Thus the longer arm of a chromosome 21 would be specified as 21q. This convention is necessary to record which arm of a chromosome is involved in a translocation or deletion. The *5p−* designation, for example, indicates that the shorter arm of chromosome 5 is shorter than normal. If all the other chromosomes are of normal length, it also indicates a deletion in this arm. Such a deletion in the terminal part of the shorter arm of chromosome 5 is a defect that leads to severe mental retardation. Infants with this uncommon defect also have distinctive facial features, and when they cry they sound so much like the mewing of a cat that the condition is known as the *cri du chat syndrome*. The 5p− condition constitutes an example of *structural* abnormality of a chromosome, as distinct from a *numerical* anomaly affecting chromosome number. The 5p+ designation would denote that the shorter arm of chromosome 5 was longer than normal due to translocation of part of another chromosome.

Anomalies Arising at the Somatic Cell Level

Two kinds of numerical aberrations can also arise at the somatic cell level. In *polyploidy* (Gr. *polys,* many), each cell contains more than two haploid sets of chromosomes, yet its chromosome number remains an exact multiple of the haploid number. *Tetraploid* cells, for example, possess twice the diploid number of chromosomes. The second kind of anomaly is a condition called *aneuploidy* (Gr. *an,* without, meaning without being an exact multiple). Here the chromosome number is irregular due to some earlier error in the segregation of daughter chromosomes. The consequence of such an error is that the chromosome number does *not* correspond to an exact multiple of the haploid number.

As we have seen, aneuploidy can also originate in an offspring at the germ cell level, leading to chromosome numbers such as 45 and 47. Polyploidy, too, can arise at the germ cell level, but this almost invariably results in spontaneous abortion. Even if triploid fetuses are born, which can happen, they are not able to survive.

Polyploidy Arising in Somatic Cells.   Although polyploidy arising in somatic cells represents a chromosomal anomaly in the sense that it is a deviation from the typical (diploid) chromosome number, it does not seem to be associated with any functional disturbance. Thus it is a normal occurrence for certain kinds of body cells to become polyploid, and such cells continue to function in a normal manner. The most extreme case of polyploidy is the megakaryocyte, the immediate precursor of blood platelets, which attains up to 64 times the haploid number of chromosomes. The hepatocyte population of the liver develops a lesser degree of polyploidy, which is manifested by fairly large nuclei with multiple nucleoli (Fig. 3-22). It is widely believed that polyploidy is an outcome of failure of the two chromatids of each chromosome to separate at anaphase, an error termed *nondisjunction,* with the result that both sets of daughter chromosomes remain in the equatorial region of the cell where the nuclear membrane reassembles and encloses them all in the same nucleus. However, alternative mechanisms by which polyploidy could arise have also been proposed. For example, in the epithelial lining of the urinary bladder, the chromosomes of binucleate cells that enter mitosis might all regroup into a single nucleus that thereby gains the tetraploid number of chromosomes.

Polyploid cells themselves are also able to undergo mitosis (Fig. 3-23).

Aneuploidy Arising in Somatic Cells.   Studies of mammalian cells growing in culture strongly suggest that there may be some sort of inherent limitation on the total number of times a normal somatic cell can divide, at least under the culture conditions employed. Cell populations obtained from an older individual, for instance, have been found to undergo fewer divisions *in vitro* than those taken from a younger individual do. This apparent limitation on the total proliferative potential of somatic cells is thought to constitute a kind of programmed senescence and could well be an important factor that determines the overall lifespan of an individual. Although seemingly determined for various types of normal cells (cells such as stem cells and lymphocytes may constitute an exception), this limitation is not inescapable. Repeated passaging of somatic cells from one culture to another (subculturing) can lead to the emergence of cell lines that seem to have the potential for multiplying forever. However, time and time again, chromosomal analysis has shown that the cells in such easily propagated cultures have acquired an aneuploid chromosome number, and, to this extent, they can no longer be regarded as normal cells. Thus overextended proliferation in somatic cells seems to be associated with the risk of some genetic change that makes them less responsive to factors that would ordinarily regulate their proliferation or curtail their reproduction. Furthermore, such a change somehow seems to set the stage for the eventual emergence of aneuploidy.

Aneuploidy Is Common in Cancer Cells.   As might be expected, a high incidence of aneuploidy is characteristic of malignant cells that undergo more or less continuous proliferation. It is believed that a malignancy arises when a somatic cell undergoes some genetic change that permits it to proliferate under conditions that would normally restrain its continuing multiplication. Furthermore, any accompanying loss of regulation of some specialized function that the cell or its progeny may perform can conflict with the needs of the body as a whole.

Because the transformation of a normal cell into a cancer cell is a genetic change, cancer cells are able to pass on their malignant and invasive properties to all their progeny. Moreover, unless a malignant tumor is entirely removed through surgery or totally destroyed by some other means, its cells may become disseminated by way of the blood or lymph to parts of the body distant from its site of origin. At such sites the cancer cells can set up new foci of destructive and invasive growth called *metastases* (Gr. *meta,* beyond; *stasis,* stand), and by this means cancer cells can overwhelm the body. By no longer responding to influences that ordinarily restrain cellular proliferation, cancer cells would go on multiplying forever if they did not have to succumb on death of their host.

Cancer cells so commonly exhibit aneuploidy that the detection of this condition in somatic cells of an otherwise chromosomally normal individual may indicate that these are cancer cells. However, the absence of aneuploidy in

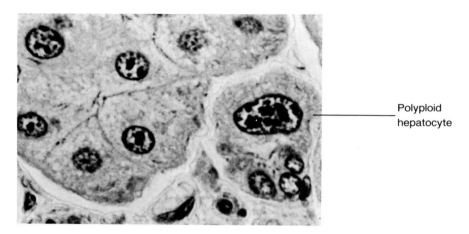

Fig. 3-22. Photomicrograph of the liver, showing a polyploid hepatocyte. Its nucleus is much larger and contains more nucleoli than that of the diploid hepatocytes seen on the left.

such cells does not preclude the possibility that they might be cancer cells, because not all malignant cells are aneuploid. The chances of their evolving toward an aneuploid chromosome number nevertheless seem to increase with their continuing multiplication. Thus aneuploidy arising at the somatic cell level may represent some ultimate outcome of the genetic changes that release cells from constraints on cellular proliferation. More will be said about the nature of such changes when we consider oncogenes in Chapter 5.

Example of a Structural Chromosome Anomaly Arising at the Somatic Cell Level. Patients with chronic myelogenous leukemia, a malignant disease in which there is an overproduction of certain white cells of the blood, char-

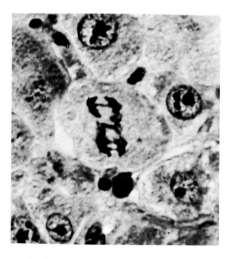

Fig. 3-23. Photomicrograph of regenerating liver (rat). Double the usual (diploid) number of anaphase chromosomes are arranged on a common spindle, indicating that this is probably a tetraploid cell dividing.

acteristically possess in the chromosome complement of their bone marrow cells a unique chromosome, which, because it was discovered in Philadelphia, is referred to as the *Philadelphia* chromosome, *Ph[1]*, or *Ph*. It represents a chromosome 22 in which almost half of the long arm is missing. Chromosome banding techniques have revealed that the missing part almost always becomes translocated onto a chromosome 9. Moreover, a tiny part of chromosome 9 also becomes translocated to the chromosome 22, so that this is actually a *reciprocal translocation*. The total number of chromosomes is nevertheless unaffected. The Philadelphia chromosome can be found in the majority of patients with chronic myelogenous leukemia and has become a valuable cytogenetic marker that is helpful in diagnosis of the disease. Although this particular chromosomal aberration is associated with the evolution of chronic myelogenous leukemia and perhaps other types of leukemia as well, its true significance remains a mystery. Because the Philadelphia chromosome arises at the somatic cell level, it is *not inherited* from one generation to another, nor is it present in every cell of the body. Further information about this chromosome can be found in the discussion of how myeloid and lymphoid cells are related in Chapter 9.

To complete our discussion on chromosomes, we shall next consider the only known circumstance in which a chromosome stays fully condensed once mitosis has ended. This can furnish potentially useful information about an individual's sex chromosome constitution without it being necessary to prepare a karyotype.

SEX CHROMATIN

Sex Chromatin Was First Noticed in Nerve Cells of Female Cats. During the course of an investigation into the effects of nerve stimulation on the microscopic appearance of the nerve cell body, Barr and Bertram noticed a small round mass of chromatin, originally

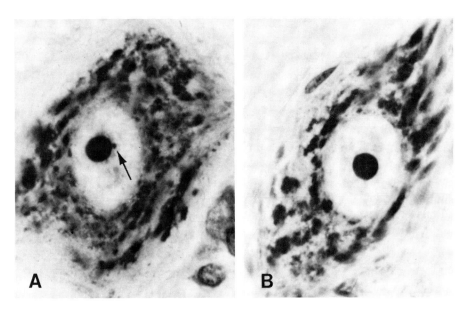

Fig. 3-24. Oil-immersion photomicrograph of nerve cells (in the anterior horn of the spinal cord) from two different cats. The pale appearance of the nuclei is due to almost all of their chromatin being extended, and the nucleolus is very large and prominent in both cells. Barr and Bertram noticed that in nerve cells taken from female cats (*A*), a little round body could be found close to the nucleolus. This can be seen at the end of the arrow. The little body was not found in the nucleus of such cells taken from male animals (*B*). (Barr ML, Bertram LF, and Lindsay HA: Anat Rec 107:283, 1950)

described by Cajal, in the nerve cells of certain cats (Fig. 3-24*A*) but not others (Fig. 3-24*B*). Laboratory records showed that this tiny mass, now known as *sex chromatin*, was present in females but not males. The inference that it would be possible to predict the sex of a cat by examining LM sections turned out to be true for humans, too. Soon a suitable method was devised whereby cells scraped from the lining of a cheek (the *buccal mucosa*) could be prepared and stained for sex chromatin, and this now provides a very rapid and straightforward means of determing whether an individual's somatic cells contain masses of sex chromatin (also referred to as *Barr bodies*).

By establishing the presence or absence of sex chromatin in typical somatic cells, it is possible to predict whether an individual possesses more than one X chromosome in each cell. Furthermore, by counting the individual small masses of sex chromatin in representative interphase cells, the total number of X chromosomes per cell can be determined. The basis for such a determination is as follows.

The X chromosome bears a variety of different genes, more than 50 of which are not in the least involved in sex determination and are just as essential to males as females (conceptuses require at least one X chromosome to be viable). Yet only one X chromosome is expressed in diploid somatic cells during interphase. Any additional X chromosomes seem to be largely unnecessary and are almost completely genetically inactivated, each appearing as a discrete mass of condensed chromatin (sex chromatin). Thus the total number of X chromosomes in a diploid cell is equal to its *number of masses of sex chromatin plus one.*

The Presence of Sex Chromatin in Cells Can Be Clinically Significant. Whenever the clinical significance of the presence of sex chromatin is being evaluated, it should always be remembered that its occurrence does not in itself indicate that an individual is female any more than its absence proves that an individual is male. As already noted, a person's sex is determined not by the number of X chromosomes he possesses but by whether the testis-determining Y chromosome is also present. Thus an XXY individual (the most common form of Klinefelter syndrome) is phenotypically male even though he has two X chromosomes in every diploid somatic cell. On the basis of sex chromatin interpretation alone, such a male would be indistinguishable from a normal female (XX) in possessing a mass of sex chromatin in each cell. Conversely, a female with Turner syndrome (XO) would be sex chromatin-negative like a normal male. A female with the XXX constitution would exhibit two sex chromatin masses per cell. Thus sex chromatin determination is a simple and effective diagnostic tool for detecting abnormalities of X chromosome number. In addition to its strictly medical use, it is also employed at major international athletics meetings to establish the chromosomal sex of the competitors.

The Microscopic Appearance of Sex Chromatin Depends on the Cell Type. In nerve cells, the sex chromatin constitutes a tiny, round basophilic mass that is generally situated close to the prominent spherical nucleolus (Fig. 3-24*A*). In most other cell types, it has a convex shape and

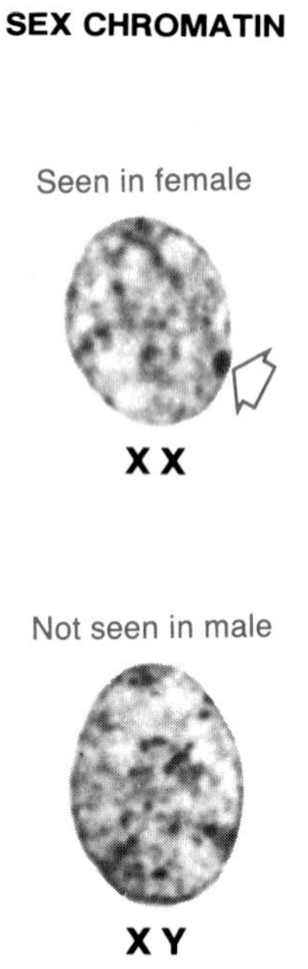

SEX CHROMATIN

Seen in female

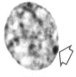

X X

Not seen in male

X Y

Fig. 3-25.   Photomicrograph of epithelial cells of the oral mucosa, stained for sex chromatin with cresyl-echt violet (oil immersion). The arrow indicates a mass of sex chromatin. (Moore KL, Barr ML: Lancet 2:57, 1955)

is attached to the inner aspect of the nuclear envelope (Fig. 3-25), but in neutrophils it takes the form of the *drumstick appendage,* a small additional lobe of the segmented nucleus (see Fig. 8-11).

The Buccal Smear Chromatin Test.   The laboratory procedure for determining whether an individual's cells contain any sex chromatin is extremely simple. Whole buccal epithelial cells are obtained by gently scraping the inside of a cheek with a spatula. They are then smeared thinly on a slide, fixed, and stained with cresyl violet. Each mass of sex chromatin appears as a darkly stained chromatin granule adhering to the nuclear envelope (Fig. 3-25). About 1 μm in diameter, it can be seen under oil immersion in whole cells and even in nuclei cut in an appropriate plane of section.

Although more intensely basophilic and somewhat larger and smoother edged than the usual kind of chromatin granule, a sex chromatin mass is substantially smaller than the nucleolus, with which structure a beginner may occasionally confuse it on initial observation. Also, students sometimes mistake bacteria colonizing the buccal epithelium for masses of sex chromatin because such bacteria also stain with cresyl violet. Furthermore, the student will find that sex chromatin can be identified with certainty only if it happens to be oriented so that it lies at the periphery of the nucleus, as seen in Figure 3-25. Cells should not be scored as chromatin-positive unless they manifest sex chromatin in such a position.

To ascertain whether sex chromatin is present or absent, it is essential to examine many interphase nuclei and to bear in mind that even where present, it would not be recognizable in every nucleus because of unsuitable orientation. Also, it disappears transiently in the S phase. Another problem is that discrete chromatin masses closely resembling sex chromatin are occasionally seen even in nuclei that lack such chromatin. A sex chromatin determination therefore requires the close scrutiny of up to 100 nuclei, from which the proportion of chromatin-positive cells can be estimated. With a trained eye, individual sex chromatin masses can be seen in 20% to 70% of buccal epithelial cells obtained from individuals with more than one X chromosome. "False-positive" chromatin granules resembling, yet not representing, masses of sex chromatin are found in up to 15% of cells of individuals having only one X chromosome.

Females Manifest Sex Chromosome Mosaicism.   In diploid somatic cells (and certain prenatal stages of oogenesis) all but one of the X chromosomes are almost completely inactive. This achieves *dosage compensation,* meaning that gene products encoded by the X chromosome are produced in equal amounts in the two sexes.

In the somatic cells of a normal female, the maternally and paternally derived X chromosomes have a more or less equal chance of becoming inactive sex chromatin. Random inactivation occurs during early embryonic life, probably around the early blastocyst stage of development. Thereafter it is fixed, so that once an X chromosome has become inactivated in any given cell, it is this X chromosome that is perpetuated as the sex chromatin in all the descendants of that cell.

Use of an Enzymatic Marker Expressed After Inactivation of an X Chromosome Can Establish Whether a Cell Population Is of Clonal Origin.   The repeating pattern of sex chromatin inheritance found in somatic cells that have undergone inactivation of an X chromosome also furnishes a convenient marker suitable for investigating whether a given cell population is *clonal,* meaning derived from a single cell. The marker most widely used for human cells is an enzyme called *glucose-6-phosphate dehydrogenase (G-6-PD),* the gene for which resides on the X chromosome. This gene exists in alternate forms (*alleles*) that code for slightly different electrophoretic variants of the same enzyme; the two most common variants are designated the A and B forms of the enzyme. As a consequence of inactivation of one of the X chromosomes, any given cell of a female who is *heterozygous* for this particular enzyme (Gr. *heteros,* other; denoting a female who possesses not just the one allele but its counterpart as well) will consistently express one allele or the other, but not both. Thus any given population of her cells that exclusively produces the A form of the enzyme must have arisen from a single cell that also produced this particular isoenzyme, and any population producing only the B form must likewise represent clonal descendants of a single cell that expressed the allele for the B form. On the other hand, a mixed cell population that synthesizes both forms of the enzyme cannot possibly represent the clonal progeny of a single cell. Utilization of G-6-PD to detect clonal populations has provided substantial evidence that certain leukemias and other myeloproliferative disorders develop clonally; in other words, the altered cells represent the progeny of a single changed cell.

Hence normal females are *mosaic* with respect to their sex chromatin. Chromosomally normal females are made up of two different kinds of cell populations existing as two admixed groups, one population expressing the maternal X and the other expressing the paternal X chromosome.

This mosaicism of females with respect to their two X chromosomes has certain implications regarding the expression of X-linked traits. The coat color of cats and mice, for example, is determined by their X chromosome, and the mottled coat color of heterozygous female tortoiseshell cats (and mice) bears witness to underlying mosaicism for this trait. Similarly, the internal surface of the back of the eye (the *ocular fundus*), as seen through an ophthalmoscope, can present a speckled appearance in women who are heterozygous for the sex-linked condition *ocular albinism* (lack of melanin pigment in the eye). An example of body-wide manifestation of X chromosome mosaicism is seen in the sex-linked dominant disorder *familial ectodermal dysplasia*, the congenital underdevelopment of ectodermal (and associated) derivatives (from the Gr. *dys*, disordered; and *plassein*, to form). A woman who is heterozygous for the *anhidrotic* form of this condition is unable to sweat from certain localized areas of her skin (*anhidrosis* meaning a deficient production of sweat). Failure to produce sweat is due to the inadequate development of sweat glands in such patches of skin. The mosaic nature of the disorder is emphasized by the finding that there is no correlation between the anhidrotic areas in sets of twin sisters manifesting this condition. Lastly, we should note that because certain chromosomal aberrations are associated with a *nonrandom* distribution of the inactivated X chromosome (presumably due to selection), they can result in full expression of X-linked disorders in women as well as men.

SELECTED REFERENCES

Cell Cycle and Cell Renewal

BASERGA R: The cell cycle. N Engl J Med 304:453, 1981

BASERGA R: Multiplication and Division in Mammalian Cells. The Biochemistry of Disease: A Series of Monographs, 6. New York, Marcel Dekker, 1976

BERTALANFFY FD, LAU C: Cell renewal. Int Rev Cytol 9:357, 1962

CAIRNIE AB, LALA PK, OSMOND DG (eds): Stem Cells of Renewing Cell Populations. New York, Academic Press, 1976

CLARKSON B, BASERGA R (eds): Control of Proliferation in Animal Cells. Cold Spring Harbor Conferences on Cell Proliferation, Vol. 1. Cold Spring Harbor, New York, Cold Spring Harbor Laboratory, 1974

GOSS RT: Turnover in cells and tissues. In Prescott DM, Goldstein L, McConkey E (eds): Advances in Cell Biology, Vol 1. New York, Appleton-Century-Crofts, 1970

HOWARD A, PELC SR: Synthesis of deoxyribonucleic acid in normal and irradiated cells and its relation to chromosome breakage. Heredity (Suppl) 6:261, 1953

LEBLOND CP, WALKER BE: Renewal of cell populations. Physiol Rev 30:255, 1956

MAZIA M: The cell cycle. Sci Am 230(1):54, 1974

POTTEN CS (ed): Stem Cells: Their Identification and Characterisation. Edinburgh, Churchill Livingstone, 1983

PRESCOTT DM: Reproduction of Eukaryotic Cells. New York, Academic Press, 1976

ROELS H: Hyperplasia versus atrophy—Regeneration versus repair. In Glynn LE (ed): Tissue Repair and Regeneration. Handbook of Inflammation, Vol 3, p 243. Amsterdam, Elsevier/North-Holland Biomedical Press, 1981

STANNERS CP, TILL JE: DNA synthesis in individual L-strain mouse cells. Acta Biochem Biophys 37:406, 1960

Radioautography (Autoradiography)

KOPRIWA BM: A reliable standardized method for ultrastructural electron microscopic radioautography. Histochimie 37:1, 1973

KOPRIWA BM, LEBLOND CP: Improvements in the coating technique of radioautography. J Histochem Cytochem 10:269, 1962

LEBLOND CP, WARREN KB (eds): The Use of Radioautography in Investigating Protein Synthesis. New York, Academic Press, 1965

ROGERS AW: Techniques of Autoradiography, 3rd ed. Amsterdam, Elsevier, 1979

SALPETER MM, SZABO M: Sensitivity in electron microscopic autoradiography. I: Effect of radiation dose. J Histochem Cytochem 20:425, 1972

SCHULTZE B: Autoradiography at the Cellular Level. Physical Technics in Biological Research, Vol 3B. New York, Academic Press, 1969

WILLIAMS MA: Autoradiography and immunocytochemistry. In Glauert AM (ed): Practical Methods in Electron Microscopy, Vol 6, Part 1. Amsterdam, North Holland, 1978

WILLIAMS JR, VAN DEN BOSCH H: High resolution autoradiography with stripping film. J Histochem Cytochem 19:304, 1971

Mitosis

ALBERTS B, BRAY D, LEWIS J, et al: The cell nucleus. In Molecular Biology of the Cell, p 646. New York, Garland Publishing, 1983

BORGERS M, DEBRABANDER M (eds): Microtubules and Microtubule Inhibitors. Amsterdam, North Holland, 1975

BRINKLEY BR, STUBBLEFIELD E: Ultrastructure and interaction of the kinetochore and centriole in mitosis and meiosis. In Prescott DM, Goldstein L, McConkey E (eds): Advances in Cell Biology, Vol 1. New York, Appleton-Century-Crofts, 1970

EVANS HJ: Chromosome aberrations induced by ionizing radiations. Int Rev Cytol 13:221, 1962

FORER A: Actin filaments and birefringent spindle fibers during chromosome movements. In Goldman R, Pollard T, Rosenbaum J (eds): Cell Motility, Book C, Microtubules and Related Proteins. Cold Spring Harbor Conferences on Cell Proliferation, Vol 3, p 1273, 1976

FULTON C: Centrioles. In Reinert J, Ursprung H (eds): Origin and Continuity of Cell Organelles, Vol 2, p 170. New York, Springer-Verlag, 1971

INOUÉ S: Cell division and the mitotic spindle. J Cell Biol 91:131s, 1981

KIHLMAN BA: Molecular mechanisms of chromosome breakage and rejoining. Adv Cell Mol Biol 1:59, 1971

MARGOLIS RL, WILSON L, KEIFER BI: Mitotic mechanism based on intrinsic microtubule behaviour. Nature 272:450, 1978

MCINTOSH JR: Microtubule polarity and interaction in mitotic spindle function. In Schweiger HG (ed): International Cell Biology 1980–1981, p 359. Berlin, Springer-Verlag, 1981

MCINTOSH JR: Mitosis and the cytoskeleton. In Subtelny S, Green

PB (eds): Developmental Order: Its Origin and Regulation, p 77. New York, Alan R Liss, 1982

NIKLAS RB: Chromosome movement: Current models and experiments on living cells. In Inoué S, Stephens RE (eds): Molecules and Movement, Vol 30, p 97. Society for General Physiologists Series. New York, Raven Press, 1975

PICKETT–HEAPS JD, TIPPIT DH, PORTER KR: Rethinking mitosis. Cell 29:729, 1982

SCHROEDER TE: Dynamics of the contractile ring. In Inoué S, Stephens RE (eds): Molecules and Movement, Vol 30, p 305. Society for General Physiologists Series. New York, Raven Press, 1975

STEVENS HOOPER C: Use of colchicine for measurement of mitotic rate in the intestinal epithelium. Am J Anat 108:231, 1961

SZOLLOSI D: Cortical cytoplasmic filaments of cleaving eggs: A structural element corresponding to the contractile ring. J Cell Biol 44:192, 1970

WOLFF S: Chromosome aberrations. In Hollaender A (ed): Radiation Protection and Recovery. New York, Pergamon Press, 1960

Chromosome Identification and Chromosomal Anomalies

BRODSKY WV, URYVAEVA JV: Cell polyploidy: Its relation to tissue growth and function. Int Rev Cytol 50:275, 1977

CASPERSSON T, ZECH L (eds): Chromosome Identification—Technique and Applications in Biology and Medicine. Nobel Symposium 23 in Medicine and Natural Sciences, 1973

CASPERSSON T, ZECH L, JOHANSSON C, MODEST E: Identification of human chromosomes by DNA-binding fluorescent agents. Chromosome, 30:215, 1970

COMINGS DE: Chromosome organization. Postgrad Med J (Supp 2) 52:17, 1976

COMINGS DE: Mechanisms of chromosome banding and implications for chromosome structure. Annu Rev Genet 12:25, 1978

EMERY AEH (ed): Antenatal Diagnosis of Genetic Disease. Edinburgh, Churchill Livingstone, 1973

FRIEDMANN T: Prenatal diagnosis of genetic disease. Sci Am 225:34, November, 1971

HERMAN CJ, LAPHAM LW: Neuronal polyploidy and nuclear volumes in the cat central nervous system. Brain Res 15:35, 1969

KESSLER S, MOOS RH: Behavioral manifestations of chromosomal abnormalities. Hosp Pract 8:131, 1973

LAMPERT F: The chromosomal basis of sex determination. Int Rev Cytol 23:277, 1968

MARSDEN M, LAEMMLI UK: Metaphase chromosome structure: Evidence for a radial loop model. Cell 17:849, 1979

MCKUSICK V: The mapping of human chromosomes. Sci Am 224:104, April 1971

MCKUSICK VA, RUDDLE FH: The status of the gene map of the human chromosomes. Science 196:390, April, 1977

NOWELL PC, HUNGERFORD DA: A minute chromosome in human chronic granulocytic leukemia. Science 132:1197, 1960

OHNO S: Major Sex Determining Genes. Berlin, Springer-Verlag, 1979

Paris Conference (1971), Supplement (1975): Standardization in human cytogenetics. Birth Defects: Original Article Series, XI: 9, 1975. The National Foundation, New York (Also in: Cytogenet. Cell Genet 15:201, 1975)

SCHENDL W: Banding patterns on chromosomes. Int Rev Cytol (Suppl) 4:237, 1974

SUMNER AT: The nature and mechanisms of chromosome banding. Cancer Genetics and Cytogenetics 6:59, 1982

THERMAN E: Human Chromosomes. Structure, Behaviour, Effects. New York, Springer-Verlag, 1980

THOMPSON JS, THOMPSON MW: Genetics in Medicine, 3rd ed. WB Saunders, 1980

VALENTINE GH: The Chromosome Disorders. An Introduction for Clinicians, 3rd ed. Philadelphia, JB Lippincott, 1975.

Sex Chromatin

BARR ML: The significance of the sex chromatin. Int Rev Cytol 19:35, 1966

KLINE AH, SIDBURY JB, RICHTER CP: The occurrence of ectodermal dysplasia and corneal dysplasia in one family. J Pediatr 55:355, 1959

LYON MF: Gene action on the X-chromosome of the mouse. Nature 190:372, 1961

MOORE KL (ed): The Sex Chromatin. Philadelphia, WB Saunders, 1966

4

The Cytoplasm

The various specialized functions of the interphase cell are carried out by its *cytoplasm*, which is the part of the cell designed to perform most of its principal metabolic activities. The energy required for such activities is derived mainly from the oxidation of foodstuffs in the cytoplasm. Hence cells must always have access to (1) oxygen for oxidative metabolism, (2) nutrients that can yield energy, and (3) chemical building blocks that can support cell growth and maintenance and the synthesis of secretory products. To carry out a broad range of different functions, the cytoplasm is equipped with several different kinds of *cytoplasmic organelles,* specialized intracellular structures that, like body organs, are designed to perform specific tasks. These intracellular structures lie in a *cytoplasmic matrix,* also known as the *cytosol.* The third major component of the cytoplasm is a complex system of interconnected skeletal elements (microtubules and various types of filaments), collectively known as the *cytoskeleton,* that internally supports the cytoplasm as a whole.

Cellular Membranes and Their Functional Significance. Metabolic reactions would be unable to proceed in an orderly and efficient manner if all the enzymes and substrates in the cell were allowed to intermingle freely with each other. Furthermore, many of the resulting reactions would be inappropriate to the needs of the cell and some would doubtless be harmful. Intracellular membranes are therefore incorporated into the cytoplasm in such a way as to subdivide it into discrete *cytoplasmic compartments.* The components within any given compartment are able to interact with one another, but they remain segregated from other constituents of the cytoplasm. The cell membrane (plasmalemma) likewise segregates the cytoplasm from the external environment of the cell, and the nuclear envelope segregates the nuclear contents from the surrounding cytoplasm. Cytoplasmic membranes also segregate the cell's secretory products from the rest of the cytoplasm.

In many instances, the marked efficiency with which enzyme–substrate interactions occur within the cell is due to the fact that the enzyme is incorporated into a membrane as an integral part of the membrane structure. It therefore comes as no surprise that a substantial number of cytoplasmic organelles have walls that are membranous. Classed as *membranous organelles,* to set them apart from *nonmembranous organelles* and *cytoplasmic inclusions,* these organelles are listed in Table 4-1. The *nonmembranous organelles,* which possess no bounding membrane of their own and lie surrounded by cytosol or associated with other membranes, will be described after we have dealt with the membranous organelles. Other materials that may be present in the cytoplasm, but that are not considered an essential part of the cell's metabolic equipment or physical makeup, include stored foodstuffs and pigments of various kinds. Classed as *cytoplasmic inclusions,* these substances will be dealt with at the end of this chapter.

CYTOPLASMIC MATRIX

The terms *cytoplasmic matrix* and *cytosol* are both commonly used to describe the *nonorganelle component of cytoplasm* occupying the intracellular spaces between organelles and inclusions. This part of the cytoplasm contains many soluble proteins, including the proteins from which organelles are assembled and the soluble enzymes involved in intermediary metabolism. Also contained in the cytosol are the substrates and products of many different enzymatic reactions. Small molecules and ions that increase the efficiency of certain metabolic reactions and contribute to the unique intracellular environment of cells are additional important constituents of the cytosol.

The more or less featureless appearance of this component as seen in conventionally stained electron microscope (EM) sections, as well as extensive use of the term *cytosol,* has tended to convey the idea that this component is the liquid part of the cytoplasm and, moreover, has given rise to the widespread impression that it is unstructured as well as fluid. However, there is a dearth of evidence to substantiate this view, particularly at the molecular level, and

Table 4-1   Components of the Cell Cytoplasm

Cytoplasmic Organelles

A. *Membranous organelles*
Cell membrane or plasmalemma (including the cell coat and microvilli)
Mitochondria
Rough-surfaced endoplasmic reticulum (rER)
Golgi apparatus
Secretory vesicles (granules)
Lysosomes
Coated vesicles
Endosomes
Peroxisomes
Smooth-surfaced endoplasmic reticulum (sER)
B. *Nonmembranous organelles*
Ribosomes (free ribosomes and polysomes)
Microtubules
Centrioles ⎤ assembled
⎥ from
Cilia and flagella ⎦ microtubules
Filaments

Cytoplasmic Inclusions

A. *Stored foods*
Glycogen
Fat (lipid)
B. *Pigments* (occasionally present)
1. *Exogenous*
Carotene
Carbon particles
2. *Endogenous*
Hemoglobin
Hemosiderin
Bilirubin
Melanin
Lipofuscin (lipochrome pigment)

Other

Cytoplasmic matrix (cytosol)

several observations are actually at variance with it. First, organelles do not have a random distribution in the cytoplasm, as would be expected if the cytosol were fluid. Also, they behave as if they were held in position instead of being freely suspended in the cytosol. Next, the improved resolution and increased depth of field attained with the high-voltage EM have disclosed the presence of a so-called *microtrabecular lattice* in the cytoplasmic matrix of whole tissue culture cells (Wolosewick and Porter).

Initial misgivings that this lattice might represent some kind of preparation artifact (*e.g.,* aggregated soluble protein) became less of a concern after its presence was consistently demonstrated in cells prepared by critical-point drying, a technique that counteracts the usual tendency of the cytoplasm to collapse as a result of surface-tension forces. Furthermore, it soon became evident that this lattice is seen just as clearly in unfixed cells prepared by freeze-drying or freeze-substitution as in fixed cells submitted to conventional fixation with glutaraldehyde followed by postfixation with osmic acid. The further observation that its microtrabeculae are readily extracted by nonionic detergents under conditions known to stabilize the cytoskeletal elements of the cell indicates that their protein composition is unrelated to that of the cytoskeleton (Porter and Tucker).

The interconnected microtrabeculae, which are roughly 6 nm thick, constitute an apparently contractile three-dimensional network that is presumed to represent part of the gel structure of the matrix. This network is thought to be involved in holding organelles in position and also in redistributing them through the cytoplasmic ground substance (matrix). Its discovery strongly suggests that the cytoplasmic matrix does indeed have its own characteristic and dynamic internal conformation. Even the soluble unpolymerized constituents of the cytosol that presumably occupy the interstices of the microtrabecular lattice may be linked or bound to it in some way. Enzymes, for example, could be held in an appropriate position for efficient processing of their substrates, mimicking the way enzymes are oriented in membranes. Hence there are reasons to believe that constraints exist on the movement of almost everything in the cytoplasm, and the notion of the cytoplasmic matrix being (1) an unstructured and homogeneous intracellular supernatant composed of freely diffusing molecules, or (2) the exclusively fluid part of the cytoplasm in which the organelles are freely suspended is no longer tenable.

CELL MEMBRANE

The *cell membrane, plasma membrane,* or *plasmalemma* is the outer membrane of the cell. Contrary to what might be shown by most diagrams, cross sections of this membrane cannot be distinguished with the light microscope (LM) because the membrane is only 8 nm to 10 nm thick, which is well below the limit of resolution of the LM. However, in hematoxylin and eosin (H & E) sections, some pink color can sometimes be observed where a "sandwich" of two contiguous cell membranes follows an oblique course with respect to the plane of section. Seen through the entire depth of section, such a slanting expanse of cell membrane may manifest enough stained protein to give a general impression of its position (see Plate 1-1C).

The Cell Membrane Appears to Be Trilaminar in the EM.
As is the case with any membrane observed in an EM section, the cell membrane is seen distinctly only where it has been cut in a perpendicular plane, as in the EM sections shown in Figures 4-1 and 4-2. In micrographs that have been taken at low magnification, the membrane is seen as a single electron-dense line. However, with the better resolution obtained at higher magnifications, it has a characteristic *trilaminar* (three-layered) appearance, il-

lustrated in Figures 4-1, *top,* and 4-2. This pattern of staining is also often described as a *unit membrane* because it corresponds to the repeating unit seen in myelin, the membrane-derived fatty insulation surrounding nerve fibers that was initially used for EM studies of the cell membrane. Again, it should be emphasized that only a true transverse section of the membrane will show this classic unit-membrane appearance. Oblique sections provide such an indistinct image that, in most cases, the membrane will not be recognized. This is worth remembering when a membrane cannot be seen where one was expected, because it could, in fact, be there, but its presence may be virtually impossible to discern because of an unfavorable plane of section. This is just as true for the intracellular membranes, which exhibit a similar trilaminar appearance in high-resolution micrographs and are believed to be fundamentally similar to the cell membrane in general molecular organization. There are, however, some differences between the external and internal membranes of the cell. Thus the internal membranes are almost imperceptibly thinner (roughly 7 nm across), and each has its own particular molecular composition and characteristic enzyme complement appropriate to the needs of the organelle to which it belongs. Also, the cell membrane is different from the other membranes in the cell in that it possesses a unique outer region made up entirely of carbohydrate chains. This part of the cell membrane constitutes an external coating, known as the *cell coat* or *glycocalyx* (Gr. *glykys*, sweet; *kalyx*, cup of a flower), and is evident in Figures 4-1, *top,* and 4-2.

The Constructional Basis of the Cell Membrane Is a Lipid Bilayer. Much of our current knowledge about the molecular composition of the cell membrane was surmised from investigations of its manifold functional attributes. An early discovery that threw some light on the matter was the observation that living cells underwent marked volume changes whenever they were immersed in a solution of different osmotic strength, because this indicated that they were each enclosed by a membrane that had differential permeability characteristics. Further work revealed that their covering membrane was not directly permeable to macromolecular substances in aqueous solution and showed that their osmotic uptake of water was due to a relatively high content of cytoplasmic proteins. A subsequent key observation was that lipid-soluble substances had the capacity to permeate the cell membrane more rapidly than most water-soluble substances, a finding that led to the hypothesis that the cell membrane is partly lipid in nature. The electrical properties of this membrane also pointed to the presence of lipids, because it was found that in the living state, the cell membrane manifests a high impedance, in marked contrast to the cytoplasm. Furthermore, electrical measurements revealed a difference in potential across the cell membrane that could only be accounted for if this membrane possessed the capacity to regulate the transmembrane passage of ions. Direct evidence of the presence of lipids was eventually obtained as a result of studies in which an acetone extract of lipids prepared from erythrocytes (which possess a cell membrane but only negligible amounts of internal membranes) was floated on a water surface. This procedure yielded a monomolecular phospholipid film, the surface area of which turned out to be almost exactly twice the total area of cell

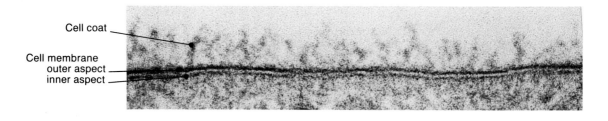

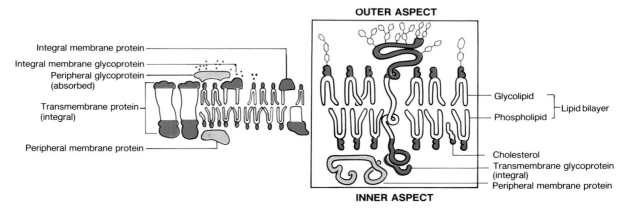

Fig. 4-1. Electron micrograph of the cell membrane (*top*) with a schematic diagram of its molecular organization (*bottom*). (*Micrograph*, courtesy of M. Weinstock)

membrane that was extracted. An inescapable conclusion now borne out by other evidence is that the lipid constituents of the cell membrane are arranged in the form of a *bimolecular layer* commonly referred to as a *lipid bilayer*.

The Molecular Structure of the Cell Membrane

Because it is well known that lipids are extremely osmiophilic, it might be thought that the two electron-dense lines characterizing the unit membrane (Fig. 4-1, *top*) would correspond fairly closely to the two phospholipid layers in the lipid bilayer. However, careful measurements have shown that this is not actually the case. Instead, it seems to be the charged (polar) groups on phospholipid and protein molecules, indicated in color in Figure 4-1, that bind EM stains. The interpretation is far from clear because it is known that only a single electron-dense line is obtained following very brief exposure to osmic acid, whereas more prolonged exposure results in the usual trilaminar pattern. After initial binding to the central lipid bilayer, the stain probably diffuses to sites where it is more permanently bound. Hence the trilaminar staining is essentially an artifact that should not be interpreted as corresponding in any precise way to the molecular structure of the cell membrane shown in the bottom part of Figure 4-1.

The *lipid bilayer* is made up of phospholipids and cholesterol (Fig. 4-1). These molecules are oriented with their nonpolar or *hydrophobic* portion (*i.e.*, the part that does not associate with water) in the central core of the membrane and their polar or *hydrophilic* region (*i.e.*, the part that associates with water) in contact with the aqueous phase at either the intracellular surface or the extracellular surface of the membrane (Fig. 4-1). The presence of cholesterol in the lipid bilayer is believed to have a stabilizing effect on the membrane and to increase its rigidity by enabling its phospholipid molecules to pack together more closely.

Cell Membrane Proteins Are Arranged in Two Different Ways. Charged water-soluble molecules and ions are unable to pass through a lipid bilayer, hence the need for *membrane proteins*, a second major constituent of the cell membrane that accounts for approximately half its weight. Therefore, an essential role played by some of these protein molecules is to furnish *transmembrane channels* for the passage of certain ions and molecules present in aqueous solution. According to the currently favored *fluid-mosaic* model put forward by Singer and Nicholson in the early 1970s, protein molecules are not arranged as any continuous layer in the cell membrane. Instead, the majority are able to drift independently in its lipid bilayer like icebergs drifting in the sea. Furthermore, the protein molecules are arranged in two different ways with respect to the lipid bilayer. Some extend all the way from one side of the cell membrane to the other. Such proteins constitute one type of *integral* or *intrinsic* membrane protein (Fig. 4-1), so called because disruptive treatment using a solvent or detergent is needed to extract these proteins from the membrane. The proteins that constitute the second group of cell membrane proteins are less firmly attached to the membrane

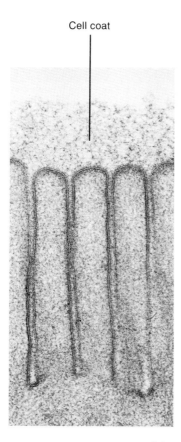

Cell coat

Fig. 4-2. Electron micrograph (×75,000) of the cell coat of an absorptive epithelial cell of the small intestine (cat). The cell surface projections seen below the cell coat are microvilli. (Courtesy of S. Ito)

and need only mild treatment with a salt solution of relatively low ionic strength before becoming dissociated from it. Such proteins can be bound to either aspect of the membrane and are generally held there by weak electrostatic forces. To denote their more peripheral position in the membrane, they are called *peripheral* or *extrinsic* membrane proteins (Fig. 4-1). Each molecule of integral membrane protein possesses at least one hydrophobic region that is intimately associated with the nonpolar hydrocarbon chains of phospholipid molecules situated in the core of the membrane. This charge-free portion of the molecule is shown free of blue color in Figure 4-1. Such a molecule also has hydrophilic regions that lie in intimate association with the polar regions of the phospholipid molecules. Polar regions are indicated in color in Figure 4-1. Some integral protein molecules are known to span the entire lipid bilayer, but others are situated in its inner or outer layer only (Fig. 4-1). Peripheral membrane protein molecules (Fig. 4-1) lack the nonpolar regions that would be necessary to anchor their central portion in the nonpolar central core of the lipid bilayer. Hence they are much more loosely bound through interactive forces between polar groups.

Some Integral Membrane Proteins Are Visible in the EM. Some of the integral membrane protein molecules that span the thickness of the cell membrane are of such substantial dimensions that with special preparative measures they can be visualized directly in the EM. They are most clearly demonstrated by a combination of two preparative techniques for transmission electron microscopy called *freeze-fracturing* and *freeze-etching.** The procedure involved is illustrated in Figure 4-3, and Figure 4-4 shows some typical results. As may be seen by comparing Figure 4-4A with Figure 4-3, *top*, freeze-fracturing discloses the presence of numerous globular *intramembranous particles*, 5 nm to 10 nm in diameter, embedded in the lipid bilayer of the cell membrane. Such particles are essentially missing after digestion with a proteolytic enzyme such as trypsin,

---

* *Freeze-Fracturing and Freeze-Etching.* In combination, these constitute a much used preparative procedure that has the capacity to reveal details of the interior of the membrane as well as its surface topography. A small tissue sample is rapidly frozen in a block of ice using liquid nitrogen and then is fractured against a knife edge (Fig. 4-3A). When the frozen tissue splits, the fracture commonly occurs transversely along the hydrophobic central plane of a cellular membrane (*i.e.*, between the two constituent layers of its lipid bilayer) (Fig. 4-3A). Such a fracture can split an intracellular membrane just as readily as the cell membrane. The next step is to apply a vacuum to the fractured tissue for a short period while it is still in the frozen state. This causes the superficial layer of ice to evaporate, leaving the intact membrane surface exposed as well (Fig. 4-3B). Removal of the layer of ice is referred to as etching, so the surface of the specimen exposed by evaporation is called its *etched surface* and the surface exposed by fracturing is called its *fractured surface* (Fig. 4-3, *top*).

A replica of the various surfaces thus exposed (*i.e.*, the fractured and etched surfaces of the specimen and the etched surface of the ice) is then prepared by depositing a thin film of heavy metal such as platinum and a reinforcing film of carbon on them. This is done in such a way that the vaporized metal is directed at an angle, so that a metal coating builds up on the near side of any high points in the replica (Fig. 4-3C). The far side remains almost free of platinum, and because the metal is applied at an angle, a shadow is produced that indicates the height and shape of any protrusions. However, in this case, the shadows are places where the layer of platinum is extremely thin or missing, so they are *less* electron dense than the remainder of the replica. Special printing in reverse contrast is necessary to convert the white (electron-lucent) shadows into the black ones that we are accustomed to seeing. This method of showing up surface topography in relief is termed *shadowing* (Fig. 4-3C). Before the specimen is examined in the EM, the tissue is digested away and the replica of its various surfaces (Fig. 4-3D) is washed and mounted on a grid. Fixation and embedding are not necessary, and relatively large expanses of membrane are readily observed.

As may be seen in Figure 4-4, the results can be quite striking. Figure 4-4A shows an erythrocyte prepared in this manner. Intramembranous particles, described in the text and indicated in the top part of Figure 4-3, are clearly seen in the face view of the fractured surface shown in Figure 4-4A. The three-dimensional appearance of the nerve fiber on the left in Figure 4-4B is due to the fracture plane passing through several different membranes. Shadowing shows the surface features of this replica to considerable advantage and provides a three-dimensional image in some ways comparable to that obtained with the SEM, except that, in this case, many of the surfaces seen are fractured surfaces.

(*Text continues on p. 80.*)

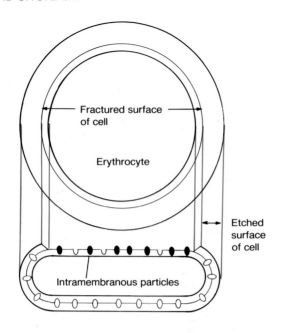

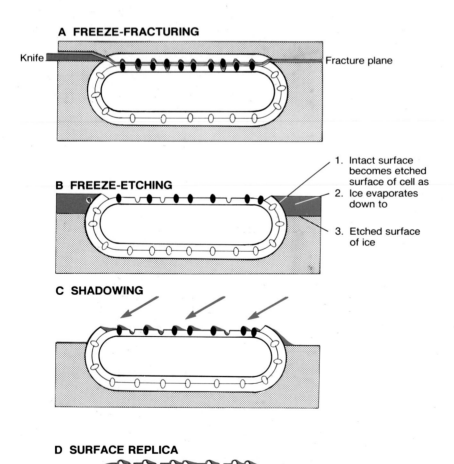

Fig. 4-3. Diagrams illustrating the procedure for preparing a freeze-fracture-etch replica of the cell membrane. The various surfaces of an erythrocyte that are exposed by this technique are indicated in the diagram at top. For details, see footnote on freeze-fracturing and freeze-etching.

Fig. 4-4. (*A*) Freeze-fracture-etch replica of the cell membrane of an erythrocyte. Note the intramembranous particles exposed in the fracture plane. The smooth surface seen between these particles represents the central plane of the lipid bilayer. (*Inset*) Part of the replica seen under higher magnification. This micrograph and inset should be compared with Figure 4-3, top. (*B*) Freeze-fracture-etch replica of a nerve fiber that lies in close association with the cell membrane of another cell, the cytoplasm of which is seen at bottom right. A second nerve fiber with two bulbous varicosities runs parallel to the freeze-fractured nerve fiber and can be seen on its right-hand side. However, this second nerve fiber lies *beneath* the expanse of cell membrane exposed in the fracture plane. Intramembranous particles are visible on the cytoplasmic and fractured surfaces of these cell membranes. (*A* and *inset*, courtesy of P. Seeman; *B*, courtesy of L. Arsenault)

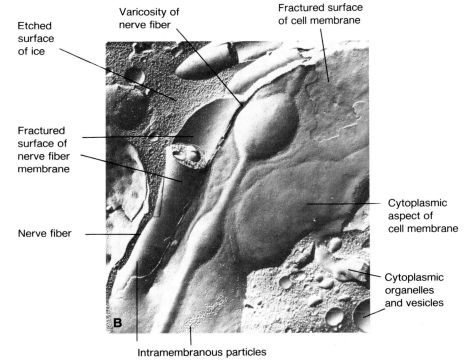

and, in general, the biochemical data relating to membrane composition and organization support the hypothesis that they correspond in some way to particles of integral membrane protein. In addition, biochemical studies show that some integral membrane proteins become labeled no matter whether it was the outer surface or the inner surface of the cell membrane that was exposed to the label. Hence it now seems probable that, in many cases, intramembranous particles represent integral membrane protein molecules (or aggregates of such molecules) that extend all the way across the membrane. Accordingly, such proteins are often referred to as *transmembrane proteins*. Some of these proteins enclose aqueous *transmembrane channels* through which certain ions and small molecules move into or out of the cell. Furthermore, a relatively large proportion of these proteins have oligosaccharide chains attached to their outward-facing end and are therefore really *transmembrane glycoproteins* (Fig. 4-1). Cell membrane enzymes and transport proteins responsible for facilitated or active transport through the cell membrane are believed to be transmembrane proteins or at least component parts of such proteins. There is some evidence that certain transmembrane proteins are indirectly anchored to cytoskeletal elements beneath the cell membrane.

The Cell Membrane Is Not a Symmetrical Structure. As can be seen in Figure 4-1, the molecular organization of the cell membrane is *asymmetrical*. Its marked asymmetry is partly due to the fact that the cell coat is present on the outer surface of the cell only. The cell coat consists primarily of oligosaccharide chains that are attached to the outer end of (1) the majority of outward-facing protein molecules and (2) some outward-facing lipid molecules in the cell membrane (Fig. 4-1). The molecules bearing these chains represent membrane *glycoproteins* and *glycolipids*, respectively. An additional factor rendering the lipid bilayer asymmetric is that its two constituent layers have substantially different lipid compositions. Also, different proteins can be present in the inner and outer parts of the membrane, and, in the case of cell membrane receptors, the region of the receptor molecule that actually interacts with the external signaling molecules has to be present on the outer surface of the cell membrane.

Occasionally, it is possible to observe asymmetry of the cell membrane directly in the EM, especially if one takes into consideration the presence of the cell coat (see Fig. 4-2). Even in cells with a less highly developed cell coat, it may be possible to see differences between the inner and outer electron-dense laminae. Thus in the surface cells of the epithelial lining of the urinary bladder, the outer part of the cell membrane is provided with densely staining plaques that give it an appearance that is different from the inner aspect of the membrane facing the cytoplasm.

The Cell Coat of Some Kinds of Cells Is Recognizable in the EM. The carbohydrate-containing outer region of the cell membrane generally is not prominent and is barely discernible in electron micrographs unless special staining has been used. There are, nevertheless, a few cell types in which it is highly developed. It can, for example, be seen to advantage on the apical surface of absorptive cells lining the small intestine (Fig. 4-2). The cell coat overlying this surface of the cells, which is covered with minute, fingerlike surface protrusions known as microvilli, is particularly thick because several of the enzymes required to complete the digestive process are so-called brush-border enzymes, which are cell-surface glycoproteins with branched oligosaccharide chains that extend up into the cell coat. This cell coat material appears as a fuzzy layer made up of fine, loosely meshed filaments of low electron density that correspond to such branched oligosaccharide chains (Figs. 4-1 and 4-2). In other cell types, it appears as a much thinner layer of similar fuzzy material (Fig. 4-1, *top*). Chemical studies indicate that the cell coat is largely made up of sialic acid–containing glycoproteins, including some that are adsorbed together with proteoglycans from the extracellular matrix. Many are integral membrane glycoproteins that are firmly anchored in the lipid bilayer of the cell membrane, as indicated in Figure 4-1. Their branched oligosaccharide chains, together with the part of the protein molecule to which they are attached, project out into the cell coat. The carbohydrate chains of cell membrane glycolipids also contribute to this material to some extent. Thus there is an intimate relationship between the cell coat and the remainder of the cell membrane. If the cell coat is enzymatically removed, the cell remains viable and regenerates a new one, but damage to any other part of the cell membrane generally results in cell death.

Experimental evidence indicates that the specific carbohydrate makeup of the exposed oligosaccharide chains in the cell coat confers a unique surface specificity on different types of cells, and this cell coat material is accordingly believed to play a key role in cell recognition during morphogenesis. Furthermore, one of the known ways by which foreign cells such as those of organ transplants are recognized and ultimately rejected as a result of immune responses is through specific recognition of foreign integral membrane glycoproteins on their cell surface.

The Cell Membrane Has Many Important Functions. As well as having antigenic specificity and a putative role in cell recognition, the cell membrane is the part of the cell that determines which constituents are able to enter or leave the cytoplasm. It is, for example, impermeable to macromolecules such as proteins and prevents their escape from the cytoplasm. Yet because it is permeable to many kinds of small molecules, dissolved gases, and ions, it permits the entry of nutrients, oxygen, and essential ions and, at the same time, allows carbon dioxide and other metabolic wastes to leave unhindered. Some of these substances cross the cell membrane by diffusing in a direction that depends solely on their concentration gradient. However, other constituents have to be transported *against* their concentration gradient, for which purpose the cell membrane is equipped with specific *active transport* mechanisms.

These transport mechanisms are active in the sense that the cell has to consume metabolic energy in order to transport the substance in the required direction. One of the best-known examples is the *sodium* (or *sodium–potassium*) *pump,* which is believed to be the specific function of a transmembrane protein in the cell membrane. It is actually a reciprocating mechanism that brings in potassium ions from outside the cell at the same time that it transfers sodium ions from the cell interior to the intercellular fluid. Other specific membrane transport proteins bring amino acids and glucose into the cell. There are also other ways of bringing external materials into the cytoplasm, which we shall consider in connection with lysosomes. We should also mention that in nerve cells and muscle cells, the cell membrane is adapted to conduct waves of depolarization.

Finally, of particular relevance to medicine is the role the cell membrane plays in receiving chemical messages from other cells. Such messages range from long-distance calls (*e.g., hormonal* signals) to direct communications from neighboring cells (*e.g., neurotransmitter* signals). The cell has the capacity to detect molecules of a given type in its immediate vicinity because some of its integral membrane proteins are specific recognition molecules called *cell-surface receptors.* The molecular configuration of a part of each cell-surface receptor enables it to interact specifically with molecules of one particular type. Many instances are now known in which such interaction brings about an immediate response or influences the course of action of the cell. During morphogenesis, for example, the receptors on the surface of different kinds of cells probably need to be involved in a continual exchange of information about the kinds of cells situated in their immediate environment. Now that it has been established that almost all body functions are hormonally regulated, it is quickly becoming evident that many kinds of diseases can be a direct result of the fact that responding cells have nonfunctional receptors or receptors with insufficient binding or internalization capacity for the cells to respond. Function can also be impaired if antibodies against cell-surface receptors are produced. Thus in myasthenia gravis, an autoimmune condition that leads to general weakening of the skeletal muscles, there is a loss of acetylcholine receptors in the muscle cell membranes at neuromuscular junctions (see Chap. 15). Receptors will be discussed again later in this chapter when we describe receptor-mediated endocytosis.

The Lipids in the Cell Membrane Behave As a Fluid. Experimental procedures whereby a cell from a given species can be induced to fuse with a cell from another species are now known. If such a fusion is brought about at body temperature, the cell membrane proteins that are characteristic of one species rapidly intermingle with their counterparts from another species, and as a consequence, it soon becomes impossible to tell which parts of the resulting hybrid cell surface were derived from each cell (Frye and Edidin). From this and from other observations made on living cells and artificial membranes, it is now evident that at body temperature, the phospholipid molecules in the lipid bilayer exist in a mobile liquid–crystal state, with the result that, to some extent, the lipid bilayer behaves as a *fluid.* The cholesterol molecules that are also present are nevertheless thought to impart a certain degree of stiffness to the lipid component. Some membrane protein particles are able to drift in the plane of the membrane whereas others are stationary. The proteins that remain fixed in position are believed to be anchored in some manner that restricts their lateral mobility in the cell membrane.

CELL FRACTIONATION

Ultrastructural investigation and radioautography at the EM level have done much to elucidate the detailed structure of the cell and to demonstrate which of its organelles participate in specific metabolic functions. More thorough characterization of the functional role of each type of organelle requires its isolation in sufficient quantity for biochemical analysis. An outline of the process of *cell fractionation,* through which this is achieved, appears in Figure 4-5.

In the first step, the cells are disrupted in a sucrose solution or some other medium that preserves organelles and prevents their aggregation. Some organelles remain intact, but cytoplasmic membranes break up into fragments that tend to form into rounded vesicles of variable dimensions. The cell homogenate is then submitted to a series of centrifugations of increasing velocity and duration, a procedure called *differential centrifugation.* Different organelles sediment at different speeds according to their size, density, and shape. The sediment is called a *pellet.* Large, dense structures such as nuclei sediment first, whereas smaller, less dense structures such as vesicles forming from the endoplasmic reticulum require higher speeds and longer times to sediment. Thus nuclei sediment at a relatively slow speed while cytoplasmic organelles remain suspended. Mitochondria and lysosomes sediment at somewhat higher speeds, and at sustained high speeds, even ribosomes will form a pellet. Such pellets can be examined in the EM to assess their degree of purity. All fractions remain contaminated, to some extent, with other organelles, but if sufficient purity has been obtained, the fractions can be submitted to biochemical analysis to determine the chemical composition and enzymatic activities of the organelles they contain.

In a somewhat different procedure called *density gradient centrifugation,* the homogenate is centrifuged through a series of sucrose solutions of different density. During centrifugation, each type of organelle becomes positioned at a level at which its density is equivalent to that of the suspending solution. Such a procedure can separate organelles that are similar in size but different in density.

Microsomes. In the early days of cell fractionation, before the morphological characteristics of the different organelles became known through electron microscopy, the term *microsome* (meaning a small body) was introduced to denote tiny structures that could be sedimented from cell homogenates by centrifugation. This has led to a misconception that there are organelles called microsomes in cells. It is now known that microsomes are mixtures of fragments of organelles that each have their own special name. Hence microsomes are not specific organelles even though this may be implied by those unfamiliar with the fine structure of the cytoplasm.

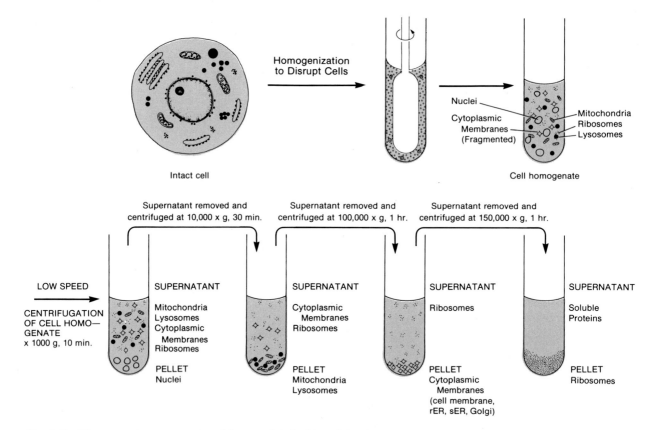

Fig. 4-5.   Diagrammatic representation of the steps involved in cell fractionation.

MITOCHONDRIA

Most of the energy required by the cell to sustain its various metabolic activities is released from nutrients through the process of intracellular oxidation. This oxidation process occurs in the cell's *mitochondria* (Gr. *mitos*, thread; *chondrion*, granule), membranous organelles that received their name because of their predominantly threadlike appearance in the LM (Fig. 4-6). Mitochondria house the chains of enzymes responsible for respiratory metabolism. These enzymes catalyze reactions that furnish the cell with most of its *adenosine triphosphate* (ATP), an important energy-rich compound that can yield its extra energy by transferring one of its energetic terminal phosphate groups to another molecule and thereby becoming adenosine diphosphate (ADP). Within mitochondria, another phosphate group is added to ADP, which thereupon regains its high-energy phosphoanhydride bonds and becomes ATP. Because mitochondria produce ATP and are responsible for providing most of the energy needed by the cell, they are often likened to the powerhouses of the cell.

Mitochondria are ovoid or elongated threadlike structures that are approximately 0.5 µm to 1 µm in diameter and roughly 5 µm to 10 µm in length. The number of mitochondria in cells differs in relation to their energy require-ments. Thus a small lymphocyte has only a few, whereas a hepatocyte possesses approximately 1000. It is common for most of the mitochondria to be situated close to the parts of the cell that have the highest energy requirements. Furthermore, under a phase-contrast microscope, it can be seen that in living cells growing *in vitro* (Fig. 4-6), the mitochondria are constantly moving and changing in shape.

In the EM it can be seen that mitochondria are bounded by *two* unit membranes (*i.e.*, an outer membrane and an inner one; shown in Fig. 4-7). These membranes are separated from each other by a narrow *intermembranous space*. Each mitochondrial membrane is about 7 nm thick and hence is slightly thinner than the cell membrane. The outer mitochondrial membrane is fairly permeable to most small molecules and ions; hence it permits their free passage into or out of the mitochondrion. The inner membrane, on the other hand, is highly selective with respect to its permeability. In addition to being virtually impermeable to ions, it can actively transport metabolites into or out of the central matrix-filled compartment of the organelle. Furthermore, it is characterized by a number of folds known as *cristae* that project like shelves into the interior of the organelle (Fig. 4-7). The number, size, and shape of mitochondrial cristae vary appreciably in different cell types. Thus in some cells, they extend about halfway across the interior, whereas

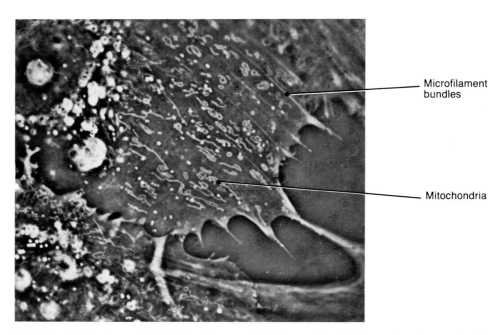

Microfilament bundles

Mitochondria

Fig. 4-6. Photomicrograph of a living hamster cell in tissue culture (oil immersion, phase contrast) showing its threadlike mitochondria. Microfilament bundles (which will be considered under Filaments) can also be distinguished. (Cormack DH, Ambrose EJ: J Royal Microscop Soc 81:11, 1962)

in muscle cells, most extend all the way across the organelle. The number of cristae seen in mitochondria is directly related to the energy requirements of cells. In some cell types the cristae are very numerous, and in certain cells they are tubular in form instead of shelflike. The interior of the mitochondrion is filled with a *mitochondrial matrix* of slightly higher electron density than the surrounding cytoplasm. Electron-dense *matrix granules,* interpreted as cation accumulations and consisting primarily of calcium phosphate, can sometimes be observed in this matrix (Fig. 4-7). The presence of matrix granules testifies to the marked capacity of mitochondria for accumulating calcium ions in their matrix, a property that helps to maintain a characteristically low level of calcium ions in the cytosol.

Mitochondria are renewed on a continuous basis throughout the cell cycle. In rat hepatocytes, for example, they are renewed in approximately 10 days. It is believed that this is achieved through fission, meaning that a partition develops across the middle of the mitochondrion, which can just be discerned on the right-hand side of Figure 4-8, and the two halves then separate along this partition.

Mitochondrial Structure Is Related to the Enzymatic and Electrochemical Activities That Bring About Oxidative Phosphorylation. Mammalian cells utilize an oxygen-independent pathway to degrade glucose as far as pyruvate (and in certain cases as far as lactate) within their cytosol. However, this anaerobic *glycolytic pathway* produces less ATP than *oxidative phosphorylation,* the oxygen-dependent (aerobic) pathway that normally comes into ef-

fect once pyruvate has been produced through glycolysis. The series of reactions that constitutes this second pathway occurs within mitochondria. Pyruvate is taken in through both membranes to the mitochondrial matrix, which is where the enzymes of the citric acid cycle (known also as the tricarboxylic or Krebs cycle) are situated. These enzymes catalyze a number of different reactions involved in the breakdown of the various end products of (1) glycolysis, (2) fatty acid metabolism, and (3) amino acid metabolism. Within the mitochondrial matrix, glycolytic end products are gradually oxidized to carbon dioxide by the enzymes of the citric acid cycle. During this process, there is a release of hydrogen atoms, some of which become transferred to nicotinamide adenine dinucleotide (NAD) and others to flavin adenine dinucleotide (FAD), coenzymes that are both derived from vitamins of the vitamin B complex. The electrons of the hydrogen are then passed along a series of respiratory enzymes called flavoproteins and cytochromes, and ultimately they combine with protons and oxygen to form water. The energy obtained from this transfer of electrons along a series of electron carriers is finally utilized to generate ATP from ADP and inorganic phosphate. Because the reactions involved in electron transport are closely coupled with those of phosphorylation, ATP is produced in an extremely efficient manner. Hence it is not surprising that the various enzymes involved in electron transport and oxidative phosphorylation are intimately associated with one another and form integrated *functional complexes* on the inner mitochondrial membrane and its cristae. The

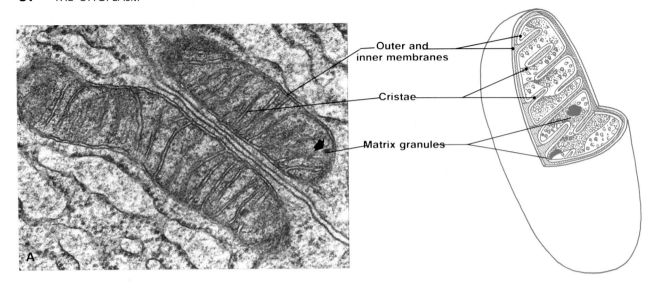

rER with
attached
ribosomes

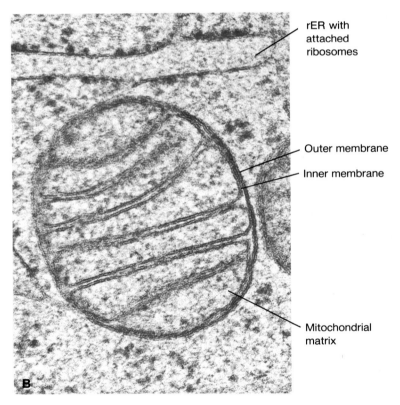

Outer membrane

Inner membrane

Mitochondrial
matrix

Fig. 4-7. (*A*) Electron micrograph (×86,000) and interpretive drawing of mitochondria in the tracheal epithelium of a rat. The arrow in the micrograph indicates a matrix granule in the mitochondrial matrix. The two parallel lines seen between the mitochondria represent the cell membranes of two contiguous cells separated by an intercellular gap. (*B*) Higher magnification electron micrograph of a mitochondrion in a Chinese hamster ovary cell prepared by freeze-substitution. This method preserves the unit-membrane appearance of the inner and outer mitochondrial membranes and also that of the rough-surfaced endoplasmic reticulum, a cisterna of which is seen at the top of the micrograph. (*A*, courtesy of M. Weinstock; *B*, courtesy of L. Arsenault)

ATP thus produced passes out through both mitochondrial membranes and is extensively employed by the remainder of the cell as an immediate source of metabolic energy.

If a preparation of mitochondrial cristae is immersed in a small pool of EM stain, it is possible to achieve a reverse form of EM staining known as *negative staining,* the ad-

vantage of which is that it discloses the surface features of structures *outlined* by the stain. Negative staining has demonstrated very clearly that the inner surface of the inner mitochondrial membrane is covered with tiny spherical projections that are 9 nm in diameter and are supported on narrow stalks. These projections are called *inner mem-*

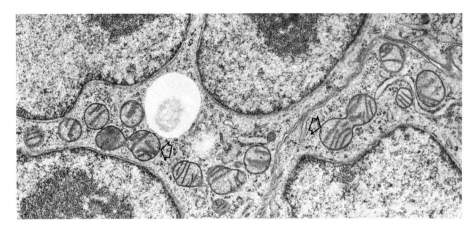

Fig. 4-8. Electron micrograph (×15,000) of adjacent cells containing mitochondria, two of which (*arrows*) have an appearance consistent with the process of division. The one on the right has a barely discernible, narrow, clear transverse band extending across its central constriction, lessening the likelihood of alternative interpretations. (Courtesy of L. Arsenault)

brane spheres or *elementary particles,* and they are believed to represent an enzyme known as F_1, which couples electron transport to the phosphorylation of ADP.

Thus there are fundamental differences in both structure and function between the two limiting membranes of the mitochondrion. The intermembranous space, too, has specific functions. Besides harboring several enzymes that are able to utilize the ATP produced in the mitochondrial matrix, this space is believed to provide a closed compartment into which protons can be pumped by the inner mitochondrial membrane. According to the *chemiosmotic hypothesis* advanced by Mitchell, the first application of electron transfer along the respiratory chain occurs when protons are pumped across the inner mitochondrial membrane from its inner to its outer aspect. This results in a proton gradient representing stored energy. The energy subsequently retrieved when the protons flow back in the reverse direction is utilized by ATP synthetase to phosphorylate ADP.

Mitochondria Appear to Be Descended from Aerobic Bacteria. With regard to the evolutionary origin of mitochondria, it is of considerable interest that these organelles contain both DNA and RNA. They also contain ribosomes that are slightly different from the other ribosomes of the cell. Thus mitochondria possess the basic requirements of an independent existence. Furthermore, it has been established that mitochondrial DNA, RNA, and ribosomes are all similar in form to their counterparts in bacteria. In addition, it is now evident that mitochondrial DNA directs the synthesis of some mitochondrial proteins. The genetic information coding for most mitochondrial proteins nevertheless resides in the cell nucleus, suggesting that mitochondrial genes have become integrated into the cell's own genome. The realization that mitochondria are semiauton-

omous organelles resembling bacteria has engendered the theory that they originated as aerobic bacteria that became incorporated into evolving animal cells, endowing them with a highly efficient means of extracting energy from foodstuffs through oxidative metabolism.

RIBOSOMES

Ribosomes are rounded ribonucleoprotein particles, 20 nm to 30 nm in diameter (Fig. 2-13), that are present in the cytoplasm both in an unbound state as free particles and also in a bound state, attached to the rough-surfaced endoplasmic reticulum (rER). These particles, which are composed entirely of rRNA and ribosomal proteins, are classified as *nonmembranous organelles* because they themselves possess no membranous component (see Table 4-1). Because unbound ribosomes are the simplest organelles that participate in protein synthesis, they will be described first.

Due to their small size, ribosomes are indistinguishable at the LM level. The color of the cytoplasm of cells seen in H & E sections can nevertheless give some impression of their relative abundance. Thus in cells that are actively synthesizing proteins, the cytoplasm is either tinged with blue or is definitely blue. Termed *cytoplasmic basophilia,* such staining is largely due to the strong affinity of rRNA for hematoxylin (the chemical basis of basophilic staining was discussed in Chap. 1 under Histological Staining). Basophilic components can be distributed diffusely through the cytoplasm, or they can be restricted to certain parts of it. Diffuse cytoplasmic basophilia generally indicates that there is an abundance of free ribosomes in the cytoplasm. Intense localized basophilia, on the other hand, generally indicates sites where there are regions of rER. However,

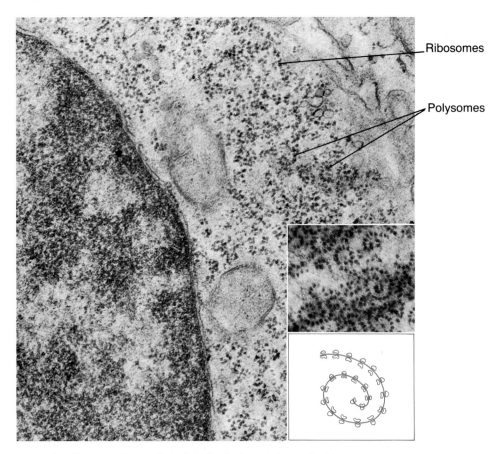

Ribosomes

Polysomes

Fig. 4-9. Electron micrograph (×40,000) of a basophilic erythroblast (rat) showing free ribosomes and polysomes in its cytoplasm. (*Insets*) Polysomes under higher magnification and interpretive diagram showing ribosomes attached to a molecule of mRNA. (*Large micrograph,* courtesy of A. Jézéquel; *upper inset,* courtesy of E. Yamada)

this is only a broad generalization because free ribosomes are almost always plentiful in the same regions as the rER, and the rER of some cells is so extensive that it renders all of the cytoplasm basophilic. Diffuse basophilia is often seen in rapidly proliferating cells, including embryonic and malignant cells. Because they need to synthesize cytoplasmic proteins very actively, such cells commonly possess enough free ribosomes to impart a diffuse basophilia to their cytoplasm. Diffuse cytoplasmic basophilia becomes quite noticeable in basophilic erythroblasts, which are erythrocytic precursors that actively synthesize the cytoplasmic protein hemoglobin. Thus after staining with a blood stain, the cytoplasm of basophilic erythroblasts appears as a uniform bluish color (see Plate 9-1*B*), and in the EM it can be seen that their cytoplasm contains an abundance of free ribosomes (Fig. 4-9).

The formation and subunit composition of ribosomes and also their functional importance have already been dealt with in Chapter 2 in connection with nucleolar genes and protein synthesis. Besides existing as separate entities, each of which is assembled from a large subunit and a small subunit (for details, see Lake), ribosomes can be strung together like beads on a string. Known as *polysomes* or *polyribosomes,* such strings of ribosomes represent transitory arrangements in which several ribosomes have become attached to a molecule of mRNA. In cases in which this mRNA molecule is relatively long, the polysome is fairly easy to recognize in the EM because its connecting strand of mRNA commonly forms a spiral (Fig. 4-9, *inset*).

The functional role of ribosomes is to provide the intracellular sites where amino acid molecules are linked together to form polypeptide chains as outlined in Chapter 2. The genetic information transcribed into each mRNA molecule is put into effect as this molecule progresses through the ribosome. After part of the molecule has passed through one ribosome, its leading 5′ end becomes attached to another ribosome that then begins to translate the same genetic information into a second and identical polypeptide chain. In this manner, a whole series of ribosomes can become attached to the same mRNA molecule, whereupon each of these ribosomes can assemble a polypeptide chain in the short time (approximately 30 seconds) it would take to synthesize only one. Because the number of ribosomes that can become attached to an mRNA molecule is a function of the length of this molecule, the number of ribosomes in a polysome provides a rough estimate of the relative length of the polypeptide chain that is being synthesized.

Whereas the ribosomes and polysomes that are involved in translating the mRNA molecules that are coding for cytoplasmic proteins lie free in the cytoplasm, those involved in translating mRNA molecules for secretory or lysosomal proteins are bound to the rER, which has a membranous component and is therefore classified as a membranous organelle.

ROUGH-SURFACED ENDOPLASMIC RETICULUM (rER)

Regions of the cytoplasm that exhibit an intense local basophilia are commonly sites that contain abundant *rough-surfaced endoplasmic reticulum* (rER). This membranous organelle is most prominent in cells that elaborate secretory proteins or glycoproteins. As an example, we shall describe the digestive enzyme-producing cells of the pancreas, which, because they are arranged in the form of spherical secretory units called *acini* (L. *acinus*, grape), are termed pancreatic *acinar cells*. In the middle of each acinus, there is a lumen that opens into a duct, but this lumen (Fig. 4-10) is seldom seen because of the plane of section. Secretory proteins are released by way of the luminal (apical) border of the cell into the lumen of the acinus (Fig. 4-11). The nucleus lies near the broad basal end of the cell, and the cytoplasm between the nucleus and the basal border of the cell characteristically contains an abundance of rER, which renders it intensely basophilic (Figs. 4-10 and 4-11). Other types of protein-secreting cells that possess a highly developed rER include fibroblasts (see Fig. 7-14) and osteoblasts (see Fig. 12-9), which are the cells that produce the organic intercellular substances of connective tissue and bone, respectively. Another example is the plasma cell (see Fig. 7-20), which synthesizes humoral antibody.

The Endoplasmic Reticulum Consists of Two Different Regions. In the early days of electron microscopy, before methods could be devised for preparing EM sections, Porter and his associates investigated the EM appearance of the attenuated marginal cytoplasm of cells grown in tissue culture. In such cells, they observed a lacelike network that appeared to consist of strands and vesicles and called it the *endoplasmic reticulum* (ER). The word *reticulum* indicated that these strands and vesicles were arranged in the form of a network (L. *rete*, net), and the word *endoplasmic* was used to denote that they were located within the cytoplasm (Gr. *endon*, within).

Later it became possible to study the endoplasmic reticulum in EM sections, whereupon it was found that this network is made up of ramifying, smooth-surfaced membranous *tubules* (the *smooth-surfaced endoplasmic reticulum*

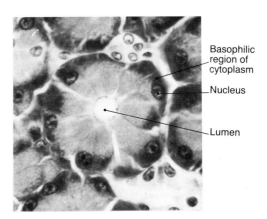

Fig. 4-10. Photomicrograph of a pancreatic acinus, showing cytoplasmic basophilia in the base of its acinar cells (H & E).

or sER) and comparatively large, parallel, flattened membranous sacs called *cisternae*, the limiting membrane of which is studded with ribosomes (Fig. 4-12). This ribosome-studded region of the endoplasmic reticulum is termed the *rough-surfaced endoplasmic reticulum* (rER). The content of its cisternae, which are interconnected with one another (see Fig. 2-3) and also with the sER, can appear slightly electron dense. The outer membrane of the nuclear envelope, which is also studded with ribosomes, is considered to be part of the rER, with which it lies in direct continuity (see Figs. 2-2, *inset*, and 2-3). The narrow cisternal lumen that is present between the inner membrane and outer membrane of the nuclear envelope accordingly is considered to be an extension of the lumen of the rER (Fig. 2-3).

Lysosomal Enzymes As Well As Secretory Proteins Are Segregated from the Remainder of the Cytoplasm. A certain amount of rER is required at some stage by virtually all kinds of cells, even those that are not secretory, for the synthesis and segregation of lysosomal enzymes. These enzymes possess hydrolase activity and are therefore potentially dangerous, so the cell segregates them from the remainder of its cytoplasm along with its secretory proteins. In contrast to the cytoplasmic proteins synthesized on free ribosomes, secretory proteins and lysosomal enzymes become segregated in the lumen of the rER during the course of being synthesized. Moreover, they remain segregated by cytoplasmic membranes until they are released from the cell or are utilized for some other purpose.

Most of the ribosomes bound to the rER are also components of polysomes. Ribosomes become attached to the *outer* surface of the rER membrane by way of their large subunit (Figs. 2-3 and 4-12), an orientation that gives them free access to the various constituents required for protein synthesis. Their growing polypeptide chain extends down a channel in the ribosome and then passes right through the rER membrane, entering the lumen of the rER (Fig. 4-12, *bottom*).

Lumen of acinus

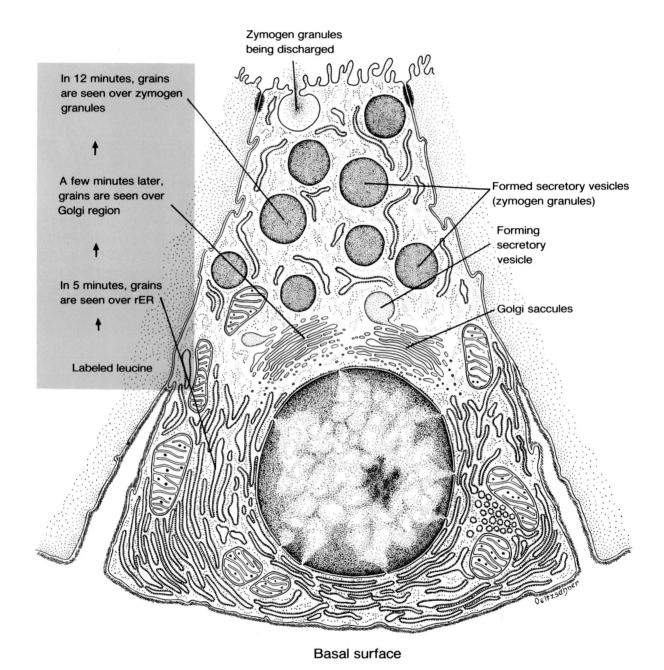

Zymogen granules
being discharged

In 12 minutes, grains
are seen over zymogen
granules

↑

A few minutes later,
grains are seen over
Golgi region

↑

In 5 minutes, grains
are seen over rER

↑

Labeled leucine

Formed secretory vesicles
(zymogen granules)

Forming
secretory
vesicle

Golgi saccules

Basal surface

Fig. 4-11. Diagram of an acinar cell of the pancreas, showing the sites where grains are seen in EM radioautographs prepared from samples of tissue taken at different times after injecting an animal with tritiated leucine. (Courtesy of C. P. Leblond)

A Signal Hypothesis Could Explain Why Ribosomes That Are Synthesizing Secretory or Lysosomal Proteins Are Selectively Bound to the rER. The question arises as to why, depending on which type of protein is being synthesized, certain polysomes become bound to the rER membrane while others remain free in the cytoplasm. According to the *signal hypothesis* proposed by Blobel and Sabatini, a theory that is now firmly supported by experimental evidence, initially all polysomes are free in the cytoplasmic matrix, but ribosomes engaged in the synthesis of those proteins that need to be segregated become attached to the rER membrane soon after protein synthesis begins. Attachment occurs because as soon as synthesis begins, every kind of protein molecule (or constituent polypeptide chain) destined to be segregated by the cell incorporates an initial *signal sequence* at its amino-terminal end. This initial sequence, which is 15 to 30 amino acid residues in length, is characterized by having hydrophilic amino acids at its beginning and end but hydrophobic amino acids in its middle. This is the same arrangement that is found in transmembrane proteins (see Fig. 4-1). This initial signal sequence provides the means whereby such protein molecules bind to receptors on the rER membrane (Fig. 4-12, stage 1), as explained in the following section.

There is evidence that binding of the signal sequence to the rER membrane is mediated by a *signal recognition protein* (or *polypeptide complex*) that is present in the cytosol (Walter and Blobel). Ribosomes that have begun to synthesize a polypeptide chain possessing a signal sequence are thought to become attached to the rER membrane by way of this signal recognition protein. Furthermore, when this recognition protein becomes associated with the signal sequence on the nascent polypeptide chain, it temporarily arrests translation and hence delays the synthesis of what might prove to be a harmful protein until this protein can be segregated from the cytosol. The rER membrane is believed to possess receptors for signal recognition protein that enable it to bind the appropriate ribosomes through bridging by this protein, and such binding enables suspended translation to resume. Two integral membrane glycoproteins of the rER membrane called *ribophorins* also participate in securing these ribosomes to the rER by binding to their large subunits. Thus the rER has one set of receptors capable of interacting indirectly with nascent polypeptide chains that possess a signal sequence and a second set of receptors capable of interacting directly with the ribosomes that are building up these chains.

A second important role of the initial signal sequence on the nascent protein molecule (or nascent constituent polypeptide chain) is that its characteristic distribution of hydrophilic and hydrophobic amino acid residues enables the protein molecule to become inserted into the rER membrane, whereupon the entire molecule crosses the membrane and enters the lumen of the rER (Fig. 4-12, stages 1 and 2). Its signal sequence is then removed by a signal peptidase that is present in the lumen of the rER (Fig. 4-12, stage 3). Loss of the signal sequence and accompanying conformational changes (Fig. 4-12, stage 4) make it impossible for such a molecule to escape from this membrane-bounded compartment by the reverse route, and the protein remains segregated by intracellular membranes until released or otherwise utilized by the cell.

The rER Is a Site of Incorporation of Integral Membrane Proteins and Membrane Lipids. It is thought that integral membrane protein and glycoprotein molecules are inserted into the rER membrane in the same way, except that instead of passing all the way through the membrane, they extend only partially through it. In the case of transmembrane protein molecules that are of considerable length, portions of the molecule may first extend into the lumen of the rER and then pass back out again before reentering it, weaving back and forth across the lipid bilayer of the membrane in a more complex configuration that has been likened to stitching. Membrane phospholipids and cholesterol are also incorporated in the rER.

The rER Is a Site of Modification of Segregated Proteins. Once the proteins synthesized by membrane-bound ribosomes of the rER have become segregated within the lumen of this organelle, certain modifications may occur in the protein molecule. Following removal of the signal sequence, the molecule may fold up because of the formation of S-S bonds (Fig. 4-12, stage 4), a configurational change that helps to keep segregation unidirectional. Also, glycoprotein precursors acquire the core sugars N-acetylglucosamine and mannose in the lumen of the rER.

From the rER, membrane-segregated proteins are delivered by means of small membranous transfer vesicles (intermediate vesicles) to the Golgi apparatus (Fig. 4-13), where they may undergo further chemical modification. The secretory proteins are then packaged into secretory vesicles (granules) and are delivered to the cell surface, from which they are released.

GOLGI APPARATUS

In 1898 the Italian neurologist Camillo Golgi, working with a microscope and little more than could be found in a poorly equipped kitchen, made an observation that started him on the road to sharing a Nobel prize many years later. He fixed some pieces of brain tissue in a bichromate solution, after which he impregnated the tissue with a silver salt. Under the microscope, he observed in the cell body of the tissue's nerve cells a network of darkly stained material that he described as the reticular apparatus of the cell. Although not always seen as a network, the same cytoplasmic organelle was later found to be present at some stage in virtually all cells of the body. Now known as the *Golgi apparatus* or *Golgi complex*, it is also often referred to simply as the *Golgi*. Considerable variation between different cell types has become evident in the position, shape, and relative size of this organelle. In cells with a markedly polarized secretory pathway (*e.g.*, acinar cells of the pancreas), the Golgi complex lies between the nucleus and the apical surface of the cell from which the secretion is released (Fig. 4-14). Component parts of the Golgi complex are more generally distributed in the cytoplasm of cells that have a less polarized secretory pathway.

A pale-staining area of cytoplasm is sometimes noticeable in H & E sections, generally near the nucleus of a cell. Termed a *negative Golgi image,* this lighter area indicates the site where the Golgi apparatus is present. It is seen to advantage in secretory cells such as osteoblasts (Fig. 4-15). This pale area is seen in actively secreting cells because the Golgi region lacks ribosomes, in marked contrast to the

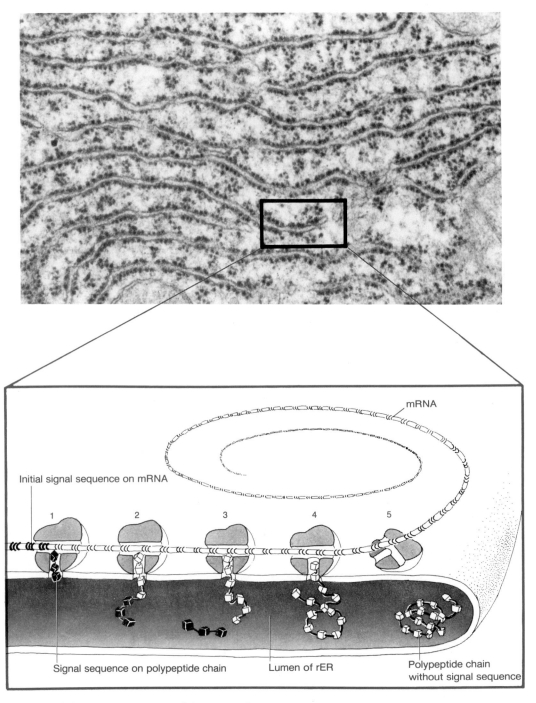

Fig. 4-12. Schematic representation of the process of protein synthesis being carried out by ribosomes bound to the rER, according to the signal hypothesis of Blobel and Sabatini. This series of diagrams depicts the main events that are taking place in the cisterna of rER indicated in the electron micrograph above. Five stages are shown in the binding of a ribosome, the synthesis of a polypeptide chain, and the segregation of this chain as a secretory product. See text for details. (*Micrograph,* Cardell R: Anat Rec 180:309, 1974)

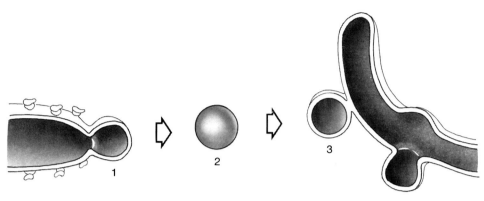

After budding from the rER (1), transfer
vesicles (2) fuse with the first Golgi
saccule (3)

Fig. 4-13. Schematic diagram showing the role of transfer vesicles in the delivery of membrane-segregated proteins from the rER to the Golgi apparatus.

cytoplasm surrounding it, which in secretory cells contains abundant rER and is therefore strongly basophilic.

The main structural unit of the Golgi apparatus is a flattened membranous vesicle described as a *Golgi saccule.* Shaped like a saucer, this saccule has a smooth-surfaced limiting membrane that does not bind ribosomes (Fig. 4-11). Golgi saccules are arranged in *Golgi stacks* that contain from three to ten saccules that are stacked like saucers (Figs. 4-16, 4-17, and 4-18). The saccules at the top and bottom of the stack are fenestrated, and in some kinds of cells, the windowlike perforations (fenestrae) in the bottom saccule are so extensive that it is more accurately described as a *network of anastomosing tubules.* The saccular contents have a relatively low electron density (Fig. 4-17A). Most cell types possess several stacks of Golgi saccules, and studies of rel-

atively thick (3 μm) sections under the high-voltage EM have clearly demonstrated that in some cell types, the saccules in each stack are interconnected with those of other stacks by a complex network of anastomosing tubules (Fig. 4-16). Hence individual Golgi stacks are not entirely independent even though they may seem to be isolated from one another in thin sections. Instead, they generally constitute part of an elaborate ramifying network termed the *Golgi complex.* Thus nerve cells possess multiple Golgi stacks that form an elaborate reticulated Golgi complex around the nucleus as first described by Golgi. Many other kinds of cells have a single Golgi network that is located on one side of the nucleus.

Each stack of saccules in the Golgi complex possesses (1) a forming face termed its *cis* (L., on this side of, near) *face* that is generally convex in shape, and (2) a maturing face termed its *trans* (L., beyond) *face* that is generally con-

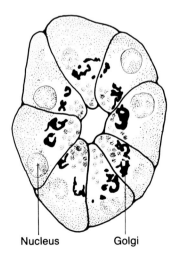

Fig. 4-14. Drawing of a pancreatic acinus specifically stained to demonstrate the position of the Golgi apparatus in pancreatic acinar cells.

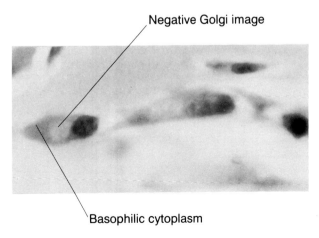

Negative Golgi image

Basophilic cytoplasm

Fig. 4-15. Photomicrograph of osteoblasts, showing a pale negative Golgi image in their basophilic cytoplasm (H & E).

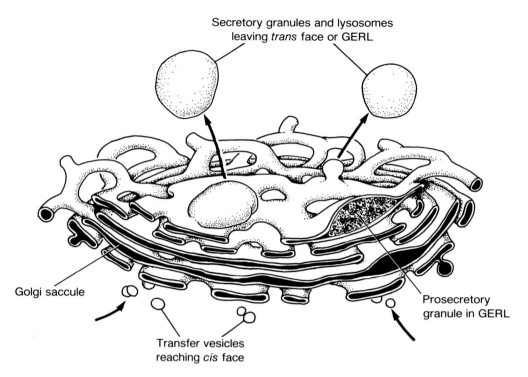

Secretory granules and lysosomes
leaving *trans* face or GERL

Golgi saccule

Transfer vesicles
reaching *cis* face

Prosecretory
granule in GERL

Fig. 4-16. Diagram of a Golgi stack and GERL, showing their relation to transfer vesicles, secretory granules, and lysosomes.

cave. As shown in Figure 4-16, the *cis* face at the bottom of the stack commonly has a number of small *transfer vesicles* associated with it. The *trans* face, on the other hand, is characterized by being associated with much larger *secretory vesicles*. In markedly polarized secretory cells (*e.g.,* pancreatic acinar cells), the *cis* face of the stack lies adjacent to the portion of rER that is situated in the base of the cell, and the *trans* face lies near the apical surface of the cell from which the secretion is released (Fig. 4-11). The Golgi is unable to synthesize proteins because its membrane lacks bound ribosomes; hence the proteins present in the Golgi membrane must be synthesized in the rER. Additional membrane is brought to the *cis* face of each Golgi stack by *transfer veiscles* (known also as *intermediate vesicles*) that bud from the rER and fuse with the lowermost saccule in the stack (Fig. 4-13). The *cis* face of the stack is accordingly often referred to as its forming face. While new membrane is being added to the *cis* face, older membrane is being removed from the *trans* face in the form of membranous walls of secretory vesicles and lysosomes (Fig. 4-16).

To counteract depletion of the membranous walls of saccules on the *trans* face as a result of formation of secretory vesicles and lysosomes, it has been suggested that saccules so depleted could be replaced by saccules moving up from below. As a compensatory measure, because the saccule on the *cis* face receives additional membrane from transfer vesicles, it might move up one level in the stack and a new saccule might start forming beneath it. Such ongoing replacement of the saccules would result in their steady

translocation from the *cis* to the *trans* face and could account for the steady turnover of Golgi membrane that has been found to occur in the Golgi stack.

A Major Role of the Golgi Apparatus Is to Modify Secretory Products. Proteins that enter the lumen of Golgi saccules have all been synthesized and segregated from the cytosol by the rER. Once transported to the Golgi apparatus in transfer vesicles, some of them then undergo further chemical modification. *Glycosylation* of glycoprotein molecules, for example, begins in the rER but is not completed until these molecules reach the Golgi apparatus. This is because only the Golgi membrane has the *glycosyltransferase* enzymes necessary to complete the process of incorporating sugars into the forming glycoprotein molecules.

The first direct experimental evidence that implicated the Golgi apparatus in this glycosylation process was obtained during a radioautographic study of mucus secretion in intestinal goblet cells. Leblond and his associates observed that tritiated glucose or tritiated galactose injected into an experimental animal rapidly became localized in the Golgi region of its goblet cells. Extending their observations to include other types of secretory cells as well, they subsequently observed that tritiated mannose became incorporated into secretory glycoproteins while such secretory products were still present in the lumen of the rER. Tritiated galactose, fucose, or sialic acid, on the other hand, were incorporated exclusively in the lumen of Golgi saccules. Thus core sugars (first N-acetylglucosamine, then mannose) are added in the rER, but terminal sugars (*e.g.,* sialic acid) are not added until glycoproteins reach the Golgi apparatus. This is the only intracellular site where carbohydrate side chains can be completed through the stepwise glycosyltransferase-mediated addition of specific sugars. Hence the saccules on the *trans* side of a Golgi stack have a higher carbohydrate content than the saccules on the *cis* side. The oligosaccharide chains of cell membrane glycoproteins that contribute to the cell coat are similarly built up by the glycosyltransferases in Golgi saccules before being transported by way of secretory vesicles and other kinds of vesicles to the cell surface. The oligosaccharide chains of cell membrane glycolipids are also thought to be completed in the Golgi.

A second type of chemical modification known to occur in Golgi saccules that was likewise discovered through the application of radioautography is the *sulfation* of secretory products. Radioautographic studies showed that radioactive sulfate administered *in vivo* rapidly became localized in the Golgi region of goblet cells and chondroblasts. As in the case of glycosyltransferases, the *sulfotransferase* enzymes responsible for the sulfation process appear to be integral membrane proteins of the Golgi membrane. Thus when the secretory product is a sulfated glycoprotein (*e.g.,* mucus) or a sulfated glycosaminoglycan (*e.g.,* chondroitin sulfate), sulfation of the secretory product takes place in the Golgi apparatus.

What Is the Route Taken by Segregated Products As They Pass Through the Golgi Apparatus? Besides modifying secretory products, the Golgi apparatus is able to sort out the various segregated proteins that enter its saccules, with the result that the secretory products of the cell become sequestered in secretory vesicles while its acid hydrolases become packaged into lysosomes. It is thought that this sorting-out process is brought about in a sequential manner as the segregated products move through the *cis* Golgi saccules toward the *trans* side of the Golgi stack.

There is an increasing amount of biochemical and histochemical evidence that suggests that the Golgi stack may contain as many as three different functional subcompartments. In the *cis* Golgi saccules, extra mannose residues are trimmed from oligosaccharide chains of glycoprotein precursor molecules that have been synthesized by the rER. N-Acetylglucosamine residues are then added in the more central saccules of the stack, which are sometimes referred to as the *medial* compartment of the Golgi. Lastly, the terminal sugars galactose and sialic acid are added in the *trans* Golgi compartment. Clearly, then, it is necessary for the glycoprotein precursor molecules to progress through the stack in a *cis* to *trans* direction. Yet the question of how they proceed from saccule to saccule is not resolved. There are essentially two possibilities.

In the first place, three-dimensional investigation of the elaborate Golgi complex present in Sertoli cells of the testis has established that it is made up of (1) sheetlike *saccular regions* that correspond to Golgi stacks and (2) tubular *intersaccular regions* consisting of anastomosing smooth-surfaced tubules that interconnect neighboring stacks of saccules (Rambourg et al). Furthermore, the saccules comprising the saccular regions are fenestrated at their periphery. The Golgi complex also possesses a *trans* tubular network and a tightly anastomosing *cis* tubular network that, for some inexplicable reason, is selectively osmiophilic in many kinds of cells. Saccular regions with associated anastomosing networks of tubules have also been demonstrated by means of negative staining in Golgi fractions of disrupted hepatocytes (Sturgess et al). The pattern of anastomosis in the tubules that constitute the intersaccular regions of the Golgi complex is elaborate. Besides interconnecting saccules that belong to adjacent stacks, it is likely that these anastomosing tubules provide a number of direct or indirect channels of communication between saccules situated at different levels within the same stack. Such parallel conduits could enable segregated proteins to pass either laterally from a given level in one stack to a more distal level in a different stack or distally from a given level in a stack to a more distal level in the same stack. The processing and sorting-out of segregated products that takes place in the Golgi apparatus could therefore depend on the progression of its luminal contents from one saccule to another, either as a result of lateral interchange between its component stacks or because of straightforward progression through the same stack. Any integral membrane proteins of the rER that are added to the Golgi membrane from transfer vesicles are thought to be returned to the rER by way of coated vesicles, many of which have been observed budding from Golgi saccules. Coated vesicles will be described later in this chapter in connection with receptor-mediated endocytosis.

The second way in which segregated products might be able to proceed from a given level to a different level in a Golgi stack, either in the same stack or in a different stack, is by *vesicular transport.* This could be brought about by coated vesicles or by transfer vesicles of some other description. Indeed, evidence has recently been obtained that a vesicular transport mechanism operates between Golgi stacks when these are maintained in a suitable cell-free system (Rothman). It may be that tubular transport through anastomosing intersaccular channels is restricted to those cell types that possess an elaborate Golgi complex and that vesicular transport operates in cell types that have a Golgi apparatus of simpler design. Or both mechanisms might operate in tandem, their respective contributions depending on local conditions or cell type. In any event, there is no evidence that the movement of secretory products from the *cis* to the *trans* face depends on the formation of new saccules at the *cis* face, and measurements of relative turnover rates indicate that Golgi membrane constituents move independently of segregated secretory products.

Cytochemical Staining Discloses Where Individual Golgi Enzymes Are Located. Histochemical EM studies

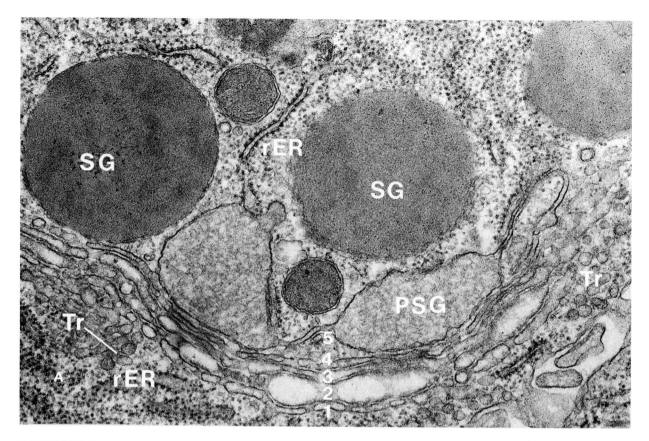

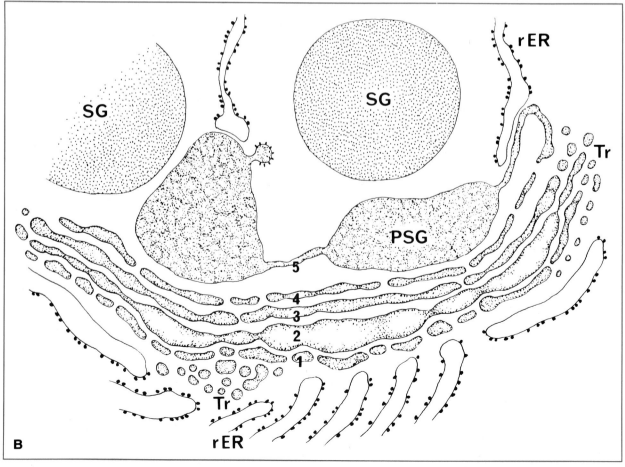

show very clearly that the different Golgi enzymes are located at different levels in the Golgi stack.

Specific phosphatases, for example, have been demonstrated by incubating extra-thick EM sections with an appropriate phosphate-yielding substrate in the presence of lead ions. Lead phosphate, the reaction product, is extremely electron dense and hence is readily identifiable in electron micrographs. Thus in Figure 4-18*B*, which shows a Golgi stack histochemically stained for nucleoside diphosphatase, the reaction product can be seen in the five saccules on the *trans* side (labeled *tGS*), but it is absent from the saccules on the *cis* side (*cGS*). Although the specific locations of many of the enzymes present in Golgi stacks have now been determined (see Table 4-2), the functional significance of this consistent pattern of localization remains to be elucidated. The markedly polarized distribution of these enzymes is believed to reflect the complex sequence of events whereby the various secretory products, lysosomal constituents, and membrane components of the cell are independently processed prior to leaving the Golgi apparatus.

Histochemical and biochemical indications that there is a strict functional compartmentalization within the Golgi stack are becoming increasingly difficult to reconcile with the earlier concept of a progressive *trans*-directed shift of the saccules comprising the stack. It seems unlikely that distinctive enzymatic distributions would be retained by the various subcompartments if their respective positions were to keep changing. Because a unique enzyme complement is evidently retained by each type of saccule, the idea that there is a vesicular transport mechanism to carry luminal contents from one saccule to another currently seems to be an attractive proposition. Such a mechanism would also enable membrane constituents to transfer from one saccule to another without the need for radical changes in membrane composition.

The Golgi Sorts and Packages Its Segregated Proteins into Two Distinct Intracellular Compartments. The proteins that reach the *cis* face of a Golgi stack following their synthesis and segregation by the rER include secretory proteins, glycoprotein precursors, and lysosomal hydrolases. A key function of the Golgi apparatus is to sort out the secretory products and to package them as *secretory granules*. At the same time, it manages to segregate the acid hydrolases and to sequester these in membranous organelles called *lysosomes*. Unlike secretory granules, lysosomes are mostly utilized by the cell for its own purposes.

In recent years, it has been determined that acid hydrolases become tagged with their own specific recognition marker, a molecular label that enables the cell to distinguish this particular class of enzymes from all its other proteins. It is now established that *mannose-6-phosphate* groups are generated in a terminal position on the oligosaccharide chains of all glycoprotein molecules that are destined for delivery to lysosomes. Furthermore, there are indications that the phosphorylation process required to generate the mannose-6-phosphate marker takes place within the *cis* compartment of the Golgi stack. It has been suggested that a receptor-mediated sorting process then delivers all molecules bearing the mannose-6-phosphate marker to the corresponding sites on the *trans* side of the stack that lysosomes will bud from. Immunocytochemical studies of secretory cells and absorptive cells have recently revealed that their intracellular receptors for mannose-6-phosphate are restricted to the saccules on the *cis* side of their Golgi stacks (see Table 4-2). This makes it seem likely that the sorting-out process by which lysosomal hydrolases are segregated from secretory products mainly involves the saccules on the *cis* side of the stack, not the saccules on the *trans* side as formerly assumed (Brown and Farquhar).

The validity and clinical importance of this so-called "postal code" hypothesis, namely that lysosomal enzyme molecules are each individually tagged with their own intracellular address label, are both clearly manifested in *I-cell disease*, a hereditary condition that is characterized by multiple lysosomal enzyme deficiencies and that results from a failure of acid hydrolases to acquire the mannose-6-phosphate marker necessary for directing them to the right destination. Because the lysosomal nature of these essential enzymes goes undetected, instead of being routed to lysosomes for internal use by the cell, they are exported along with its secretory proteins. The basis of this defect appears to be a deficiency in the phosphorylation of mannose. Indeed, it was by comparing cells from patients who had I-cell disease with cells from normal individuals that the existence of the mannose-6-phosphate recognition marker first came to light.

Fig. 4-17. (*A*) Electron micrograph (×37,500) of part of a secretory cell of rat parotid gland, showing a Golgi stack and adjacent organelles. (*B*) Diagram of the Golgi stack in *A*. Near the lower margin, the ends of associated cisternae of rER along the *cis* face of the stack may be seen; these ends lack ribosomes. Transfer vesicles (*Tr*) can be seen between the cisternae of rER and the *cis* face of the Golgi. The first Golgi saccule (*1*) is heavily fenestrated; the second is distended. The third and fourth are flattened, and the fourth is more fenestrated than either the second or the third. The fifth element (at the top of the stack) is the GERL. It extends along the *cis* face in a less regular manner than the Golgi saccules, and it is irregularly distended so as to form prosecretory granules (*PSG*). These eventually become released as secretory granules (*SG*). The regions of cisternae of rER that come into intimate contact with the GERL are also free of ribosomes. (*A*, courtesy of A. R. Hand, from Leblond CP, Bennet G: In Brinkley BR, Porter KR [eds]: International Cell Biology 1976–1977, p 326. New York, Rockefeller Press, 1977; *B*, courtesy of C. P. Leblond)

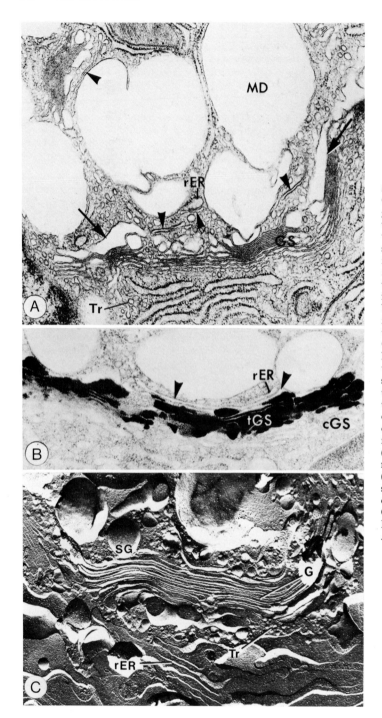

Fig. 4-18. (*A*) Electron micrograph (×20,000) of the Golgi–GERL region of a mucus-secreting cell (sublingual gland of rat). This highly developed Golgi stack is made up of nine Golgi saccules (*GS*). Large mucous secretory vesicles (*MD*) are associated with the *trans* face of the stack, and transfer vesicles (*Tr*) are associated with its *cis* face. The arrows at left and right indicate dilatations of *trans* Golgi saccules that are distended because they contain accumulating secretory product. The four arrowheads indicate the narrower GERL cisterna, which is bounded by a slightly thicker membrane and lies at some distance from the *trans* face, in close apposition to a cisterna of the rER (*labeled*). (*B*) Electron micrograph (×22,000) of a Golgi stack in a similar cell. This section has been reacted histochemically for the enzyme nucleoside diphosphatase, which is clearly confined to the five saccules on the *trans* side of the stack (*tGS*). The arrowheads indicate the GERL, the last element on the *trans* face, which does not contain this enzyme. A small cisterna of the rER (*labeled*) lies in close apposition to the GERL. Like the GERL, the saccules on the *cis* side of the stack (*cGS*) fail to react positively for this particular phosphatase. (*C*) Freeze-fracture replica (×16,000) of a Golgi stack, showing the general topography of the region illustrated in *A* and *B*. Transfer vesicles (*Tr*) are bringing secretory protein to the *cis* face of the stack from the rER, and secretory granules (*SG*) are budding from the *trans* face of the stack. (*A* and *B*, Hand AR, Oliver C: In Cantin M [ed]: Cell Biology of the Secretory Process, p 148. Basel, S Karger, 1984; *C*, courtesy of L. Arsenault)

The Golgi Apparatus Is the Main Center of Membrane Traffic Within the Cell. In recent years, it has also become evident that the Golgi apparatus plays a central role in directing and redirecting the various kinds of internal membrane traffic in the cell. Thus it serves as a major distribution center for newly synthesized membrane constituents such as integral membrane glycoproteins of the cell

membrane, and it redirects much of the recycled membrane that returns to it in the form of coated vesicles. As already mentioned, the turnover of Golgi membrane constituents does not depend on the *trans*-directed flow of secretory products passing through the Golgi. Integral membrane proteins, for example, have been found to turn over more slowly than secretory proteins. This difference in respective

Table 4-2   Some Representative Enzyme and Receptor Locations Within the Golgi Stack and GERL

A. Localized

Cis Side	Intermediate Saccules	*Trans* Side	GERL
Mannose-6-phosphate receptors	Nicotinamide adenine dinucleotide phosphatase	Acid phosphatase Thiamine pyrophosphatase Nucleoside diphosphatase Galactosyltransferase	Acid phosphatase Cytidine monophosphatase

B. Unlocalized

5′-Nucleotidase
Adenylate cyclase

turnover rates is not surprising because secretory proteins are synthesized *de novo*, but membrane proteins are reutilized extensively by the cell. Thus the Golgi apparatus is considered to be the main intracellular site where reusable constituents retrieved from redundant membrane are recycled along with membrane constituents that have been newly synthesized by the rER. The fact that Golgi saccules possess a number of enzymes capable of bringing about chemical modification has led to the additional suggestion that they may be able to repair or to modify such membrane constituents before these are reutilized.

The Golgi Apparatus Plays a Role in Both Lipoprotein Secretion and Prohormone Processing. Like secretory proteins and glycoproteins, secretory *lipoproteins* are packaged into secretory granules on the *trans* side of the Golgi. Saccules become distended with lipoprotein particles destined for secretion, as can be seen in the bottom half of Figure 19-17, which shows the cytoplasm of a hepatocyte engaged in the synthesis and secretion of plasma lipoproteins.

We should also mention that the Golgi apparatus is implicated in the intracellular processing of *peptide hormone precursors,* meaning that it participates in the production of the active form of these hormones, which is brought about by mild intracellular proteolysis. Two examples of peptide hormones that are derived from precursor molecules through such processing are parathyroid hormone and insulin.

The GERL

In certain cell types, most of which actively elaborate secretory products, the farthest element on the *trans* side of the Golgi stack possesses its own unique complement of phosphatases. The distinctive nature of this Golgi-associated structure was first brought to the attention of cell biologists by Novikoff, who devised the acronym *GERL* for it. The location and morphology of the GERL both indicate that it is closely related to the Golgi apparatus (*G* for Golgi). Also, it is known that (1) segregated proteins can enter the GERL lumen from Golgi saccules, and (2) prosecretory vesicles (granules) can develop from bulbous distensions that form at the perimeter of the GERL (Fig. 4-17). Furthermore, tubular connections have been traced between the GERL and the uppermost saccule in the Golgi stack, which is consistent with the idea that tubular channels may serve to deliver secretory products to the GERL from the Golgi saccules below. Alternatively, a vesicular transport mechanism could deliver segregated secretory products from the Golgi saccules to the GERL.

The *E* and the *R* in GERL denote that this structure is also intimately associated with cisternae of the rER. It is evident that ribosome-free regions of the rER membrane lie closely apposed to the GERL (Fig. 4-17), and some cisternae of the rER seem to project into its fenestrations. It was initially thought that cisternae of the rER might open directly into the GERL, but so far there is no definitive proof that such openings exist. Also, if there were any direct exchange of luminal contents between the rER and the GERL, it seems likely that such an exchange would be vesicle mediated instead of taking place through unregulated openings.

The *L* in GERL stands for lysosomes. The GERL contains acid phosphatase, an acid hydrolase present in lysosomes, and lysosomes commonly arise as bulbous distensions of the GERL in cells that possess this element in their Golgi stacks.

In some cell types, the GERL has the form of an anastomosing tubular network, whereas in others it is a relatively flat, fenestrated saccule with local dilatations (Figs. 4-17 and 4-18). Its limiting membrane appears slightly thickened when compared with that of the rER or Golgi (Fig. 4-18*A*). Also, the GERL may lie at some distance from the Golgi stack (Fig. 4-18*A*).

Neither the functional significance of the close association of the GERL with the rER and most distal *trans* Golgi saccule nor the precise role of the GERL in the production of lysosomes has been elucidated. It is conceivable that the GERL may provide a more direct route for certain enzymes synthesized in the rER to reach the sites from which lysosomes and secretory vesicles arise. Pres-

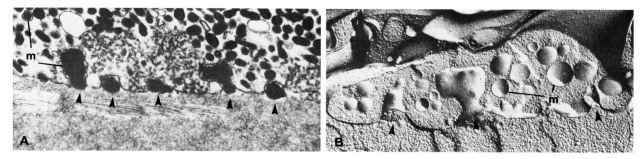

Fig. 4-19. (*A*) Electron micrograph (×21,000) of a neurosecretory axon terminal showing secretory granules being released by exocytosis. The limiting membranes (*m*) of secretory granules become part of the cell membrane as the granular contents are extruded (*arrowheads*). (*B*) Freeze-fracture replica (×28,000) of a similar neurosecretory axon. Limiting membranes (*m*) can be distinguished in some of the secretory granules, and the contents of three of the granules are in the process of being released by exocytosis (*arrowheads*). (Courtesy of L. Arsenault)

ent evidence indicates that when a GERL is present, it receives the luminal contents of Golgi saccules before these are delivered to secretory vesicles or lysosomes. Hence the GERL could represent a sort of mixing bowl or secondary sorting center for segregated enzymes reaching it from two distinct sources. However, it is still uncertain whether the GERL represents an integral part of either the Golgi apparatus or the rER, or whether it represents a separate compartment with its own distinct identity.

SECRETORY VESICLES (GRANULES)

When seen in LM sections, *secretory vesicles* have the appearance of granules because their protein content coagulates during fixation; hence they are more commonly referred to as *secretory granules.* Through convention it has become customary to refer to them as granules at the EM level as well, despite the fact that their content is not solid in the living state and that they are really *vesicles* bounded by a unit membrane (Fig. 4-19). The secretory proteins elaborated by actively secreting cells such as acinar cells of the pancreas are stored in a suitably concentrated condition as secretory granules that are ready to be discharged whenever needed. The comparatively large secretory granules in such cells attain a diameter of approximately 1.5 μm and are often described as *zymogen granules* because they contain enzymes, some in precursor form. It is sometimes possible to see zymogen granules quite clearly in H & E sections because they stain a vivid red due to their high protein concentration.

With the EM it is possible to recognize certain stages in the derivation of secretory granules. Thus the rims of saccules at the *trans* face of Golgi stacks and also the GERL (if present) can dilate locally to form *prosecretory granules* (Fig. 4-17), so called because they represent secretory granules at their earliest stage of formation before they have budded off as separate structures. Their content is less electron dense than that of secretory granules because it is still not completely condensed (Fig. 4-17*A*). Once prosecretory

granules bud off, their size may decrease as a result of extraction of fluid from their lumen. Hence the earliest free granules are sometimes referred to as *condensing vacuoles,* which is a potentially confusing term because *vacuole* (L. *vacuus,* empty) means a small *space* or *cavity,* whereas the structure is a membranous vesicle.

The mechanism by which secretory products are released at the cell surface is termed *exocytosis* (Gr. *ex,* out of or away from; *osis,* process). It involves fusion of the outer surface of the secretory vesicle with the inner (intracellular) surface of the cell membrane. The cell membrane then opens at the site of fusion, discharging the content of the vesicle to the exterior of the cell (Fig. 4-19). However, not all the vesicular structures that arise from the *trans* face of a Golgi stack or from the GERL are destined to discharge their contents by exocytosis at the cell surface. Some of these structures are lysosomes, which, as we shall see, have a very important role within the cell.

LYSOSOMES

Lysosomes are spherical membranous organelles, the diameters of which are so small (only 0.2 μm to 0.4 μm) that they are difficult to resolve in the LM. The number of lysosomes per cell varies substantially according to cell type. The most remarkable feature of this particular organelle, however, is that it contains a surprisingly large number of *acid hydrolases,* the enzymatic activities of which are maximal at the acid *p*H maintained in the lysosomal interior, a *p*H of approximately 5. This important group of enzymes is potentially capable of destroying virtually all the major macromolecular constituents of the cell; hence it has to be segregated from the remainder of the cell by the lysosomal membrane.

In contrast to the organelles thus far described, the LM provided no direct evidence for the existence of lysosomes. The existence of such organelles in the cytoplasm was first postulated in 1955 by de Duve from biochemical data. Shortly before that time, de Duve and his associates were examining the enzyme content of fractions separated from rat liver cell homogenates by differential centrifugation (Fig. 4-5). They were particularly interested in investigating the enzymes in the fractions that contained mitochondria. By refinements of the centrifugation procedures, they managed to obtain a fraction which, although similar to mitochondria in sedimentation characteristics, contained enzymes different from those of mitochondria. In this fraction, they unexpectedly found a number of hydrolytic enzymes, including acid phosphatase. They then performed biochemical experiments that led them to postulate that the hydrolytic enzymes would be contained in vesicles about 0.4 μm in diameter, and that each of these vesicles would be limited by a membrane that prevented the enzymes from reacting with substrates in the cytoplasm. Realizing that the little bodies in this fraction were not mitochondria but, instead, a new type of cytoplasmic organelle, they proposed the name *lysosome* for this organelle.

Identification of Lysosomes with the EM

Subsequently, the fractions containing acid phosphatase were examined in the EM. As was anticipated, lysosomes proved to be membranous organelles approximately 0.5 μm in diameter. Since that time, Novikoff and others have studied lysosomes in a great variety of cells by combining the histochemical test for acid phosphatase with electron microscopy.

Of the large number of hydrolases present in lysosomes (phosphatases, proteases, nucleases, lipases, phospholipases, glycosidases, and sulfatases), *acid phosphatase* remains the enzyme that is most readily detected histochemically. Lysosomes encountered in conventionally stained electron micrographs appear as in Figure 4-20*A*, in which their limiting unit membrane and glycoprotein-rich, moderately electron-dense content can be distinguished. The more electron-dense structures seen in their vicinity in this micrograph are secondary lysosomes, which will be described in the following sections.

The formation of lysosomes resembles that of secretory granules. Their various hydrolases, almost all of which are glycoproteins, are initially synthesized in the rER and then carried to the *cis* face of a Golgi stack by transfer vesicles. The Golgi stack then sorts them out from secretory products through a recognition process involving their mannose-6-phosphate marker, as explained earlier in this chapter in the section on the Golgi apparatus. On reaching the *trans* face of the stack, the hydrolytic enzymes enter bulbous dilatations of the periphery of its uppermost saccules or GERL, and these dilatations then bud off as lysosomes (Fig. 4-16).

Lysosomal hydrolases are utilized by the cell (1) to degrade any exogenous particulate matter or macromolecular constituents that it may have ingested from its immediate environment, and (2) to dispose of any macromolecular cellular constituents or organelles that are no longer useful to the cell. This is achieved in such a way that the lysosomal enzymes are generally prevented from leaking into the cytoplasmic matrix. However, in situations that cause a substantial drop in oxygen tension (*hypoxia*), these destructive enzymes can escape through the lysosomal membrane and then begin acting on the remainder of the cell. Once liberated from the cell itself, they may even start degrading other macromolecules in the general vicinity of the cell if conditions are acidic. Massive leakage of hydrolytic enzymes from lysosomes is the cause of *autolysis,* a commonly encountered form of postmortem degeneration that spoils the microscopic detail of histological sections.

To explain how the cell uses its intracellular hydrolases to digest any particulate matter it may have taken into its cytoplasm, it is now necessary to introduce some terms that are used to describe the various stages of uptake.

A lysosome that buds from the *trans* face or GERL saccule of a Golgi stack is termed a *primary lysosome* (Figs. 4-20 and 4-21, shown at *left*). The degradative enzymes segregated within primary lysosomes are used to dispose of exogenous materials, deteriorating organelles, and useless substances arising within the cell. Once a primary lysosome has fused with another vesicle containing material from any of these sources, the resulting vesicle (which, of course, contains the material to be digested as well as lysosomal enzymes) is referred to as a *secondary lysosome* (Figs. 4-20 and 4-21).

We shall next consider what happens when cells take up particles or macromolecular compounds from their surroundings.

The Cell Employs Its Lysosomal Hydrolases As an Internal Demolition System

In general, the only water-soluble substances that can permeate the cell membrane directly are those that are relatively low in molecular weight (below 400 daltons) and lack a high molecular charge. Compounds of higher molecular weight can nevertheless be brought into the cell through *endocytosis* (Gr. *endon,* within; *osis,* process), the general term for any process whereby the cell engulfs materials from its surroundings. When the material being ingested is some kind of particulate matter or macromolecular complex, the process is more often referred to as *phagocytosis* (Gr. *phagein,* to eat). *Pinocytosis* is a second form of endocytosis in which the material being engulfed is a small sample of the extracellular fluid (Gr. *pinein,* to drink).

Phagocytosis. In *phagocytosis,* the cell takes up particles or macromolecular aggregates from its surroundings as depicted at the top right of Figure 4-21. A particle that comes into contact with the cell surface is engulfed and surrounded on all sides by cell membrane, with the result that it becomes contained in a *phagocytic vesicle.* This membranous vesicle then detaches from the cell membrane and sinks deeper into the cytoplasm; it is referred to as a *phagosome* (Fig. 4-21).

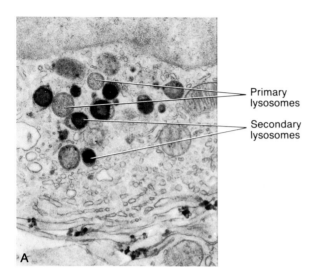

A

Primary
lysosomes

Secondary
lysosomes

Fig. 4-20. (*A*) Electron micrograph (×18,000) of primary and secondary lysosomes in a rat macrophage. The pale area seen at the top of the illustration is part of the nucleus. (*B*) Electron micrograph of a primary lysosome from a follicular cell of the thyroid. (*C*) Electron micrograph (×90,000) of a multivesicular body (the limiting membrane of which is indicated by the *arrow*). (*A*, courtesy of C. Nopajaroonsri and G. Simon; *B*, courtesy of C. P. Leblond; *C*, Friend DS, Farquhar MG: J Cell Biol 35:357, 1967)

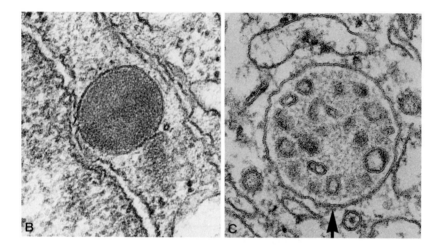

B

C

Invagination of the cell membrane during any form of endocytosis results in its *outer* half becoming the *inner* half of the vesicular membrane. The inner aspect of the portion of cell membrane that forms the membranous walls of the vesicle nevertheless continues to face the cytoplasmic matrix. Hence there is essentially *no change in orientation* of the cell membrane, and what might initially seem to be inside-out reversal of this membrane as a result of endocytosis is more apparent than real.

The fate of phagosomes and their contents is most clearly established in neutrophils, which are leukocytes that actively phagocytose bacteria when these infect the body. Once a phagosome enters the cytoplasm, it fuses with a primary lysosome and is thereafter referred to as a *secondary lysosome* (Fig. 4-21). Additional primary lysosomes can also fuse with the secondary lysosome, and several secondary lysosomes can coalesce with one another. The hydrolytic enzymes contributed by the primary lysosomes serve to degrade the engulfed material. Whatever remains following enzymatic digestion inside the secondary lysosome constitutes a *residual body* (Fig. 4-21). Residual bodies

may eventually be extruded from the cell by *exocytosis* (Fig. 4-21).

Lysosomes Are Directly Implicated in Certain Inflammatory Conditions. It is becoming increasingly evident that in addition to the role played by lysosomal enzymes in protecting the body from infectious bacteria, they themselves can exacerbate certain kinds of inflammatory lesions. Thus the liberation of acid hydrolases and other active constituents from the azurophil lysosomal granules of neutrophils is thought to be a contributing factor in the massive tissue destruction that characterizes purulent (pus-forming) inflammatory lesions. One way in which these constituents escape to the exterior of the cell is through premature leakage from phagocytic vesicles that have formed but have not yet had enough time to seal off completely, as depicted in Figure 4-21.

Another clinical problem that directly concerns lysosomes results from the chronic inhalation of *silica* particles and certain other kinds of dusts. In *silicosis*, silica particles are engulfed by lung macrophages, but they resist all attempts at enzymatic degradation because they are inorganic. Furthermore, they can damage the various membranes of the cell, including the membranous walls of secondary lysosomes and also the cell membrane. Destructive en-

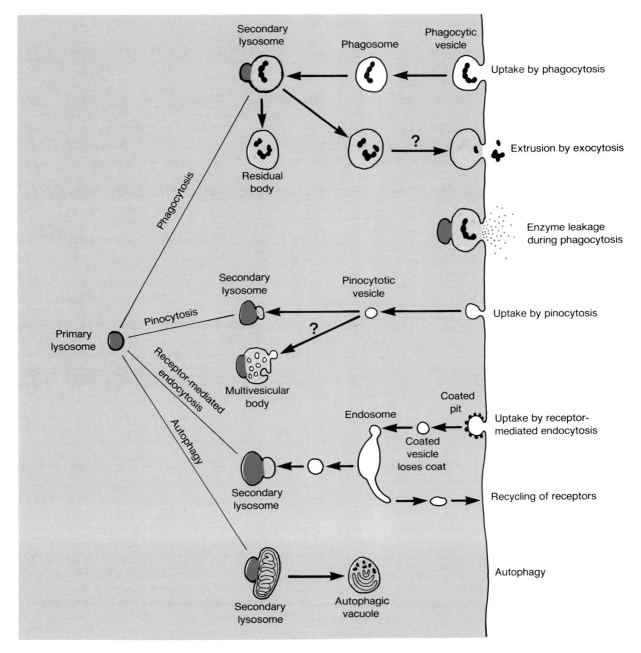

Fig. 4-21. Schematic representation of the various forms of participation of primary lysosomes in the intracellular disposal of ingested materials and obsolete organelles. For details, see text.

zymes leak from the secondary lysosomes into the cytoplasmic matrix and eventually reach the surrounding tissues as well. Resulting death of the macrophages that phagocytosed the silica particles leads to liberation of their ingested particles, which are then ingested by other macrophages in a futile and never-ending attempt to clear them from the lungs.

Lysosomes are also involved in the pathogenesis of *gout*, a condition in which crystals of monosodium urate become deposited in joint tissues. When neutrophils attempt to phagocytose these crystals, their lysosomal granular constituents are liberated in large enough amounts to elicit a painful acute inflammatory reaction that is commonly localized in the metatarsophalangeal joint of the great toe.

The fate of materials that enter the cell by *pinocytosis* (Fig. 4-21) is still unclear. There are indications that some become localized within structures known as *multivesicular bodies* (Figs. 4-20 and 4-21) that contain hydrolytic enzymes and are accordingly considered a type of secondary lysosome.

These two long-established forms of endocytosis are now known to be supplemented by a third form of endocytosis that is characterized by being highly specific because it is mediated by cell-surface receptors.

Receptor-Mediated Endocytosis. Cells are thought to obtain many of their necessary macromolecular substances through pinocytosis. However, such uptake is nonspecific and the amount brought into the cytoplasm depends on the concentration in the external medium. In some cases, macromolecular substances are taken up in a highly selective manner by a much less fortuitous mechanism called *receptor-mediated endocytosis.* The selectivity of this process is due to the possession of cell-surface *receptors* that pick up certain macromolecular substances whenever these substances become available in the cell's microenvironment. Substances that bind selectively to cell-surface receptors are termed *ligands* (L. *ligare,* to bind). Once bound to their specific receptors, ligands can be rapidly internalized by receptor-mediated endocytosis; their concentration in the external medium does not determine their rate of uptake. More than 20 different macromolecular compounds are now known that can enter cells by means of this more efficient form of endocytosis. Such compounds include various kinds of regulatory and signaling molecules as well as essential constituents that are required for cellular growth and function. In some cases, the receptors dissociate from the internalized ligand–receptor complexes, escape lysosomal degradation, and are reutilized for trapping more ligand. In other cases, both the receptor and the ligand are degraded, with the result that endocytosis leads to a net decrease in the number of surface receptors, a phenomenon known as *down-regulation.*

Coated Pits and Coated Vesicles. Almost all receptor-mediated endocytosis occurs at sites on the cell surface known as *coated pits,* which are shallow surface indentations where a fibrous protein called *clathrin* is intimately associated with the cytosol-facing aspect of the cell membrane (Figs. 4-22 and 4-23). It is thought that new coated pits are always being formed and that they then invaginate, with the result that, at any given moment, they occupy about 1% or 2% of the cell's total surface area. The clathrin-containing coating remains applied to the underside of the cell membrane during the process of invagination and pinches off so as to form a *coated vesicle* (Fig. 4-23), but it becomes detached before this vesicle fuses with a lysosome or any other membranous organelle.

In vitro studies indicate that this coating is a basketlike polygonal framework composed of pinwheel-shaped subunits termed *triskelions* that contain clathrin complexed with another protein of lower molecular weight. The unique three-pronged construction of its clathrin-containing subunits (illustrated in Fig. 4-23C) enables them to assemble spontaneously into a curved lattice made up of hexagons with some pentagons. The final outcome of assembly is the formation of a hollow spherical latticework that resembles a geodesic dome (Figs. 4-22 and 4-23). When pentagons are introduced into a hexagonal lattice, the initially planar lattice gradually becomes curved, its curvature increasing with the proportion of pentagons added. Thus what started out as a planar arrangement ultimately becomes transformed into a hollow closed sphere. Growth of the clathrin latticework, accompanied by the gradual incorporation of pentagons into its predominantly hexagonal arrangement, is therefore believed to facilitate the invagination and pinching off of vesicles of cell membrane during receptor-mediated endocytosis.

Clathrin-coated vesicles can also be seen budding from the rER, from Golgi saccules, and from secretory vesicles that are undergoing condensation (*i.e.,* condensing vacuoles). They have been found to participate in a number of different forms of intracellular transport, including the pathways by which (1) secretory proteins are transferred to Golgi saccules from the rER, (2) membrane constituents reach the cell membrane from the Golgi complex, (3) lysosomal enzymes gain access to lysosomes from Golgi saccules, and (4) immunoglobulins taken up at absorptive surfaces are transported across the cell to secretory surfaces. Because coated vesicles also participate in receptor-mediated endocytosis and recovery of excess membrane from secretory surfaces, they clearly represent a very heterogeneous class of membranous organelles. Hence it would appear that clathrin lattices are utilized to a marked degree to bring about the formation of membranous vesicles from cytoplasmic membranes. Coated vesicles formed in this manner play important roles both in delivering luminal contents from one membranous organelle to another and in conserving cytoplasmic membrane.

Low-Density Lipoproteins. Among the more important macromolecular compounds internalized through the mechanism of receptor-mediated endocytosis are the *low-density lipoproteins* (LDL), which represent an important source of the cholesterol needed for synthesis of most cellular membranes. Detailed studies in fibroblasts have shown that the amount of LDL internalized is a function of the proportion of surface LDL receptors that become intimately associated with coated pits (Goldstein et al.). Relevant here are the *genetic hyperlipoproteinemias,* a group of genetically distinct disorders of lipid metabolism characterized by elevated lipid and lipoprotein levels in the plasma. One such disorder clearly illustrates the clinical importance of the close association between LDL receptors and coated pits. Even though the total numbers and binding characteristics of the LDL receptors on cells of individuals expressing this particular defect seem normal, LDL is not internalized because these receptors lack an affinity for coated pits and therefore fail to become trapped there. Almost any kind of defect in LDL receptors or LDL metabolism creates a health hazard, because an individual's inability to remove LDL from the bloodstream at an adequate rate results in elevation of the plasma cholesterol levels, and this heightens the risk of developing atherosclerotic lesions in the walls of arteries (see Chap. 16).

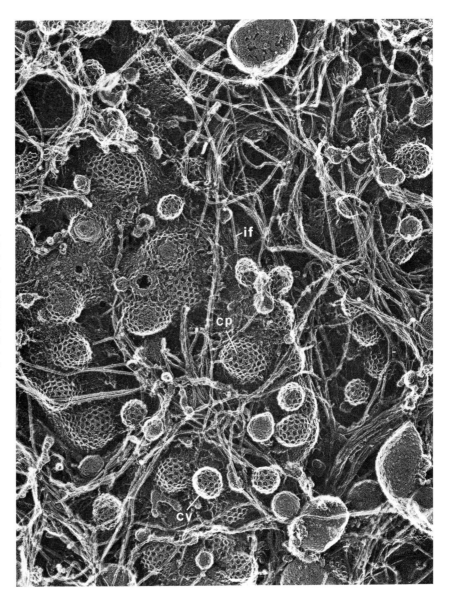

Fig. 4-22. Electron micrograph of a replica made of the inner (cytoplasmic) aspect of the cell membrane of a mouse hepatocyte. This fragment of cell membrane was prepared using a special quick-freeze, deep-etch, and rotary shadowing method that preserves and exposes the clathrin-containing basketwork of coated pits (*cp*) and coated vesicles (*cv*) as well as a number of intermediate filaments (*if*) of the cell membrane-associated cytoskeleton. (Hirokawa N, Heuser J: Cell 30: 395, 1982)

The general picture emerging from experimental studies of receptor-mediated endocytosis is that ligand internalization is a direct consequence of the active formation of coated vesicles from coated pits. In many cases, the ligand–receptor complexes formed on absorptive surfaces are initially random in their distribution. However, while drifting laterally in the cell membrane, they soon encounter coated pits, whereupon they begin to collect in these and are then internalized through the formation of coated vesicles (Fig. 4-23). In other cases, for example the LDL receptors on fibroblasts, the receptors stay preferentially distributed in coated pits at all times; this does not require them to be complexed with their ligand.

Endosomes. The cell is able to deal with internalized ligand–receptor complexes in a number of different ways. In certain cases, the complex is simply shuttled across the cell so that the same ligand can be released by exocytosis from some other part of the cell surface. Examples of such a pathway include (1) the transplacental exchange of maternal antibodies from the mother's plasma to the fetus *in utero*, and (2) the transepithelial route by which neonates receive maternal antibodies from ingested breast milk by way of their intestinal epithelial cells.

Under other circumstances, the ligand may be submitted to degradation by lysosomal enzymes. Yet this is not usually the next stage of ligand processing. In most instances, the ligand is first delivered to an intermediate *prelysosomal compartment* commonly referred to as an *endosome* (Fig. 4-21). This is an acidic membrane-bounded compartment that lacks the high concentration of hydrolytic enzymes present in lysosomes. Recent evidence indicates that the interior

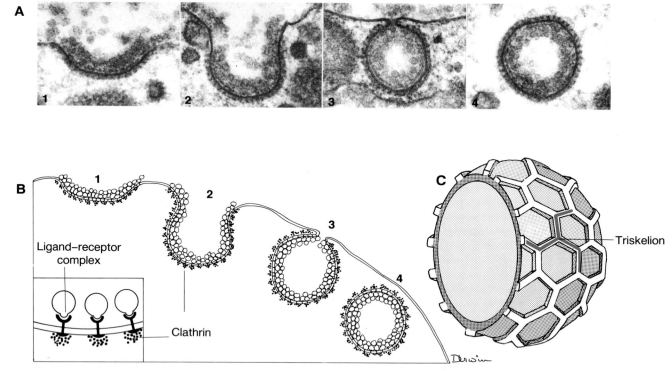

Fig. 4-23. (*A*) Series of electron micrographs (×53,000) illustrating the process of formation of a coated pit (*1* and *2*) and its invagination to form a coated vesicle (*3* and *4*). Large lipoprotein particles are seen here being ingested through receptor-mediated endocytosis by a hen oocyte (staining enhanced with tannic acid). (*B*) Comparable series of interpretive diagrams. (*Inset*) Cell membrane receptors for lipoprotein become closely associated with the clathrin-containing latticework of a coated pit. (*C*) Diagram of a coated vesicle. The highly characteristic latticework enclosing this type of vesicle is made up of hexagons, with some pentagons. One of the triskelions (the clathrin-containing subunits from which the lattice is constructed) is indicated in blue. (*A,* Perry MM, Gilbert AB: J Cell Sci 39:257, 1979)

of endosomes furnishes an acidic nondegradative intracellular environment in which *ligands can become dissociated from their receptors.* Receptors thus recovered can be returned to the cell surface to be used again (Fig. 4-21).

Whereas some receptors are conserved in this manner and reutilized (*e.g., LDL* receptors), others undergo degradation by lysosomal hydrolases along with their bound ligand, which results in their down-regulation (*e.g.,* receptors for *epidermal growth factor*). In the case of the iron-carrying transport protein *transferrin,* both the ligand and its receptor remain intact and both are returned to the cell membrane. The details are as follows. *Ferrotransferrin* (a transferrin molecule carrying two Fe^{3+} ions) is taken up by receptor-mediated endocytosis, whereupon it donates its iron to the cell. Still membrane-bound as a ligand–receptor complex, the protein (now *apotransferrin, i.e.,* transferrin devoid of iron) then returns to the cell membrane and is subsequently released through exocytosis.

Endosomes are thought to convey ligand–receptor complexes received from coated vesicles that have shed their coats (Fig. 4-21) to the general vicinity of the *trans* Golgi saccules and GERL, where many steps in the complicated task of segregating and redirecting ligands, receptors, and cellular membrane are believed

to occur. Roughly 200 nm to 400 nm in diameter and with contents that are relatively electron lucent, endosomes vary from being vesicular (or multivesicular) to tubular in shape. Fusion is common between endosomes. They seem to form all the time, serving as little membranous containers that shuttle back and forth between the superficial cytoplasm and the reticular *trans* Golgi and lysosomal region. Their migration toward the Golgi–lysosomal zone is saltatory and apparently guided by microtubules. Because the complicated sequence of events whereby several different ligands entering the cell by way of the same endocytic vesicle have to be sorted out and directed toward appropriate intracellular destinations begins in the acidic endosomal compartment, these membranous vesicles are also sometimes described as *sorting vesicles* or *receptosomes.* It seems likely that they constitute a series of prelysosomal compartments that bring about progressive dissociation of ligands from their receptors and sequester these ligands. Thus ingested glycoproteins bearing terminal galactose groups have been localized in the luminal contents of the vesicular portion of endosome-derived vesicles that then fuses with a primary lysosome (Fig. 4-21). The unloaded receptors, on the other hand, remain membrane-bound and accumulate in the tubular portion of endosome-derived vesicles before returning to the surface (Fig. 4-21). In addition to endosomes that are vesicular and tubular, there are some that are multivesicular,

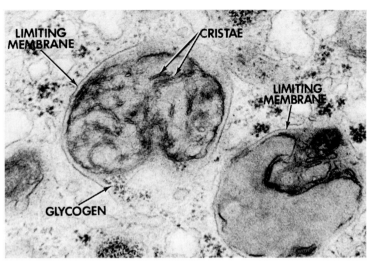

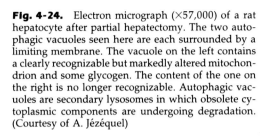

Fig. 4-24. Electron micrograph (×57,000) of a rat hepatocyte after partial hepatectomy. The two autophagic vacuoles seen here are each surrounded by a limiting membrane. The vacuole on the left contains a clearly recognizable but markedly altered mitochondrion and some glycogen. The content of the one on the right is no longer recognizable. Autophagic vacuoles are secondary lysosomes in which obsolete cytoplasmic components are undergoing degradation. (Courtesy of A. Jézéquel)

but the functional significance of multivesicular endosomes is still unclear.

Autophagy. Besides using its lysosomal enzymes to purge itself of useless ingested materials, the cell utilizes these same acid hydrolases to dispose of its own worn-out organelles and superfluous endogenous products such as an excess of secretory granules. It may also employ these enzymes to extract biologically active compounds from inactive precursors (*e.g.*, in liberating thyroid hormone from thyroglobulin). The intracellular disposal of deteriorating organelles is called *autophagy* (Gr. *autos*, self + *phagein*, to eat). When the cellular component to be eliminated is an excess of secretory granules, the autophagic process is more often referred to as *crinophagy* (Gr. *krinein*, to separate).

Mitochondria, fragments of rER, and other organelles that have deteriorated and are of no further use to the cell become enclosed and segregated from the remainder of the cytoplasm by an intracellular membrane thought to be derived from the endoplasmic reticulum. Like phagosomes, these organelle-segregating vesicles fuse with primary lysosomes, and, as a consequence, their contents are submitted to hydrolytic digestion (Fig. 4-21). The resulting structures, known as *autophagic vacuoles* or *cytolysosomes,* contain an assortment of organelles at various stages of degradation; hence they exhibit a wide variety of appearances in the EM. Remnants of membranes can often be recognized because they persist longer than other components (Fig. 4-24). The contents of autophagic vacuoles may eventually be extruded from the cytoplasm by exocytosis. If they remain in the cell for a very long time, they may accumulate lipid products and a pigment called *lipofuscin*, which will be described later in this chapter.

Lysosomal Storage Diseases. The clinical importance of lysosomal enzymes in the everyday metabolic activities of body cells is exemplified by a substantial number of dif-

ferent (although relatively rare) diseases that result from specific deficiencies in lysosomal function. In each of these so-called *lysosomal storage diseases,* a specific compound produced by the cell, such as a complex lipid product or glycogen, remains incompletely degraded (catabolized) by lysosomal enzymes. As a result, this compound builds up in the cytoplasm and soon begins to interfere with cell function. It has been shown that such accumulation is not due to overproduction. The problem lies in the lysosomes, which are deficient in some specific enzymatic activity that they would normally otherwise possess. Furthermore, this absence of a particular enzymatic function is the result of a genetic defect that, in almost all of these diseases, is inherited as an autosomal recessive trait. Genetic counseling and early antenatal detection, together with the option of therapeutic abortion, now serve to safeguard against perpetuation of these diseases.

Tay-Sachs disease is one of the most progressively debilitating and ultimately lethal disorders in this major group of genetic diseases. It is caused by the deficiency of a specific acetylhexosaminidase required to degrade a ganglioside produced by neurons. Because this particular lysosomal enzymatic activity is lacking, the secondary lysosomes in neurons, including those of the brain, become filled with concentric electron-dense laminae representing the ganglioside that the cells are unable to degrade (Fig. 4-25). As their cytoplasm becomes increasingly filled with residual bodies packed with this undigested material, the neurons are unable to function properly. Essential brain functions become impaired and untimely death in infancy ensues.

PEROXISOMES

Initially called *microbodies* because of their comparatively small diameter (generally less than 1 μm), *peroxisomes* are membrane-bounded organelles of somewhat inconsistent shape, size, and enzyme content that constitute a popu-

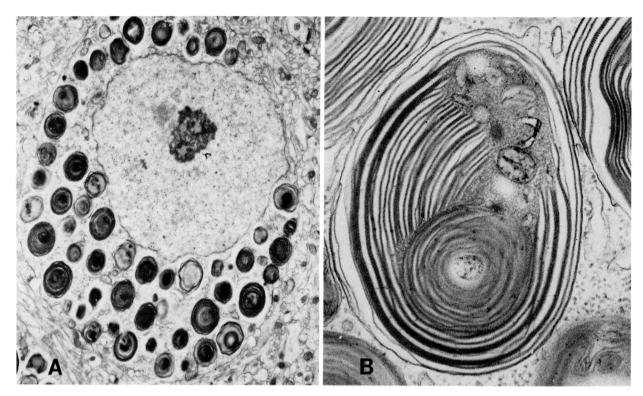

Fig. 4-25. Membranous residual bodies in nerve cells of a patient with Tay-Sachs disease. (*A*) Micrograph (×8000) of a neuron from the cerebral cortex, packed with membranous residual bodies composed of concentric, electron-dense laminae. (*B*) Micrograph (×70,000) of a membranous residual body from a brain cell of this patient. These laminated dense bodies are a distinctive feature of the brain cells of patients with Tay-Sachs disease. (Terry RD, Weiss M: J Neuropath Exp Neurol 22:18, 1963)

lation of tiny vesicles distinct from lysosomes. They are known as peroxisomes because they contain peroxide-forming enzymes and catalase and are involved in the formation and degradation of intracellular hydrogen peroxide. This hydrogen peroxide participates in certain metabolic reactions and is utilized by phagocytic cells to kill ingested microorganisms. However, because it is deleterious to certain other enzymatic reactions, its levels need to be regulated to maintain normal metabolic activity.

Peroxisomes vary appreciably in size and appearance depending on species and cell type. They are relatively large in hepatocytes and kidney cells but are sufficiently small in absorptive cells of the intestine to warrant being called *microperoxisomes*. In human cells, their moderately electron-dense content is homogeneous and has a finely granular appearance, but in many other species, it also possesses a more electron-dense, semicrystalline core of variable appearance called a *nucleoid* (see Fig. 19-18). Such a core is absent from liver peroxisomes prepared from reptiles, birds, and man, which are species that lack *urate oxidase* (*uricase*), an enzyme that degrades urates. Furthermore, nucleoids extracted from liver peroxisomes of all species possessing such cores are rich in this particular enzyme. Hence the core seen in peroxisomes is believed to be a crystalline (or semicrystalline) array of urate oxidase.

It is now clearly established that peroxisomes play a direct role in lipid metabolism, and it has been suggested that they may be involved in the production of glucose from lipids. Thus experimental studies in animals indicate that hypolipidemic drugs, which are employed clinically to reduce elevated blood levels of lipid and cholesterol, can significantly increase the number of peroxisomes present in hepatocytes. Hepatocyte peroxisomes, like mitochondria, are able to break down fatty acids by β-oxidation, and hypolipidemic drugs have been found to induce a substantial (tenfold) rise in the level of β-oxidative enzymes in peroxisomes.

The oxidase enzymes in peroxisomes (urate oxidase, D-amino acid oxidase, and α-hydroxyacid oxidase) produce hydrogen peroxide, whereas catalase converts this product to oxygen and water. Catalase can also utilize hydrogen peroxide to oxidize a variety of different substrates within the cell, including alcohols. The comparatively large spherical to ovoid peroxisomes in hepatocytes may therefore help their sER and mitochondria to metabolize ingested alcohol.

Little is known about the formation of peroxisomes except that (1) they are commonly seen in the immediate vicinity of the endoplasmic reticulum and (2) urate oxidase and catalase are both synthesized as free proteins in the

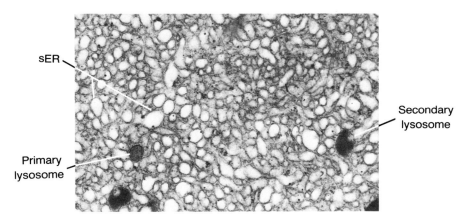

Fig. 4-26. Electron micrograph (×15,400) of part of a steroid-producing cell from the zona reticularis of human adrenal cortex, showing interconnected tubules of smooth endoplasmic reticulum (*sER*) that follow a tortuous course through the cytoplasm. (Courtesy of M. J. Phillips)

cytosol prior to reaching the lumen of peroxisomes. Apparent continuities between the peroxisome membrane and smooth-surfaced regions of the endoplasmic reticulum have been interpreted as indicating that peroxisomes may develop as small local dilatations of the endoplasmic reticulum that bud directly from the endoplasmic reticulum and accumulate such enzymes within their lumen.

SMOOTH-SURFACED ENDOPLASMIC RETICULUM (sER)

The second region of the endoplasmic reticulum is called the *smooth-surfaced endoplasmic reticulum* (sER). It differs from the rER in that (1) its limiting membrane is smooth (*i.e.*, not studded with ribosomes) and (2) it consists of tubules that branch and anastomose in an irregular manner (Fig. 4-26). It is nevertheless continuous with the rER, and its integral membrane proteins are synthesized by the rER. The amount of sER present in the cytoplasm varies with cell type; it is prominent only in a few cell types. Being devoid of ribosomes, the sER does not impart any cytoplasmic basophilia and it is unable to synthesize proteins. Its main functions are to elaborate certain other cell constituents and to degrade potentially cytotoxic compounds, as outlined below.

Lipids Are Synthesized by the sER. The sER is the site of intracellular synthesis of lipids and cholesterol derivatives and hence is fairly prominent in those cells that elaborate lipids, lipoproteins, or steroids (the latter being related chemically to cholesterol). The absorptive cells in the epithelial lining of the small intestine constitute an example of a cell type that can synthesize *lipids* in its sER and then export them from its surface. These cells are able to absorb breakdown products of fat digestion and then recombine them as lipids (fats) in their sER. The tiny droplets of fat thus formed are later secreted by the cells into the adjacent tissue fluid, whereupon they are known as *chylomicrons.*

These fat droplets drain along with tissue fluid into lymphatics and eventually they reach the bloodstream by way of the lymph.

The lipid portion of *plasma lipoprotein* molecules is synthesized by the sER of hepatocytes whereas the protein portion is synthesized by the rER of the same cells. The sER is also prominent in cells that secrete *steroid hormones,* particularly the hormone-secreting cells of the adrenal cortex (Fig. 4-26).

The sER Detoxifies Drugs. It is well established that drugs are detoxified in the liver, and studies with the EM indicate that the sER is very much involved. For example, when barbiturates such as phenobarbital are given to experimental animals, the amount of sER present in their hepatocytes increases greatly. A more extensive sER is able to detoxify the drug faster. The sER is believed to detoxify many drugs, including alcohol. The sensitivity or resistance of each individual to a prescribed dose of drug depends in part on the time it takes for the drug to be degraded and rendered inactive. This in turn depends on the amount of sER in the hepatocytes of the individual when the drug was administered.

The sER Is Involved in Hepatic Glycogen Metabolism. When glycogen is present, it exists as unsegregated deposits in the cytoplasmic matrix. In hepatocytes, such deposits are commonly found in close proximity to the sER. Thus in Figure 4-27, tubules of sER extend through a region where glycogen is present. There is evidence that glycogen synthase phosphatase and phosphorylase phosphatase, two phosphoprotein phosphatases involved in the regulation of hepatic glycogen metabolism, are closely associated with the sER (Margolis et al). Also, glucose-6-phosphatase, one of the several enzymes required to break down glycogen into glucose, is known to be associated with the endoplasmic reticulum of these cells.

The sER Can Regulate the Intracellular Distribution of Calcium Ions. As will become clear in Chapter 15, muscular contraction is regulated by the local concentration

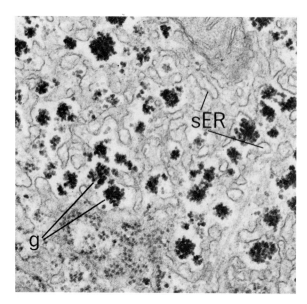

Fig. 4-27. Electron micrograph (×38,500) of a rat hepatocyte containing glycogen (*g*) that lies in close proximity to tubules of the sER. (Cardell R: Int Rev Cytol 48:221, 1977)

of calcium ions in the contractile elements of the muscle cell. The intracellular distribution of calcium ions in skeletal muscle cells and cardiac muscle cells is known to be regulated by their very elaborate sER, which intimately surrounds each of their individual contractile elements (see Fig. 15-16). Termed the *sarcoplasmic reticulum,* the sER of the muscle cell is able to release stored calcium ions from its lumen and thereby bring about a contraction, after which it sequesters them again, and this induces a relaxation. Enzymes that can pump calcium ions into the lumen of the sarcoplasmic reticulum are present in its membrane, and other proteins with the capacity to bind calcium ions are situated inside the reticulum. In other cell types, however, most of the intracellular calcium is thought to be stored within mitochondria.

We shall now go on to consider the *nonmembranous organelles* of the cytoplasm. Free ribosomes and polysomes were dealt with in connection with protein synthesis; the next organelles to be described are the various elements that make up the *cytoskeleton,* so called because in many ways its constituent elements serve as the skeleton and muscles of the cell.

MICROTUBULES

Microtubules are slender tubular structures of unfixed length with a constant outer diameter of 25 nm (Fig. 4-28). If cut in cross section, they appear as tiny circles with a lumen that is less electron dense than their walls (Fig. 4-28A). After special EM staining, it can be seen that each

microtubule is made up of 13 longitudinal, rodlike *protofilaments,* a unique construction that reflects its underlying pattern of organization of constituent subunits. With suitable staining, it is sometimes possible to see this characteristic plan of construction quite clearly in the component microtubules of centrioles (see Fig. 3-10, *left*) and also in cilia (see Figs. 4-33 and 4-34, *bottom right*). At the LM level, cytoplasmic microtubules are best demonstrated by immunofluorescent staining using fluorescent-labeled antibody to tubulin, which is their chief protein constituent (Fig. 4-29).

The Tubulin in Microtubules Is in Equilibrium with Soluble Tubulin. Not all the tubulin in the cell is present in the form of microtubules. Some of it is also always present in soluble form as a cytoplasmic protein. Actually, soluble tubulin itself is made up of two structurally similar peptides (α-tubulin and β-tubulin) that are associated with each other as a dimer. Shaped like a shell enclosing two peanuts (Fig. 4-34), the tubulin dimer represents the subunit from which microtubules are assembled. Moreover, once tubulin dimers have been incorporated into a microtubule, they remain in dynamic equilibrium with the dimers that constitute the cytoplasmic pool of free tubulin. *In vitro* studies indicate that tubulin dimers are (1) preferentially incorporated at one end of the microtubule, and (2) preferentially lost from its other end, dissociating at a faster rate than they are added. Furthermore, when certain steady-state conditions are maintained *in vitro,* the net amount of assembly occurring at the growing end of the microtubule compensates for the net amount of disassembly taking place at the other end, with the result that there is a steady translocation of constituent tubulin subunits toward the end that is preferentially dissociating. Such intrinsic displacement mechanisms are often described as molecular *treadmilling.* However, it seems somewhat doubtful whether the conditions found in living cells would permit such treadmilling of tubulin subunits to occur. It is nevertheless well established that except for the microtubules of cilia, flagella, centrioles, and basal bodies, microtubules represent labile structures that have a tendency to break down into their constituent tubulin subunits. Furthermore, these tubulin subunits are continually being reincorporated into existing microtubules as well as being assembled into new ones.

Microtubule Assembly Is a Regulated Process. Polymerization of tubulin to form microtubules is initiated at sites called *microtubule-organizing centers* that can be present almost anywhere in the cytoplasm but are most numerous in the immediate vicinity of the centrioles. This is known because if colchicine is applied and subsequently removed, new cytoplasmic microtubules begin to assemble in the pericentriolar region. Also, when a cell divides and its tubulin subunits are utilized to produce spindle microtubules instead of cytoplasmic microtubules, subsequent reassembly of its cytoplasmic microtubules occurs in close association with the pericentriolar microtubule-organizing centers of the daughter cells. The polymerization and depolymerization of tubulin dimers are both closely regulated so that microtubules form only in the necessary locations and on the appropriate occasions. There are indications that certain *microtubule-associated proteins,* which are so called because of their intimate association with microtubules, participate in regulating microtubule assembly.

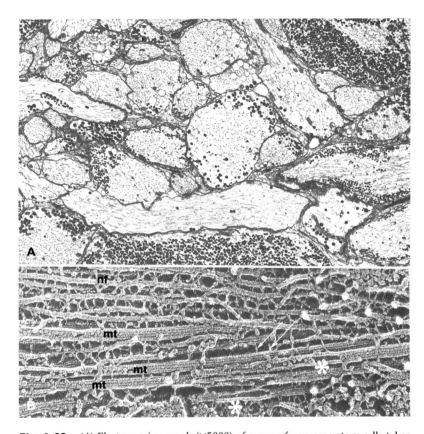

Fig. 4-28. (*A*) Electron micrograph (×5000) of axons of neurosecretory cells taken at a magnification that discloses their numerous microtubules. The microtubules can be seen cut in longitudinal section (*bottom* of micrograph) and cross section (*center*). The round electron-dense granules seen in a peripheral position in these axons are neurosecretory granules. (*B*) Electron micrograph (×179,000) of a replica made of the interior of an unfixed saponin-treated frog axon, showing microtubules (*mt*) stabilized by taxol together with neurofilaments (*nf*). This axon was prepared using a special quick-freeze, deep-etch, and rotary shadowing method that preserves and exposes the intricate system of cross-connections that exists between its neurofilaments and microtubules (*arrows*). The asterisks indicate sites where tubulin subunits are discernible on the internal surface of microtubules that have broken open and unrolled. Longitudinal ridges on the external surface of the microtubules correspond to protofilaments. (*A*, courtesy of L. Arsenault; *B*, Hirokawa N: J Cell Biol 94:129, 1982; by permission of The Rockefeller University Press)

The Cell Utilizes Its Microtubules in Several Ways. Because cytoplasmic microtubules are relatively rigid but are capable of bending, they provide internal support for the cell and represent its main skeletal element. Moreover, their distribution has a profound effect on cell morphology, and it accounts for many kinds of bizarre cell shapes. Cytoplasmic microtubules are also believed to facilitate the intracellular transport of organelles, particles, and macromolecules along specific routes through the cytoplasm. Their role in transporting such components has been likened to that of railroad tracks guiding the movement of trains. This capacity for directing intracellular transport is particularly important in the extremely long cytoplasmic process that extends from the cell body of nerve cells. The microtubules within such a process (Fig. 4-28*A*) are able to direct the intracellular transport of materials synthesized in the cell body so that these will eventually reach the tip of the process.

It should also be remembered that microtubules are essential for the process of segregation of daughter chromosomes at mitosis. As noted in Chapter 3, assembly of the interpolar microtubules separates the centriole pairs, and continued elongation of these microtubules lengthens the mitotic spindle. A further role of microtubules, which will be considered in subsequent sections, is to generate sliding forces between the adjacent doublet microtubules of cilia. These forces are harnessed by the cilium and are utilized to generate ciliary motility.

Certain Drugs Affect Microtubule-Dependent Functions. Mitosis and other processes that depend on the

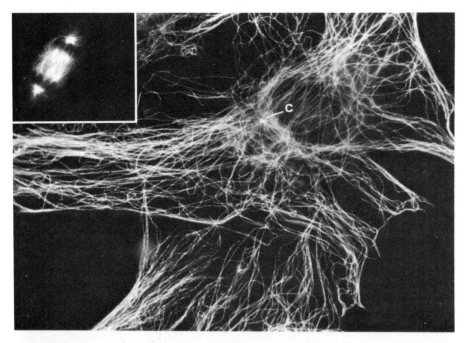

Fig. 4-29. Immunofluorescence photomicrograph of a mouse embryo fibroblast in tissue culture (oil immersion). Antibody to microtubule protein (tubulin) was employed to demonstrate the distributions of cytoplasmic microtubules during interphase (*large photomicrograph*) and spindle microtubules during anaphase (*inset*). The nucleus of the interphase cell lies toward the top right corner of the large photomicrograph; the centrioles (C) appear as a brightly fluorescent spot to the lower left of the nucleus. Both the mitotic spindle and the centrioles are evident in the anaphase cell (*inset*); the two sets of daughter chromosomes appear dark against the fluorescing microtubules of the spindle. During mitosis, the cytoplasmic microtubules seen during interphase are absent. (Courtesy of J. A. Connolly)

participation of microtubules are profoundly, but nevertheless reversibly, perturbed by the alkaloids *colchicine*, *vinblastine*, and *vincristine*. These drugs bind to the soluble tubulin subunits from which new microtubules are ordinarily assembled. The inhibitory effect of such binding on the assembly process was discussed in Chapter 3 under Drugs That Block Mitosis. As noted above, microtubules are always losing and reacquiring constituent tubulin dimers. All three of these drugs inhibit the reincorporation of tubulin dimers. The resulting uncompensated loss of tubulin subunits occurring primarily at the net disassembly end of microtubules eventually eliminates these structures from the cytoplasm. Hence colchicine treatment *destroys cytoplasmic microtubules.* Accordingly, in addition to being used to block mitosis in the preparation of chromosomes for cytogenetic studies (Chap. 3), colchicine is used clinically to treat acute attacks of gout. It is so efficient at destroying cytoplasmic microtubules that it diminishes neutrophil migration into inflammatory foci and thereby helps to ameliorate the intense acute inflammation associated with this condition (see Chap. 8).

As well as being present as individual entities, microtubules constitute the chief structural components of the next group of cytoplasmic organelles to be described. Centrioles, the structure of which was dealt with briefly in Chapter 3 and is illustrated in Figure 3-10, also belong to this microtubule-containing group of nonmembranous organelles and will be considered again when we describe the basal bodies of cilia.

CILIA AND FLAGELLA

Cilia are motile, hairlike processes almost 10 μm long with a diameter of about 0.2 μm. They extend from the luminal border of most of the surface cells in the wet epithelial lining of certain internal passages and cavities, notably those in the upper part of the respiratory tract. As many as several hundred cilia can be present on each cell, as becomes strikingly evident if these cells are observed in the scanning electron microscope (Fig. 4-30). Besides being made up of *ciliated cells*, the epithelial lining of the upper part of the respiratory tract contains numerous mucus-secreting cells that are known as *goblet cells* because their content of mucous secretory vesicles gives them a characteristic gobletlike shape (Fig. 4-31). After the mucus in

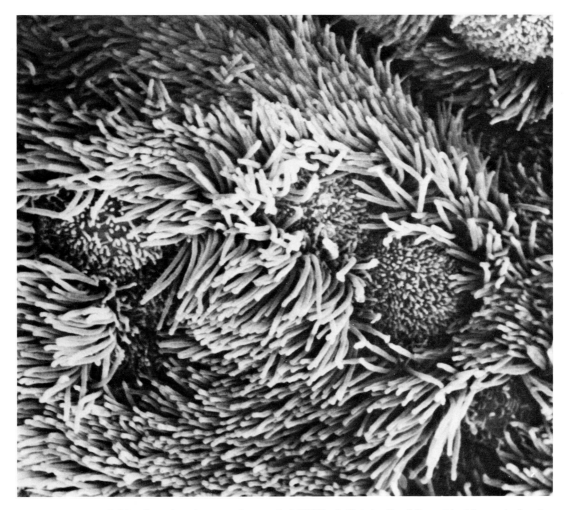

Fig. 4-30. Scanning electron micrograph (×7000) of ciliated cells of the oviduct (mouse), showing the surface appearance of ciliated cells. A few nonciliated cells can also be seen; these have microvilli on their surface. (Courtesy of Dirksen ER: In Hafez ESE [ed]: Scanning Electron Microscopic Atlas of Mammalian Reproduction, Tokyo, Igaku Shoin, 1975)

these cells has been discharged by exocytosis, it serves to trap any particulate matter settling out of the inhaled air. It forms a sticky protective coating that is continually swept over the surface of the epithelium in one direction only by sequential beating of the underlying cilia. These underlying cilia can just be individually discerned under the LM (Fig. 4-31), and with special staining it is even sometimes possible to see that every cilium has a tiny associated structure known as a *basal body* at its base (Figs. 4-32 and 4-34, *upper left*).

The Basal Bodies of Cilia and Flagella Are Derived from Centrioles.   Under the EM, basal bodies exhibit a structure identical to that of *centrioles,* described in Chapter 3 under Mitosis and illustrated in Figure 3-10. Like centrioles, they are tiny cylindrical structures 0.5 μm long and 0.2 μm in diameter with nine longitudinal triplet microtubules in their walls (see Fig. 3-10). A nonciliated cell in

G_1 possesses two centrioles, which are present in close association with each other and commonly are situated near the middle of the cell. In preparation for ciliogenesis, cylindrical structures called *centriolar organizers* form near this original pair of centrioles. Numerous *procentrioles* (immature centrioles) then assemble around the centriolar organizers. The multiple centrioles that are formed in this manner are all potentially capable of generating cilia. They migrate to a level just below the luminal border of the cell and become basal bodies, whereupon microtubules grow from the outward-facing (distal) end of each basal body to produce a cilium. Anchoring *rootlets* subsequently form at the proximal end of the basal body (Figs. 4-32 and 4-33); generally, this is the end that contains the axial cartwheel component described in connection with Figure 3-10. In addition, a small striated structure called a *basal foot* extends laterally from the basal body, as may be seen on careful

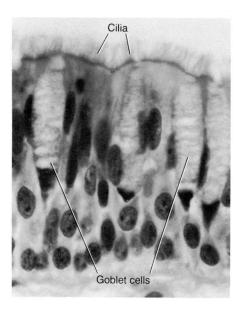

Fig. 4-31. Photomicrograph of the pseudostratified ciliated columnar epithelium with goblet cells that lines the trachea. Individual cilia can just be discerned on the luminal border of the ciliated cells. The goblet cells are producing mucus.

inspection of the basal body on the right-hand side of Figure 4-32.

Could One Function of Centrioles Be to Detect Signals? Hypotheses about the nature of centriolar involvement in development of the mitotic spindle currently focus on the role of pericentriolar microtubule-organizing centers rather than on that of the centrioles themselves. This role of centriole-associated microtubule-organizing centers in initiating microtubule assembly is clearly an important feature of ciliogenesis also. However, in contrast to centriolar involvement in the formation of a mitotic spindle, which is only a temporary structure, each centriole-derived basal body remains permanently associated with the cilium (or flagellum) it produces. This raises the question of whether it might continue to serve some useful purpose after producing the cilium. Calculations by Albrecht–Buehler have shown that on purely theoretical grounds, centrioles (and therefore basal bodies) would be perfectly designed for receiving exogenous directional signals. Furthermore, a pair of centrioles arranged perpendicular to each other potentially would be capable of receiving spatial signals from any given direction and could discriminate the altitude as well as the latitude of the signal source. The nature of these directional signals is still totally unknown, but several observations suggest that this hypothesis amounts to something more than sheer speculation.

First, motile cells need to be able to sense their direction of movement. *In vitro*, it is common for such cells to develop a single

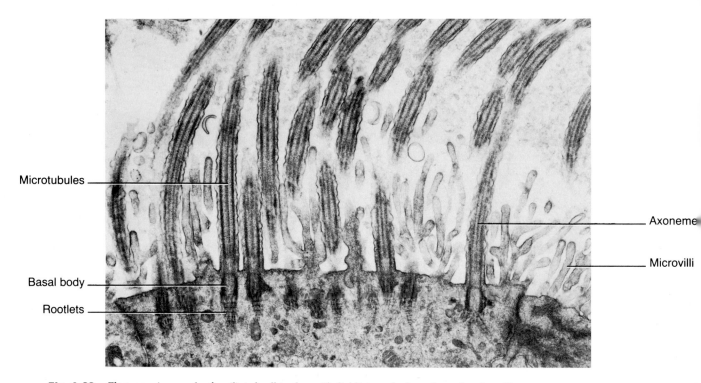

Fig. 4-32. Electron micrograph of a ciliated cell in the epithelial lining of a bronchus, showing cilia and microvilli on its luminal border. (Sturgess J: In Quinton P, Martinez R [eds]: Fluid and Electrolyte Transport in Exocrine Glands in Cystic Fibrosis. San Francisco, San Francisco Press, 1982)

position in the cell is a primary determinant of the cytoskeletal arrangement within the cell. Such observations are consistent with the hypothesis that the centrioles may play a role in determining the direction of cell migration as well as determining cell polarity.

A second reason for the belief that basal bodies might retain some signal-detecting function is that the stimulus-sensing portions of most of the major sensory receptors, including those situated in the organs of special sense, are derived either wholly or in part from modified cilia. Foremost among these receptors are the photoreceptors of the eye and the hair cells of the ear. Also, modified cilia constitute the stimulus-sensing part of the olfactory receptors present in the nasal cavities. Hence the basal bodies of such cilia are in a logical position to collect signal energy and to facilitate its transduction into optic, acoustic, vestibular, or olfactory afferent nerve impulses.

The Ciliary Shaft (Axoneme) Generates Two Different Kinds of Strokes.   During ciliogenesis, the two innermost microtubules of each triplet microtubule in a basal body grow out of the basal body and become peripheral microtubules of a cilium. The outermost microtubule in each triplet microtubule of the basal body does not increase in length. As a result, the shaft of a cilium (termed its *axoneme*) possesses nine peripheral *doublet* microtubules (Figs. 4-33 and 4-34). In addition, two *singlet* microtubules are present in its middle (Figs. 4-33 and 4-34). Thus the axoneme has nine peripheral doublets and two central singlets, and is surrounded by cell membrane (Figs. 4-33*B* and 4-34), whereas the basal body has nine peripheral triplets, no central singlets, and is surrounded by cytoplasmic matrix. As described in the caption accompanying Figure 4-34, a highly complex system of separate interconnections exists between the peripheral doublets and the central singlets. The functional role of most of these linkages seems to be to harness forces generated by the microtubules so that they can be used by the axoneme for tasks such as propelling a sheet of mucus. Measurements have shown that particles caught in nasal mucus can be moved by as much as 6 mm or more per minute by this mechanism.

While cilia are executing their forceful forward beat, which is termed their *effective stroke*, they are straight and relatively rigid. They then bend and execute a *recovery stroke* that allows them to regain their starting position. The force of the effective stroke can transport a mucous coating forward, and the gentler recovery stroke that follows permits cilia to slide back under it, avoiding the problem of moving it back again afterward. The plane in which the cilium executes its beats is its plane of symmetry (*i.e.,* the central plane lying perpendicular to a line drawn between its two central singlets) (Fig. 4-34, *upper right*).

The energy required for ciliary activity is derived from ATP through the ATPase activity of a protein called *dynein* that forms short hooklike arms on each peripheral doublet of the axoneme (Fig. 4-33 and 4-34). ATP-induced sliding of the doublets relative to one another generates the forces that bring about the beating of cilia, and complex interconnections between the peripheral doublets and central

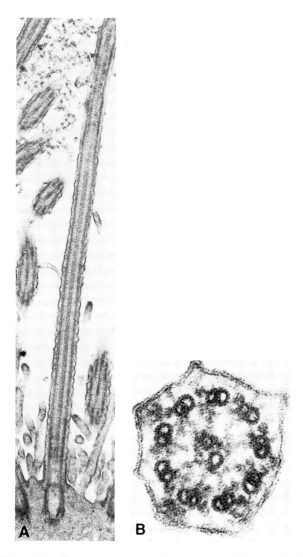

Fig. 4-33. Electron micrographs of a cilium cut in (*A*) longitudinal section and (*B*) transverse section, obtained from ciliated epithelial lining cells of a bronchus. This figure may be compared with Figure 4-34, which illustrates some of the details that can be seen. (*A,* courtesy of J. Sturgess; *B,* Sturgess J, Turner TAP: In Chernick V, Kendig E [eds]: Respiratory Diseases in Childhood. Philadelphia, WB Saunders, 1982)

rudimentary and nonmotile *primary cilium* that, together with its associated basal body, is generally oriented so that it points in the direction in which the cell is heading. The other centriole is generally oriented parallel to the cell's substrate, giving the impression that centrioles and basal bodies could represent some kind of signal-detector device. Furthermore, only cells that are motile or potentially capable of migrating possess centrioles. These include all motile types of animal cells but exclude the stationary cells of higher plants. Evidence is accumulating that the centrioles of migrating endothelial cells (the lining cells of blood vessels and lymphatics) become preferentially located in their leading half, and that their

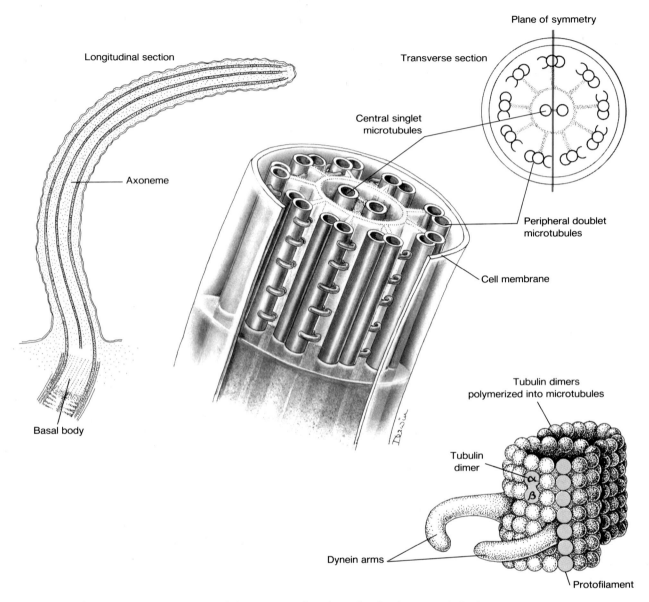

Fig. 4-34. Diagrammatic representation of the structure of a cilium (for details, see text). In the peripheral doublet microtubules, the microtubule that is provided with dynein arms is made up of 13 rod-shaped protofilaments, each consisting of tubulin dimers arranged end to end, that extend the entire length of the microtubule (*bottom right*). Its companion microtubule has only 10 or 11 protofilaments of its own and has to share the remainder with the other microtubule (*bottom right*). A rigid radial spoke connects each doublet to an inner sheath that surrounds the two central singlet microtubules (*center* and *top right*). There are also flexible nexin linkages between adjacent doublets, but for simplicity these have been omitted. (Courtesy of J. Sturgess and T. A. P. Turner)

singlets (illustrated in Figs. 4-33 and 4-34) apply the forces that are generated to bend the whole axoneme.

Spermatozoa have a tail with a structure that is basically similar to that of a ciliary axoneme except for the fact that it has some additional components and is much longer than a cilium. Known as a *flagellum* (L. for whip) because it executes a characteristic whiplike motion during swimming

movements, it possesses nine peripheral doublets and two central singlets as a cilium does.

FILAMENTS

The last group of nonmembranous organelles to consider are called *filaments.* The words *fiber, fibril,* and *filament* all

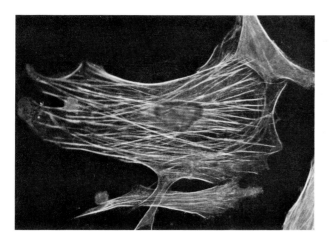

Fig. 4-35. Immunofluorescence photomicrograph of a mouse embryo fibroblast in tissue culture (oil immersion). Antibody to tropomyosin was employed to demonstrate the distribution of bundles of tropomyosin-containing actin microfilaments in the cytoplasm. These bundles lie just below the cell membrane and are more common on the side of the cell attached to the substrate. (Courtesy of L. Subrahmanyan and A. Jorgensen)

mean elongated threadlike structures. In practice these terms are used in microscopy to refer to threadlike structures of decreasing diameters. The words themselves, however, have no precise connotations regarding size. If, for example, such structures can be seen with the unaided eye or under the low power of the LM, they are referred to as *fibers.* Those resolved only under the high power of the LM are generally termed *fibrils.* The larger of the structures resolved only by the EM are usually also termed *fibrils,* whereas those of smaller diameter are termed *filaments.* Cytoplasmic *filaments* constitute a heterogeneous group of threadlike structures that are distinct from microtubules and can only be seen in the EM. However, in some cells, they are arranged in bundles or networks that are large enough to be seen under the higher powers of the LM in suitable preparations (Fig. 4-35).

Three different categories of filaments have now been identified: (1) *microfilaments,* which correspond to the *thin filaments* present in muscle cells; (2) *thick filaments,* which are present in muscle cells and may also exist in a more temporary or labile form, as much shorter filaments, in other cell types as well; and (3) *intermediate filaments,* a heterogeneous class of filaments that are so called because their diameter is intermediate between that of thin and thick filaments.

Microfilaments

Microfilaments are slender rods with a diameter of 6 nm to 7 nm (Fig. 4-36). They are composed of *actin,* generally in association with another protein called *tropomyosin* and, in the thin filaments of muscle cells at least, other proteins

that confer on them a sensitivity to the local concentration of calcium ions. The *thin filaments* of skeletal and cardiac muscle cells, which correspond to the *microfilaments* in other types of cells, are known to contain the regulatory protein *troponin* as well as actin and tropomyosin. These additional proteins mediate calcium ion regulation of the interaction between actin and myosin.

Thick Filaments

The thick filaments in muscle cells are noticeably thicker than the thin filaments and have a more variable diameter (12 nm to 16 nm). They are composed of the protein *myosin.* There is evidence that myosin is also present in the cytoplasm of nonmuscle cells, but it is still unclear whether this protein exists as microfilament-associated thick filaments as in muscle cells. It is widely acknowledged that thick filaments of some description could, in fact, exist in all kinds of cells, but so far this has not been conclusively demonstrated. It is possible that, in most situations, such filaments are relatively scarce and too short for easy recognition (conceivably being only the length of a myosin dimer), or perhaps they are being missed because they are transitory structures or represent extremely labile arrangements that are difficult to preserve.

Contractile Filaments Can Be Arranged Differently in Different Cell Types

It has long been established that the thick and thin filaments of muscle cells, their so-called *contractile filaments,* are arranged so that interaction between them generates muscular contractions. It is now believed that a basically similar mechanism operates at the periphery of nonmuscle cells and that this contractile mechanism generates forces that are utilized by the cell for various forms of cell motility. The structural basis of contractility is considered briefly in the following section.

Contractile Filaments Have a Characteristic Arrangement in Striated Muscle Cells. In skeletal and cardiac muscle cells, which are characterized by being striated, the contractile filaments are arranged as cylindrical components, known as myofibrils, that extend from one end of the cell to the other. Myofibrils are made up of identical segments called sarcomeres that are joined together end to end as a long series by their strong interconnecting elements, which are termed Z lines. The top part of Figure 15-5 shows that one half of the thin filaments in a sarcomere are attached to each of its Z lines, from which they extend as far as the middle third of the sarcomere. The thick filaments extend through the middle two thirds of the sarcomere with the two sets of thin filaments interdigitated between them (see Fig. 15-5, *top*). When the muscle cell is stimulated to contract, the two sets of thin filaments are drawn farther in between the thick filaments until they almost meet; the thick filaments remain fixed in position (see Fig. 15-5, *bottom*). This sliding action, the energy for which comes from the splitting of ATP, draws the two Z lines closer together. The net result of such shortening of all the sarcomeres along the length of each myofibril

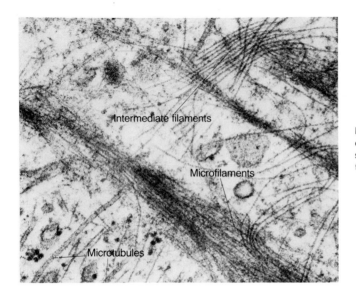

Fig. 4-36. Electron micrograph of a region of the cytoplasm of an endothelial cell from pig aorta growing in tissue culture, showing microfilaments, intermediate filaments, and microtubules. (Courtesy of V. I. Kalnins)

is contraction of the whole cell. More details about muscular contraction will, of course, be given when we deal with skeletal muscle in Chapter 15.

Other Arrangements of Contractile Filaments Are Found in Other Cell Types. EM studies have now confirmed the presence of microfilaments in an overwhelming number of different cell types, especially within the peripheral (cortical) zone of cytoplasm just under the cell membrane. Moreover, evidence is accumulating that some of these microfilaments are indirectly linked to the cell membrane. In some cell types, cytoplasmic microfilaments become organized into large bundles that are commonly referred to as *stress fibers.* These well-defined bundles can sometimes be seen *in vitro* when living cells are examined under a phase-contrast microscope (see Fig. 4-6), and they become strikingly evident after immunofluorescent staining for actin or tropomyosin (Fig. 4-35). At present, it seems that several different attachment proteins could be involved in linking the superficial end of these prominent microfilament bundles to so-called *focal contact* areas where the cell membrane adheres to the underlying substrate.

The contractile activities that result from interaction between microfilaments and associated myosin range from changes in the general shape of the cell to cytoplasmic constriction during cell division. An arrangement of parallel microfilaments, termed a contractile ring, appears under the cell membrane in the midregion of the cell during telophase. Contractile activity of the filaments in this ring, which encircles the cell at the bottom of its developing cleavage furrow, deepens this furrow and eventually constricts the cell into two halves.

Cytochalasins Interfere with Microfilament-Mediated Functions by Preventing Microfilament Assembly. In 1969, when Schroeder treated some dividing marine eggs with *cytochalasin,* a drug derived from certain fungi, he noticed that the contractile ring under the developing cleavage furrow became disorganized and the furrow

failed to form properly. As a result, the treated eggs did not constrict into two and each egg had two nuclei. The cause of this finding has now been established as cytochalasin-induced disassembly of the microfilaments in the contractile ring as a direct consequence of interruption of their assembly process.

The fungus-derived alkaloid *phalloidin* is a second drug that can interfere with microfilament-mediated functions; its main effect is to inhibit cell migration. However, in this case, the action of the drug is to *inhibit* the disassembly of microfilaments, which locks them into a static rather than a dynamic arrangement.

Microfilament bundles are also present in the cores of cell-surface projections known as microvilli, described in the following section.

Contractile Filaments Have a Characteristic Arrangement in Microvilli. The luminal surface of absorptive cells, such as those of the epithelium that lines the small intestine, exhibits a thin superficial layer of extremely fine, perpendicular striations that are barely discernible under the LM. Such a surface is termed a *striated border,* another name for which is *brush border.* Under the EM, it can be seen that this border is made up of *microvilli* (L. *villus,* tuft of hair), which are tiny fingerlike processes about 0.1 μm in diameter that project from the cell surface (Figs. 4-2, 4-37, 4-38, and 4-39). The vast numbers of microvilli comprising such borders greatly expand the area over which absorption takes place. Almost all cell types have at least a few microvilli on their free surfaces, but this is not always obvious.

As illustrated in Figures 4-38 and 4-39, each microvillus contains a bundle of crosslinked microfilaments that extends down the central core of the microvillus into the underlying cytoplasmic matrix. At the tip of the microvillus, the microfilaments are anchored to the cell membrane in much the same way as thin filaments are anchored to the Z lines at either end of a sarcomere of skeletal muscle (Fig. 4-38, *left*). In the cortical region of cytoplasm just under the microvilli, myosin is also present.

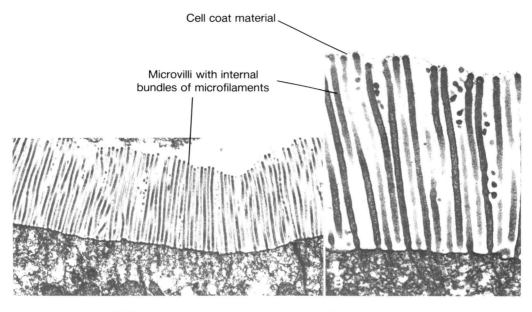

Cell coat material

Microvilli with internal
bundles of microfilaments

Fig. 4-37. (*A*) Electron micrograph (×7000) of the striated border of an absorptive epithelial cell. (*B*) Higher magnification shows its microvilli and its superficial covering of cell coat material. At the bottom of the micrograph, bundles of microfilaments can just be discerned extending down from each microvillus toward the terminal web. (Courtesy of L. Arsenault)

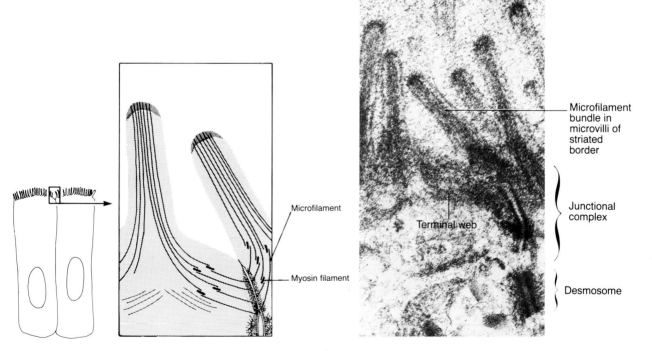

Microfilament

Myosin filament

Microfilament
bundle in
microvilli of
striated
border

Junctional
complex

Terminal web

Desmosome

Fig. 4-38. Diagrammatic representation and electron micrograph of the striated border of intestinal absorptive epithelial cells, showing a tentative interpretation of the manner in which the microfilament bundles, which are present in their apical microvilli, are arranged with respect to their terminal web. Sliding of these microfilaments past myosin, depicted here as short filaments, is believed to affect the height of the microvilli. (*Micrograph,* courtesy of D. Murray and A. Pittaway)

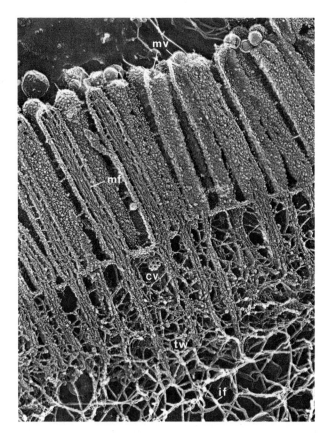

Fig. 4-39. Electron micrograph (×97,000) of a replica made of the striated border of an intestinal absorptive epithelial cell. This striated border was prepared using a special quick-freeze, deep-etch, and rotary shadowing method that preserves and exposes the bundle of actin-containing microfilaments (*mf*) in each microvillus (*mv*). These microfilaments extend down as far as the terminal web (*tw*), beneath which the cytoplasm contains a coarser network of thicker intermediate filaments (*if*). (Hirokawa N, Tilney LG, Fujiwara K, Heuser JE: J Cell Biol 94:425, 1982; by permission of The Rockefeller University Press)

It has been shown that under experimental conditions, the actin and myosin can be induced to interact and thereby change the overall height of the striated border. The height of striated border microvilli has also been found to change *in vivo* under fasting conditions and when cells migrate from crypts to villi, but this is considered to be more likely a reflection of some variation in the relative rates of assembly and disassembly of their component microfilaments. One arrangement of microfilaments and myosin that could account for striated border contractility is depicted in Figure 4-38, *left*. However, recent findings suggest that this model is really an oversimplification of what is turning out to be a highly complex arrangement. For an up-to-date account of work on the cytoskeleton of the striated border, the reader is referred to Mooseker et al.

Finally, a note of caution. It is not uncommon for beginners to mistake microvilli for cilia. A glance at Figure 4-32 will show how they can be distinguished from each other. Microvilli are shorter than cilia and lack a basal body and internal microtubules. Instead of microtubules, a microfilament bundle is seen in the core of microvilli.

Intermediate Filaments

Intermediate filaments are intermediate between microfilaments and thick filaments in diameter (Fig. 4-36); the range is approximately 7 nm to 11 nm. Because of their diameter, they are also referred to as *10-nm filaments*. Less is known about this category of filaments, but it is evident that it represents a very heterogeneous group of filaments made up of several different proteins that may turn out to have a variety of different functions. Table 4-3 lists the five main classes of intermediate filaments together with some cell types in which they have been demonstrated.

The intracellular localization of intermediate filaments suggests that, in many cases, they supplement microtubules in providing support and maintaining the shape of the various parts of the cell. The role of some classes of intermediate filaments seems to be to transmit pull and to ensure an equal distribution of tensile forces throughout the cell. Thus in smooth (*i.e.*, nonstriated) muscle cells, bundles of intermediate filaments transmit the pull of contraction to their sites of attachment on the cell membrane. Another example is the strong cablelike bundles of prekeratin filaments (tonofilaments) that are anchored to the cell membrane of keratinocytes in the epidermal layer of the skin. These filaments are believed to distribute tensile stresses equally throughout the keratinocyte so that it can withstand a certain amount of rough treatment. Referred to as tonofibrils, such bundles of prekeratin filaments are even large enough to be seen under the LM (see Fig. 17-5A). EM studies of the axon (the nerve fiber that propagates the impulses generated by a neuron) have established the presence of numerous fine crosslinkers interconnecting the neurofilaments, microtubules, and membranous organelles in the axon (Fig. 4-28B). Such crosslinkers are not associated with any other type of intermediate filament.

CYTOPLASMIC INCLUSIONS

Stored Foods

Of the three basic foodstuffs (carbohydrates, fats, and proteins), only carbohydrate and fat are stored in the cell as inclusions.

Carbohydrate is stored chiefly in hepatocytes and, to a lesser extent, in muscle cells and other cells. In every case, it is stored in the form of *glycogen* as free deposits in the cytoplasmic matrix. In H & E sections, glycogen is seen only as clear rough-edged spaces (see Fig. 1-12). In electron micrographs, it can appear in two different forms. *α-Particles*, found for example in chondrocytes and hepatocytes, are rosettes of moderately electron-dense particles (Fig. 4-40). *β-Particles*, found for example in muscle cells, are single discrete particles that are a little larger than a ribosome (Fig. 4-41).

Fat (lipid) is stored by the fat cells of adipose tissue (adipocytes) and the fat-storing cells of the liver (lipocytes).

Table 4-3 Comparative Distribution of the Main Classes of Intermediate Filaments

Classes of Filaments	Cell Types
1. Prekeratin (cytokeratin) (= tonofilaments)	Epithelial cells
2. Desmin (skeletin)	Muscle cells
3. Neurofilament	Neurons
4. Glial filament	Astrocytes, ependymal cells, Schwann cells, pituicytes
5. Vimentin (decamin)	Mesenchymal derivatives including endothelial cells, muscle cells, neuroectodermal derivatives including early differentiating neurons and most kinds of glial cells, immature cells, and many kinds of cells growing *in vitro*

Under certain conditions, it accumulates in other cells as well, especially in hepatocytes (see Fig. 1-13). In these cells, it is present in the form of free cytoplasmic droplets that lack a limiting membrane. The appearance of lipid droplets in H & E sections was described in Chapter 1 and is illustrated in Figure 1-13.

Pigments

Observation of normal or abnormal coloration of the various parts of the body, and knowledge of the basis for such color, can be of considerable use to the medical student. Sometimes one of the chief factors in the clinical diagnosis of a disease is the changed color of some part of the body. Color can be even more important to the pathologist than to the clinician because mention of any change in color is routinely included in reports of the gross appearance of diseased organs taken at operation or autopsy.

Color in any tissue is mainly due to the kind and amount of pigment it contains. Pigments are traditionally classified as inclusions even though in certain disease states, pigments derived from cells are present intercellularly as well as within cells. There are, of course, many colorless cellular constituents that appear colored after they have been treated with a stain, but these are not pigments. To be classified as a *pigment*, a substance has to possess some color of its own in its natural state. Hence pigments do not require any staining to be seen. They can nevertheless be colored further and, in some cases, differently by histological stains or histochemical procedures.

All pigments can be classified as either *exogenous* or *en-*

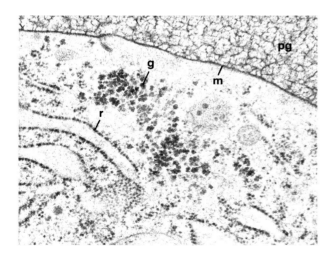

Fig. 4-40. Electron micrograph (×25,000) of part of a hypertrophied chondrocyte, showing multiparticulate rosettes of glycogen (*g*) stored in its cytoplasm. Glycogen particles have a larger diameter than ribosomes (*r*), which can be seen here bound to the rER. The extracellular material attached to the external surface of the cell membrane (*m*) is the proteoglycan network (*pg*) in cartilage matrix, preserved by freeze-substitution. (Courtesy of L. Arsenault)

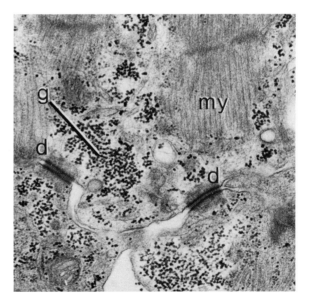

Fig. 4-41. Electron micrograph (×25,500) of part of a rat cardiac muscle cell that is storing glycogen (*g*) as single discrete particles. Also seen are myofibrils (*my*), which are the contractile elements of the cell, and desmosomes (*d*), which are the cell junctions that hold these cells together. (Courtesy of I. Taylor)

dogenous in origin. *Exogenous pigments* (Gr. *ex*, out; *genein*, to produce) are those that have been generated outside the body and subsequently taken into it by some route. *Endogenous pigments* (Gr. *endon*, within) are generated within the body from nonpigmented precursors.

Exogenous Pigments.   *Carotene* is the pigment that gives carrots their bright orange color. The carotenes are a family of fat-soluble compounds that, when taken up from foods, color body components containing fat. A familiar example is the yellow of an egg yolk, which is caused by the carotene absorbed by chickens from the food they eat. The color of butter is likewise due to the carotene in cow's milk. In dissecting the body, it is common to find that human fat tissue appears quite yellow because of its carotene content.

Several forms of carotene are provitamins and may be converted into vitamin A in the body, which is one good reason for eating fresh vegetables or drinking vegetable juices. Occasionally, however, individuals do not practice moderation in this respect. It is possible to eat so many carrots or tomatoes, or to drink so much vegetable juice, that the skin of the body takes on a yellow (or even reddish) color due to its great content of carotene. The condition caused by excessive consumption of carotene is called *carotenemia* (meaning carotene in the blood), and individuals with this condition may, at first glance, be thought to have jaundice. It is an unusual condition in adults, but it is sometimes seen in babies given too much vegetable juice.

Inhaled *dusts* can be a cause of coloration of the lungs, and it is common to find that the lungs of heavy smokers are blackened by a dense accumulation of carbon particles from the tobacco smoke they have been inhaling. Such particles are present in highly phagocytic alveolar macrophages in the walls of the lung alveoli.

Certain *minerals* taken by mouth or absorbed through the body surface can also lead to pigmentation. For example, an accumulation of silver can cause a gray pigmentation of the body, and absorbed lead can impart a blue line to the gums. *Tattoo marks* are made of inorganic pigments driven deeply into the skin with needles, where some of them become fixed in position within cells that, under the EM, appear to be dermal fibroblasts (Lea and Pawlowski). A fibroblast that contains deposits of tattoo ink particles may be seen in Figure 7-14.

Endogenous Pigments.   The most abundant endogenous pigment in the body is *hemoglobin*, the iron-containing pigment of erythrocytes that has the important function of transporting oxygen throughout the body. After four months, erythrocytes wear out and are destroyed by macrophages, whereupon their hemoglobin is degraded to two other endogenous pigments: hemosiderin, which contains iron; and bilirubin, which is free of iron. Hemosiderin is formed in secondary lysosomes from the iron-storing protein ferritin.

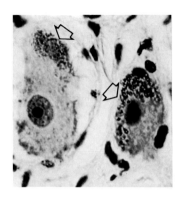

Fig. 4-42.   Photomicrograph of the cell bodies of two ganglion cells. The arrows indicate granules of lipofuscin (lipochrome pigment) in their cytoplasm.

The iron-containing pigment *hemosiderin* is golden brown and is often noticeable in spleen sections, where it is present in macrophages that are disposing of worn-out erythrocytes. The amount of hemosiderin normally present in macrophages of the spleen, bone marrow, and liver becomes greatly increased at these sites in disease states that are characterized by accelerated erythrocyte destruction.

The other pigment, *bilirubin*, is yellowish-brown. Because it contains no iron and is of no further use to the body, it is removed from the bloodstream by the liver and is voided by way of the bile. Bile is a yellow-to-brown fluid secreted by the liver, and it is stored and concentrated in the gallbladder. Eventually, it passes into the intestine, where it plays an important role in digestion and absorption. Its content of bilirubin becomes oxidized to biliverdin, which is green. However, only a small amount of biliverdin is present normally, so human bile is yellow to brown.

The brown-to-black pigment present in the skin, hair, and eyes is *melanin*. This pigment exists in two different forms called *eumelanin* and *phaeomelanin*, the colors of which are brownish-black and reddish-yellow, respectively. Redheads and blondes produce phaeomelanin. Increased amounts of melanin are formed in the skin as a direct response to the ultraviolet radiation in sunlight, and this pigment is responsible for dark skin color in black races. Melanin is also present in the substantia nigra, a part of the brain. The cells that synthesize melanin are called melanocytes. They contain tyrosinase, an enzyme that produces the colorless intermediate dopa (dihydroxyphenylalanine) from the amino acid tyrosine and then converts this intermediate into melanin.

Finally, very long-lived cells, such as neurons and cardiac muscle cells, tend to accumulate a pigment that is called *lipofuscin* (L. *fuscus*, brown) because of its lipid nature and golden brown color. Because it is a colored lipid material, this pigment is also often referred to as *lipochrome pigment*. Lipofuscin deposits are sometimes quite noticeable in LM sections (Fig. 4-42). They represent a normal end product of wear and tear that resists digestion by lysosomal enzymes and that therefore accumulates in the form of residual bodies (Fig. 4-21).

SELECTED REFERENCES

Cell Biology and Organelles

BÜCHER T, SEBALD W, WEISS H (eds): Biological Chemistry of Organelle Formation. New York, Springer-Verlag, 1980

DEDUVE C, BEAUFAY H: A short history of tissue fractionation. J Cell Biol 91:293s, 1981

FLICKINGER CJ, BROWN JC, KUTCHAI HC, OGILVIE JW: Medical Cell Biology. Philadelphia, WB Saunders, 1979

GALL JG, PORTER KR, SIEKEVITZ P (eds): Discovery in cell biology. J Cell Biol 91:1s, 1981

HOLTZMAN E, NOVIKOFF AB: Cells and Organelles, 3rd ed. Philadelphia, Saunders College Publishing, 1984

HOPKINS CR: Structure and Function of Cells. London, WB Saunders, 1978

Fine Structure of Cells and Tissues

FAWCETT DW: The Cell, 2nd ed. Philadelphia, WB Saunders, 1981

KESSEL RG, KARDON RH: Tissues and Organs: A Text-Atlas of Scanning Electron Microscopy. San Francisco, WH Freeman, 1979

PORTER KR, BONNEVILLE MA: An Introduction to the Fine Structure of Cells and Tissues, 4th ed. Philadelphia, Lea & Febiger, 1973

Cytoplasmic Matrix

PORTER KR, TUCKER JB: The ground substance of the living cell. Sci Am 244 No 3:56, 1981

WEBER K, OSBORN M: The molecules of the cell matrix. Sci Am 253 No 4:110, 1985

Cell Membrane

ALBERTS B, BRAY D, LEWIS J et al: The plasma membrane. In Molecular Biology of the Cell, p 255. New York, Garland Publishing, 1983

BRETSCHER MS: The molecules of the cell membrane. Sci Am 253 No 4:100, 1985

FOX CF: The structure of cell membranes. Sci Am 226:30, 1972

FRYE LD, EDIDIN M: The rapid intermixing of cell surface antigens after formation of mouse-human heterokaryons. J Cell Sci 7: 319, 1970

LOFTAN R, NICOLSON GL: Plasma membranes of eukaryotes. In Schwartz LM, Azar MM (eds): Advanced Cell Biology, p 129. New York, Van Nostrand Reinhold, 1981

LUCY JA: The fusion of cell membranes. Hosp Prac September, 1973

NICOLSON GL, GIOTTA G, LOTAN R et al: The membrane glycoproteins of normal and malignant cells. In Brinkley BR, Porter KR (eds): International Cell Biology 1976–1977. New York, Rockefeller University Press, 1977

NICOLSON GL, POSTE G: The cancer cell: Dynamic aspects and modifications in cell surface organization. Parts I and II. N Engl J Med 295:197, 1976; 295:253, 1976

PINTO DA SILVA P, BRANTON D: Membrane splitting in freeze-etching. J Cell Biol 45:598, 1970

RAMBOURG A, LEBLOND CP: Electron microscope observations on the carbohydrate rich cell coat present at the surface of cells in the rat. J Cell Biol 32:27, 1967

ROBERTSON JD: Membrane structure. J Cell Biol 91:189s, 1981

SINGER SJ: Proteins and membrane topography. Hosp Prac, May, 1973

SINGER SJ, NICOLSON GL: The fluid mosaic model of the structure of cell membranes. Science 175:720, 1972

Mitochondria

ERNSTER L, SCHATZ G: Mitochondria: A historical review. J Cell Biol 91:227s, 1981

GOODENOUGH U, LEVINE R: The genetic activity of mitochondria and chloroplasts. Sci Am 223:22, November, 1970

HINKLE PC, MCCARTY RE: How cells make ATP. Sci Am 238 No 3: 104, 1983

MARGULIS L: Symbiosis and evolution. Sci Am 225:48, August, 1971

MITCHELL P: Keilin's respiratory chain concept and its chemiosmotic consequences. Science 206:1148, 1979

TEDESCHI H: Mitochondria: Structure, Biogenesis and Transducing Functions. Cell Biology Monographs, Vol 4. Wein, Springer-Verlag, 1976

WHITTAKER PA, DANKS SM: Mitochondria: Structure, Function, and Assembly. New York, Longman, 1979

Ribosomes, Rough-Surfaced Endoplasmic Reticulum, and Protein Synthesis

ALBERTS B, BRAY D, LEWIS J et al: The endoplasmic reticulum. In Molecular Biology of the Cell, p 335. New York, Garland Publishing, 1983

BLOBEL G: Synthesis and segregation of secretory proteins: The signal hypothesis. In Brinkley BR, Porter KR (eds): International Cell Biology 1976–1977. New York, Rockefeller University Press, 1977

DAVIS BD, TAI PC: The mechanism of protein secretion across membranes. Nature 283:433, 1980

DEPIERRE JW, DALLNER G: Structural aspects of the membrane of the endoplasmic reticulum. Biochim Biophys Acta 415:411, 1975

JAMIESON JD, PALADE GE: Production of secretory proteins in animal cells. In Brinkley BR, Porter KR (eds): International Cell Biology 1976–1977. New York, Rockefeller University Press, 1977

LAKE JA: The ribosome. Sci Am 245 No 2:84, 1981

LEBLOND CP, WARREN KB: The Use of Radioautography in Investigating Protein Synthesis. New York, Academic Press, 1965

NONOMURA Y, BLOBEL G, SABATINI D: Structure of liver ribosomes studied by negative staining. J Mol Biol 60:303, 1971

PALADE GE: Intracellular aspects of the process of protein secretion. Science 189:347, 1975

SIEKEVITZ P, ZAMECNIK PC: Ribosomes and protein synthesis. J Cell Biol 91:53s, 1981

WALTER P, BLOBEL G: Translocation of proteins across the endoplasmic reticulum, III. Signal recognition protein (SRP) causes signal sequence-dependent and site-specific arrest of chain elongation that is released by microsomal membranes. J Cell Biol 91:557, 1981

Golgi Apparatus and GERL

ALBERTS B, BRAY D, LEWIS J et al: The Golgi apparatus. In Molecular Biology of the Cell, p 355. New York, Garland Publishing, 1983

BENNETT G: Role of the Golgi complex in the secretory process. In Cantin M (ed): Cell Biology of the Secretory Process, p 102. Basel, S Karger, 1984

BROWN WJ, FARQUHAR MG: The mannose-6-phosphate receptor for lysosomal enzymes is concentrated in *cis* Golgi cisternae. Cell 36:295, 1984

DUNPHY WG, ROTHMAN JE: Compartmental organization of the Golgi stack. Cell 42:13, 1985

FARQUHAR MG: Intracellular membrane traffic: Pathways, carriers, and sorting devices. In Fleischer S, Fleischer B (eds): Methods in Enzymology, Vol 98, Biomembranes Part L, p 1. New York, Academic Press, 1983

FARQUHAR MG, PALADE GE: The Golgi apparatus (complex)—(1954–1981)—from artifact to center stage. J Cell Biol 91:77s, 1981

HAND AR: Morphology and cytochemistry of the Golgi apparatus of rat salivary gland acinar cells. Am J Anat 130:141, 1971

HAND AR, OLIVER C: The role of the GERL in the secretory process. In Cantin M (ed): Cell Biology of the Secretory Process, p 148. Basel, S Karger, 1984

LEBLOND CP, BENNETT G: Role of the Golgi apparatus in terminal glycosylation. In Brinkley BR, Porter KR (eds): International Cell Biology 1976–1977. New York, Rockefeller University Press, 1977

NEUTRA M, LEBLOND CP: Synthesis of the carbohydrate of mucus in the Golgi complex, as shown by electron microscope radioautography of goblet cells from rats injected with ^{3}H-glucose. J Cell Biol 30:119, 1966

NOVIKOFF AB, MORI M, QUINATANA N, YAM A: Studies of the secretory process in the mammalian exocrine pancreas. I. The condensing vacuoles. J Cell Biol 75:148, 1977

NOVIKOFF AB, NOVIKOFF PM: Cytochemical contributions to differentiating GERL from the Golgi apparatus. Histochem J 9:525, 1977

NOVIKOFF PM, YAM A: Sites of lipoprotein particles in normal rat hepatocytes. J Cell Biol 76:1, 1978

RAMBOURG A, CLERMONT Y, HERMO L: Three-dimensional architecture of the Golgi apparatus in Sertoli cells of the rat. Am J Anat 154:455, 1979

RAMBOURG A, CLERMONT Y, MARRAUD A: Three-dimensional structure of the osmium-impregnated Golgi-apparatus as seen in the high voltage electron microscope. Am J Anat 140:27, 1974

ROTHMAN JE: The Golgi apparatus: Two organelles in tandem. Science 213:1212, 1981

ROTHMAN JE: The compartmental organization of the Golgi apparatus. Sci Am 253 No 3:74, 1985

Lysosomes

ALBERTS B, BRAY D, LEWIS J et al: Lysosomes and peroxisomes. In Molecular Biology of the Cell, p 367. New York, Garland Publishing, 1983

BAINTON D: Sequential degranulation of the two types of poly-

morphonuclear granules during phagocytosis of microorganisms. J Cell Biol 58:249, 1973

BAINTON DF: The discovery of lysosomes. J Cell Biol 91:66s, 1981

BAINTON DF, NICHOLS BA, FARQUHAR MG: Primary lysosomes of blood leukocytes. In Dingle JT, Dean RT (eds): Lysosomes in Biology and Pathology, Vol 5. Amsterdam, North Holland, 1976

BRADY RO: Hereditary fat metabolism diseases. Sci Am, August, 1973

BROWN WJ, FARQUHAR MG: The mannose-6-phosphate receptor for lysosomal enzymes is concentrated in *cis* Golgi cisternae. Cell 36:295, 1984

DINGLE JT, JAQUES PJ, SHAW IH (eds): Lysosomes in Biology and Pathology, Vol 6. Frontiers of Biology, Vol 48. Amsterdam, Elsevier/North-Holland Biomedical Press, 1979

HIRSCH JG: Lysosomes and mental retardation. Quart Rev Biol 47:303, 1972

HOLTZMAN E: Lysosomes: A Survey. Cell Biology Monographs Vol 3. Wein, Springer-Verlag, 1976

NOVIKOFF AB: Lysosomes: A personal account. In Hers G, Van Hoof F (eds): Lysosomes and Storage Diseases, p 1. New York, Academic Press, 1973

Endocytosis and Coated Vesicles

ANDERSON RGW, KAPLAN J: Receptor-mediated endocytosis. In Satir BH (ed): Modern Cell Biology, Vol 1. New York, Alan R Liss Inc, 1983

DAUTRY-VARSAT A, LODISH HF: How receptors bring proteins and particles into cells. Sci Am 250 No 5:52, 1984

GOLDSTEIN JL, ANDERSON RGW, BROWN MS: Coated pits, coated vesicles, and receptor-mediated endocytosis. Nature 279:679, 1979

GOLDSTEIN JL, ANDERSON RGW, BROWN MS: Receptor-mediated endocytosis and the cellular uptake of low density lipoprotein. In Membrane Recycling. Ciba Foundation Symposium 92:77, 1982

GOLDSTEIN JL, BROWN MS, ANDERSON RGW: The low-density lipoprotein pathway in human fibroblasts. Biochemical and ultrastructural correlations. In Brinkley BR, Porter KR (eds): International Cell Biology 1976–1977. New York, Rockefeller University Press, 1977

HEUSER J, EVANS L: Three dimensional visualization of coated vesicle formation in fibroblasts. J Cell Biol 84:560, 1980

Peroxisomes

DEDUVE C: Microbodies in the living cell. Sci Am No 5 248:74, 1983

KINDL H, LAZAROW PB (eds): Peroxisomes and glyoxysomes. Ann NY Acad Sci 386:1, 1982

Smooth Endoplasmic Reticulum

BLACK WH: The development of smooth surfaced endoplasmic reticulum in adrenal cortical cells of fetal guinea pig. Am J Anat 135:381, 1972

CARDELL RR: Smooth endoplasmic reticulum in rat hepatocytes during glycogen deposition and depletion. Int Rev Cytol 48:221, 1977

CARDELL RR, JR, BADENHAUSEN S, PORTER KR: Intestinal triglyceride absorption in the rat. An electron microscopical study. J Cell Biol 34:123, 1967

HIGGINS JA, BARRNETT RJ: Studies on the biogenesis of smooth endoplasmic reticulum membranes in livers of phenobarbital treated rats. J Cell Biol 55:282, 1972

KAPPAS A, ALVARES AP: How the liver metabolizes foreign substances. Sci Am 232:22, June, 1975

MARGOLIS RN, CARDELL RR, CURNOW RT: Association of glycogen synthase phosphatase and phosphorylase phosphatase activities with membranes of hepatic smooth endoplasmic reticulum. J Cell Biol 83:348, 1979

Microtubules

BORGERS M, DEBRABANDER M (eds): Microtubules and Microtubule Inhibitors. Amsterdam, North Holland, 1975

DUSTIN P: Microtubules. Berlin, Springer-Verlag, 1978

DUSTIN P: Microtubules. Sci Am 243(2):67, 1980

GOLDMAN R, POLLARD T, ROSENBAUM J (eds): Cell Motility. Book C. Microtubules and Related Proteins. Cold Spring Harbor Conferences on Cell Proliferation, Vol 3. Cold Spring Harbor, NY, Cold Spring Harbor Laboratory, 1976

MARGOLIS RL, WILSON L: Microtubule treadmills—possible molecular machinery. Nature 293:705, 1981

OLMSTED JB, BORISY GG: Microtubules. Ann Rev Biochem p 507, 1973

TILNEY LG, BRYAN J, BUSCH DJ et al: Microtubules: Evidence for 13 protofilaments. J Cell Biol 59:267, 1973

YAMADA KM, SPOONER BS, WESSELS NK: Axon growth: Roles of microfilaments and microtubules. Proc Natl Acad Sci USA 66: 1206, 1970

Cilia, Flagella, and Centrioles

ALBRECHT-BUEHLER G: Does the geometric design of centrioles imply their function? Cell Motility 1:237, 1981

BROKAW CJ, VERDUGO P (eds): Mechanism and Control of Ciliary Movement. Progress in Clinical and Biological Research, Vol 80. New York, Alan R Liss, 1981

GIBBONS IR: Structure and function of flagellar microtubules. In Brinkley BR, Porter KR (eds): International Cell Biology 1976–1977. New York, Rockefeller University Press, 1977

KALNINS VI, PORTER KR: Centriole replication during ciliogenesis in the chick tracheal epithelium. Z Zellforsch 100:1, 1969

OLMSTED JB: Microtubules and Flagella. In Brinkley BR, Porter KR (eds): International Cell Biology 1976–1977. New York, Rockefeller University Press, 1977

SLEIGH MA (ed): Cilia and Flagella. London, Academic Press, 1974

STRACHER A (ed): Muscle and Nonmuscle Motility, Vol 2. New York, Academic Press, 1983

SUMMERS KE, GIBBONS IR: Adenosine triphosphate-induced sliding of tubules in trypsin treated flagella of sea urchin sperm. Proc Natl Acad Sci USA 68:3092, 1971

WHEATLEY DN: The Centriole: A Central Enigma of Cell Biology. New York, Elsevier, 1982

WOLFE J: Basal body fine structure and chemistry. Adv Cell Molec Biol 2:151, 1972

Filaments

GILBERT D: 10 nm Filaments. Nature 272:577, 1978

GOLDMAN R, POLLARD T, ROSENBAUM J (eds): Cell Motility. Book A.

Motility, Muscle and Non-muscle Cells and Book B Actin, Myosin and Associated Proteins. Cold Spring Harbor Conferences on Cell Proliferation, Vol 3. Cold Spring Harbor, NY, Cold Spring Harbor Laboratory, 1976

GROSCHEL-STEWART U, DRENCKHAHN D: Muscular and cytoplasmic contractile proteins. Coll Relat Res 2:381, 1982

HIROKAWA N: Cross-linker system between neurofilaments, microtubules, and membranous organelles in frog axons revealed by the quick-freeze, deep-etching method. J Cell Biol 94:129, 1982

HIROKAWA N, TILNEY LG, FUJIWARA K, HEUSER JE: Organization of actin, myosin, and intermediate filaments in the brush border of intestinal epithelial cells. J Cell Biol 94:425, 1982

HUXLEY HE: The relevance of studies on muscle to problems of cell motility. In Cell Motility Book A Motility, Muscle and Non-muscle Cells. Cold Spring Harbor Conferences on Cell Proliferation, Vol 3. Cold Spring Harbor Laboratory, 1976

INOUÉ S, STEPHENS RE (eds): Molecules and Cell Movement. Society of General Physiologists Series, Vol 30. New York, Raven Press, 1975

MCINTOSH JR (ed): Modern Cell Biology, Vol 2: Spatial Organization of Eukaryotic Cells. New York, Alan R Liss, 1983

MOOSEKER MS, BONDER EM, CONZELMAN KA et al: Brush border cytoskeleton and integration of cellular functions. J Cell Biol 99: 104s, 1984

POLLARD TD: Cytoplasmic contractile proteins. In Brinkley BR, Porter KR (eds): International Cell Biology 1976–1977. New York, Rockefeller University Press, 1977

STEINERT PM, JONES JCR, GOLDMAN RD: Intermediate filaments. J Cell Biol 99:22s, 1984

TAYLOR DL: Dynamics of cytoplasmic structure and contractility. In Brinkley BR, Porter KR (eds): International Cell Biology 1976–1977. New York, Rockefeller University Press, 1977

TILNEY LG: Actin: Its association with membranes and the regulation of its polymerization. In Brinkley BR, Porter KR (eds): International Cell Biology 1976–1977. New York, Rockefeller University Press, 1977

WESSELS NK: How living cells change their shape. Sci Am 225:76, 1971

Cytoplasmic Inclusions

BIAVA C: Identification and structural forms of human particulate glycogen. Lab Invest 12:1179, 1963

CRICHTON RR: Ferritin: Structure, synthesis, and function. N Engl J Med 284:1413, 1971

FRANK AL, CHRISTENSEN AK: Localization of acid phosphatase in lipofuscin granules and possible autophagic vacuoles in interstitial cells of the guinea pig testis. J Cell Biol 36:1, 1968

LEA PJ, PAWLOWSKI A: Human tattoo: Electron microscopic assessment of epidermal epidermo-dermal junction and dermis. Int J Dermatol (in press)

MALKOFF D, STREHLER B: The ultrastructure of isolated and in situ human cardiac age pigment. J Cell Biol 16:611, 1963

REVEL JP: Electron microscopy of glycogen. J Histochem Cytochem 12:104, 1964

SENIOR JR: Intestinal absorption of fats. J Lipid Res 5:495, 1964

5

Cellular Differentiation and Proliferation

TERMINOLOGY AND PRINCIPLES OF CELLULAR DIFFERENTIATION

CELLULAR PROLIFERATION IS INTRINSICALLY REGULATED IN NORMAL CELLS BUT NOT IN NEOPLASTIC CELLS

Oncogenes Have the Potential to Transform Normal Cells into Neoplastic Cells

Cellular Proliferation Is Also Extrinsically Regulated

Growth Regulators

EMBRYONIC DEVELOPMENT OF THE FOUR BASIC TISSUES

All of the many different types of cells found in the human body originate from a single cell, the fertilized ovum. As the embryonic cells arising from the fertilized ovum increase in number, they embark on orderly programs of differentiation that result in development of the various tissues of the body. In this chapter, we shall describe the fundamental pattern of tissue development that emerges, but before doing so, it is necessary to introduce and explain some basic terms and principles.

TERMINOLOGY AND PRINCIPLES OF CELLULAR DIFFERENTIATION

The *potentiality* of a cell is the sum total of all its latent capabilities, including every capability that will ever be expressed by the progeny of that cell but that cell itself may not yet have had occasion to manifest. Hence a cell's potentiality denotes its capacity for giving rise to cells of other types. The fertilized ovum, for example, is *totipotential* because it is the ancestral cell from which every kind of cell in the body is derived. But for how many cell generations does totipotentiality persist in its descendants?

Commonly, the two daughter cells resulting from the cell's first mitotic division adhere to one another, and both contribute to the subsequent development of an embryo. But occasionally after this division, the two daughter cells separate and each develops into an embryo; this, of course, results in the development of identical twins and shows that after one division, both daughter cells retain totipotentiality. Furthermore, the first four cells all may occasionally separate, resulting in the birth of identical quadruplets. Very rarely, five identical quintuplets are born—all of which shows that through the first three mitotic divisions, the cellular descendants of the fertilized ovum can retain totipotentiality. But if daughter cells remain together and cell division continues, the formation of a clump of cells called a *morula* (L. *morus,* mulberry) (see Fig. 5-1A) is soon formed. The cells of the clump destined to become body cells become different from one another, generally more or less imperceptibly, and in so doing cease to be totipotential. Cells with diminished potentiality that become different from their cells of origin are described as having undergone some degree of *differentiation*. Thus as a result of differentiation, cells gain new attributes but lose some of their former potentiality. The characteristic properties of each distinctive type of cell in the body reflect which particular genes are being expressed by that type of cell in postnatal life. The distinctive structural and functional features of the majority of differentiated cell types, often referred to as their *phenotype* (Gr. *phainein*, to show; *typos*, type), remain relatively stable under ordinary circumstances. Certain types of cells do, however, undergo limited changes in phenotypic expression, and this is referred to as *phenotypic modulation* (L. *modulatus*, regulated or arranged). Phenotypic modulation can occur without any accompanying loss of potentiality.

There is one notable exception to the generalization that cells arising from the fertilized ovum undergo differentiation and thereupon lose some of their potentiality: the cells that are destined to be *germ cells* retain their totipotentiality.

Thus among the cells of the early female embryo, there are certain cells that do not undergo any differentiation. As the embryo develops, these cells proliferate and migrate in large numbers to the developing ovaries, where, after puberty, they begin to develop further into mature female germ cells. That such cells retain totipotentiality is demonstrated not only by their capacity for producing ova that develop into embryos if fertilized but also by the fact that on occasion a diploid germ cell precursor may give rise to a multi-tissue ovarian tumor in the total absence of any fertilization. Such a tumor, which is called a *teratoma* (Gr. *teras*, monster), commonly becomes large enough to require surgical excision. The cut surface of a teratoma discloses a hodgepodge of the various kinds of tissues normally found in the body. Bits of skin, hair, ill-formed teeth, and pieces of bone and cartilage may all be present, along with some nervous tissue, parts of eyes, and so on. Obviously, the cell from which the tumor arose was totipotential, but the cells and tissues that arose from it failed to develop in the orderly manner that characterizes normal embryonic development. A teratoma can similarly arise from a totipotential germ cell precursor in the testis.

It is now accepted that every cell in the body has the same gene complement. When totipotential cells give rise to committed cells with restricted potentialities, the appropriate genes are maintained in a transcriptionally active state while the remainder are selectively inactivated. This is one of the main reasons why over 90% of the chromatin in the interphase nucleus is present in the condensed state.

Cytoplasmic Factors Are Believed to Play a Role in Cell Determination. There is a certain amount of experimental evidence to suggest that conditions in the cell cytoplasm play a role in acquisition and maintenance of the differentiated state. Unlike the meticulous segregation of mitotic chromosomes, which ensures that both daughter cells will receive precisely the same gene complement, the cytoplasm of a cell does not always divide equally in either a quantitative or a qualitative sense. It has long been known that the daughter cells arising at the earliest stages of embryonic development receive unequal amounts of cytoplasm. Moreover, the daughter cells that receive different portions of the cytoplasm of the fertilized ovum differentiate into different kinds of cells.

It is often assumed that if the daughter cells that result from later developmental or postnatal divisions become different from each other, this difference is due to their being exposed to different microenvironments. However, there is reason to suspect that this is not always the sole factor involved. For example, it has been established that in the grasshopper, when a neuroblast (nerve cell progenitor) divides, one of its daughter cells differentiates into a neuron whereas the other daughter cell remains a neuroblast. In an experiment reported in 1953, Carlson inverted a neuroblast mitotic spindle so that the chromosomes that would ordinarily have reached one pole would segregate to the other pole instead, and vice versa. However, this manipulation made no difference to the outcome: the cell expected to become a neuroblast still became a neuroblast, and the cell expected to differentiate still became a neuron. The implication of this finding is that here again, qualitative differences exist between the regions of cytoplasm at the two poles of the dividing cell, and that the cytoplasmic conditions passed on to one of the daughter cells are conducive to terminal neuronal differentiation whereas those passed on to the other daughter cell are essentially unchanged.

Steroid hormone levels and other microenvironmental influences nevertheless exert important effects on gene expression in postnatal life. Cells that are environmentally responsive are described as being *competent*. Cells that do not alter their phenotype in response to environmental influences are described as *determined* or *committed* cells.

The keratinizing cells of the epidermis (the epithelial part of the skin), for example, are cells that are *determined*. This occasionally creates an awkward situation when the plastic surgeon transplants skin from one site on the body to another. At its new site, the piece of transplanted skin continues to manifest the same features (for example, hair) that it had at its former site. However, if tissue that gives rise to a particular kind of skin is transplanted to some other site on the embryo, it produces skin of the type that would be expected to develop at the transplantation site. The cells of such tissue, being *competent*, respond to environmental influences that alter gene expression and make it different from tissue left at its normal site on the embryo.

Finally, because each progressive step in differentiation is accompanied by a certain loss of potentiality, differentiating cells become increasingly determined. Like differentiation, determination occurs in steps. Hence all end cells are determined, but not all determined cells are end cells. Even stem cells are determined because the number of different cell types they can produce is limited.

It is not difficult to accept that the daughter cells of a cell that has become determined would be similarly determined, but little is known about the mechanism whereby such determination is passed on from one cell generation to the next. It seems improbable that the active genes in the mother cell give rise directly to the active genes in the daughter cells because all the nuclear DNA has to be replicated, and in the process, all the genes on every DNA molecule, including genes that have been inactivated as condensed chromatin, become replicated. A more likely explanation is that the specific gene-regulatory proteins made by the mother cell continue to exert identical effects on the daughter cells. Thus continuation of each specific line of determination may be due to the gene-regulatory proteins that are present in the cytoplasm of the mother cell when it divides.

Evidence confirming that the intracytoplasmic environment retains a profound influence on gene expression comes from cell fusion experiments and studies in which the nucleus of one kind of cell is introduced into the enucleated cytoplasm of another kind of cell (*i.e.*, one that is differently determined). For example, if an erythrocyte nucleus of a chick (a species in which erythrocytes retain their nucleus) is introduced into the cytoplasm of some other type of cell taken from the chick, rat, or man, its inactive globin genes are reexpressed. The pattern of cytoplasmic regulation of gene expression is, however, somewhat unpredictable, because fusion of an entire rat myoblast (muscle cell precursor) with an entire mouse fibroblast leads to the production of a cell hybrid that is fibroblastlike, but introduction of a rat myoblast nucleus into enucleated cytoplasm of a mouse fibroblast produces a cell hybrid that, after fusing with other similar cells, differentiates into a muscle fiber (Ringertz et al). The latter result could simply reflect the fact that the cytoplasm of a differentiated fibroblast does not contain enough regulatory protein to redirect determination toward a fibroblastlike phenotype, or it might indicate that certain forms of determination are more stable and less susceptible to experimental manipulation than others.

We shall next consider the relation between cellular differentiation and cellular proliferation and address the subject of neoplasia, which will be of particular interest to those studying medicine.

CELLULAR PROLIFERATION IS INTRINSICALLY REGULATED IN NORMAL CELLS BUT NOT IN NEOPLASTIC CELLS

When discussing cell renewal in Chapter 3, we noted that, as a general rule, the higher the level of differentiation that a cell attains, the less likelihood there is that it will retain the capacity for mitosis. Indeed, certain types of very highly differentiated cells have totally relinquished all capacity for proliferation. There must therefore be some intrinsic mechanism within the cell that determines its extent of growth and proliferation, without which the body presumably would become too large and inefficient. Moreover, if such intrinsic regulation were to become inoperative, a cell would continue to proliferate until its progeny encroached too far on some vital part of the body. This is evidently what happens in *cancer*.

Cancers are more accurately described as *neoplasms* (Gr. *neos*, new; *plassein*, to form), a term that denotes the important fact that they represent growths of *new* (*i.e., abnormal*) cells in the body. Because neoplasms may form lumps, they are commonly referred to as *tumors* (L. *tumere*, to swell) even though swellings result from other causes as well (*e.g.*, a bump on the head, which becomes distended with fluid exudate). Hence most of the swellings seen by general practitioners are not neoplasms. Furthermore, some tumors are benign overgrowths that are not invasive. The present discussion concerns *malignant* tumors, which are more dangerous because they are invasive and can spread.

It is perhaps not surprising that continuously proliferating cancer cells rarely approach the level of differentiation attained by their normal counterparts. Indeed, microscopic assessment of the level of differentiation attained by different cancers is one of the criteria used to predict their relative malignancy. Thus the constituent cells of many types of malignant tumors are described as exhibiting *anaplasia* (Gr. *ana*, up, backward), which means that they appear less differentiated than their normal counterparts, and certain malignant tumors are described as being *undifferentiated*. In general, then, the differentiation of neoplastic cells is impaired, but their proliferation is unrestricted.

Neoplastic cells also manifest deficient regulation of their movement *in vitro*. Normal cells maintained *in vitro* eventually establish enough intercellular adhesions to stabilize all movement, a phenomenon known as *contact inhibition of movement*. Such contact inhibition, to a variable extent, is lacking in neoplastic cells, which never stop climbing over normal cells when both are grown *in vitro*. Furthermore, normal cells eventually stop dividing under *in vitro* conditions; their saturation density depends on the serum concentration in the culture medium. Such *density-dependent inhibition of growth* is considered to be a manifestation of growth-factor dependency and an indication that these factors eventually become depleted from the medium. Because neoplastic cells exhibit an autonomous pattern of growth, their proliferative capacity is not restricted by the availability of such factors and they continue to proliferate indefinitely, piling up on the floor of the culture vessel.

Malignant transformation is believed to be a consequence of critical genetic changes in the cell. Suggestions as to what these critical changes could be include the rearrangement of certain genes, the occurrence of one or more criticalpoint mutations, or any combination of such changes that might lead to the loss of normal regulation of cellular proliferation. The proliferative capacity of normal human cells appears to be limited to a maximum of about 50 population doublings, as determined for human embryonic fibroblasts grown *in vitro* (Hayflick). However, mutants capable of more sustained proliferation will occasionally emerge from normal cell populations growing *in vitro*. Moreover, many agents that are mutagenic when tested in bacteria are also carcinogenic when tested in laboratory animals, suggesting that in certain cases at least, carcinogenesis may be traced to some kind of mutation. However, the extensive damage done to DNA by mutagens would be expected to create an enormous number of different variants, only a small surviving fraction of which would ever progress as far as expressing malignant behavior.

Another known cause of malignant transformation is infection with *oncogenic viruses* (Gr. *onkos,* mass or tumor), which include both *DNA tumor viruses* and *RNA tumor viruses.* Genes of DNA tumor viruses become integrated directly into the genome of the cells they infect. In the case of RNA tumor viruses, however, DNA copies of the viral RNA must first be produced by means of a viral enzyme called *reverse transcriptase,* and these copies then become integrated into the genome of the infected cells. But how can active expression of a cancer-causing viral gene induce malignant transformation? The answer to this question is finally beginning to come to light in the case of RNA tumor viruses. It now appears that each of these viruses carries an activated transforming gene known as an *oncogene* that it derived from cells it infected. Hence the transforming genes carried by RNA tumor viruses are actually of *cellular* origin. The relevance and importance of this remarkable class of cellular genes to medical cell biology warrant the following further discussion.

Oncogenes Have the Potential to Transform Normal Cells into Neoplastic Cells

Powerful new gene transfer techniques and molecular cloning methods now make it possible to characterize the specific base sequences of individual genes. Furthermore, it has recently been established that a number of vertebrate genes possess *transforming* (*oncogenic*) potential, meaning that the cells that express them may undergo malignant transformation. Once acquired, the transformed state can then be inherited as a dominant trait with the result that all the progeny of the transformed cell are malignant, too.

It is now evident from *in vitro* studies that tumor cell DNA has the capacity to transform normal cells into permanently malignant cells. The dominant transforming sequences responsible for such malignant transformation are termed *oncogenes*. Detailed base sequence analysis has disclosed extensive homology between (1) cellular dominant transforming genes (*c-oncogenes*) identified in the DNA of specific types of vertebrate tumor cells and (2) viral dominant transforming genes (*v-oncogenes*) identified in specific types of RNA tumor viruses. Both of these classes of transforming genes seem to have arisen from the same small repertoire of normal ancestral cellular genes, which are accordingly termed *proto-oncogenes*. The transduction of proto-oncogenes into RNA tumor viruses was an evolutionary development that turned out to have far-reaching consequences because it was the study of these viruses that first brought the tumorigenic potential of oncogenes to light.

The normal nontransforming roles of most cellular oncogenes are still largely unknown, but because these particular genes are evidently of ancient origin and were conserved throughout evolution to the vertebrates, it is widely believed that their normal functions must have been of vital importance to the organism. Evidence is now accumulating that the gene products of cellular oncogenes play key roles in regulating cellular proliferation.

Inappropriate Expression of Oncogenes Can Result in Malignant Transformation. Although every different type of cell in the body receives an identical gene complement, each individual cell type expresses its own particular gene combination. Gene expression by any given type of cell may also vary over the lifetime of an individual because some genes are active at certain stages but not at others. Thus genes required for the rapid embryonic development of a tissue could become less active during adult life in accordance with an orderly program of prenatal development and postnatal function. Furthermore, the reactivation of such genes is postnatal life could prove highly detrimental to the complex internal organization of the body. What then might reactivate oncogenes in adult life, and why would this aberrant oncogene expression lead to the development of a tumor?

Various types of chromosomal aberrations are known to occur in malignant cells; those most frequently reported are translocations and aneuploidy. In the present context, translocations could be very significant. It has been found that if a cellular oncogene becomes translocated to a site where DNA is being transcribed very actively, its expression comes under the influence of the new set of genes and transcriptional control elements now situated in its vicinity. For example, transposition of an inactive *c-myc* oncogene to a transcriptionally active immunoglobulin gene-bearing domain on another chromosome can activate (derepress) this oncogene and lead to the malignant transformation of cells of the B-lymphocyte lineage. Oncogene translocation can also be found in some cases of chronic myelogenous leukemia. Such examples suggest that oncogenes can be activated postnatally by chromosomal rearrangements that fortuitously enhance their transcription. Aneuploidy might also be expected to interfere with the normal regulation of cellular proliferation in cases in which the loss or gain of entire chromosomes results in a critical loss, overproduction, or imbalance of essential growth regulators or their receptors.

It is now known that oncogenes manifest their latent transforming potential under two different sets of circumstances. First, the antecedent proto-oncogene may have undergone a *mutation* that results in some crucial *qualitative* change in the structure and function of the gene product. Such a structural alteration in the gene has been shown to be the case in development of carcinoma of the human bladder. In this case, the active oncogene (*ras*) differs from the proto-oncogene from which it arose by only a simple point mutation that results in a single amino acid substitution in its gene product (Reddy et al; Tabin et al). Certain other malignancies are characterized by increased postnatal levels of the oncogene product caused by enhanced gene expression. Such a *quantitative* change in oncogene expression can reflect either a specific *enhancement* of transcriptional activity or an *amplification* of the total number of oncogene copies present in the cell. Thus in the case of tumors arising from cells of the B-lymphocyte lineage, sustained oncogene expression can be the result of translocation of an oncogene to the vicinity of the enhancer region of an active immunoglobulin domain. Such rearrangement effectively deregulates the oncogene *c-myc*, leading to an increase in its expression. In acute promyelocytic leukemia and certain other tumors, on the other hand, there is evidence that excessive oncogene expression is an outcome of 30- to 50-fold amplification of the number of oncogene copies per cell.

Aberrant or unregulated postnatal expression of oncogenes somehow deranges the manner in which cellular proliferation is regulated, setting the stage for a malignancy to develop. Yet there is ample evidence to indicate that tumorigenesis is a multistage process. Postnatal oncogene activation may therefore represent only one of the crucial steps that ultimately lead to the development of cancer. The extent to which oncogene expression is involved in development of the many different forms of human cancer and the essential nature of such involvement are naturally issues that are currently of great concern.

The Roles of Cellular Oncogenes in Normal Cells Remain to Be Elucidated. Although the expression of some oncogenes appears to be specific to certain cell types, the oncogenes *c-ras* and *c-myc* are expressed by a variety of different tumors, indicating their more general involvement in malignant transformation. The recent discovery that these two widely detected oncogenes can collaborate with each other in the course of tumorigenesis has led to the view that autonomously growing tumors may arise from precancerous growths as a consequence of specific forms of cooperative or complementary gene expression. Furthermore, all tumors that arise from different stages of a given cell lineage do not necessarily express the same oncogenes. It is interesting that *c-myc*, the oncogene expressed in promyelocytic leukemia cells, reverts to the inactive state if these cells are induced to undergo terminal differentiation into mature granulocytes. Furthermore, oncogenes are expressed differentially during normal prenatal and early postnatal development in the mouse. Also, the level of expression of *c-ras* increases when the liver undergoes regeneration in the rat. Finally, the gene products encoded by certain human oncogenes have sequences in common with a cell-cycle regulator of yeast. Such observations are now interpreted as indicating that in normal cells, cellular oncogenes play a fundamental role in regulating cellular growth and proliferation. A regulatory role of such extreme importance would, of course, explain the extent to which these particular genes have been conserved over the course of evolution. Indeed, several of them have now been traced back to *Drosophila* and even to yeast.

Accordingly, cellular oncogenes are thought of as a family of genes collectively responsible for the normal intrinsic regulation of cellular proliferation. Their products range from growth factors and responding transducers that are associated with the cytoplasmic aspect of the cell membrane to nuclear matrix components that could be involved in regulating gene transcription. Hence cellular proliferation is believed to be regulated by the components of a *mitogenic pathway*, which is an interactive network or chain of command incorporating cellular oncogene products that extends all the way from the cell surface to the interior of the nucleus.

There is already a substantial basis for speculation as to what the normal roles of certain cellular oncogenes might be. For example, the polypeptide gene product of *c-sis* (which is the cellular counterpart of the oncogene carried by simian sarcoma virus) manifests a marked degree of structural homology and functional similarity to the platelet-derived growth factor (PDGF) released from platelet granules during blood clotting (Doolittle et al; Waterfield et al). PDGF is a potent mitogen for many different kinds of mesenchymally derived cells and is believed to play a key role in repair processes. If responsive cells were to begin producing inappropriate endogenous levels of such growth regulators, this could lead to autonomous (*autocrine*) stimulation of their own proliferation. Transforming polypeptide growth factors isolated from tumor cells show extensive amino acid–sequence homology with EGF, an epidermal growth factor that regulates the proliferation of epidermal cells (Marquardt et al). Furthermore, the protein encoded by the viral oncogene of avian erythroblastosis virus is closely similar to a portion of the EGF receptor. The gene product encoded by the *ras* oncogene complexes with the transferrin receptor and has been localized to the cytoplasmic aspect of the cell membrane. Transferrin is an iron-binding protein that acts as a growth regulator. Because transferrin receptors are found on proliferating normal cells as well as on malignant cells, it is possible that aberrant expression of the *ras* oncogene may interfere with normal growth regulation by way of the transferrin receptor.

It is particularly interesting that the products of several oncogenes are so closely similar to growth regulators or their cell-surface receptors. Moreover, a minor structural alteration or inappropriate increase in the level of expression of any gene that codes for a growth regulator or its receptor could conceivably enable a cell to escape from the normal constraints on its proliferation, enabling it to take on a totally autonomous existence. These studies on oncogenes also suggest that there may be fewer common molecular pathways leading to oncogenesis than formerly supposed.

Summary. A heterogeneous family of cellular genes called oncogenes manifests the potential for malignant transformation. Untimely postnatal expression or overexpression of one or more of these genes can lead to the development of a malignancy, ostensibly through failure or deregulation of the normal constraints on cellular proliferation. Oncogene expression in some malignancies is a reflection of augmented transcription. In other cases, there is a slight qualitative alteration in the molecular composition of the oncogene product that presumably interferes with its normal regulatory function in the cell. There are indications that cellular oncogenes may be involved in regulating cellular proliferation during normal development and growth of the body.

Next, we shall briefly consider some of the extrinsic mechanisms by means of which the body continuously regulates the size of its various cell populations and organs.

Cellular Proliferation Is Also Extrinsically Regulated

A characteristic of the body that has long been recognized is the truly remarkable stability of its internal environment. To a large extent this stability is dependent on adequate proliferative control of the cell populations that make up its various tissues, organs, and body systems. For example, the required numbers of each individual type of cell in the blood have to be maintained even though all blood cells ultimately need to be replaced when they deteriorate or die. In other words, cell production has to compensate exactly for cell loss. Also, the various organs of the body need to be kept fairly constant in size to maintain appropriate levels of function. How, then, are the respective numbers and functional activities of the various types of specialized cells regulated? In many instances, changes in the level of demand for their respective functional activities, including any requirements for more cells, are monitored and signaled to them by cells of a different type. Commonly, this is achieved through some type of humoral mechanism mediated by either a hormone or a growth regulator.

Growth Regulators

Cellular proliferation is subject to extrinsic regulation by *growth regulators* produced elsewhere in the body. More is currently known about mitogenic growth regulators than about proliferation inhibitors. Some polypeptides and proteins known to act as mitogenic growth stimulators are (1) *epidermal growth factor* (EGF), the effectiveness of which is potentiated by (2) the hormone *insulin,* in addition to which there are (3) *platelet-derived growth factor* (PDGF), (4) *fibroblast-derived growth factor* (FDGF), (5) *nerve growth factor* (NGF), and (6) a small group of *insulin-like growth factors.* Research in the field of growth regulation is progressing rapidly and is yielding information that has broad implications for medical cell biology. For a representative survey of investigative advances in elucidating the roles and modes of action of growth regulators, see Mozes et al. In addition to the growth regulators just mentioned, blood cell progenitors, of which there are numerous different kinds, require their own complex system of specific growth regulators to enable them to produce the necessary population size of each type of blood cell and still maintain the appropriate balance between cell renewal and differentiation. Discussion of this group of regulators will be deferred until we deal with myeloid tissue in Chapter 9.

Less is known about proliferation inhibitors, but they appear to play a particularly important role in those tissues and organs with populations of cells that are not in active cycle. Regeneration studies of organs such as the liver have provided clear-cut evidence that the total mass of their constituent cell populations is regulated with great precision. For example, investigations in experimental animals have shown that the surgical removal of up to two thirds of the liver is followed by rapid and precise restoration of this organ to its former mass.

A number of different growth regulators are believed to participate in liver regeneration. There is also a concept known as the *chalone hypothesis* (Gr. *chalan,* to relax), the first experimental evidence for which was reported by Bullough and Laurence, who were working on epidermis in the 1960s. According to this hypothesis, mitotic activity can be shut down in organs or tissues by a tissue-specific proliferation inhibitor termed a *chalone* that is produced by the *same* tissue. Thus a chalone is essentially a hypothetical endogenous growth inhibitor, the local levels of which are believed to decline as further mitotic activity becomes necessary (*e.g.,* during healing or regeneration). It is not known whether the chalone would inhibit mitosis directly or indirectly. The quest for chalones is beset with difficulties, and the evidence for their existence is equivocal. Furthermore, the number of studies that document enough screening to show that the proliferation inhibitor is absolutely tissue specific is remarkably small. Nevertheless, a cytosolic *hepatic proliferation inhibitor* that could represent a chalone has recently been isolated from rat liver and purified to homogeneity (Iype and McMahon). It is a protein with a molecular weight of 26,000 daltons that specifically inhibits the DNA synthesis and proliferation of normal rat hepatocytes, but does not have this effect on transformed liver cells. However, from an operational point of view, it would be difficult to distinguish between a locally acting chalone and a long-range negative regulator that passes into the circulation and rapidly reaches target cells in all regions of the liver by way of its rich blood supply.

The evidence for chalones is controversial and difficult to evaluate. Despite claims to the contrary, it is often stated that neither the existence nor the specificity of chalones has ever been proved satisfactorily. The main problem lies in demonstrating the properties that distinguish a chalone from any other kind of negative growth regulator, the existence of which has never seriously been doubted. In any event, there seems to be no reason to assume that tissue-specific chalones represent exclusive or even primary regulators of cellular proliferation. Proliferative control evidently requires a multiplicity of growth regulators, some positive and some negative. Intrinsic as well as extrinsic regulation is obviously important because the extrinsic mechanisms that normally regulate cellular proliferation fail to do so in neoplastic disease.

EMBRYONIC DEVELOPMENT OF THE FOUR BASIC TISSUES

This last part of the chapter deals with the developmental origins of the four basic tissues, namely, epithelium, connective tissue, nervous tissue, and muscle tissue. It is intended primarily for readers who have not yet studied embryology. We shall begin by tracing the embryonic origins of the three *germ layers* that give rise to these basic tissues.

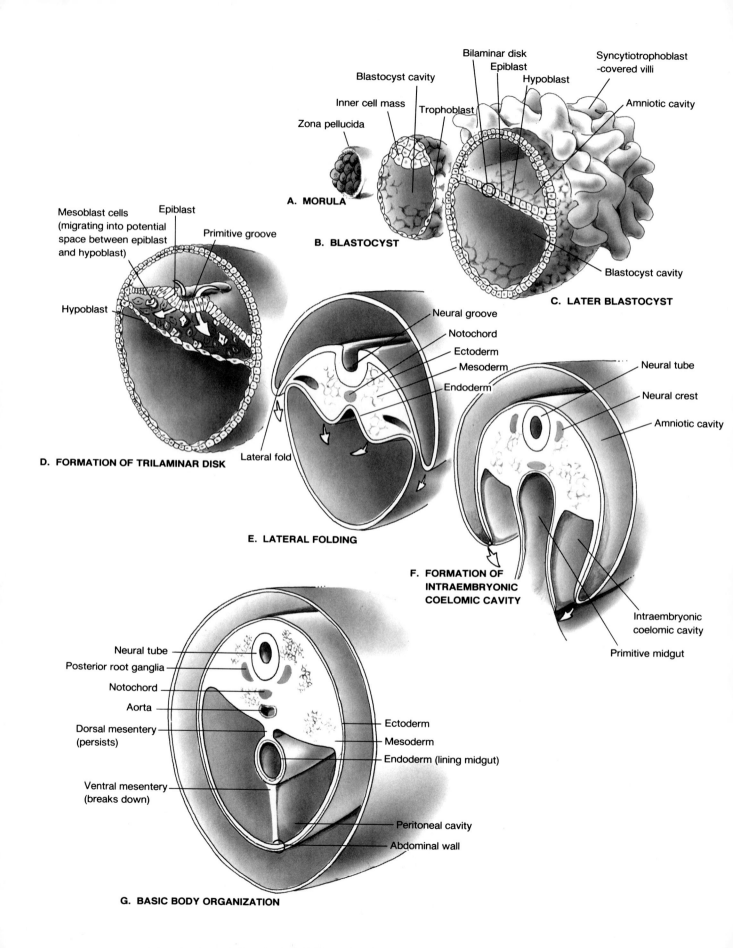

Zona pellucida

Inner cell mass

Blastocyst cavity

Trophoblast

A. MORULA

Bilaminar disk
Epiblast
Hypoblast

Syncytiotrophoblast -covered villi

Amniotic cavity

B. BLASTOCYST

Blastocyst cavity

C. LATER BLASTOCYST

Mesoblast cells (migrating into potential space between epiblast and hypoblast)

Epiblast

Primitive groove

Hypoblast

D. FORMATION OF TRILAMINAR DISK

Neural groove
Notochord
Ectoderm
Mesoderm
Endoderm

Lateral fold

E. LATERAL FOLDING

Neural tube
Neural crest
Amniotic cavity

F. FORMATION OF INTRAEMBRYONIC COELOMIC CAVITY

Intraembryonic coelomic cavity

Primitive midgut

Neural tube
Posterior root ganglia
Notochord
Aorta
Dorsal mesentery (persists)

Ectoderm
Mesoderm
Endoderm (lining midgut)

Ventral mesentery (breaks down)

Peritoneal cavity
Abdominal wall

G. BASIC BODY ORGANIZATION

Synopsis of Embryonic Development. The fertilized ovum or *zygote* undergoes a series of divisions (*cleavages*) that lead to the development of a solid spherical mass of cells termed a morula (Fig. 5-1A). When continuing mitosis causes the morula to enlarge, it develops a central cavity and becomes a hollow sphere called a *blastocyst* (Fig. 5-1B), at which stage *implantation* in the uterine wall occurs. Prior to implantation, the blastocyst develops an *inner cell mass* that will give rise to the embryo, and a thin outer shell of cells called the *trophoblast* that contributes to the placenta (Fig. 5-1B). The zona pellucida (Fig. 5-1A) persists until implantation but then degenerates. At the time of implantation, the trophoblast develops two layers, an inner *cytotrophoblast* and an outer *syncytiotrophoblast* consisting of fused trophoblast cells, solid protrusions of which grow invasively into the uterine lining (Fig. 5-1C).

At this stage, the inner cell mass has developed an internal *amniotic cavity* (Fig. 5-1C). Furthermore, the part of the inner cell mass that now comprises the floor of the amniotic cavity has differentiated into a *bilaminar* (two-layered) *embryonic disk* (Fig. 5-1C), the upper layer of which is termed the *epiblast* (Gr. *epi*, upon) and the lower layer is termed the *hypoblast* (Gr. *hypo*, under). The *epiblast* appears to give rise to all three embryonic *germ layers*, namely *ectoderm*, *mesoderm*, and *endoderm*. The fate of the cells that constitute the hypoblast layer of the bilaminar disk is less certain. The next important stage is formation of a *trilaminar embryonic disk*, which is made up of the three germ layers (Fig. 5-1D). This process is known as *gastrulation*. At a medial site on the epiblast termed the *primitive groove*, epiblast cells migrate (1) between the epiblast and hypoblast and (2) into the hypoblast itself. The cells that migrate between the two layers give rise to embryonic *mesoderm* (Gr. *mesos*, middle; *derma*, skin). The cells that enter the hypoblast become embryonic *endoderm* (Gr. *entos*, inside). The cells that remain in the epiblast give rise to embryonic *ectoderm* (Gr. *ektos*, outer). Embryonic mesoderm gives rise to a number of important structures and tissues, including the *notochord* (Fig. 5-1E), around which the vertebrae subsequently develop, and the many different kinds of ordinary and special connective tissues (including the skeletal tissues, blood cells, and the blood cell–forming tissues), as well as muscle tissue, the kidneys, and the gonads. Multipotential mesoderm-derived cells that are still undifferentiated are often described as *mesenchymal* cells (Gr. *enchyma*, infusion). The lining membranes of the digestive and respiratory tracts, together with their associated glands (which include the liver and pancreas) and also the lining of the urinary bladder, are endoderm derived. Both the epidermis of the skin (including such appendages as hair and nails) and the nervous system are derived from ectoderm.

Following gastrulation, the next important stage in embryonic development is the differentiation of *neuroectoderm* accompanied by formation of the neural tube and separation of the neural crest, which we shall describe when we outline the development of the nervous system. At this stage, an embryonic body cavity termed the *intraembryonic coelom* also begins to develop in the mesoderm (Fig. 5-1E and F). The basic structure of the body is established by a process of lateral folding of the trilaminar embryonic disk. On both sides of the embryo, a *lateral fold* containing a lateral expansion of the amniotic cavity grows down toward the ventral midline (Fig. 5-1E and F), whereupon the two folds fuse with each other and establish the basic body plan (Fig. 5-1G). The *peritoneal cavity* is one of the body cavities derived from the intraembryonic coelom, and the *abdominal wall* arises from the inner part of the lateral fold (Fig. 5-1F and G).

Before considering the four basic tissues that subsequently develop from the three germ layers of the embryo, we should point out that classification of these tissues is based on their respective microscopic structure and functions, not on their embryonic origin. Nevertheless, it so happens that most epithelial tissue develops from ectoderm and endoderm, but this is not entirely so because some epithelial tissue is mesoderm derived. Connective tissue arises from mesoderm. Muscle tissue is derived almost entirely from mesoderm, but a small amount of it arises from ectoderm. Nervous tissue is derived from ectoderm, but in the peripheral nervous system, it is admixed with mesoderm-derived connective tissue. Muscle tissue is similarly a composite of muscle cells and connective tissue.

Epithelial Tissue (Epithelium). From its derivation, the word *epithelium* (Gr. *epi*, upon; *thele*, nipple) means something that covers nipples (the nipples referred to in this context are the tiny capillary-containing papillae of connective tissue that project into the translucent epithelium of the lips and give them their color). From this beginning, the term *epithelium* came to be used for all the covering and lining membranes of the body that are composed of contiguous cells. The epithelial part of the skin (its outer part) develops from ectoderm. The epithelial lining of the digestive tract is derived from endoderm, whereas that enclosing the peritoneal cavity arises from mesoderm. Epithelium of mesodermal origin (*e.g.*, the membrane that lines the peritoneal cavity) is more often referred to as *mesothelium* even though it is also a true epithelium. An exception is the mesoderm-derived epithelium that lines the blood vessels, lymphatics, and heart, which, through convention, has come to be known as *endothelium*. Distinctions based on embryonic origin are made not because there are any characteristic differences in microscopic structure between similar ectoderm-, mesoderm-, or endoderm-derived epithelia, but because mesoderm-derived epithelia can behave differently under pathological conditions, particularly when they are involved in malignant disease.

All epithelial membranes are made up of contiguous cells that are joined together by cell junctions, as will be described in the next chapter. They are all supported by con-

---

Fig. 5-1. Diagrammatic survey of human embryonic development, illustrating derivation of the three germ layers from the inner cell mass and subsequent establishment of the basic plan of the body as a result of lateral folding of the embryonic disk. For details, see text.

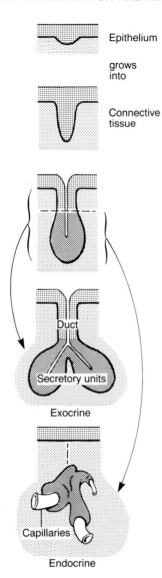

Fig. 5-2. Schematic diagram showing the process by which epithelial tissue gives rise to exocrine and endocrine glands.

Exocrine glands (Gr. *ex*, out or away from; *krinein*, to separate) deliver their secretion onto the surface from which the gland developed, in other words, *outside* the substance of the body. All exocrine glands therefore have a *duct* system that conveys their secretion from their secretory units to some surface (Fig. 5-2). Most *endocrine* glands develop in the same way except that the counterpart of the duct system breaks down, with the result that endocrine glands have no ducts (Fig. 5-2). Such glands are entirely made up of islands of secretory cells embedded in connective tissue and closely associated with its capillaries (Fig. 5-2). Their secretory product enters these capillaries and is carried throughout the body by the bloodstream. Endocrine secretions are generally referred to as *hormones* (Gr. *hormaein*, to arouse to activity or spur on) because they have profound physiological effects on other cells.

Connective Tissue. Connective tissue develops from *mesenchyme*, a derivative of mesoderm. Because it develops from the middle germ layer, it is in the right position to nourish and support the epithelial membranes and glands that arise from ectoderm, mesoderm, and endoderm. The heart and blood vessels are also formed from mesenchyme; hence *the vessels in which blood circulates are confined to connective tissue.* To a large extent, connective tissue consists of the nonliving *intercellular substances* produced by certain of its cells. Cartilage and bone, as well as ligaments, tendons, and fasciae, develop from mesenchyme and represent types of connective tissue that consist chiefly of intercellular substances. In these tissues, the principal function of con-

nective tissue, the capillaries of which nourish their cells. Some epithelial membranes contain cells that elaborate secretions onto the free surface of the membrane. An example is the epithelial lining of the intestine, which is always kept wet. However, there are sites where the need for secretions cannot be met by cells of the membrane itself. Furthermore, the need to produce a secretion can be out of keeping with the other functions of the membrane. In such cases, cells grow down from the membrane into the underlying developing connective tissue of the embryo as illustrated in Figure 5-2. Here they form structures that have come to be known as *glands*, because some of the first ones observed were acorn shaped (L. *glans*, acorn).

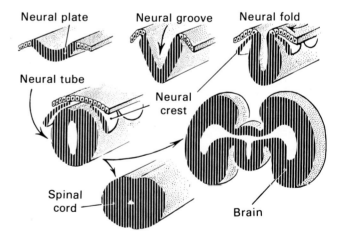

Fig. 5-3. Diagrammatic summary of the development of the central nervous system. The axial mid-dorsal ectoderm of the embryo forms a neural plate that deepens into a neural groove. When the edges of this groove (the neural folds) fuse dorsally to form the neural tube, some of the neuroectodermal cells become detached and form the neural crest. In the head region, the neural tube gives rise to the brain, and in the remainder of the body it gives rise to the spinal cord.

nective tissue cells is to elaborate intercellular substances. However, there are also other kinds of connective tissue that are essentially cellular and whose cells are concerned with other functions, such as defending the body against infectious microorganisms and other foreign agents. Among these cells are the leukocytes of the blood. All blood cells, as well as all blood vessels, are of mesenchymal origin.

Nervous Tissue.   At an early stage of development called *neurulation,* the mid-dorsal ectoderm becomes depressed along the axial midline of the embryo, forming the *neural plate* (Fig. 5-3). This plate then deepens into a *neural groove* (Figs. 5-1E and 5-3), the edges of which grow toward each other and fuse, with the result that the groove becomes a *neural tube* lying just below the dorsal surface of the embryo (Figs. 5-1F and 5-3). This tube extends from the head region into the tail of the developing embryo. In the head region, its walls thicken and develop into the *brain* (Fig. 5-3). The remainder of the neural tube gives rise to the *spinal cord* (Fig. 5-3). At both sites, the neuroectodermal cells in its walls give rise to *neurons* and their supporting *glial* cells (Gr. *glia,* glue). A small and irregular flattened mass of neural tissue becomes detached along the line of fusion of the neural folds. Known as the *neural crest* (Figs. 5-1F and 5-3), this mass gives rise both to the *spinal ganglia* (Gr. *ganglion,* a knotlike mass) that develop bilaterally along the developing spinal cord (Fig. 5-1G) and to the *autonomic ganglia.* It also contributes to the *cranial ganglia.* These three types of ganglia also contain neurons and supporting glial cells.

From the cell bodies of the neurons situated in the developing neural tube and ganglia, cytoplasmic processes called *nerve fibers* grow out into mesenchyme that has begun to differentiate into connective tissue. Meanwhile, certain neurons migrate to other parts of the body. Each nerve fiber acquires a sheath of delicate connective tissue, and bundles of nerve fibers become grouped together as *nerves,* in which the nerve fibers are collectively ensheathed with connective tissue.

Muscle Tissue.   Muscles are composed of muscle cells that are known as *muscle fibers* because of their elongated shape. Individual muscle fibers are surrounded by delicate connective tissue that provides them with a rich blood supply. In addition, bundles of muscle fibers and also entire muscles are wrapped with even stronger connective tissue. These various connective tissue wrappings merge with one another at the ends of the muscle and provide attachments to the tendons or other connective tissue structures on which the muscle pulls. Both the muscle fibers and their various orders of connective tissue wrappings are regarded as integral components of muscle tissue, and both are derived from mesoderm.

In the chapters that follow, each of these four basic tissues and their various subtypes will be described separately.

SELECTED REFERENCES

Cellular Differentiation and Embryonic Development of the Four Basic Tissues

ALBERTS B, BRAY D, LEWIS J et al: Molecular Biology of the Cell, pp 435–449. New York, Garland Publishing, 1983

GURDON JB: The Control of Gene Expression in Animal Development. Cambridge, MA, Harvard University Press, 1974

HAYFLICK L: The cell biology of aging. J Invest Dermatol 73:8, 1979

HAYFLICK L: The cell biology of human aging. Sci Am 242 No 1: 58, 1980

MOORE KL: The Developing Human: Clinically Oriented Embryology, 3rd ed. Philadelphia, WB Saunders, 1982

RINGERTZ NR, LINDER S, ZUCKERMAN SH: Analysis of differentiation by fusion of cells and cell fragments. In Schweiger HG (ed): International Cell Biology 1980–1981, p 512. Berlin, Springer-Verlag, 1981

SAUNDERS GF (ed): Cell Differentiation and Neoplasia. New York, Raven Press, 1977

Cellular Proliferation, Growth Regulation, and Neoplastic Transformation*

BISHOP JM: Cancer genes come of age. Cell 32:1018, 1983

BUICK RN, POLLACK MN: Perspectives on clonogenic tumor cells, stem cells, and oncogenes. Cancer Res 44:4909, 1984

BULLOUGH WS: Chalone control systems. In Lobue J, Gordin AS (eds): Humoral Control of Growth and Differentiation. New York, Academic Press, 1973

CAIRNS J: The origin of human cancers. Nature 289:353, 1981

CHAGANTI RSK: Significance of chromosome change to hematopoietic neoplasms. Blood 62:515, 1983

COOPER GM: Cellular transforming genes. Science 218:801, 1982

CROCE CM, KLEIN G: Chromosome translocations and human cancer. Sci Am 252 No 3:54, 1985

DE KLEIN A, VAN KESSEL AG, GROSVELD G et al: A cellular oncogene is translocated to the Philadelphia chromosome in chronic myelocytic leukemia. Nature 300:765, 1982

DOOLITTLE RF, HUNKAPILLAR MW, HOOD LE et al: Simian sarcoma virus *onc* gene, v-*sis,* is derived from the gene (or genes) encoding a platelet-derived growth factor. Science 221:275, 1983

DOWNWARD J, YARDEN Y, MAYES E et al: Close similarity of epidermal growth factor receptor and v-*erb-B* oncogene protein sequences. Nature 307:521, 1984

FARBER E: Chemical carcinogenesis. N Engl J Med 305:1379, 1981

FINKEL T, COOPER GM: Detection of a molecular complex between ras proteins and transferrin receptor. Cell 136:1115, 1984

GILLIES SD, MORRISON SL, OI VT, TONEGAWA S: A tissue-specific transcription enhancer element is located in the major intron of a rearranged immunoglobulin heavy chain gene. Cell 33:717, 1983

HELDIN C-H, WESTERMARK B: Growth factors: Mechanism of action and relation to oncogenes. Cell 37:7, 1984

HOUCK JC (ed): Chalones. Amsterdam, North Holland, 1976

---

* For references on hematopoietic growth regulators, see Selected References, Chapter 9.

KLEIN G: The role of gene dosage and genetic transpositions in carcinogenesis. Nature 294: 313, 1981

KLEIN G: Specific chromosomal translocations and the genesis of B-cell–derived tumors in mice and men. Cell 32:311, 1983

LAND H, PARADA LF, WEINBERG RA: Cellular oncogenes and multistep carcinogenesis. Science 222:771, 1983

LAND H, PARADA LF, WEINBERG RA: Tumorigenic conversion of primary embryo fibroblasts requires at least two cooperating oncogenes. Nature 304:596, 1983

LEDER P, BATTEY J, LENOIR G et al: Translocations among antibody genes in human cancer. Science 222:765, 1983

MARQUARDT H, HUNKAPILLER MW, HOOD LE et al: Transforming growth factors produced by retrovirus-transformed rodent fibroblasts and human melanoma cells: Amino acid sequence homology with epidermal growth factor. Proc Natl Acad Sci USA 80:4684, 1983

MAUER HR: Chalones: Specific regulators of eukaryote tissue growth. In Talwar GP (ed): Regulation of Differentiated Function in Eukaryote Cells. New York, Raven Press, 1975

MOZES LW, SCHULTZ J, SCOTT WA, WERNER R (eds): Cellular Responses to Molecular Modulators. Miami Winter Symposia, Vol 18. New York, Academic Press, 1981

REDDY EP, REYNOLDS RK, SANTOS E, BARBACID M: A point mutation is responsible for the acquisition of transforming properties by the T24 human bladder carcinoma oncogene. Nature 300:149, 1982

STILES CD: The molecular biology of platelet-derived growth factor. Cell 33:653, 1983

TABIN CJ, BRADLEY SM, BARGMANN CI et al: Mechanism of activation of a human oncogene. Nature 300:143, 1982

VANDE WOUDE GF, LEVINE AJ, TOPP W, WATSON JD (eds): Cancer Cells 2: Oncogenes and Viral Genes. Cold Spring Harbor, NY, Cold Spring Harbor Laboratory, 1984

WATERFIELD MD, SCRACE GT, WHITTLE N et al: Platelet-derived growth factor is structurally related to the putative transforming protein p28^{sis} of simian sarcoma virus. Nature 304:35, 1983

WEINBERG RA: Oncogenes and the molecular biology of cancer. J Cell Biol 97:1661, 1983

WEINBERG RA: A molecular basis of cancer. Sci Am 249 No. 5:126, 1983

PART THREE

THE TISSUES OF THE BODY

The third portion of this book deals with the microscopic structure and general functions of the four basic tissues and their various subtypes. In addition, it contains information relating to the immune system, the nervous system, and the musculoskeletal system and therefore serves as an introduction to Part Four, which describes the systems of the body.

6

Epithelial Tissue

Almost all body surfaces are covered or lined* by continuous sheets of cells termed *epithelial membranes* or *epithelia*. Such cellular sheets are also able to invaginate into the underlying connective tissue, where the epithelial cells differentiate into secretory cells or duct cells and constitute structures known as *epithelial glands* (see Fig. 5-2). Epithelial membranes and glands constitute the two broad subdivisions of *epithelial tissue*, which represents the simplest of the basic tissues. As noted under Epithelial Tissue in Chapter 5, epithelial tissue can develop from each of the three germ layers of the embryo (ectoderm, mesoderm, or endoderm).

To study the different types of epithelial membranes and glands, it is necessary to discuss and examine sections of organs and structures that incorporate various other tissues as well. However, at this stage, there is no reason for anyone new to the subject to feel compelled to learn the detailed structure and points of recognition of the entire organ or structure. Such matters and the specific functions of the component parts of the structure will be considered in Part Four, after we have dealt with the tissues. Beginning students will find that the best way to attain a general comprehension of the way such body parts are constructed and function is to learn histology a step at a time, beginning with the cell and then proceeding to the simplest of the four basic tissues.

EPITHELIAL MEMBRANES

Epithelial membranes are continuous sheets of cells with contiguous cell borders that have characteristic specialized sites of close contact called *cell junctions*, which will be

---

* A *lining* is a membrane that covers the *inner* surface of a hollow structure. The term *covering* is used for the *outer* surface of a structure but can also be used with reference to an internal surface, provided it refers to the surface and not to the structure itself. The term *covering* should also be used for any component that projects into a lumen from an internal surface (even if this covering constitutes part of a lining) because it is the *outer* surface of the component that projects from the surface. Thus the ovaries are described as having a *covering* of simple cuboidal epithelium that is continuous with the simple squamous mesothelial *lining* of the peritoneal cavity.

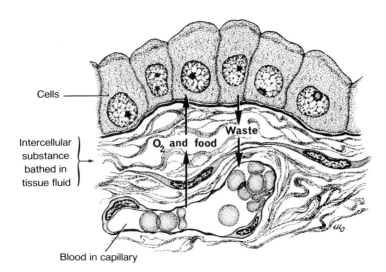

Cells

Intercellular
substance
bathed in
tissue fluid

O₂ and food

Waste

Blood in capillary

Fig. 6-1. Diagram of an epithelial membrane illustrating the functional dependence of its cells on the underlying connective tissue, the tissue fluid of which provides the cells with their oxygen and nutrients and serves as the medium through which their metabolic wastes diffuse into capillaries.

described later in this chapter. Such membranes, which can be one or more cells thick (see Fig. 6-3), contain *no capillaries*. Nutrients and oxygen therefore have to reach their cells from capillaries situated in the underlying loose connective tissue by diffusion through the intercellular substances of connective tissue (Fig. 6-1). These intercellular substances also provide support for the membrane. Epithelia are attached to the underlying connective tissue by a component known as a *basement membrane*, which is a layer of intercellular material of complex composition that is distributed as a thin layer between the epithelium and the connective tissue. This material is not very evident in hematoxylin and eosin (H & E) sections (see Fig. 6-4), but it can often be seen to advantage in sections stained by the PAS reaction (Fig. 6-2). The nature and composition of the basement membrane will be discussed in Chapter 7.

Functional Importance of Epithelia. The most obvious function of epithelial membranes is that of protecting the connective tissue they cover. Furthermore, some of their cells can also be secretory or absorptive in function. For example, secretory cells may be interspersed between other supporting cells of the membrane as depicted in Figure 6-3D. In this instance, the secretory cells produce mucus, a viscous fluid that flows over the entire membrane surface and keeps it wet and slippery.

In addition to providing protection, some epithelial membranes are adapted to carry out selective absorption. Thus in the epithelial lining of the small intestine, absorptive cells take up appropriate substances from the lumen of the digestive tract but leave the unwanted materials behind. The absorbed substances then pass into the body, where they are taken into the blood or lymph. In a similar fashion, the epithelial walls of the kidney tubules selectively resorb useful constituents of urinary filtrate and thereby prevent loss of useful substances from the body via the urine. Very thin epithelial membranes allow fluid to pass through them and can act as dialysis membranes, allowing water and ions but not macromolecules to diffuse across them.

The protection afforded by epithelial membranes is of two general kinds. Certain membranes have to withstand a great deal of wear and tear. For example, the esophagus, through which chewed food passes into the stomach, requires a highly protective lining that is several cells thick. Such protection is of even more importance in animals that make a habit of swallowing chewed-up bones. The other kind of protection is required to counteract the drying out of cells at body surfaces exposed to air. In the skin, such protection is afforded by a multilayered epithelial membrane, the outer layers of which have become transformed into tough *keratin* (see Fig. 6-8). The keratin constitutes a relatively impervious outer layer that protects the underlying cells from dehydration and also prevents the body from soaking up water when immersed in it. The thick epithelial membrane of the skin and its tough outer layer of keratin also render it suitably protective against wear and tear. Hence calluses developing at sites subjected to excessive wear consist primarily of keratin.

In the respiratory tract, protection against drying out is achieved in a completely different manner. The epithelial lining of the nasal passages is richly provided with secretory cells that produce mucus and thereby prevent it from drying out. In addition, numerous small glands lying deep to the membrane produce secretions that help to keep it wet. These secretions are delivered by way of ducts that open onto its free surface. The epithelial lining of the passages that conduct air to the lungs is similarly provided with glands that produce secretions to help prevent it from drying out. In the respiratory portion of the lungs, where an interchange of oxygen and carbon dioxide takes place between the blood in pulmonary capillaries and the air in lung alveoli (air sacs), it is essential for the alveolar lining to be thin enough for gases to diffuse efficiently between blood and air. In this case, the tissue fluid produced by the pulmonary capillaries exudes through the thin epithelial lining of the alveoli and serves to keep their inner surface wet.

From the foregoing examples, it is clear that epithelial membranes are functionally adapted in a wide variety of ways. Furthermore, their microscopic structure often provides reliable clues about their respective functions. We shall now consider the microscopic features and functions of the different kinds of epithelial membranes present in the body. These membranes are broadly subdivided into three classes according to the number of cell layers of which they are constructed. An epithelial membrane that consists

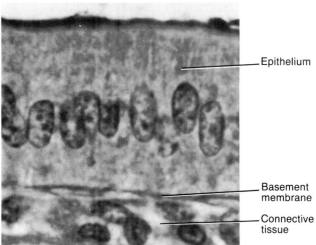

Epithelium

Basement membrane

Connective tissue

Fig. 6-2. Photomicrograph of simple columnar intestinal epithelium (PAS stain). The stained layer on the free surface of the epithelium is mucus. The basement membrane under the epithelium is also PAS-positive because of its glycoprotein content.

of only a single layer of cells is termed a *simple epithelium* (Fig. 6-3*A, B,* and *C*). An epithelium that is two or more cells thick is called a *stratified epithelium* (Fig. 6-3*E, F,* and *G*). If some of its cells reach from the base of the membrane to its free surface but others reach only partway to the surface, the membrane is described as a *pseudostratified epithelium* (Fig. 6-3*D*); this is because transverse sections of the membrane may give the false impression that it is made up of several layers of cells.

Simple Epithelia

Simple Squamous Epithelium.   An epithelial membrane that consists of a single layer of flattened cells (Fig. 6-3*A*) is termed a *simple squamous epithelium* (*squamous* means scalelike). The cytoplasm of its cells may be too attenuated to be discerned clearly in light microscope (LM) sections. The thin-walled portion of kidney tubules, seen in the renal medulla, is composed of this type of epithelium (Fig. 6-4*A*). Simple squamous epithelium cannot always be counted on to show to advantage in kidney sections, so the endothelial lining of blood vessels or the mesothelial lining of the major body cavities (pleural, pericardial, or peritoneal) is sometimes studied instead. Despite their special names, endothelium and mesothelium are both unexceptional examples of simple squamous epithelium. Organs that are invaginated into major body cavities are covered by a serosal layer of mesothelium, and the thin film of fluid present in such cavities facilitates independent movements of the organs that project into them. Mesothelium can be prepared as a flat mount, making it possible to obtain an *en face* (face-on) view of its free surface.

Simple Cuboidal Epithelium.   Described as *cuboidal* only because its cells appear square in cross section, this type of single-layered epithelium is actually made up of cells that have a hexagonal lateral outline (Fig. 6-3*B*). One of

the few sites where simple cuboidal epithelium is present is the ovary, where it constitutes the epithelial covering of that organ. Another site is the renal medulla, where it lines the small ductlike collecting tubules (Fig. 6-4*B*).

Simple Columnar Epithelium.   This type of epithelium is made up of a single layer of tall cells (Fig. 6-3*C* and *D*) that again fit together in a hexagonal pattern. In its unspecialized form, these cells are all similar in microscopic appearance. The principal function of unspecialized simple columnar epithelium is to protect wet body surfaces. In addition, it can elaborate watery secretions. Epithelium of this type lines the minor ducts of glands (see Fig. 6-21).

In *simple secretory columnar epithelium,* the columnar cells are all specialized to secrete mucus in addition to being protective. Sites where this type of epithelium is present include the lining of the stomach and the lining of the cervical canal of the uterus (Fig. 6-4*C*). All its component cells look alike and exhibit a foamy appearance in H & E sections. Mucus does not stain with hematoxylin or eosin, so in H & E sections the region of cytoplasm superficial to the nucleus appears pale and vacuolated (Fig. 6-4*C*). With PAS staining, however, the mucous secretory vesicles in these cells stain similarly to those in goblet cells.

A simple columnar epithelium that is made up of *absorptive cells* as well as *secretory cells* lines the intestine. To facilitate absorption, this membrane is only one cell thick. It is nevertheless subject to daily abrasion, and to resist wear and tear, its free surface has to be coated with slippery mucus. Accordingly, interspersed with cells that are specialized for absorption, there are many *goblet cells* that secrete protective mucus. As noted in Chapter 4, mucus-secreting cells that lie interspersed with cells of some other kind, such as absorptive cells, assume the shape of a goblet because the region of cytoplasm packed with mucous secretory vesicles can expand and assume a bowllike shape by indenting the cytoplasm of the other cells adjacent to

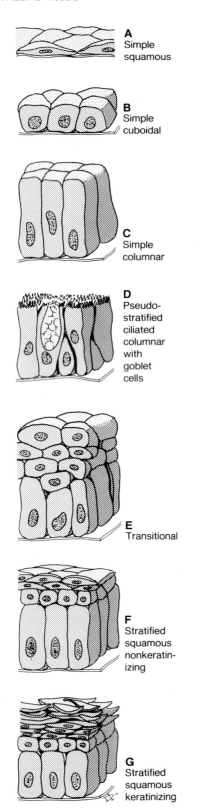

A
Simple
squamous

B
Simple
cuboidal

C
Simple
columnar

D
Pseudo-
stratified
ciliated
columnar
with
goblet
cells

E
Transitional

F
Stratified
squamous
nonkeratin-
izing

G
Stratified
squamous
keratinizing

Fig. 6-3.   Diagrammatic representation of the seven main types of epithelial membranes.

it. The nucleus of the goblet cell lies in its narrow stemlike portion, close to its base (see Fig. 6-6).

On the luminal surface of the absorptive cells of the intestinal epithelium, there is a special border that has a refractive index that is different from the rest of the cell. Under the LM, fine perpendicular striations can be discerned in this border; hence it is called a *striated border* (see Fig. 18-32B). This type of epithelium is therefore called *simple striated columnar epithelium with goblet cells*. With the electron microscope (EM), it can be seen that striated borders are composed of large numbers of *microvilli,* which are minute fingerlike processes projecting up from the luminal surface of the cell (see Figs. 4-2, 4-37, and 4-39).

Yet another combination of cells found in simple columnar epithelium is that of *ciliated cells* interspersed with *goblet cells.* Ciliated cells have already been described in detail under Cilia and Flagella in Chapter 4. Beating of their cilia propels a coating of mucus along the free surface of the membrane. *Simple ciliated columnar epithelium with goblet cells* is found in certain parts of the upper respiratory tract, but its distribution is more limited than that of pseudostratified ciliated columnar epithelium with goblet cells.

Pseudostratified Epithelia

Pseudostratified Ciliated Columnar Epithelium. In pseudostratified epithelia, all the cells lie in contact with the basement membrane but they do not all reach the surface (Fig. 6-3D). Pseudostratified ciliated columnar epithelium with goblet cells lines most of the upper respiratory tract (Fig. 6-5). All the tall cells bordering on the free surface of this type of epithelium are either ciliated cells or goblet cells. The basal cells (*i.e.*, those cells that do not reach all the way to the surface) serve as stem cells for the two kinds of taller cells, providing replacements for these when they are lost from the membrane.

Goblet cells have the EM characteristics depicted in Figure 6-6. The narrow stemlike basal portion of the cell contains a highly developed rough-surfaced endoplasmic reticulum (rER) as well as the nucleus. Superficial to the basal portion, there is a prominent cup-shaped Golgi complex. The protein moiety of the secretory glycoprotein mucus is synthesized in the rER, and as it passes through the Golgi saccules, it undergoes further glycosylation. Membrane-bounded mucous secretory vesicles fill the wide superficial portion of the cell, and a few microvilli are present on its apical surface (Fig. 6-6). Supplemented by copious secretions from underlying glands, the mucus released from goblet cells forms a substantial coating or *mucous blanket* over the entire internal surface of the respiratory passages. This sticky mucous blanket serves as an efficient dust-catcher and thoroughly moistens the inspired air. Ciliary action continually moves it upward to the pharynx, and it is then swallowed or expelled.

We shall find that in the male reproductive system, the type of epithelium lining the ductus epididymis is *noncili-*

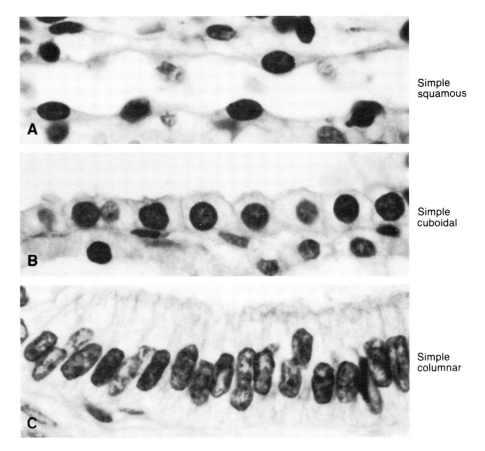

Fig. 6-4. Photomicrograph of three types of simple epithelium. Simple squamous epithelium (*A*) and simple cuboidal epithelium (*B*) are from nephron and collecting tubule of rabbit kidney medulla; simple columnar epithelium (*C*) is from the canal of the uterine cervix.

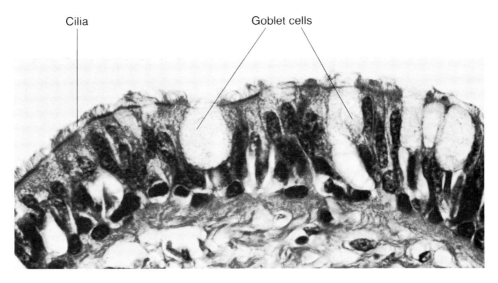

Fig. 6-5. Photomicrograph of pseudostratified ciliated columnar epithelium with goblet cells (bronchial lining). Basal cells that are not tall enough to reach its free surface are present in this type of epithelium. (Courtesy of J. Sturgess)

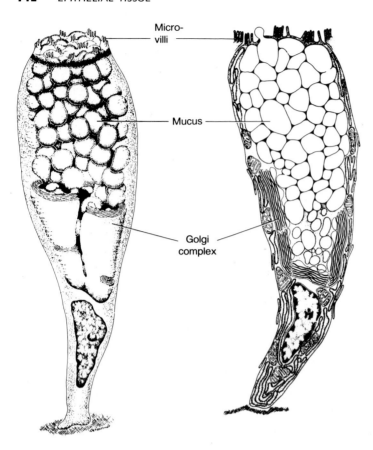

Micro-
villi

Mucus

Golgi
complex

Fig. 6-6. Interpretive diagram and electron micro-scopic drawing of a goblet cell (Courtesy of C. P. Le-blond)

ated pseudostratified columnar epithelium without goblet cells.

Stratified Epithelia

Stratified epithelia (*i.e.,* membranes that are two or more cells thick) are better suited to withstand wear and tear than simple epithelia are. However, because of their strat-ified structure, they are not as efficient at absorption. Fur-thermore, they are ill-adapted for secretory functions. When necessary, secretions must therefore be provided by as-sociated accessory glands that open onto the free surface of the membrane by way of ducts.

Stratified Columnar Epithelium.   Generally not exceeding two cells in thickness, this type of epithelium is primarily protective in function. Whereas ducts of moderate size are commonly lined by simple columnar epithelium, most larger ducts are lined by stratified columnar epithelium. There are also a few sites where stratified columnar epi-thelium is ciliated.

Stratified Squamous Nonkeratinizing Epithelium.   This type of epithelial membrane (Figs. 6-3F and 6-7) is common on wet surfaces that are subject to considerable wear and tear at sites where absorptive function is not required. The

secretions necessary to keep such surfaces wet have to come from appropriately situated glands. Sites lined by this type of epithelium include the esophagus and the floor and sides of the oral cavity (which are moistened by saliva) and also the vagina (which is kept moist by cervical mucus). Begin-ners occasionally misconstrue the term stratified squamous epithelium as meaning that this type of epithelium is made up of successive layers of squamous cells. As may be seen in Figure 6-3F, the basal layer adjacent to the basement membrane is, in fact, composed of cells that are essentially columnar. Just above this layer, the cells are polyhedral (many-sided), and it is only toward the free surface of the membrane that the cells take on a squamous shape.

Stratified Squamous Keratinizing Epithelium.   This type of epithelium (Figs. 6-3G and 6-8) closely resembles strat-ified squamous nonkeratinizing epithelium except that its more superficial cells become transformed into a tough nonliving layer of *keratin* that is tightly attached to the underlying living cells. The epithelial part of the skin (the *epidermis*) provides a good example of stratified squamous keratinizing epithelium (Fig. 6-8). In skin, keratin serves several purposes. It is virtually waterproof and hence pre-vents evaporation from the cells beneath it; likewise, it keeps the body from imbibing water in the bathtub. Because it is tough and resilient, it protects the underlying epithelial

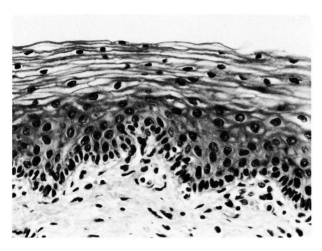

Fig. 6-7. Photomicrograph of stratified squamous nonkeratinizing epithelium (lining of monkey vagina). (Courtesy of C. P. Leblond)

cells from wear and tear, and being impervious to bacteria, it constitutes a first line of defense against infection. Over the soles of the feet and the palms of the hands, stratified squamous epithelium is thicker and the keratin in particular is very thick; this helps to withstand the great wear to which these surfaces are exposed. This type of epithelium will be described in detail when we consider the epidermis in Chapter 17.

Transitional Epithelium. When stretched, transitional epithelium has an appearance similar to stratified squamous nonkeratinizing epithelium. When it is not stretched, however, its more superficial cells appear markedly rounded rather than squamous (Figs. 6-3E and 6-9). Such a design allows this type of membrane to withstand stretch without its component cells pulling apart from one another. Hence transitional epithelium is well suited for lining tubes and hollow viscera that are subject to distension; classic examples include the ureters and urinary bladder (Fig. 6-9).

Many of the surface cells in the transitional epithelium of the urinary bladder are either polyploid or multinucleated. Binucleate cells as well as polyploid nuclei are seen in the superficial layers of this epithelium during the embryonic development of the mouse. Hence it is thought that when the binucleate cells divide, their chromosomes regroup in such a way that the two daughter cells both acquire a single nucleus containing twice the former number of chromosomes.

It is difficult to decide whether transitional epithelium should be classified as a stratified or a pseudostratified epithelium. If one regards any contact at all between the component cells and the basement membrane as being sufficient grounds for including an epithelium in the pseudostratified category, it might be argued that transitional epithelium should be relegated to that particular class of epithelial membranes. If, however, the presence of many cell layers in the epithelium is considered a more important criterion, then it might be argued that transitional epithelium should be considered a multilayered epithelium, similar in many important respects to other stratified epithelia. This particular epithelium is especially difficult to classify because, as first indicated by LM observations and then confirmed by scanning electron microscopic studies of the epithelial lining of the human urinary bladder, many of the cells above the basal layer of the epithelium (if not all of them) have long, thin cytoplasmic processes (pedicles) that extend down to the basement membrane. These cells are therefore anchored to the basement membrane along with the basal cells. Another difficulty in classifying this type of epithelium is deciding whether to classify it in the multilayered conformation seen when the bladder is empty or in the attenuated state seen when the bladder is distended with urine.

CELL JUNCTIONS

Along the contiguous borders of epithelial cells there are *cell junctions,* which are sites where some kind of special contact can be recognized between the cells. There are three main types of cell junctions, each of which is designed according to a different principle. In the first type, which is found only in epithelial tissue and is known as the *tight* or *occluding junction,* the contiguous cell membranes are

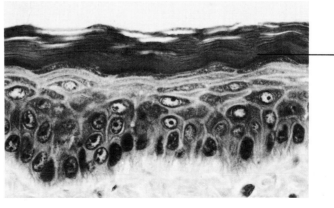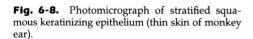
Keratin

Fig. 6-8. Photomicrograph of stratified squamous keratinizing epithelium (thin skin of monkey ear).

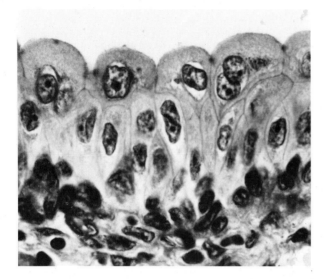

Fig. 6-9. Photomicrograph of transitional epithelium (epithelial lining of urinary bladder of dog). In this nondistended state, the rounded surface cells bulge into the lumen. Multinucleated surface cells can be seen at upper left and upper right.

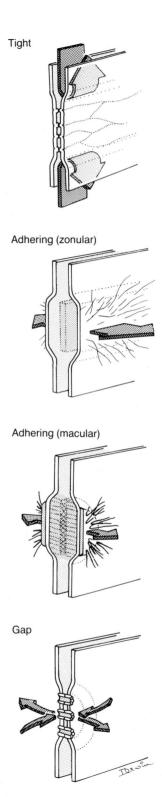

Fig. 6-10. Diagrammatic representation of the structure of the four major types of cell junctions present between epithelial cells. Details are given in the text.

fused together by an anastomosing system of occluding ridges that constitute a seal between the cells (Fig. 6-10). The second type of cell junction is known as the *adhering junction* because it represents a site of extra-strong adhesion between contiguous cells. Adhering junctions are not restricted to epithelial tissue; they maintain strong adhesion between cardiac muscle cells as well. As we shall see, there are two different kinds of adhering junctions that each have their own particular role in maintaining intercellular adhesion (Fig. 6-10). The third type of junction, which is again not unique to epithelial tissue, is called the *gap junction* because a narrow intercellular gap is present between the contiguous cell membranes in this kind of junction. However, the gap is bridged by a number of tiny tubular passageways that represent channels of direct communication between the interiors of neighboring cells (Fig. 6-10). A few investigators prefer to use the term *nexus* (L. for bond) for this type of junction in order to emphasize that it is essentially a *communicating junction* (*i.e.,* a link in a functional chain). The problem with the term *gap junction* is that it is a purely morphological term devoid of any information relating to function.

Three additional expressions are incorporated into the names of the various types of cell junctions. These expressions denote the overall *shape* of the junction. A junction that extends around the entire perimeter of the cell like a belt, as illustrated on the left of Figure 6-12, is described as a *zonula* (L. for belt). However, if the junction occupies only a strip or patch of the cell surface, it is called a *fascia* (L. for band). Finally, a junction that is small and circular

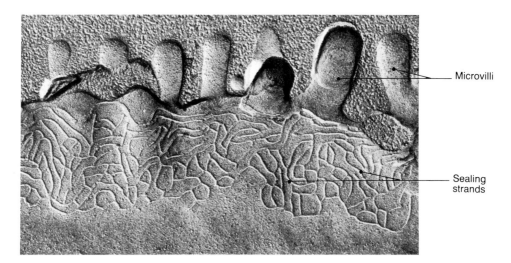

Microvilli

Sealing
strands

Fig. 6-11. Electron micrograph (×50,000) of a freeze-fracture replica that shows part of a continuous tight junction (zonula occludens) on a lateral border of an epithelial lining cell of the intestine (*Xenopus* tadpole). This multistranded system of sealing ridges effectively occludes the intercellular space along the junction. (Hull BE, Staehelin LA: J Cell Biol 68:688, 1976)

(*i.e.*, spotlike) in outline (see Fig. 6-12) is described as a *macula* (L. for spot).

Tight Junctions

In situations in which it is necessary to maintain an effective seal between epithelial cells, the lateral margins of contiguous cells are fused together along a system of surface ridges (Figs. 6-10, 6-11, and 6-12). In some cases, these ridges extend around the entire perimeter of each cell very near its apical (luminal) surface (Fig. 6-12). They comprise a continuous beltlike junction that is generally described as a *continuous tight* (or *occluding*) *junction* but that is also called a *zonula occludens*. The matching surface ridges seen on contiguous cells (Fig. 6-10) are assembled from integral membrane protein particles. The currently accepted interpretation is that complementary or interacting protein particles of the two apposed cell membranes establish mutual contact and become interlocked across the intercellular gap like the teeth of a zipper. This results in the formation of a number of sealing strands that occlude the intercellular space (Staehelin and Hull). Furthermore, it has been found that the number of sealing strands that make up a continuous tight junction varies with the location of the junction; the most effective seal is provided by the wide multistranded type of tight junction seen, for example, between intestinal epithelial cells (Fig. 6-11). These are the important occluding junctions that prevent the inappropriate macromolecular substances present in the intestinal contents from gaining direct access to the intercellular spaces, and

they also prevent the loss of macromolecular compounds into the intestinal contents as a result of passage in the reverse direction (Fig. 6-10). The physiologically essential role of continuous tight junctions in providing a tight seal was confirmed experimentally when it was demonstrated that they prevent electron-dense markers from entering the intercellular space from the lumen of the intestine and vice versa.

A more speculative function of zonular tight junctions is that they could play a role in restricting the lateral mobility of membrane proteins that are specific to particular domains of the cell surface. Certain proteins are found exclusively in particular areas of the cell membrane (*e.g.*, the part apposed to a lumen or to a blood vessel). There must therefore be some device to prevent them from intermingling with the proteins in other parts of the cell membrane as a result of lateral diffusion in the plane of the membrane.

Fascia occludens junctions are similar to zonula occludens junctions except that they are strip-shaped or band-shaped and hence do not comprise a continuous belt around the entire perimeter of the cell. Fascia occludens junctions characterize the endothelial lining of blood vessels; the capillaries of the brain, however, are exceptional in that their endothelial cells are joined by continuous (zonular) tight junctions. The seal effected by the fascia type of occluding junction is interrupted because it is restricted to specific areas of the cell perimeter. It is therefore *incomplete*. In subsequent chapters, we shall find that it is this arrangement that enables capillaries to produce tissue fluid. Furthermore, it provides leukocytes with the escape route they require when they enter connective tissue from venules during the acute inflammatory reaction.

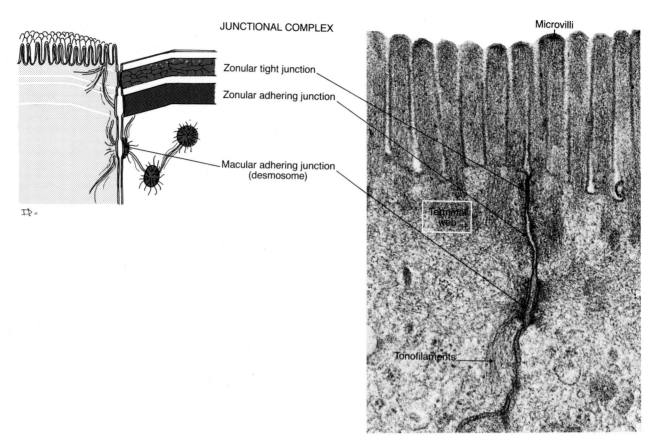

JUNCTIONAL COMPLEX

Zonular tight junction

Zonular adhering junction

Macular adhering junction
(desmosome)

Microvilli

Terminal web

Tonofilaments

Fig. 6-12. Explanatory diagram and electron micrograph of the three types of cell junctions that make up a junctional complex, showing their respective positions relative to the microvillus-covered luminal surface of absorptive epithelial cells of the intestinal lining. The level of the terminal web is also indicated. Details are given in the text. (Electron micrograph, courtesy of E. Horvath and D. Murray)

Adhering Junctions

The adhering junctions that strongly bond contiguous epithelial cells together are of two different types. The first type, present for example between intestinal epithelial cells, is termed the *zonula adherens*. Like the zonula occludens, this type of adhering junction extends around the entire perimeter of the cell. It, too, lies close to the luminal border of the cell, at a level just below the zonula occludens on each lateral border (Fig. 6-12). At a level just below these two parallel beltlike junctions, spotlike (*macular*) adhering junctions are also present. Representing the second type of adhering junction, macular adhering junctions are scattered around the perimeter of the cell in the form of a discontinuous row (Fig. 6-12). This characteristic arrangement of the three specified kinds of junctions is called a *junctional complex* (Fig. 6-12). Because the beltlike zonula adherens junction occupies the middle (intermediate) position of the junctional complex, it is also commonly referred to as an *intermediate junction*. Another name for the same type of beltlike junction is *belt desmosome*. It has a com-

paratively wide (20 nm) intercellular gap that is filled with fine filamentous material of moderately low electron density and undetermined composition. This intercellular filamentous material is believed to constitute a strong bond between the apposed cell membranes (Figs. 6-10 and 6-12). The zonular adhering junction is a major site where cytoplasmic microfilaments are anchored to the cell membrane; hence its primary role seems to be the prevention of cell separation during various contractile activities involving the contractile filaments associated with the luminal border and its microvilli.

The actin-containing microfilaments that are anchored to the zonular adhering junction are mostly arranged in the form of a prominent circumferential band encircling the whole cell. This band is situated in the peripheral cytoplasm, just deep to the zonula adherens on the lateral borders of the cell. When this marginal band contracts, it constricts the luminal surface of the cell. Such contraction, in conjunction with the strong cell-to-cell adhesion maintained at this level by the zonular adhering junction, is believed to play an important role in the morphogenesis of epithelially derived organs (*e.g.*, in bringing about the invagination of neural plate neuroectoderm to form the neural tube). It is also probably responsible for decreasing the diameter of any discontinuities that may occur in epithelial membranes as a result of cell damage. A diminution of the luminal surface area of the cells around the periphery of such a lesion would effect a net reduction in the overall diameter of the discontinuity. Other putative functions ascribed to the zonular adhering junction include (1) maintenance of tension in the membrane and (2) apical constriction of its component cells so that their microvilli fan out and provide regions of cell membrane between the bases of their microvilli with freer access to the luminal contents (Mooseker et al).

The second type of adhering junction is called a *desmosome* (Gr. *desmos*, band or ligament; *soma* body), *spot desmosome*, or *macula adherens* to reflect the fact that its shape is circular and spotlike (L. *macula*, spot). It constitutes part of the junctional complex but is also present elsewhere on contiguous cell surfaces (Fig. 6-12). In this type of junction, bundles of *tonofilaments* (a type of intermediate filament composed of prekeratin) are anchored to a disklike *plaque*, which is a mass of electron-dense material that adheres to the cytoplasmic aspect of each apposed area of cell membrane (Figs. 6-10 and 6-13). An electron-dense line is also seen extending along the midline of its relatively wide (30 nm) glycoprotein-containing intercellular gap (Fig. 6-13). The structural basis for this prominent line is still somewhat speculative, but a currently accepted interpretation is that it represents interconnecting or interwoven portions of filamentous intercellular elements called *transmembrane linkers* (indicated in Fig. 6-10) that extend across the intercellular gap and secure the apposed regions of cell membrane to each other (Staehelin and Hull).

The fine structure of the desmosome is a clear indication that it plays a major role in maintaining adequate adhesion between contiguous cell borders. Its associated tonofilaments are arranged so that the tensile forces they transmit become distributed from one cell to the next over a substantial area of epithelial membrane. Moreover, its transmembrane linkers evidently constitute some kind of special arrangement that resists cell separation caused by such forces. Desmosomes are most abundant in epithelial membranes that are adapted to withstand wear and tear (*e.g.,* stratified squamous keratinizing epithelium). In the deep layers of the epidermis, desmosomes are so numerous that the keratinocytes they join exhibit a prickly appearance after they shrink on fixation (see Fig. 17-5). However, desmosomes are not exclusive to epithelial tissue; the same type of junction (but with associated intermediate filaments that are not made of prekeratin) is present between muscle cells of the heart.

The *hemidesmosome* (Gr. *hemi*, half), a variant of the spotlike adhering junction, has the structure of only half a desmosome. This type of junction bonds epithelial cells to their underlying basement membrane, and it is particularly well developed under the basal layer of the epidermis (Fig. 6-14).

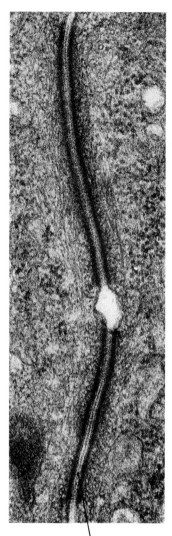

Electron-dense line

Fig. 6-13. Electron micrograph of spot desmosomes (macula adherens junctions) between epithelial cells (lining epithelium of chick trachea). Extending along the midline of the intercellular gap in this type of junction is a thin electron-dense line. The electron-lucent gap is flanked on either side by a much thicker electron-dense line representing plaque material that adheres to the cytoplasmic aspect of the apposed cell membranes. Bundles of tonofilaments arranged parallel to the cell membrane are discernible in the peripheral cytoplasm of the cells at either side of the junction. Their role is to transmit and distribute tensile forces from one site of cellular attachment to another. (Courtesy of V. I. Kalnins)

Gap Junctions (Nexuses)

The term *gap junction* is now favored because it emphasizes the difference in cross-sectional appearance between communicating junctions and sealing junctions. However, this difference is not particularly evident in routine EM sections,

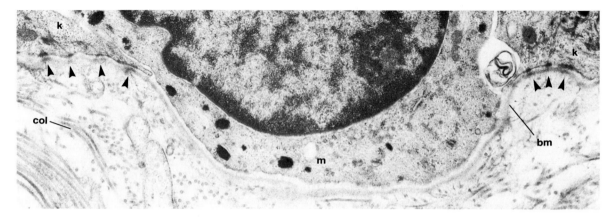

Fig. 6-14. Electron micrograph of a part of the epidermal–dermal border (biopsy of human skin), showing hemidesmosomes (*arrowheads*) attaching the basal surface of keratinocytes (*k*) to the underlying basement membrane (*bm*). The fibrils present in the underlying connective tissue are collagen fibrils (*col*). Part of a melanocyte (*m*) is seen at center. (Courtesy of P. Lea)

and many of the junctions first identified as tight junctions were subsequently found to be gap junctions. Nevertheless, in suitable high-resolution micrographs of gap junctions cut in transverse section, it can be discerned that the cell membranes are not fused together as in tight junctions but are separated by an unusually narrow intercellular gap of about 3 nm—hence the term *gap junction*. Like desmosomes, gap junctions are spotlike in outline; they do not form zonulae.

Much of our present knowledge about the gap region in these junctions was gained from the use of applied electron microscopic methods. An early experimental approach was to introduce an electron-dense heavy-metal marker (lanthanum hydroxide) into the intercellular space bordering on a gap junction. This marker infiltrated the intercellular space between the two cell membranes and negatively stained (*i.e.*, outlined) a series of tiny structural elements traversing the gap region in the junction (Fig. 6-10). Further information about the fine structure of the gap region came from use of the freeze-fracture-etch technique (Fig. 4-3) discussed in connection with the cell membrane in Chapter 4. Fractures passing through the gap region revealed the presence of tiny tubular channels that extend across the narrow intercellular gap and connect the external surfaces of the apposed cell membranes. These studies clearly indicated that the structures negatively stained by lanthanum were cylindrical in shape with an open channel roughly 2 nm in diameter extending down their middle (Fig. 6-10). Fluorescent dyes of low molecular weight (less than 1500 daltons) and uncharged permeability probes with molecular dimensions not exceeding 2 nm are able to pass freely between cells that are interconnected by gap junctions.

The structures outlined by lanthanum are therefore believed to be the walls of tiny *interconnecting passageways* that directly link the interiors of contiguous cells (Fig. 6-10). Known as *connexons*, they are made up of integral membrane protein particles of each of the apposed cell membranes. These particles interlock across the narrow gap region and constitute the walls of numerous cylindrical communication channels (Fig. 6-10). On each cell membrane, the protein particles appear as rings of six dumbbell-shaped sub-

units that enclose one half of the central channel. A slight left-hand twist in the way the subunits are arranged keeps the central channel open. However, the subunits can also assume a more perpendicular orientation that closes off the channel and prevents direct cell-to-cell communication by way of its lumen. It has also been found that the channel discriminates against negatively charged molecules, suggesting the presence of negatively charged molecules in its walls.

The multiple communication channels in gap junctions enable ions and small molecules including amino acids, sugars, nucleotides, and steroids to pass directly from one cell to another without the need for such constituents to enter the intervening intercellular space. The use of permeability probes has shown that water-soluble molecules with molecular weights of up to 1000 daltons can pass freely from cell to cell whereas nucleic acids, proteins, and other macromolecules cannot. Cyclic adenosine monophosphate (cAMP) not only passes unimpeded through gap junctions but also increases gap junction permeability through the creation of new gap junctions as well as through the addition of extra connexons to preexisting gap junctions. Because cAMP is the intracellular mediator or "second messenger" in many different hormonal responses, such induction of gap junctions by cAMP is considered to be an important means of propagating the message from cell to cell to amplify the response.

A clearly demonstrated factor that regulates opening and closing of the permeability channels in gap junctions is the *intracellular* concentration of free *calcium ions*. Under physiological conditions, intracellular calcium levels are kept well below those of tissue fluid, and this maintains the permeability channels in the open configuration. However, critical cell damage results in a massive influx of extracellular calcium ions that, in turn, causes these channels to close. The role of such a sealing-off mechanism in preserving the integrity of the living cells in a damaged epithelial membrane is fairly obvious. At the periphery of the site of damage (commonly a focus of cell death or a tiny tear in the membrane), the intracellular calcium levels in damaged cells become elevated. This then has the immediate effect of sealing off their gap junctions and preventing loss of essential ions and small molecules from neighboring undamaged cells by way of open permeability channels of gap junctions. The same mechanism preserves the integrity of undamaged cells in epithelial glands such as the liver, as well as in other tissues provided with gap junctions, in situations in which these cells lie in proximity to cells that become damaged. Gap junctions are also sensitive to *p*H; their electrical conductivity (which is a function of their ionic permeability) decreases as the H^+ concentration rises in the cytoplasm.

Physiological Implications of Gap Junctions. As already noted, gap junctions permit direct cell-to-cell transfer of low–molecular weight nutrients, and they ensure widespread dissemination of molecular intracellular signals. They can also play an essential role in conducting electrical signals from cell to cell. This latter property, which is a consequence of the flow of ions through their aqueous conducting channels, keeps epithelial cells electrically coupled. More importantly, it plays a key role in conducting waves of depolarization throughout the heart in a pattern that brings about the contraction of its various component parts in the appropriate working sequence. Gap junctions similarly conduct waves of depolarization from one smooth muscle cell to another in visceral smooth muscle. Furthermore, at electrical synapses (which operate on an entirely different principle from the chemical synapses that represent the vast majority of synaptic connections in the nervous system), they transmit nerve impulses directly and without delay.

Gap junctions are also commonly present between embryonic cells, particularly during the early stages of development. Their presence is thought to indicate a requirement for direct metabolic coupling between embryonic cells, together with the need for a direct cell-to-cell transfer of nutrients. Another hypothesis is that these communicating junctions play a vital role in relaying cell recognition signals, positional information, or other signals required to direct the normal course of development of the embryo. The presence of gap junctions between the cells of epithelial membranes also has implications with regard to the transfer of nutrients from epithelial cells situated near the capillaries in the underlying connective tissue to cells that have to survive in a less advantageous position.

THE TERMINAL WEB

The narrow transverse zone of cytoplasm that lies just beneath the striated border of an intestinal absorptive cell is reinforced with a dense network of intermediate filaments.

Some microfilaments and what appear to be a few very short myosin filaments are present here as well. Because this zone is so rich in filaments and has a texture that is weblike, it is known as the *terminal web* (Figs. 4-39 and 6-12). At the periphery of the terminal web, microfilaments are anchored to the cell membrane along the zonula adherens. The microfilaments in the cores of the microvilli that make up the striated border extend down as far as the terminal web, where they are thought to interact with associated myosin as outlined in connection with microvilli in Chapter 4 and illustrated in Figure 4-38. Many of the tonofilaments present in the terminal web are anchored to spot desmosomes; some of these junctions belong to the junctional complex and others lie elsewhere on the cell surface (Fig. 6-12). For further information about the organization of the brush border and terminal web, see Mooseker et al.

CELL RENEWAL IN EPITHELIA

There are basically two different arrangements for cell renewal in epithelia. In simple epithelia that are not specialized (*i.e.*, simple squamous, simple cuboidal, and unmodified simple columnar epithelia), all the cells of the epithelium retain the capacity for mitosis. However, epithelia containing specialized cell types that cannot divide are provided with stem cells that have the capacity to produce their different kinds of specialized cells (stem cells were described under Cell Renewal in Chap. 3). In simple columnar epithelium, the stem cells lie protected below the general surface of the epithelium in small glandular invaginations called crypts. In pseudostratified epithelium, the stem cells are present in the basal cell population that lies between its taller, nondividing cells. In stratified epithelium, the stem cells are present in the basal layer. Their progeny cells differentiate and cease dividing as they become displaced toward the free surface of the epithelium.

A damaged epithelial membrane repairs itself very readily. This repair process is partly dependent on regeneration through mitosis, but it is also partly a consequence of migration of the nearby surviving cells into the bare area. Compensatory proliferation generally occurs at a short distance behind the migration front. In situations in which large areas of skin become denuded, epidermal stem cell reserves located in the deeper parts of hair follicles and sweat glands act as a supplementary source of new epidermal cells.

EPITHELIAL GLANDS

Epithelial glands represent the second major subdivision of epithelial tissue. They are broadly classified as *exocrine* or *endocrine*. The development of these two different categories of glands, including the basis on which they are

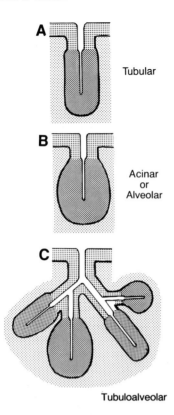

A — Tubular

B — Acinar or Alveolar

C — Tubuloalveolar

Fig. 6-15. Diagrammatic representation of three of the arrangements found in exocrine glands. (*A* and *B*) Simple glands have a duct that does not branch. (*C*) Compound glands have a branching duct system. Glands may have (*A*) tubular or (*B*) acinar or alveolar secretory units. Some compound glands (*C*) possess both kinds of secretory units.

distinguished, is illustrated in Figure 5-2 and was described in Chapter 5 under Embryonic Development of the Four Basic Tissues.

Exocrine Glands

Goblet cells are often regarded as unicellular mucus-secreting *exocrine glands* rather than as an integral component of *epithelial membranes*. All multicellular exocrine glands have two major epithelial components: (1) groups of specialized cells called *secretory units* that produce their secretions, and (2) tubular *ducts* that convey these secretions to an epithelially covered surface. The duct cells may also alter the concentration or composition of the secretion, but the important constituents of the secretion are generally proteins or glycoproteins that have been synthesized by the secretory cells. Exocrine glands can be classified in at least four different ways, as described in the following sections.

Simple and Compound Glands.   A gland that has only a *single unbranched duct* is termed a *simple gland* (Fig. 6-15*A*

and *B*). If it has a *branched duct system* leading from a number of secretory units, it is called a *compound gland* (Fig. 6-15*C*). Compound glands are much larger than simple glands. One of the few examples of a simple gland that has a distinguishable secretory unit and an easily recognized duct is the sweat gland (see Fig. 17-8). The unbranched but coiled secretory portion of the gland lies deep in the skin. It opens into a duct of approximately the same diameter that follows a more or less coiled course to the skin surface (see Fig. 17-1*A*).

Many compound glands are large enough to be termed *organs*. Both the liver and the pancreas are large compound glands with extensive branching duct systems. The duct system of a large compound gland can be likened to a tree. The main duct is like the trunk of a tree. Smaller ducts extend from the trunk like branches and, in turn, give rise to smaller and smaller branches. These eventually terminate at secretory units, the products of which they drain away to the site where the main duct (corresponding to the trunk) opens on some surface. For example, the main ducts of the pancreas and liver both deliver secretions into the small intestine.

Tubular, Acinar, and Alveolar Glands.   If the secretory unit or units of a gland are tubular (Fig. 6-15*A*), the gland is called a *tubular gland*. But if the secretory units are more rounded, the gland is said to be an *acinar* (L. *acinus*, grape or berry) or an *alveolar* (L. *alveolus*, little hollow sac) *gland*. Although in the past some distinction was made between acini and alveoli, now they are all usually called *alveoli*, except those in the pancreas, which, because of custom, are still termed *acini*. If glands contain both tubular and alveolar secretory units, or units that have some characteristics of each, they are called *tubuloalveolar glands* (Fig. 6-15*C*).

Mucous, Serous, and Mixed Glands.   *Mucous glands* produce the viscous glycoprotein secretion *mucus. Serous glands* commonly secrete enzymes in their wheylike, watery secretions (L. *serum*, whey). Both mucous and serous secretions can be produced by the same gland, in which case the gland is termed a *mixed gland* because it possesses both kinds of secretory units. In H & E sections, serous units, mucous units, and mixed secretory units with serous and mucous secretory cells contributing to the same unit can be distinguished from one another as described in the following sections.

Acinar secretory cells such as those of the pancreas appear more or less triangular in outline (Fig. 6-16). In *serous secretory units*, the wide base of these secretory cells exhibits an intense basophilia because of an abundance of rER. It also houses the cell's large spherical nucleus (Fig. 6-16). Eosinophilic *zymogen granules* are sometimes quite prominent in the apical cytoplasm of the acinar cells of such enzyme-secreting serous glands. These granules represent secretory vesicles that contain enzymes, some of which are

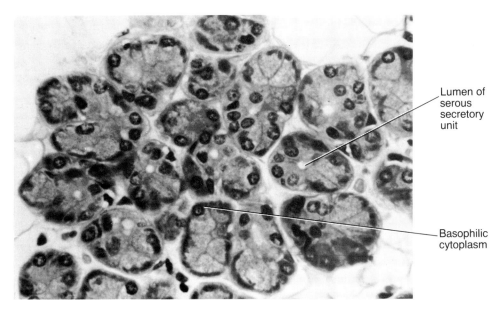

Fig. 6-16. Photomicrograph of serous secretory units in the parotid gland.

in precursor form. The secretory pathway of enzyme-se-creting cells was described in Chapter 4 and is illustrated Figure 4-11. In the regions of their lateral cell borders that lie adjacent to the lumen of the acinus, there are prominent junctional complexes. At numerous sites along their contiguous borders, there are also spot desmosomes and gap junctions.

In H & E sections, *mucous secretory units* appear extremely pale compared with serous secretory units (Fig. 6-17). The nucleus of their constituent mucus-secreting cells is relatively small, and it is also generally flattened, appearing to be pressed against the base of the cell. The remainder of the cell is pale and vacuolated because of its content of mucous secretory vesicles (Fig. 6-17). This stored mucus

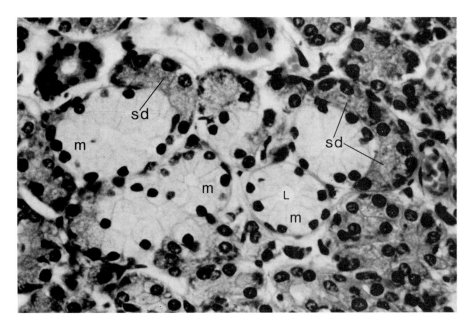

Fig. 6-17. Photomicrograph of serous, mucous, and mixed secretory units in the submandibular gland. A few serous units made up solely of serous cells can be seen at bottom right. Mucous secretory units consisting entirely of mucus-secreting cells (*m*) are extremely pale-staining, making their lumen (*L*) difficult to discern. Mixed secretory units are capped by a serous demilune (*sd*).

can be clearly demonstrated by the PAS procedure, which stains glycoproteins.

Both serous and mucous secretory units are present in mixed glands that produce *seromucous* secretions. Most mixed glands also contain a number of *mixed secretory units* made up of mucous and serous secretory cells arranged in such a way that both types of cells secrete into the same lumen. Mixed secretory units are mostly made up of mucus-secreting cells, but, in addition, a small cap of serous secretory cells is present on one side of the unit. This cap is termed a *serous demilune* (L. *demidius*, half; *luna*, moon) because it resembles a crescent moon when cut in cross section (Fig. 6-17). In the EM, it can be seen that the serous secretion it produces reaches the lumen of the secretory unit by way of narrow *intercellular canaliculi.*

Interposed between the secretory cells and the basement membrane that surrounds the secretory units of exocrine glands, there are epithelial cells with long branched processes that cradle the secretory unit like a loose basket. These cells are best demonstrated through the use of appropriate histochemical techniques (Fig. 6-18). When they contract, they squeeze the secretion from the secretory unit into the duct system. Because such cells are contractile and yet are derived from epithelial tissue, they are called *myoepithelial cells* (Gr. *mys*, muscle).

Merocrine and Holocrine Glands. Exocrine glands can also be classified according to how the secretory cells release their secretion. In a *merocrine gland,* the secretion is released by exocytosis (*i.e.,* by fusion of the membranous walls of secretory vesicles with the cell membrane; see Fig. 4-11). Almost all exocrine glands are of this type. A now familiar example of a merocrine gland is the acinar component of the pancreas. However, the flask-shaped sebaceous glands that open into hair follicles release their secretion in a completely different manner. In this case, entire cells are sacrificed in producing the secretion. This type of gland is therefore described as *holocrine* (Gr. *holos,* all). As the progeny of the cells that constitute the gland's lining layer become displaced toward its interior, they accumulate intracellular lipid droplets, appearing pale and vacuolated (Fig. 6-19). As the lipid-laden cells move away from the investing connective tissue that provides them with necessary nutrients, they die and thereupon disintegrate. *Sebum,* the oily secretion that results from their disintegration, helps to maintain the suppleness of the skin and hair.

In the histological literature, reference is also occasionally made to *apocrine glands.* This term dates back to early LM observations that suggested that in certain glands (the so-called apocrine sweat glands, for example), the secretory cells part with portions of their superficial cytoplasm and cell membrane during the process of releasing their secretion. However, this impression has not been substantiated by EM observations. The only kind of gland that might be considered to be apocrine (but even this is contentious) is the mammary gland. Claims have been made that its secretory cells lose tiny fragments of cell membrane, and possibly even minute amounts of apical cytoplasm, as investments of the lipid droplets

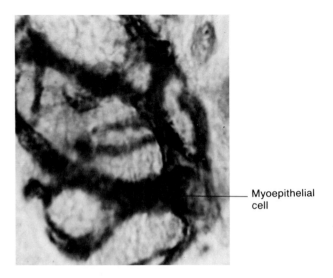

Myoepithelial cell

Fig. 6-18. Photomicrograph of a myoepithelial cell with its contractile processes wrapped around a secretory unit (section of rat submandibular gland, histochemically stained for alkaline phosphatase). (Leeson CR: Nature 178:858, 1956)

that they release during milk secretion. Now largely outdated, the idea of apocrine secretion is no longer useful, and almost all the glands once described as apocrine are now considered to be merocrine.

All Compound Exocrine Glands Have the Same General Plan of Organization. The *epithelial* components of a compound exocrine gland (*i.e.,* its secretory units and ducts) comprise its *parenchyma* (Gr. for something poured in), whereas its supporting *connective tissue* (and also its blood vessels and nerve fibers) constitutes its *stroma* (Gr. for something laid out to lie on). The whole gland is enclosed by a tough *capsule* constructed of fibrous connective tissue. Fibrous connective tissue *septa* that are continuous with its fibrous capsule support it internally and subdivide its parenchyma. In large compound glands such as the liver, the segments of parenchyma that are separated in this manner constitute anatomically distinct *lobes.* In smaller compound glands, however, these segments can only be seen at the microscopic level; hence they are called *lobules. Interlobar septa* separate lobes whereas *interlobular septa* (Fig. 6-20) separate lobules. The fibrous septa support the main branches of the duct system and converge toward the site where the main duct leaves the gland. *Interlobular ducts* extending along the fibrous interlobular septa are generally fairly prominent in sections (Fig. 6-20). *Intralobular ducts,* which lie *within* lobules, have a smaller lumen and a thinner epithelial lining. Furthermore, they are embedded in substantially lesser amounts of connective tissue. These two kinds of ducts may be compared in Figures 6-20 and 6-21. The delicate connective tissue situated between the secretory units of the gland constitutes the remainder of the stroma. It contains numerous capillaries that provide the secretory cells with nutrients and oxygen. The larger blood vessels supplying the gland enter or leave it by way of its

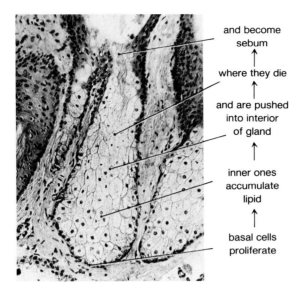

Fig. 6-19. Photomicrograph of a sebaceous gland of the skin, illustrating the stages by which a holocrine secretion is produced. Sebaceous glands open into hair follicles.

and become sebum

↑

where they die

↑

and are pushed into interior of gland

↑

inner ones accumulate lipid

↑

basal cells proliferate

fibrous connective tissue septa; they can readily be distinguished from interlobular ducts because they are lined with squamous cells whereas the ducts are lined with columnar cells.

Control of Secretory Activity. In exocrine glands, the process of secretion is elicited by nerve impulses and also by certain hormones. However, the secretory activity of glands, unlike the activity of one's skeletal muscles, is not under voluntary nervous control. People cannot voluntarily stop themselves from sweating or prevent their mouths from becoming dry if they become nervous while making a speech. The nervous control of the secretory activity of exocrine glands is mediated by what is termed the involuntary or *autonomic* division of the nervous system, which functions more or less automatically, except that it is also affected by emotional states as explained in connection with the Adrenal Medulla in Chapter 22.

The hormonal control of the secretory activity of exocrine glands is seen, for example, in the gastrointestinal tract. The presence of certain foods in the stomach causes an appropriate hormone to be secreted into the bloodstream; this then instructs certain glands farther down the tract to secrete digestive juices so that when the contents of the intestinal tract arrive there, they will be further digested.

Endocrine Glands

The structure of most endocrine glands is relatively simple because these glands have *no ducts*; they secrete into the bloodstream instead. Small groups of secretory cells are arranged around the comparatively wide capillaries that are present in the delicate connective tissue between these cells (see Fig. 5-2, *bottom*). A tough *capsule* of fibrous connective tissue encloses the whole gland, and in many instances, projections of fibrous connective tissue extend into the interior of the gland as *trabeculae* (L. for small beams). These strong beamlike components, which again provide internal support and convey blood vessels into the substance of the gland, can impart a lobular appearance to the gland when it is seen in section.

The secretory products of endocrine glands are called *hormones*. However, hormones are also produced by secretory cells that are scattered throughout other parts of the body (in the brain and throughout the digestive tract),

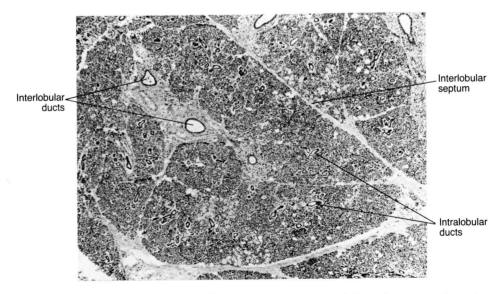

Interlobular ducts

Interlobular septum

Intralobular ducts

Fig. 6-20. Low-power photomicrograph showing the general organization of a compound exocrine gland (parotid).

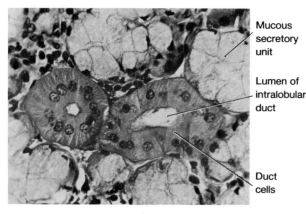

Mucous
secretory
unit

Lumen of
intralobular
duct

Duct
cells

Fig. 6-21.   Photomicrograph of intralobular ducts in a mucous gland.

so they do not represent exclusive products of endocrine glands. Also, a gland that secretes a useful substance into the bloodstream is sometimes referred to as endocrine even if this substance is not a hormone. For example, the liver (which is the exocrine gland that secretes bile into the intestine) is often cited as being partly endocrine because it also releases glucose into the bloodstream. The pancreas is also partly exocrine, secreting digestive enzymes into the intestine, and partly endocrine, secreting the hormones insulin and glucagon into the bloodstream.

Endocrine glands characteristically *store* the hormone they secrete. In most cases, the hormone accumulates *intracellularly* as secretory granules that are ready to be discharged by exocytosis. Indeed, it has been ascertained that the amount of insulin stored in the secretory granules of β cells of pancreatic islets would cause the blood sugar level to plummet to a fatally low level if the contents of these granules were ever to be liberated into the bloodstream all at the same time.

An altogether different storage arrangement is found in the thyroid gland. Here, an inactive macromolecular precursor known as thyroglobulin is first produced, and this precursor then serves as a continuing source of thyroid hormone. The iodinated form of thyroglobulin is stored *extracellularly* in the central lumen of thyroid follicles, which are spherical storage units with walls composed of the cells that produce thyroid hormone. These cells first secrete thyroglobulin into the follicular lumen and then produce thyroid hormone from the stored precursor.

The body has a variety of different endocrine glands; most possess secretory cells of more than one type. Regulation of their secretory activities is a somewhat complex matter, but in most cases, the general principle underlying their regulation is *negative feedback.* Feedback mechanisms are able to compensate very precisely for alterations in the rates at which cells carry out their specific functions. A straightforward example of such an arrangement is the hormonal mechanism that maintains the blood calcium level within its normal limits. Any significant decline in

the blood calcium level stimulates certain endocrine cells to release a hormone (parathyroid hormone) that sets in motion a set of compensatory processes capable of restoring the blood calcium level to its normal range. However, rising calcium levels then begin to exert a negative feedback on these cells so that release of the hormone is terminated when the blood calcium level returns to its normal range.

SELECTED REFERENCES

Cell Junctions

ALBERTS B, BRAY D, LEWIS J ET AL: Cell junctions. In Molecular Biology of the Cell, p 682. New York, Garland Publishing, 1983

CLAUDE P, GOODENOUGH DA: Fracture faces of zonulae occludentes from tight and leaky epithelia. J Cell Biol 58:391, 1973

FAWCETT DW: Junctional specializations. In The Cell, 2nd ed, p 124. Philadelphia, WB Saunders, 1981

GILULA NB: Gap junctions and cell communication. In Brinkley BR, Porter KR (eds): International Cell Biology 1976–1977. New York, Rockefeller University Press, 1977

GILULA NB: Junctions between cells. In Cox RP (ed): Cell Communication, p 1. New York, John Wiley & Sons, 1974

HERTZBERG EL, LAWRENCE TS, GILULA NB: Gap junctional communication. Annu Rev Physiol 43:479, 1981

HULL BE, STAEHELIN LA: Functional significance of the variations in the geometrical organization of tight junction networks. J Cell Biol 68:688, 1976

LENTZ T, TRINKAUS JP: Differentiation of the junctional complex of surface cells. J Cell Biol 48:455, 1971

LOEWENSTEIN WR: Permeability of the junctional membrane channel. In Brinkley BR, Porter KR (eds): International Cell Biology 1976–1977. New York, Rockefeller University Press, 1977

MCNUTT NS, WEINSTEIN RS: The ultrastructure of the nexus. A correlated thin-section and freeze-cleave study. J Cell Biol 47:666, 1970

MCNUTT NS, WEINSTEIN RS: Membrane ultrastructure at mammalian intercellular junctions. Prog Biophys Mol Biol 26:47, 1973

OVERTON J: Experimental manipulation of desmosome formation. J Cell Biol 56:636, 1973

PAPPAS GD: Junctions between cells. Hosp Prac, August, 1973

REVEL JP: Morphological and chemical organization of gap junctions. Electron Microscopy 1978, Vol 3, p 651. Papers presented at Ninth International Congress on Electron Microscopy. Toronto, Microscopical Society of Canada, 1978

STAEHELIN LA: Structure and function of intercellular junctions. Int Rev Cytol 39:191, 1974

STAEHELIN LA, HULL BE: Junctions between living cells. Sci Am 238: 140, May, 1978

WEINSTEIN RS, MCNUTT NS: Cell junctions. N Engl J Med 286:521, 1972

Terminal Web

HIROKAWA N, TILNEY LG, FUJIWARA K, HEUSER JE: Organization of actin, myosin, and intermediate filaments in the brush border of intestinal epithelial cells. J Cell Biol 94:425, 1982

MOOSEKER MS, BONDER EM, CONZELMAN KA ET AL: Brush border cytoskeleton and integration of cellular functions. J Cell Biol 99: 104s, 1984

7

Loose Connective Tissue and Adipose Tissue

With this chapter we begin the study of a group of interrelated tissues that are classed under the general heading connective tissues because they are all derivatives of the embryonic tissue mesenchyme. The tissues that make up this connective tissue group are (1) loose connective tissue, (2) adipose tissue (fat tissue), (3) blood cells, (4) the blood cell–forming tissues, (5) dense ordinary connective tissue, (6) cartilage, and (7) bone.

LOOSE CONNECTIVE TISSUE

Loose connective tissue (also known as *areolar tissue*) permeates almost every part of the body, providing intimate support for blood vessels and nerves of all sizes. It is also the usual arena for the process of inflammation, which commonly occurs when some part of the body is invaded by pathogenic microorganisms. One of its most obvious roles is to hold together and nourish the other tissues of the body. It is able to carry out these functions because it produces relatively abundant amounts of *intercellular substances*.

The intercellular components of loose connective tissue fall into two different classes: (1) *intercellular fibers* made of fibrous proteins, and (2) an *amorphous intercellular component* made up of nonfibrous macromolecular intercellular substances arranged in the form of a shapeless gel (Gr. *a*, without; *morphē*, form). Strong fibers made of the fibrous protein *collagen* are able to resist stretch. Fibers made of the protein *elastin*, on the other hand, elongate passively if stretched and then recoil when released. Collagen is also a major constituent of the basement membranes found along the interface between loose connective tissue and its adjoining tissues.

The amorphous intercellular component of loose connective tissue is a gelatinous *ground substance* or *intercellular matrix* that fills the interstitial gaps between its component cells and capillaries. Because this amorphous component has the structure of a gel, it is riddled with countless submicroscopic intermolecular spaces that act as a reservoir for interstitial (tissue) fluid. The vast amounts of tissue fluid held in these interstices in its gel structure (1) facilitate the diffusion of oxygen and nutrients from the capillaries in loose connective tissue to the cells in the various tissues of the body, and (2) promote effective diffusion of metabolic by-products in the reverse direction (see Fig. 1-2). Hence two distinctive features of loose connective tissue are that (1) its cells are separated from one another fairly widely by intercellular substances, and (2) amorphous ground substance represents a major constituent of its intercellular substances. In the latter respect, loose connective tissue differs from dense ordinary connective tissue, which is primarily a fibrous tissue.

As will become increasingly evident when we consider the various kinds of cells that are present in this tissue, loose connective tissue also plays an important defensive role in the mounting of the acute inflammatory reaction and immune responses. Additional cell types involved in the acute inflammatory reaction and immune responses will be described in subsequent chapters.

CONNECTIVE TISSUE FIBERS

A microscopic preparation that shows the fibers in loose connective tissue to considerable advantage can easily be made from a small piece of subcutaneous connective tissue taken from a laboratory animal. A small tissue sample is removed from the superficial fascia under the skin, stretched out flat to make a preparation called a *spread*, and then fixed and suitably stained to reveal its various components (Fig. 7-1). A glance at Figure 7-11 will provide a preview of the intercellular fibers and a variety of different cell types that may be seen in such a preparation.

The *collagen fibers* can be recognized by their relatively large diameter and by the fact that they are somewhat acidophilic. By employing a trichrome stain (*e.g.*, Mallory,

van Gieson, or Masson stain), it is possible to distinguish them clearly from the other tissue components that stain pink with hematoxylin and eosin (H & E) (*e.g.*, muscle fibers). Collagen fibers are characteristically thick and unbranched, with a diameter of 2 μm to 10 μm, and in spreads they commonly appear wavy (Fig. 7-1; see also Fig. 7-11). Careful focusing under the microscope discloses that they are made up of smaller *collagen fibrils* (Fig. 7-1). Such fibers are made of type I collagen (see Table 7-1); the difference between type I collagen and the other types of collagen will be explained later in this chapter.

Collagen is a tough protein. Hence if meat contains a high proportion of collagen, it is tough to eat. Lengthy cooking nevertheless produces a tender stew because prolonged boiling eventually converts all the collagen into a much softer hydrated product called gelatin. Furthermore, collagen can be made into leather. Following removal of the epidermis and hair from the hide of an animal, the collagen in the hide (present mostly in the dense ordinary connective tissue layer of the dermis) is treated with a tanning agent that increases its resistance to deterioration.

Elastic fibers are comparatively thin (up to 1 μm in diameter), are less wavy than collagen fibers, and are branched (Fig. 7-1; see also Fig. 7-11). Whereas unfixed collagen fibers are white, unfixed elastic fibers appear slightly yellow. In stained spreads, elastic fibers may appear red or reddish-brown if a more selective stain such as orcein has been used. However, after H & E staining, they rarely acquire a deep enough pink color to be distinguishable in spreads or sections. One of the few sites where elastin can be discerned in routine sections is in the walls of arteries. The reason for this is that the elastin here is present as laminae as well as fairly large fibers.

Fibers of a third type, known as *reticular fibers*, are also present, but these fibers are not sufficiently prominent to be recognizable with routine staining even in connective tissue spreads. They represent *collagen fibrils* that are arranged as narrow bundles 0.5 μm to 2 μm in diameter; these bundles are coated with glycoprotein and polysaccharide-containing proteoglycan, which are macromolecular intercellular substances of complex molecular composition that we shall describe when we consider the amorphous component of connective tissue. Compared with collagen fibers, reticular fibers are fine and delicate; furthermore, they branch extensively to form a delicate supporting network (L. *rete*, net). Reticular fibers provide intimate support for capillaries, nerve fibers, and muscle fibers. In addition, they are closely associated with the connective tissue side of basement membranes. They also serve as fine supporting elements for the parenchymatous cells of major glands such as the liver and for the free populations of blood-forming cells in myeloid and lymphatic tissues.

Although reticular fibers cannot be discerned in connective tissue spreads or routine H & E sections, their pres-

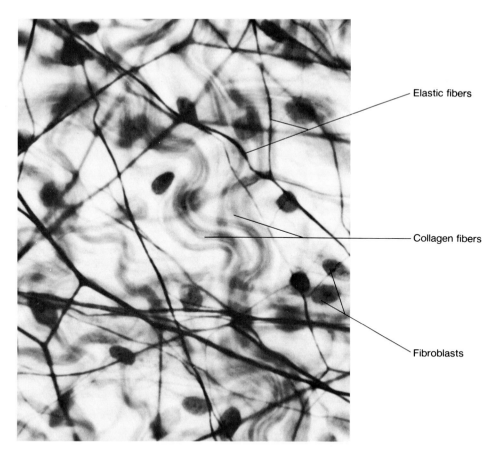

Fig. 7-1. Photomicrograph of loose connective tissue (prepared as a spread and stained with Weigert's hematoxylin, eosin, and resorcin-fuchsin).

ence in tissues such as the hematopoietic tissues can be clearly demonstrated by impregnation with silver, which stains them black (Fig. 7-2). Collagen fibers, on the other hand, stain yellow to brown. The basis of the silver impregnation technique is that the tissue is treated first with a reducible silver salt and then with a reducing agent. The reducing agent acts like a photographic developer, reducing the silver salt to metallic silver, which appears black. The glycoprotein in the coating of reticular fibers also renders them PAS-positive. This represents yet another way of distinguishing them from collagen fibers because the macromolecular carbohydrate content of collagen fibers is insufficient for them to be stained by the PAS procedure. Reticular fibers contain type III collagen (see Table 7-1). In loose connective tissue, they are believed to be produced by fibroblasts, but in the hematopoietic tissues, they appear to be produced by *reticular cells.*

Before we describe the fine structure of intercellular fibers and explain how their structure is related to the way they are formed, it is necessary to present some essential background information on the five main types of collagen.

Collagen

Molecular Structure of the Various Types of Collagen. Collagen molecules are relatively long (approximately 300 nm) and narrow (approximately 1.5 nm). Each molecule consists of three polypeptide chains wound together in the form of a triple helix. Termed α *chains*, these polypeptide chains are made up of repetitive sequences of three amino acids. Five different types of collagen have now been characterized, each of which has its own particular combination of constituent α chains, and several other types of collagen are known to exist as well. The main tissue distributions of these five types of collagen are listed in Table 7-1. In type I collagen, which is characteristic of ordinary connective tissue, bone, and dentin, there is a minor difference in amino acid composition and amino acid sequence between one of the α chains and the other two, which are identical. Each of the molecules of the various other types of collagen is made up of three identical α chains that are distinctive for each collagen type. In certain tissues, however, type V collagen appears to be made up of two different kinds of α chains.

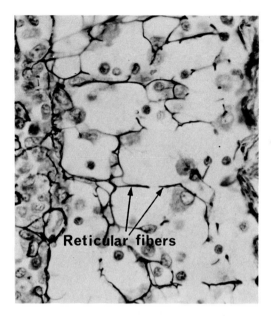

Fig. 7-2. Photomicrograph of reticular fibers in a section of lymph node (PA-silver stain). (Courtesy of Y. Clermont)

Whereas fibrils of type I collagen aggregate into substantial collagen fibers, type II collagen, which is characteristic of cartilage and the vitreous body of the eye, remains in the form of fine fibrils that stay widely dispersed. Type IV collagen, which is apparently confined to basement membranes, produces a fine-woven meshwork instead of forming fibrils or fibers. It has a higher content of carbohydrate side chains and also of the hydroxylated amino acids hydroxylysine and hydroxyproline than the other types of collagen.

The composition of the collagens is unusual for proteins in that the collagens contain a high proportion of proline and glycine, and it is unique in that a substantial number of their proline and lysine residues undergo posttranslational hydroxylation. Although the functional role of the hydroxyproline groups is still a matter of conjecture, advantage can be taken of their relative abundance. For example, it is possible to predict whether a given cell type has the potential to produce collagen by determining whether it produces an enzyme that can hydroxylate proline. Moreover, elevated hydroxyproline levels in the urine reflect an accelerated rate of collagen breakdown in the body. Clinical conditions that are characterized by an excessive resorption of bone, which is a tissue that contains abundant collagen, are generally detectable by this means.

Hydroxylation of proline is promoted by *vitamin C*, which maintains the enzyme prolyl hydroxylase in its active state. Inadequate amounts of vitamin C in the diet can therefore result in the formation of collagen that is not strong enough, and this is a hallmark of the condition *scurvy*. Clinical manifestations of scurvy include capillary bleeding into the skin, accompanied by a generalized fragility of blood vessels and also connective tissue deterioration that becomes particularly noticeable in the gums. The teeth may even loosen in their alveoli because of degeneration of the collagen in the periodontal ligaments that attach the teeth to the alveolar bone. A further complication of scurvy is that wound healing may become impaired. In addition, there are skeletal manifestations of the disease; these will be described in Chapter 12.

The functional significance of the hydroxylysine content of collagen is better understood. First, it participates in the formation of the crosslinks between collagen molecules that give collagen fibers their remarkable strength. Second, it provides collagen molecules with sites of attachment for short carbohydrate chains that are made up of glucose, galactose, or of both of these sugars.

Table 7-1   Distributions and Origins of the Five Types of Collagen

Collagen Type	Principal Tissue Distribution	Cells of Origin
I	Loose and dense ordinary connective tissue; collagen fibers	Fibroblasts and reticular cells; smooth muscle cells
	Fibrocartilage	
	Bone	Osteoblasts
	Dentin	Odontoblasts
II	Hyaline and elastic cartilage	Chondrocytes
	Vitreous body of eye	Retinal cells
III	Loose connective tissue; reticular fibers	Fibroblasts and reticular cells
	Papillary layer of dermis	
	Blood vessels	Smooth muscle cells; endothelial cells
IV	Basement membranes	Epithelial and endothelial cells
	Lens capsule of eye	Lens fibers
V	Fetal membranes; placenta	Fibroblasts
	Basement membranes	
	Bone	
	Smooth muscle	Smooth muscle cells

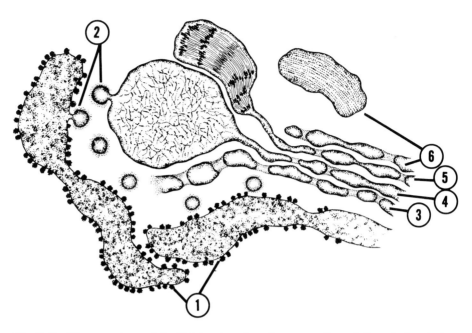

Fig. 7-3. Diagram of part of the Golgi region of a collagen-secreting cell. From bottom to top, note (*1*) cisternae of rER studded with ribosomes; (*2*) transfer vesicles, one of which is budding from a cisterna and another is fusing with a distended portion of a Golgi saccule; (*3*) the first saccule of a stack of Golgi saccules at upper right; (*4*) the second saccule with a distended portion filled with entangled threads; (*5*) the third saccule with a distended portion filled with parallel threads, and (*6*) the fourth saccule, and above it a structure with discrete striations, which is a distended portion that has separated from it; here the parallel threads have aggregated. This structure is a secretory vesicle, and its contents will be released at the cell surface. (Courtesy of M. Weinstock and C. P. Leblond)

Procollagen Secretion. Collagen is produced from a precursor protein called *procollagen* that is synthesized by the rough-surfaced endoplasmic reticulum (rER). The α chains of a procollagen molecule are similar to those of a collagen molecule except that they are extended by a 10-nm–long propeptide at their carboxy-terminal end and a 15-nm–long propeptide at their amino-terminal end. It has been established that a complete pro-α chain can be synthesized in approximately 5 or 6 minutes and that hydroxylation of its proline and lysine residues commences within a few minutes of their incorporation. Glycosylation of hydroxylysyl and other residues also takes place as soon as these pro-α chains enter the lumen of the rER.

Further information about collagen synthesis has been derived from radioautographic studies of tritiated proline incorporation in fibroblasts and odontoblasts (the cells that produce dentin in teeth). The pro-α chains synthesized by the rER (which is labeled *1* in Fig. 7-3) are carried by transport vesicles (labeled *2* in Fig. 7-3) to *cis* Golgi saccules, peripheral distensions of which contain fine entangled threads representing pro-α chains (shown at level *4* in Fig. 7-3). Distensions of saccules in the upper levels of Golgi stacks (level *5* in Fig. 7-3) contain threads that appear straighter and more parallel in arrangement, and by the time the secretory product reaches secretory vesicles (as-

sociated with level *6* in Fig. 7-3), rigid parallel threads representing triple helices of procollagen can be discerned. Radioactivity can be found in these cylindrical vesicles approximately 35 minutes after administering the labeled precursor (Weinstock and Leblond).

Once these procollagen molecules are released from secretory vesicles by exocytosis and enter the intercellular space, the action of carboxy-terminal and amino-terminal peptidases causes the propeptide extension sequences to split off from both of their ends, producing collagen molecules. The collagen molecules are then believed to undergo spontaneous self-assembly into collagen fibrils, but basement membrane type IV collagen is an exception. Procollagen synthesis, secretion, and processing are essentially similar in fibroblasts, osteoblasts, and odontoblasts, all of which produce collagen.

The *propeptide extension sequences* of pro-α chains are believed to play a major role both in facilitating the intracellular association of these chains into triple helices and in preventing premature assembly of such helices into collagen fibrils within the cell. The clinical importance of pro-α chain processing by extracellular peptidases is clearly illustrated by Ehlers–Danlos syndrome type VII, an inherited connective tissue disorder characterized by unusually soft skin, hyperextensibility of joints, and congenital dislocation of the hip. In this genetic disorder, the substitution of an amino acid at

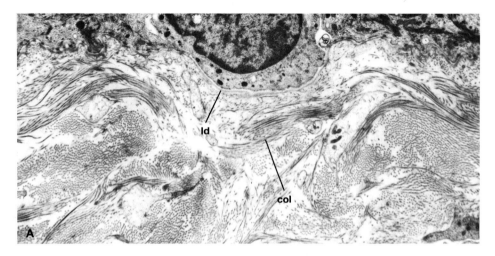

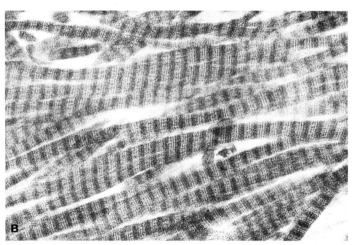

Fig. 7-4. (*A*) Electron micrograph of the superficial region of the dermis, showing collagen fibrils (*col*) in the vicinity of the epidermal–dermal border at low magnification (biopsy of human skin). The inner border of the epidermis and its underlying basement membrane (the lamina densa of which is labeled *ld*) extend across the top of the micrograph. (*B*) Electron micrograph (×37,000) illustrating the characteristic staining pattern of the collagen fibril (osteoid tissue of rat). (*A,* courtesy of P. Lea, *B,* courtesy of L. Arsenault)

the cleavage site for amino-terminal procollagen peptidase interferes with collagen fibrillogenesis. Furthermore, it is widely believed that the main reason why type IV collagen does not self-assemble into collagen fibrils is because it is resistant to extracellular processing by procollagen peptidases.

Collagen Fibrils Have a Distinctive Axial Periodicity That Reflects Their Unique Pattern of Assembly. Collagen fibrils (Figs. 7-4 and 7-5) are formed in the extracellular space from collagen molecules that self-assemble according to the staggered molecular arrangement shown diagrammatically in Figure 7-5*A*, in which collagen molecules are represented as arrows. As each collagen molecule becomes incorporated into the parallel array, it extends beyond its neighbor by one quarter of its length. Furthermore, a tiny gap region becomes incorporated at each intermolecular position (Fig. 7-5*A*). The location and precise transverse alignment of the gap regions become evident after *negative staining* (a method outlined in Chap. 4 under Mitochondria) because the electron microscope (EM) stain

enters the intermolecular spaces in the fibril (compare Fig. 7-5*A* with Fig. 7-5*B*, which shows a fibril with its gap regions demonstrated by negative staining). Hence the gap regions appear *more* electron dense with negative staining. Moreover, a repeating unit (*period*) made up of one dark segment plus one light segment is evident in such a preparation. A similar periodicity is obtained with conventional EM staining, but it is reversed because there is less material in the gap regions to take up the stain and the gap regions therefore appear to be *less* electron dense (compare Fig. 7-5*B* with Fig. 7-5*C*, which shows a fibril stained in the conventional manner). Furthermore, superimposed on this basic periodicity is an additional complex pattern of narrow transverse lines (Fig. 7-4) that reflects the transverse alignment of charged amino acids in the collagen molecules. Hence collagen fibrils can be specifically recognized in the EM by their distinctive *axial periodicity* (repeating pattern of light and dark segments). This 64-nm periodicity reflects the unique pattern of incorporation of collagen molecules into the fibril.

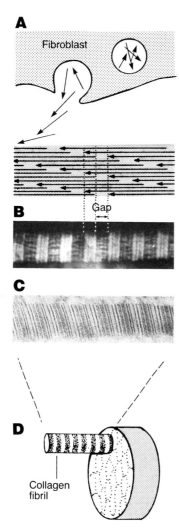

A

Fibroblast

B

Gap

C

D

Collagen
fibril

Fig. 7-5. Diagram summarizing the formation and periodicity of collagen fibrils. Collagen molecules (*arrows*) from fibroblasts undergo extracellular assembly (*A*), becoming incorporated into the component fibrils of collagen fibers (*D*). The electron micrographs illustrate collagen fibrils after (*B*) negative staining and (*C*) conventional staining. See text for details. (*B*, courtesy of A. Howatson and J. Almeida; *C*, courtesy of H. Warshawsky)

EM studies have shown that reticular fibers are also made up of fibrils that exhibit the characteristic axial periodicity of collagen fibrils. When they are impregnated with a silver salt, most of the silver becomes deposited in a polysaccharide-rich coating that covers the exterior of reticular fibers, the carbohydrate content (4%) of which is approximately 10 times higher than that of collagen fibers.

Collagen Degradation.   Collagen can be broken down extracellularly and at neutral *p*H by collagenases produced by fibroblasts, macrophages, and neutrophils. In addition, it is susceptible to the proteolytic action of the lysosomal elastase of neutrophils and macrophages. Furthermore, ly-

sosomal cathepsins (cathepsins B and N) have collagenolytic activity at the low *p*H that characterizes secondary lysosomes. It is therefore likely that collagen degradation is partly extracellular and partly an intracellular process.

Elastin

Elastic Fibers Are Built Around a Microfibrillar Scaffold.   Elastin, too, is assembled extracellularly from a soluble precursor protein called *tropoelastin*. Elastic fibers differ from collagen fibers in that they are not made up of fibrils, nor do they exhibit axial periodicity. Furthermore, in order to assemble elastic fibers the cell must also produce fibrils of another type called *microfibrils* (Fig. 7-6). These additional fibrils are necessary because elastin is an *amorphous* protein that, unless molded into fibers, becomes deposited as *laminae* (sheets). Such elastic laminae, along with elastic fibers, are produced by the smooth muscle cells in the walls of blood vessels. Hence bundles of microfibrils are required as a scaffolding that molds the secreted tropoelastin into roughly cylindrical fibers, and as a result, both tropoelastin and the microfibrillar glycoprotein (which is chemically distinct from elastin and collagen) become incorporated into elastic fibers. Accordingly, the generally pale-staining interior of an elastic fiber (Fig. 7-6) represents the amorphous protein elastin. Enclosing and embedded within this principal component of the fiber are the microfibrils that served as its scaffolding while it was being formed (Fig. 7-6B). Approximately 11 nm in diameter, they stain more darkly than the elastin, outlining the perimeter of the fiber (Fig. 7-6).

In certain respects, the amino acid composition of elastin is similar to that of collagen. However, the proportion of charged amino acids is considerably lower, and although elastin is rich in proline and glycine, it contains little hydroxyproline and lacks hydroxylysine. Furthermore, it contains two unique amino acid derivatives called *desmosine* and *isodesmosine* that crosslink the tropoelastin molecules in elastin. Lysyl oxidase, an enzyme that links the lysine groups of four tropoelastin molecules together during the formation of elastin, is present in the extracellular space. Elastin is believed to be made up of crosslinked flexible peptide chains that, by entering into labile interactions, can cause transient changes in the internal configuration of the protein (Partridge). EM studies of purified elastin indicate that it contains interwoven bundles of paired filaments running roughly parallel to the long axis of the fiber (Gotte).

AMORPHOUS GROUND SUBSTANCE

In addition to the three types of connective tissue fibers, the interstitial space of loose connective tissue contains a relative abundance of *amorphous ground substance* (see Fig. 7-7). This component constitutes a biochemically complex and highly hydrated semisolid gel. The macromolecular organic content of this gel is present in such low concentration that it hardly stains at all. For this reason, the presence of amorphous ground substance in hematoxylin and

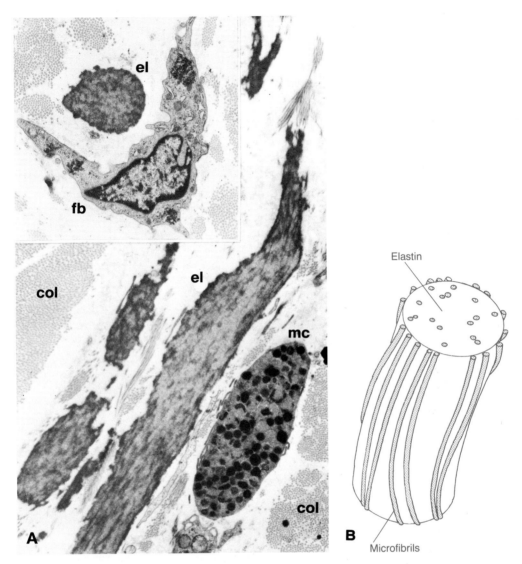

Fig. 7-6. (*A*) Electron micrograph of the superficial region of the dermis, showing elastic fibers (*el*) cut in longitudinal section (biopsy of human skin). Darker-stained microfibrils are also discernible in these fibers. Collagen fibrils cut in cross section (*col*) and part of a heavily granulated mast cell (*mc*) are also present in this section. (*Inset*) Electron micrograph of an elastic fiber (*el*) cut in transverse section (from the same source). Darker-stained microfibrils can be seen inside the fiber and at its periphery. A fibroblast (*fb*) is also present. (*B*) Diagram illustrating the structure of an elastic fiber. The microfibrils shown here constituted a scaffolding for the fiber while it was forming. (*A*, courtesy of P. Lea, *inset*, courtesy of P. Lea and A. Pawlowski)

eosin (H & E) sections or spreads is generally overlooked. Furthermore, this component becomes distorted and finally collapses during the dehydration stages of tissue processing. Its presence is nevertheless still sometimes detectable in skin sections in the papillary layer of the dermis, which is an easily recognized layer of loose connective tissue that lies immediately below the epidermis (see Fig. 17-4). This superficial layer of connective tissue also has numerous blood capillaries and comparable lymphatic capillaries. The

functional significance of the close association between these two kinds of vessels and relatively large amounts of amorphous ground substance will become clear when we discuss the formation of tissue fluid and lymph.

Another point worth emphasizing is that the relative proportion of amorphous ground substance in connective tissue decreases with age. Compared with collagen and elastin, it is abundant in the fetus and the newborn. The fact that its relative contribution diminishes throughout life is particularly noticeable in the skin, which gradually becomes thinner and more wrinkled with advancing old age. Hence when a physician requests a patient's age, he is sometimes obliged to seek confirmation of the patient's answer by observing the general appearance of the patient's skin.

The amorphous component of connective tissue contains a class of macromolecular compounds formerly called *acid mucopolysaccharides* (*muco-* describing their slippery mucuslike nature, and *acid* denoting a preponderance of acidic carbohydrate groups in their polysaccharide chains) but now termed *glycosaminoglycans*. This more recent name reflects the chemical composition of their polysaccharide (*glycan*) chains. The *glycosamino-* part of the term indicates that the linear polysaccharide chain is made up of *repeating disaccharides*, each containing a uronic acid linked to a hexosamine (amino sugar) residue. Some glycosaminoglycans are, in turn, complexed with proteins as *proteoglycans*.

Hyaluronic acid, the principal glycosaminoglycan, constitutes a highly hydrated gel that holds vast amounts of tissue fluid in its interstices. Its repeating disaccharide unit is made up of N-acetylglucosamine linked to glucuronic acid. The unbranched polysaccharide chain of the hyaluronic acid molecule (one end of which may be attached to a peptide) is extremely long, and in aqueous solution, it is irregularly folded and occupies a relatively huge domain (400 nm in diameter). Furthermore, it is believed that hyaluronic acid and the other macromolecular constituents of the amorphous ground substance constitute a macromolecular meshwork. The interstices of this meshwork are filled with tissue fluid, which is the aqueous phase of the gel. As we shall describe later in this chapter, there is an upper limit to the volume of fluid that can be accommodated in such a gel, so in situations in which excess tissue fluid is produced, it forms pools of free fluid in the midst of the gel.

In addition to hyaluronic acid (which is unsulfated), a number of *sulfated glycosaminoglycans* (Table 7-2) are present in the amorphous intercellular component of the different types of connective tissues, particularly in cartilage and bone that have not yet become calcified. In addition to helping to hold the tissue fluid necessary for diffusion, some of the sulfated glycosaminoglycans exist as very firm gels that are capable of providing support. The most obvious example is cartilage matrix. The only reason for listing all the sulfated glycosaminoglycans here is that a number of them are also present in relatively small amounts in the amorphous ground substance of loose connective tissue.

Proteoglycans. Under normal physiological conditions, the glycosaminoglycans other than hyaluronic acid (*i.e.*, the sulfated glycosaminoglycans) become covalently bound as side chains to an axial *core protein* prior to secretion. The resulting *proteoglycan*, with its integral glycosaminoglycan chains, is a very large macromolecule that somewhat resembles a centipede when seen in the EM (see inset of Fig. 7-9).

Table 7-2 Extracellular Sulfated Glycosaminoglycans

Glycosaminoglycan	Repeating Disaccharide Unit
Heparan sulfate	N-acetylglucosamine and glucuronic or iduronic acid
Chondroitin-4-sulfate Chondroitin-6-sulfate	N-acetylgalactosamine and glucuronic acid
Dermatan sulfate	N-acetylgalactosamine and glucuronic or iduronic acid
Keratan sulfate	N-acetylglucosamine and galactose

Proteoglycans differ from glycoproteins (small quantities of which also contribute to the ground substance) in that they are of substantially greater molecular size and possess numerous glycosaminoglycan chains that are invariably made up of a continuously repeating disaccharide unit (which is specified in Table 7-2). These chains are entirely different from the much shorter oligosaccharide chains on glycoprotein molecules because glycoprotein side chains are made up of a variety of different sugar residues that are not linearly arranged as repeating disaccharide groups. The molecular structure of proteoglycans and the aggregates that they form will be described in further detail when we consider cartilage matrix in Chapters 11 and 13. The important point here is that proteoglycans are complex macromolecules largely composed of sulfated glycosaminoglycans. The single long polysaccharide chain of hyaluronic acid could also be attached to a peptide or small protein, but such an arrangement would still differ from glycosaminoglycan attachment to a core protein; hence hyaluronic acid is not classed as a proteoglycan.

Staining Methods for Glycosaminoglycans. Although sulfated glycosaminoglycans are sufficiently polyanionic (acidic) to take up some hematoxylin in H & E sections of cartilage matrix, their concentration in the amorphous ground substance of loose connective tissue is too low for effective staining by this means. Staining methods that can indicate their presence in this tissue include the use of high-affinity cationic (basic) stains (*e.g.*, alcian blue). Alternatively, a metachromatic (Gr. *meta*, beyond; *chroma*, color) cationic stain that stains glycosaminoglycans a color different from that of the stain itself can be used. Toluidine blue, for example, is a blue stain that imparts a purple color to glycosaminoglycans. This difference in color is thought to be a result of close packing of the dye molecules that become adsorbed to closely spaced anionic sites along the glycosaminoglycan molecule. A third way of demonstrating glycosaminoglycans is to take advantage of their marked affinity for colloidal iron. When applied at low *p*H, colloidal ferric iron binds fairly specifically to the anionic groups on glycosaminoglycans; the second step in the procedure is then to stain for this adsorbed iron. However, the only unequivocal way to ascertain which polyanionic constituents are being stained by any of these procedures is to include the appropriate series of enzyme-treated controls.

Unlike glycoproteins, neither glycosaminoglycans nor proteoglycans are PAS-positive. This is because the 1,2-glycol groups in uronic acids require more time for oxidation to aldehyde by periodic acid than is generally allowed in the PAS procedure. Hence it is possible, by histochemical means, to distinguish between the proteoglycans and the glycoproteins in the amorphous component of connective tissue. Because glycoproteins lack a preponderance of acidic (anionic) groups, they do not show the cationic staining and metachromasia exhibited by glycosaminoglycans. However, they are marginally detectable in the ground substance through use of the PAS procedure, which stains them a very faint magenta.

The Fluid Content of Amorphous Ground Substance.
The interstitial fluid (tissue fluid) that bathes connective tissue is retained by the amorphous intercellular component of this tissue. The fluid is held there primarily by the extended hydrophilic glycosaminoglycan chains of proteoglycans. These chains entangle with those of neighboring molecules and constitute an interconnecting network. The interstices of this network have a considerable capacity for holding tissue fluid. However, between the extensive domains occupied by the proteoglycan molecules, there are fine tortuous channels through which tissue fluid, with its dissolved nutrients and gases, can permeate. These channels permit a limited circulation of tissue fluid through the macromolecular meshwork, and as it circulates, there is probably some interchange between the fluid sequestered in the interstices of the gel and the relatively free tissue fluid that circulates slowly through the channels. Substances of low molecular weight are able to diffuse freely through the tissue fluid present throughout the gel. The source and fate of this essential fluid will be considered in the following discussion.

Tissue Fluid and Lymph. Capillaries are lined by squamous *endothelial cells* with lateral borders that are fused to each other at tight junctions. In most regions of the body, these junctions are of the *fascia occludens* type, described under Cell Junctions in Chapter 6. Because this type of junction extends only partway around the perimeter of the cell, there are slitlike intercellular spaces between the junctions where no special arrangement exists to maintain an effective seal. However, these clefts are so narrow that under normal conditions, they permit only small molecules and ions to pass between the cells. The intercellular passage of proteins and other macromolecular substances is impeded.

To explain why such an arrangement would lead to the continuous production of tissue fluid, we should point out that the blood vessels of smallest caliber offer the greatest resistance to blood flow and therefore have the greatest effect in lowering the hydrostatic pressure of the blood flowing through them. By the time blood is delivered to capillaries from arterioles (the finest branches of the arterial tree), its pressure has been considerably reduced, and this pressure continues to drop along the course of each capillary. The hydrostatic pressure in the arterial half of the

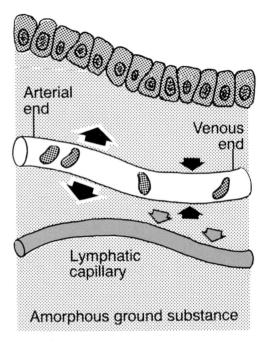

Fig. 7-7. Schematic diagram depicting the mechanism of formation of tissue fluid. Much of the tissue fluid produced by the arterial part of a capillary is resorbed by the venous part of the vessel (*black arrows*). The excess (*blue arrows*) enters lymphatic capillaries and drains away as lymph. Protein that accumulates in the interstitial space also drains away in the lymph.

capillary is nevertheless sufficient to force a certain amount of the fluid portion of blood, depleted of its macromolecular content, through the narrow slits between the endothelial cells. *Tissue fluid* is the dialysate of blood that is thereby formed. However, the macromolecules retained in the fluid portion of blood (*blood plasma*) then exert an osmotic pressure that opposes this hydrostatic pressure and serves to draw fluid back into the capillary. Even so, in the arterial half of the capillary, the resulting osmotic pressure of its contents remains less than the hydrostatic pressure; hence tissue fluid (plasma depleted of most of its protein) is *produced* (Fig. 7-7). In the venous half of the capillary, however, the situation is reversed because resistance of the narrow lumen to the flow of blood further reduces the hydrostatic pressure to a level that is below the osmotic pressure, and, as a result, fluid is *resorbed* (Fig. 7-7). This arrangement therefore leads to the continuous production and resorption of tissue fluid, promoting a steady circulation of tissue fluid through the fine aqueous channels in the gel structure of the ground substance.

A further point to be emphasized is that the volume of tissue fluid produced by the arterial part of a capillary exceeds the volume of fluid that is resorbed by its venous part. The surplus is drained away through an independent set of thin-walled vessels comparable to blood capillaries and termed *lymphatic capillaries*. The clear, watery fluid that collects in them is called *lymph* (L. *lympha,* clear water), and it is composed of tissue fluid in which interstitial protein has accumulated. From the lymphatic capillaries (Fig. 7-7), lymph drains by way of lymphatic vessels into lymphatic ducts that empty into large veins at the root of the neck; hence it is eventually added back to the blood (for further details about these vessels, see Chap. 16).

Causes of Edema

Under certain physiological and pathological conditions, tissue fluid or fluid exudate is produced in amounts that exceed the total volume resorbed at the venous end of blood capillaries and drained away by way of lymphatic capillaries. The resulting accumulation of tissue fluid leads to recognizable swelling of connective tissue, a condition known as *edema* (Gr. *oidema,* a swelling). Clinical confirmation of edema can be obtained by applying gentle fingertip pressure to the site where it is suspected. If there is an excess of tissue fluid in the tissue, a depressed pit will be left for some time because the applied pressure will squeeze free tissue fluid out of the region and into its surroundings. Hence this condition is often described as *pitting edema.* Because the amount of pressure applied is insufficient to displace normal amounts of tissue fluid from the gel structure of the ground substance, a depression is only seen if tissue fluid is present in excess.

It might seem likely that the increased hydrostatic pressure of the tissue fluid or fluid exudate in edematous (swollen) connective tissue would cause its lymphatic capillaries to collapse, thereby interfering with lymphatic drainage. However, this does not happen because the endothelial cells that line lymphatic capillaries have *anchoring fibers* that extend into the surrounding tissue (see Fig. 16-28). The more distended with interstitial fluid the tissue becomes, the greater the tension exerted by these fine collagen fibrils on the walls of the vessel, with the result that the lumen of the vessel is kept open.

The quantity of interstitial fluid or fluid exudate that accumulates in the edematous tissue depends to a marked degree on the subtype of connective tissue that is involved. Whereas loose connective tissue offers minimal resistance to being spread apart from within, dense ordinary connective tissue (*e.g.,* a tendon) is comparatively resistant to such expansion. At most sites, edema tends to be self-limiting because the more swollen a tissue becomes, the more it resists further distension. Prolonged standing in hot weather can cause a physiological edema of the lower extremity. Edema is also one of the cardinal signs of the acute inflammatory reaction, which will be described in Chapter 8 when we consider neutrophils. Some other causes of edema that may be encountered in medical practice are described in the following sections.

1. *The Venous Return May Become Impaired.* Any marked venous compression or occlusion (*e.g.,* as a result of venous thrombosis) can impair the venous drainage of the capillary

bed of a given region and can cause the capillary blood pressure to rise along the entire length of the affected capillaries. This leads to an increase in the rate of production of tissue fluid and a decrease in its rate of resorption at the venous end of these capillaries. Excess amounts of tissue fluid that are not able to drain away as lymph then accumulate as pools of free fluid in the gel structure of the ground substance, causing a local or regional edema. Widespread edema can develop as a complication of cardiac failure, which occurs when the heart fails to pump out blood as fast as this is being returned by way of veins.

2. *Lymphatics May Become Obstructed.* Blockage of lymphatics causes regional edema for two reasons. First, the lymphatics fail to return the normal volume of excess tissue fluid to the blood circulatory system. Second, obstructed lymphatics cannot drain away the small but still significant amounts of plasma protein that escape from blood capillaries even under normal conditions. As the interstitial concentration of proteins rises in the tissue fluid, the osmotic pressure differential between tissue fluid and the plasma in the venous portion of a capillary declines. As a result, the amount of tissue fluid resorbed by that part of the capillary also declines. The marked persistent lymphedema that characterizes the tropical disease *elephantiasis* is a striking example of the effect of chronic lymphatic obstruction by parasitic worms. Such allusion to an elephant certainly conveys the enormously swollen appearance of the affected part of the body.

3. *The Permeability of Capillaries May Be Increased.* Capillary permeability is known to increase markedly at sites of extensive burns and also following crush injury. Leakage of plasma by the damaged capillaries in and around such sites can reduce the blood volume to such an extent that the amount of blood returning to the heart becomes inadequate for the heart to continue to pump efficiently. This, in turn, can lead to further complications, as students will find later in their studies when they address the clinical problem of shock. Furthermore, because blood cells are not lost along with the leaking plasma, they become more concentrated in the plasma that remains. This effect, which is termed *hemoconcentration,* can be corrected through the intravenous administration of blood plasma.

To complete our discussion of the intercellular components that are associated with loose connective tissue, we shall now describe basement membranes.

BASEMENT MEMBRANES

The extensive interface between connective tissue and the various tissues that it supports and nourishes (namely epithelial, nervous, and muscle tissue) is characterized by the presence of a thin layer of specialized intercellular matrix called a *basement membrane.* This extracellular layer is so called because the first site where it was noticed was immediately beneath the basal surface of epithelial membranes. Under the light microscope (LM), the basement membrane appears homogeneous and PAS-positive because of its glycoprotein content (see Fig. 6-2). Electron micrographs nevertheless reveal the presence of a moderately electron-dense layer, seldom more than 100 nm

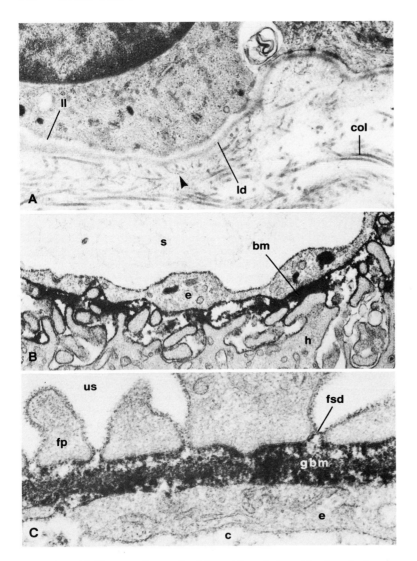

Fig. 7-8. (*A*) Electron micrograph of the epidermal–dermal border of a human skin biopsy, showing the basement membrane under the epidermis. Its lamina densa (basal lamina) is labeled ld and its lamina lucida is labeled ll. Arrowhead indicates associated reticular fibers of its third layer, the lamina fibroreticularis. Collagen fibrils (*col*) are also present in the superficial region of underlying dermal connective tissue. (*B*) Electron micrograph of part of the border of a rat liver sinusoid, showing the basement membrane–like material (*bm*) that supports the walls of the vessel. This material constitutes a discontinuous supporting element that lies between the endothelial lining (*e*) of the sinusoid (*s*) and the adjacent microvillus-covered surface of hepatocytes (*h*). It is stained immunocytochemically as a result of an *in vivo* injection of laminin antibody conjugated to horseradish peroxidase (*HRP*). (*C*) Electron micrograph of part of the wall of a glomerular capillary of rat kidney, showing the glomerular basement membrane (*gbm*) lying between (1) foot processes (*fp*) of the glomerular epithelium and (2) endothelial cells (*e*) that line the fenestrated glomerular capillary (*c*). The urinary filtrate produced by the capillary passes first through the glomerular basement membrane and then through filtration-slit diaphragms (*fsd*) between adjacent foot processes before gaining access to the urinary space (*us*). As in (*B*), the basement membrane glycoprotein laminin is demonstrated by immunocytochemical staining, using injected antilaminin conjugated to HRP. The peroxidase reaction product (which is electron dense) is present throughout the entire thickness of the glomerular basement membrane, extending from the endothelium to the foot processes. It also appears to be localized on the basement membrane–associated surfaces of both the foot processes and the endothelial cells. (*A*, courtesy of P. Lea, *B* and *C*, courtesy of D. R. Abrahamson and J. P. Caulfield)

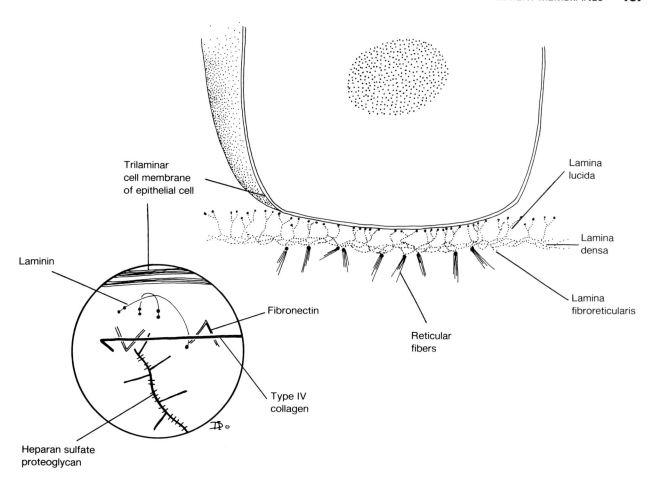

Fig. 7-9. Diagrammatic representation of the basement membrane under an epithelial membrane. Details of its molecular composition (*inset*) are discussed in the text.

thick, that follows the contours of the cell surface at a distance of up to 60 nm from the cell membrane (Fig. 7-8*A*). This electron-dense layer was first given the name *basal lamina*. However, subsequent indiscriminate use of the terms *basement membrane* and *basal lamina* caused confusion because whereas these two terms were initially thought to denote the same structure observed at the LM and EM levels, respectively, it is now clear that the electron-dense layer seen in the EM represents only a part of the basement membrane. Fortunately, new terms that avoid this problem have now emerged. These will be described in the following paragraph.

The electron-dense layer formerly known as the basal lamina is now called the *lamina densa* (Figs. 7-8*A* and 7-9). It varies in thickness from 20 nm to 300 nm, depending on its location. On either side of the lamina densa, there is a less distinct electron-lucent layer that is often referred to as a *lamina rara*. The convention has been to call the lamina rara on the connective tissue side the *lamina rara interna* and the electron-lucent layer on the cellular side, the *lamina rara externa*. However, even this nomenclature

presents some difficulties when it comes to describing the glomerular basement membrane of the kidneys. As a result, a third terminology has recently been introduced to overcome the problem of deciding which side is internal and which side is external. The electron-lucent layer on the cellular side, with a thickness of 10 nm to 50 nm, is now known as the *lamina lucida* (Figs. 7-8*A* and 7-9). The third layer, which is variable in appearance and is comparatively ill-defined, is called the *lamina fibroreticularis* because typically it lies in intimate association with reticular fibers of the underlying connective tissue (Figs. 7-8*A* and 7-9).

Oblique or horizontal sections through the lamina densa reveal that it contains a very fine meshwork of type IV collagen. Unlike type I and type III collagen, type IV collagen is not characteristic of loose connective tissue (see Table 7-1). This delicate network of type IV collagen, together with some of the constituent glycoproteins of the basement membrane, is, in fact, a product of the cell that the basement surrounds or underlies. In contrast, the reticular fibers of the lamina fibroreticularis contain type III collagen, which is an interstitial connective-tissue product, so this part of the basement membrane is clearly transitional to connective tissue. There is also some type V collagen on the connective tissue side of some basement membranes. The nature of the lamina lucida is less firmly established. Suitable EM preparations show that it is traversed by delicate cords that extend from the lamina densa to the cell membrane as depicted in Figure 7-9. These cords are believed to be essentially similar to the anastomosing cords that make up the lamina densa except that they are loosely arranged instead of being closely packed as a tight network. It has recently been established that the anastomosing cords seen both in the lamina densa and, to a lesser extent, in the lamina lucida possess an axial core filament made up of *type IV collagen* and that this filament is encased by a sheath containing the adhesive glycoprotein *laminin* (Inoué et al). Immunocytochemical studies have confirmed that laminin is a universal major constituent of basement membranes (Figs. 7-8*B* and *C*).

As depicted in the inset of Figure 7-9, molecules of *laminin* become preferentially bound to type IV collagen. Another domain on these crucifix-shaped molecules interacts with a laminin receptor in the cell membrane, so an important role of laminin is evidently to attach cells to the basement membrane. In addition, laminin has an affinity for (1) heparan sulfate, which is present in basement membranes as heparan sulfate proteoglycan (Fig. 7-9, *inset*), and (2) other glycosaminoglycans. Another high–molecular weight constituent of basement membranes is the adhesive glycoprotein *fibronectin*. This is essentially a V-shaped molecule that has collagen-binding domains on both arms (Fig. 7-9, *inset*). In addition to binding to many different kinds of macromolecules that include collagen (particularly type III collagen), proteoglycans, heparin, other glycosaminoglycans, and fibrin, fibronectin interacts with a cell membrane receptor; hence it promotes cellular adhesion and the spreading of cells over the basement membrane. Thus fibronectin has a dual role: attaching the basement membrane to its underlying mat of reticular fibers and acting in conjunction with laminin to promote cellular adhesion to the basement membrane.

In addition to these two reasonably well-characterized glycoproteins and also to a sulfated, but less well-characterized, glycoprotein called *entactin*, basement membranes contain a substantial quantity of *heparan sulfate proteoglycan* (Fig. 7-9, *inset*). All of these macromolecular compounds seem to be constituents of the sheath that surrounds the axial filament in the so-called cords observed in the basement membrane. Recent studies of the ultrastructure of basement membranes by Inoué et al and by Laurie et al provide evidence for further morphological organization into (1) hollow rod-shaped structures termed *basotubules* that are composed of a plasma component of extracellular amyloid deposits called *amyloid P*, and (2) tiny paired structures called *double pegs* that apparently represent *nidogen*, a basement membrane protein that enhances integration of basement membrane components (Timpl et al).

In addition to being present under epithelial cells, basement membranes are found along the boundary between loose connective tissue and (1) muscle fibers, and (2) the Schwann cell investment of peripheral nerve fibers. Basement membranes are also found in association with the basal surface of endothelial cells and around adipocytes (fat cells) despite the fact that both of these cell types are components of connective tissue itself because they are derived from mesenchyme.

The most obvious functional roles of basement membranes are to bond cells to the underlying or surrounding connective tissue and to provide these cells with flexible support. These functions are particularly evident in the lens capsule, a highly developed basement membrane that besides having to support the lens has to be able to change its shape every time the eye accommodates for distant vision. Basement membranes are freely permeable to substances of low molecular weight but impede the passage of macromolecules. This property is utilized to particular advantage in the glomerular capillaries of the kidneys. Indeed, the single most important factor that prevents loss of plasma protein into the urine is selective filtration through the glomerular basement membrane. A more speculative role of basement membranes, for which there is accumulating experimental evidence, is that they act as substrates capable of directing cell growth and migration during morphogenesis, regeneration, and repair.

CELLS OF LOOSE CONNECTIVE TISSUE

The forerunner of loose connective tissue is the embryonic tissue *mesenchyme*, which is so called because it was thought to arise exclusively from mesoderm, the middle germ layer of the embryo. It is now known that although almost all mesenchyme is mesodermal in origin, in the head region some of it arises from neural crest. Mesenchyme is characterized by having a population of widely spaced, pale-staining stellate cells with long interconnecting cytoplasmic processes. These cells lie embedded in a gelatinous amorphous ground substance (Fig. 7-10) that begins to contain very fine intercellular fibers as development proceeds. All the cells of loose connective tissue arise directly or indirectly from embryonic mesenchymal cells.

Postnatal loose connective tissue contains a variety of different cell types with activities that range from the production of intercellular substances to the mounting of inflammatory and immune responses. Figure 7-11 shows the seven types of connective tissue cells most commonly encountered in this tissue; each is described in turn in the remainder of the chapter. However, this figure is a composite drawing based on many different spreads and sections, so not all these cell types could be found in a single field. Some of these cell types develop in connective tissue itself, whereas others arise from mesenchyme situated elsewhere in the body and subsequently enter loose connective tissue via the bloodstream.

Endothelial Cells

Endothelial cells develop from the embryonic mesenchymal cells that surround (1) groups of developing blood cells

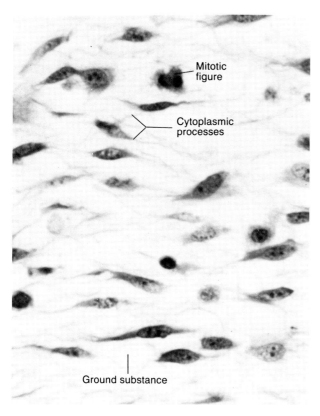

Mitotic figure

Cytoplasmic processes

Ground substance

Fig. 7-10.   Photomicrograph of mesenchyme (embryonic connective tissue).

(*i.e., blood islands*) or (2) tiny pools of tissue fluid that accumulates in mesenchyme. When the lateral borders of these cells become joined to one another, wide capillarylike tubes are formed, and this marks the beginning of development of the blood vascular system.

In LM sections, the only part of endothelial cells that can be identified with certainty is their nucleus. In electron micrographs, however, it can be seen that their attenuated cytoplasm is wrapped around the lumen of the vessel as depicted in Figure 7-12. In capillaries and other small blood vessels of loose connective tissue, there are *tight junctions* between the lateral borders of endothelial cells. As noted above in the section on Tissue Fluid and Lymph, in most regions of the body, these junctions are strip-shaped (*i.e., fascia occludens* junctions); hence the capillaries that supply most parts of the body possess intercellular slits through which tissue fluid is able to pass. However, in certain sites where it is necessary for the permeability of capillaries to be supplemented, the endothelial cells are provided with round, windowlike areas that are 60 nm to 80 nm in diameter. These are called *fenestrae* (L. for windows). Such extra-permeable capillaries are called *fenestrated capillaries* (Fig. 7-12B); capillaries that lack fenestrae are termed *continuous capillaries* (Fig. 7-12A). Although fenestrae were initially thought to be perforations through the cytoplasm

of endothelial cells, EM studies have shown that they are not really unguarded openings. In almost every case, they are covered by a delicate and selectively permeable *diaphragm* (see Fig. 16-20A) that is seldom distinguishable in electron micrographs unless suitable precautions have been taken to preserve its integrity or appropriate methods such as freeze-fracture have been employed to demonstrate its presence. The only fenestrated capillaries that seem to lack diaphragms are the extremely permeable glomerular capillaries that produce urinary filtrate in the kidneys, but in this case, there is a thick glomerular basement membrane to provide the necessary selective permeability (see Fig. 7-8C caption and Fig. 21-11). Endothelial cells line the entire circulatory system, constituting a continuous squamous epithelium termed *endothelium* that produces a basement membrane. Both types of blood capillaries are therefore supported by a basement membrane that lies external to their endothelium (Fig. 7-12). Seen face-on, endothelial cells commonly appear to be long and narrow (generally up to 50 μm long and 15 μm wide).

Other features of endothelial cells that can be observed in electron micrographs of capillaries include the presence of numerous endocytotic pits and vesicles (see Fig. 16-19), contractile filaments, a few mitochondria, and relatively small amounts of rER and sER (smooth-surfaced endoplasmic reticulum). Characteristic rodlike granules in the cytoplasm of endothelial cells have also been described (Weibel and Palade).

The fact that endothelial cells retain the capacity to divide facilitates maintenance of the lining layer of the circulatory system and enables new capillaries to sprout from the existing endothelium whenever the need arises. Endothelial cells play an important role in facilitating the exchange of substances across capillary walls, and they provide the intercellular slits through which tissue fluid passes. In addition, they produce type III collagen and proteoglycans, which are interstitial connective tissue constituents. The fact that they also differentiate from mesenchyme and give rise to tumors classified as being of connective tissue origin are further reasons for considering endothelial cells as a component of connective tissue. Although the convention has been to view them strictly as squamous epithelial cells, few would disagree that from a developmental and functional point of view, they belong to connective tissue.

Pericytes

Pericytes are pale-staining connective tissue cells with long, slender cytoplasmic processes that lie immediately external to the endothelium of (1) blood capillaries and (2) the small venules into which capillaries empty. Called *pericytes* because of their perivascular position (Gr. *peri*, around), these cells lie scattered along the course of the vessel with their processes wrapped around the basal surface of its endothelium. Their position relative to the endothelium is such

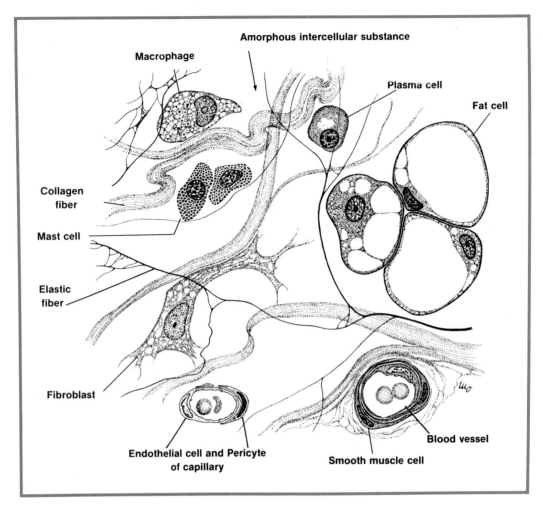

Fig. 7-11. Diagrammatic representation of the cells and fibers of loose connective tissue. These microscopically identifiable components lie embedded in amorphous ground substance and are continuously bathed with tissue fluid produced by capillaries.

that they are insinuated into the basement membrane of the vessel (Fig. 7-12; see also Figs. 14-26, 16-19, and 16-22).

There is substantial evidence that pericytes retain enough mesenchymal potentiality in adult life to give rise to both fibroblasts and smooth muscle cells. Their comparatively undifferentiated appearance, broad potentiality, pale staining, and stellate shape are all consistent with the hypothesis that they represent residual mesenchymal cells that remain available for the repair of connective tissue and damaged blood vessels whenever the need arises. For example, connective tissue repair requires the formation of arterioles and venules that possess smooth muscle cells in their walls (Fig. 7-11, *blood vessel*). It is now established that pericytes can produce the smooth muscle cells that appear under such conditions. Finally, during the repair of wounds, there is extensive proliferation of fibroblasts, which are the cells that produce the intercellular substances of loose connective tissue. *In vitro* evidence indicates that

fibroblasts mature enough to have formed intercellular substances are still able to divide. It is nevertheless questionable whether mature fibroblasts could serve as the source of all the new fibroblasts that participate in the repair process. It is now believed that capillary-associated pericytes, proliferating along with endothelial cells in the repair process, serve as progenitor cells for such fibroblasts (Ross et al).

Fibroblasts

Fibroblasts (L. *fibra*, fiber; Gr. *blastos*, germ) are the cells that produce the fibers and amorphous ground substance of ordinary connective tissues. At the stage when they are actively producing intercellular substances, they either possess wide cytoplasmic processes (Fig. 7-13, *middle*) or appear spindle-shaped (Fig. 7-13, *bottom*). Their abundant cytoplasm is markedly basophilic and their nucleoli are

by fibroblasts for the secretion of procollagen, proteoglycans, tropoelastin, and the microfibrillar glycoprotein that becomes incorporated into elastic fibers. The steps in protein synthesis and secretion are essentially similar to those described in Chapter 4, with the minor difference that in fibroblasts, the secretory process is not polarized. In other words, fibroblasts are able to release their secretory products from any part of their cell surface, not just from an apical surface as in epithelial cells. The fine structure of the fibroblast, illustrated in Figure 7-14, is typical of a cell that secretes proteins very actively.

Whereas the collagen-forming role of fibroblasts is extremely well known, it is not as widely appreciated that fibroblasts also produce collagenase and can therefore break down collagen, including residual collagen that is left behind when bone matrix is resorbed. Hence it is possible for collagen to be present within fibroblasts, but it is always confined to phagosomes or secondary lysosomes and is not present within secretory organelles. Fibroblasts are therefore capable of producing new collagen and breaking down existing collagen, both at the same time.

Macrophages

The macrophages of loose connective tissue, sometimes also referred to as *histiocytes,* are relatively large free phagocytic cells with a diameter of approximately 12 μm that engulf particulate matter and submit it to lysosomal

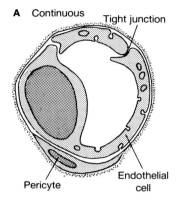
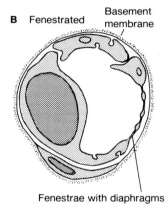

Fig. 7-12. Schematic representation of (*A*) continuous and (*B*) fenestrated capillaries, showing the relative positions and general features of their endothelial cells and pericytes. See text for details.

generally prominent, indicating active protein synthesis (Fig. 7-13). The same cells become less active during adult life and are then often referred to as *fibrocytes.* The flattened ovoid nucleus of a fibrocyte contains chromatin that is much more condensed, and its cytoplasm is less basophilic than that of a fibroblast. However, because it has been found that adult fibrocytes can still take up labeled proline, a collagen precursor, it seems likely that they continue to secrete small amounts of intercellular substances throughout life. Fibrocytes seem to be unable to divide; hence connective tissue repair is effected by ingrowth of young fibroblasts derived primarily from pericytes.

It should be kept in mind that the fibroblast is not the *only* kind of cell that forms intercellular substances. Thus the collagen and proteoglycans in cartilage and bone matrix are produced by chondroblasts and osteoblasts, respectively. Furthermore, the reticular fibers of the hematopoietic tissues are produced by reticular cells. In addition, it is now clear that smooth muscle cells form elastin in the walls of blood vessels. Other special dental connective tissue cells (odontoblasts and cementocytes) produce intercellular substances of the tooth.

The secretory pathway for procollagen that was described earlier in this chapter and is illustrated in Figure 7-3 is used

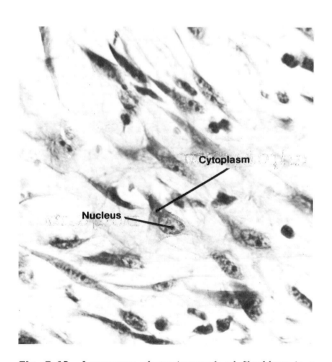

Fig. 7-13. Low-power photomicrograph of fibroblasts in a healing wound. These cells have basophilic cytoplasm and are actively synthesizing intercellular substances.

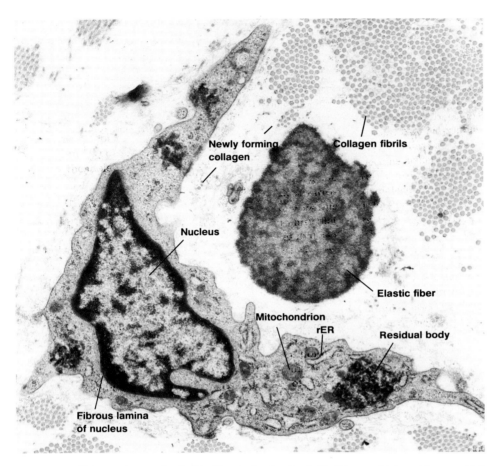

Fig. 7-14. Electron micrograph of a fibroblast in the dermis of skin (biopsy of tattooed human skin). Distended cisternae of rough-surfaced endoplasmic reticulum (*rER*) and residual bodies containing aggregates of tattoo ink particles are prominent in its cytoplasm. The fibrous lamina of its nucleus can just be discerned. (Courtesy of P. Lea)

hydrolysis. Macrophages are classified as connective tissue cells because they represent a normal component of loose connective tissue and they are derived from mesenchyme. However, macrophages also constitute an essential component of other tissues and organs, notably the hematopoietic tissues and the liver. Connective tissue macrophages have a round to oval or angular shape, and their dark-staining nucleus, which is generally eccentric in position, commonly has the shape of an indented oval or kidney bean (Fig. 7-15). Sometimes the relatively large particles that these cells have phagocytosed obscures their nucleus, but even if their nucleus cannot be seen, the presence of extraneous particles within a rather large cell generally indicates that it is a macrophage of some kind. The process of phagocytosis was described in Chapter 4 in the section on Lysosomes. Engulfed particles (including such experimental markers as particles of India ink or trypan blue dye) pass into the cytoplasm in phagosomes that then fuse with primary lysosomes. Hydrolytic enzymes from the primary

lysosomes attack and degrade organic macromolecules in the ingested material. When seen in the EM, macrophages typically manifest phagocytosed material present in phagosomes, together with an assortment of various kinds of secondary lysosomes including residual bodies that contain indigestible remains (Fig. 7-16). A few cisternae of rER and a prominent Golgi apparatus are also present. The surface of macrophages generally has an irregular appearance because of the presence of pseudopodia, surface folds, and microvilli.

Among the various duties carried out by the macrophages in loose connective tissue are the elimination of certain kinds of infectious microorganisms, clearance of the cellular debris resulting from the acute inflammatory reaction that follows infection or trauma, and ingestion of the daily accumulation of exogenous particulate matter that clutters up the lungs of heavy smokers. The main function of the macrophages in the spleen is to dispose of worn-out blood cells, whereas the macrophagelike dendritic cells in lymph

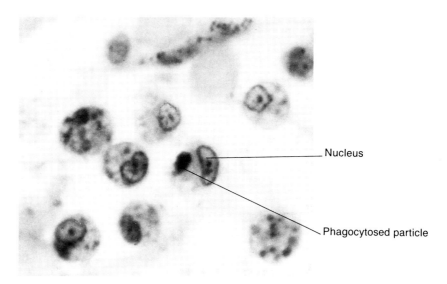

Fig. 7-15. Photomicrograph of a group of macrophages that are phagocytosing cellular debris at a site of acute inflammation. Macrophages can be recognized by their bean-shaped nucleus and large ingested particles.

nodes seem to be able to process ingested antigens ready for subsequent presentation to lymphocytes. In addition to these various phagocytic functions, there is evidence that macrophages represent the cellular source of (1) complement proteins and (2) a number of important hematopoietic growth regulators. (Information about hematopoietic regulators can be found in Chap. 9; complement proteins will be considered later in this chapter.) Because the macrophages of the body carry out such a variety of functions, they are believed to represent a very heterogeneous population.

Antibody Molecules Can Facilitate Phagocytosis.   It is now known that at least two different conditions can render macrophages more efficient at phagocytosing microorganisms. Under the first of these conditions, which leads to the production of what are termed *activated macrophages,* macrophages are influenced by a *migration inhibitory factor* that is released by antigen-stimulated regulatory T-lymphocytes. (This factor and its effects on macrophages will be discussed in Chap. 10.) The other condition known to enhance the phagocytosis of microorganisms by macrophages is the existence of any preformed antibody (immunoglobulin) molecules that are directed against specific antigens on the surface of these microorganisms. One end of the immunoglobulin molecule, which in its monomeric form is shaped like a Y, is called its *Fc* end (*F* for fragment and *c* for crystallizable, *i.e.,* the part of the molecule that will crystallize if it is split off by a proteolytic enzyme). The Fc portion of the immunoglobulin molecule corresponds to the tail region of the Y-shaped molecule, whereas the antigen-combining sites are situated on its two arms. These arms retain their antigen-binding specificity after controlled proteolytic digestion of the immunoglobulin molecule, so

they are termed the *Fab* portion of the molecule (*f*ragment, *a*ntigen-*b*inding). Macrophages possess cell-surface receptors for the Fc end of antibody molecules of the immunoglobulin G (IgG) class and accordingly bind such molecules to their surface (for a description of the various classes of immunoglobulin, see Chap. 10). Because of this arrangement, antibody molecules become bound to macrophages in such a way that their opposite end (*i.e.,* their antigen-combining end) is exposed at the cell surface. If any such molecules are directed against surface antigens of infectious microorganisms, they enable the macrophage to recognize those specific microorganisms and facilitate its attachment to them, augmenting phagocytosis. Moreover, the presence of surface Fc receptors on the macrophage enables it to attach itself to microorganisms that have already become coated with antibody because the antibody molecules bound to the microorganisms are oriented with their Fc end facing outward.

In addition to Fc receptors, macrophages possess surface receptors for C3, the third component of complement. *Complement is a self-assembling series of plasma proteins that has the ultimate potential to inflict lethal damage on cells by way of their cell membrane (see Chap. 8 under Neutrophils). Because complement can become bound to antibody-coated microorganisms, C3 receptors can also facilitate phagocytosis. Moreover, C3 is a chemotactic factor, meaning that it has the selective capacity to attract certain cells, and it is known that macrophages are attracted toward chemotactic factors.*

Macrophages also play an important role in facilitating immune responses, as will be discussed in Chapter 10.

The precursor cell that becomes a macrophage is the *monocyte,* a type of leukocyte (white blood cell). Monocytes migrate from the bloodstream into loose connective tissue,

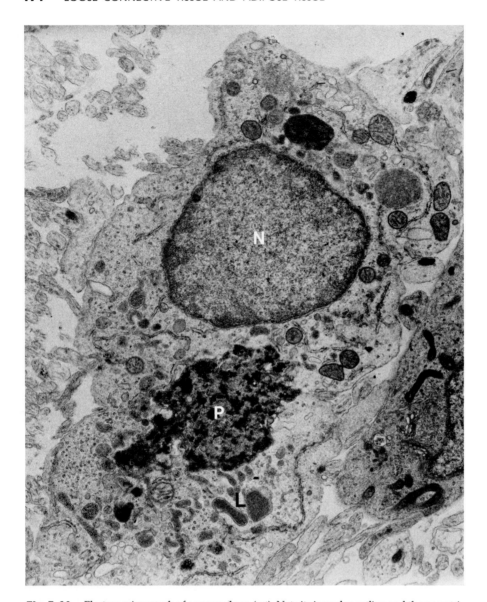

Fig. 7-16. Electron micrograph of a macrophage (rat). Note its irregular outline and the eccentric position of its nucleus (*N*). Directly beneath the nucleus, a prominent dark phagosome (*P*) can be seen. Its content appears to be a remnant of the nucleus of a phagocytosed cell. Farther below are various types of dense bodies, and at bottom center, a group of lysosomes (*L*) can be seen. Some of these lysosomes (the ones just above the letter *L*) seem to be elongating toward the phagosome. The rER is not prominent in macrophages. (Imamoto K, Leblond CP: J Comp Neurol 180:139, 1978)

where they undergo a direct transformation into macrophages. Hence macrophages represent immigrant cells that develop in loose connective tissue from mesenchyme-derived blood cells. They retain the capacity for cell division and remain viable in loose connective tissue for several months. Under certain conditions, macrophages and their precursors (monocytes) fuse and form very large multinucleated cells called *foreign body giant cells* that are able to act as a barrier between comparatively large masses of

foreign material and the remainder of the body (Fig. 7-17). Giant cells of this type are common in *tuberculosis*. The central region of the tubercular lesion undergoes necrosis, leaving an outer shell of viable fused cytoplasm with a highly characteristic spherical arrangement of macrophage nuclei at its periphery (Fig. 7-17A). In addition, foreign body giant cells are seen in chronic nodular lesions called *granulomas* (Fig. 7-17B). *Osteoclasts,* which are large multinucleated cells that are specialized to break down bone

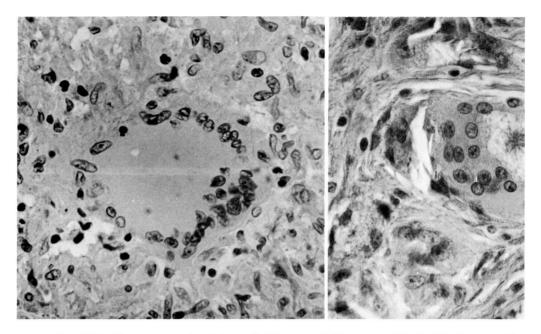

Fig. 7-17. Photomicrographs of giant cells. The one at left is typical of the kind that forms in sites infected with the tubercle bacillus. The one at right, of which only a portion is shown, is seen in what is termed a nonspecific granuloma. (Courtesy of T. Brown)

matrix, are also formed through the fusion of monocytes, but they are believed to represent an essentially independent line of differentiation.

Plasma Cells

Plasma cells have long been classified as connective tissue cells because they are often found in the loose connective tissue of certain parts of the body. It has since been established that they are descendants of mesenchyme-derived B-lymphocytes that enter this tissue. Furthermore, it is now clear that plasma cells are also very numerous in lymphatic tissue (particularly the spleen and lymph nodes), so these cells can be thought of as belonging to both loose connective tissue and lymphatic tissue.

Plasma Cells Play a Key Role in the Acquisition of Immunity. In view of the rapid advances now being made in contemporary immunology, it seems almost incredible that until 40 years ago the functional role of plasma cells, the existence of which had been recognized for many years, was virtually unknown. To discuss the role of these cells in immunity, we need to introduce some more terms.

The word *immunity* (L. *immunis*) means *safe* or *exempt* from infection. *Immunology*, the science of immunity, began when it was discovered that individuals who had recovered from communicable diseases were, in most instances, safe from getting the same disease under similarly infectious conditions. This, of course, raised the question of why having one bout of the disease protected the individual from having other bouts of the same disease.

It was then established that the individual developing immunity

had certain proteins, termed *antibodies*, in his blood plasma that reacted specifically with the kind of organism responsible for the disease and in such a way as to render these organisms innocuous should they enter his body again.

Much was learned about antibodies before their cellular origin was determined; for example, it was learned that they were a type of globulin, a particular kind of protein in the blood plasma. Accordingly, antibodies are now usually referred to as *immunoglobulins*. Moreover, it was discovered that they were specific for the infecting organism, and tests were devised for their detection. In some cases, antibodies would be formed when killed disease organisms, or organisms otherwise treated to prevent them from propagating, were injected as *vaccines*, and so it became possible to *immunize* individuals against certain communicable diseases. Nevertheless, the cellular source of antibodies was still unknown, even though by then pathologists and histologists were already very familiar with the appearance of plasma cells and knew that they were seen at sites exposed to infection, especially the loose connective tissue present beneath wet epithelial linings.

By means of a suitable immunofluorescence technique, Coons and his associates, in 1955, showed that the antibody produced in response to an injected antigen originated from plasma cells. This was the first direct evidence that *plasma cells represent the cellular source of circulating immunoglobulins (humoral antibodies).* An *antigen* (Gr. *anti,* against; *gennan,* to produce) is a substance against which something is produced—in this case, a specific antibody. However, in order to act as an antigen, the substance must be *macromolecular* and it must reach *immunologically responsive cells* of the appropriate antigenic specificity by way of one of the body fluids. Most antigens are proteins or lipopolysac-

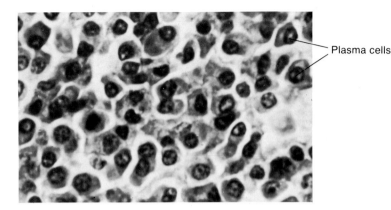

Plasma cells

Fig. 7-18. Photomicrograph of a group of plasma cells in the loose connective tissue below the epithelial covering of a tonsil. Their basophilic cytoplasm and negative Golgi region can easily be discerned.

charide-protein complexes of high molecular weight, and there are very few antigens with a molecular weight of less than 5000 daltons. In order to incite antibody formation, the macromolecular substance must also be *foreign to the body*. In other words, it must differ in molecular structure from the molecules produced by the body during the normal course of events. Any different kind of immunogenic macromolecular substance (*foreign antigen*) that is introduced into the body may elicit the production of a *specific antibody* that is capable of combining with that particular substance in a highly specific manner. Substances that can act as foreign antigens include macromolecules released by infecting microorganisms such as viruses, bacteria, and protozoa. Antigens of inhaled pollens and dusts sometimes gain access to loose connective tissue through tiny breaks in the epithelial lining of the respiratory tract, whereupon they, too, can act as foreign antigens. Finally, there are a few chemical compounds of low molecular weight called *haptens* that can elicit antibody formation by combining with a carrier protein. The changed configuration of the carrier macromolecule results in the production of an antibody with antihaptenic activity.

The preceding section will serve as general background for the remainder of this chapter and several chapters that follow. We shall now go on to consider some structural features of plasma cells that become evident at the LM and EM levels.

The LM features of mature plasma cells make them quite easy to identify in H & E sections. Unless plasma cells are crowded or compressed by their surroundings, as in Figure 7-18, they are rounded in outline and about 15 μm in diameter (Fig. 7-19). Their spherical-to-ovoid nucleus generally lies eccentrically in the cell (Fig. 7-19), and its clumps of peripheral condensed chromatin can so resemble the numerals on a dial that it is often described as having a clockface appearance. If its nucleolus can be distinguished, this appears very large (Fig. 7-19). Further characteristics of plasma cells are that they exhibit an intense cytoplasmic basophilia and commonly show a distinct negative Golgi image (Fig. 7-19). These are additional indications of active protein secretion.

The marked secretory activity of plasma cells is just as obvious at the EM level. Their cytoplasm contains an abundance of ribosomes, which accounts for their intense cytoplasmic basophilia. As may be seen in Figure 7-20, it also contains a very prominent rER, cisternae of which become widely dilated with segregated immunoglobulin (Ig). Once the Ig heavy and light chains that make up each Ig molecule have been synthesized, they undergo covalent interchain linkage while still within the rER. Glycosylation of these Ig molecules commences in the rER and is completed in the Golgi complex. A steady supply of secretory vesicles rapidly carries the Ig secretory product from the prominent Golgi complex of the cell to all parts of the cell surface, where it is then promptly liberated. Hence plasma cells do not store their Ig in secretory vesicles for any length of time. Association of monomeric Ig molecules into dimers or pentamers (which occurs during the secretion of IgA

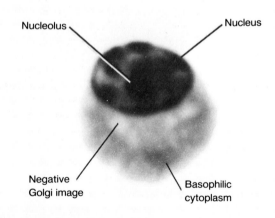

Nucleolus

Nucleus

Negative Golgi image

Basophilic cytoplasm

Fig. 7-19. Oil-immersion photomicrograph of a plasma cell from the large intestine. Note the characteristic features of a plasma cell: the clockface appearance of the nucleus due to peripheral chromatin granules; a prominent nucleolus; basophilic cytoplasm; and a negative Golgi image. This cell has a rounded outline because it was not compressed by the surrounding tissue.

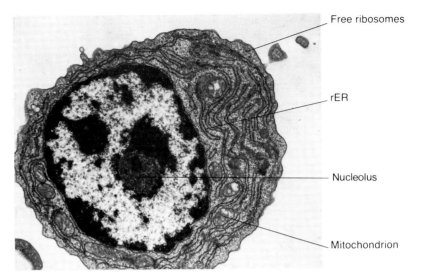

Free ribosomes

rER

Nucleolus

Mitochondrion

Fig. 7-20. Electron micrograph showing the characteristic features of a plasma cell. (Hay JB, Yamashita A, Morris B: Lab Invest 31:276, 1974)

and IgM, respectively) has already taken place by the time the Ig is released by exocytosis at the cell surface. The entire process of Ig synthesis and secretion is completed in about 20 minutes. An additional morphological characteristic of mature plasma cells is that they sometimes contain *Russell bodies*, which are dense bodies or inclusions that are 2 μm to 3 μm in diameter. The significance of these inclusions, however, is not known.

The Ig secreted into the interstitial space by the plasma cells of loose connective tissue (including some that is produced by *plasmablasts*, their immediate precursors) reaches the lymph by way of tissue fluid. Ig secreted by the plasmablasts and plasma cells of lymph nodes also passes into the lymph. The lymph, in turn, delivers the Ig from both of these sources to the bloodstream. However, under normal conditions, only the Ig reaches the blood; hence plasma cells are not observed in the peripheral blood. In the spleen, plasma cells are provided with more direct access to the blood (see Chap. 10).

Antibodies that circulate in the bloodstream are called *humoral antibodies* (L. *humor*, liquid). There is also a cell-mediated type of immunity that is not dependent on humoral antibodies. We shall deal with this second type of immunity in Chapter 10. The factors involved in causing plasma cells to develop from B-lymphocytes will also be considered in that chapter.

Mast Cells

Mast cells are relatively large rounded or ovoid cells that contain numerous spherical, membrane-bounded secretory granules. Where present in dense ordinary connective tissue, they may appear more fusiform. Their spherical-to-ovoid nucleus is generally obscured by their substantial content of dark-staining secretory granules (see Figs. 7-7 and 7-21). With appropriate staining, mast cells are fairly

conspicuous in connective tissue spreads, particularly where they lie scattered along capillaries and other small blood vessels. These are sites where many mast cells are preferentially distributed (Fig. 7-21A). However, in H & E sections, these cells are less prominent and are easily missed.

At the EM level, the outline of mast cells appears somewhat irregular (Fig. 7-22). The cytoplasm contains numerous mitochondria (Fig. 7-22) and a small amount of sER; some rER and a prominent Golgi apparatus are also present (Fig. 7-22). The most noticeable feature of the cytoplasm, however, is its content of relatively large secretory granules (about 0.2 μm to 0.8 μm in diameter); each is enclosed within a unit membrane (Fig. 7-22, see also Fig. 7-6A, *lower right*). The internal appearance of these granules is somewhat variable. They may contain electron-dense lamellae, crystalline lattices, or densely packed fine amorphous particles (Fig. 7-22). Empty vacuoles, which indicate granular discharge, and a few disintegrating granules may also be present (Fig. 7-22).

Mast cell granules contain *heparin*, which is a sulfated glycosaminoglycan, and *histamine*, which is a potent mediator of certain types of allergic responses and a primary mediator of the acute inflammatory reaction. In rats and mice, but not in man, mast cell granules also contain another vasoactive amine called serotonin (*vasoactive* denoting that it can affect the diameter of blood vessels). In man, serotonin is present in blood platelets but not in mast cells. Due to the considerable content of the glycosaminoglycan heparin in mast cell granules (heparin represents approximately 25% of their total content), mast cell granules stain *metachromatically* (see above under Staining Methods for Glycosaminoglycans).

Whereas heparin obtained from other sources prevents blood from clotting, the heparin isolated from human mast cell granules is a poor anticoagulant. The functional significance of the heparin in mast cells is therefore unsettled. However, it is known that hep-

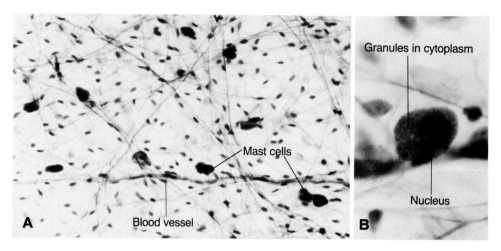

Fig. 7-21. Photomicrograph of mast cells in loose connective tissue under (*A*) low power and (*B*) high power (subcutaneous connective tissue spread stained with Weigert's hematoxylin, eosin, and resorcin-fuchsin). A number of these cells lie scattered along small blood vessels.

arin acts as a cofactor for lipoprotein lipase, an enzyme involved in fat metabolism, and that this enzyme is bound to the surface of capillary endothelium, so it is conceivable that the heparin is more involved in promoting the clearing of plasma lipids than in acting as an anticoagulant. Also, heparin is known to possess anticomplement activity. However, it now seems likely that the heparin in mast cell granules is, in fact, present in the form of heparin proteoglycan and that the primary function of this macromolecular complex may be to provide a granular matrix that is capable of ionic binding of the other granular constituents.

It should also be mentioned here that there is a remarkably close structural and functional resemblance between the mast cells of loose connective tissue and blood basophils, the rarest type of leukocyte. The only substantial differences are that in mast cells the nucleus is rounded whereas in basophils it is generally bilobed and that these two cell types are found in two quite different tissues. The pharmacologically active constituents in their granules appear to be identical, but the main glycosaminoglycan in the proteoglycan matrix of human basophil granules is reported to be chondroitin sulfate rather than heparin. Basophil granules nevertheless seem to be discharged by the same kind of mechanism as mast cell granules. Although it has not yet been ascertained how the mast cells of loose connective tissue are related developmentally to blood basophils, there is *in vitro* evidence from experimental animals that both kinds of cells are formed from precursors that are generated in myeloid tissue (red bone marrow) and that the progenitors of mast cells and basophils can arise from multipotential hematopoietic stem cells. *In vitro* studies also indicate that mast cells are fully differentiated cells that do not undergo self-renewal. Hence it is evident that mast cells represent a population of immigrant cells that reach loose connective tissue by way of the bloodstream.

Before going on to discuss the functional significance of the histamine that accounts for an additional 10% or so of

the content of mast cell granules, we should briefly explain how mast cells are involved in anaphylaxis and other immediate hypersensitivity reactions.

Histamine Is Released from Mast Cell Granules in Immediate-Type Hypersensitivity Reactions. It is now established medical practice to secure a measure of protection against a number of potentially fatal major infectious diseases by injecting a vaccine prepared from the causative microorganisms. This vaccine is modified in such a way as to avoid transmission of the disease without destroying the antigenicity of the disease-causing microorganisms. This preventive approach to the control of infectious diseases, sometimes described as a *prophylactic* measure (Gr. *prophylaxis*, to be on guard), has been remarkably successful. Smallpox, for example, has now been eradicated from the human population worldwide and no longer menaces mankind as a highly contagious and devastating disease. However, although an individual's first exposure to a given antigen will generally elicit immunity against that antigen, subsequent exposure to the same antigen will, on occasion, have deleterious or even lethal consequences for the individual concerned. Termed *anaphylaxis* because it was initially thought to be the converse of prophylaxis, the adverse reaction elicited by subsequent exposure to the antigen is, in fact, an extreme form of allergic response.

Anaphylaxis is particularly easy to demonstrate in guinea pigs. If an initial injection of an antigen is followed approximately 2 weeks later by a second injection of the same antigen, the animal will go into *anaphylactic shock*. This state is manifested by severe difficulty in breathing and acceleration of the heart rate; indeed, the animal may die because of a total inability to breathe. The reason for this respiratory difficulty is that the smooth muscle in the walls of bronchioles, which are the tubes of small diameter that deliver air to the lungs, contracts to such an extent that the bronchiolar lumen becomes too constricted for a sufficient volume of air to pass into or out of the lungs.

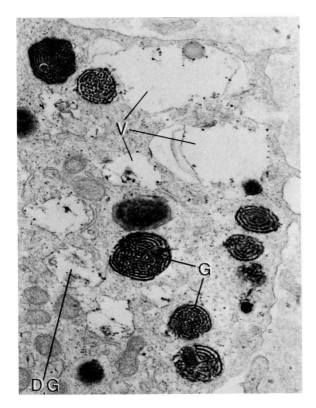

Fig. 7-22. Electron micrograph of a partly degranulated mast cell in loose connective tissue beneath the epithelial lining of the stomach. Cytoplasmic processes project from the border of the cell. Note the large typical granules (*G*), the disintegrating granules (*DG*), and the empty vacuoles (*V*) left in the cytoplasm where some of its granules have been discharged. (Steer HW: J Anat 121: 395, 1976)

Another effect observed in anaphylaxis is that thin-walled vessels such as venules and capillaries become dilated and leaky, allowing plasma to escape from them. As a result, blebs of fluid may form in the loose connective tissue immediately under the epidermis. Such a cutaneous manifestation of an immediate hypersensitivity reaction is called *urticaria.*

Soon after histamine was discovered, it was found that many of the symptoms observed in anaphylactic shock could be reproduced by injecting a guinea pig with histamine. This indicated a causal relationship between contact with antigen and the release of histamine.

Histamine, a vasoactive amine derived from the amino acid histidine, exerts a profound effect on visceral smooth muscle and the smooth muscle in the walls of the cardiac and pulmonary arteries, causing these two kinds of smooth muscle to contract. However, it causes all other arterial smooth muscle to relax, so that distributing arteries and small arterioles dilate. A further effect of histamine is that it elicits contraction of the endothelial cells that line venules, causing them to undergo slight separation where their lateral borders are not joined at tight junctions of the fascia occludens type. The same mechanism of induced widening

of the intercellular slits, which allows immunoglobulins and other plasma proteins to leak from these vessels, occurs during the first phase of the acute inflammatory reaction, which will be described in Chapter 8. Histamine also has a number of other effects in the body that we shall not consider here. For further information about mast cells and histamine, see Beaven.

Mast Cell Degranulation Is Triggered by the Interaction of Antigen with Surface-Bound IgE.   Mast cells degranulate and liberate the contents of their granules (1) if a *specific antigen–antibody interaction* occurs at their surface, or (2) in response to *direct damage* (*e.g.,* as a result of trauma and even during the fixation stage of tissue processing). The immunological basis for degranulation is described in the following sections.

As in macrophages, the cell membrane of mast cells is provided with *Fc receptors.* However, the only antibodies for which these receptors have a high affinity is a class of immunoglobulins called *immunoglobulin E (IgE),* one of the five classes of Ig that will be described in Chapter 10. This relatively minor class of immunoglobulins binds to blood basophils as well as to mast cells. Certain individuals produce antibodies of the IgE class when antigens from pollen or dust enter their body by way of tiny breaks in the epithelium that lines their respiratory tract. Other individuals produce IgE directed against antigens that similarly gain access to the body by way of the lining of their digestive tract. Any of the IgE molecules that are thereby formed can become bound, irrespective of their antigenic specificity, to the Fc receptors on mast cells or basophils. Furthermore, these antibody molecules become bound with their Fab end exposed at the mast cell or basophil surface. Accordingly, once an antigen has elicited the production of a specific antibody of the IgE class, mast cells that become primed with this particular antibody are able to recognize the same antigen as soon as it reenters the body. Furthermore, if the antigen is polyvalent, it can bridge the preformed IgE molecules that have become bound to the Fc receptors on these cells. Mast cells degranulate and liberate their histamine and other allergic and inflammatory mediators when a polyvalent antigen crosslinks IgE molecules that are bound to their Fc receptors.

Because surface-bound IgE molecules enable strategically positioned mast cells to respond to foreign antigens even before such antigens enter the lymph or blood, mast cells are also generally the first cells to respond to pathogenic microorganisms and certain kinds of parasites when these gain access to the body by way of a discontinuity in a mucosal epithelium or a lesion on the body surface. Mast cells therefore represent an important part of the body's defense mechanism for eliminating infectious organisms. Yet certain individuals also overreact in a seemingly needless manner to foreign antigens that are apparently harmless. These people are referred to as *allergic* individuals.

An IgE-mediated response to a foreign antigen that involves primarily mast cells is generally manifested as an *immediate hy-*

persensitivity reaction (allergy). For example, even the tiniest amount of ragweed pollen, which is prevalent in the air at the time when hay is cut, can cause anyone who is allergic to its antigen to develop *hay fever*, a condition that is characterized by a runny nose, bouts of sneezing, and itchy eyes. These are probably already familiar symptoms of *allergic rhinitis* (an example of a mucosal *immediate hypersensitivity reaction*) that are rapidly induced by the histamine released from mast cells. There are literally hundreds of different allergy-causing antigens (*allergens*) to which allergy sufferers are exposed in everyday life. Such people respond to specific allergens by secreting IgE. Together with plasma cells that produce secretory immunoglobulin (IgA), IgE-secreting plasma cells lie preferentially distributed in the loose connective tissue layer adjacent to the wet epithelial linings of the respiratory and digestive tracts. This, of course, is only to be expected because these are the sites where foreign antigens are repeatedly gaining access to the body.

The severity of most allergic symptoms can generally be alleviated by administering an *antihistamine*. An antihistamine does not prevent the release of histamine, but it does occupy the histamine receptors on the responding cells and thereby limits the effectiveness of the amount of histamine that is liberated. Furthermore, antihistamines are now widely available that can alleviate allergic and anaphylactic manifestations without interfering with gastric secretion, an essential body function also mediated by histamine. Another therapeutic approach is to use a *desensitization* procedure. The rationale on which such procedures are at least partly based is that an extended course of subcutaneous injections of minute but gradually increasing doses of the allergy-causing antigen will eventually elicit production in local lymph nodes of another class of immunoglobulin called IgG (also described in Chap. 10). IgG, the class of antibody most commonly·produced as a result of any sustained immunization procedure, shows no tendency to bind preferentially to the surface of mast cells or basophils, nor does it facilitate the release of their histamine. IgG can nevertheless compete with IgE for binding sites on the allergen. Once the production of specific IgG has begun, the IgG molecules are able to combine with the allergen before it has a chance to reach the surface-bound IgE on mast cells and basophils. Histamine release and the resulting allergic symptoms are thereby avoided.

Roughly 20% of all people tested are hypersensitive to one or more antigens that present no problems for the remainder of the population. There seems to be a genetic basis for the development of hypersensitivities, but the mechanism involved remains to be elucidated. It has been suggested that either the predisposition to produce IgE or a heightened responsiveness to potentially allergenic antigens might be inherited.

Systemic Anaphylaxis. On occasion, a systemic (body-wide) anaphylactic reaction may be encountered in an individual who has produced substantial amounts of IgE in response to a sensitizing antigen that is present, for example, in a wasp sting or antibiotic. Sometimes a patient does not know or forgets that he has had effective prior contact with a particular antigen; hence the physician should watch any patient given an injection of penicillin or tetanus antitoxin, for example, to see if he has developed a hypersensitivity to it. Any indication that the patient may be going into anaphylactic shock must be dealt with promptly. Systemic anaphylaxis is a consequence of mas-

sive body-wide release of histamine and other mediators of immediate-type hypersensitivity reactions from both mast cells and basophils. Because such a profound reaction can lead to cardiovascular collapse, it is potentially fatal.

Mast Cells Also Liberate Other Chemical Mediators of Allergic and Inflammatory Reactions. Mast cells constitute the direct or indirect source of an ever-lengthening list of potent chemical mediators of allergic and acute inflammatory reactions. These mediators include *histamine* and several other granule-associated, preformed mediators, including *eosinophil chemotactic factors of anaphylaxis* (ECF-A), *neutrophil chemotactic factor* (NCF), some lysosomal *hydrolases*, and an assortment of other enzymes. In addition to these so-called primary mediators, mast cells liberate a number of substances that are generated when their granules are discharged. Known as secondary mediators, these include *slow-reacting substance of anaphylaxis* (SRS-A), *platelet activating factor* (PAF), and several *prostaglandins*, a family of arachidonic acid derivatives with a broad spectrum of biological activities.

ECF-A is so named because when it is released from mast cell granules, it attracts *eosinophils*, a type of leukocyte. Such selective attraction of cells toward a specific compound is termed *chemotaxis* (Gr. *taksis*, an orderly arrangement). ECF-A is actually a group of small and intermediate-sized peptides that evidently attract neutrophils as well as eosinophils. *NCF* is a protein that specifically attracts neutrophils. The consequences of liberation of such chemotactic factors will be dealt with in Chapter 8, but one notable repercussion is that the eosinophils dampen the inflammatory effects of the mast cell–derived mediators by producing several enzymes that are capable of degrading them. *SRS-A* is a sulfate-containing ester of low molecular weight. It effects are similar to those of histamine. However, whereas histamine exerts rapid but short-lasting effects on both smooth muscle and vascular permeability, SRS-A has a more sustained effect and hence is called a slow-reacting substance. *PAF*, which is believed to be a group of phospholipids, can trigger the aggregation and degranulation of platelets. For further information about mast cell mediators, see Austen, and Austen and Orange.

ADIPOCYTES AND ADIPOSE TISSUE

Fat cells, which are also known as *adipocytes*, occur either singly or in small groups in loose connective tissue (see Fig. 7-11). In addition to such isolated groups of fat cells, entire regions of connective tissue (subcutaneous fat tissue, for example) are specialized for fat storage. Such regions are lobular in organization and are referred to as *adipose tissue (fat tissue)*. The main role of this special type of connective tissue is to store lipid, which is the principal source of chemical energy in the body. Other cells that share this fat-storing function are the fat-storing cells of myeloid tissue and the lipocytes of the liver. Hepatocytes and a few other kinds of cells are also able to store lipid, but if lipid accu-

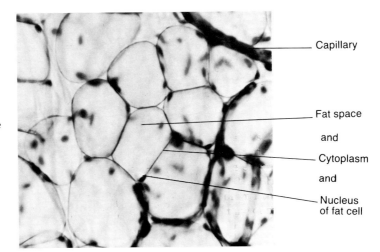

Fig. 7-23. Photomicrograph of adipose tissue (white fat) prepared as a whole mount.

Capillary

Fat space

and

Cytoplasm

and

Nucleus
of fat cell

mulates in excessive amounts, it begins to interfere with the essential functions of these cells.

Adipocytes arise from pericapillary mesenchymal cells that occupy the same relative position in the embryo. Whereas mature adipocytes produce very little collagen, adipocyte precursors produce type I and type III collagen, and this has been cited as evidence that adipocyte precursors might develop from the same mesenchyme-derived progenitors as fibroblasts.

Although the lipid stored by adipocytes is not retained in H & E sections, its presence in frozen sections can easily be demonstrated through the use of a fat stain such as a Sudan dye (see Fig. 1-13B). As lipid droplets accumulate in the common type of adipocyte (*i.e.*, a cell of white fat) they coalesce, with the result that a large central droplet is formed and is surrounded by a remarkably thin rim of cytoplasm (Figs. 7-11 and 7-23). A mature, well-filled adipocyte therefore has the typical appearance of a signet ring; its flattened nucleus corresponds to the signet and its pale-stained rim of cytoplasm represents the ring (Fig. 7-11). In H & E sections, the fat cells of adipose tissue and large isolated groups of adipocytes in connective tissue may even exhibit a chicken-wire appearance because of the large empty space formerly filled with lipid that is left within each adipocyte (Fig. 7-23). The diameter of an adipocyte that has become filled with stored lipid is generally between 70 μm and 120 μm, but it can be up to five times larger in people who are obese.

The lobules of adipose tissue into which its fat cells are packed are demarcated by supporting septa of loose connective tissue. Capillaries and sympathetic nerve fibers, both of which become intimately associated with adipocytes, are brought into adipose tissue in these septa. Within the lobules, the adipocytes are supported by a stroma that contains collagen fibers and a network of reticular fibers with fibroblasts and abundant capillaries (Fig. 7-23) in its interstices. This stroma, which commonly also contains

some mast cells, accounts for about 5% of the total mass of the tissue.

The thin rim of cytoplasm of an adipocyte that is storing its full complement of lipid is only 1 μm to 2 μm thick; hence many of its organelles are displaced to the perinuclear region where there is more cytoplasm (Fig. 7-24B). Free ribosomes, both types of endoplasmic reticulum, a Golgi region, and numerous mitochondria can all be found in adipocytes. Mitochondria are prominent (Fig. 7-24B) and are important to the function of fat cells, as will become apparent in the following section on Adipose Tissue. In addition to lipid, some stored glycogen is sometimes present in these cells. For some reason that is not yet clear, there is a basement membrane between the adipocyte and its surrounding stroma.

New Adipocytes Can Be Generated at Any Time During Postnatal Life. *In vitro* studies indicate that cell division does not occur in fully differentiated adipocytes that are lipid-laden (*i.e.*, typical fat cells with a single large lipid droplet in their cytoplasm). However, such cells are long-lived, so anyone born with a large number of adipocytes still runs the risk of becoming obese as a result of overeating. Furthermore, postnatal adipose tissue contains immature adipocytes and residual adipocyte precursors (Fig. 7-24A) from which additional adipocytes can arise (*e.g.*, as a result of hormonal stimulation by estrogen). Fat deposition accompanied by expansion of the existing adipocyte population as a result of proliferation of adipocyte precursors can occur as a consequence of high caloric intake during excessive breast-feeding. It can also occur at or around the time of puberty as a result of stimulation by estrogen. In addition, an increase in the amount of fat tissue is sometimes encountered during late adolescence and in middle-aged individuals who are already fat.

Recent *in vitro* findings indicate that lipid-filled adipocytes may also become depleted of lipid and elongate into cells that resemble

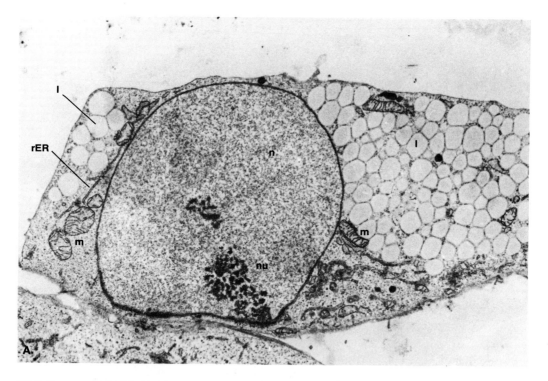

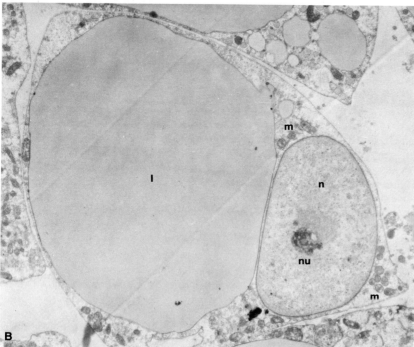

Fig. 7-24. (*A*) Electron micrograph of part of a differentiating adipocyte precursor growing *in vitro*. Fusiform in shape, this cell has a large pale-staining ovoid nucleus (*n*) and prominent nucleoli (*nu*). Accumulating lipid droplets (*l*), together with mitochondria (*m*) and a small amount of rough-surfaced endoplasmic reticulum (*rER*), are present in its cytoplasm. (*B*) Electron micrograph, taken at a lower magnification (×4000), of a differentiating adipocyte precursor grown *in vitro* and isolated by flotation. This cell contains a single large central lipid droplet (*l*), a more flattened nucleus (*n*) that still has a prominent nucleolus (*nu*), and a number of mitochondria (*m*). Its microscopic appearance is now beginning to resemble that of an adipocyte, which would exhibit a flatter nucleus, a larger central lipid droplet, and an even thinner rim of cytoplasm. (*A*, courtesy of RLR Van; *B*, Green H, Meuth M: Cell 3:127, 1974, copyright by MIT Press)

Mesenchymal progenitor → Adipocyte precursor → Immature adipocyte accumulates lipid → Mature adipocyte becomes laden with stored lipid

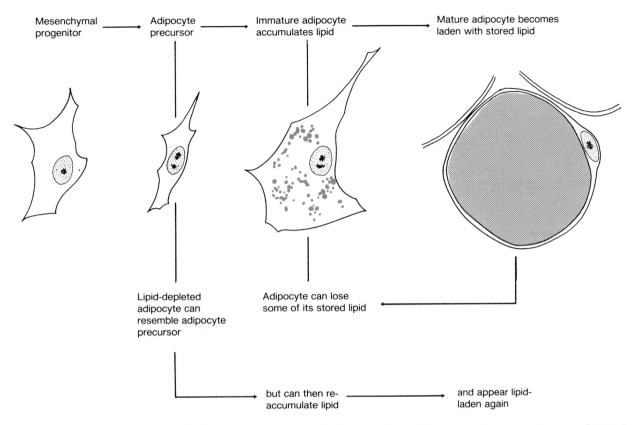

Lipid-depleted adipocyte can resemble adipocyte precursor

Adipocyte can lose some of its stored lipid

but can then re-accumulate lipid → and appear lipid-laden again

Fig. 7-25. A tentative scheme of adipocyte differentiation, maturation, and subsequent changes in shape and lipid content based on *in vitro* studies of adipocyte progenitors.

adipocyte precursors not only in appearance but also in replicative potential (Fig. 7-25). It has been suggested that this change reflects reversion of the fully differentiated adipocyte to an earlier or less mature but fully committed stage that is still capable of proliferation and subsequent full expression of the adipocyte phenotype (see Roncari and Van, and Van). According to this view, cells that have completed a full round of adipocyte differentiation and lipid accumulation may lose their lipid and still be able to replicate and then undergo further adipocyte expression. Steady-state conditions in the adult may therefore depend on a dynamic equilibrium between (1) precursor replication and adipocyte differentiation and maturation and (2) adipocyte death and lipid depletion of adipocytes, leading to their reversion to cells with the characteristics seen in immature adipocytes. Finally, although there appear to be several different ways of producing supplementary fat cells, the only known way of getting rid of them again is by *lipectomy* (*adipectomy*) (*i.e.*, surgical excision of excess subcutaneous fat tissue). However, this is not the ideal solution because adipocytes situated elsewhere in the body can increase in size (*hypertrophy*) and in number (undergo *hyperplasia*) to make up the deficit.

ADIPOSE TISSUE

White Fat and Brown Fat Constitute Two Different Subtypes of Adipose Tissue. The body contains two different kinds of adipose tissue, *white fat* and *brown fat*. Al-

most all human adipose tissue is *white fat,* which despite its name is generally cream-colored or yellow because of its carotene content. *Brown fat* is comparatively scanty in man but relatively abundant in certain other mammals. In life it has a brown color because of its very rich capillary blood supply and because its cells contain numerous mitochondria and are therefore rich in cytochromes (mitochondrial enzymes that, like hemoglobin, have a colored component). Brown fat is primarily concerned with the regulation of body temperature in the newborn, and in a number of species that hibernate, it also serves as a source of heat production during arousal from hibernation. A few more details about brown fat are given at the end of this chapter.

White Fat

White fat comprises 10% to 20% of the body weight in adult males and 15% to 25% in adult females. Collectively, it constitutes a relatively large diffuse organ that metabolically is very active; it is primarily engaged in the uptake, synthesis, storage, and mobilization of neutral lipid. As a result of this mobilization, the caloric content of the lipid stored in white fat can be made available as fuel to cells in other parts of the body. At body temperature, the lipid in adipocytes is present as oil. It consists of triglycerides, each made up of three molecules of fatty acid esterified to glycerol. Triglycerides have the highest caloric content of all food; hence the fat in adipocytes represents a comparatively lightweight store of high-calorie fuel. Moreover, subcutaneous white fat provides those of us who live in a cold climate with a certain amount of comforting thermal insulation. In addition, it serves as an excellent filler for various cervices in the body structure and provides cushions on which certain parts of the body can rest.

Each adipocyte synthesizes the lipid it stores from chemical building blocks brought to it by way of the bloodstream. The fat in the diet, as well as carbohydrates and proteins, can provide these building blocks.

The Fate of Fat in the Diet. Neutral fats (triglycerides) consumed in the diet are digested chiefly by the enzyme *lipase*, which is secreted by the pancreas into the duodenum. Its action is facilitated by bile, which is secreted by the liver into the same site. Bile components help to emulsify the fat so that the action of the lipase is more effective. As a result of digestion, some fat is broken down to fatty acids and glycerol, while the remainder is broken down only as far as monoglycerides. The fatty acids are absorbed through the luminal border of the absorptive epithelial cells lining the intestine. Within these cells, glycerol phosphate is synthesized and combined in the sER with fatty acids, forming new triglycerides. Monoglycerides, too, are absorbed and recombined with fatty acids in the sER to form triglycerides.

Details about fat absorption are given in Chapter 18, but here we should mention that newly reconstituted triglyceride (neutral fat) is transported to the lateral borders of the intestinal epithelial cells in vesicles that bud from the sER in which it is formed. Thus the fat droplets within intestinal epithelial cells are enclosed by membrane derived from the sER. When they reach the cell membrane, however, these membrane-bound droplets fuse with it and discharge their contents as naked droplets into the intercellular space between each epithelial cell and the next. In this manner, the fat droplets soon gain access to the tissue fluid beneath the epithelium and travel with it as it drains into the lymphatic capillaries in the underlying connective tissue. After a fatty meal, the droplets of newly synthesized fat may be numerous enough to make the lymph milky in appearance; indeed, if a great deal of fat has been consumed, even the blood plasma may become milky when the lymph reaches the bloodstream. Because this milky appearance of the "juice" (lymph) from the lymphatics was found to be caused by the presence of tiny fat droplets approximately 1 μm in diameter, the droplets were termed *chylomicrons* (Gr. *chylos*, juice; *micros*, small). In addition to triglycerides, chylomicrons contain phospholipids, cholesterol ester, and some protein, which is complexed with the lipid as lipoprotein.

As the blood containing chylomicrons passes through capillaries, the chylomicrons become exposed to *lipoprotein lipase*, an enzyme produced by adipocytes that also becomes bound in stable form to the surface of the endothelial lining

cells of these vessels. This enzyme breaks down their triglycerides into fatty acids and glycerol again. When this happens in a capillary in fat tissue, the fatty acids may be absorbed by a fat cell and may be combined with glycerol phosphate synthesized by the fat cell.

After chylomicrons have been cleared from the blood, there is still lipid in the blood in the form of *lipoproteins* (lipid complexed with protein), which are produced chiefly by the liver and are synthesized in part from lipid obtained from chylomicrons absorbed by that organ. The lipoproteins serve as a source of fatty acids for the body cells. Fatty acids are obtained locally by cells because of the local action of lipoprotein lipase on the lipoproteins brought to cells by way of the capillaries.

The Lipid in Adipocytes Is Formed from Fatty Acids of Chylomicrons and Lipoproteins in the Plasma. Most of the lipid in adipocytes is derived from this source in the following manner. Under the action of lipoprotein lipase, free fatty acids are released from the chylomicrons or very low-density lipoprotein (VLDL) of blood and pass into the cells of adipose tissue. Within fat cells, fatty acids are rapidly reconverted into triglycerides by means of a coupling reaction involving glycerol phosphate; this substance is available only from the glucose metabolism occurring in the fat cell. The glycerol released from the breakdown of the triglycerides coming to the cell cannot be recombined with the fatty acids because adipose tissue lacks the enzyme (glycerol kinase) essential for this to happen; hence the glycerol phosphate required to produce triglycerides within fat cells depends on carbohydrate being metabolized in the same cell.

Unlike the situation in the absorptive epithelial cells of the intestine, the lipid droplets in adipocytes are not enclosed by a unit membrane. However, the fat droplets of adipocytes are sometimes seen to be covered by an investing array of parallel microfilaments. New fat first appears in the cytoplasm in the form of very fine droplets that can be isolated from homogenates of fat cells, constituting what biochemists call *liposomes*. Their diameter varies from being half to twice that of chylomicrons, which they somewhat resemble when seen in the EM.

The Fates of Carbohydrate and Protein in the Diet. In the intestine, carbohydrates are broken down by enzymes to monosaccharides, whereas proteins are degraded to amino acids. These products are absorbed through the epithelial cells of the intestine and reach the blood circulation; they, too (particularly glucose), can serve as building blocks for fat. Both glucose and amino acids pass through the cell membranes of fat cells by means of specific transport mechanisms.

Lipids Can Be Formed from Glucose or Amino Acids. As mentioned in Chapter 4 in connection with mitochondria, glucose is broken down in the cytoplasmic matrix by a series of reactions termed *glycolysis*, and the products of glycolysis are oxidized by enzymes within the mitochondria to provide most of the energy required by the cell. However, certain products of the breakdown of both glucose and amino acids in the cytoplasmic matrix can be converted to long-chain fatty acids which, as already explained, are combined with newly synthesized glycerol phosphate to become triglycerides.

Fat Is Broken Down Again in Fat Cells, Releasing Fatty Acids That Other Body Cells Use for Fuel. When calorie intake is restricted for any reason, the energy requirements of the cells of the body are met by drawing on the food reserve stored in fat cells. Furthermore, under the influence of a lack or an excess of certain hormones (which will be described in the following sections), fatty acids are released from fat cells and used for fuel. The mechanism by which fat is broken down depends on the action of another enzyme system called *tissue lipase,* which is distinct from the lipoprotein lipase system. The tissue lipase system consists of a hormone-sensitive triglyceride lipase and a monoglyceride lipase.

Under ordinary conditions, the triglyceride lipase remains inactive and must be activated before it is able to break down triglyceride molecules. This activation occurs following the interaction of a lipolytic hormone (*e.g.,* epinephrine or norepinephrine) with its specific receptor on the cell surface. As a result of this interaction, the levels of intracellular cyclic adenosine monophosphate (cAMP, a nucleotide that acts as a chemical messenger to tell the cell it has been stimulated by a hormone) rise, and this is thought to be responsible for the activation of tissue lipase. The functioning of this system breaks down triglycerides at the surface of the lipid droplet, and the fatty acids thereby released are either metabolized or pass through the cell membrane of the adipocyte to enter the capillary circulation. In the bloodstream they bind to albumin, which acts as a carrier, and are thereby transported to the cells that utilize them for fuel.

Further Metabolic Functions of Adipose Tissue. Besides storing lipids and releasing the constituent fatty acids for use as a fuel, adipocytes accumulate cholesterol and bind, internalize, and degrade low-density lipoprotein (LDL). Adipocytes thereby help to remove circulating LDL, elevated levels of which are atherogenic (see Chap. 4 under Receptor-Mediated Endocytosis).

Adipose Tissue Is Affected by Sex Hormones, Insulin, Epinephrine, and Norepinephrine. These hormones (the last of which is also a neurotransmitter) have profound effects on adipose tissue. For example, because the level of the sex hormone *estrogen* and also the pattern of distribution and degree to which estrogen receptors are expressed influences the sites where adipose tissue will accumulate, fat distributions are often noticeably different in females and males. Two hormones with important effects on the metabolic activities of adipocytes are insulin, produced by the pancreas, and epinephrine, produced by the adrenal medulla. Whereas *insulin* promotes glucose uptake and hence fat storage by adipocytes, *epinephrine* promotes the breakdown and mobilization of this stored fat. In addition to being released as an adrenal medullary hormone, *norepinephrine* is the neurotransmitter released at the adipocyte-associated terminals of postganglionic fibers of the sympathetic nervous system (a division of the autonomic nervous system, which will be described in Chap. 14). Norepinephrine has the same lipolytic effect on adipose tissue as epinephrine does.

Insulin Effects on Adipocytes. The quantity of insulin liberated into the bloodstream is continuously geared to the glucose level of the blood. Thus the consumption of carbohydrates leads to the release of more insulin. Among its other effects, insulin promotes several reactions in adipocytes that enable them to synthesize and store more lipid. These reactions include (1) accelerated glucose uptake, (2) augmented conversion of glucose into triglyceride, and (3) increased lipoprotein lipase activity, leading to (4) accelerated intracellular delivery of fatty acids from chylomicrons and lipoprotein lipid. Insulin also retards lipid mobilization by depressing the action of enzymes that promote lipid breakdown.

Epinephrine and Norepinephrine Effects on Adipocytes. The quantities of epinephrine norepinephrine liberated into the bloodstream by the adrenal medulla depend on the degree to which the adrenals are being stimulated by sympathetic nerve impulses. Release of these two hormones is maximal under emergency conditions, but it also becomes elevated in certain emotional states. The amount of norepinephrine liberated from sympathetic nerve terminals at the periphery of adipocytes is similarly dependent on their degree of sympathetic stimulation. Both of these catecholamines have a profound effect on adipocyte metabolism. Their primary effect is to stimulate the formation of more cAMP, an ATP-derived nucleotide that mediates the effects of many different hormones. The cAMP, in turn, augments the activity of tissue lipase, with the result that fatty acids are produced in increased amounts from the stored triglycerides. LDL uptake is also enhanced.

Much of our knowledge about the action of epinephrine and norepinephrine on adipose tissue comes from the study of brown fat, the essential features of which are described in the following section.

Brown Fat

The most significant feature of this second subtype of adipose tissue is that it is thermogenic and can *generate body heat.* The arrangement of lipid droplets in the cells of brown fat is *multilocular,* meaning that lipid is always stored in the form of *multiple* droplets (L. *locus,* place or site) and not as a large central droplet. This arrangement differs from the characteristic *unilocular* arrangement seen in the lipid-laden adipocytes of white fat. The cells of brown fat are smaller than those of white fat, yet their mitochondria are larger and more numerous. This relative abundance of mitochondria in brown fat is clearly related to its role as a heat-producing tissue. The cells of brown fat are richly supplied with postganglionic sympathetic nerve fibers.

Only a small amount of brown fat persists after the perinatal period in man. It is mostly confined to the interscapular subcutaneous fat tissue, but it can also be found in the mediastinum and along the aorta.

SELECTED REFERENCES

Intercellular Substances and Fibroblasts

ALBERTS B, BRAY D, LEWIS J ET AL: The extracellular matrix. In Molecular Biology of the Cell, p 692. New York, Garland Publishing, 1983

DUANCE VC, BAILEY AJ: Biosynthesis and degradation of collagen. In Glynn LE (ed): Tissue Repair and Regeneration. Handbook of Inflammation, Vol 3, p 51. Amsterdam, Elsevier/North Holland Biomedical Press, 1981

GABBIANI G, RUNGGER–BRÄNDLE E: The fibroblast. In Glynn LE (ed): Tissue Repair and Regeneration. Handbook of Inflammation, Vol 3, p 1. Amsterdam, Elsevier/North Holland Biomedical Press, 1981

GOSPODAROWICZ D, FUJII DK: The extracellular matrix and the control of cell proliferation and differentiation. In Mozes LW, Schultz J, Scott WA, Werner R (eds): Cellular Responses to Molecular Modulators. Miami Winter Symposia, Vol 18, p 113. New York, Academic Press, 1981

GOTTE L: Molecular morphology of elastin. In Robert AM, Robert L (eds): Biology and Pathology of Elastic Tissues. Frontiers of Matrix Biology, Vol 8, p 33. Basel, S Karger, 1980

HALL DA: The Aging of Connective Tissue. New York, Academic Press, 1976

HAY ED (ed): Cell Biology of the Extracellular Matrix. New York, Plenum Press, 1981

HEINEGÅRD D, PAULSSON M: Structure and metabolism of proteoglycans. In Piez KA, Reddi AH (eds): Extracellular Matrix Biochemistry, p 277. New York, Elsevier, 1984

KEWLEY MA, STEVEN FS, WILLIAMS G: The presence of fine elastic fibrils within the elastic fiber observed by scanning electron microscopy. J Anat 123:129, 1977

KLEINMAN HK, KLEBE RJ, MARTIN GR: Role of collagenous matrices in the adhesion and growth of cells. J Cell Biol 88:473, 1981

MONTES GS, BEZERRA MSF, JUNQUEIRA LCU: Collagen distribution in tissues. In Ruggeri A, Motta PM (eds): Ultrastructure of the Connective Tissue Matrix, p 65. Boston, Martinus Nijhoff, 1984

PARTRIDGE SM: The lability of elastin structure and its probable form under physiological conditions. In Robert AM, Robert L (eds): Biology and Pathology of Elastic Tissues. Frontiers of Matrix Biology, Vol 8, p 3. Basel, S Karger, 1980

PIEZ KA, REDDI AH (eds): Extracellular Matrix Biochemistry. New York, Elsevier, 1984

RAMACHANDRAN GN, REDDI AH (eds): The Biochemistry of Collagen. New York, Plenum, 1976

REDDI AH (ed): Extracellular Matrix Structure and Function. UCLA Symposia on Molecular and Cellular Biology, New Series, Vol 25. New York, Alan R Liss, 1985

ROSS R: Connective tissue cells, cell proliferation and synthesis of extracellular matrix—a review. Philos Trans R Soc Lond [Biol] 271:247, 1975

ROSS R, BORNSTEIN P: Elastic fibers in the body. Sci Am 224 No 6: 44, 1971

RUGGERI A, MOTTA PM (eds): Ultrastructure of the Connective Tissue Matrix. Boston, Martinus Nijhoff, 1984

SNODGRASS MJ: Ultrastructural distinction between reticular and collagenous fibers with an ammoniacal silver stain. Anat Rec 187:191, 1977

TEN CATE AR, DEPORTER DA, FREEMAN E: The role of fibroblasts in the remodeling of periodontal ligament during physiologic tooth movement. Am J Orthod 69:155, 1976

WEINSTOCK M, LEBLOND CP: Synthesis, migration and release of precursor collagen by odontoblasts as visualized by radioautography after ^{3}H-proline administration. J Cell Biol 60:92, 1974

Basement Membranes

DAVIES P, ALLISON AC, CARDELLA CJ: The relation between connective tissue cells and intercellular substances, including basement membranes. Philos Trans R Soc Lond [Biol] 271:363, 1975

DODSON JW, HAY ED: Secretion of collagenous stroma by isolated epithelium grown in vitro. Exp Cell Res 65:215, 1971

FURCHT LT: Structure and function of the adhesive glycoprotein fibronectin. In Satir BH (ed): Modern Cell Biology, Vol 1, p 53. New York, Alan R Liss, 1983

HAKOMORI S, FUKUDA M, SEKIGUCHI K, CARTER WG: Fibronectin, laminin, and other extracellular glycoproteins. In Piez KA, Reddi AH (eds): Extracellular Matrix Biochemistry, p 229. New York, Elsevier, 1984

INOUÉ S, LEBLOND CP, LAURIE GW: Ultrastructure of Reichert's membrane, a multilayered basement membrane in the parietal wall of the rat yolk sac. J Cell Biol 97:1524, 1983

KEFALIDES NA: Chemical properties of basement membranes. Int Rev Exp Pathol 10:1, 1971

LAURIE GW, LEBLOND CP, INOUÉ S ET AL: Fine structure of the glomerular basement membrane and immunolocalization of five basement membrane components to the lamina densa (basal lamina) and its extensions in both glomeruli and tubules of the rat kidney. Am J Anat 169:463, 1984

REALE E: Electron microscopy of the basement membranes. In Ruggeri A, Motta P (eds): Ultrastructure of the Connective Tissue Matrix, p 192. Boston, Martinus Nijhoff, 1984

TIMPL R, DZIADEK M, FUJIWARA S ET AL: Nidogen: A new self-aggregating basement membrane protein. Eur J Biochem 137:455, 1983

Endothelial Cells

WEIBEL ER, PALADE GE: New cytoplasmic components in arterial endothelia. J Cell Biol 23:101, 1964

Macrophages

CARR I: The biology of macrophages. Clin Invest Med 1:59, 1978

CARR I: The Macrophage. A Review of Ultrastructure and Function. New York, Academic Press, 1973

CLINE MJ: The White Cell. Cambridge, Harvard University Press, 1975

PAGE RC: The macrophage as a secretory cell. Int Rev Cytol 52: 119, 1978

PEARSALL NN, WEISER RS: The Macrophage. Philadelphia, Lea & Febiger, 1970

Plasma Cells

DEPETRIS S, KARLSBAD G, PERNIS B: Localization of antibodies in plasma cells by electron microscopy. J Exp Med 117:849, 1963

MOVAT HZ, FERNANDO NVP: The fine structure of connective tissue. II. The plasma cells. Exp Mol Pathol 1:535, 1962

RIFKIND RA, OSSERMAN EF, HSU KC, MORGAN C: The intracellular distribution of gamma globulin in a mouse plasma cell tumor as revealed by fluorescence and electron microscopy. J Exp Med 116:423, 1962

Mast Cells

AUSTEN KF: Biological implications of the structural and functional characteristics of the chemical mediators of immediate-type hypersensitivity. In The Harvey Lectures, Series 73, p 93. New York, Academic Press, 1979

AUSTEN KF, ORANGE RP: Bronchial asthma: The possible role of the chemical mediators of immediate hypersensitivity in the pathogenesis of subacute chronic disease. Am Rev Respir Dis 112: 423, 1975

BEAVEN MA: Histamine (first part). N Engl J Med 294:30, 1976

BEAVEN MA: Histamine (second part). N Engl J Med 294:320, 1976

DENBURG JA, MESSNER H, LIM B ET AL: Clonal origin of human basophil/mast cells from circulating multipotent hemopoietic progenitors. Exp Hematol 13:185, 1985

FERNANDO NVP, MOVAT HZ: The fine structure of connective tissue. III. The mast cell. Exp Mol Pathol 2:450, 1963

MOTA I: The behaviour of mast cells in anaphylaxis. Int Rev Cytol 15:363, 1963

SELYE H: The Mast Cells. Washington, Butterworth, 1965

SMITH DE: The tissue mast cell. Int Rev Cytol 14:327, 1963

WENDLING F, SHREEVE M, McLEOD D, AXELRAD A: A self-renewing, bipotential erythroid/mast cell progenitor in continuous cultures of normal murine bone marrow. J Cell Physiol 125:10, 1985

Adipocytes and Adipose Tissue

BROWN MS, GOLDSTEIN JL: How LDL receptors influence cholesterol and atherosclerosis. Sci Am 251 No 5:58, 1984

CAHILL GF, RENOLD AE: Adipose tissue—A brief history. In Angel A, Hollenberg CH, Roncari DAK (eds): Adipocyte and Obesity. New York, Raven Press, 1983

GOLDSTEIN JL, BASU SK, BROWN MS: Receptor-mediated endocytosis of low-density lipoprotein in cultured cells. In Fleischer S, Fleischer B (eds): Methods in Enzymology, Vol 98, Biomembranes, Part L, p 241. New York, Academic Press, 1983

RONCARI DAK, VAN RLR: Adipose tissue cellularity and obesity: New perspectives. Clin Invest Med 1:71, 1978

SENIOR JR: Intestinal absorption of fats. J Lipid Res 5:495, 1964

SHELDON H: The fine structure of adipose tissue. In Rodahl K, Issekutz B (eds): Fat As a Tissue, p 41. New York, McGraw-Hill, 1964

SHELDON H, ANGEL A: Some considerations on the morphology of adipose tissue. In Meng HC (ed): Proc Internat Symp on Lipid Transport, p 155. Springfield, IL, Charles C Thomas, 1964

SMITH RE, HOCK RJ: Brown fat: Thermogenic effector of arousal in hibernation. Science 140:199, 1963

THOMPSON JF, HABECK DA, NANCE SL, BEETHAM KL: Ultrastructural and biochemical changes in brown fat in cold exposed rats. J Cell Biol 41:312, 1969

VAN RLR: Human adiposity and the fat cell precursor. Näringsforskning Arg 26:86, 1982

VAN RLR, RONCARI DAK: Complete differentiation in vivo of implanted cultured adipocyte precursors from adult rats. Cell Tissue Res 225:557, 1982

WOOD EN: An ordered complex of filaments surrounding the lipid droplets in developing adipose cells. Anat Rec 157:437, 1967

8

Blood Cells

Blood cells represent a category of *free* connective tissue cells that are not attached to other cells or held in position by intercellular substances. They are produced by the hematopoietic tissues (which will be described in the following chapters), and on entering the bloodstream they become suspended in *blood plasma,* the fluid portion of the blood. Blood cells are broadly subdivided into (1) *red blood cells* or *erythrocytes* (Gr. *erythros,* red), which appear red because of their hemoglobin content; (2) *white blood cells* or *leukocytes* (Gr. *leukos,* white), which if packed together appear white; and (3) *blood platelets,* which are tiny fragments of cytoplasm.

Aside from blood platelets (which are only parts of cells), mature erythrocytes are the only cells in the body that lack a nucleus. Although erythrocytes possess a nucleus during their development, they extrude it before they enter the circulation. In contrast, leukocytes retain their nucleus, which eventually assumes a characteristic shape for each type of leukocyte. Platelets are not whole cells but cell membrane–covered fragments of cytoplasm that are liberated from megakaryocytes, which are exceptionally large cells situated in myeloid tissue (red bone marrow). These cell fragments nevertheless perform very important functions.

Whereas erythrocytes and platelets carry out important functions in the blood, most kinds of leukocytes perform their specialized duties after they have left the bloodstream and have entered loose connective tissue. Hence leukocytes are blood cells chiefly in the sense that they use the blood as a means of transport.

Blood Films Are Used for the Microscopic Study of Blood Cells and Platelets. Although blood cells can be identified in sections, they are seen to better advantage if they are spread out very thinly on a slide before being fixed and stained. Such a preparation is called a *blood film.*

To obtain blood for making a blood film, a cleansed finger or earlobe is punctured lightly and the first drop of blood is wiped away with sterile gauze because it becomes too large. Then a tiny drop wells up from the puncture. Although blood films are made in different ways in different laboratories, one way is to touch the tiny drop with a clean slide, avoiding contact with the skin, so that most of the drop adheres to the slide a short distance from one end. A second slide is then lowered onto the first at an angle of about 30° (Fig. 8-1A) so that one end just touches the front edge of the drop of blood. This slide is then pushed steadily forward using only light pressure so that the blood is drawn out (not pushed) into a thin film. The angle at which the slide is held affects the thickness of the film: the greater the angle, the thicker the film. Thicker films are also obtained if the spreading is done rapidly. Moreover, each film is generally thicker where the drop first spreads out (Fig. 8-1B).

The film is fixed and then stained with a blood stain. Although there are several different blood stains, all are generally used as a single solution. They contain polychromed derivatives of a red acid stain such as eosin and a blue basic stain such as methylene blue. The blood cells illustrated in the color plates of this edition are all stained with Wright's blood stain, which confers the colors described in this chapter and in Chapter 9. Sufficient blood stain isused to cover the film, followed by an acidic buffer (pH 6.5) to dilute the stain and adjust the colors. After rinsing and drying, the film can be mounted under a coverslip.

ERYTHROCYTES

Erythrocytes (red blood cells) are the most common type of blood cell; they are from 500 to 1000 times more numerous than leukocytes. In absolute numbers, there are about 5 million erythrocytes per cubic millimeter of blood.

The human erythrocyte has the shape of a *biconcave disk* (Fig. 8-2), but other shapes are found in other species. In certain diseases, erythrocytes with altered shapes can be seen (Fig. 8-3B), hence determining the shapes of erythrocytes is of diagnostic importance. The diameter of erythrocytes is usually measured in blood films (Fig. 8-1). Because they have the shape of a biconcave disk, they lie flat on the slide, so drying does not greatly affect their size. In normal blood, the diameter of erythrocytes has a mean value of 7.2 μm and does not vary by much more than 0.5 μm from this mean value. Thus a glance at the size distribution of erythrocytes (which is called a Price–Jones curve) reveals any abnormalities of size that might occur.

An erythrocyte smaller than 6 μm in diameter is termed a *microcyte* (Gr. *mikros*, small), as illustrated in Figure 8-3B, whereas an erythrocyte larger than normal (from 9 μm to 12 μm in diameter) is termed a *macrocyte* (Gr. *makros*, large), also illustrated in Figure 8-3B. Thus a shift in size range toward smaller erythrocytes is called a *microcytic* condition, and toward bigger ones, a *macrocytic* condition (see Fig. 8-5). In some conditions, both microcytes and macrocytes may be present concurrently (Fig. 8-3B).

With the introduction of electronic counting instruments in hematology laboratories, it is now common practice to measure the red cell volume instead of size, because the volume of the red cell has diagnostic significance. Accordingly, the terms microcyte and macrocyte have come to mean erythrocytes of smaller and larger volume, respectively.

The factors determining and maintaining the highly

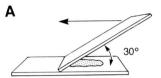
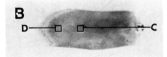
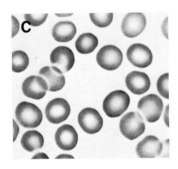
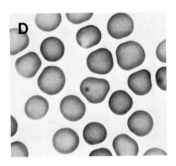

Fig. 8-1. (*A*) Diagrammatic representation of the standard procedure for preparing a blood film. (*B*) Photograph of a stained blood film, indicating a good site (C) and a poor site (D) for observing erythrocytes. (*C*) Photomicrograph of field C, where a few erythrocytes just overlap. (*D*) Photomicrograph of field D, where the erythrocytes are spread too sparsely for their pale centers to show clearly.

characteristic shape of an erythrocyte are the particular molecular constituents of its cell membrane and the constitution of the colloidal complex with which it is filled. Moreover, these constituents confer pliability and elasticity so that the red cell can undergo deformation as required in passing through networks of vessels that have a small lumen.

About 66% of the content of the erythrocyte is water and about 33% is the protein *hemoglobin*. This protein contains a protein moiety, *globin*, joined to the pigment *heme*. Although only only 4% of hemoglobin actually consists of heme, its combination with globin results in a combined entity (hemoglobin) that is colored; hence hemoglobin, too, is spoken of as a pigment. A small amount of

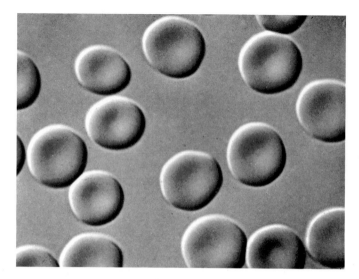

Fig. 8-2.   Photomicrograph of erythrocytes in a fresh preparation, as seen under an interference microscope. (Bessis M: Living Blood Cells and Their Ultrastructure. New York, Springer-Verlag, 1973)

other protein, several enzymes, and some lipid also exist in the cell along with hemoglobin.

It may seem curious that erythrocytes containing only a soft jelly would maintain their biconcave shape, and that the molecular constitution of the jelly could be an important factor in making the cell assume this shape. However, the fact is that a change in the chemical constitution of hemoglobin can be responsible for causing the cells to take on a different shape. For example, there is a disease (called *sickle cell anemia*) in which the erythrocytes may assume the form of sickles. In this form, they are destroyed easily, and so individuals with this disease do not have enough erythrocytes and suffer from *anemia* (a subject that will be dealt with in more detail later in this chapter). In 1949 Pauling and his colleagues discovered that hemoglobin in sickle cells was slightly different from normal and the difference was sufficient to make the cells assume a shape different from a biconcave disk when the hemoglobin is deoxygenated. Hereditary factors are responsible for the condition; hence this disease exemplifies how an altered base sequence in a DNA molecule, resulting in the substitution of one amino acid (valine) for the usual one (glutamic acid) in the hemoglobin molecule, can cause disease.

Erythrocytes sometimes adhere to one another via their broad surfaces and thereby form arrangements that resemble piles of stacked coins (Fig. 8-4). Called *rouleaux* (Fr. for rolls), such arrangements are believed to be due to surface-tension forces. Their presence may indicate that the plasma globulin levels are elevated, although they are occasionally also seen at sites where the circulation is slow. The stacked arrangement is only temporary; its constituent erythrocytes separate without any harmful effects.

In electron microscopic (EM) sections, the cytoplasmic content of erythrocytes appears more or less uniformly electron dense (see Fig. 16-19). Until a day or two after erythrocytes have entered the circulation, they are still relatively immature. At this early stage, a few ribosomes and occasionally even a few small mitochondria may be discernible in their cytoplasm. Later, however, there is little else in their cytoplasm but hemoglobin, which in the con-

centration present in **mature erythrocytes** is fairly electron dense in appearance **because of its iron** content (see Fig. 16-19). The **characteristic biconcave shape** of erythrocytes can also sometimes **be recognized in an** EM section (see Fig. 14-26).

The cell **membrane of the erythrocyte** prevents the escape of hemoglobin **into the plasma. It also exhibits selectivity** with regard to **the passage of ions. Some electron micro**scopic **features of the erythrocyte** membrane are illustrated in Figure 4-4*A*.

Blood Group Antigens.   Certain integral membrane glycoproteins and glycolipids of the erythrocyte cell membrane have oligosaccharide chains that carry *blood group antigen* specificity. A major group of erythrocyte antigens are those belonging to the *ABO system*. Anyone who lacks antigen A on his erythrocytes possesses agglutinating antibody to antigen A in his plasma. Conversely, those who lack antigen B on their red cells produce anti-B. Those in blood group AB, however, possess both of these antigens on their erythrocytes and produce neither antibody; hence they are universal recipients. Individuals in blood group O have neither A nor B antigen on their erythrocytes and are universal donors; in other words, their erythrocytes are tolerated by anyone who might need a transfusion. Before carrying out a blood transfusion, it is necessary to match the ABO-group antigens of the donor to those of the recipient because mismatching can result in agglutination and lysis (*hemolysis,* which is described in the following section) of the donor erythrocytes (*i.e.,* a *hemolytic transfusion reaction*). The *Rh* antigen is another blood group antigen that is of considerable clinical importance because unless special measures are taken, an Rh-negative mother may begin to produce antibody to Rh antigen if she is bearing an Rh-positive fetus. Transplacental exchange of the maternal antibody may then lead to lysis of the fetal erythrocytes, which is detrimental to the fetus.

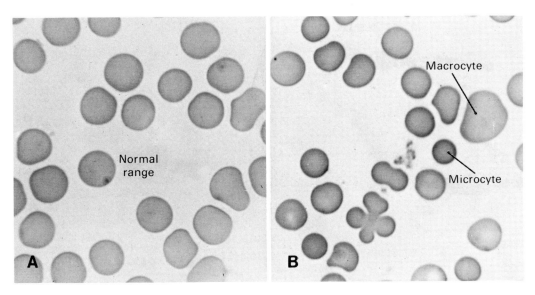

Fig. 8-3. Photomicrographs showing (*A*) normal-sized erythrocytes and (*B*) macrocytic and microcytic erythrocytes (rabbit). Poikilocytes (erythrocytes with abnormal shapes) can also be seen in *B*.

The Appearance of Erythrocytes Is Altered by Solutions of Different Osmotic Strengths. The osmotic strength of blood plasma is equal to that of erythrocytes; hence the plasma is described as being *isotonic* (Gr. *iso*, equal; *tonos*, tension) with them. In plasma, then, there is no tendency for erythrocytes to take up water from the plasma or vice versa. It is possible to prepare a salt solution that is *isotonic* with erythrocytes. A solution with a salt concentration lower than that of erythrocytes is termed *hypotonic* (Gr. *hypo*, under), whereas one of greater concentration is termed *hypertonic* (Gr. *hyper*, above or over). Erythrocytes are fairly resistant to minor changes in osmotic strength, but in a solution that is sufficiently *hypotonic*, they swell and assume a spherical shape. Another phenomenon then occurs: their membrane becomes incapable of retaining hemoglobin, and this escapes into the surrounding fluid, coloring it. This is known as *hemolysis* (Gr. *lysis*, solution). The cell membrane remains to constitute what is termed the *ghost* of the cell.

Hemolysis can be induced by means other than hypotonic solutions. Certain chemicals, particularly lipid solvents, exert a hemolytic effect. Snake venom, a potent source of lipolytic enzymes, is a hemolytic agent. The plasma of some species hemolyzes the erythrocytes of others. Antibodies made by injecting the erythrocytes of one animal into a genetically dissimilar one will hemolyze the erythrocytes of the first; this phenomenon involves the fixing of complement, which will be explained later in this chapter.

It should also be mentioned, however, that some hemoglobin release is normal in sites such as the spleen, where worn-out red cells are always being phagocytosed by macrophages.

The erythrocytes in any given sample of blood are not all equally susceptible to hemolysis. Erythrocytes are therefore described as varying in their *fragility* (*i.e.,* their susceptibility to hemolysis). Because the fragility of erythrocytes can become altered in certain disease states, fragility determinations are of diagnostic value.

If erythrocytes are suspended in a *hypertonic* solution, osmotic withdrawal of water results in their irregular shrinkage and the formation of notches and indentations in their outlines. Such erythrocytes are described as *crenated* (L. *crena*, notch).

Erythrocytes Are Involved in Body-wide Transport of Oxygen and Carbon Dioxide. In the lungs, the hemoglobin in erythrocytes readily combines with oxygen and becomes *oxyhemoglobin*. The oxyhemoglobin subsequently yields its oxygen to the body tissues, and the deoxygenated blood returns to the lungs to become reoxygenated. Erythrocytes are also involved in the transport of carbon dioxide from the tissues to the lungs; this function is dependent on their content of the enzyme *carbonic anhydrase*.

Erythrocytes have to be able to take up and yield their oxygen and carbon dioxide very rapidly. To facilitate this, their surface area is increased by their biconcave shape, which provides a surface area that is 20% to 30% greater than that of a sphere containing the same amount of hemoglobin. This unique shape also reduces the distance over which blood gases have to diffuse. Because the human red cell contains no nucleus, its interior is entirely filled with hemoglobin; furthermore, its rounded edges and resilient properties render it resistant to damage and provide the flexibility necessary for it to negotiate capillary bifurcations.

A major reason why hemoglobin is confined within cells is that erythrocytes, in addition to their content of hemoglobin, contain a

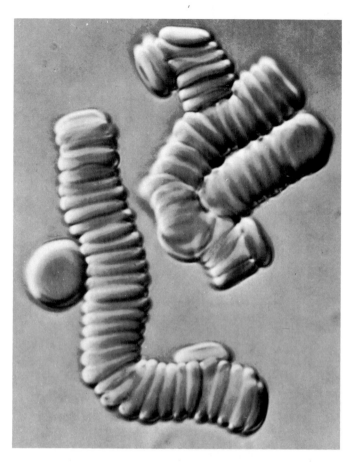

Fig. 8-4. Photomicrograph of erythrocytes adhering to one another and forming rouleaux in a fresh preparation, as seen under an interference microscope. (Bessis M: Living Blood Cells and Their Ultrastructure. New York, Springer-Verlag, 1973)

number of enzymes that keep hemoglobin in the reduced state in which it carries oxygen. These enzymes must be kept in intimate association with the hemoglobin to maintain it in its reduced form. Furthermore, in comparison with the other macromolecules in the body, hemoglobin molecules are relatively small; hence if they were free in the plasma, they would leak across the endothelial lining of the blood vascular system. Once hemoglobin does become free in the plasma, it soon escapes into the tissues and also enters the urine. In a virulent form of malaria known as blackwater fever, for example, so many erythrocytes can become damaged by the malarial parasite that the urine can become tea-colored.

The oxyhemoglobin of erythrocytes in the capillaries near the body surface imparts a pink color to the cheeks and a variable degree of redness to the lips and mucous membranes. The depth of color imparted depends on a number of different factors, including the proportion of such capillaries that are open at any given time in the local capillary bed, the proximity of these vessels to the surface, the transparency of the overlying tissue, and the proportion of oxyhemoglobin present in the blood.

Cyanosis. Deoxygenated hemoglobin has a bluish tinge. Under ordinary circumstances, insufficient amounts of deoxygenated hemoglobin are formed as blood passes through capillaries for this blue color to become evident. However, exposure to severe cold can cause the local capillary microcirculation in the lips to shut down to such an extent that the level of deoxyhemoglobin in the superficial capillaries rises and its blue color then begins to show.

In certain diseases, the process of oxygenation in the lungs is seriously impaired, and as a result, blood with a considerable content of deoxyhemoglobin is delivered to capillaries all over the body. A sufficient absolute amount of deoxyhemoglobin can impart a blue color to all surfaces of the body that are normally pink or red. Such a widespread change in color is termed *cyanosis* (Gr. *kyanos*, blue).

Carbon Monoxide Poisoning. Hemoglobin also has a very high affinity for carbon monoxide. Furthermore, this odorless gas becomes bound to hemoglobin much more strongly than oxygen does. As a result, anyone who breathes air that contains even a low level of carbon monoxide accumulates increasing amounts of it that become bound to his hemoglobin and render the hemoglobin unavailable for the transport of oxygen. This can happen even in a parked car if the engine is kept running to keep the heater going because the weather is cold. Because hemoglobin that has taken up carbon monoxide is bright red, the cherry-red color of the lips of the carbon monoxide victim belie the fact that his body tissues are starved of oxygen.

The Oxygen-Carrying Capacity of the Blood Can Be Directly Determined from a Small Blood Sample. In medical practice, it is sometimes necessary to establish whether a patient's blood can carry the required amount of oxygen. Aside from relatively rare instances in which

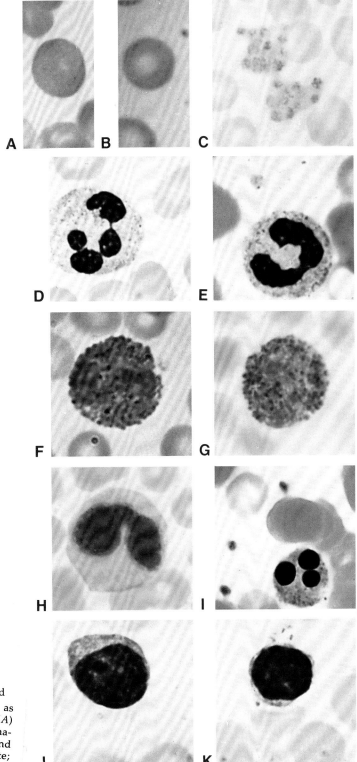

Plate 8-1. Erythrocytes, platelets, and leukocytes as seen in a peripheral blood film (Wright's blood stain). (*A*) Polychromatophilic erythrocyte; (*B*) erythrocyte (mature); (*C*) platelets; (*D*) neutrophil (mature); (*E*) band neutrophil; (*F*) eosinophil; (*G*) basophil; (*H*) monocyte; (*I*) degenerating neutrophil; (*J*) large lymphocyte; (*K*) small lymphocyte.

the patient's hemoglobin is chemically altered, it is obvious that the oxygen-carrying capacity of his blood could be diminished by the presence of (1) an insufficient number of erythrocytes in the peripheral blood, (2) an insufficient concentration of hemoglobin per erythrocyte, or (3) both of these factors combined. Two laboratory tests for detecting such deficiencies determine (1) the number of erythrocytes per cubic millimeter of blood, and (2) the amount of hemoglobin per 100 ml of blood.

Erythrocyte Counting. A small sample of blood is measured out and diluted using a specially designed pipet. Following dilution and mixing, a few drops of the diluted blood are run into a *hemocytometer*. This is a ruled slide with a surface that is divided into squares of given sizes for counting different kinds of blood cells (see Fig. 8-10*B*). Because the volume of diluted blood placed above each ruled square is known, the number of erythrocytes per cubic millimeter of blood can readily be calculated from the number of erythrocytes counted in each square. However, because this method is extremely time-consuming, hematology laboratories routinely use electronic counting instruments that can perform large batches of blood counts in a short period.

Hematocrit Estimation. Another rapid way to determine whether the patient's blood contains a normal complement of erythrocytes is to estimate the *packed red cell volume* from a small blood sample by submitting it to centrifugation. This procedure is known as *hematocrit* determination (Gr. *haima*, blood; *krino*, to separate) because it involves separating the blood cells from the plasma. Erythrocytes account for almost all the packed-cell volume. The hematocrit is the volume occupied by the erythrocytes expressed as a percentage of the total volume of the blood sample.

Hemoglobin Estimation. Several methods are also available for estimating hemoglobin content from a single drop of blood. From the small measured sample, the total amount of hemoglobin per 100 ml of blood is calculated.

A red cell count of 4 to 5 million erythrocytes per cubic millimeter of blood is considered normal for women, whereas from 4.5 to 5.5 million is normal for men. Normal hematocrit values are approximately 41% for women and approximately 47% for men. Women normally have approximately 13.5 g of hemoglobin and men normally have approximately 15 g of hemoglobin per 100 ml blood.

Anemias

If the amount of hemoglobin in the circulating blood is significantly reduced from its normal level, the patient is suffering from *anemia* (Gr. meaning without blood). A lack of hemoglobin can be due either to a lack of erythrocytes or to a lack of hemoglobin itself.

Human erythrocytes have a lifespan of only 100 to 120 days. They must then be removed to prevent them from disintegrating and cluttering up the circulatory system. Worn-out erythrocytes are removed from the bloodstream by the macrophages in the spleen, assisted by those of the bone marrow and liver. To compensate for such destruction, new erythrocytes need to be generated and delivered to the blood at the same rate. Under conditions in which erythrocyte depletion outweighs erythrocyte production, an anemia develops. Anemias can result from (1) accelerated removal or wholesale destruction of erythrocytes (*e.g.,* through hemolysis) (2) severe blood loss (*e.g.,* through hemorrhage) or (3) insufficient erythrocyte production.

To determine whether the problem lies in the rate of erythrocyte production or in the rate of erythrocyte destruction, useful information can be gained from what is termed the *reticulocyte count.*

The Reticulocyte Count. Almost all the erythrocytes in a stained blood film have a clear pink color (Plate 8-1*B*). However, 1% to 2% of the erythrocyte population may appear slightly larger and exhibit a bluish tinge (Plate 8-1*A*). Such erythrocytes are described as *polychromatophilic erythrocytes* (red cells that become stained many colors; Plate 8-1*A*). We shall now explain what causes the blue tinge in a red cell.

The nucleated precursor cells giving rise to erythrocytes are larger cells called *erythroblasts* that synthesize the hemoglobin later found in their progeny, the erythrocytes. For synthesizing hemoglobin, they have abundant polysomes that render their cytoplasm diffusely basophilic (see Plate 9-1*B*). However, they divide several times in forming erythrocytes, and in so doing, the polysome complement becomes divided so that there are only enough polysomes in immature erythrocytes to impart a trace of basophilia to the cytoplasm.

Polychromatophilic erythrocytes are difficult to identify in films stained with ordinary blood stains. A much better way to identify the cells is to stain them with brilliant cresyl blue. This stain may be mixed with a fresh drop of blood and a blood film made that may be subsequently stained with an ordinary blood stain. Brilliant cresyl blue reacts in a curious manner with the rRNA that persists and produces a threadlike blue structure that sometimes looks like a wreath (Fig. 8-5), but if the rRNA is scanty, it may constitute no more than a few scattered dots. Because this appearance was thought to indicate some kind of reticular network in the cytoplasm, such cells were called *reticulocytes*. This name persists even though the network is now known to be an artifact due to the staining procedure. The *reticulocyte* is, of course, the same cell as a polychromatophilic erythrocyte seen after staining with an ordinary blood stain (Plate 8-1*A*). The use of radioautography following administration of labeled amino acid has shown that reticulocytes are still capable of a significant level of protein synthesis, so they would also contain some mRNA and tRNA in addition to rRNA.

The rRNA present in reticulocytes liberated from the bone marrow into the circulation soon fades away; it remains only for about 2 days in immature erythrocytes.

Precise data about the numbers of reticulocytes released from the bone marrow into the circulation under normal conditions are not easily ascertained. However, because

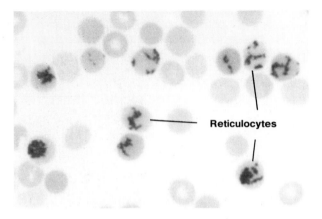

Fig. 8-5. Photomicrograph showing reticulocytes in a film of peripheral blood (rabbit). The wreathlike network in reticulocytes demonstrated by staining with brilliant cresyl blue represents their residual cytoplasmic RNA. The reticulocyte count of this experimental animal has been increased by prior bleeding.

the storage space in the marrow is not correspondingly increased when erythrocyte production is increased, more reticulocytes are liberated into the blood. Thus the reticulocyte count rises when more erythrocytes are produced, and reticulocyte counts can be used to monitor the rate of red cell production.

Under otherwise normal circumstances, any condition that causes an increased rate of erythrocyte destruction (or loss by hemorrhage) is compensated for by an increase in the rate of erythrocyte production. So if, for example, the reticulocyte count remains high day after day, it can be assumed that the rate of destruction of erythrocytes is increased, or that erythrocytes are being lost from the circulation in some other fashion. In other words, the reticulocyte count can be used not only to provide information about the rate of erythrocyte production but also, in conjunction with daily erythrocyte counts, about the rate of erythrocyte destruction or loss.

Anemias Can Be Classified as Hypochromic or Hyperchromic. Sooner or later, the medical student must learn how to decide whether a blood film indicates a *hypochromic microcytic anemia* or a *macrocytic anemia* or some other kind of blood disorder designated by this type of terminology. What do these terms mean?

Macrocytes and microcytes have already been defined. If in any anemia the erythrocytes tend to be substantially larger than normal, the anemia is said to be *macrocytic;* if smaller than normal, *microcytic;* and if of normal size, *normocytic.* The terms *hyperchromic, normochromic,* and *hypochromic* refer to the total amount of hemoglobin in the red cells, which is what accounts for their depth of color in films.

Because an erythrocyte has the shape of a biconcave disk, it is thinner in the middle than at the edge, and so its central region stains lighter than its periphery (Fig. 8-1C).

However, this appearance is seen only in the proper part of a well-made film that is just thick enough for occasional cells to partly overlap one another (Fig. 8-1C). The lighter staining central area cannot be seen properly where the cells are spread too thinly (Fig. 8-1D).

If the central pale area represents roughly a third of the diameter of the erythrocyte and the peripheral region shows fairly intense staining (Fig. 8-6B), the erythrocytes are said to be *normochromic* (normal in color). Some anemias are characterized by a reduction in the number of erythrocytes, but such cells that are present are normochromic; hence they are said to be *normochromic anemias.* However, in a much more common type of anemia, the erythrocytes exhibit enlarged central pale areas and poorly stained peripheral zones (Fig. 8-6A). The cells altered in this way are said to be *hypochromic* (undercolored); hence the anemias with which they are associated are called *hypochromic anemias.* In still other anemias, there are fewer cells than normal but these are well filled with hemoglobin. It is doubtful whether red cells can be overfilled, and so the reason these anemias are called *hyperchromic* is that the cells are generally larger and, because they are well filled, they take on a deeper color (Fig. 8-6C).

Films of normal blood usually exhibit an occasional erythrocyte of abnormal shape. The general term for such a cell is a *poikilocyte* (Gr. *poikilis,* manifold). In the anemias, poikilocytes are common; hence, anemic blood is often said to exhibit *poikilocytosis* (Fig. 8-3B). In some anemias, the abnormal shape is named more specifically—for example, the type in which erythrocytes tend to be shaped like sickles, which has already been mentioned.

Different Types of Anemia Result from Deficiencies in Iron or Vitamin B_{12}. In any given anemia, knowing whether the hemoglobin content is reduced to a greater or lesser extent than the erythrocyte count can help to indicate the possible cause of the anemia. For example, iron is an essential constituent of hemoglobin, and so when iron is deficient, the production of hemoglobin is reduced. However, iron is not as necessary for the production of erythrocytes as it is for the formation of hemoglobin, so in iron-deficiency anemias, the hemoglobin content of blood is reduced to a greater extent than the number of erythrocytes. Hence the cells are poorly filled with hemoglobin and the anemia is said to be of the *hypochromic* type (Fig. 8-6A).

On the other hand, certain dietary factors (vitamin B_{12} and folic acid) seem to be more necessary for the production of erythrocytes than for the production of hemoglobin. When either of these substances is lacking, there is more difficulty in producing erythrocytes than in producing hemoglobin. Hence erythrocytes produced under these conditions are filled to capacity with hemoglobin, and the anemia is of the *hyperchromic macrocytic* type (Fig. 8-6C). The anemias in this category are all caused by a deficiency of either vitamin B_{12} or folic acid. An example is *pernicious anemia,* which results from a failure to secrete *intrinsic factor,* a constituent glycoprotein of gastric juice that is necessary

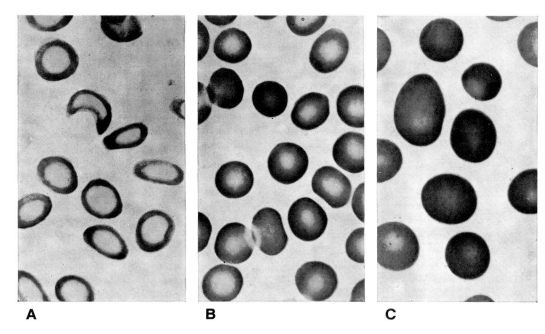

Fig. 8-6. Photomicrograph showing (*A*) microcytic hypochromic erythrocytes in an iron-deficiency anemia (fewer and smaller erythrocytes exhibiting a larger central pale area); (*B*) normal erythrocytes (normal numbers of normocytic normochromic erythrocytes); and (*C*) macrocytic hyperchromic erythrocytes in pernicious anemia (fewer and larger erythrocytes that have the appearance of being overfilled with hemoglobin).

for the absorption of vitamin B_{12} from the intestine. Dietary supplements of this vitamin are ineffective in treating pernicious anemia because the vitamin cannot be absorbed from the gut. However, marked improvement is generally obtained if this vitamin is administered by injection. The anemia recurs only if these injections are discontinued.

Erythrocyte Production Is Stimulated by Erythropoietin

A glycoprotein hormone called *erythropoietin* augments erythrocyte production by promoting proliferation and maturation of the later stages of the erythrocytic series. This action will be discussed in Chapter 9.

PLATELETS

Blood platelets, which are also known as *thrombocytes* (Gr. *thrombus*, clot), are comparatively small, disk-shaped fragments of granule-containing cytoplasm with a diameter of approximately 2 μm to 3 μm. These fragments become detached from very large cells called *megakaryocytes* that are present in red bone marrow. Furthermore, they are produced in such a manner that each fragment becomes invested with a covering membrane (see Chap. 9). Platelets have no nuclear component; hence they are not whole cells. Their numbers in peripheral blood vary from 150,000 to

400,000 per cubic millimeter. Their microscopic appearance in a stained blood film is shown in Figure 8-7 and Plate 8-1C, but before we go on to describe their structure, we should discuss some of their very important functions.

Platelets Play a Key Role in the Arrest of Bleeding (Hemostasis)

When someone sustains a laceration, blood flows from cut or otherwise damaged vessels. However, unless these vessels are relatively wide, the flow of blood soon dwindles and ceases. Although other factors also operate to achieve this end—for example, vasoconstrictor substances such as serotonin may induce contraction of the circular layer of smooth muscle in the vessel wall and thereby constrict the lumen of the vessel—the main reason for cessation of bleeding is that platelets settle and adhere to the inner surface of the vessel wall in the vicinity of the cut. More and more platelets then adhere to those that have already attached themselves to the vessel lining, and the resulting accumulation of platelets progressively restricts the size of the opening through which blood is escaping. This process of *platelet aggregation* leads to a buildup of platelets on the wall of the damaged vessel and eventually results in the formation of a *platelet (hemostatic) plug.*

Platelet aggregation is normally accompanied by the formation of *fibrin*, a fibrous protein derived from the plasma precursor *fibrinogen* through an elaborate clotting

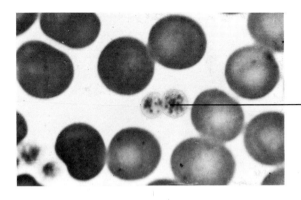

— Platelets

Fig. 8-7. Photomicrograph of two blood platelets in a film of peripheral blood, showing their central granulomere and surrounding hyalomere. Their diameter is substantially smaller than that of an erythrocyte.

mechanism known as *blood coagulation.* Thus blood coagulation can be initiated by platelet aggregation. However, it is not only when blood vessels are cut that platelets adhere to their lining. A common degenerative change that is a part of the aging process is *arteriosclerosis* (Gr. *sclerosis,* hardening; *i.e.,* hardening of the arteries). In this condition, the endothelial lining of arteries is generally affected in such a way that it no longer presents a smooth uninterrupted surface to flowing blood. As a consequence, platelets come into contact with certain intercellular components of the arterial wall to which they readily adhere. (The details will be given later in this chapter). Platelets can build up at such a site and, together with fibrin that forms in association with them as a result of coagulation, may occlude the lumen of a vessel. If the occluded vessel is a coronary artery and a portion of the heart muscle is thereby deprived of its necessary oxygen supply, the individual will experience an *acute coronary attack.* If a similar process occurs in an artery that supplies the brain, the individual will suffer a *stroke.* Further information about platelet involvement in arterial occlusion can be found in Chapter 16.

The essentials of the mechanism of blood clotting that are described in the following discussion are intended for students who have not yet had the opportunity to study physiology, which deals with the subject of blood coagulation much more thoroughly.

The Mechanism of Blood Coagulation. Whereas the process of *aggregation* is associated with flowing blood, the process of *coagulation* can also take place in stationary blood (*e.g.,* it can yield a blood clot in a test tube). Coagulation can also occur in extravasated blood, which is blood that has escaped from vessels into the body tissues. Thus the breaking of a bone tears a number of vessels and causes blood to leak into the soft tissues in the immediate vicinity of the fracture site. As in a test tube, blood that escapes from the vascular system produces an extensive meshwork of fibrin, entrapping erythrocytes that subsequently disintegrate.

The reason why blood remains uncoagulated in blood vessels and yet clots soon after it is removed is a complicated matter that involves a host of different factors. For a comprehensive account of the mechanism of blood coagulation

that includes a discussion of the many factors involved, see Mustard and Packham, 1979. The following section will present only a very brief overview of this complex process.

One of the proteins present in blood plasma is *fibrinogen.* Under ordinary conditions, fibrinogen exists in solution. Also present is a plasma globulin called *prothrombin,* which, under ordinary conditions, is inactive. However, damaged tissues liberate a coagulation factor known as *tissue thromboplastin* (factor III). Although many other coagulation factors are also involved, release of tissue thromboplastin triggers conversion of *prothrombin* to *thrombin,* and this, in turn, causes soluble *fibrinogen* to polymerize into insoluble *fibrin.* Because tissue thromboplastin (factor III) comes from the damaged tissue, it is referred to as an *extrinsic* factor (*i.e.,* a factor that does not originate from blood itself).

The coagulation mechanism, however, can also be triggered by an *intrinsic* platelet factor III (phospholipid) that orginates from blood platelets. When a platelet plug begins to form on the inner surface of a degenerating artery or cut vessel, the extrinsic and intrinsic factors operate jointly, leading to coagulation. Hence coagulation commonly takes place at sites of platelet aggregation.

Platelets that adhere to the inner surface of a blood vessel aggregate into a mass that is termed a *white thrombus* because it is white in the fresh state. A white thrombus forms only in flowing blood, whereas a *red thrombus* forms when stationary blood coagulates. Aggregation, then, leads to the formation of a white thrombus consisting primarily of fused platelets. Coagulation, on the other hand, leads to the formation of a red thrombus consisting of fibrin threads with enmeshed erythrocytes.

Now that we have dealt briefly with coagulation, we shall consider how the microscopic structure of platelets is related to the functions they perform.

Platelet Structure

Microscopic Appearance of Platelets. If observed in vessels in which blood is circulating, platelets appear as individual oval biconvex disks. In blood films, however, the platelets may aggregate unless precautions are taken (Plate 8-1C). Seen under oil immersion, platelets are generally flat and rounded in appearance (Fig. 8-7) because they tend to spread out on a glass surface. Their outer region stains a transparent pale blue (Plate 8-1C) and is called the *hyalomere* (Gr. *hyalos*, glass; *meros*, part). Their more central part is called the *granulomere* because it contains purple-colored material that generally looks like granules (Plate 8-1C).

Platelet Counting. To count platelets as individual entities, it is necessary to obtain a blood sample using laboratory supplies that have been treated with an anticoagulant (*e.g.*, heparin or citrate). One way to do a platelet count is to lyse the erythrocytes and then count the platelets that remain using a hemocytometer and a phase-contrast microscope. A faster method now used in hematology laboratories is to count the platelets with an automated electronic counter.

Fine Structure of Platelets. The EM discloses the presence of a circumferential ring of supporting microtubules that helps to maintain the biconvex discoid shape of the circulating platelet (Figs. 8-8 and 8-9). Microfilaments are also present at the platelet periphery. These filaments are believed to participate in the release reaction and in clot retraction, which are processes that we shall be considering when we deal with platelet function. Another feature of the platelet seen at the EM level is that it possesses two different systems of channels. One system is known as the *surface-connected open canalicular system* because it is made up of tubules that communicate with the platelet surface (Figs. 8-8 and 8-9). Longitudinal and transverse sections of these tubules (Fig. 8-8, *left*) have an inner surface that is characterized by the presence of cell coat material similar to that present on the outer surface of the platelet (Fig. 8-8). The canaliculi of the surface-connected open canalicular system are also relatively wide and tortuous, as can be seen on the left-hand side of Figure 8-8, where many have been cut in transverse section. Accordingly, this system represents a tubular labyrinth of invaginated surface membrane that ramifies through the cytoplasm and provides a major conduit for the release of a number of important secretory substances to the exterior of the platelet.

The second tubular system is termed the *dense tubular system* because the lumen of its component tubules contains a material that is moderately electron dense (Figs. 8-8 and 8-9). This is a closed system of somewhat narrower membranous tubules that appears to be derived from the endoplasmic reticulum. The detailed functional role of this particular part of the platelet has not yet been fully elucidated, but its lumen can sequester calcium ions that are involved in regulating the platelet's internal contractile activities, and there are histochemical indications that this system may also be involved in prostaglandin synthesis. The fact that there are regions in the platelet where tubules belonging to each of its tubular systems come into close apposition with each other suggests that there may be some functional link between these two systems.

Glycogen particles are present either in small groups or as larger aggregates (Fig. 8-8). A few mitochondria (Fig. 8-8), ribosomes, and dense bodies (Fig. 8-8), alternatively known as dense or very dense granules, are also present. In addition, platelets contain various other kinds of granules (Fig. 8-8). Certain of these granules contain lysosomal hydrolases and are thought to represent platelet *lysosomes*. However, the majority of colored granules seen in the light microscope (LM) are secretory granules called α-*granules*. These are membrane-bounded secretory granules that appear round to oval in electron micrographs and measure 0.2 μm to 0.3 μm in diameter (Fig. 8-8). Their content of finely particulate material contains a large number of substances involved in platelet function that are believed to have been synthesized by the megakaryocyte. Such substances include platelet factor 4 (which possesses antiheparin activity), factor V (a blood coagulation factor), fibrinogen, and PDGF (platelet-derived growth factor). PDGF is a mitogenic glycoprotein that induces proliferation in several different cell types, including smooth muscle cells, connective tissue cells such as fibroblasts, and also certain glial cells. PDGF seems to play a key role both as a chemoattractant and as a mitogen in the recruitment of cells for the repair of tissues during wound healing. It is also widely believed to be implicated in the pathogenesis of atherosclerosis (see also Chap. 16).

In electron micrographs, the markedly electron-dense content of platelet *dense bodies* (otherwise known as *dense* or *very dense granules*) may lie eccentrically with respect to its surrounding membrane as a result of extraction or uneven shrinkage (Fig. 8-8). It has been determined that the serotonin content of platelets is proportional to the number of dense bodies they contain. *Serotonin* (5-hydroxytryptamine) is a tryptophan-derived amine that is produced by enteroendocrine cells of the digestive tract (see Chap. 18). Platelets take up this amine from the bloodstream and store it in their dense bodies. It is a pharmacologically potent vasoactive substance that, if released, causes the smooth muscle cells in the walls of blood vessels of most parts of the body to contract. In addition to serotonin, the dense bodies of platelets store the catecholamine epinephrine as well as calcium, adenosine triphosphate (ATP), and adenosine diphosphate (ADP). Accordingly, they are often referred to as *amine storage granules*. The functional significance of the presence of some of these constituents will become apparent shortly. Platelets also possess a few catalase-containing peroxisomes with smaller dimensions than the other three kinds of granules.

Finally, we should add that there are indications from *in vitro* studies that in addition to playing a major secretory role, platelets have the potential to engulf various kinds of particulate matter by phagocytosis.

Platelet Function

Platelet Adherence Can Trigger the Release Reaction. Under normal conditions, circulating platelets do not adhere to the endothelial lining of blood vessels. However, any interruption in the continuity of this lining as a

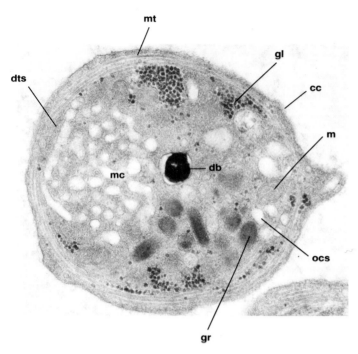

Fig. 8-8. Electron micrograph (×30,000) of a blood platelet. A group of granules (*gr*) is seen at lower right, and a prominent marginal ring of microtubules (*mt*) supports its periphery. Other discernible features of its cytoplasm include the open canalicular system (*ocs*) that opens onto its surface, a tubule belonging to its dense tubular system (*dts*), its cell coat (*cc*), mitochondria (*m*), glycogen particles (*gl*), and a dense body (*db*). In the region labeled *mc* (membrane complex), there is an intimate association between the open canalicular system and the dense tubular system. (White JG: In Cantin M (ed): Cell Biology of the Secretory Process, p 546. Basel, S Karger, 1984)

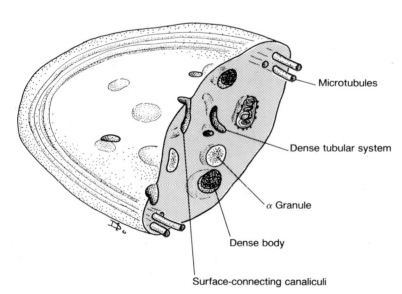

Fig. 8-9. Drawing of a blood platelet, illustrating its internal structure and principal organelles as seen at the EM level.

result of injury or disease can bring platelets into contact with other tissues or tissue components as well. It has been known for some time that if *collagen* is exposed to flowing blood, platelets will adhere to it. In the presence of calcium ions, platelets also adhere to exposed basement membrane and the microfibrils associated with the elastin in blood vessel walls.

Next, it has been shown that platelet adhesion (to collagen, for example) sets in motion a process designated the *release reaction* by Grette. This reaction culminates in discharge of the constituents in the various kinds of platelet granules, including the dense bodies. These granules all move away from the periphery of the platelet as a result of contractile activity of its microfilaments and associated myosin, and their contents are thereupon liberated into the surface-connected tubular system that opens onto the platelet surface (Figs. 8-8 and 8-9). The release reaction is triggered by a wide variety of substances, including collagen, epinephrine, thrombin, ADP, antigen–antibody complexes, and many other compounds. To initiate the release reaction, these substances merely have to come into contact with the surface membrane of the platelet.

ADP is liberated in the release reaction from the dense bodies of platelets that adhere to collagen, for example. This ADP is then instrumental in bringing about further adhesion of other platelets to those that have already adhered. Newly formed thrombin as well as serotonin liberated by the release reaction also promotes platelet aggregation. Within a few minutes, a platelet plug is thereby formed that becomes large enough to seal off the hole in the wall of the bleeding vessel. The platelets that contribute to this plug subsequently degenerate, and the defect in the vessel wall is eventually repaired with intercellular substances by fibroblasts. Accompanied by capillaires, these fibroblasts migrate into the repair site and convert the thrombus into loose connective tissue. Such replacement is termed *organization* of the thrombus.

Platelets Play a Key Role in Clot Retraction. A platelet plug that has formed in a cut vessel soon undergoes *clot retraction*. This process can also occur in a thrombus that has formed in an uncut vessel, and it even takes place in blood that has coagulated in a test tube. Such retraction can reduce the volume of the clot by as much as 90% of its initial volume. Clot retraction depends on the presence of both platelets and fibrin, as we shall now explain.

Following aggregation and thrombus formation, platelets undergo a profound change in appearance. This change is often referred to as *platelet activation*. Until platelets become activated, they are the least deformable of all the circulating blood elements because their periphery is supported by a fairly rigid marginal ring of microtubules. However, they also possess a number of contractile filaments located just under their surface membrane. The activation of platelets is accompanied by a marked change of shape from a disk-like structure to a spiny sphere with long, thin pseudopodia. The remaining granules also come to occupy a more central

position in the platelet. Meanwhile, the marginal bundle of microtubules becomes disorganized and additional microfilaments are produced as a result of polymerization of soluble actin. Furthermore, short myosin filaments are detectable among the microfilaments. Interaction between the two types of filaments is believed to be responsible for bringing about retraction of the clot. The contractile activity of platelets apparently enables them to pull on the fibrin threads to which they are attached, with the result that the fibrin threads become gathered together into a substantially smaller volume.

Platelet Production Is Stimulated by Thrombopoietin

When serum obtained from animals that have undergone a severe blood loss is injected into normal animals, it causes an elevation of the platelet count. (*Serum* is the term used for the plasma constituents that are still present after blood has coagulated.) It is therefore believed that in response to severe blood cell depletion, a humoral regulator is produced that stimulates platelet formation in bone marrow. Called *thrombopoietin* or *thrombopoietic stimulatory factor*, this putative regulator seems to be a glycoprotein, but its cellular source is not established and its precise action has not been elucidated. Because its effects are not manifested for several days, it probably augments the production of megakaryocytes and increases the rate at which they mature. The presence of such a regulatory factor has been demonstrated in the serum of patients who experience a platelet deficiency that is due to reduced numbers of megakaryocytes in their bone marrow (Hoffman et al). Because the activity of this regulatory factor is generally measured as an effect on megakaryocyte colony formation, another designation employed for it is *Meg-CSA*, which denotes megakaryocyte colony-stimulating activity.

Platelet Lifespan

Unless platelets participate in hemostasis, their average life expectancy is approximately 8 to 10 days. At the end of this period, they are phagocytosed by macrophages, primarily those situated in the spleen. The spleen also serves as a storage organ for platelets. Studies using platelets tagged with a radioisotope indicate that at any given time, roughly one third of the total platelet population is held in the spleen as a storage pool.

Any marked decrease in the rate of platelet production (*e.g.*, as a consequence of overcrowding of normal bone marrow cells by invading tumor cells) is accompanied by a fall in the platelet count. There are also situations in which platelets are generated in normal numbers but are then prematurely withdrawn from circulation. Such conditions can generally be remedied by surgical removal of the spleen, which is the primary site of phagocytic removal of platelets. The term used for a *platelet deficiency* is *thrombocytopenia*

(Gr. *penia,* poverty). Such a deficiency leads to a tendency to develop hemorrhages for no apparent reason; these hemorrhages may occur in the skin, a mucous membrane, or elsewhere in the body.

LEUKOCYTES

The microscopic appearance of leukocytes in a blood film shows surprisingly little evidence of the fact that in life, they are actively motile cells that perform their most important functions outside the bloodstream. Numbering 5000 to 9000 per cubic millimeter of blood, leukocytes can be classified into five different types according to their specific staining characteristics, nuclear morphology, and respective functions (Table 8-1). On the basis of their LM appearance, leukocytes are also broadly subdivided into two more general categories: (1) *granular leukocytes* and (2) *nongranular leukocytes,* so called because they lack conspicuous cytoplasmic granules when seen at the LM level. However, even nongranular leukocytes may contain a few inconspicuous granules in their cytoplasm.

Each of the three types of granular leukocytes is named according to the staining reaction of its characteristic cytoplasmic granules. One type has specific granules that become colored by acid stains such as eosin; these cells are called *eosinophils* or *acidophils* (Plate 8-1F). Leukocytes with granules that have an affinity for basic stains are termed *basophils* (Plate 8-1G). Those with specific granules that are neither markedly acidophilic nor basophilic are termed *neutrophils* (Plate 8-1D and E). Neutrophils are alternatively known as *polymorphs,* an abbreviation of *polymorphonuclear leukocytes.* This name distinguishes them not by the color of their specific granules but by the shape of their nucleus, which exhibits a variety of different appearances because it can be made up of anywhere from one to five lobes. An abbreviation that is often used for the lengthy name polymorphonuclear leukocyte is *PMN-leukocyte.*

The nongranular leukocytes are of two main types. *Lymphocytes* (Plate 8-1J and K) are found in lymph as well as in blood. *Monocytes* are the largest nongranular leukocytes (Plate 8-1H).

Like erythrocytes, leukocytes express a number of clinically important antigens on their cell surface. A group of such antigens that are of particular relevance to transplantation biology and medicine are the HLA antigens.

HLA Antigens. Leukocytes possess a rather complicated system of major transplantation antigens called the *HLA system* (*h*uman *l*eukocyte-*a*ssociated antigens). Also often referred to as *major histocompatibility antigens* because they are encoded by a gene complex called the *m*ajor *h*istocompatibility *c*omplex or *MHC,* HLA antigens are integral membrane glycoproteins that are present in the cell membrane and that, in a mismatched situation, are likely to elicit a graft-rejection response (the nature of which we

Table 8-1   Classification of Leukocytes

Granular Leukocytes	Nongranular Leukocytes
Neutrophils (polymorphs, PMNs)	Lymphocytes
Eosinophils	Monocytes
Basophils	

shall consider in Chap. 10). The same HLA antigens are expressed on the other nucleated cells of the body and also on platelets, but they are not detectable on mature erythrocytes. The chances that an organ transplant will survive are greatly increased if the HLA antigens of the transplant donor match those of the recipient.

Leukocyte Counting.   It is often possible to learn a good deal about a patient's medical condition by carefully examining a peripheral blood film. First, the presence of *abnormal blood cells* is associated with certain disease states. Second, a determination of the *relative proportions* of the different types of leukocytes (which is called a *differential leukocyte count*) provides information that can be of diagnostic significance. However, to arrive at a diagnosis, it is just as important to know whether the *total number* of leukocytes (called the *total leukocyte count*) is normal. A standard procedure for obtaining the total leukocyte count is described in the following section.

A blood-cell pipet is used to measure out a small sample of blood. This sample is then diluted in the pipet with an appropriate volume of counting fluid that has been specially formulated to lyse the erythrocytes and stain the leukocyte nuclei. The total number of leukocytes per cubic millimeter of blood is calculated from the average number of leukocyte nuclei present per large square of a hemocytometer (Fig. 8-10). In hematology laboratories, total leukocyte counts are carried out in large batches using an automated electronic counter. However, differential counts require the recognition of each individual type of leukocyte and still must be done manually.

Studying the Different Kinds of Leukocytes in a Blood Film.   Because there are approximately 1000 erythrocytes for every leukocyte, it may take a great deal of searching to find a particular kind of leukocyte in a blood film. Under low power, however, the leukocytes appear as scattered blue dots in a sea of red cells. A common procedure is first to spot the blue-stained nucleus of a leukocyte under low power and then to switch to high-dry or oil-immersion before trying to identify the leukocyte.

A blood film is generally somewhat thicker at the end from which it was spread (Fig. 8-1B). However, although leukocytes are more numerous in this thicker part, they do not stain sharply. They appear to much better advantage in the thinner part of the film, but they are less numerous here than might be expected. Because they are somewhat larger than erythrocytes, they are drawn toward

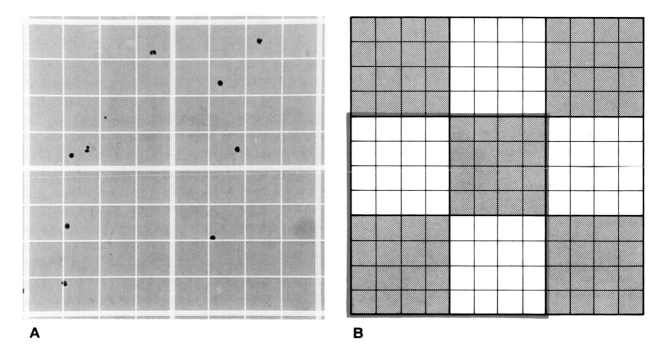

Fig. 8-10. (*A*) Photomicrograph of leukocytes prepared for a total leukocyte count in a hemocytometer. Leukocytes are counted in the large squares (1 mm square) bounded by triple lines, four of which may be seen in this photomicrograph. (*B*) Diagram of a hemocytometer grid, indicating in blue the five large squares (1 mm square) that are actually used for counting leukocytes. The area photographed in *A* is outlined in blue.

the edges of the film as well as toward its very end. When brought to either of these positions, leukocytes generally appear distorted and may even break open. It is therefore necessary to observe leukocytes in the thinner part of the film, where they are more difficult to find. To see good examples of each type of leukocyte, it may be necessary to observe several different blood films.

The Differential Count. Because the various types of leukocytes are not of equal size, they do not become distributed evenly throughout the film. This makes it more difficult to estimate the relative incidence of the different types of leukocytes. A truly representative sample cannot be obtained by observing any one part of the film. Instead, a systematic field-by-field examination of the entire film is necessary.

In attempting to recognize the different types of leukocytes, much time can be saved if one *avoids* the following:

1. *Examining Degenerating Leukocytes.* In blood films, there are always a few disintegrating, damaged, or degenerating leukocytes. Trying to guess what they might have been can be entertaining, but it is a waste of time. For reference purposes, a degenerating neutrophil is shown in Plate 8-1*l*.
2. *Confusing Clumps of Platelets with Leukocytes.* Unless special preventive precautions are taken, platelets can aggregate and may even look a little bit like a leukocyte to an inexperienced observer (Plate 8-1*C*).
3. *Examining Cells That Are Too Difficult to Classify.* The beginning student should not attempt to identify leukocytes that he can-

not recognize easily. Such attempts should be deferred until he has gained more experience.

As will become evident from the following description of the five different types of leukocytes, the microscopic appearance of both the cytoplasm and the nucleus can provide helpful clues about the cell's identity.

Neutrophils (Polymorphs)

Fifty to seventy percent of the leukocytes in the peripheral blood are neutrophils. In absolute numbers, 3000 to 6000 neutrophils per cubic millimeter of blood is considered normal. Hence neutrophils are the most common type of leukocyte present in a blood film.

Before assuming their mature form and entering the bloodstream, neutrophils pass through a series of developmental stages in myeloid tissue (red bone marrow). Most of the neutrophils that gain access to the bloodstream of healthy individuals have already matured. In certain disease states, however, the peripheral blood film is characterized by the presence of larger numbers of *immature* neutrophils; hence it is also necessary to know how to recognize immature neutrophils.

The average duration of granulocyte circulation in the bloodstream is estimated to be approximately 10 hours. Granulocytes then leave the small blood vessels (primarily venules) at random and enter connective tissue, where they carry out useful functions for another day or two.

In blood films, mature neutrophils are from 12 μm to 15 μm in diameter. The segmented nucleus of most neutrophils consists of two to five lobes interconnected by fine strands of chromatin (Plate 8-1D). Their nucleoli cannot be distinguished. In mature neutrophils, sex chromatin (where present) can sometimes be seen as a separate tiny lobe known as a *drumstick appendage* (Fig. 8-11). The cytoplasm of mature neutrophils contains two kinds of granules. The true neutrophilic granules in many preparations are so fine that they are difficult to resolve with the LM; hence all that may be seen is that the cytoplasm has a granular appearance. Commonly, these granules either have or impart to the cytoplasm a lavender (lilac) color. Granules larger than the specific neutrophilic granules are also seen; these are reddish-purple (Plate 8-1D). Because this color is imparted to them by methylene azure, which is one of the basic dyes in a blood stain, they are called *azurophilic granules*. As we shall see when we study the formation of granular leukocytes, the first granules that appear in cells of this lineage are of the azurophilic type; only later do true neutrophilic granules appear, and, when they do appear, they are first seen in the Golgi region of the developing cells.

Immature Forms.   During the development of neutrophils, the nucleus becomes increasingly indented so that it acquires a horseshoe shape, whereupon the cell is given the name *band* (or *stab*) *neutrophil* (Plate 8-1E). Under normal conditions, the horseshoe-shaped nucleus of the band form becomes segmented to divide the nucleus into two or more lobes before the cell is released into the bloodstream from bone marrow; accordingly, under normal conditions not more than 1% or 2% of band forms are seen in films. But if there is a great need for neutrophils in the blood (as will be explained in connection with inflammation below), more band forms and even some metamyelocytes are released into the bloodstream, and these are seen in blood films.

Mature Neutrophils.   An EM section of a mature neutrophil is too thin to reveal as many nuclear lobes as can be seen in a blood film. Whereas there is much condensed chromatin along the inner surface of the nuclear envelope, the more central region of each lobe appears paler in EM sections because it consists primarily of extended chromatin (Fig. 8-12). The cytoplasm contains a few mitochondria and a small Golgi apparatus, but its most striking feature is its content of membrane-bounded granules. As already noted, these are of two different types: *azurophilic granules* and *specific granules*. The azurophilic granules are less numerous but slightly larger than the specific granules; their diameter is approximately 0.4 μm. They are round or oval and more electron dense than the specific granules. Furthermore, their formation precedes that of the specific granules. The specific granules are somewhat smaller (up to 0.3 μm in diameter), but they are much more numerous.

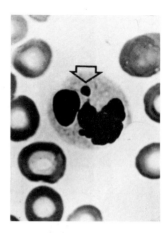

Fig. 8-11.   Photomicrograph of a mature neutrophil that is exhibiting sex chromatin, as seen in a film of peripheral blood. The sex chromatin (*arrow*) is identifiable as a drumstick appendage.

Neutrophil Granules Contain Substances That Destroy Bacteria.   The *azurophilic granules* of a neutrophil correspond to its *lysosomes*. They contain a number of different proteolytic, lipolytic, and carbohydrate-degrading enzymes and also several other *acid hydrolases*. In addition, they contain a peroxidase that is termed *myeloperoxidase* because it characterizes granulocytes that are derived from myeloid tissue. This enzyme is believed to potentiate the bacteriocidal activity of *hydrogen peroxide*, which is also produced by the cell. Several *cationic (basic) proteins* with bacteriocidal activity are also present in these lysosomal granules.

The more numerous *specific granules* contain comparatively few substances. These include *collagenase* and an iron-binding protein called *lactoferrin*, so called because it is an iron-binding protein that was first recognized in milk (L. *lac*, milk; *ferrum*, iron). This protein chelates ferric iron with such high affinity that it can deprive phagocytosed bacteria of the iron they need for further growth; hence it is bacteriostatic. A second property of lactoferrin is that it can inhibit the production of granulocyte-macrophage colony stimulating factor (GM-CSF) by macrophages (Broxmeyer et al). GM-CSF (see Chap. 9) is a hematopoietic regulatory factor that, if produced in sufficient quantity, stimulates *in vitro* formation of neutrophil–monocyte/macrophage colonies. Hence it has been suggested that lactoferrin may serve as one of the negative feedback regulators of neutrophil production.

Both types of neutrophil granules fuse with phagosomes, whereupon their combined resources can effectively destroy any bacteria that the neutrophil may have engulfed by phagocytosis.

Neutrophils Perform a Key Role in the Acute Inflammatory Reaction

Acute inflammation is a generally localized process that is set into motion when living tissues are affected by an in-

Segmented nucleus

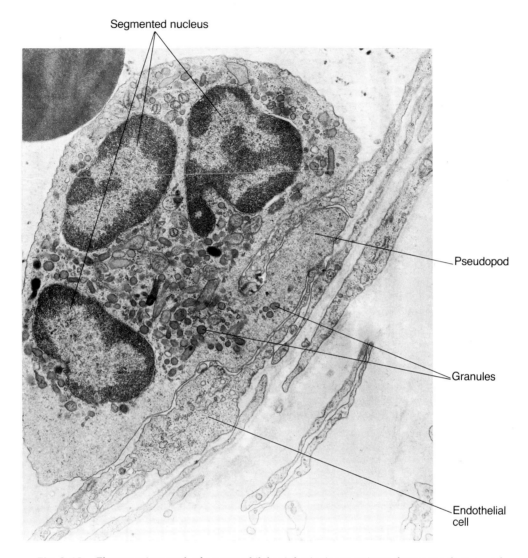

Pseudopod

Granules

Endothelial cell

Fig. 8-12. Electron micrograph of a neutrophil that is beginning to emigrate from a venule at an early stage of the acute inflammatory reaction (rat). This cell has inserted a pseudopod between endothelial cells of the venule. Its variously sized granules and segmented nucleus are characteristic of the mature neutrophil. Pericyte processes can be seen external to the endothelium. (Movat HZ: In Movat HZ (ed): Inflammation, Immunity and Hypersensitivity. Cellular and Molecular Mechanisms, 2nd ed. Hagerstown, Harper & Row, 1979)

jurious agent. It acts not only to eliminate or neutralize the injurious agent or curb its damaging effects but also to repair any damage that may have been caused. It is frequently described as consisting of three consecutive phases—injury, reaction, and repair.

The injurious agents that elicit acute inflammation are many and varied. Body tissues may be invaded by bacteria, viruses, protozoa, or multicellular pathogenic organisms. Acute inflammation can also be a result of physical injury (*e.g.,* from heat, cold, radiation, or chemicals). A similar inflammatory reaction can even be elicited by endogenous substances that are produced in the body itself, as in gout (which will be described later in this chapter).

As long ago as 200 A.D., the *classic signs and symptoms* of acute inflammation were recognized as redness, heat, swelling, pain, and loss or impairment of function. As we shall see, these characteristics are due to microscopically detectable changes in connective tissue that primarily affect its terminal vascular bed.

To record the occurrence of acute inflammation in any given part of the body, the suffix *-itis* is added to the name of the body part where inflammation is detected. Virtually

Table 8-2   Typical Examples of Inflammatory Conditions

Condition	Site of Inflammation
Appendicitis	Appendix
Arthritis	Joints
Cholecystitis	Gallbladder
Colitis	Colon
Cystitis	Urinary bladder
Glomerulonephritis	Renal glomeruli
Laryngitis	Larynx
Nasopharyngitis	Nose and throat
Sinusitis	Nasal sinuses
Tonsillitis	Tonsils

all parts of the body can be affected by inflammation; some representative examples are given in Table 8-2. Such examples serve to emphasize how much discomfort and illness can be traced to inflammation. A basic familiarity with this process is therefore a great asset to medical students.

Microscopic Features of the Acute Inflammatory Reaction.   Anyone who has had the unpleasant experience of driving a bacterially contaminated sharp object such as a dirty sliver through the epidermis of a finger and down into the underlying connective tissue (Fig. 8-13A) will doubtless have noticed that without appropriate management, the surrounding tissue becomes inflamed. Such acute inflammation is manifested by the penetrated region becoming red, warm, swollen, and tender to the touch. These signs are usually accompanied by a general disinclination to use the finger whenever this can be avoided (impaired function). The microscopic basis for these characteristic changes will now be explained.

Previous discussion has portrayed capillaries as simple loops that receive blood from arterioles and then deliver it to venules. In fact, the terminal vascular bed is not as simple as this because, as can be seen in Figure 16-21, arterioles also connect with venules by way of thin-walled bypass channels, and some of the capillaries in a network arise from the proximal portion of such channels. Because smooth muscle cells are present in the walls of both the arterioles and the proximal portion of the bypass channels, both of these kinds of vessels are involved in regulating blood flow through capillaries.

All of the component capillaries in the terminal vascular bed of a damaged region open up because of (1) dilatation of the arterioles that supply them and (2) relaxation of their precapillary sphincters (see Fig. 16-21). The resulting transitory increase in local blood flow is soon followed by an overall slowing of the flow rate. At this stage the endothelium lining the venules becomes leaky, as explained under Mast Cells in Chapter 7. As a result, plasma escapes through the widened intercellular slits. These slits are present at the margins of contiguous endothelial cells, between the sites where these cells are joined to one another by fascia occludens (tight) junctions. Plasma can also leak directly across any endothelial cells that may have been damaged (*e.g.*, as a result of a burn). Such movement of plasma from venules into the amorphous ground substance of loose connective tissue is often described as *exudation*. It brings infecting microorganisms into direct contact with any immunoglobulin that may have been produced as a result of prior exposure to the same microorganism or its antigens. Another consequence of exudation is that small pools of excess interstitial fluid begin to accumulate in the amorphous ground substance of the affected region. The resulting *edema* often causes tenderness because of pressure on sensory nerve endings. In addition, certain inflammatory mediators elicit pain through direct stimulation of afferent nerve endings that are sensitive to pain-inducing stimuli.

Once blood flow has slowed and exudation has started, *neutrophils* begin to adhere to the endothelial lining of venules. This change in their position is termed *margination*. By inserting pseudopodia between contiguous endothelial cells, neutrophils make tiny temporary openings between these cells and then squeeze through such openings (Fig. 8-12). Such penetration of the vessel wall is called *diapedesis* (Gr. *dia*, through; *pedesis*, leaping). Once neutrophils have succeeded in escaping from venules, they migrate to sites where bacteria are multiplying and rapidly phagocytose and destroy them (Fig. 8-13). Some of the mechanisms that are involved will now be described.

Neutrophils Dispose of Infecting Bacteria.   The fatal attraction that some bacteria have for neutrophils seems to have a *chemotactic* basis, meaning that a chemical gradient attracts these cells toward their prey. Bacteria are known to elaborate several substances that can exert such an effect on neutrophils. However, there is now much evidence that neutrophils are also attracted to sites where an antibody has combined with an antigen of the infectious agent to form an antigen–antibody complex. Furthermore, the presence of such complexes enhances phagocytic activity in neutrophils. However, the reason antigen–antibody complexes attract these cells is that such complexes fix and activate what is termed *complement*.

Complement is a series of approximately 20 plasma proteins that interact sequentially and become activated when an antibody combines with an antigen. The various components of complement combine with the antigen–antibody complex in an ordered sequence, and, as they do so, various biological effects result.

The immunological processes of a given individual can identify only certain sites on foreign organisms or cells as antigenic, and these (termed *antigenic sites*) are the sites with which antibody combines. In those foreign cells where the antigenic sites lie spaced fairly closely together (as in

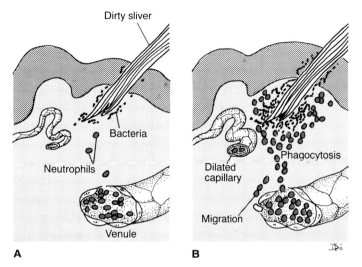

Fig. 8-13. Diagrammatic representation of the role of neutrophils in the acute inflammatory reaction. (*A*) Neutrophils migrate from congested, dilated venules. (*B*) On reaching multiplying bacteria introduced through injury, the neutrophils engulf them by phagocytosis.

bacteria and cells such as erythrocytes from donors of a different blood type), the combining of antibody also initiates the binding of complement to these sites. This in itself is sufficient to cause certain kinds of cells to lyse, an effect called *complement-mediated lysis*. But even if lysis does not ensue, several biologically active substances are formed and released from the various complement proteins during the process of complement fixation and activation. For example, it has long been known that certain substances present in plasma can, by attaching to bacteria, make it easier for neutrophils to phagocytose bacteria; such substances are therefore called *opsonins* (Gr. for something to eat). It was already known that antibodies could be formed against bacterial antigens, so for a long time it was thought that antibodies themselves were responsible for the opsonizing effect. However, it is now known that the opsonizing effect is mainly due to split products released from complement when it becomes attached to the antigen–antibody complex. Complement and specific cleavage products of its components can greatly enhance the neutrophil's capacity to detect and phagocytose bacteria. This is because neutrophils (also monocytes, macrophages, and B-lymphocytes) are endowed with cell-surface receptors for C3, the third component of complement, as well as receptors for the Fc end of immunoglobulin. We might also add here that viral inactivation by antibody is a different matter because complement is not involved.

The action of the lysosomal hydrolases from neutrophil granules is by no means limited to the destruction of phagocytosed bacteria. Under certain circumstances, these enzymes are liberated from neutrophils in quantities sufficient to increase the overall severity of the acute inflammatory reaction quite markedly. For example, the inflammation that is associated with acute attacks of *gout* (see below) and with the chronic disease *rheumatoid arthritis* is initiated by substances that continue to be produced in the body—urate crystals in gout and antigen–antibody complexes in rheumatoid arthritis. Each of these conditions is characterized by extensive and sustained phagocytosis of the offending substance by neutrophils. Moreover, phagocytic activity can be so vigorous that lysosomal hydrolases escape to the exterior of the cell as a result of premature leakage from phagocytic vesicles that have not yet had time to seal off completely (see Fig. 4-21).

In the next section, we shall discuss a drug that has the potential to reduce the intensity of the acute inflammatory reaction through a direct action on neutrophils.

Neutrophils Are the Culprits in Painful Attacks of Acute Gouty Arthritis. *Gout* is a metabolic disorder that has a familial tendency. It is characterized by insufficient excretion of *uric acid* (the end product of human purine metabolism), which therefore accumulates in the bloodstream. An unfortunate outcome of elevated uric acid levels is that tiny crystals of *monosodium urate* become deposited in joint tissues. Clinically, the most common manifestation of gout is an *acute arthritis* (inflammation of a joint), and the joint that typically is most affected is the first metatarsophalangeal joint of the great toe. Yet the extreme tenderness and pain experienced in a severe episode of gout are not due to the urate crystals themselves. The inflammation, which is termed *acute gouty arthritis*, is, in fact, incited and aggravated by the numerous *neutrophils* that invade the affected tissues and ingest the urate crystals.

The first anti-inflammatory agent found to alleviate acute attacks of gouty arthritis was *colchicine*, which is now well known to be very effective in eliminating cytoplasmic microtubules (described under Mitosis in Chap. 3 and Microtubules in Chap. 4). There are indications that such destruction of cytoplasmic microtubules reduces the motility of neutrophils, rendering them less able to invade the joint tissues. The administration of colchicine also appears to diminish the liberation of enzymes known to aggravate inflammation. Furthermore, it suppresses the release of an inflammation-eliciting glycoprotein that is otherwise liberated in response to the ingestion of urate crystals. Although colchicine is effective at subduing acute episodes of gouty arthritis, its usefulness in this regard is limited by its broad spectrum of antimicrotubule activity. Today, gout can be controlled by means of other drugs that either decrease the formation of uric acid or facilitate its excretion. Colchicine is nevertheless still employed as an effective preliminary medication to obtain rapid relief of acute attacks of gouty arthritis.

Vasoactive Inflammatory Mediators. The local redness and local increased temperature that characterize sites of acute inflammation are due to increased amounts of blood flowing through the local terminal vascular bed. The increased blood flow is, in turn, due to dilatation of the arterioles and venules that determine the volume of blood circulating through this vascular bed. The associated swelling is the result of plasma exudation from venules. Yet it is not necessary for any of these vessels to be affected directly by the inflammatory agent itself. The immediate cause of such changes is the local action of what are termed the *chemical mediators* of the acute inflammatory reaction. *Histamine* is a vasoactive amine that is liberated from the mast cells in and near the affected region. A host of other chemical mediators are also involved; their formation involves interactions between plasma proteins and peptides that are far beyond the scope of this chapter. An important group of vasoactive peptides are called *kinins*. In addition to increasing vascular permeability and bringing about vasodilation and leukocyte emigration into the tissues, kinins can elicit pain. Certain *complement* cleavage products and *prostaglandins* (fatty acids first isolated from seminal fluid) are also believed to play a role in mediating the acute inflammatory response. Another potent chemical mediator is *SRS-A*, the slow-reacting substance of anaphylaxis (see Chap. 7 under Mast Cells). For further information on mediators of the inflammatory process, see Movat, and Rodnan et al.

Monocytes and Macrophages Are Also Participants in the Acute Inflammatory Reaction. The emigration of neutrophils from venules is accompanied by a closely similar margination and diapedesis of monocytes. On entering the tissues, monocytes transform into macrophages. Initially, the macrophages participate jointly with the neutrophils in the removal of microbes by phagocytosis. A few days later, however, they dominate the picture because they have a longer lifespan than neutrophils. Furthermore, macrophages are attracted to certain strains of bacteria that neutrophils ignore, and they are able to phagocytose the cellular debris that remains when the inflammation subsides.

The ensuing phase of repair requires the formation of fibroblasts that are probably derived mainly from pericytes scattered along small blood vessels. These fibroblasts restore the intercellular substances in the region. New capillaries bud from the existing vessels and grow into the reparative tissue, with the result that it soon becomes well vascularized. Damaged epithelial tissue regenerates as described in Chapter 6.

Neutrophils Contribute to the Formation of Pus and Pyrogens. The accumulated dead neutrophils and other tissue-breakdown products that are formed in infected wounds contribute to the formation of a creamy yellow, semifluid material called *pus*. If the infected wound is open to the surface, the pus can drain of its own accord or can be absorbed into a dressing. If, however, the pus accumulates below a surface, it can form an *abscess* that may require surgical incision to promote drainage.

Certain breakdown products of neutrophils and bacterial endotoxin are known as *pyrogens* (Gr. *pyr*, fire; *gennan*, to produce) because after they are absorbed into the body and carried to the thermostatlike temperature regulatory center in the hypothalamus, they affect it in such a way that the body temperature becomes elevated and the patient develops a *fever*. Another such product, which will be described in the following section, has an effect on the bone marrow.

Leukocytosis and Neutrophilia. Many kinds of severe infections are accompanied by a rise in the total number of leukocytes per cubic millimeter of blood. Such a rise is called a *leukocytosis* (Gr. *osis*, process; a suffix that when incorporated into a hematological term denotes a process that results in some kind of *increase*). When a leukocytosis is entirely due to a rise in the neutrophil count, it is more precisely described as a *neutrophilia*. The term used for a *lowered* neutrophil count is *neutropenia*.

In response to bacterial endotoxin, a *leukocytosis-inducing factor (neutrophil-releasing factor)* is produced that stimulates the release of mature neutrophils from the bone marrow. Along with the large numbers of mature neutrophils that are stored in the bone marrow, increased numbers of *immature neutrophils* are released into the circulation in response to this factor. Accordingly, in many types of acute bacterial infections, the total leukocyte count of the peripheral blood rises and a differential leukocyte count reveals that this rise is due to increased proportions of *band neutrophils* and their immediate precursors (*neutrophilic metamyelocytes*, which will be described in Chap. 9).

In tabulating the numbers of neutrophils seen in a peripheral blood film, it is conventional to enter band forms and metamyelocytes on the left and more mature forms (with two to five lobes) on the right. Accordingly, if it can be seen from an ongoing series of blood films from a patient that the proportion of immature cells is *increasing*, this is described as a *shift to the left*. If, on the other hand, the proportion of immature forms is *decreasing*, this is called a *shift to the right*. In general, a shift to the *left* indicates that the infection is *progressing* whereas a shift to the *right* signals that recovery is underway.

Eosinophils

From 1% to 4% of the leukocytes in a peripheral blood film are eosinophils. In absolute numbers, 120 to 350 eosinophils per cubic millimeter of blood is considered normal. However, the eosinophil count of peripheral blood may fluctuate, and furthermore it can manifest a diurnal variation (L. *diurnus*, daily) because it tends to be somewhat

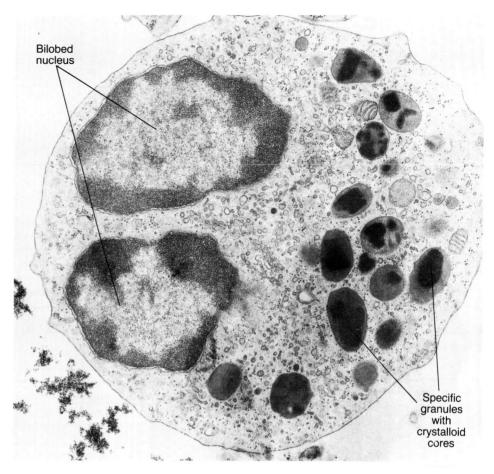

Bilobed
nucleus

Specific
granules
with
crystalloid
cores

Fig. 8-14. Electron micrograph of an eosinophil. Its bilobed nucleus and distinctive specific (lysosomal) granules are highly characteristic of the eosinophil. A few mitochondria are also visible in the cytoplasm. (Courtesy of H. Z. Movat)

higher in the early hours of the morning than in the early hours of the afternoon.

Eosinophils have a diameter of between 12 μm and 17 μm in blood films; hence they are marginally larger than neutrophils. Their nucleus is typically bilobed and nucleoli are absent (Plate 8-1*F* and Fig. 8-14). The condensed chromatin of an eosinophil stains less intensely than that of a neutrophil (Plate 8-1*F*). The cytoplasm of an eosinophil is characterized by the presence of large refractile granules that have a red or reddish-purple color in a well-stained blood film (Plate 8-1*F*).

In electron micrographs, it can be seen that, as in neutrophils, the condensed chromatin is peripherally distributed along the inner surface of the nuclear envelope (Fig. 8-14). The chief feature of the cytoplasm is its content of highly characteristic *specific* granules. These membrane-bounded granules are ovoid (0.5 μm to 1.5 μm long and 0.3 μm to 1 μm wide) with electron-dense crystalloid cores (Fig. 8-14) that consist chiefly of basic proteins. Their crystalloid cores have different shapes in different species. The

specific granules of eosinophils contain large amounts of peroxidase and many of the hydrolytic enzymes found in the azurophilic granules of neutrophils; hence in eosinophils, the specific granules are regarded as lysosomes. Mature eosinophils also contain some smaller spherical granules that lack crystalloid cores. These smaller granules are particularly rich in acid phosphatase and arylsulfatase. The only other prominent organelles in eosinophils are their Golgi apparatus and mitochondria; the other organelles have only minor representation. As in neutrophils, Fc and C3 receptors are present in the eosinophil cell membrane.

Eosinophils are produced and subsequently held in reserve in the bone marrow. When they leave the bone marrow, they spend a few hours circulating in the bloodstream (their half-life in the blood is approximately 8 hours.). Like neutrophils, they then leave the circulatory system as motile cells, entering connective tissue to carry out useful functions for a few more days. This results in a preferential distribution of eosinophils in the innermost loose connective tissue layer of the intestine, skin, and lungs.

Eosinophils Have a Regulatory Role in Allergic Inflammation. Whereas there is *in vitro* evidence to suggest that eosinophils may not be quite as efficient as neutrophils in phagocytosing and destroying microorganisms, it has long been recognized that they are somehow involved in immediate-type hypersensitivity reactions because eosinophils increase in number not only at the sites of such reactions but also in the peripheral blood of people with allergies. Furthermore, the hormone *cortisol (hydrocortisone)*, known to depress allergic reactions, has a similar effect on the number of circulating eosinophils. Indeed, the normal diurnal variation in the eosinophil count is believed to reflect diurnal changes in the level of cortisol secretion by the adrenal cortex. Cortisol reduces the eosinophil count by enhancing eosinophil diapedesis and diminishing the release of eosinophils from the marrow.

Eosinophils are commonly present in the nasal secretions of allergic individuals who suffer from hay fever (allergic rhinitis) and in the sputum of patients who have asthma. Moreover, it has been shown experimentally that eosinophils are attracted to free antigen–antibody complexes that they thereupon phagocytose. It has been suggested that eosinophils may play a role in dampening down and eventually terminating local inflammatory reactions that are of allergic origin. This suggestion is based on the fact that eosinophil granules contain several enzymes that are capable of degrading chemical mediators of the acute inflammatory reaction. Thus eosinophil arylsulfatase can degrade SRS-A, the slow-reacting substance of anaphylaxis liberated by mast cells and basophils when they degranulate. Eosinophils, and also neutrophils, produce a histaminase that can inactivate histamine. Furthermore, eosinophils and neutrophils are both attracted toward ECF-A, which are the eosinophil chemotactic factors of anaphylaxis that are liberated by degranulating mast cells and basophils. Eosinophils are also chemotactically attracted toward sites of histamine release. Once the eosinophils are present, they phagocytose and digest the released mast cell granules. Such lines of evidence suggest that eosinophils have a local regulatory function in controlling the severity of acute allergic inflammation.

Eosinophils Are Involved in the Destruction of Helminth Parasites. An elevated eosinophil count in the peripheral blood (*eosinophilia*) can also be an indication that an individual is infested with certain types of parasites. Eosinophils are thought to play an important defensive role against such infestations. One kind of parasite that is now known to be attacked by eosinophils is the schistosomula, the larval stage of *Schistosoma*. This is a species of helminth worm that invades the bloodstream and then matures in the liver before migrating to a venule situated close to the lumen of the gut or urinary bladder, from which its eggs are able to pass into the feces or urine. In this particular case, it has been established that eosinophils are able to discharge the contents of their granules onto the surface of parasites that have become opsonized. The major basic protein present in the specific granules of eosinophils seems to be involved both in securing cellular attachment to the parasite and in inflicting lethal damage. It seems likely that a concerted effort involving immunoglobulin E (IgE), complement, mast cells, and eosinophils is necessary to combat helminth parasites. These parasites would first trigger any mast cells that had become sensitized with preformed IgE to liberate their inflammatory mediators. The released mediators would then recruit eosinophils capable of inflicting complement-dependent lethal damage on the parasite. For further information, see Kay, and Sullivan.

Basophils

Basophils constitute only approximately 0.5% of peripheral blood leukocytes. This means that there are only about 40 basophils per cubic millimeter of blood; hence to find one in a blood film it may be necessary to examine several hundred leukocytes in more than one film. These cells have a diameter of 10 μm to 12 μm and are therefore about the same size as neutrophils (compare Plate 8-1D and G). Their nucleus is generally bilobed (Plate 8-1G), although it can be further segmented, and it stains less deeply than that of a neutrophil. However, it is not always possible to see these characteristics in a blood film because the nucleus of a basophil can be entirely obscured by the abundant dark blue granules in the cytoplasm (Plate 8-1G). The large membrane-bounded granules of basophils have a diameter of up to 0.5 μm. They are metachromatic and essentially similar to mast cell granules. Chemical mediators liberated when basophils degranulate include histamine, SRS-A, and ECF-A. However, it is not clear whether human basophil granules contain heparin; it has been suggested that their metachromatic staining properties may be due to the presence of chondroitin sulfates instead. The cell-surface receptors on basophils closely resemble those on mast cells (see Chap. 7), and the mechanism of degranulation appears to be the same in both cell types.

Basophils, like eosinophils, tend to leave the bloodstream under the influence of certain hormones, for example, cortisol. Also, they can accumulate at sites of certain kinds of allergic inflammation (*e.g.*, in allergic contact dermatitis), and there are indications that they may be able to release their mediators a little at a time in such allergic conditions.

The cell membrane of basophils is provided with Fc receptors that have a high affinity for plasma *IgE* molecules. If circulating basophils become sensitized with an IgE that is directed against a polyvalent antigen and then encounter that particular antigen in the blood, they liberate their inflammatory mediators directly into the bloodstream. A large-scale systemic release of such mediators from blood basophils as well as from mast cells can have disastrous consequences because it can result in a widespread vascular collapse that leads to death (*systemic anaphylaxis*).

Are Basophils Related to Mast Cells? It is becoming increasingly apparent that only minor and relatively trivial differences exist between blood basophils and mast cells of connective tissue. Such differences would include the fact that basophils have a nuclear morphology and life span that are more similar to those of eosinophils than those of mast cells, which possess a spherical or ovoid nucleus and are comparatively long-lived. Also, mast cells are not found in the peripheral blood. A simple hypothesis that would explain the remarkable resemblance between basophils and mast cells is that both cell types might be derived from the same myeloid precursors. Recent studies have shown that histamine-containing cells are a normal component of the clonal hematopoietic mixed colonies that grow *in vitro* from human multipotential hematopoietic stem cells (Denburg et al), but it is not yet possible to distinguish whether these cells belong to the basophil or the mast cell series, or whether they represent a common precursor for both of these lineages. It is of interest that in the bone marrow of patients with chronic myelogenous leukemia or agnogenic myeloid metaplasia (which are two separate myeloproliferative disorders), there are cells with ultrastructural features that are essentially intermediate between these two cell types (Zucker–Franklin). This observation has led to the suggestion that an earlier bipotential cell may serve as a common progenitor for both of these cell types. If such a bipotential cell exists, it could perhaps give rise to (1) mast cell precursors that migrate into loose connective tissue and differentiate into mast cells and (2) basophil precursors that complete their maturation within myeloid tissue and then circulate as basophils in the peripheral blood.

Lymphocytes

Lymphocytes comprise 20% to 50% of the blood leukocytes; hence in a peripheral blood film, there are roughly half as many lymphocytes as neutrophils. In absolute numbers, there are 1500 to 4000 lymphocytes per cubic millimeter of blood. In addition to being a normal component of blood, lymphocytes are present in the lymph, hence their name. Broadly speaking, peripheral blood lymphocytes fall into two different size ranges. Most are 6 μm to 9 μm in diameter and are called *small lymphocytes* (Plate 8-1K). However, a low proportion of blood lymphocytes are noticeably larger (9 μm to 15 μm in diameter), and these cells are commonly referred to as *large* lymphocytes (Plate 8-1J). The functional meaning of this size difference is by no means clear, but the distinction is still useful because an increase in the number of large lymphocytes can have diagnostic significance (as, for example, in the recognition of acute viral infections and certain forms of immunodeficiency). Lymphocytes are included in the nongranular category of leukocytes because they lack prominent cytoplasmic granules when seen in the LM. However, roughly 10% contain tiny reddish-purple–staining (azurophilic) granules that represent their lysosomes.

In many cases, the spherical nucleus of a *small lymphocyte* can be seen to have a small indentation on one side. Almost all its chromatin is condensed; hence the nucleus is relatively small and its nucleoli are obscured by condensed chromatin (Plate 8-1K). In comparison with other leukocytes, a small lymphocyte possesses remarkably little cytoplasm. Even after the cell has been spread out in a blood film, only a narrow rim of slightly basophilic cytoplasm is visible (Plate 8-1K). In LM sections, the cytoplasm of a small lymphocyte can hardly be seen at all. Living lymphocytes are motile and can squeeze between the endothelial cells of blood vessels. They are able to migrate through other kinds of wet epithelial membranes as well.

In electron micrographs of small lymphocytes, free ribosomes can readily be seen in the cytoplasm. A few mitochondria, sparse cisternae of rER, and a small Golgi apparatus also can sometimes be discerned, but in general, cytoplasmic organelles are scant (Fig. 8-15). Hence compared with granular leukocytes, small lymphocytes appear relatively undifferentiated. Yet some of these cells will give rise to highly differentiated effector cells of the immune reponse after they have become stimulated by antigen.

A *large lymphocyte* has a nucleus that is slightly larger than that of a small lymphocyte. Again, the nucleus may either be spherical or have a small indentation on one side (Fig. 8-1J). Some initial difficulty may occasionally be experienced in distinguishing between a large lymphocyte and a monocyte, which it can superficially resemble. However, a large lymphocyte is generally slightly smaller than a monocyte and has a less copious amount of cytoplasm, and although its nucleus may exhibit a small indentation, it is never as kidney-shaped as that of a monocyte (compare J with H in Plate 8-1). Compared with a small lymphocyte, on the other hand, a large lymphocyte has more cytoplasm and a generally comparable degree of cytoplasmic basophilia (compare J with K in Plate 8-1). At the EM level, it can also be seen that the cytoplasm of a large lymphocyte possesses a somewhat fuller complement of organelles that includes larger numbers of mitochondria and free ribosomes, more cisternae of rER, and a Golgi apparatus that is slightly larger (Fig. 8-16). Remarkably little is known about the population of large lymphocytes present in peripheral blood. Their functional significance is still very much a matter of conjecture. It is widely assumed that they represent a relatively unimportant and heterogeneous class of cells that includes some circulating progeny cells of antigen-activated lymphocytes together with some poorly differentiated cells that will probably turn out not to belong to the lymphocyte lineage at all.

On the basis of their functional properties, small lymphocytes are classified into two main groups called *B-lymphocytes* and *T-lymphocytes* (or *B-cells* and *T-cells*). In postnatal life, B-lymphocytes differentiate in myeloid tissue whereas T-lymphocytes differentiate in the thymus. However, their microscopic appearance is identical, making other methods necessary to distinguish between them. Some major distinguishing characteristics are listed in Table 8-3. The functional properties and various other features of these two different types of lymphocytes, including their respective roles in immune responses, will be discussed in Chapter 10 when we deal with lymphatic tissue and the immune system. In addition to B- and T-lymphocytes, there is a class of so-called *null cells* that do not fit into either category because they lack definitive B- or T-cell markers. Although it has been determined that certain subpopula-

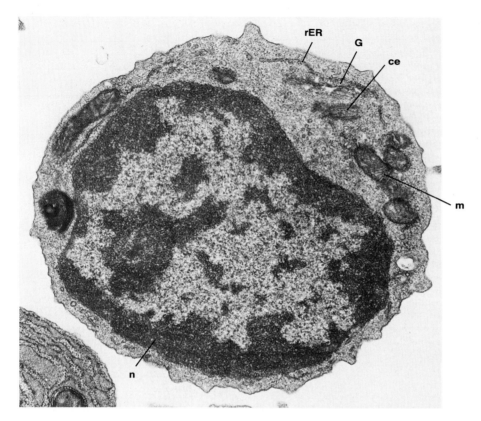

Fig. 8-15. Electron micrograph (×22,000) of a small lymphocyte (T-lymphocyte). Its nucleus (*n*), which contains a great deal of condensed chromatin, occupies much of the cell volume. Many free ribosomes, a small amount of rough-surfaced endoplasmic reticulum (*rER*), mitochondria (*m*), a small Golgi region (*G*), and one of the centrioles (*ce*) are distinguishable in the cytoplasm. (Waterhouse PD, Anderson PJ, Brown DL: Exp Cell Res 144:367, 1983)

tions of null cells manifest cytotoxic activity, their relationship to B- and T-lymphocytes has not yet been elucidated. The null cell population also contains hematopoietic progenitor cells and stem cells that have the potentiality to produce other types of blood cells, in other words, hematopoietic cells that are not really lymphocytes at all.

Monocytes

Monocytes comprise from 2% to 8% of the blood leukocytes. In absolute numbers, there are approximately 200 to 600 monocytes per cubic millimeter of blood. Typical monocytes can usually be recognized in a blood film without too much difficulty. However, a variable degree of resemblance may be seen between monocytes and large lymphocytes, particularly if these lymphocytes are atypical. Monocytes are from 12 μm to 20 μm in diameter and are therefore usually the largest leukocytes seen in a blood film (Plate 8-1*H*). Their nucleus is somewhat variable in appearance. It ranges from being a deeply indented ovoid shape or roughly kidney-shaped to having the form of a wide horseshoe (Plate 8-1*H*). It may even become twisted or folded over on itself as an artifact of blood film prepa-

ration. Its chromatin is less condensed and therefore lighter staining than that of lymphocytes (compare *H* with *J* and *K* in Plate 8-1). Nucleoli, although present, are not usually discernible in a blood film. Compared with the other leukocytes, monocytes have a copious amount of cytoplasm that stains a characteristic pale grayish-blue color (Plate 8-1*H*). Fine pinkish-purple (azurophilic) granules can also sometimes be discerned in the cytoplasm, but specific granules are lacking.

At the EM level, it can be seen that in monocytes the nucleus possesses more of an indentation than is found in lymphocytes (Fig. 8-17). There is a good deal of peripheral condensed chromatin, and more centrally, some extended chromatin and two or more nucleoli may be seen (Fig. 8-17). In the cytoplasm, there is a fairly prominent Golgi apparatus (Fig. 8-17, labeled *G*). Other distinctive features of the cytoplasm include a moderate content of ribosomes and polysomes, a small amount of rER, and a number of small mitochondria. Small dense granules that are 0.3 μm to 0.6 μm in diameter are also present; they represent lysosomes and correspond to the fine azurophilic granules seen at the LM level. The surface of monocytes tends to be irregular because of its small projecting processes (Fig.

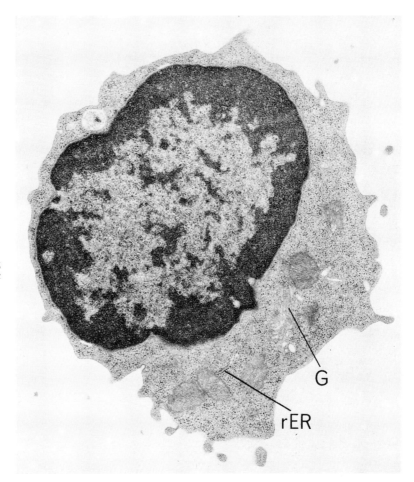

Fig. 8-16. Electron micrograph of a large lymphocyte. In its cytoplasm, rough-surfaced endoplasmic reticulum (*rER*) and a Golgi region (*G*) can be seen. (Everett NB, Perkins WD: Hemopoietic stem cell migration. In Cairnie AB, Lala PK, Osmond DG (eds): Stem Cells of Renewing Cell Populations, p 229. New York, Academic Press, 1976)

Table 8-3   Some Distinctive Features of the Two Main Types of Peripheral Blood Lymphocytes

	B-Lymphocytes	T-Lymphocytes
Distinctive Surface Determinants		
Surface (membrane) immunoglobulin (sIg)	Present	Absent
C3 receptor	Present	⎱ Absent from certain subsets
Fc receptor	Present	⎰ but present on others
Sheep erythrocyte receptor	Absent	Present
Thy 1 antigen (mouse)	Absent	Present
T (OKT) antigen (man)	Absent	Present
Preferential Mitogenic Responses		
Bacterial lipopolysaccharide (LPS)	Yes	No
Concanavalin A (Con A)	No	Yes
Phytohemagglutinin (PHA)	Yes/No*	Yes

* Not in the mouse

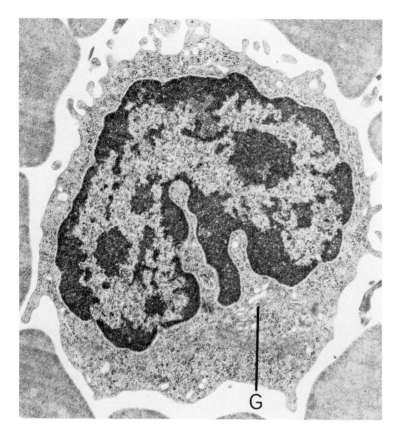

G

Fig. 8-17. Electron micrograph of a monocyte. Note the eccentric position of its bean-shaped nucleus, and its Golgi region (G). (Everett NB, Perkins WD: Hemopoietic stem cell migration. In Cairnie AB, Lala PK, Osmond DG (eds): Stem Cells of Renewing Cell Populations, p 230. New York, Academic Press, 1976)

8-17, *top*). As in macrophages, the monocyte cell membrane is provided with Fc and C3 receptors.

A very important functional role of monocytes is that they serve as immediate precursors for macrophages. There are also indications that circulating monocytes have the capacity to phagocytose bacteria, viruses, and antigen–antibody complexes from the bloodstream. However, the phagocytic activity of circulating monocytes is probably not as great as that of tissue macrophages. As already noted, monocytes migrate in increased numbers from venules to sites of acute inflammation. Under ordinary circumstances, monocytes have a half-life in the circulation of up to 3 days, after which they leave the bloodstream in a random manner. They are able to transform directly into a variety of different kinds of macrophages, including those of loose connective tissue, the hematopoietic tissues, the central nervous system (*microglia*), the liver (*Kupffer cells*), the lungs (*alveolar macrophages*), and the peritoneal, pleural, and synovial cavities. In addition, monocytes are able to fuse and thereby form either *foreign body giant cells* or *osteoclasts*.

SELECTED REFERENCES

Comprehensive

BESSIS M: Living Blood Cells and Their Ultrastructure. New York, Springer-Verlag, 1973

CLINE MJ: The White Cell. Cambridge, MA, Harvard University Press, 1975

WILLIAMS WJ, BEUTLER E, ERSLEV AJ, LICHTMAN MA: Hematology, 3rd ed. New York, McGraw-Hill, 1983

Erythrocytes

BESSIS M: Corpuscles. Atlas of Red Blood Cell Shapes. Berlin, Springer-Verlag, 1974

BESSIS M, WEED RI, LEBLOND PF (eds): Red Cell Shape—Physiology, Pathology, Ultrastructure. New York, Springer-Verlag, 1973

SURGENOR D: The Red Blood Cell, 2nd ed, Vols 1 and 2. New York, Academic Press, 1974

Platelets

GORDON JL (ed): Platelets in Biology and Pathology. Research Monographs in Cell and Tissue Physiology, Vol. 1. Amsterdam, Elsevier/North-Holland, 1976

GORDON JL (ed): Platelets in Biology and Pathology, 2. Research Monographs in Cell and Tissue Physiology, Vol 5. Amsterdam, Elsevier/North-Holland, 1981

GRETTE K: Relaxing factor in extracts of blood platelets and its function in the cells. Nature 198:488, 1963

HOFFMAN R, MAZUR E, BRUNO E, FLOYD V: Assay of an activity in the serum of patients with disorders of thrombopoiesis that stimulates formation of megakaryocytic colonies. N Engl J Med 305: 533, 1981

HOVIG T: The ultrastructural basis of platelet function. In Baldini MG, Ebbe S (eds): Platelets: Production, Function, Transfusion and Storage. New York, Grune & Stratton, 1974

MUSTARD JF, PACKHAM MA: Factors influencing platelet function: Adhesion, release and aggregation. Pharmacol Rev 22:97, 1970

MUSTARD JF, PACKHAM MA: The reaction of the blood to injury. In Mozat HZ (ed): Inflammation, Immunity and Hypersensitivity. Molecular and Cellular Mechanisms, 2nd ed, p 558. Hagerstown, Harper & Row, 1979

MUSTARD JF, PACKHAM MA, KINLOUGH–RATHBONE RL: Platelets and atherosclerosis. In Miller NE (ed): Atherosclerosis: Mechanisms and Approach to Therapy, p 29. New York, Raven Press, 1983

ROSS R: Atherosclerosis: A problem of the biology of arterial wall cells and their interactions with blood cell components. Arteriosclerosis 1:293, 1981

ULUTIN ON, JONES JV (eds): Platelets—Recent Advances in Basic Research and Clinical Aspects. International Symposium. Amsterdam, Excerpta Medica, 1975

WEISS JH: Platelet physiology and abnormalities of platelet function. N Engl J Med 293:531, 1975

WHITE JG: The secretory process in platelets. In Cantin M (ed): Cell Biology of the Secretory Process, p 546. Basel, S Karger, 1984

WHITE JG: The ultrastructure and regulatory mechanisms of blood platelets. In Lasslo A (ed): Blood Platelet Function and Medicinal Chemistry, p 15. New York, Elsevier Biomedical, 1984

ZUCKER MB: The functioning of blood platelets. Sci Am 242 No 6: 86, 1980

Granular Leukocytes, Acute Inflammation, and Immediate Hypersensitivity

AUSTEN KF: Biological implications of the structural and functional characteristics of the chemical mediators of immediate-type hypersensitivity. In The Harvey Lectures, Series 73, p 93. New York, Academic Press, 1979

AUSTEN KF, ORANGE RP: Bronchial asthma: The possible role of the chemical mediators of immediate hypersensitivity in the pathogenesis of subacute chronic disease. Am Rev Respir Dis 112: 423, 1975

BAINTON DF, ULLYOT JL, FARQUHAR MG: The development of neutrophilic polymorphonuclear leukocytes in human bone marrow: Origin and content of azurophil and specific granules. J Exp Med 134:907, 1971

BASS DA: The functions of eosinophils. Ann Intern Med 91:120, 1979

BEAVEN MA: Histamine (first of two parts). N Engl J Med 294:30, 1976

BEAVEN MA: Histamine (second of two parts). N Engl J Med 294: 320, 1976

BEESON PB, BASS DA: The Eosinophil. Major Problems in Internal Medicine, Vol 14. Philadelphia, WB Saunders, 1977

BROXMEYER HE, DE SOUSA M, SMITHYMAN A ET AL: Specificity and modulation of the action of lactoferrin, a negative feedback regulator of myelopoiesis. Blood 55:324, 1980

DENBURG JA, MESSNER H, LIM B ET AL: Clonal origin of human basophil/mast cells from circulating multipotent hemopoietic progenitors. Exp Hematol 13:185, 1985

FARQUHAR MG, BAINTON DF: Cytochemical studies on leukocyte granules. Proc 4th Int Cong Histochemistry and Cytochemistry, p 25. Kyoto, Society for Histochemistry and Cytochemistry, 1972

KAY AB: The role of the eosinophil in physiological and pathological processes. In Thompson RA (ed): Recent Advances in Clinical Immunology, No 2, p 113. Edinburgh, Churchill Livingstone, 1980

KLEBANOFF SJ, CLARK RA: The Neutrophil: Function and Clinical Disorders. New York, Elsevier/North Holland, 1978

KOKUBUN Y (ed): Phagocytosis. Baltimore, University Park Press, 1979

MOVAT HZ: The acute inflammatory reaction. In Movat HZ (ed): Inflammation, Immunity and Hypersensitivity. Cellular and Molecular Mechanisms, 2nd ed, p 1. Hagerstown, Harper & Row, 1979

MOVAT HZ (ed): Inflammation, Immunity and Hypersensitivity. Molecular and Cellular Mechanisms, 2nd ed. Hagerstown, Harper & Row, 1979

MOVAT HZ: The Inflammatory Reaction. Amsterdam, Elsevier, 1985

PARWARESCH MR: The Human Basophil. Morphology, Origin, Kinetics, Function and Pathology. Berlin, Springer-Verlag, 1976

RODNAN GP, SCHUMACHER HR, ZVAIFLER NJ (eds): Primer on the Rheumatic Diseases, 8th ed, p 16. Atlanta, Arthritis Foundation, 1983

RYAN GB, MAJNO G: Acute Inflammation. Am J Pathol 86:183, 1977

SULLIVAN TJ: The role of eosinophils in inflammatory reactions. In Brown E (ed): Progress in Hematology, Vol 11, p 65. New York, Grune & Stratton, 1979

WEISSMAN G (ed): Handbook of Inflammation, Vol 2. The Cell Biology of Inflammation. Amsterdam, Elsevier/North-Holland, 1980

ZUCKER–FRANKLIN D: Ultrastructural evidence for the common origin of human mast cells and basophils. Blood 56:534, 1980

ZWEIFACH BZ, GRANT L, MCCLUSKEY RT (eds): The Inflammatory Process, 2nd ed, Vols 1 to 3. New York, Academic Press, 1974

Nongranular Leukocytes*

BENACERRAF B: Regulatory T lymphocytes and their antigen receptors. In Pernis B, Vogel HJ (eds): Regulatory T Lymphocytes, p 3. New York, Academic Press, 1980

LEVITT D, COOPER MD: Expression and function of B-lymphocyte receptors. In Bearn AG, Choppin RW (eds): Receptors and Human Diseases, p 98. New York, Josiah Macy, Jr Foundation, 1979

NICHOLS BA, BAINTON DF, FARQUHAR MG: Differentiation of monocytes. Origin, nature and fate of their azurophil granules. J Cell Biol 50:498, 1971

REINHERZ EL, SCHLOSSMAN SF: The characterization and function of human immunoregulatory T lymphocyte subsets. Immunology Today, April:69, 1981

REINHERZ EL, SCHLOSSMAN SF: The differentiation and function of human T lymphocytes. Cell 19:821, 1980

REINHERZ EL, SCHLOSSMAN SF: Regulation of the immune response—inducer and suppressor T-lymphocyte subsets in human beings. N Engl J Med 303:370, 1980

SKELLY RR, POTTER TA, AHMED A: Lymphocyte antigens and receptors. In Atassi MZ, van Oss CJ, Absolom DR (eds): Molecular Immunology. A Textbook, p 597. New York, Marcel Dekker, 1984

VAN FURTH R (ed): Mononuclear Phagocytes. Philadelphia, FA Davis, 1970

VOGLER LB, GROSSI CE, COOPER MD: Human lymphocyte subpopulations. In Brown EB (ed): Progress in Hematology, Vol XI, p 1. New York, Grune & Stratton, 1979

---

* See also references on Lymphocytes listed under Selected References, Chapter 10.

9

Myeloid Tissue

Hematopoietic Tissues.   Blood cells are highly specialized cells that can already carry out their respective functions by the time they enter the bloodstream. Under ordinary conditions, they do not circulate until proliferation is completed and they reach the necessary level of maturation. Hence dividing blood cells are rarely seen in a normal peripheral blood film. If any are found, they are almost always lymphocytes or cells of the monocyte-macrophage lineage, because both kinds of cells are able to reenter the bloodstream, even after they have been stimulated to divide on leaving the confines of the blood circulatory system.

In this chapter and in Chapter 10, we shall be considering how the vast numbers of specialized blood cells required to maintain essential blood cell functions are produced on a daily basis. Furthermore, it will soon become apparent that although the blood cell–forming tissues are conventionally subdivided into myeloid tissue and lymphatic tissue, the radical distinction that was once made between these two forms of the tissue is gradually becoming less useful as our knowledge of them increases.

The process by which blood cells are formed is called *hematopoiesis* (Gr. *hemato*, blood; *poiein*, to make), so the tissues in which new blood cells are produced are known as the *hematopoietic* (the short form of which is *hemopoietic*) *tissues*. The two major subdivisions of hematopoietic tissue are (1) *myeloid tissue* and (2) *lymphatic tissue*. The hematopoietic tissue in which erythrocytes, platelets, and most kinds of leukocytes are produced in man is known as *myeloid tissue* (Gr. *myelos*, marrow) because it corresponds to the *red bone marrow* that is present in the medullary cavities of certain bones. Lymphocytes, however, are more numerous in the lymph nodes, spleen, and thymus, so it has become customary to classify these particular organs as *lymphatic tissue*. B-Cells, a major class of small lymphocytes, are nevertheless produced exclusively in *myeloid tissue*. Also, prenatally in man (and postnatally as well as prenatally in the mouse and rat), the *spleen* serves as a site of active myeloid hematopoiesis even though it is still regarded as a lymphatic organ. Moreover, the human spleen and liver, both of which are organs that play a major role in fetal hematopoiesis, retain a lifelong ability to regenerate blood cells of the myeloid (*i.e.*, nonlymphoid) lineages. However, this latent capacity is generally expressed only under abnormal conditions (*e.g.*, in severe hemolytic anemia). Any such myeloid differentiation that occurs at some site in the body other than bone marrow is described as *extramedullary hematopoiesis*.

Red Bone Marrow Is Hematopoietically Active. In adult life, human bone marrow is present in two distinct forms. At sites where the marrow remains hematopoietically active, it produces so many erythrocytes that it has a bright red color; hence it is known as *red marrow. Yellow marrow* is markedly different because instead of producing new blood cells, it stores fat. Its yellow color is due to the carotene that is present in the fat that accumulates in its abundant fat-storing cells. During active growth of the skeleton, red marrow is progressively replaced by yellow marrow in most of the long bones. In adult life, red marrow is restricted in distribution to the pelvis, ribs, and sternum, the bodies of vertebrae, the bones that comprise the vault of the skull, and the cancellous bony regions present both at the proximal end (*i.e.,* proximal epiphysis) of each femur and humerus and also within some short bones. Hence to obtain a representative sample of active bone marrow cells for clinical evaluation, it is necessary to aspirate them by needle from one of their major sources, generally either the sternum or the crest of the ilium.

When the demand for erythrocyte replacement is markedly increased, as happens for example in a severe hemolytic anemia, there can be a progressive resubstitution of red marrow for yellow marrow. The factors that regulate interconversion of these alternative forms of bone marrow are not yet fully elucidated. However, local temperature appears to play a decisive role. Thus if yellow marrow from a rabbit's tibia is transplanted to a subcutaneous site on the animal's abdominal wall where the local temperature is barely 4°C higher, the effects of a higher environmental temperature act synergistically with a long-lasting hematopoietic stimulus in bringing about reconversion to red marrow (Bigelow and Tavassoli). Hence the total amount of red marrow in the body evidently depends on current hematopoietic demands, but its skeletal distribution seems to be a reflection of the prevailing local temperature.

Myeloid tissue is basically made up of (1) a very heterogeneous population of *developing blood cells* that lie suspended but not fixed in (2) a *connective tissue stroma.* The free marrow cells represent a continuously renewing cell population with the capacity to provide a lifelong supply of new blood cells. Their proliferation and differentiation are affected by the microenvironmental influence of the stromal elements of bone marrow, which include a variety of different types of connective tissue cells that are held in place by a delicate meshwork of collagen fibers and reticular fibers. The stroma of myeloid tissue is also provided with characteristically wide yet thin-walled venous vessels termed *sinusoids* that constitute a route of direct access for newly formed blood cells to enter the circulation. Postnatal production of human blood cells of the myeloid series normally occurs in red marrow that is confined within the nonexpandable medullary cavities of particular bones. It has been suggested that chronic crowding of the available space by the ever-expanding population of differentiating blood cells that is present in these cavities could promote penetration of the flimsy walls of sinusoids by actively motile maturing blood cells.

CONNECTIVE TISSUE STROMA

Sinusoids

The stroma of myeloid tissue is normally so densely populated with differentiating blood cells that sinusoids are not always readily discernible in sections of bone marrow. In an active marrow, these vessels commonly appear as fairly wide oval areas that are filled with erythrocytes and are bounded by endothelial cells (Fig. 9-1). The sinusoids are easier to distinguish if the developing blood cell population in the intervening stroma is experimentally depleted (Fig. 9-2). The sinusoids in the medullary cavity of a long bone are predominantly radial in their orientation, and they anastomose freely. Much of the blood that enters them comes from capillaries that have already supplied the bone cortex with oxygen and nutrients. The wide collecting sinusoids into which these sinusoids drain empty, in turn, into a large central sinusoid from which most of the blood leaves by way of (1) the main (nutrient) veins accompanying the nutrient artery or arteries of the bone, and (2) metaphyseal emissary veins.

The sinusoids of myeloid tissue are lined with a layer of *fenestrated endothelium* that is supported by delicate reticular fibers (Fig. 9-2). Surrounding the endothelium, there is a tenuous basement membrane that is markedly discontinuous and generally rather difficult to discern in electron micrographs. Occluding junctions are present between the endothelial cells, but they are less extensive than those of capillaries. Another feature of the sinusoidal endothelial cells is that they exhibit numerous coated pits and vesicles as well as a wide assortment of diaphragm-closed fenestrae, pits, and channels that bear witness to a very active macromolecular exchange between blood plasma and the stromal microenvironment. Electron microscope (EM) tracer studies have also demonstrated a transcellular transport mechanism that can rapidly transfer small blood-borne particles to the perisinusoidal extravascular spaces.

Many of the particles that are taken up along the luminal border of the endothelial cells are quickly released from the basal border of these cells. However, small particles of inert material are sometimes retained by these endothelial cells for a considerable time. In a few species, such as the rabbit, sinusoid-associated *macrophages* are apparently able to extend their pseudopodia through (rather than between) these endothelial cells to reach into the sinusoidal lumen (as may be seen in Fig. 9-3, at *upper right*). Sooner or later, then, any extraneous particulate matter taken up by myeloid tissue from the bloodstream through either of these mechanisms ends up in its highly phagocytic macrophages. Its macrophages also engulf extruded red cell nuclei and actively devour any newly forming blood cells that are defective. In most species, however, sinusoid-associated macrophages of the spleen play a more important role than those of myeloid tissue in removing particulate material and defective or senescent blood cells from the circulation. Before it became evident from EM studies that actively phagocytic macrophages are so closely associated with the fenestrated endothelial cells that line the sinusoids, it was thought that all this extraneous material was taken up solely by the endothelial cells,

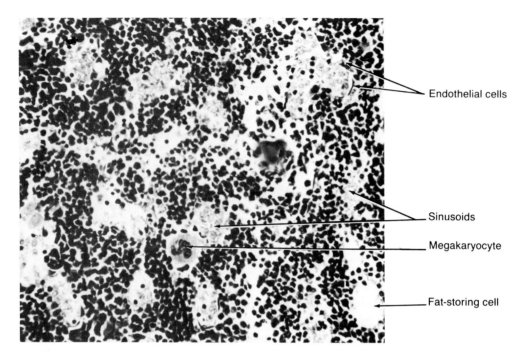

Endothelial cells

Sinusoids

Megakaryocyte

Fat-storing cell

Fig. 9-1. Photomicrograph of red bone marrow (low power).

which were initially called *reticuloendothelial cells* because of an exaggerated impression of the extent of their phagocytic activity.

There are indications that maturing blood cells are readily deformable and are able to squeeze their way into the sinusoids of myeloid tissue through temporary transendothelial *migration pores* that they create in the region of attenuated cytoplasm near the periphery of the endothelial cells. Hence it seems that their access to the sinusoids of myeloid tissue is a selective process that requires active blood cell motility. Furthermore, although the nucleus of a maturing leukocyte is readily deformable, that of a maturing erythrocyte is not. Accordingly, any forming red cell that tries to squeeze through a migration pore when still nucleated will lose its nucleus in the attempt. Hence nucleated human erythrocytes are not normally seen in the peripheral blood.

External to the endothelium there is a discontinuous and apparently retractable adventitial layer made up of reticular (reticulum) cells, which are a type of stromal cell that we shall describe in the next section.

Stromal Cell Types in Myeloid Tissue

In addition to *endothelial cells* and a widely distributed population of acid phosphatase-positive, monocyte-derived *macrophages,* the stromal cells of myeloid tissue include ordinary *fibroblasts* and similar reticular cell–derived fibroblastic cells with the capacity to secrete collagen of more than one type and also fibronectin. Such collagen-produc-

ing cells are the probable source of the substantial collagen fibers that (1) reinforce the walls of the medullary blood vessels in the marrow cavity and (2) provide a certain amount of internal support for the stroma as a whole. Studies of mouse bone marrow also indicate the presence of fibroblastic stromal cells that have osteogenic potential. Because such cells manifest features that are common to both fibroblasts and osteoblasts, they may represent some kind of intermediate or precursor cell type with the potential to express properties that are characteristic of either cell lineage. However, their potential for producing bone tissue does not seem to be quite so important as their putative role in the local regulation of proliferation and differentiation of myeloid cells, which will be discussed in the following section.

Also present in the stroma of myeloid tissue are a variable number of *fat-storing cells* (Fig. 9-1). These cells are believed to represent reticular cell progeny that have entered an extended phase of lipid accumulation and storage. The *reticular (reticulum) cells* of myeloid tissue are large and irregularly shaped, substrate-adherent (fixed) cells derived from mesenchyme. They are called *reticular* cells because they produce a network of delicate *reticular fibers* (L. *rete,* net). Although still far from being adequately characterized, it is known that they are capable of secreting both type I and type III collagen (see Table 7-1). Other distinguishing characteristics include the fact that they can be stained histochemically for either acid or alkaline phosphatase, depending on the species, and that their progeny have mod-

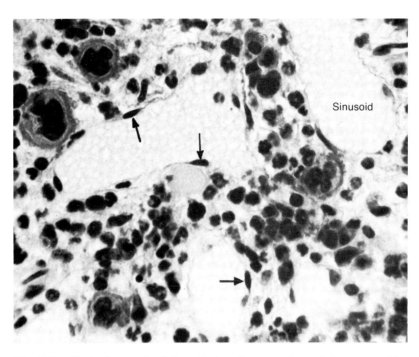

Fig. 9-2. Photomicrograph of sinusoids in red marrow (mouse) demonstrated by depleting the hematopoietic cells with a lethal dose of total body radiation. Arrows indicate the nuclei of endothelial lining cells of the sinusoids.

erate phagocytic potential. These otherwise pale-staining and nondescript cells are not at all easy to identify in marrow sections stained with hematoxylin and eosin (H & E). However, some of their progeny cells tend to accumulate lipid, a role that becomes particularly noticeable in yellow marrow. As in adipocytes (fat cells), these fat-laden stromal cells are easily recognized in H & E sections by the presence of a large, rounded empty space that indicates the position of their extracted fat droplet (Fig. 9-1).

It has been established *in vitro* that lipid accumulation within such stromal cells of myeloid tissue is enhanced by addition of the glucocorticoid hormone cortisol (hydrocortisone), yet insulin is without effect. Lipid accumulation by the adipocytes of adipose tissue, on the other hand, is more sensitive to insulin than to cortisol. Such a difference in target cell responsiveness suggests that these cells could represent two distinct cell types. This is why some investigators prefer to use the less committal term *fat-storing cells* instead of *marrow adipocytes.* It has been suggested that the fat-storing cells in myeloid tissue could serve as a local energy reserve or have additional functions that go beyond simply occupying space that is not being used to produce blood cells. This would help to explain the observation that the fat reserves in bone marrow are preferentially spared under conditions of acute total starvation. However, it seems that yellow marrow is even better protected in this regard. Furthermore, fat-containing cells are invariably observed in marrow cultures that are engaged in sustained and productive hematopoiesis, although the significance of their presence is still not entirely clear (see Tavassoli).

We can summarize most of the foregoing discussion by saying that the stromal cells of myeloid tissue include endothelial cells, macrophages, and fibroblastic reticular cells, and that lipid tends to accumulate in adipocytelike, stromal fat-storing cells that are believed to be a derivative of the stromal reticular cells.

Experimental Evidence Indicates That Stromal Cells of Myeloid Tissue Can Exert a Local Regulatory Influence on Hematopoietic Differentiation. The various stromal cell functions of myeloid tissue have not yet been fully elucidated and currently are matters of intensive investigation. Pioneering studies of ectopic transplants of bone tissue, bone marrow, or spleen cells have nevertheless established that myeloid tissue develops only after the *appropriate stroma* has been laid down, for example in a newly forming or an artificially evacuated medullary cavity. After the necessary supporting stroma has formed or has been reconstituted, its interstices become seeded by circulating multipotential hematopoietic stem cells. These are the stem cells from which blood cells of all types arise.

One of the first groups of investigators to demonstrate the presence of fibroblastic cells with osteogenic potential in the stroma of mouse bone marrow was that of Friedenstein et al, whose experiments showed that the transplantation of such stromal cells could pave the way for successful transference of the specific microenvironment of myeloid tissue. It was therefore proposed that the stromal cells of myeloid tissue provide a *specific microenvironmental influence* that promotes sustained and regulated proliferation and differentiation of multipotential hematopoietic stem

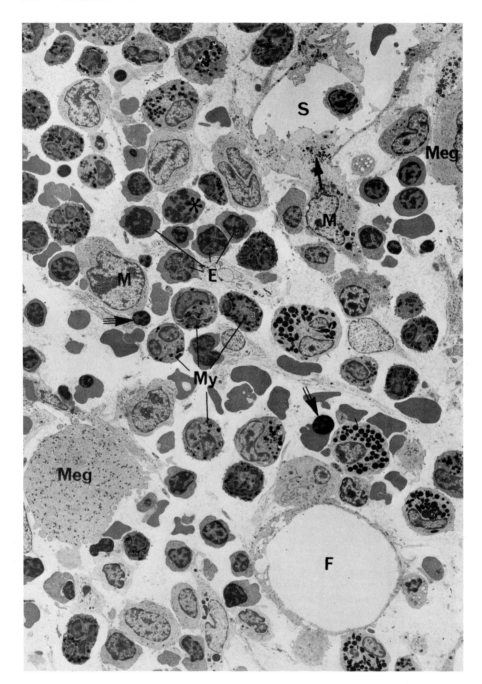

Fig. 9-3. Low-power electron micrograph ($\times$1700) showing the general appearance of myeloid tissue following intravenous injection of colloidal carbon into a rat to demonstrate macrophages (*M*). At upper right, a macrophage is extending a large pseudopodium (indicated by *arrow*) up into the lumen of a sinusoid (*S*). Phagocytosed carbon particles are visible within this pseudopodium. Another macrophage (*M*), left of center, is phagocytosing a nucleus (indicated by *arrow*) probably recently extruded from a normoblast in the island of developing erythroid cells (*E*) above center. Note the increasing electron density in the developing erythroid cells (*E*), due to accumulation of hemoglobin. A cell at the top of the island (indicated by *asterisk*) is in mitosis. Below the erythroid island, developing cells of the granulocytic series (*My*) may be seen. At bottom, a megakaryocyte (*Meg*) at left and a fat cell (*F*) at right are evident. Just above the fat cell, a normoblast is extruding its nucleus (arrow). (Courtesy of S. Luk and G. Simon)

cells and their progeny. This stromal influence constitutes an essential part of what is termed the *hematopoietic inductive microenvironment* of myeloid tissue, although whether the microenvironment is really inductive as opposed to permissive for particular lines of differentiation is a question that we shall have to address later in this chapter. A great deal of experimental work has subsequently been done in long-term marrow cultures, using a novel culture method devised by Dexter. The success of this method depends on the establishment of a long-lasting multilayer that is made up of several different types of adherent stromal cells. In addition to supporting proliferation and differentiation of the various kinds of hematopoietic progenitors (which will be described later in this chapter), Dexter cultures permit multipotential hematopoietic stem cells to undergo several months of self-renewal. Studies using these cultures are bringing to light some of the reasons why myeloid differentiation is so dependent on the presence of stromal cells of myeloid tissue (see Allen and Dexter). Such studies are gradually disclosing the complexities of an interacting network of close-range factors and factor-producing stromal cells that are involved in the local regulation of stem cell proliferation. Some of these factors are believed to be produced by the fibroblastic reticular cells whereas other factors seem to come from the macrophages. Close-range regulation of proliferation and differentiation through intimate association or direct contact of hematopoietic cells with reticular cells and macrophages therefore seems a likely proposition at this time. This functional dependence of the hematopoietic cell population on the stromal component of myeloid tissue clearly needs to be taken into account in the clinical management of myeloproliferative disorders such as aplastic anemia and the various forms of leukemia.

We shall now focus our attention on the various classes of hematopoietic cells that are present in myeloid tissue, beginning with ancestral hematopoietic stem cells.

HEMATOPOIETIC DIFFERENTIATION

There Are Three Broad Categories of Hematopoietic Cells. Early hematopoietic cells are comparatively undifferentiated; hence they all tend to have a similar appearance under the microscope. However, there is much experimental and clinical evidence to indicate that hematopoietic cell populations contain three broad categories of cells. Those in the first two categories are morphologically unrecognizable and therefore require appropriate indirect assay methods for their study. These three major cellular compartments are represented in Figure 9-4. The first compartment is a reserve pool of *self-renewing stem cells*. The second compartment represents an intermediate category that is made up of the various types of *differentiating progenitor cells*. The earliest progenitors have a broad spectrum of potentialities whereas the latest progenitors in the hierarchy are committed to specific cell lineages (Fig. 9-4). The third compartment in the hematopoietic cell population is made up of *fully functional mature blood cells* and their various derivatives, including blood platelets. All the cells in the third compartment except B- and T-lymphocytes were fully described in Chapter 8; B- and T-lymphocytes

will be considered in further detail in Chapter 10. The remainder of this chapter therefore deals with the various types of hematopoietic stem cells and progenitors.

Multipotential Hematopoietic Stem Cells

It is now known that all types of blood cells are ultimately derived from a class of ancestral hematopoietic stem cells called *multipotential hematopoietic stem cells*, the cells of origin that are represented at the top of the differentiation scheme shown in Figure 9-4. In addition to being able to give rise to blood cells of every kind, these ancestral stem cells are potentially capable of very extensive proliferation. Accordingly, they represent a lifelong potential source of new blood cells that counteracts depletion of the hematopoietic cell population by maintaining an intrinsic capacity for self-renewal. Following the discovery of multipotential hematopoietic stem cells, a number of years passed before anything was learned about the various types of hematopoietic progenitors. These cells remained essentially uncharacterized until suitable *in vitro* techniques were devised for their study. In the following discussion, we shall first consider how multipotential hematopoietic stem cells were discovered.

The Multipotential Hematopoietic Stem Cells of Mice Have the Capacity to Produce Large Mixed Colonies in the Spleen. The chromosome damage inflicted by a lethal dose of ionizing radiation is generally manifested as an abnormal mitotic division that is rarely able to proceed to completion (this was discussed under Mitosis in Chap. 3). The tissues that are most severely affected are those that undergo a rapid rate of cell turnover. Granular leukocytes, for example, only circulate for an average of 10 hours. To prevent their numbers from decreasing, it is necessary for them to be replaced by the bone marrow as quickly as they leave the bloodstream. The same is true of platelets. Erythrocytes, on the other hand, last for 4 months; hence any radiation-induced decline in their rate of production takes more time to become apparent. Accordingly, in the few days following whole-body exposure to a lethal dose of radiation, there is a marked decline in the neutrophil and platelet count of the peripheral blood. Lymphocyte proliferation and the production of new lymphocytes are similarly curtailed; hence the production of plasma cells in response to antigens is also markedly diminished.

Primarily because of this failure to produce new neutrophils and new antibody-forming cells, the body becomes unable to ward off infections. Moreover, because the epithelial cells that line the intestine are normally lost at a rapid rate and must be replaced, another immediate and serious effect of lethal doses of total-body radiation is that the intestinal lining cells are not replaced as quickly as they are lost. As a result, patches of the intestinal mucosa become denuded even though the cells that persist flatten out in an attempt to cover such areas. The denuded areas soon become invaded by bacteria and, because the body has lost

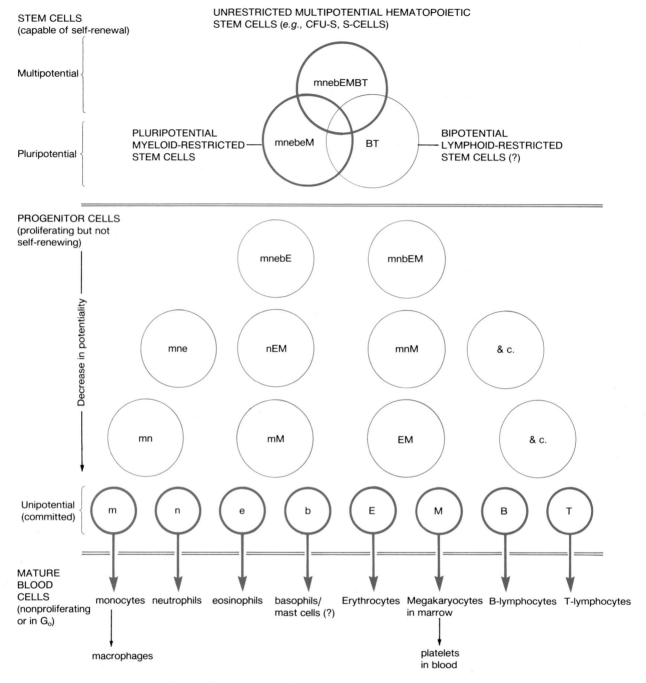

Fig. 9-4. A currently favored scheme of hematopoietic differentiation based on assaying the potentialities of myeloid and lymphatic stem cells and progenitors. The bottom row of the diagram indicates the meaning of the various abbreviations that are used.

its chief means of resisting infection and also its capacity to produce platelets for preventing hemorrhages from denuded sites along the intestine, death rapidly ensues.

Yet a lethally irradiated mouse that is given a sufficient number of nonirradiated bone marrow cells in the form of an intravenous transfusion will survive. It survives because multipotential hematopoietic stem cells from the transfused marrow settle in its hematopoietic tissues and repopulate them with donor-derived hematopoietic cells. The engrafted multipotential hematopoietic stem cells soon produce enough new granular leukocytes and platelets to ward off the infections and hemorrhages that would otherwise kill the animal. Furthermore, the capacity of the recipient animal for producing new antibody-forming cells is restored.

The series of experimental investigations that established the important characteristics of multipotential hematopoietic stem cells began with the observation that the spleen of the recovering mice develops a countable number of small nodules that project from its surface (see references for Till, McCulloch, and coworkers). LM sections disclosed that these nodules represent large colonies of hematopoietic cells that include differentiating cells of the erythroid and granulocytic series and, in some cases, megakaryocytes as well. To investigate whether these so-called *spleen colonies* were clonal in origin, repopulation studies were carried out using marked bone marrow cells that had been individually tagged with a unique chromosomal marker so that their progeny cells could be recognized under the microscope. Such markers are generated by exposing the cells to a sublethal dose of radiation that is sufficient to produce a microscopically identifiable chromosomal abnormality without impairing cell function or proliferative capacity. The result of these studies was that nearly all the dividing cells in each spleen colony possessed the same chromosomal marker. It was concluded that each spleen colony arises from a single multipotential cell. The self-renewing ancestral stem cell that gives rise to a spleen colony is accordingly designated *CFU-S* (CFU for *colony-forming unit* and S for *spleen*).

By assaying the capacity of nucleated peripheral blood cells for spleen colony formation, it has been established that relatively low numbers of multipotential hematopoietic stem cells circulate in the bloodstream (approximately four out of every 1×10^5 nucleated peripheral blood cells are CFU-S). These multipotential stem cells have also been found in hematopoietic organs other than myeloid tissue.

During Prenatal Development, Multipotential Hematopoietic Stem Cells Migrate from the Yolk Sac to the Liver, Spleen, and Bone Marrow. Multipotential hematopoietic stem cells develop in the embryonic yolk sac from mesenchymal cells of its blood islands. The first organ to become seeded with hematopoietic stem cells that leave the yolk sac is the liver. The spleen and bone marrow then become seeded with stem cells from the liver. After birth, red bone marrow constitutes the chief site where the pool of multipotential hematopoietic stem cells is maintained.

Certain Morphological Similarities Exist Between Multipotential Hematopoietic Stem Cells and Small Lymphocytes. There is no certain way of identifying multipotential hematopoietic stem cells on the basis of their microscopic appearance. However, it is known that these cells are quite small (7 μm to 7.5 μm in diameter) and that they constitute only a minor cell population (0.6% to 0.8% of the total nucleated cell population in mouse bone marrow). Further information about the morphology of multipotential hematopoietic stem cells comes from raising their relative incidence in myeloid tissue by experimental means. By treating mice with antiproliferative drugs and then separating their bone marrow cells using density gradient centrifugation, van Bekkum and his coworkers were able to raise the proportion of assayable CFU-S in myeloid cell suspensions to a maximal concentration of 30%. This procedure enabled them to recognize and characterize the enriched cell population in the EM and hence to arrive at a detailed morphological description of the type of cell that is believed to correspond to CFU-S and presumably its early descendants as well. Their study was subsequently broadened to include the early myeloid cells of the rat, monkey, and man.

An example of the prospective stem cell type that they described is illustrated in Figure 9-5. It bears a certain resemblance to the small lymphocyte in that it possesses a very thin rim of cytoplasm and manifests an undifferentiated appearance. Its sparse cytoplasm contains remarkably few organelles other than abundant free ribosomes and a few small mitochondria. However, its rounded nucleus is a little more irregular in outline than that of the small lymphocyte and its indentations are not quite as deep. Also, the chromatin is more extended and more evenly dispersed than that of a lymphocyte (compare Fig. 9-5 with Fig. 8-15). Nucleoli are very large and prominent (Fig. 9-5). Although a small Golgi apparatus, occasional cisternae of rER, and lysosomes are present in small lymphocytes, these organelles have not been observed in the prospective stem cells. Hence there are a few reproducible but minor morphological differences that distinguish prospective multipotential hematopoietic stem cells from small lymphocytes in a stem cell–enriched population of myeloid cells seen in EM section. However, there are no known morphological criteria for distinguishing between multipotential hematopoietic stem cells and their early descendants because these are all early cells that are poorly differentiated. Instead of relying on morphology alone, it is necessary to recognize such cells by other characteristics, such as their respective proliferative capacity, potentiality, and capacity for self-renewal.

Multipotential Hematopoietic Stem Cells Are the Cells Responsible for Repopulating Hematopoietic Tissue. Permanent repopulation of the bone marrow following a lethal dose of whole-body radiation depends on its being seeded by an adequate number of multipotential hematopoietic stem cells. These ancestral stem cells are believed to be able to self-renew indefinitely so that they can persist throughout life. Under normal circumstances, however, they are not required to proliferate as extensively as might be thought because along their various lines of differentiation, there are other more restricted orders of stem cells that can also proliferate very extensively. Nevertheless, these lower orders of stem cells are probably unable to maintain their operational numbers for an indefinite period, and hence they probably need occasional replenishment from multipotential hematopoietic stem cells to supplement their population size.

Hematopoietic Progenitor Cells

At some point along each line of hematopoietic differentiation, it is conventional to begin referring to the cells as progenitor cells instead of orders of stem cells. The term *progenitor cell* (L. for parent or ancestor) is generally reserved for a cell that is capable of proliferation and further

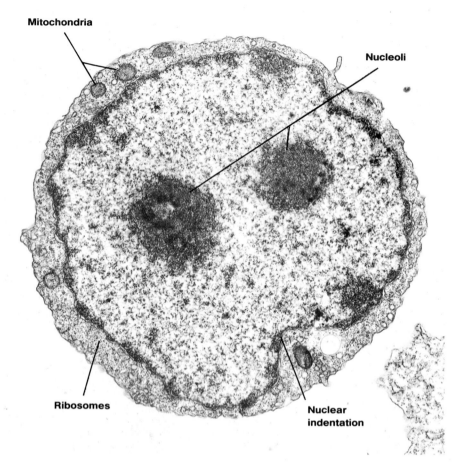

Mitochondria

Nucleoli

Ribosomes

Nuclear indentation

Fig. 9-5. Electron micrograph of a prospective multipotential hematopoietic stem cell obtained from the bone marrow of a Rhesus money. For a description, see text. (Courtesy of D. W. van Bekkum)

differentiation but that has a somewhat limited or virtually no detectable capacity for self-renewal. However, recent findings suggest that, in some cases, progenitor cells may retain the capacity for apparently limitless self-renewal under optimal *in vitro* conditions, making the criteria for the distinction between progenitor cells and stem cells difficult to define (Wendling et al). Thus the fertilized ovum is considered to be an example of a progenitor cell because it is the predecessor of all body cells, but it is not considered to be a stem cell because it does not possess an apparently limitless capacity for self-renewal nor does it persist as the same kind of cell throughout adult life.

Whereas mouse multipotential hematopoietic stem cells (CFU-S) possess sufficient proliferative potential to produce very large (*i.e.*, macroscopically visible) mixed colonies in the spleen of lethally irradiated mice, no comparable assay exists for the equivalent ancestral stem cells in man. However, a successful alternative approach has been to cultivate colony-forming hematopoietic cells in tissue culture in order to establish which types of cells they produce in the colonies

they generate. A number of years after the appropriate conditions for growing progenitor cells were devised, it became evident that under optimal conditions, cells manifesting limited self-renewal (*i.e.*, stem cells) could produce *in vitro* colonies as well. These conditions included the use of a semisolid medium that kept the progeny of proliferating hematopoietic cells closely associated with one another instead of allowing them to disperse. It soon became evident that hematopoietic colonies would form in such a culture medium provided that it also contained a specific regulatory factor called *colony stimulating factor* (CSF). The cell from which each of these colonies arose was designated *CFU-C*, the C indicating that it had the capacity to form a colony in culture. Hence the first type of hematopoietic cell from which colonies could be grown *in vitro* was CFU-C (Ichikawa et al, Bradley and Metcalf). Subsequent studies showed that this progenitor gives rise to both neutrophil granulocytes and monocytes, so it has now been renamed *CFU-GM*. Further details of this cell will be given later in this chapter.

When the hormone erythropoietin (which promotes erythrocytic differentiation) was used in place of CSF, another type of myeloid progenitor produced smaller colonies of cells that synthesized hemoglobin and underwent full differentiation into erythrocytes (Stephenson et al). These progenitors are called *CFU-E*, the E denoting the erythrocytic line of differentiation. CFU-E is a large, motile, and rapidly proliferating cell that does not appear to synthesize hemoglobin in detectable amounts until it is exposed to erythropoietin. It then stops moving, and its program of hemoglobin synthesis and morphological differentiation begins. From this point on, no more than six divisions occur before the cells in the colony lose their nucleus and become erythrocytes.

Further work on erythroid cultures established the existence of an earlier erythroid progenitor that produces numerous colonies of hemoglobin-synthesizing cells that are either scattered or fused together as a single large mass (Axelrad et al). Such a mass is termed an *erythropoietic burst* and the progenitor that gives rise to it is called *BFU-E* (for *erythropoietic burst-forming unit*).

BFU-E is smaller than CFU-E and has a much greater proliferative capacity. There are early and late types of BFU-E that have slightly different properties. BFU-E can give rise to a large number of CFU-Es, each of which produces a number of erythrocytes, so this achieves great amplification of the initial cell number. Erythropoietin is known to promote proliferation and differentiation of CFU-E into morphologically recognizable erythrocyte precursors. Another regulatory factor called BPA (*burst-promoting activity*) acts at the BFU-E level. Erythropoietin sensitivity is thought to develop at the late BFU-E level, with the result that erythropoietin becomes the primary regulator at the CFU-E level. These two regulators will be considered again in the section on Hematopoietic Regulators.

Recent work on the regulation of proliferation and differentiation of hematopoietic progenitor cells has had the predictable result that a much broader range of progenitor cells is now recognized. However, recent progress has also served to focus attention on an inherent difficulty in interpretation, namely, that of knowing whether the kinds of progeny that arise from a progenitor cell really manifest the entire range of potentialities of that cell, or whether they only mirror those potentialities that can be expressed under the particular *in vitro* conditions that are being employed. The extent to which such essentially artificial conditions simulate actual conditions in the *in vivo* microenvironment will determine how much of the cell's total potentiality becomes evident. Some of the gaps in our present knowledge regarding the interrelationships between the different hematopoietic progenitors can therefore be attributed to a lack of familiarity with the essential factors that are necessary to guarantee expression of their full potentiality. To fill in such gaps, it is still necessary to seek indirect information from the study of hematopoietic disorders.

Do Myeloid Cells Follow Any Particular Differentiation Pattern? Until fairly recently, *in vitro* findings appeared to support the contention that hematopoietic progenitors underwent an orderly and obligatory series of progressive restriction steps in their potentiality, enabling a family tree to be constructed in which the parents, grandparents, and great-grandparents of each type of blood cell could be charted in relation to the ancestral multipotential hematopoietic stem cell from which they were descended. This led to the concept that specific types of blood cells had mutual progenitors that were only distantly related to the mutual progenitors of other types of blood cells. However, Ogawa and his coworkers have now shown that the range of possible combinations of potentialities in such intermediate hematopoietic progenitors is far broader than was formerly realized (Ogawa et al and Suda et al), making it seem likely that virtually any combination of potentialities is possible. The former concept of a rigidly predetermined pattern of stepwise increasing restriction of (1) cell potentiality and (2) the potential for self-renewal, characterized by a clearly defined sequence of parent–progeny relationships, is therefore giving way to the alternative proposal, for which there is growing acceptance, that such potentialities begin to be lost in an entirely random (stochastic) manner. The finding of only a fixed number of specific combinations in earlier studies could readily be explained if the culture conditions that were used were only favorable to the growth of certain types of colonies. The contention that the progressive restriction in potentiality is essentially a stochastic process is supported by statistical analysis of the relevant data. A representation of some of the combinations that have been reported in the recent literature is included in Figure 9-4, which illustrates in a general way how such a random loss of potentiality is thought to occur.

The early *in vitro* studies of CFU-C, CFU-E, and BFU-E soon led to the development of more sophisticated culture media that incorporated further essential factors and permitted fuller expression of potentiality in terms of colony formation. Such improvements were richly rewarded by the successful *in vitro* growth of a wide variety of different uni-, bi-, tri-, and pluripotential hematopoietic progenitors. These improvements have, in turn, provided assay systems for characterizing the specific factors that regulate the proliferative activity of these hematopoietic progenitors. As a result, a plethora of such factors are now known. Those seeking detailed information about these regulators will find it in the next section; for a more comprehensive review, see Schrader.

Another exciting development in this field is that Nakahata and Ogawa, and also others, have been able to produce *in vitro* colonies consisting of relatively undifferentiated (*blast*) cells from cells that they consider to be multipotential hematopoietic stem cells. These colonies contain daughter cells that are capable of generating multilineage colonies, which is an indication that the cell of origin is not only multipotential but also is capable of self-renewal. Such self-renewing multipotential cells are designated *S-cells* (Fig. 9-4) to denote their capacity for forming *stem cell* colonies, and they appear to be very closely related to CFU-S, which is the type of multipotential hematopoietic stem cell that can give rise to spleen colonies in mice. This finding and a number of other observations now make it seem unlikely that any one known type of multipotential hematopoietic stem cell represents the single ancestral cell type from which all other hematopoietic cells are derived. Instead, there seems to be a *class* of multipotential hematopoietic stem cells of which CFU-S and S-cells are only examples, and although these two cell types represent the earliest hematopoietic stem cells recognized so far, there could be other even more primitive hematopoietic stem cells for which no appropriate assay system has yet been devised.

The overall pattern of hematopoietic differentiation that is emerging, then, is one of a continuum of (1) random and progressive nonreversible restriction of potentiality accompanied by (2) an eventual loss of the capacity for self-renewal (generally, but not necessarily invariably, the arbitrary cutoff point for loss of an extensive capacity for self-renewal is the border line between hematopoietic stem cells and progenitors), culminating in (3) total commitment and, with the exception of lymphocytes and certain cells of the monocyte-macrophage lineage, (4) loss of proliferative capacity followed by (5) terminal maturation with eventual transition into functional end cells (Fig. 9-4, *bottom*).

Hematopoietic Regulators. The proliferation and differentiation of hematopoietic progenitor cells are closely coordinated by humoral regulators; the best characterized of these regulators is the glycoprotein hormone erythropoietin. Appropriate regulation of the proliferative activity of the later cells in the progenitor cell compartment enables the body's various blood cell requirements to be adjusted on an individual, day-to-day basis. Under ordinary circumstances, the earliest hematopoietic progenitors and the stem cells capable of generating them only participate to a minor extent. Under emergency conditions, however, these earlier cells serve as an essential source of the vast numbers of new blood cells that are suddenly needed. Multipotential hematopoietic stem cells are required for the permanent repopulation and full functional recovery of hematopoietic tissues that undergo massive destruction as a result of drug cytotoxicity or radiation damage. They are also the cells responsible for full recovery of hematopoietic function after bone marrow transplantation. Far less is known about how these multipotential stem cells are regulated, but we shall need to consider them next to maintain a logical order of presentation.

Through the use of Dexter cultures, it has been established that in mouse myeloid tissue, *CFU-S* is subject to close-range regulation by both a stimulator and an inhibitor of DNA synthesis. The presence of a CFU-S survival-enhancing factor has also been demonstrated. The source of these three factors appears to be the stromal cells in the adherent layer of these cultures.

Whereas certain regulatory factors are lineage specific, others have been found to affect multiple lineages. A broadly acting regulator called *interleukin 3* (IL3), for example, seems able to sustain the self-renewal and differentiation of various early stages of hematopoiesis as well as to support the differentiation of a broad range of myeloid progenitors. The source of IL3 is believed to be activated T-lymphocytes.

A colony-forming stem cell called *CFU-GEMM* produces an *in vitro* colony that contains cells of all myeloid lineages. The word *myeloid* is used in this context to denote the lines of differentiation that lead to the formation of all kinds of blood cells except B- and T-lymphocytes, which belong to the *lymphoid* lineages instead. Recent evidence for the additional presence of T- and B-lymphocytes in these colonies strongly suggests that such stem cells may actually be unrestricted in potentiality. A reticular fibroblastic stromal cell line isolated from myeloid tissue is known to produce an inhibitor of CFU-GEMM.

The tri- and bipotential myeloid progenitors *CFU-MIX* (which produces mixed, partly erythroid colonies made up of two or three lineages) and *CFU-C* (which gives rise to neutrophils and monocytes/macrophages and is accordingly also known as *CFU-GM*) appear to be influenced also by stimulators made by endothelial cells. Regulators with CFU-C stimulatory activity (often collectively referred to as CSA or CSF, denoting colony stimulatory activity or factor) are also produced by myeloid reticular stromal cells, monocytes, macrophages, fibroblasts, and T-lymphocytes. Furthermore, macrophages can induce other cells to release hematopoietic stimulators, and reticular stromal cells, monocytes, and macrophages can also release hematopoietic inhibitors. In regulation that is as complex as this, one can only hope to remember a few broad generalities, for example the fact that CFU-C is subject to dual stimulatory and inhibitory regulation by close-range as well as long-range stimulatory and inhibitory factors, with monocytes and macrophages playing a central role in the regulatory process.

A specific stimulatory factor derived from T-lymphocytes has also been identified that stimulates proliferation and differentiation of the unipotential progenitor *CFU-EO*, which gives rise to eosinophils. Stromal reticular cells produce a specific stimulatory factor for *CFU-M*, the unipotential progenitor of monocytes/macrophages. A reversible inhibitor of DNA synthesis has recently been discovered that is specific for *BFU-E*, an early unipotential progenitor of erythrocytes already described previously in this chapter. BFU-E also responds to a stimulatory factor and survival potentiator called *BPA* (denoting *burst-promoting activity*) made by T-lymphocytes, monocytes, marrow stromal cells, and endothelial cells that may, in fact, prove to be identical to IL3.

Finally, *erythropoietin* stimulates proliferation and differentiation of the late erythroid progenitor CFU-E and probably all except the initial stages of BFU-E. This glycoprotein hormone is known to be produced by the kidneys and liver, but its cellular source or sources remain uncertain.

Damaged or worn-out erythrocytes are always being removed from the circulating blood. If erythrocyte depletion lowers the blood hemoglobin concentration sufficiently to result in an oxygen deficit in the body tissues, the kidneys sense this lowered oxygen tension and respond to it by releasing erythropoietin. The action of this hormone is to stimulate the proliferation and differentiation of unipotential erythroid progenitors (primarily CFU-E) in myeloid tissue, with the result that these progenitors give rise to he-

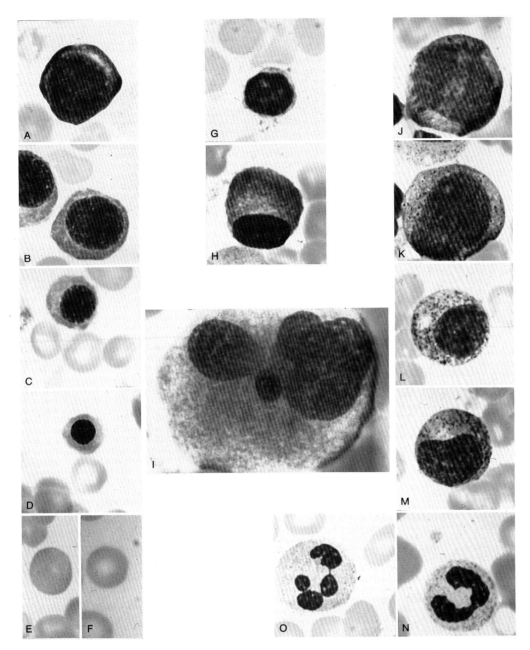

Plate 9-1. Photomicrographs of some stages of erythrocytic, leukocytic, and megakaryocytic maturation that can be recognized morphologically in a marrow film (Wright's blood stain) (A) Proerythroblast; (B) basophilic erythroblast; (C) polychromatophilic erythroblast; (D) normoblast; (E) polychromatophilic erythrocyte; (F) mature erythrocyte; (G) small lymphocyte; (H) plasma cell; (I) megakaryocyte; (J) myeloblast; (K) promyelocyte; (L) neutrophilic myelocyte; (M) neutrophilic metamyelocyte; (N) band neutrophil; (O) mature neutrophil.

moglobin-synthesizing cells that then go on to produce erythrocytes.

Erythropoietin levels, and hence erythrocyte production, become markedly depressed in experimental animals that have been hypertransfused with enough erythrocytes to raise their erythrocyte count far above normal. Under these conditions, the number of CFU-Es drops considerably, but because BFU-Es do not decline to the same extent, there are enough of them to give rise to new CFU-Es as soon as erythropoietin production resumes.

In view of the fact that committed myeloid progenitors seem to be generated on a random basis and are then either amplified or inhibited from proliferating through the appropriate release of regulatory factors, some refinement of the original concept of a *hematopoietic inductive microenvironment* needs to be made. This environment would now perhaps be more accurately called a *hematopoiesis-regulating microenvironment.*

Most of our information about hematopoiesis comes from the study of myeloid lines of differentiation. Although there is much evidence that B- and T-lymphocytes are derived from the same multipotential hematopoietic stem cells as myeloid cells are, not much is known about how this is actually achieved. One idea is that they might arise directly from the multipotential stem cells; another is that they, too, might be derived from the multipotential stem cells through a stochastic process of progressive restriction of their potentiality. The rather minimal evidence in favor of the existence of a restricted class of *lymphatic stem cells* that are capable of producing both B- and T-lymphocytes (Fig. 9-4) will be reviewed in the following section, along with the evidence for a common origin between B- and T-lymphocytes and the other types of blood cells.

How Are the Myeloid and Lymphoid Lineages Interrelated? Early studies of the spleen colonies that developed from CFU-Ss bearing specific chromosomal markers clearly established that these stem cells could give rise to granular leukocytes, erythrocytes, and megakaryocytes. Until recently, however, the evidence regarding lymphocyte formation within spleen colonies was somewhat inconclusive. Yet there was little doubt that lymphatic tissues as well as myeloid tissue became repopulated following transfusion of irradiated mice with bone marrow suspensions containing CFU-S. Indeed, unique chromosomal markers induced in CFU-S could later be found in cells of lymphatic tissue as well as in those of myeloid tissue, suggesting that lymphocytes were derived from CFU-S (Wu et al).

Any lingering doubts that lymphocytes are descendants of CFU-S were largely dispelled when it was realized that B-lymphocytes arose in myeloid tissue and not in lymphatic tissue as formerly supposed. Further evidence for a common origin of the myeloid and lymphoid lineages has come from studies of the *Philadelphia chromosome* (Ph[1]), which is present in the hematopoietic cells of patients with chronic myelogenous leukemia (CML). In addition to being found in representative cells of virtually all the myeloid lineages, this characteristic chromosome, described under Chro-

mosomal Anomalies in Chapter 3, can also be detected in cells of the B-lymphocyte lineage. Furthermore, Ph[1] can be found in the undifferentiated (blast) cells of approximately 25% of patients diagnosed as having the adult form of acute lymphocytic leukemia. These observations are consistent with a malignant transformation occurring at the level of the multipotential hematopoietic stem cell and then becoming manifested in the lymphoid as well as the myeloid progeny. Strain-specific and cell-type–specific genetic markers that do not depend on chromosome damage or malignant transformation for their detection have borne out the conclusion that myeloid tissue contains normal multipotential self-renewing stem cells that are capable of producing lymphoid as well as myeloid progeny.

Much useful information has been gained through use of the enzyme *glucose-6-phosphate dehydrogenase* (G-6-PD) as a clonal marker, as described in connection with Sex Chromatin in Chapter 3. From a series of investigations on CML patients heterozygous for G-6-PD, Fialkow concluded that the transformed leukemic stem cell could give rise to both B- and T-lymphocytes. Although circulating T-lymphocytes sampled during clinical remission did not belong to the leukemic clone, this could be explained if long-lived T-lymphocytes that arose prior to emergence of the leukemic clone (or that were otherwise derived independently of it) predominated at the time of sampling. T- and B-lymphocytes have also been found to belong to the same clone as the myeloid cells of a similarly heterozygous patient who had *sideroblastic anemia* (Gr. *sideros*, iron), a form of anemia that is characterized by an abnormal iron distribution in cells of the erythroid series (Prchal et al). Also, a detailed analysis of the various types of cells present in individual clonal multilineage colonies growing *in vitro* from peripheral blood cells of normal volunteers who were heterozygous for G-6-PD revealed that they can contain T-lymphocytes in addition to myeloid cells (Messner et al). There are therefore a number of independent lines of evidence that multipotential hematopoietic stem cells capable of producing both myeloid and lymphoid progeny exist in man as well as in the mouse.

On the issue of whether there are separate orders of restricted lymphoid and myeloid stem cells, there is less general agreement. There is certainly less evidence for the existence of bipotential lymphoid-restricted stem cells than for pluripotential myeloid-restricted stem cells. Stem cells fitting the latter description are involved in *polycythemia vera*, a myeloproliferative disorder characterized by overproduction of erythrocytes. A study using the clonal marker G-6-PD revealed that in this disorder, neither B- nor T-lymphocytes belonged to the same clone as the erythrocytes and the other affected myeloid lineages, indicating that the affected stem cell level was myeloid-restricted. It is also possible that normal colony-forming cells capable of giving rise to multilineage myeloid colonies but not lymphocytes *in vitro* might include some myeloid-restricted cells. However, perhaps the most convincing argument for the existence of myeloid-restricted stem cells comes from repopulation studies of mice transfused with chromosomally marked bone marrow cells. Using such a system, Abramson et al traced individual unique radiation-induced chromosomal markers to (1) myeloid cells together with B- and T-lymphocytes, (2) myeloid cells only, or (3) T-lymphocytes only. This suggested the existence of multipotential hematopoietic stem cells, myeloid-restricted stem cells, and T-lymphocyte–restricted stem cells, respectively. In a subsequent study, Jones–Villeneuve and Phillips transfused irradiated mice with cells from Dexter cultures and, by tracing a strain-specific marker chromosome, investigated the respective capacities of these cells for repopulating (1) myeloid tissue and (2) lymphatic tissue of the host. The results indicated that (1) the two repopulating capacities were sometimes dissociated from each other, and (2) the capacity to produce T-lymphocytes was highly correlated with the capacity to produce B-lymphocytes. A logical interpretation of these findings would be that the conditions furnished by the Dexter cultures were conducive to the growth of bipotential lymphoid stem cells as well as to that of multipotential hematopoietic stem cells. Taken in conjunction with each other, these last two investigations provide a certain amount of indirect evidence for the existence of (1) *myeloid-restricted* and (2) *lymphoid-restricted* stem cells in addition to (3) *unrestricted* multipotential hematopoietic stem cells (Fig. 9-4).

Even though the experimental evidence for bipotential lymphoid-restricted stem cells as forerunners of both B- and T-lymphocytes is quite meager, there seems to be a general willingness to accept this idea from a conceptual point of view. It is possible that the elusive nature of lymphoid stem cells is simply a result of not knowing the optimal experimental conditions for promoting their self-renewal and ensuring expression of their dual potentiality.

In due course, the progeny of hematopoietic progenitor cells reach the stage of becoming morphologically identifiable under the microscope. The earliest microscopically recognizable cells are still immature and are accordingly often described as *blood cell precursors*. The precursors then undergo a maturation process whereby they become fully functional *blood cells*.

Morphologically Recognizable Stages of Erythropoiesis

The earliest erythrocytic precursor that is microscopically distinguishable is the *proerythroblast*. This is a relatively large cell that ranges from 12 μm to 15 μm in diameter. In marrow films, the chromatin in its large spherical nucleus is finely granular and there are commonly two prominent nucleoli. The cytoplasm is noticeably basophilic (Plate 9-1*A*). As the proerythroblast continues to differentiate, increasing numbers of diffusely distributed ribosomes and polysomes intensify this basophilia.

The progeny of proerythroblasts are called *basophilic erythroblasts*. In marrow films, these cells are slightly smaller than proerythroblasts. Their spherical nucleus is smaller and its chromatin is more condensed. Their cytoplasm is diffusely basophilic (Plate 9-1*B*) because of the presence of abundant polysomes where globin chains of hemoglobin are being synthesized (see Fig. 4-9). Development of the other cytoplasmic organelles is minimal.

Cells at the next stage of erythroid differentiation are called *polychromatophilic erythroblasts*. The polychromatophilic color observed in marrow films results because the polysomes take up the basic stains present in the blood stain whereas the hemoglobin that is being synthesized takes up eosin. The net result is that the cytoplasm appears a muddy-gray or bluish-pink color (Plate 9-1*C*). The nucleus of the polychromatophilic erythroblast is somewhat

smaller than that of a basophilic erythroblast, and its coarse chromatin granules are aggregated, making the nucleus appear very basophilic. No nucleoli are visible at this stage. The polychromatophilic erythroblast is the last cell in the erythroid series to divide.

At the next stage of maturation, which is termed the *normoblast,* the dark-staining nucleus becomes small and pyknotic (Plate 9-1*D*). It is actively extruded while the cytoplasm is still slightly polychromatophilic, resulting in the formation of a *polychromatophilic erythrocyte* (Plate 9-1*E*). As described in connection with Anemias in Chapter 8, the polychromatophilic erythrocyte is more easily recognized as a *reticulocyte* with the polysomes that are still present in its cytoplasm showing up in the form of a reticulum (see Fig. 8-5).

There is evidence to suggest that nuclear extrusion by the normoblast is an active process that is brought about by the contractile activity of a ring of microfilaments that develops in association with the nucleus prior to enucleation (Repasky and Eckart). Once extruded, the nucleus is generally phagocytosed by a stromal macrophage, as may be seen in Figure 9-3 at middle left (the *arrow* indicates a phagocytosed nucleus). Tiny remnants of nuclear material are nevertheless occasionally left behind in erythrocytes; these remnants are called *Howell–Jolly bodies.*

The human body is very economical with respect to its utilization of iron. The iron obtained through the phagocytic destruction of worn-out erythrocytes by macrophages of the spleen and bone marrow is reutilized for the synthesis of new hemoglobin.

Morphologically Recognizable Stages of Granulopoiesis

The first stage of granulocytic differentiation that can be recognized under the microscope is the *myeloblast*. This is a large rounded cell that is 15 μm to 20 μm in diameter in a marrow film. Its slightly basophilic rim of cytoplasm is largely devoid of granules (Plate 9-1*J*). Its spherical nucleus is very large, with finely dispersed chromatin and two or more prominent nucleoli.

The next stage in the granular leukocyte series, called the *promyelocyte,* is generally the first stage that histology students can recognize in a marrow film. However, because the only granules formed at this stage are azurophilic granules that are not of different (*i.e., specific*) types, it is not possible to distinguish between the three different types of promyelocytes (neutrophilic, eosinophilic, and basophilic promyelocytes). Promyelocytes nevertheless appear as very large cells (larger than even the myeloblast) with a slightly coarser chromatin texture, prominent nucleoli, and a more copious, slightly basophilic cytoplasm that contains a number of purple-colored azurophilic granules (Plate 9-1*K*).

At the promyelocyte stage, then, all neutrophil granules are of the azurophilic type (Plate 9-1*K*, and Fig. 9-6). In

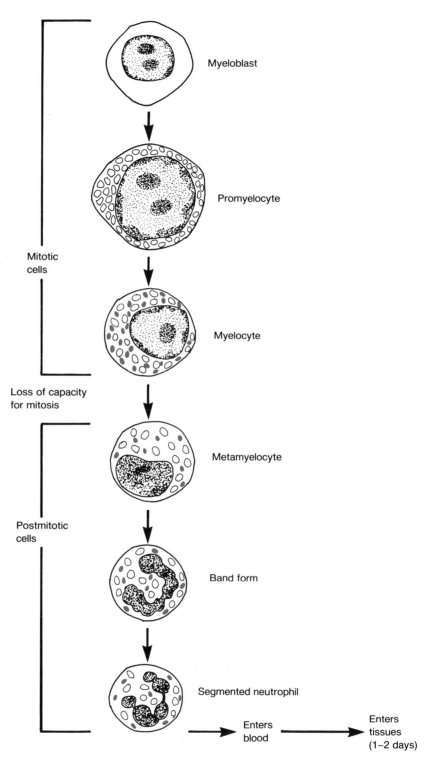

Fig. 9-6. Schematic diagram of maturation in the neutrophil series. Azurophilic granules appear at the promyelocyte stage, and specific granules (shown in blue) appear at the myelocyte stage. (Based on Bainton et al)

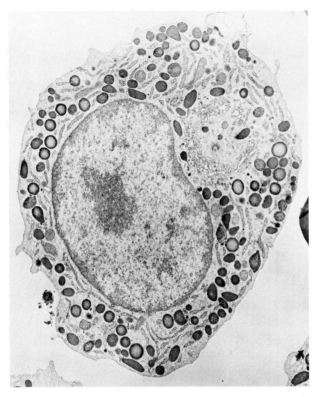

Fig. 9-7. Electron micrograph (×15,000) of a promyelocyte, histochemically reacted for the enzyme peroxidase. The only granules formed at this time are peroxidase-positive; these are lysosomes and correspond to the azurophilic granules seen with the LM. Note the well-developed Golgi at the indentation of the nucleus. (Bainton DF, Ullyot JL, Farquhar MG: J Exp Med 134: 907, 1971)

the EM, it can be seen that these granules are either spherical or ovoid (Fig. 9-7). Cisternae of rough-surfaced endoplasmic reticulum lie scattered in the cytoplasm, and a prominent Golgi complex is situated close to the slight indentation of the nucleus, as can be seen in Figure 9-7. Production of these Golgi-derived azurophilic granules, which are peroxidase-positive and represent lysosomes, soon ends, and their numbers dwindle during subsequent maturation toward the mature granulocyte (see references for Bainton, Farquhar, and coworkers).

The next stage of granulocytic maturation, the formation of the *myelocyte*, involves a noticeable reduction in cell size as well as a change in the appearance of the nucleus and cytoplasm (Plate 9-1L). Whereas the nucleus of a promyelocyte is only slightly indented (Fig. 9-7), the more ovoid nucleus of the myelocyte develops a deeper indentation and it assumes a more eccentric position within the cell (Plate 9-1L and Fig. 9-6). Generally, such a cell is not called a myelocyte until it contains approximately a dozen granules in its cytoplasm. However, myelocytes that are more

mature may become fairly heavily loaded with granules. The specific granules that appear at this stage (shown in *blue* in Fig. 9-6) enable three different types of myelocytes to be distinguished, with neutrophilic myelocytes predominating (Plate 9-1L). The three different types of myelocytes then go on to mature into the three different types of granular leukocytes; the capacity for mitosis is lost at the myelocyte stage (Fig. 9-6).

From the neutrophilic myelocyte stage on, Golgi-derived specific neutrophilic granules (shown in *blue* in Fig. 9-6) begin to accumulate. These specific granules are smaller, less electron dense, and rounder than the azurophilic granules; furthermore, they are not peroxidase-positive (Bainton, Farquhar, and coworkers).

A characteristic feature of the following stage of maturation, which is called the *metamyelocyte* (Gr. *meta*, beyond), is that its nucleus becomes more or less kidney-shaped. Again, three separate types of metamyelocytes are recognized based on the color of their specific granules. The appearance of a neutrophilic metamyelocyte is shown in Plate 9-1M. Continuing maturation in each granulocyte series leads to further diminution in cell size and additional changes in nuclear shape, first to the *band* (horseshoe) form (Plate 9-1N) and then to the *segmented* (lobed) form that characterizes the mature granulocyte (Plate 9-1O and Plate 8-1F and G).

A large pool of mature neutrophils is held in reserve in myeloid tissue. Bacterial endotoxin is known to trigger release of these reserve cells into the peripheral blood.

Eosinophil Formation. The first stage of the eosinophil series to become microscopically recognizable is the eosinophilic myelocyte. By the metamyelocyte stage, the slightly indented nucleus has developed a constriction that subsequently deepens until the nucleus becomes subdivided into two lobes interconnected by a thin strand (see Plate 8-1F). The maturation of an eosinophil also involves progressive condensation of its chromatin, but the depth of nuclear staining in a mature eosinophil remains less than that in a mature neutrophil (compare F with D in Plate 8-1). The lysosomal specific granules of eosinophils develop in the same way as the lysosomes of other kinds of cells do (Bainton and Farquhar).

Basophil Formation. The nucleus of a basophilic myelocyte undergoes less change than occurs in the formation of a neutrophil. At the metamyelocyte stage, it may develop irregular constrictions, but it generally becomes bilobed. The chromatin of the basophil remains incompletely condensed and stains relatively lightly. In contrast, the specific granules stain very deeply, and where present over the nucleus, they tend to obscure it. Unlike the lysosomal specific granules of the eosinophil, the specific granules of the basophil represent secretory granules.

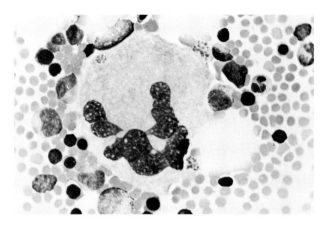

Fig. 9-8. Photomicrograph of a megakaryocyte in a marrow film, showing its huge size in comparison with erythrocytes and its large, multilobed nucleus.

Morphologically Recognizable Stages of Formation of Nongranular Leukocytes

Morphologically recognizable precursors of nongranular leukocytes cannot be distinguished as readily as those of granulocytes, even at their later stages of differentiation. The microscopically distinguishable precursors of monocytes are called monoblasts and promonocytes. Monocytes mature from promonocytes and only divide under unusual circumstances. In contrast to neutrophils, large numbers of mature monocytes are not retained as a reserve pool in the bone marrow.

Hematologists are able to recognize lymphocytic precursors called lymphoblasts and prolymphocytes, but it requires a great deal of training to be able to distinguish these cells from other precursors in myeloid tissue that have a similar microscopic appearance. In a marrow film, it should nevertheless be possible to recognize (1) small lymphocytes that represent their progeny cells (Plate 9-1G) and (2) plasma cells that represent progeny cells of antigen-stimulated B-lymphocytes (Plate 9-1H).

Megakaryocyte Maturation and Platelet Formation

Megakaryocytes are extremely large cells with a large, dark-staining nucleus that is made up of a number of interconnected lobes (Fig. 9-8 and Plate 9-1I). This nuclear morphology is a result of polyploidy; most megakaryocytes have eight times the diploid chromosome number. In addition to their huge nucleus, megakaryocytes possess a great deal of cytoplasm. The function of these cells is to produce blood platelets, which are liberated fragments of cytoplasm that circulate in the peripheral blood.

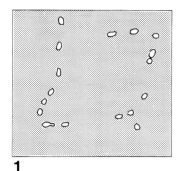

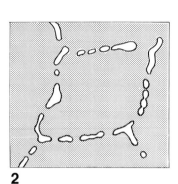

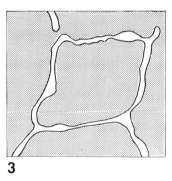

Fig. 9-9. Diagram showing how a platelet is formed from the cytoplasm of a megakaryocyte through the development and fusion of cytoplasmic vesicles to form platelet demarcation channels.

In marrow sections, megakaryocytes are much larger than any other marrow cells (see Figs. 9-1 and 9-2). If observed in only a single plane of focus, a megakaryocyte with a multilobed nucleus may appear to be a multinucleated cell. Careful focusing will nevertheless disclose that what seem to be separate nuclei are interconnected. Megakaryocytes can thereby be distinguished from osteoclasts, which are large multinucleated cells that are sometimes present on bone surface (see Fig. 12-14). Osteoclasts can generally be recognized by their proximity to bone tissue, but by focusing on nuclei, any osteoclasts that seem to lie within the marrow can be distinguished from megakaryocytes.

Megakaryocytes are end cells that become polyploid by undergoing *endoreduplication*, which means chromosomal

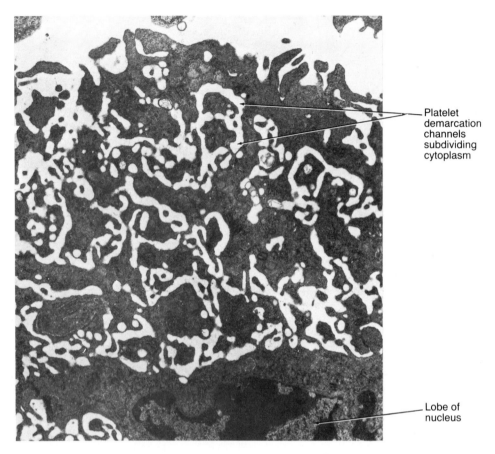

Platelet
demarcation
channels
subdividing
cytoplasm

Lobe of
nucleus

Fig. 9-10. Electron micrograph of part of a megakaryocyte (mouse) showing the formation of platelet demarcation channels, along which its cytoplasm will fragment to produce platelets. (Courtesy of V. I. Kalnins)

replication that is not followed by division of the cytoplasm. Furthermore, when they undergo nuclear division, their daughter chromosomes do not segregate into separate nuclei, and this results in the formation of a single, multilobed polyploid nucleus. This unique process is termed *endomitosis.* Increased ploidy is an essential prerequisite for the maturation of megakaryocyte cytoplasm that leads to the production of platelets. As noted in connection with platelets in Chapter 8, there is evidence that megakaryocyte maturation and platelet production are promoted by a humoral regulator called thrombopoietin.

Polyploid megakaryocytes develop a complex and anastomosing internal membrane system that subdivides their cytoplasm into numerous portions, each with its own limiting membrane. The process begins with the extensive development of membranous vesicles that are arranged as depicted in Figure 9-9. The cytoplasmic portions that become demarcated in this manner are approximately the size of a platelet. The individual vesicles fuse with their neighbors (Fig. 9-9) and are apparently able to establish

continuity with the cell membrane so that the cytoplasm becomes riddled with surface-connected anastomosing *platelet demarcation channels* (Fig. 9-10). In this way, platelets are able to separate from the megakaryocyte and still retain a covering membrane.

Observations made with the scanning electron microscope and time-lapse studies performed *in vitro* support an early observation that megakaryocytes are also able to extend cytoplasmic processes (now termed *proplatelet processes* or *platelet ribbons*) into the lumen of myeloid tissue sinusoids. Platelets are therefore probably able to pinch off from the tips of these processes as well. Hence platelets are presumably liberated a few at a time from proplatelet processes before being produced by terminal fragmentation of the entire cytoplasm.

SELECTED REFERENCES

General

TAVASSOLI M, YOFFEY JM: Bone Marrow Structure and Function. New York, Alan R Liss, 1983

WRIGHT DG, GREENBERGER JS: Long-Term Bone Marrow Culture. Kroc Foundation Series, Vol 18. New York, Alan R Liss, 1984

Myeloid Stroma and Sinusoids

BIGELOW CL, TAVASSOLI M: Studies on conversion of yellow marrow to red marrow by using ectopic bone marrow implants. Exp Hematol 12:581, 1984

DE BRUYN PPH: Structural substrates of bone marrow function. Seminars in Hematology 18:179, 1981

FRIEDENSTEIN AJ: Precursor cells of mechanocytes. Int Rev Cytol 47:327, 1976

FRIEDENSTEIN AJ, CHAILAKHYAN RK, LATSINIK NV ET AL: Stromal cells responsible for transferring the microenvironment of the hemopoietic tissues. Transplantation 17:331, 1974

LICHTMAN MA: The relationship of stromal cells to hemopoietic cells in marrow. In Wright DG, Greenberger JS (eds): Long-Term Bone Marrow Culture. Kroc Foundation Series, Vol 8, p 3. New York, Alan R Liss, 1984

TAVASSOLI M: Marrow adipose cells and hemopoiesis: An interpretive review. Exp Hematol 12:139, 1984

TAVASSOLI M, FRIEDENSTEIN A: Hemopoietic stromal microenvironment. Am J Hematol 15:195, 1983

WEISS L: The structure of bone marrow. Functional interrelationships of vascular hematopoietic compartments in experimental hemolytic anemia: An electron microscope study. J Morphol 117:467, 1965

WEISS L: The hematopoietic microenvironment of the bone marrow: An ultrastructural study of the stroma in rats. Anat Rec 186:161, 1976

WEISS L, CHEN LT: The organization of hematopoietic cords and vascular sinuses in bone marrow. Blood Cells 1:617, 1975

ZAMBONI L, PEASE D: The vascular bed of the red bone marrow. J Ultrastruct Res 5:65, 1961

Hematopoietic Stem Cells and Progenitors and Their Regulators

ABRAMSON S, MILLER RG, PHILLIPS RA: The identification in adult bone marrow of pluripotent and restricted stem cells of the myeloid and lymphatic systems. J Exp Med 145:1567, 1977

ADAMSON JW, FIALKOW PJ, MURPHY S ET AL: Polycythemia vera: Stem cell and probable clonal origin of the disease. N Engl J Med 295:913, 1976

ALLEN TD, DEXTER TM: The essentials of the hemopoietic microenvironment. Exp Hematol 12:517, 1984

AXELRAD A, CROIZAT H, ESKINAZI D ET AL: Gene controlled negative regulation of DNA synthesis in erythropoietic progenitor cells. J Cell Physiol (Suppl) 1:165, 1982

AXELRAD AA, MCLEOD DL, SUZUKI S, SHREEVE MM: Regulation of the population size of erythropoietic progenitor cells. In Differentiation of Normal and Neoplastic Hemopoietic Cells, p 155. Cold Spring Harbor, NY, Cold Spring Harbor Laboratory, 1978

BECKER AJ, MCCULLOCH EA, TILL JE: Cytological demonstration of the clonal nature of spleen colonies derived from transplanted mouse marrow cells. Nature 197:452, 1963

BEKKUM VAN DW, VAN DEN ENGH GJ, WAGEMAKER G ET AL: Structural identity of the pluripotential hemopoietic stem cell. Blood Cells 5:143, 1979

BRADLEY TR, METCALF D: The growth of mouse bone marrow cells in vitro. Aust J Exp Biol Med Sci 44:287, 1966

BROXMEYER HE, DE SOUSA M, SMITHYMAN A ET AL: Specificity and modulation of the action of lactoferrin, a negative feedback regulator of myelopoiesis. Blood 55:324, 1980

CORMACK D: Time-lapse characterization of erythrocytic colony-forming cells in plasma cultures. Exp Hematol 4:319, 1976

DENBURG JA, MESSNER H, LIM B ET AL: Clonal origin of human basophil/mast cells from circulating multipotent hemopoietic progenitors. Exp Hematol 13:185, 1985

DEXTER TM: The message in the medium. Nature 309:746, 1984

DEXTER TM, SPOONCER E, VARGA J ET AL: Stromal cells and diffusible factors in the regulation of haemopoietic cell development. In Killmann SA, Cronkite EP, Muller–Berat CN (eds): Haemopoietic Stem Cells, p 303. Copenhagen, Munksgaard, 1983

EVERETT NB, PERKINS WD: Hemopoietic stem cell migration. In Cairnie AB, Lala PK, Osmond DG (eds): Stem Cells of Renewing Populations. New York, Academic Press, 1976

FAUSER AA, MESSNER HA: Identification of megakaryocytes, macrophages and eosinophils in colonies of human bone marrow containing neutrophilic granulocytes and erythroblasts. Blood 53:1023, 1979

FIALKOW PJ: Cell lineages in hematopoietic neoplasia studied with glucose-6-phosphate dehydrogenase cell markers. J Cell Physiol (Suppl) 1:37, 1982

FIALKOW PJ: Hierarchal hematologic stem cell relationships studied with glucose-6-phosphate dehydrogenase enzymes. In Killmann SA, Cronkite EP, Muller–Berat CN (eds): Haemopoietic Stem Cells, p 174. Copenhagen, Munksgaard, 1983

FIALKOW PJ, DENMAN AM, JACOBSON RJ, LOWENTHAL MN: Chronic myelocytic leukemia: Origin of some lymphocytes from leukemic stem cells. J Clin Invest 62:815, 1978

FIALKOW PJ, JACOBSON RJ, PAPAYANNOPOULOU T: Chronic myelocytic leukemia: Clonal origin in a stem cell common to the granulocyte, erythrocyte, platelet and monocyte/macrophage. Am J Med 63:125, 1977

FOWLER JH, WU AM, TILL JE ET AL: The cellular composition of hemopoietic spleen colonies. J Cell Physiol 69:65, 1967

HEATH DS, AXELRAD AA, MCLEOD DL, SHREEVE MM: Separation of the erythropoietin-responsive progenitors BFU-E and CFU-E in mouse bone marrow by unit gravity sedimentation. Blood 47:777, 1976

ICHIKAWA Y, PLUZNIK DH, SACHS L: In vitro control of the development of macrophage and granulocyte colonies. Proc Natl Acad Sci USA 56:488, 1966

ISCOVE NN, SIEBER F: Erythroid progenitors in mouse bone marrow detected by macroscopic colony formation in culture. Exp Hematol 3:32, 1975

JOHNSON GR, METCALF D: Pure and mixed erythroid colony formation in vitro stimulated by spleen conditioned medium with no detectable erythropoietin. Proc Natl Acad Sci USA 74:3879, 1977

JONES–VILLENEUVE E, PHILLIPS RA: Potentials for lymphoid differentiation by cells from long term cultures of bone marrow. Exp Hemat 8:65, 1980

DE KLEIN A, VAN KESSEL AG, GROSVELD G ET AL: A cellular oncogene is translocated to the Philadelphia chromosome in chronic myelocytic leukemia. Nature 300:765, 1982

LORD BI: Haemopoietic stem cells. In Potten CS (ed): Stem Cells: Their Identification and Characterization, p 118. Edinburgh, Churchill Livingstone, 1983

MAK TW, MCCULLOCH EA (eds): Cellular and Molecular Biology of Hemopoietic Stem Cell Differentiation. New York, Alan R Liss, 1982 (also published as J Physiol (Suppl 1) 1982)

MCCULLOCH EA, MAK TW, PRICE GB, TILL JE: Organization and communication in populations of normal and leukemic hemopoietic cells. Biochim Biophys Acta 355:260, 1974

MCCULLOCH EA, TILL JE: The sensitivity of cells from normal mouse bone marrow to gamma radiation in vitro and in vivo. Radiat Res 16:822, 1962

MCCULLOCH EA: Stem cells in normal and leukemic hemopoiesis. Blood 62:1, 1983

MESSNER HA, IZAGUIRRE CA, JAMAL N: Identification of T lymphocytes in human mixed hemopoietic colonies. Blood 2:402, 1981

MESSNER HA, LIM B, JAMAL N, TAKAHASHI T: Lymphoid cells in multilineage colonies. In Killmann SA, Cronkite EP, Muller–Berat CN (eds): Haemopoietic Stem Cells, p 338. Copenhagen, Munksgaard, 1983

METCALF D, MOORE MA: Haemopoietic Cells. Amsterdam, North Holland, 1971

METCALF D: The molecular biology and functions of the granulocyte-macrophage colony-stimulating factors. Blood 67:258, 1986

MONETTE FC: Cell amplification in erythropoiesis: In vitro perspectives. In Dunn CDR (ed): Current Concepts in Erythropoiesis, p 21. New York, John Wiley & Sons, 1983

MOORE MAS, METCALF D: Ontogeny of the haemopoietic system: Yolk sac origin of in vitro and in vitro colony-forming cells in the developing mouse embryo. Br J Haematol 18:279, 1970

MOORE MAS, WILLIAMS N, METCALF D: In vitro colony formation by normal and leukemic human hematopoietic cells: Characterization of the colony forming cells. J Nat Cancer Inst 50:603, 1973

NAKAHATA T, OGAWA M: Identification in culture of a class of hemopoietic colony-forming units with extensive capability to self-renew and generate multipotential hemopoietic colonies. Proc Natl Acad Sci USA 79:3843, 1982

OGAWA M, PORTER PN, NAKAHATA T: Renewal and commitment to differentiation of hemopoietic stem cells (An interpretive review). Blood 61:823, 1983

PORTER PN, OGAWA M: Erythroid burst-promoting activity (BPA). In Dunn CDR (ed): Current Concepts in Erythropoiesis, p 81. New York, John Wiley & Sons, 1983

PRCHAL JT, THROCKMORTON DW, CARROLL AJ ET AL: A common progenitor for human myeloid and lymphoid cells. Nature 274: 590, 1978

SCHRADER JW: Bone marrow differentiation in vitro. In Atassi MZ (ed): CRC Critical Reviews in Immunology, Vol 4, p 197. Boca Raton, FL, CRC Press, 1983

STEPHENSON JR, AXELRAD AA, MCLEOD DL, SHREEVE MM: Induction of colonies of hemoglobin-synthesizing cells by erythropoietin in vitro. Proc Natl Acad Sci USA 68:1542, 1971

STROME JE, MCLEOD DL, SHREEVE MM: Evidence for the clonal nature of erythropoietic bursts: Application of an in situ method for demonstrating centromeric heterochromatin in plasma cultures. Exp Hematol 6:461, 1978

SUDA T, SUDA J, OGAWA M: Single-cell origin of mouse hemopoietic colonies expressing multiple lineages in variable combinations. Proc Natl Acad Sci USA 80:6689, 1983

TILL JE: Stem cells in differentiation and neoplasia. J Cell Physiol (Suppl) 1:3, 1982

TILL JE, MCCULLOCH EA: A direct measurement of the radiation sensitivity of normal mouse bone marrow cells. Radiat Res 14:213, 1961

TILL JE, MCCULLOCH EA: Hemopoietic stem cell differentiation. Biochim Biophys Acta 605:431, 1980

WENDLING F, SHREEVE M, MCLEOD D, AXELRAD A: A self-renewing, bipotential erythroid/mast cell progenitor in continuous cultures of normal murine bone marrow. J Cell Physiol 125:10, 1985

WRIGHT EG, LORD BI, DEXTER TM, LAJTHA LG: Mechanisms of haemopoietic stem cell proliferation control. Blood Cells 5:247, 1979

WU AM, TILL JE, SIMINOVITCH L, MCCULLOCH EA: A cytological study of the capacity for differentiation of normal hemopoietic colony-forming cells. J Cell Physiol 69:177, 1967

Maturation of Erythrocytes

KRANTZ SB, JACOBSON LO (eds): Erythropoietin and the Regulation of Erythropoiesis. Chicago, University of Chicago Press, 1970

NIENHUIS AW, BENZ EJ: Regulation of hemoglobin synthesis during the development of the red cell. N Engl J Med 287:1318, 1371, 1430, 1977

REPASKY EA, ECKERT BS: The effect of cytochalasin B on the enucleation of erythroid cells in vitro. Cell Tissue Res 221:85, 1981

Maturation of Granulocytes

BAINTON DF, FARQUHAR MC: Differences in enzyme content of azurophil and specific granules of polymorphonuclear leukocytes: Cytochemistry and electron microscopy of bone marrow cells. J Cell Biol 39:299, 1968

BAINTON DF, FARQUHAR MC: Origin of granules in polymorphonuclear leukocytes: Two types derived from opposite faces of the Golgi apparatus in developing leukocytes. J Cell Biol 28:277, 1966

BAINTON DF, FARQUHAR MC: Segregation and packaging of granules in eosinophilic leukocytes. J Cell Biol 45:54, 1970

BAINTON DF, ULLYOT JL, FARQUHAR MC: The development of neutrophilic polymorphonuclear leukocytes in human bone marrow: Origin and content of azurophil and specific granules. J Exp Med 134:907, 1971

FARQUHAR MC, BAINTON DF: Cytochemical Studies on Leukocyte Granules. Proc 4th Int Cong Histochemistry and Cytochemistry, Kyoto, Japan, p 25. Published by the Soc Histochemistry and Cytochemistry, 1972

Maturation of Nongranular Leukocytes

BRAHIM F, OSMOND DG: Radioautographic studies of the production and fate of bone marrow lymphocytes and monocytes. Proc Canad Fed Biol Soc, pp 136–137, 1967

NICHOLS BA, BAINTON DF, FARQUHAR MG: Differentiation of monocytes. Origin, nature and fate of their azurophilic granules. J Cell Biol 50:498, 1971

OSMOND DG: Potentials of bone marrow lymphocytes. In Cairnie AB, Lala PK, Osmond DG (eds): Stem Cells of Renewing Cell Populations. New York, Academic Press, 1976

OSMOND DG, MILLER SC, YOSHIDA Y: Kinetic and hemopoietic properties of lymphoid cells in the bone marrow. In Haemopoietic Stem Cells. Ciba Foundation Symposium 13 (new series). Amsterdam, ASP (Elsevier, Excerpta Medica, North-Holland), 1973

Maturation of Megakaryocytes and Platelet Formation

BECKER RP, DE BRUYN PPH: The transmural passage of blood cells into myeloid sinusoids and the entry of platelets into the sinusoidal circulation; a scanning electron microscopic investigation. Am J Anat 145:183, 1976

BENTFIELD–BARKER ME, BAINTON DF: Ultrastructure of rat megakaryocytes after prolonged thrombocytopenia. J Ultrastruct Res 61:201, 1977

HOFFMAN R, MAZUR E, BRUNO E, FLOYD V: Assay of an activity in the serum of patients with disorders of thrombopoiesis that stimulates formation of megakaryocytic colonies. N Engl J Med 305:533, 1981

PENINGTON DG: The cellular biology of megakaryocytes. Blood Cells 5:5, 1979

WRIGHT JH: The histogenesis of the blood platelets. J Morphol 21:263, 1910

YAMADA E: The fine structure of the megakaryocyte in the mouse spleen. Acta Anat 29:267, 1957

10

Lymphatic Tissue and the Immune System

The second type of hematopoietic tissue is *lymphatic (lymphoid) tissue*, which is represented by a small group of organs and tissues consisting of the *thymus, lymphatic nodules (lymphoid follicles), lymph nodes,* and *spleen*. An obvious characteristic of the four forms of lymphatic tissue is that they are densely populated with lymphocytes. This is because they are involved with lymphocyte production, immune responses, or both of these processes occurring at the same time. The four forms of lymphatic tissue are often referred to as parts of the *immune system;* a *system* is a group of body components that carries out some special function for the body as a whole. In addition, lymph nodes belong to the *lymphatic system,* the part of the circulatory system that collects and drains lymph. Lymph nodes are included in this system because they are distributed at intervals along the course of the larger lymphatic vessels and because one of their principal functions is to filter the lymph that is going to be returned to the circulating blood.

As already explained in the section on Amorphous Ground Substance in Chapter 7, lymph originates as the surplus tissue fluid that blood capillaries are unable to resorb (see Fig. 7-7). After collecting in lymphatic capillaries, this excess fluid drains along an anastomosing system of *lymphatics (lymphatic vessels)* and enters the *thoracic duct* and *right lymphatic duct,* which are two large *lymphatic ducts* that open into the junctions between the subclavian and internal jugular veins on the left and right sides of the body, respectively. From the two lymphatic ducts, lymph is continuously being returned to the blood circulatory system. Prior to its reaching the bloodstream, however, lymph and any *foreign antigens* (defined in Chap. 7 under Plasma Cells) that it may contain *must pass through lymph nodes.*

Hence a lymph node situated along the course of a lymphatic that is draining a site of infection can filter bacteria from the lymph that is passing through it, thereby reducing their chances of entering the bloodstream. As a result, the node may become secondarily infected and swollen. Similarly, malignant cells may dissociate from the primary tumor of a cancer patient, gain access to a lymphatic, and be filtered out in a lymph node, whereupon they may give rise to a secondary malignant growth. A secondary malignant tumor is termed a *metastasis* (Gr. *meta,* beyond; *stasis,* stand). The spleen likewise serves as a filter for the peripheral blood. This filtering function of lymph nodes and the spleen depends on their resident population of macrophages.

Here we should also point out that because only one form of *lymphatic tissue* is intimately associated with the lymphatic system per se, it is really more precise to refer to the family of lymphatic tissues and organs as the *lymphoid tissues* or as parts of the *lymphoid system.*

Small Lymphocytes Are Recirculating Immunocompetent Cells. As will be explained later in this chapter, a key step in lymphocyte differentiation is the acquisition of a particular *antigenic specificity* by each lymphocyte. This step is known as *programming for antigen recognition,* and as a result of it, every small lymphocyte acquires the unique capacity to recognize a specific antigen. Furthermore, these cells are continuously interchanging from the bloodstream to the lymph and then back again, a process called *recirculation.* To cross over from the blood to the lymph, lymphocytes have to escape from a certain type of blood vessel mostly present in lymph nodes, whereupon they are caught up in the stream of lymph that is flowing through these nodes and subsequently are returned with it to the bloodstream. During their double path of recirculation through the body (starting in the bloodstream, then entering the lymph, then returning to the blood again), they have a high probability of encountering any foreign antigens that may have entered the body. Such an encounter can elicit an immune response. Hence the majority of lymphocytes found in the blood or lymph represent *recirculating immunocompetent cells,* which means cells with a fully developed functional capacity to recognize and respond to foreign antigens. As already noted in the preceding chapters, the small lymphocytes that are present in the blood and lymph are made up of two main classes. Those that differentiated in the *thymus* are termed *T-lymphocytes* and

those that arose in the *bone marrow* (which corresponds to the *bursa of Fabricius* in chickens) are called *B-lymphocytes.*

THE ROLE OF LYMPHOCYTES IN IMMUNE RESPONSES

The body's adaptive response to certain potentially harmful foreign macromolecular substances, infections, and other persistent sources of non-self antigens (an organ transplant obtained from an unrelated donor, for example) is to mount an *immune response.* Immune responses entail the recognition of any foreign antigens (and hence recognition of their cellular source), and they are directed toward total elimination of such antigens or their cellular source from the body. They differ from the acute inflammatory reaction and other constitutive defense mechanisms of the body (*e.g.,* nonspecific phagocytosis) mainly in that they are *highly specific.*

Immune Responses Can Be Antibody-Mediated or Cell-Mediated. There are two distinct types of immune responses. One type, already mentioned in Chapter 7 in connection with plasma cells, results in the production of *circulating immunoglobulins* and is therefore termed the *humoral antibody response.* The *plasma cells* that secrete humoral antibodies are produced by *B-lymphocytes* in response to antigen, but this type of response generally requires the help of T-lymphocytes as well. The other type of immune response is termed the *cell-mediated immune response.* It is carried out by *cytotoxic T-lymphocytes* (also known as *killer cells*) that are capable of recognizing and destroying cells with surface antigens that are detectably different from the surface macromolecules on the body's own cells. This type of response is mediated by the progeny of antigen-activated T-lymphocytes without requiring the participation of B-lymphocytes. Both types of response are triggered by an encounter between a lymphocyte and the antigen it is programmed to recognize.

Lymphocyte Activation. When a small lymphocyte comes into contact with an antigen to which it responds, it develops into a much larger cell with abundant free ribosomes and polysomes in its cytoplasm (Fig. 10-1). Its content of cytoplasmic RNA increases to such an extent that its cytoplasm becomes intensely basophilic. Then it replicates its DNA and undergoes a series of divisions that generates a clone of identically programmed cells. The antigen-induced changes that precede this clonal expansion of the lymphocyte are described as *lymphocyte activation.* An *activated lymphocyte* is an enlarged lymphocyte that has recently responded to an antigen; it can attain a diameter of up to 30 μm, thereby becoming larger than the so-called large lymphocytes of peripheral blood.

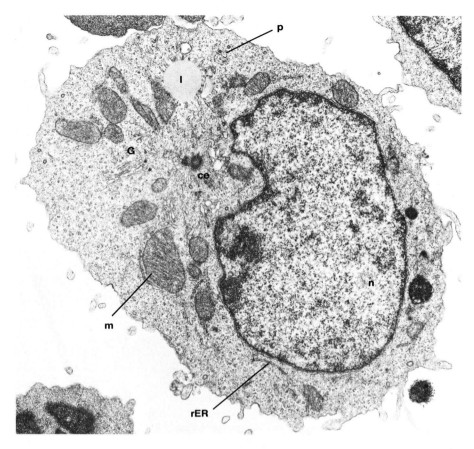

Fig. 10-1. Electron micrograph (×13,500) of an activated T-lymphocyte, obtained from mouse spleen and activated with concanavalin A. The cell is relatively large and its nucleus (*n*) contains a great deal of extended chromatin. Many free ribosomes and polysomes (*p*), together with mitochondria (*m*), a lipid droplet (*l*), a pair of centrioles (*ce*), a small amount of rough-surfaced endoplasmic reticulum (*rER*), and a prominent Golgi complex (*G*), can be distinguished in the cytoplasm. (Waterhouse PD, Anderson PJ, Brown DL: Exp Cell Res 144:367, 1983)

Mixed Lymphocyte Cultures. It is possible to take advantage of lymphocyte activation when screening for particular forms of human leukocyte antigen (HLA)-incompatibility between transplant recipients and the prospective donors (the general nature of HLA antigens was discussed under Leukocytes in Chap. 8). Thus any mismatching of certain HLA-D antigens (HLA class II antigens) will become apparent if leukocyte samples obtained from the recipient and from this prospective donor are cocultured as a *mixed lymphocyte culture* (MLC). If some of these cells enlarge and subsequently divide, indicating that antigenic differences exist between the prospective donor and recipient, histoincompability at one or more HLA loci is indicated. This kind of reaction is termed the *mixed lymphocyte reaction* (MLR), and most of the responding cells are known to be a subpopulation of T-lymphocytes.

B-LYMPHOCYTES AND THEIR INVOLVEMENT IN THE HUMORAL ANTIBODY RESPONSE

Each B-lymphocyte becomes able to recognize a particular antigen. To explain this, it is first necessary to consider what determines the specificity of an antibody molecule. An immunoglobulin molecule is made up of four polypeptide chains with a small number of attached oligosaccharide groups. Two of the four chains are *heavy chains* that are

identical to each other, and the other two are *light chains* that are identical to each other. The heavy chains are so called because they contain a larger number of amino acids than the light chains. The molecule is Y-shaped and hence it is bilaterally symmetrical. Whereas the stem of the Y is made up of parts of the two heavy chains, each arm is made up of the remainder of the heavy chain together with a light chain lying beside it.

At the tip of each arm of the Y, there is an *antigen-recognition site* that can interact specifically with an antigen. Part of each antigen-recognition site is constructed from a heavy chain and part is constructed from a light chain. The specificity of the antigen-recognition site is determined by its amino acid sequence. To denote that the antigen-recognizing specificity of different antibody molecules is due to variability in the terminal half of each arm of the Y, this part of the immunoglobulin molecule is called its *variable region*. The remainder of the molecule is called its *constant region*. The genes that code for the amino acid sequence of the variable region confer sufficient antigen-recognizing diversity on immunoglobulin molecules for them to be able to recognize virtually every antigen that enters the body.

Antibody Diversity Is Created by Gene Recombination and Somatic Mutation. The fact that the constant region of the immunoglobulin molecule is always the same suggests that the genes coding for the constant part of the molecule arose from a single primordial gene that underwent reduplication during the course of evolution. A number of separate genes coding for the variable region are inherited through the germ cells. Through genetic recombination they generate a broad range of antibody specificities that is further broadened by somatic mutation. Each B-lymphocyte progenitor expresses a gene that codes for the variable region of the light chain and also a gene that codes for the variable region of a heavy chain, generating a unique antigen-recognizing specificity. For further information about the generation of antibody specificity, see Tonegawa.

Antigenically Programmed B-Lymphocytes Play a Key Role in the Humoral Antibody Response

The particular gene combination that is established in a B-lymphocyte is a matter of chance. Thereafter, the B-lymphocyte is committed to producing immunoglobulin molecules of the same antigenic specificity; in other words, it is *antigenically determined.* Following its activation, all its progeny cells remain identically programmed, producing antibody molecules of the same specificity. Prior to activation, each B-lymphocyte bears small patches of specific surface immunoglobulin (in most cases *sIgM* and *sIgD*) on its surface. (IgM and IgD are two classes of immunoglobulin that will be described later in this chapter; the prefix s denotes that they are expressed on the cell surface.) These tiny patches of sIg enable the B-lymphocyte to recognize the particular antigen for which it is programmed. When the B-lymphocyte encounters this antigen, it becomes activated, resulting in its clonal amplification and differentiation into antibody-producing cells of the same antigenic specificity. Hence the antigen-recognition sites on a B-lymphocyte represent the cell-surface equivalent of the antibody molecules that its progeny cells will subsequently secrete.

Some of the progeny cells of an activated B-lymphocyte do not differentiate into plasma cells. Instead, they acquire more sIg and persist as an amplified population of B-lymphocytes called *B-memory cells.* These cells retain the morphological appearance of small lymphocytes and, in contrast to the B-lymphocytes of peripheral blood, which have only a short lifespan, they can remain in the lymphatic organs for long periods—hence the term B-memory cells. Furthermore, enough of them are produced to effect more immediate and more extensive production of antibody to the same antigen if they become reexposed to it. Such an amplified response is called a *secondary response.* It differs from a *primary* immune response (*i.e.*, the immune response elicited by initial contact with a given antigen) in that it is more rapid in onset and produces antibody in larger quantities. Hence the essential difference between a primary response and a secondary response is that there is a larger number of B-lymphocytes to respond to the antigen in a secondary response. All subsequent responses to the same antigen are referred to as secondary responses.

Factors Produced by T-Helper Cells Generally Are Required for an Effective B-Cell Response to an Antigen. As a general rule, a number of stringent conditions must be met before a B-lymphocyte can become activated. First, the appropriate antigen must bind to the antigen-recognition sites on its cell surface. The other requirements all involve the cooperation of a subset of T-lymphocytes known as *T-helper cells.* For a T-helper cell to assist in the activation of a B-lymphocyte, it needs to be programmed to respond to the same antigen as the B-lymphocyte. Furthermore, a factor known as *interleukin 1* (IL-1), which is produced by macrophages and other kinds of accessory cells, is known to promote the proliferation of T-helper cells of any specificity by stimulating these cells to produce another factor called *interleukin 2* (IL-2) that, in turn, induces T-cell proliferation. The result of this two-stage process is that it nonspecifically increases the population size of T-helper cells available to promote B-cell activation. (The action of IL-2 will be mentioned again when we consider lymphokines.) When the antigen combines with the receptors on a T-helper cell programmed to recognize that antigen, it triggers the release of a number of different soluble T-cell factors (*T-cell lymphokines*), several of which are now known to be required in most cases for antigen-induced B-cell activation, proliferation, and maturation to form antibody-secreting cells. A few antigens (notably bacterial polysaccharides) effectively activate B-cells without requiring the participation of T-helper cells, but these antigens constitute the exception, not the rule. Such antigens are described as *T-cell independent antigens.* Also, there are indications that T-helper cells may not be an absolute requirement for the production of antibodies of the IgM class.

To simplify matters, we shall defer detailed discussion of the specific requirements that must be met before a T-helper cell can become activated by an antigen and thereupon release the factors concerned. These precisely regulated conditions will be discussed when we deal with T-lymphocytes, the functionally heterogeneous family of thymus-derived lymphocytes to which T-helper cells belong. The following synopsis will nevertheless provide an overview of how B-cell activation, clonal expansion, and maturation of progeny cells into plasma cells seem to be effected.

It has now become evident that a series of progressive changes occurs when a B-lymphocyte becomes activated by antigen. Prior to its activation, a B-cell or T-cell exists in the G_0 (nondividing) state. However, a T-helper factor (or factors) provided by T-helper cells has the capacity to induce an antigen-stimulated resting B-lymphocyte to leave G_0 and enter the G_1 stage of the cell cycle. There are also other T-cell factors, termed replication factors, that are evidently necessary to induce effective continuing proliferation of this B-cell following its antigen-specific entry into the cell cycle. A third group of T-cell factors is believed to be responsible for inducing maturation of progeny cells of the activated B-lymphocyte into plasma cells. For further details, see Melchers and Andersson.

The Development of B-Lymphocytes.   Two stages of B-lymphocyte differentiation have now been characterized. The earliest of these is the *pre–pre-B-lymphocyte,* which is believed to represent the unipotential B-lymphoid stem cell (or a very early progenitor of the B-lymphocyte) in bone marrow. Cells at this stage of differentiation do not produce any detectable levels of immunoglobulin. The pre–pre-B-lymphocyte gives rise to cells called *pre-B-lymphocytes* that produce immunoglobulin M (IgM, which will be described later in this chapter). However, the immunoglobulin is confined to the cytoplasm of pre–B-lymphocytes without being expressed on their cell surface, so these cells are still not able to recognize or respond to specific antigens. The *B-lymphocytes* that arise from them, on the other hand, bear IgM on their surface (*sIgM*) in addition to having this so-called cIgM in their cytoplasm; hence they develop the capacity to recognize and respond to specific antigens. For further information about the differentiation of B-lymphocytes, see Levitt and Cooper, and Cooper.

We shall now go on to consider the various types of T-lymphocytes and their respective roles in the two kinds of immune responses.

T-LYMPHOCYTES AND THEIR ROLE IN IMMUNITY

The majority of the peripheral blood lymphocytes (roughly 60% to 80% of the small lymphocytes) represent long-lived recirculating T-cells. Radiation-induced chromosomal aberrations have been found in some of these cells 10 years after patients have been treated with radiation, indicating a lifespan in excess of 10 years.

During the course of differentiation in the thymus, each T-lymphocyte becomes programmed to recognize and respond to a particular antigen. However, its antigen-recognition sites, which are termed *T-cell receptors,* are not actually immunoglobulin molecules as they are in B-cells. The T-cell receptor is nevertheless made up of two polypeptide chains, each with a variable and a constant region and small oligosaccharide side chains (Yanagi et al, Hedrick et al). Furthermore, like sIg, it is firmly anchored in the cell membrane as an integral membrane protein. It is believed that the T-cell receptor recognizes its corresponding antigen in the same way that an immunoglobulin molecule does. As in B-lymphocytes, unique antigenic specificities are generated by recombination between gene segments that encode the variable regions of the receptor.

The Recognition of Foreign Antigens by T-Cells Is MHC-Restricted.   Whereas B-lymphocytes are able to recognize antigen by itself, most T-cells will only respond to a foreign antigen if it is presented to them on the surface of an *accessory cell,* which is a suitable type of macrophage or some other kind of *antigen-presenting cell.* Moreover, the antigen has to be presented along with integral cell membrane glycoproteins encoded by genes of the major histocompatibility complex (MHC). In other words, for most T-lymphocytes to become activated by an antigen, a *dual recognition process of the foreign antigen and a self-MHC an-*

tigen on the same cell surface is necessary. This unique capacity of the T-lymphocyte for recognizing such an association between two different kinds of antigens on the surface of a cell is attained during T-cell differentiation in the thymus. Perhaps not everyone would agree that education amounts to learning how to recognize two things at the same time, but the T-lymphocytes' acquisition of this useful capacity is often referred to as *thymic education.*

This requirement that the foreign antigen be presented in the context of unequivocal molecular proof of the individual's own identity increases the chances that T-lymphocytes will detect any foreign antigens that may become expressed on the surface of the body's own cells (*e.g.,* as a result of a viral infection). This mandatory requirement for documented self-identification also ensures rapid detection of foreign MHC glycoproteins on any cells that are foreign to the body, triggering a cell-mediated immune response that will eradicate them. It is not yet clear whether the T-cell receptor is able to recognize a foreign antigen and a self-MHC antigen both at the same time or whether this recognition process involves a combination of two distinct T-cell receptors. As a rule, *T-helper cells* recognize a foreign antigen in the context of a family of MHC-encoded glycoproteins called *HLA class II antigens* on the surface of *antigen-presenting cells,* whereas *cytotoxic T-cells (killer cells)* recognize a foreign antigen in the context of another family of MHC-encoded glycoproteins called *HLA class I antigens.* Hence recognition of a foreign antigen by a T-cell is described as being *MHC-restricted.*

T-Lymphocytes Consist of a Number of Different Functional Subsets

Despite their uniform microscopic appearance, T-lymphocytes do not constitute a functionally homogeneous population. Instead, they represent a number of different *functional subsets,* each with its own characteristic function, lifespan, and repertoire of antigenic surface markers by which its members can be identified (Reinherz and Schlossman). Functional competence with respect to a T-cell function is acquired during the differentiation of T-lymphocytes in the thymus.

Broadly speaking, there are two main categories of T-lymphocytes: *regulatory T-cells* and *cytotoxic T-cells (T_C cells).* The two subtypes of *regulatory T-cells* are (1) *T-helper (T_H) cells,* which are required for the induction of T-dependent B-cell responses and also for cytotoxic T-cell/T-suppressor cell activation by antigen, and (2) *T-suppressor (T_S) cells,* which can suppress both the humoral antibody response and the cell-mediated immune response. T_S cells can inhibit B-cell function directly and also by inhibiting T_H activation. Some T_S cells are antigen-specific whereas others seem to lack antigenic specificity. The *cytotoxic T-cells* are *killer cells* that carry out the cell-mediated immune response. Of the subsets of T-lymphocytes that can be identified, when activated by antigen one acts as T_H cells and another acts as either T_C cells or T_S cells.

Other subsets that have been described include *T-memory cells*, which are long-lived progeny cells of T-lymphocytes corresponding to B-memory cells, and *T-amplifier (T_A) cells*, which are less mature, short-lived T-cells that remain in the spleen and thymus without recirculating and that have been found to enhance the functional activities of B- and T-lymphocyte populations. Finally, there are *delayed hypersensitivity T-cells (T_{DH} or T_D)*. These cells play an important role in *delayed hypersensitivity reactions,* which also depend on the persistence of T-memory cells and protect the body against certain major infectious diseases including tuberculosis, syphilis, and leprosy. When activated, T_{DH} cells secrete a number of *lymphokines* (Gr. *kinesis*, movement), which are hormonelike soluble factors that affect other cells. A few lymphokines are now known to be produced by B-lymphocytes as well. T_{DH} cells are so closely similar to T_H cells that they could even represent the same cell population.

Lymphokines. Exposure of certain subsets of T-lymphocytes to antigens leads to the release of a remarkable array of lymphokines. One of these factors, *interleukin 2* (IL-2), which is alternatively known as *T-cell growth factor* (TCGF), binds to receptors that become expressed on the surface of activated T-cells of any antigenic specificity and enables them to continue to proliferate indefinitely. Other lymphokines include factors that facilitate or suppress humoral and cell-mediated immune responses (*T-helper* and *T-suppressor factors*) and that induce cellular proliferation (*mitogenic factor*), loss of macrophage mobility (*migration-inhibitory factor*, MIF), enlargement and increased phagocytic activity of macrophages (*macrophage-activating factor*, MAF), inhibition of viral replication (*interferon*), and sustained proliferation and differentiation of myeloid progenitors (*colony-stimulating factors*). T- and B-lymphocytes also produce a lymphokine called *osteoclast-activating factor* (OAF), which is a polypeptide that induces osteoclastic bone resorption (Horton et al; Chen et al). Hence T-lymphocytes play a central role in regulating a broad range of cellular processes, including several that are not strictly immunological.

The Role of Cytotoxic T-Cells in Cell-Mediated Immunity.

Once a cytotoxic T-cell specifically recognizes the antigenically different surface of a target cell, it establishes intimate contact with the cell that it is about to destroy. Such an immune response involving *cell-to-cell contact* between a lymphocyte and its target cell is described as a *cell-mediated immune response*. Unlike the situation in which killing is mediated by humoral antibody, complement is not required for killing by this type of response. The cell-mediated immune response is the primary cause of graft rejection following organ or tissue transplantation from an unrelated donor. In addition to having a primary role in transplantation immunity, cytotoxic T-cells can destroy certain disease-causing bacteria (notably the tubercle bacillus that causes tuberculosis), fungi, and virus-infected cells, thereby limiting viral replication.

Recent work on the mechanism of target cell lysis by cytotoxic T-cells (T_C cells), and also by natural killer cells (NK cells), which will be considered later in the chapter, indicate that target cell lysis by granulated forms of these cells may be due to the induction of characteristic circular porelike lesions in the target cell membrane (Podack). These lesions seem to be membrane perforations at sites where tubular complexes have been inserted into the target cell membrane. The source of the protein monomers from which these tubular complexes are assembled has been traced to the large cytoplasmic granules that characterize certain forms of cytolytic T-lymphocytes and NK cells. After such a cytolytic T-lymphocyte or NK cell establishes direct contact with a target cell, the microtubular skeleton of the cytotoxic cell becomes reoriented, bringing the Golgi complex and cytolytic granules of this cell into proximity with the contact area (for further information, see Young and Cohn). When the granules have been maneuvered into this position, their contents are discharged by exocytosis. Granule-mediated lysis at Ca^{2+}-dependent, and it is accompanied by DNA degradation that could be due to activation by incoming Ca^{2+} of a Ca^{2+}-dependent endonuclease. Hence although target cell *recognition* by a T_C cell is antigenically *specific*, the mechanism by which it is *killed* is *nonspecific*.

It is of interest that a comparable reorientation of the microtubular skeleton brings the Golgi complex into closer apposition with the site of cell-to-cell contact when an MHC-restricted T_H cell interacts with an antigen-presenting B-lymphocyte (Kupfer et al).

Transplantation Terminology. A graft made from one site on an individual to another site on the *same individual* is generally referred to as an *autograft* (Gr. *autos*, self). The same kind of graft is sometimes described as *autochthonous*, which means indigenous. A graft or transplant made from an individual to a *genetically similar individual* (*e.g.*, between identical twins or between a donor and recipient of the same inbred strain) is described as *syngeneic* (Gr. *syn*, together) or as an *isograft* (Gr. *isos*, equal). A graft made between *genetically nonidentical* members of the *same species* is termed an *allograft* (Gr. *allos*, another) and is described as *allogeneic*. The older term for this type of graft, *homograft*, is now considered inappropriate because *homos* means the *same*. A graft made between members of two *different species* is termed a *heterograft* (Gr. *heteros*, other). Another term for this type of graft is *xenograft* (Gr. *xenos*, stranger).

Allograft Rejection. Autografts and isografts usually take quite readily. However, an allograft will generally elicit an *allograft reaction (rejection response)* that can be recognized histologically by the fact that the graft and graft bed soon become heavily infiltrated with *graft rejection cells* (Fig. 10-2). The majority of these early infiltrating cells represent cytotoxic T-cells (killer cells). In most cases, they are generated in the vicinity of the graft site in local lymph nodes. They pass through the efferent lymphatics of these nodes and enter the blood circulation, where they need to make only one circuit before entering loose connective tissue. Here they migrate randomly, and those that encounter the allograft are able to recognize and destroy its cells. Many of those that miss the allograft are found in the superficial

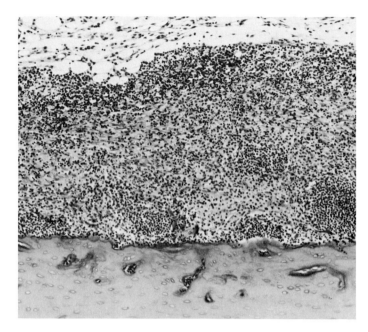

Fig. 10-2. Photomicrograph of a bone allograft undergoing an allograft reaction (rat). The dense connective tissue of the periosteum (middle third of photomicrograph) exhibits a particularly heavy infiltration of graft rejection cells. Dead bone is present at bottom. (Courtesy of F. Langer and K. Pritzker)

layer of connective tissue (lamina propria) beneath the epithelial lining of the intestine. For further information about the types of cells involved in allograft rejection, see Carpenter.

In addition to provoking a cell-mediated immune response, the foreign antigens of an allograft will activate B-lymphocytes of the recipient. This leads to the production of humoral antibodies that are directed against these antigens. However, the surface antigens on most kinds of body cells lie too far apart for complement to become fixed when antibody binds to them. Hence when humoral antibodies are produced in response to allograft antigens, they do not necessarily have a deleterious effect on the transplanted cells. Indeed, by combining with the foreign antigens on these cells, they can actually have the opposite effect. This is because surface-bound antibodies can hide surface antigens from cytotoxic T-cells and hence interfere with the recognition of foreign cells by the killer cells that have set out to destroy them. This effect of humoral antibody is known as *enhancement* because the production of antibody may actually *enhance survival of the allograft.*

Measures Can Be Taken to Reduce the Chances of Allograft Rejection. Allograft rejection is, of course, the main obstacle to success in attempts to transplant organs from one person to another. Initial crossmatching of HLA antigens of the donor to those of the recipient is important in selecting the donor. Immunosuppressive measures can then be used to suppress allograft rejection. One approach is to administer *immunosuppressive drugs* that interfere with lymphocyte proliferation, but this is not without some danger because these drugs will also reduce the recipient's capacity to ward off infections.

Surface Markers Can Be Used to Distinguish T-Lymphocytes from B-Lymphocytes. No consistent morphological differences can be recognized between T- and B-lymphocytes. However, a number of specific surface determinants, listed previously in Table 8-3, have now been identified by which these two types of lymphocytes may be distinguished from each other. Furthermore, there are distinctive T-cell markers called *OKT (T) antigens* that are characteristic for human T-lymphocytes and their various subsets.

Thus whereas B-lymphocytes possess surface (membrane) immunoglobulin (primarily sIgM with or without sIgD) that is detectable by means of suitable immunofluorescent staining, T-lymphocytes lack this marker. On the other hand, T-lymphocytes have the characteristic but unexplained property of forming *rosettes* with *sheep erythrocytes*, which means that erythrocytes obtained from a sheep will adhere to the surface of human T-lymphocytes. B-lymphocytes lack these so-called *E rosette* surface receptors for sheep erythrocytes. Other differences have not turned out to be consistent criteria for distinguishing between B- and T-lymphocytes. Thus Fc receptors and C3 receptors, which were initially thought to be distinctive surface markers for B-cells and cells of the granulocytic and monocytic lineages, are also present on certain subpopulations of T-cells and certain types of null cells (namely NK and K cells, which will be described in a subsequent section). For further discussion about these surface markers, see Vogler et al.

Additional B- and T-Cell–Associated Antigens Can Be Distinguished Through the Use of Monoclonal Antibodies. In recent years it has also become possible to detect unique surface antigens on human B-lymphocytes and T-lymphocytes by their capacity to bind *monoclonal antibodies*, which are monospecific antibodies produced by antibody-secreting hybridoma cell lines. The first step in raising a monoclonal antibody is to immunize an experimental animal with the antigen that is being studied. Then antibody-producing cells obtained from the spleen of the immunized animal are induced to fuse with *myeloma cells*, which are rapidly proliferating transformed cells that are capable of perpetuating antibody secretion (Milstein; Diamond et al). The resulting hybrid cells are called *hybridoma* cells (which is short for *hybrid-myeloma* cells). A continuous clonal cell line can then be grown from any hybridoma cell that expresses the relevant antigenic specificity. The main advantages of this technological achievement are that (1) it ensures an inexhaustible supply of antibody that has been produced under rigorously controlled conditions and (2) the antibody that it produces is *monospecific;* in other words, it lacks the unwanted specificities that so often limit the usefulness of the mixture of antibodies generally obtained as a result of an immunization procedure.

At least seven cell-surface antigens that seem to be uniquely associated with human B-cells have now been recognized through the use of mouse monoclonal antibodies. Termed *CD antigens* (for clusters of *d*ifferentiation), some (the *pan B-cell antigens*, [Gr. *pan,* all]) are present on all B-cells whereas others are expressed only at particular stages of development or during activation. Monoclonal antibodies specific for such markers are now being used in studies of B-cell differentiation and in the detection and characterization of B-cell malignancies.

In the T-cell series, monoclonal antibodies have been used to identify pan T-cell antigens and also T-subset antigens. These surface antigens include the E rosette receptor for sheep erythrocytes (CD2), which is a pan T-cell marker, the T (OKT) antigens (see Table 8-3), and several others. Each of these antigens has now been given a CD designation according to an internationally accepted nomenclature. T_H cells express T4 (CD4), and T_C/T_S cells express T8 (CD8).

Null Cells, Natural Killer Cells, and Antibody-Dependent Killer Cells.

Cells of the lymphocyte series that do not possess a characteristic set of surface markers that identifies them as either T- or B-lymphocytes are described as *null cells* (L. *nullus*, not any). Roughly 5% to 10% of the peripheral blood lymphocytes are null cells. They are believed to include certain early differentiation stages of B- and T-lymphocytes. This null cell population also includes two possibly overlapping classes of cytotoxic lymphocytes (antibody-independent *n*atural *k*iller or *NK cells* and antibody-dependent *k*iller cells or *K cells*) that, under *in vitro* conditions, have been found to manifest spontaneous inherent cytolytic activity toward (1) some but not all kinds of cancer cells, (2) certain kinds of engrafted normal cells (*e.g.,* those of transplanted bone marrow), and (3) a few microorganisms. However, there seems to be more than one type of these cells because some are null cells and others bear T-cell markers. For further information about these interesting cells, see Herberman, and Herberman and Ortaldo.

Most neoplasms that develop from lymphocytes can be classified as being of either T- or B-cell origin; those that are of neither T- nor B-cell origin are classified as *null cell* tumors.

The Development of T-Lymphocytes.

As in the case of B-lymphocytes, the antigenic specificities of T-lymphocytes are generated on a random basis as a result of somatic recombination of gene segments and do not require the participation of the antigens concerned. T-lymphocytes are produced in the thymus from T-lymphoid stem cells called *prethymocytes* or *prothymocytes*. These stem cells arise from bone marrow (also from the liver and spleen during fetal life) and migrate to the thymus, whereupon they are influenced by the thymic microenvironment, notably its epithelial reticular cells and the hormones that they produce. It appears that prethymocytes entering the thymus may have already undergone determination with respect to their antigenic specificity and functional capacity. However, they do not become immunocompetent until they have proliferated, differentiated into *thymocytes,* and emerged from the thymus as *peripheral blood T-cells.* T-cell maturation is then completed in the peripheral blood.

The differentiation pathway of T-lymphocytes has been worked out in considerable detail. Thymocyte reactivity to monoclonal antibodies has permitted distinctions to be made between an early type of thymocyte, an intermediate type of common thymocyte, and mature thymocytes of two different kinds, one corresponding to the T4 (CD4)-positive T_H subset and the other representng the T5 and T8 (CD8)-positive T_C/T_S subset. Immunological competence is acquired at the mature thymocyte stage but does not become fully developed until these cells leave the thymus as peripheral T-lymphocytes. The lymphoid cells in the thymic medulla, unlike those of the thymic cortex, are immunocompetent and similar (if not identical) to peripheral T-cells.

Before going on to describe the microscopic structure of the thymus, we shall briefly consider some current ideas about the nature of immunological tolerance and the manner in which the body remains tolerant to its self-constituents.

TOLERANCE AND AUTOIMMUNITY

Under normal conditions, the body does not mount immune responses that are directed against its own macromolecules. Yet such molecules are immunogenic if they are introduced into the body of another individual, and under unusual conditions, they may elicit an immune response in the body in which they reside. Furthermore, the effective concentration of a foreign antigen (particularly if this concentration is either very high or very low) and the particular conditions under which the antigen stimulates cells of the immune system determine whether the antigen will elicit an immune response. A specific lack of responsiveness to an antigen is called *immunological tolerance,* and immunological reactivity directed against self-macromolecules is termed *autoimmunity.*

There appear to be a number of different ways in which tolerance can be established. It is evident, for example, that it can be induced at either the T-cell or the B-cell level, although as a rule, it is more readily established at the T-cell level.

It was initially proposed by Burnet that tolerance induction at the T-cell level is due to *clonal deletion* of T-cells as a result of premature contact with the antigen for which they are programmed. However, it has subsequently been found that T-cells carrying anti–self-specificity do exist in the body, so total annihilation of the troublemakers cannot be the explanation. The idea of clonal deletion then gave way to the general belief that tolerance is entirely due to the generation of appropriately programmed T-suppressor (T$_S$) cells. This newer view is based on the finding that the spleen of a tolerant animal contains specific T$_S$ cells that, when transfused into a nontolerant animal, can render it tolerant also. However, *in vitro* studies now indicate that relatively high concentrations of antigen can also induce T-cell nonresponsiveness in a direct manner, particularly when the antigen is not presented in the usual way (*i.e.*, on the surface of antigen-presenting cells). Furthermore, T-helper clones can be rendered nonresponsive in this manner in the total absence of any suppressor cells. Hence it is not certain that T$_S$ cells are necessary for tolerance *induction.* Nor does clonal deletion seem to be involved, because following the induction of high-dose tolerance in these studies, the cloned T-helper cells remained alive and well and were responsive to IL-2. For further details, see Feldmann et al.

There is also evidence that B-cell exposure to a high concentration of antigen leads to a subsequent lack of B-cell reactivity to that particular antigen, particularly if this is done in the absence of T-helper cells in the case of a T-dependent antigen. This is especially true of B-cells obtained from newborn animals.

From the foregoing discussion, it is evident that both the availability of antigens and the circumstances under which T-lymphocytes may become exposed to them can be instrumental in determining whether an individual becomes immunologically responsive or tolerant to these antigens. In this connection, it is worth mentioning that in the thymic cortex, T-lymphocytes possessing new antigenic specificities are generated under antigen-depleted conditions. The purpose of the substantial measure of protection from circulating and lymph-borne antigens that exists awaits clarification. One idea is that it represents a safeguard against unnecessary or inappropriate clonal expansion of the newly generated T-lymphocytes. However, a second advantage of antigenic shielding during T-cell differentiation and maturation in the thymus is that it reduces the chances of exposure to antigen concentrations that are high enough to cause inappropriate high-dose tolerance. In support of this suggestion, it has been shown that tolerance to an antigen can indeed result from intrathymic injection of that antigen.

The connection between acquired tolerance to a foreign antigen and the body's natural tolerance of its own macromolecules is still being elucidated, but it is widely believed that T-suppressor cells play a key role in maintaining the tolerant state toward self-antigens. When such tolerance of the body's own macromolecules breaks down, an *autoimmune disease* (Gr. *autos,* self) develops. Autoimmunity seems to be able to develop in a number of different ways. In *chronic thyroiditis* (*Hashimoto's disease*), for example, thyroglobulin—a self-antigen that is normally secluded from the rest of the body in thyroid follicles—comes into contact with the immune system and is thereupon mistaken for a foreign antigen. If non-self-antigens such as those expressed by a drug or virus become attached to the surface of body cells, they can make these cells seem foreign to the immune system. Certain other autoimmune diseases seem to be a result of cross-reacting immune responses that eventually involve normal body components as well as the foreign antigens that elicited these responses. In short, any unusual form of recognition or case of mistaken identity of a body antigen may be manifested as an autoimmune disease. Normally, among populations of lymphocytes that are potentially reactive to self-antigens, there is a delicate balance between those that are capable of promoting autoreactivity and those that are capable of suppressing it. If this balance is upset and suppression is outweighed, autoimmunity results. For further discussion of this important group of diseases, see Rose.

THE LYMPHATIC (LYMPHOID) ORGANS

The *lymphatic (lymphoid) organs* are broadly classified as (1) *central (primary)* or (2) *peripheral (secondary).* The central lymphatic organs are the sites where new lymphocytes are autonomously produced; hence they include the bone marrow as well as the thymus. The peripheral lymphatic organs are the sites where lymphocytes respond to antigens, and they include the lymph nodes, spleen, tonsils, other mucosa-associated lymphatic tissue, and even the skin. We shall now consider the various lymphatic organs, beginning with the thymus.

THE THYMUS

The *thymus* is a somewhat triangular, bilobed lymphatic organ, most of which lies immediately posterior to the upper part of the sternum where it appears as a flattened pinkish-gray mass. Its size relative to the rest of the body is greatest at birth. Beginning at about the time of puberty, however, it begins to involute, gradually diminishing in size with advancing age yet apparently still producing some new lymphocytes. This process of involution is accelerated by adrenal corticosteroids and sex hormones. Thus oversecretion of adrenal corticosteroids as a result of disease or stress can lead to premature involution of the thymus, and a deficiency of such hormones can result in failure of the thymus to involute.

Synopsis of Development. The beginning of thymic development is marked by epithelial tubes growing into mesenchyme from the endodermal lining of the third and part of the fourth pharyngeal pouch on each side of the body. These endodermal tubes become solid cords that eventually

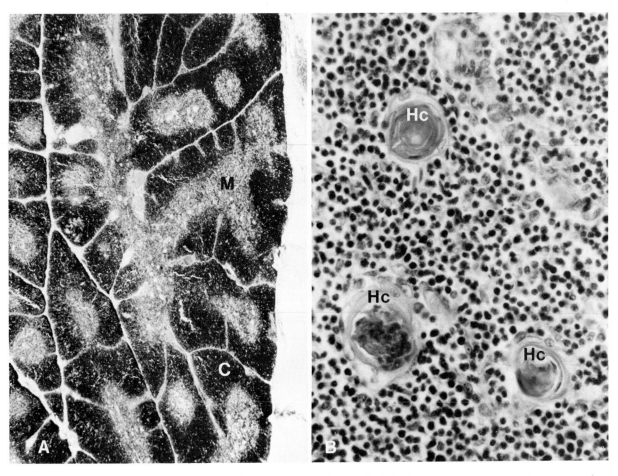

Fig. 10-3. (*A*) Very low-power photomicrograph of the thymus of a child. The septa appear as clear lines. The cortex (*C*) of the lobules is dark; the medulla (*M*) is light. The medulla of one lobule is continuous with that of another. (*B*) High-power photomicrograph of an area of medulla. Three thymic (Hassall's) corpuscles (*Hc*) are shown.

are pulled down into the thorax and lose their connection with their sites of origin. At this stage, the thymus resembles an endocrine gland because it is composed of cords of epithelial cells. These cords then develop side branches representing the core (medulla) of lobules. This arrangement of cells then begins to change. Groups of medullary epithelial cells become characteristically arranged in the form of concentric whorls called *thymic (Hassal's) corpuscles* (Fig. 10-3*B*). The presence of these structures, the flattened cells of which have a tendency to undergo a certain degree of keratinization, is a unique feature whereby a section of the thymus can generally be recognized. However, the functional significance of these structures remains undetermined. For the most part, the rest of the epithelial cells become arranged in the form of an extensive loose network of *epithelial reticular cells* (L. *rete*, net), the cytoplasmic processes of which are interconnected by desmosomes. The associated mesenchyme gives rise to a thin capsule around each lobe of the organ and thin septa that subdivide the

organ into incomplete lobules (Fig. 10-3*A*). Hence the central part of each lobule remains continuous with that of other lobules (Fig. 10-3*A, middle*) even though a lobule that has been sectioned parallel to and close to its external surface may appear completely surrounded by septa (Fig. 10-3*A, top right*). When the thymus begins to involute, adipocytes may accumulate in its septa.

The Thymus Consists of a Cortex and Medulla. The thymocyte population of each lobule is not evenly distributed; instead, it is concentrated toward the borders that abut on the capsule or septa. Dark-staining because of its dense population of developing T-lymphocytes, the peripheral part of each lobule is termed its *cortex* (L. for bark or shell). The paler staining central region of the lobule is called its *medulla* (Fig. 10-3*A*). The cortical population of developing T-lymphocytes lies freely suspended in the wide spaces between the epithelial reticular cells. It represents an intimate mixture of early, intermediate, and mature thymocytes at their various stages of differentiation and maturation. In addition, the thymus becomes infiltrated with stromal macrophages and dendritic cells; most of the latter are confined to the inner medulla. A final point about the general structure of the thymus is that unlike the arrangement found in lymph nodes, no lymphatics empty into it. Hence no lymph drains into the thymus. However, the thymus has efferent lymphatics that carry away surplus interstitial fluid and protein.

The Blood Supply of the Thymic Cortex.   The blood vessels that supply the thymic cortex are *all capillaries*. Thymic arteries extending from the inferior thyroid and internal thoracic arteries enter the thymic medulla and supply arterioles that extend along the corticomedullary junction. Injection studies in mouse thymus show that capillaries loop out from these arterioles into the thymic cortex in the form of anastomosing arcades (Raviola and Karnovsky). At the corticomedullary junction, the capillary arcades empty into medullary venules. Blood leaves the thymus by way of the inferior thyroid, internal thoracic, and left brachiocephalic veins.

The T-Lymphocytes Developing in the Thymic Cortex Are Shielded from High Concentrations of Antigens. There is experimental evidence that the microenvironment within the thymic cortex is fairly well shielded from blood-borne antigens (Raviola and Karnovsky). As already noted, a second form of antigenic protection is that the thymus *lacks afferent lymphatics* with the potential to supply antigens at even higher concentrations than are present in the blood.

To reach cortical thymocytes from the blood in a cortical capillary, a circulating antigen would have to be able to permeate the series of layers seen in Figure 10-4: (1) the endothelial lining of the vessel, (2) its basement membrane, (3) a layer of perivascular connective tissue, (4) the basement membrane of epithelial reticular cells, and (5) a continuous covering made up of these cells that represents an important part of the permeability barrier. Furthermore, macrophages are strategically located in the perivascular connective tissue in an appropriate position to intercept and remove any blood-borne antigens that may escape from a vessel. This unique combination of safeguards affords the cortical thymocytes a substantial measure of protection from circulating macromolecules, although their protection is not absolute because of possible indirect leakage from medullary venules. There are nevertheless enough anatomical barriers and perivascular macrophages to restrict access of macromolecules to the developing T-lymphocytes and to warrant use of the term *blood–thymus barrier*. The net result is that *only negligible levels of antigens reach these cells.*

The functional significance of the blood–thymus barrier remains uncertain, but some of the possibilities were discussed in the previous section on Tolerance and Autoimmunity. It is possible that if antigens were freely admitted to the thymic cortex, antigen-in-

duced clonal selection might generate huge clones of identically programmed T-lymphocytes instead of an even representation of T-lymphocytes with a broad repertoire of useful new specificities.

T-Lymphocytes Enter the Peripheral Blood from the Thymic Cortex. The thymic cortex serves as a lifelong source of T-lymphocytes, but it is most active in fetal and early postnatal life. Unlike the lymph nodes and spleen, the lymphatic tissue of which is almost nonexistent if an animal is isolated from contact with foreign antigens by being reared in a totally germ-free environment, the thymus produces T-lymphocytes continuously and its rate of lymphocyte production remains unaffected by antigen levels or the numbers of lymphocytes in the peripheral blood. Hence *the thymus produces T-cells autonomously.* In fact, so many T-cells leave the thymus that they could replace the entire blood lymphocyte population every 6 hours or so. In addition to the many T-cells that leave the thymus there are enormous numbers of these cells that die there.

One mechanism by which new antigenic specificities are known to be generated in T-lymphocytes is through somatic mutation in their rapidly proliferating progenitors. An extremely high incidence of cell death is seen in the thymic cortex; some estimates exceed 90% of the total thymocyte population. The most likely explanation of this high rate of cell death is that many of the mutants produced are nonviable.

In certain respects the thymic cortex and thymic medulla behave as if they were functionally independent of each other. Lymphoid stem cells generated in the bone marrow migrate through the walls of blood vessels situated in the outermost zone of the thymic cortex. As they and their progeny proliferate and differentiate, their progeny cells migrate from the outer cortex to the inner cortex. The T-cells that they produce can apparently leave the vicinity of the inner cortex, possibly by way of the medullary venules at the corticomedullary junction, without having to enter the substance of the thymic medulla. The T-cells characterizing the thymic medulla, on the other hand, evidently belong to the recirculating pool of T-lymphocytes and freely exchange with the T-lymphocytes in other lymphatic organs. The T-lymphocytes formed in the thymic cortex do not return to it after they have left, but recirculating immunocompetent T-lymphocytes can enter the thymic medulla, especially following T-cell activation.

Plasma cells are rarely present in the thymic cortex. This is because any B-lymphocytes that enter the cortex find themselves in an antigen-deficient environment in which they are unlikely to become activated. However, if B-cells enter the thymic medulla, they can become activated and will then give rise to plasma cells.

Thymic Hormones

It is possible to restore full immunological competence to an animal that has been thymectomized at birth by means of a thymic transplant. Such restoration is not due, as might

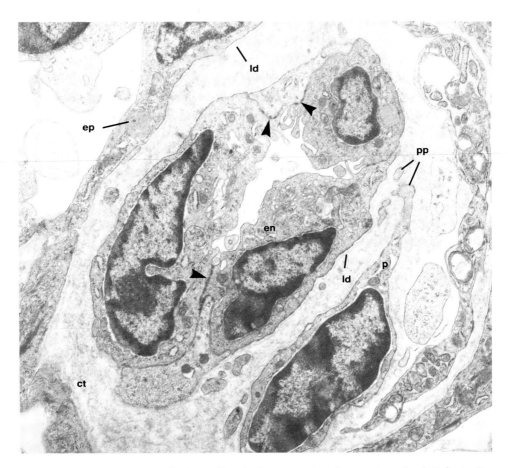

Fig. 10-4. Electron micrograph of a capillary in the cortex of rat thymus. Arrowheads indicate sites where the endothelial cells are joined by a number of tight junctions. The endothelial lining (*en*) is surrounded by its basement membrane (the lamina densa of which is labeled *ld*), a comparatively wide interstitial space containing perivascular connective tissue (*ct*), the basement membrane of epithelial reticular cells (the lamina densa of which is also labeled *ld*), and a covering of epithelial reticular cells (*ep*). A perivascular cell (*p*) that is probably a pericyte, together with its cytoplasmic processes (*pp*), is seen at lower right. (Anderson AO, Anderson ND, White JD: In Hay JB (ed): Animal Models of Immunological Processes, p 25. London, Academic Press, 1982)

be thought, to the acquisition a supplementary supply of T-lymphocytes from the transplanted thymus. This is because even with a syngeneic graft, most of the transplanted lymphoid cells die before the thymic circulation has had the chance to become reestablished. However, the epithelial reticular cells in the transplant survive, suggesting that it is these cells that play a role in the restoration of immunological competence.

This finding led to a suspicion that these cells might represent a source of humoral factors that are capable of promoting the differentiation of prethymocytes. The hypothesis was tested by transplanting thymic fragments confined within diffusion chambers into animals that had been thymectomized at birth. The pore size selected for these chambers was sufficient to permit the free passage of soluble factors but not cells. The results were as anticipated—the artificially encapsulated thymic tissue was still able to reverse the functional impairment associated with neonatal thy-

mectomy. From sections made of the residual thymic tissue in the chambers, it was evident that only a mass of epithelial reticular cells remained. It was therefore concluded that *thymic epithelial reticular cells elaborate diffusible factors that are capable of directing the differentiation of T-lymphocytes.*

These so-called *thymic hormones* produced by thymic epithelial reticular cells have turned out to be important because it is now known that T-lymphocytes differentiate from their progenitor cells under the influence of such hormones. One prospective thymic hormone secreted by these cells is a polypeptide called *thymopoietin*. Another contender is a slightly smaller polypeptide called *thymosin α_1*. Both of these polypeptides can rapidly induce the expression of T-lymphocyte surface markers on T-lymphocyte precursors.

There is also evidence that T-cell predecessors need to *pass through the thymus* before their progeny will become

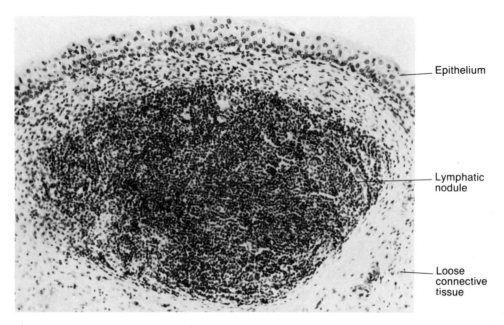

Epithelium

Lymphatic nodule

Loose connective tissue

Fig. 10-5. Photomicrograph of a lymphatic nodule lying in loose connective tissue beneath a wet epithelial membrane (urinary bladder of a dog). The epithelium above the lymphatic nodule is of the transitional type.

fully immunocompetent, possibly because T-cell differentiation is promoted by direct cellular interaction with epithelial reticular cells and close proximity to stromal macrophages. Processing by the thymic microenvironment is therefore regarded as an important stage of T-cell differentiation.

We shall next turn our attention to the peripheral (secondary) lymphatic tissues and organs, which show varying degrees of specialization toward facilitating immune responses to antigens. The simplest kind of arrangement is the solitary unencapsulated lymphatic nodule.

LYMPHATIC NODULES (LYMPHOID FOLLICLES)

In the superficial layer of loose connective tissue (*lamina propria*) that is situated beneath the wet epithelial lining of the intestine, respiratory tract, and urinary tract, it is not uncommon to find isolated aggregates of small lymphocytes (Fig. 10-5). Known as *lymphatic nodules* or *lymphoid follicles*, these roughly spherical aggregates have no limiting connective tissue capsule of their own, and hence they are described as a form of *unencapsulated lymphatic tissue*. In their simplest form, lymphatic nodules are solitary discrete structures approximately 1 mm in diameter. When observed under low power, they appear as a rounded, darkly stained mass consisting primarily of blue-stained nuclei of lymphocytes that stands out in contrast to the pale-staining background of loose connective tissue (Fig. 10-5). The out-

ermost border of the nodule is not sharply defined because there is no surrounding capsule.

Although wet epithelial membranes possess their own particular specializations for excluding inappropriate materials from the body, foci of epithelial cell death or damage and the development of minor leaks between contiguous cells can permit the access of infectious microorganisms and antigens from other sources (*e.g.,* food or pollen). The body's first line of immunological defense against any antigens or antigenic microorganisms that may succeed in entering the body by way of such discontinuities is represented by its unencapsulated lymphatic tissue. *Solitary lymphatic nodules* indicate sites where such antigens have entered the subepithelial connective tissue in concentrations sufficient to activate B-lymphocytes that are programmed to recognize them. Hence lymphatic nodules contain the clonal descendants of activated B-lymphocytes. Indeed, in lymphatic nodules that contain activated B-lymphocytes that are still in the process of enlarging and dividing, it is often possible to distinguish a lighter staining central region known as a *germinal center*. Such centers represent sites where the B-cells are still undergoing active proliferation and differentiation in response to continuing activation by an antigen or as a result of secondary exposure to an antigen; hence they indicate that immunological memory for that antigen has already been established. In addition, germinal centers are themselves believed to be a site where B-memory cells are generated.

The solitary lymphatic nodules that form and subsequently disperse in mucosal loose connective tissue represent expanded clones of B-lymphocytes; hence they correspond to the lymphatic nodules found in lymph nodes. As will be explained in the section that follows, the antigenically activated B-lymphocytes of at least certain kinds of mucosal lymphatic nodules can also serve as a source of the IgA-secreting plasma cells that are found in the lamina propria of mucosal membranes.

Solitary lymphatic nodules, then, are only temporary structures that develop in the lamina propria of mucous membranes as a result of specific antigenic stimulation of B-lymphocytes by antigens that they happen to encounter during their random wandering through this layer of loose connective tissue. The permanent peripheral lymphatic organs exhibit an increasingly complex design that facilitates B- and T-cell interaction and promotes direct contact between lymphocytes and the foreign antigens to which they can respond.

Peyer's Patches and Other Forms of Gut-Associated Lymphatic Tissue

The next level of complexity is seen in *permanent aggregates of lymphatic nodules* that can become large enough to extend down into the submucosal layer of connective tissue. Instead of being transitory, small, and solitary, such lymphatic nodules are permanent, large, multiple, and confluent. This type of organization is found in (1) the *tonsils*, which are confluent aggregates of more or less unencapsulated lymphatic tissue that are arranged in the form of an incomplete ring in the walls of the pharynx and nasopharynx and at the base of the tongue (*i.e.,* surrounding the crossover point between the digestive tract and the respiratory tract); (2) *Peyer's patches,* which are even larger masses of confluent lymphatic nodules situated in the walls of the small intestine, particularly the ileum; and (3) the *appendix,* which has extremely large masses of confluent lymphatic nodules in its walls.

Collectively, such permanent aggregates of confluent unencapsulated lymphatic nodules, together with solitary nodules of the temporary type already described, make up a large part of the *gut-associated lymphoid (lymphatic) tissue* (GALT). This lymphoid tissue, in turn, constitutes part of a more generalized *common mucosal immune system* that also includes the *bronchus-associated lymphoid tissue* (BALT).

Unlike the arrangement that we shall find in lymph nodes are not provided with afferent lymphatics or a well-defined surrounding capsule. Antigens are nevertheless able to reach them by diffusing through the lamina propria. In the case of the tonsils, Peyer's patches, and appendix, it is now clear that there is a special type of surface epithelial cell that is highly modified to keep bringing in tiny samples of intraluminal antigens so that these come into direct contact with gut-associated lymphatic tissue (Owen). Termed an *M cell* (for *m*embranelike epithelial cell) but also sometimes referred to as a FAE (*f*ollicle-*as-*

sociated *e*pithelial) cell, this is a dome-shaped cell with a basal cavity that becomes packed with so-called *intraepithelial leukocytes* (IELs), accompanied in some cases by a macrophage as well (Fig. 10-6).

The cytoplasm of an M cell is so thinly stretched that it cannot be distinguished in the LM; hence only the position of the cell is recognizable as a tiny nest of closely associated IELs. When seen in the electron microscope, the cytoplasm of the M cell appears fairly dark (Fig. 10-6*A*). Furthermore, the lateral borders of this type of cell are joined to contiguous borders of neighboring absorptive columnar cells by junctional complexes. Yet its cytoplasm contains few lysosomes, suggesting that its primary role is to transfer macromolecules across its attenuated cytoplasm instead of degrading them. In contrast to the numerous relatively long microvilli seen in the brush border on neighboring absorptive columnar cells, only tiny ridges or small numbers of short microvilli are present on the luminal surface of the M cell (Fig. 10-6*B*).

The role of the M cell is to transport representative samples of intraluminal antigens across its cytoplasm to closely associated lymphocytes and macrophages in the region of the lamina propria above confluent lymphatic nodules. Such antigen sampling is thought to be an important stage in the process of generating IgA-producing plasma cells. Secretory IgA is an effective defense mechanism that guards against infection by way of mucosal membranes. Antibodies of this class, which will be described in further detail later in this chapter, play a key role in maintaining mucosal immunity because they are able to decrease the adherence of microbes to the epithelial surface and they can neutralize viruses and bacterially produced intraluminal toxins.

The sequence of events that follows antigen sampling is clearest in the case of Peyer's patches. At the periphery of the lymphatic nodules in these aggregates, there are specialized venules called high endothelial venules (to be described later in this chapter) from which recirculating lymphocytes are able to leave the bloodstream and enter the lymphatic nodules. Those lymphocytes that enter the superficial region of the lamina propria may come into direct or indirect contact with antigen samples that are being transported there by way of M cell vesicles. Following contact with such antigens, B-lymphocytes become activated and generally undergo a certain amount of clonal expansion in the germinal centers of the lymphatic nodules within the patch. Their progeny cells then enter the efferent lymphatics of these nodules and are carried by the lymph to mesenteric lymph nodes, where they undergo further proliferation. Many of the progeny cells formed in the mesenteric lymph nodes then pass, along with the efferent lymph that leaves these nodes, to the thoracic duct lymph and enter the bloodstream. However, they subsequently leave the blood circulation and preferentially return to the lamina propria of mucosal membranes, including the same sites in the intestine from which their long itinerary began. Hence instead of giving rise directly to plasma cells, the activated B-cells in Peyer's patch nodules generate *circulating precursors of IgA-producing plasma cells.* When these precursor cells reach the right destination, they undergo final maturation into plasma cells and produce IgA that is thereupon transported across the mucosal epithelium into the gut lumen. For further information about these and other aspects of mucosal immunity, see Befus and Bienenstock, and Anderson et al.

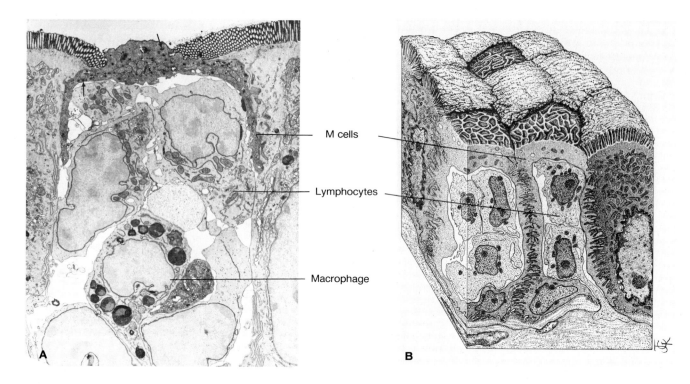

M cells

Lymphocytes

Macrophage

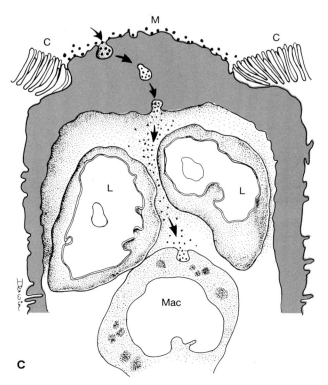

Fig. 10-6. (*A*) Electron micrograph, (*B*) three-dimensional drawing, and (*C*) interpretive schematic diagram of a portion of the epithelial covering above a lymphatic nodule in a Peyer's patch (mouse). Attenuated M cells (shown in blue and labeled M in *C*) extend as membranelike cytoplasmic bridges between the absorptive columnar epithelial cells present on either side (labeled C in *C*). Beneath the M cell shown in *A* and *C* lies a small nest of intraepithelial lymphocytes (labeled L in *C*) together with a central macrophage (*Mac*). The M cell provides a thin membranelike barrier between the lumen above and the lymphocytes in the intercellular space below. This M cell has taken up the enzyme horseradish peroxidase (HRP), an exogenous EM tracer represented by black dots in *C*, and has released it into the intercellular space below. Arrows in *A* indicate vesicles that are carrying HRP across the cell. Any macrophages (*Mac*) that may be present at this site will ingest macromolecules and particulate matter that reaches them by way of the same pathway. It is not clear whether the lymphocytes respond directly to incoming antigens in the subepithelial region or whether these antigens are carried first by cells to the germinal centers of the underlying lymphatic nodules. (*A* and *B*, Owen RL, Nemanic P: Scanning Electron Microscopy/ 1978/Vol 2:367, 1978; *C*, based on Owen RL: Gastroenterology 72: 440, 1977)

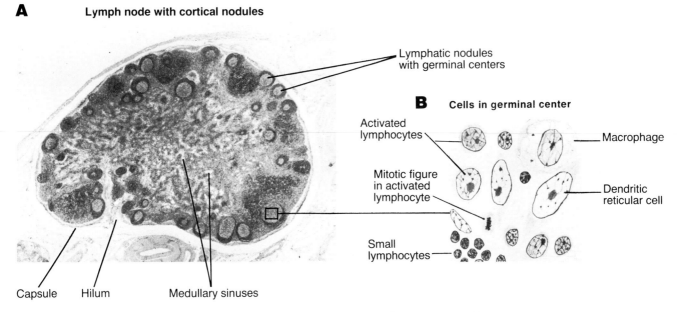

A   Lymph node with cortical nodules

Lymphatic nodules with germinal centers

B   Cells in germinal center

Activated lymphocytes

Macrophage

Mitotic figure in activated lymphocyte

Dendritic reticular cell

Small lymphocytes

Capsule   Hilum   Medullary sinuses

Fig. 10-7. (*A*) Photomicrograph of a lymph node (low power). (*B*) Drawing of some representative cells present in the germinal centers of its secondary lymphatic nodules (high power).

LYMPH NODES

Distributed along the course of the major tributaries that drain into the thoracic duct and right lymphatic duct, there are a number of kidney-shaped structures that are up to 2 cm long and are known as *lymph nodes*. These structures are relatively plentiful in the axillae and groin and also in association with the major blood vessels of the neck and mesentery.

As in the thymus, a lymph node possesses a *capsule* and has an outer *cortex* and an inner *medulla*. However, in this case, lymphocytes proliferate in the cortex and their progeny move directly into the medulla. Another difference of the cortex of a lymph node is that it is largely composed of *lymphatic nodules* (Figs. 10-7 and 10-8). Moreover, lymph nodes do not possess the epithelial reticular cell component found in the thymus.

The more complex organization of a lymph node enables it to perform two major functions. First, a large resident population of macrophages enables it to trap and remove any particulate matter that may be present in the lymph passing through it. This task is sometimes referred to as its *filtering function*. Secondly, its lymphocytes can become activated by any foreign antigens that may be present in this lymph, whereupon clonal expansion within the node contributes additional lymphocytes to the recirculating lymphocytes that leave the node by way of its efferent lymph. This is often referred to as its *lymphocyte-forming* function. Prolonged or secondary exposure to an antigen leads to the formation of germinal centers in its lymphatic nodules; however, these centers subsequently disappear

when the antigenic stimulus subsides. Moreover, depending on the type of antigenic stimulation that is involved, some of the progeny cells generated in these centers will differentiate into plasma cells whereas others will leave the node as cytotoxic T-cells. Hence there are many processes occurring in a lymph node, and not all of these would be immediately apparent to anyone observing it in histological section.

The Stromal Component of a Lymph Node

Surrounding a lymph node there is a distinct *capsule* made of dense ordinary connective tissue (Figs. 10-7 and 10-8). Because lymph nodes commonly lie in adipose tissue, some of this tissue may adhere to the capsule when the node is obtained for sectioning. Recognition of this fat tissue can help in distinguishing a section of lymph node from one of spleen, which has a smooth (serosal) surface. Some lymphatic vessels open onto the convex surface of the node whereas others leave from the deepest part of its indentation, which is termed its *hilum*. The lymphatics that convey lymph to the node are described as *afferent*, and those that carry it away are described as *efferent* (Fig. 10-8). Both kinds of lymphatics are provided with flap valves to prevent lymph from passing backward toward its site of origin. The capsule of the lymph node is thickest at the hilum, where it gives rise to connective tissue *trabeculae* (L. for small beams) that extend into the substance of the node, providing support and conveying blood vessels into the interior of the organ. Other trabeculae extend inward from the convex surface of the capsule (Fig. 10-8).

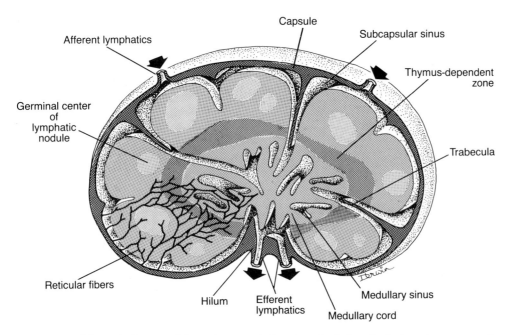

Fig. 10-8. Schematic diagram of the main parts of a lymph node. Its lymphatic tissue is represented in blue.

From the afferent lymphatics of the node, lymph drains into the *subcapsular sinus*, which is a narrow, lymph-filled space that is situated immediately beneath its capsule (Fig. 10-8). Lymph then flows into narrow channels that extend through the cortex and are accordingly known as *cortical sinuses*. These channels lead into similar medullary channels called *medullary sinuses* that deliver lymph to the efferent lymphatics draining the node (Fig. 10-8). The lymphatic sinuses are all lined by a layer of simple squamous endothelium that is either wholly or, in the case of the subcapsular sinus, partly discontinuous. Furthermore, in addition to lymph, these sinuses harbor free cells, most of which are lymphocytes and macrophages. Such cells are able to enter or leave the sinuses by passing through the gaps between their lining cells.

As in myeloid tissue, there are also stromal elements within the lymph node that serve to hold its free cells loosely in place. Its internal stroma is made up of connective tissue cells and their associated intercellular components, which are represented primarily by networks of reticular fibers that interconnect both with the capsule and with the trabeculae (Fig. 10-8). The stromal cells include macrophages, various subtypes of reticular cells, and fibroblasts.

The *macrophages* (see Fig. 10-13E) phagocytose and remove particulate matter and unwanted macromolecular constituents from the lymph before it is returned to the bloodstream. At least some types of macrophages can also facilitate immune responses, apparently by processing foreign antigens into a more immunogenic form that is more readily recognized by T-lymphocytes. It has been suggested that such enhanced immunogenicity results because traces of the ingested antigen escape complete degradation within secondary lysosomes and then become liberated from the cytoplasm by exocytosis. Such incompletely degraded macromolecules, along with undegraded antigens, can remain associated with the cell membrane of macrophages for a substantial length of time, possibly being held there through binding to preformed antibody molecules that have become attached by their Fc end to the Fc receptors on these cells (see Macrophages in Chap. 7).

Antigen molecules (both in undegraded and partly degraded form) are also believed to be displayed on the surface of other antigen-presenting cells. Notable among these is a subtype of reticular cells that is known as a *dendritic cell* or *dendritic reticular cell* because it possesses very long and apparently motile cytoplasmic processes (Gr. *dendron*, tree). This is a pale-staining, nonphagocytic type of cell that can retain foreign antigens on its surface for long periods. Like a macrophage, it presents such antigens to T-lymphocytes in the context of its own MHC-encoded self-recognition surface glycoproteins. In addition to being present in the cortex of lymph nodes, antigen-presenting cells of this type are also found in the lymphatic nodules of Peyer's patches and the white pulp of the spleen, where they evidently serve the same purpose.

The Lymphatic Component of a Lymph Node

Between the cortical sinuses, there is a meshwork of reticular fibers (Fig. 10-8) with abundant small lymphocytes

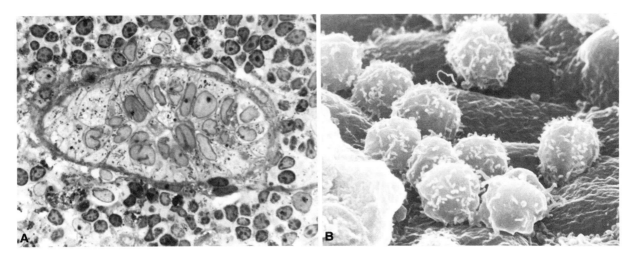

Fig. 10-9. (*A*) Photomicrograph of a postcapillary venule in a rat lymph node (semithin section, toluidine blue). The characteristic high endothelium of these vessels is specifically recognized by recirculating T- and B-lymphocytes. (*B*) Scanning electron micrograph (×875) of small lymphocytes adhering to the luminal surface of the cuboidal endothelial lining of a postcapillary venule. (*A*, Anderson ND, Anderson AO, Wyllie RG: Immunology 31:455, 1976; *B*, Anderson AO, Anderson ND: Immunology 31:731, 1976)

and a few stromal cells in its interstices. Within the medulla, there is a similar meshwork (Fig. 10-8) that is packed with small lymphocytes, a few stromal cells, and numerous plasma cells at various stages of maturation. In an antigen-stimulated lymph node, the more or less pyramidal regions of cortex that are densely populated with small lymphocytes assume a more rounded appearance (Fig. 10-7) because of the development of central pale *germinal centers* (Figs. 10-7 and 10-8). These spherical-to-ovoid accumulations of small lymphocytes so closely resemble the unencapsulated type of lymphatic nodule already described that they, too, are given the name *lymphatic nodules.* Lymphatic nodules that lack a germinal center are described as *primary*, whereas those that exhibit such a center are described as *secondary*. As in the case of a solitary unencapsulated lymphatic nodule, each lymphatic nodule in a lymph node has only a transitory existence. A narrow extension of the nodule reaches down into the medulla, where it becomes subdivided into a number of wavy columns of lymphoid cells. Termed *medullary cords,* these columns indicate sites where tortuous stromal passageways have become tightly packed with lymphoid cells (Fig. 10-8).

Extending from the lymphatic nodules of a lymph node to its medullary cords is its so-called *paracortical region* (Gr. *para,* beside). This region can be further subdivided into *mid* and *deep cortical regions.* An interesting feature of the deep cortical region is that it contains blood vessels of a special type that will now be described.

The Thymus-Dependent Zone of the Lymph Node Is Provided with High Endothelial Venules. Arteries enter the node at its hilum and then branch out in the form of

an arterial tree. Fine branches of this tree extend into the cortex of the node, where they supply arterial blood to the capillaries associated with the periphery of lymphatic nodules and other parts of the cortex. An unusual feature of the *postcapillary venules* into which these cortical capillaries empty is that they are provided with a *high endothelial lining;* hence they are commonly referred to as *high endothelial venules* or *HEVs* (Fig. 10-9). These specialized venules arch through the deep cortex near the corticomedullary junction (Fig. 10-10). The veins into which they drain accompany the arteries within the trabecular connective tissue and then leave the node at its hilum.

Whereas the postcapillary venules in other parts of the body are lined by simple squamous endothelium, the high endothelial venules (HEVs) of the lymph node are provided with a lining of simple *cuboidal* endothelium instead (Figs. 10-9 and 10-11). Recirculating T- and B-cells recognize and adhere to these high endothelial cells, whereupon they squeeze between them (Fig. 10-11) and enter the so-called *thymus-dependent zone* in the deep cortex of the node (Fig. 10-8). Hence HEVs are the sites where recirculating T- and B-cells cross over from blood to lymph in their path of recirculation through the body. For further information about these specialized vessels, see Anderson et al.

The *thymus-dependent zone* of the cortex is so named because it undergoes marked depletion following neonatal thymectomy. Its T- and B-cell composition reflects that of the peripheral blood circulating through it; hence T-cells predominate. T-Lymphocytes that encounter antigen in the lymph node generally become activated and undergo proliferation in the interfollicular (internodular) region. Fol-

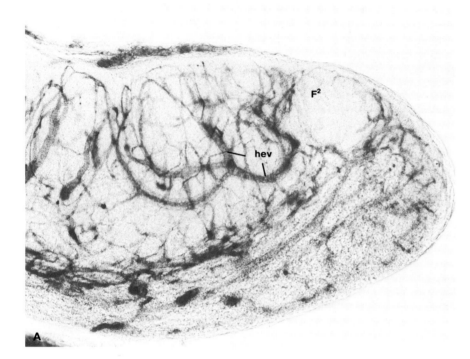

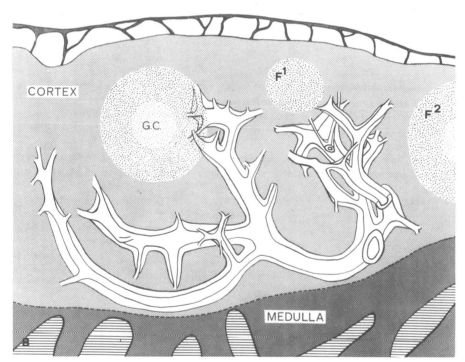

Fig. 10-10. (A) Photomicrograph of a cleared thick section of rat lymph node perfused with alcian blue, showing postcapillary venules with a high endothelial lining (high endothelial venules, *hev*) in its deep cortex. F² is a secondary lymphatic nodule. This preparation also shows that lymphatic nodules are not highly vascularized. (B) Interpretive diagram in which these postcapillary venules are indicated in white. F¹ and F² show the positions of two lymphatic nodules in the cortex; G.C. indicates the germinal center of a secondary lymphatic nodule. Part of the subcapsular sinus can be seen at the top of the diagram. (A, Anderson AO, Anderson ND: Am J Pathol 80: 387, 1975; B, Anderson AO, Anderson ND, White JD: In Hay JB (ed): Animal Models of Immunological Processes, p 25. London, Academic Press, 1982)

lowing activation, T-cells and their progeny are able to leave the node along with recirculating lymphocytes by way of its efferent lymph.

The B-lymphocytes that enter the lymph node are characterized by a different distribution. The majority of them move into the cortex of the node and make their way into its lymphatic nodules. In addition to constituting most of the cells in primary nodules, B-cells become concentrated in the so-called *follicular mantle* surrounding the germinal center of secondary nodules, and they are also present in the medullary extensions of each lymphatic nodule that comprise the medullary cords. These cords also commonly

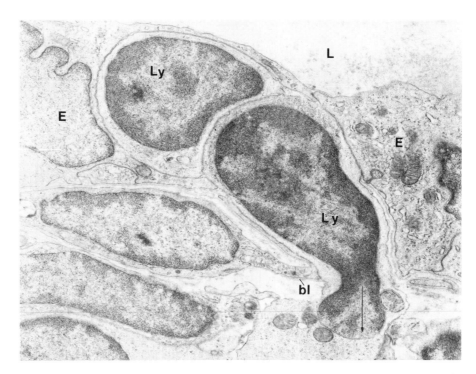

Fig. 10-11. Electron micrograph (×18,500) of part of the wall of a postcapillary venule of a lymph node (rat), showing two lymphocytes (*Ly*) passing through the wall between two endothelial cells (*E*) that line the lumen (*L*). Part of one lymphocyte (arrow), has created a gap in the basement membrane (labeled *bl*), and the cell is escaping from the vessel. (Nopajaroonsri C, Luk S, Simon GT: Am J Pathol 65:1, 1971)

contain *plasma cells* (see Fig. 10-13D) that are derived from B-cells that have become activated in the cortex. This is because the descendants of such cells move down into the medulla during the course of their differentiation and maturation. The mature plasma cells in the medulla have a limited lifespan of approximately 3 days. Because they are nonmotile, they remain within the medullary cords, but the immunoglobulin they produce passes out of the node by way of the efferent lymph. Hence mature plasma cells are relatively uncommon in lymph and are seldom encountered in the peripheral blood.

Finally, the *germinal centers* (Fig. 10-12) that are found in the secondary lymphatic nodules of lymph nodes are the sites where B-cells are undergoing active proliferation as a result of prolonged or secondary responses to antigen. They are not present before birth, and they fail to appear in animals reared in a germ-free environment. Within these centers, it is usually possible to find mitotic figures (Figs. 10-7B and 10-13A) and activated lymphocytes with basophilic cytoplasm (Figs. 10-7B and 10-13C). The same features are also seen in the germinal centers of unencapsulated lymphatic nodules. In addition to B-cells and the dendritic cells (Fig. 10-13B) already described, a few T-cells and macrophages (Fig. 10-7B) are present in germinal centers.

The immunoglobulins produced by the plasma cells of lymph nodes and the spleen, unlike those produced by the

plasma cells beneath mucosal epithelia, are primarily of the IgG class. The principal differences between IgG, IgA, and the other three classes of immunoglobulins are summarized in the following section.

There Are Five Classes of Immunoglobulins

Five distinct classes of immunoglobulins are now recognized on the basis of their different molecular sizes and composition. These are known as *IgG, IgM, IgA, IgD,* and *IgE.*

IgG. IgG is the main class of antibody that is produced as a result of a secondary humoral antibody response or prolonged immunization procedure. It accounts for approximately 75% of the total immunoglobulin in the blood plasma. IgG molecules are able to bind complement by their Fc end, and they are comparatively long-lived. Furthermore, IgG is the *only* class of maternal immunoglobulin that can be transferred across the placenta to provide the fetus with passive immunity. The fetus is unable to make antibodies of its own until about the fifth month of gestation.

IgM. Each molecule of IgM is a pentamer consisting of five IgG subunits held together in a ring structure by disulfide bonds. IgM is generally the first class of immunoglobulin to be produced in a primary humoral antibody response. It is more efficient than IgG in binding complement and in mediating antibody-dependent cytotoxic responses, but it is less efficient than IgG in neutralizing other functional macromolecules. IgM is also more likely than IgG

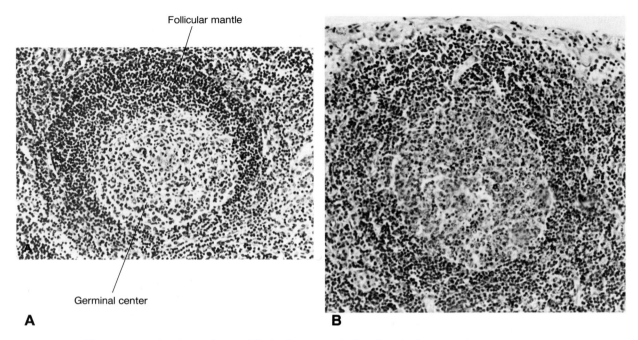

Fig. 10-12. Photomicrographs of secondary nodules in the cortex of a lymph node (low power). (*A*) A lymphatic nodule that exhibits a pale-staining germinal center and a follicular mantle containing mostly B-cells. (*B*) A lymphatic nodule with a germinal center that contains many basophilic cells. Details of some cell types present in such a center are shown in Fig. 10-13*A, B,* and *C.*

to produce antigen–antibody complexes that precipitate. Together with IgD, IgM in monomeric form is the main class of sIg expressed on B-lymphocytes.

IgA. Another major class of immunoglobulins, known as IgA, is characteristic of external body secretions such as those of the respiratory and digestive tracts and also milk and tears. In addition, it is present in the plasma, where it accounts for approximately 10% to 15% of the total immunoglobulin. In secretions, the IgA (*secretory IgA* or *SIgA*) is present mainly in the form of a dimer consisting of two IgA subunits linked by a glycopeptide *J* (joining) *chain* to a glycoprotein *secretory component* (SC). IgM, too, can become complexed with a secretory component, resulting in its secretion as a secretory immunoglobulin. The Ig subunits of IgA are made by IgA-producing plasma cells. The secretory component of IgA is a cell-surface receptor on mucosal and secretory epithelial cells that can bring about the transcellular endocytotic transport of both IgA and IgM through the cell. Following such transport, the secretory component remains permanently complexed with these immunoglobulins as they become released into a lumen through exocytosis. The role of secretory IgA in mucosal immunity was briefly discussed in connection with gut-associated lymphatic tissue earlier in this chapter.

IgD. This relatively minor class of immunoglobulins differs from IgG only with respect to fine details of molecular structure. As already noted, IgD and IgM are both present on the surface of B-lymphocytes, where they serve as antigen-recognition sites.

IgE. Although present only in low concentrations in the plasma, IgE plays a key role in mediating the immediate type of hypersensitivity reaction, described under Mast Cells in Chapter 7. This class of immunoglobulins has a high affinity for surface receptors on mast cells and basophils. Produced in response to allergens such as those of pollen and dusts, IgE molecules become attached by their Fc end to the Fc receptors on these two kinds of cells. This orientation leaves the antigen-combining sites of these molecules exposed and ready to interact with the same antigens if these reenter the body. IgE is made by plasma cells that are situated in the lamina propria under mucosal epithelia, in other words, in the same sites as the plasma cells that make IgA. The IgE molecule is monomeric and only slightly larger than the IgG molecule. Neither IgE nor IgA binds complement.

Lymph Nodes Can Vary in Microscopic Appearance

A certain amount of variation may be found among the lymph nodes in the different regions of the body. For example, in some nodes, the cortical lymphatic nodules are highly developed whereas the medulla is not. In nodes of this type, it is difficult to find medullary cords and sinuses. In nodes taken from other regions, it may be the medulla rather than the cortex that is well developed. Such nodes are suitable for studying the medullary cords. It should also be borne in mind that a single section of a lymph node may not always be very representative of its structure as a whole.

In addition to lymph nodes, most mammals possess a small number of structures that are essentially similar except that in the fresh state, their color is yellow or red instead of gray. When seen in section, these structures resemble lymph nodes, but they contain

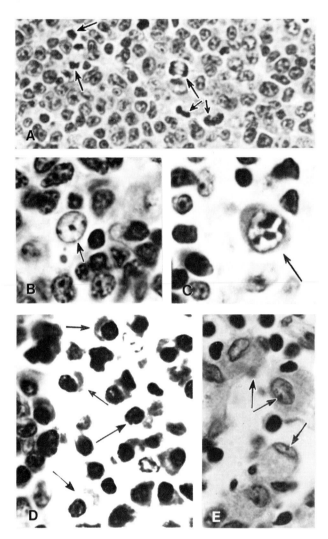

Fig. 10-13. Photomicrographs of some representative regions of a mediastinal lymph node (rat). (*A*) Active germinal center. Arrows indicate cells in mitosis. (*B*) Germinal center. Arrow indicates the nucleus of a dendritic cell; its cytoplasm is very indistinct. (*C*) Edge of a germinal center. Arrow indicates a large cell with a ring of basophilic cytoplasm that has a sharp edge. This free rounded cell is either an activated lymphocyte or a plasmablast. (*D*) Medullary cord. Arrows indicate plasma cells. Negative Golgi areas can be seen in their cytoplasm, particularly at bottom left. (*E*) Medullary sinuses. Arrows indicate macrophages.

somewhat better defined channels, some or all of which are filled with blood instead of lymph. If only some of the channels are filled with blood and others contain lymph, the structure is described as a *hemal lymph node.* If all the channels are filled with blood, it is called a *hemal node.*

It is not clear whether hemal lymph nodes or hemal nodes are always present in man, but their presence has often been described in the prevertebral peritoneal tissue, in the root of the mesentery, near the rim of the pelvis, and occasionally at other sites as well. Although there is an insufficient number of these structures in the human body to filter much blood, it is important to know of their

existence so that in the event that they are found at operation or autopsy, they are not mistaken for pathologically altered tissue.

THE SPLEEN

We have seen that diffusely distributed lymphatic nodules represent local immune responses to antigens that are present in *tissue fluid,* and that lymph nodes carry out local immune responses to antigens that have entered the *lymph.* The *spleen* is the lymphatic organ that is designed to facilitate immune responses to antigens that have gained access to the circulating *blood.* In considering what kinds of immune responses occur in the spleen, it is helpful to make some comparisons with what happens in the lymph nodes. Except in the relatively rare instance of *septicemia,* which is generalized infection of the blood, the antigen concentrations in the blood remain substantially below those in the lymph that drains from a site of infection. Lymph nodes are also more likely to be involved in cell-mediated immune responses, as in the case of immune responses to organ transplant antigens reaching regional lymph nodes via the lymph. Because the spleen receives blood from all regions of the body, its lymphocytes would only encounter low concentrations of such transplant antigens. Hence there are reasons for thinking that the spleen is primarily involved in the formation of humoral antibodies.

Purple due to its great content of blood, the spleen has roughly the same size and shape as a clenched fist. It lies in the abdomen in the shelter of the left 9th, 10th, and 11th ribs, with its long axis lying parallel to them. Because the spleen is soft in consistency, it is vulnerable to rupture in severe crushing-type injuries. Most of its surface is a smooth *serosal* surface, which means that is unattached to other organs. Its long medial recess is termed its *hilum.* Branches of the splenic artery enter the substance of the spleen at several sites along the length of the hilum. Veins and efferent lymphatics leave the spleen in association with the arterial branches that enter it. The veins unite to form the splenic vein. In contrast to the arrangement found in lymph nodes, no afferent lymphatics supply the spleen. Its *lymphatics are all efferent,* and they are all confined to the connective tissue that ensheathes its large blood vessels.

The spleen carries out two fairly major functions. First, it produces *humoral antibodies* directed against *blood-borne antigens.* Numerous plasma cells that are capable of producing very substantial quantities of immunoglobulin arise in the spleen from B-lymphocytes that become activated by blood-borne antigens. The spleen contains such a large population of plasma cells that it represents the body's chief source of humoral antibodies.

The second major function of the spleen is *to dispose of defective blood cells.* For this purpose, it possesses a very large population of resident macrophages that have ready access to the blood cells passing through it. These intensely phagocytic cells are responsible for the continuous removal

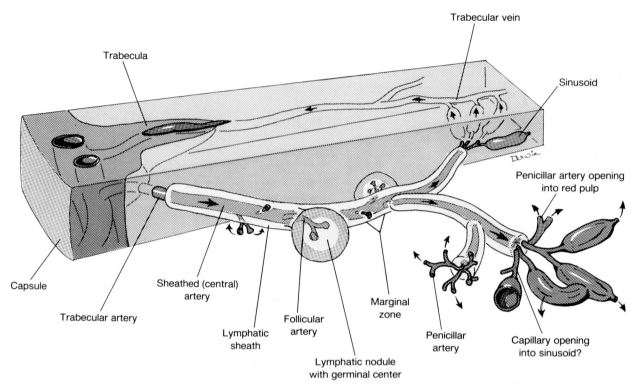

Fig. 10-14. Simplified schematic diagram of a representative portion of the spleen, showing its blood circulation and the white pulp surrounding its arterial supply. The penicillar arteries open into a reticular meshwork situated between the sinusoids of the red pulp. According to Knisely, some capillaries may open directly into sinusoids (*bottom right*). Otherwise, they all would begin as blind-ending sacs that drain into the trabecular veins. For further details and discussion, see text.

of senescent or damaged blood cells and platelets, circulating debris, and any suspended particulate matter that may be present in the blood. Iron liberated from the hemoglobin of phagocytosed erythrocytes is reutilized for the production of new erythrocytes in the bone marrow. The pigment bilirubin, also formed during hemoglobin degradation, circulates to the liver and is excreted by way of the bile. A third and more minor function of the spleen is that it can concentrate and store certain types of blood cells and also platelets. For example, approximately one third of the body's total platelet population is sequestered in the spleen at any one time. Yet the various functions of the spleen can all be carried out by the other hematopoietic tissues, so that if surgical removal of the spleen becomes necessary, it does not create any serious problems.

In fetal life, the spleen also becomes a site of active myeloid hematopoiesis, a potentiality that remains in adult life. Under conditions such as severe hemolytic anemia, the spleen can reexpress this potentiality and can engage in extramedullary hematopoiesis.

As we shall explain in the following section, the spleen can be thought of as consisting of two different components. One of these components, known as its *white pulp*, is designed to facilitate the development of immune re-

sponses. The other component, called its *red pulp*, is designed to facilitate the removal of deteriorating blood cells and platelets.

The Spleen Is Made up of White Pulp and Red Pulp. The limiting *capsule* of the spleen is composed of dense ordinary connective tissue covered by squamous mesothelium (Figs. 10-14 and 10-15). In addition to abundant collagen fibers and elastic fibers, it contains a few smooth muscle cells, yet the spleen manifests very little contractility in man. From the hilum and capsule, trabeculae of dense ordinary connective tissue extend into the substance of the spleen, bringing in blood vessels and nerves and providing substantial support (Figs. 10-14 and 10-15). The space between the trabeculae and the capsule is occupied by the *splenic pulp*. Most of the *white pulp* is represented by tiny islands up to 1 mm in diameter that are distributed through the *red pulp* (Fig. 10-15). The soft splenic pulp receives internal support from a meshwork of reticular fibers, but it is not organized into a cortex and medulla, nor is it subdivided into lobules. Histological sections disclose that the tiny is-lands of white pulp are *lymphatic nodules* mainly consisting of B-lymphocytes (Fig. 10-16). The red color of red pulp as seen in the fresh state is due to its enormous content of erythrocytes. The distinctive

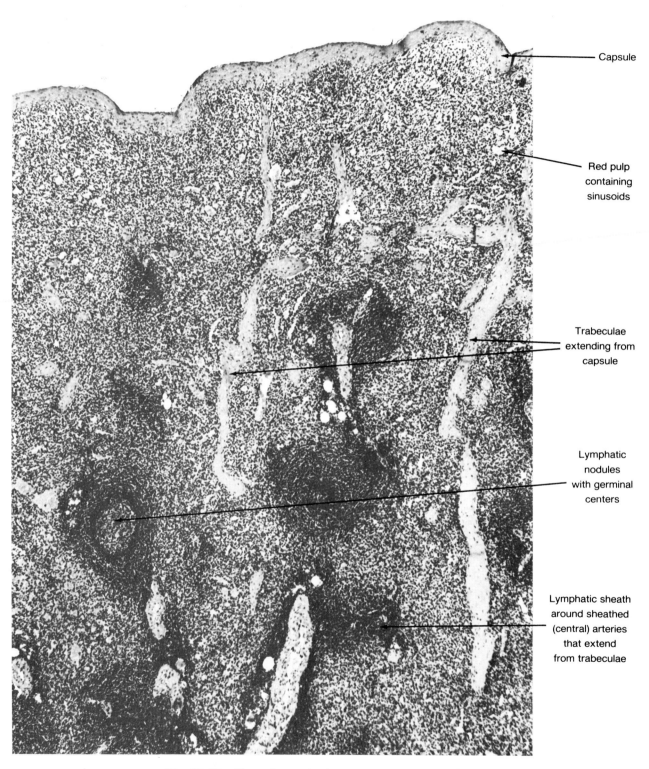

Capsule

Red pulp
containing
sinusoids

Trabeculae
extending from
capsule

Lymphatic
nodules
with germinal
centers

Lymphatic sheath
around sheathed
(central) arteries
that extend
from trabeculae

Fig. 10-15. Photomicrograph of a representative portion of the spleen (very low power). There is continuity between the trabeculae and capsule. Due to an abundance of small lymphocytes, the white pulp (periarterial lymphatic sheaths together with their associated lymphatic nodules) stains more darkly than the red pulp. Sinusoids are just discernible as pale areas in the red pulp.

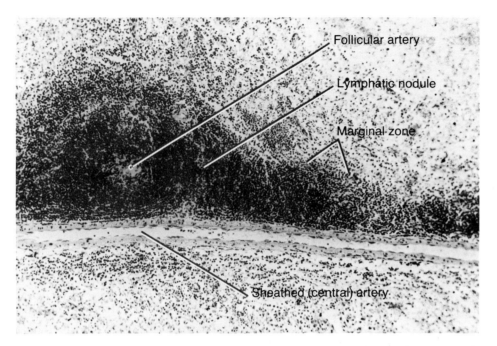

Fig. 10-16. Low-power photomicrograph of a sheathed (central) artery extending from a trabecula of the spleen. In this longitudinal section of the vessel, note the lymphatic sheath, the lymphatic nodule with its follicular artery, and the position of the border between the white pulp and the surrounding red pulp. This border is termed the *marginal zone*.

organization of the red pulp, as will be described, enables it to function as an efficient *blood filter* that can extract defective blood cells and platelets as well as remove superfluous debris and particulate matter from the blood circulation.

The Lymphatic Component of the Spleen

The irregularly branching system of splenic trabeculae conveys the branches of the splenic artery throughout the substance of the spleen. Small arterial branches extending from the trabeculae supply the splenic pulp. Associated with the extending portion of these arterial branches, there is a surrounding *lymphatic sheath* that contains a dense accumulation of small lymphocytes held in place by a supporting network of delicate reticular fibers (Figs. 10-14 and 10-15). Scattered along the course of these extending arterial branches, which are termed *sheathed* or *central* arteries, there are numerous *lymphatic nodules* (Figs. 10-14 and 10-16). Such association of lymphatic nodules with arterial vessels represents a unique feature of the spleen. Arterial branches supplying the capillaries in the lymphatic nodules are generally referred to as *follicular arteries* (Figs. 10-14 and 10-16) because lymphatic nodules are also known as *lymphoid follicles*. However, because of their small diameter, these fine arterial branches are often described as arterioles. In summary, then, the *white pulp* consists of lymphocyte-packed *lymphatic sheaths* and *lymphatic nodules* that are arranged along the small arterial branches emerging

from the trabeculae to supply the splenic pulp. We should also mention that in addition to having an abundant content of small lymphocytes, the white pulp is known to include antigen-presenting dendritic cells. Epithelial reticular cells, on the other hand, are not present in the spleen; they are unique to the thymus.

The periarterial and periarteriolar *lymphatic sheaths* become densely populated with *T-lymphocytes*. These cells assume their typical perivascular distribution after they have entered the immediate vicinity of the sheaths by way of small arterial vessels that supply the extensive interface between the white pulp and red pulp, which is termed the *marginal zone* of the spleen (Figs. 10-14 and 10-16). In contrast, the *lymphatic nodules* of the white pulp become densely populated with *B-lymphocytes*. When there is a prolonged or secondary exposure of these cells to blood-borne antigens, *germinal centers* appear within the nodules (Fig. 10-14). Proliferating and differentiating progeny of the activated B-lymphocytes in primary and secondary lymphatic nodules become progressively displaced toward the red pulp, where their maturation into antibody-secreting plasma cells is completed. Plasma cells are therefore generally quite prominent in the marginal zone and red pulp of the spleen.

The Red Pulp of the Spleen

The two main components in the red pulp of the spleen are (1) its numerous *sinusoids*, which are characteristic thin-

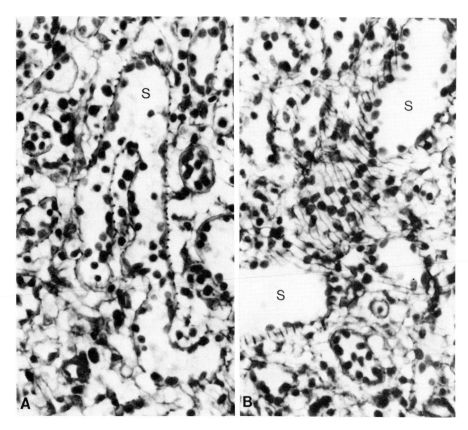

Fig. 10-17. Photomicrographs of spleen (PAS stain). (*A*) Sinusoids (*S*) are cut in longitudinal section. Their scant basement membrane is in the form of anastomosing rings that encircle the sinusoids. The rings in this plane of section appear as dark dots along the outside margin of the sinusoids, as shown at just right of center. (*B*) A sinusoid is seen in a grazing section that discloses the anastomosing rings of basement membrane surrounding it (*center*).

walled venous blood vessels with a wide lumen and large numbers of associated macrophages, and (2) its supporting meshwork of reticular fibers with their associated population of reticular cells and vast numbers of blood cells lying free in the interstices of the meshwork. Because the reticular fibers of the red pulp merge with the collagen fibers of both the capsule and the trabeculae, they provide the red pulp with delicate internal support.

How Do Blood Cells Enter and Leave the Red Pulp? Arterial blood reaches the red pulp by way of continuations of the sheathed arteries (Fig. 10-14). On approaching the red pulp, these vessels give rise to a small group of straight arterial branches known as *penicillar arteries* (L. *penicillus*, painter's brush) that are so called because they stick out at an angle like bristles from an artist's brush (Fig. 10-14). Each penicillar artery is believed to open, usually by way of two or three arterioles, into the reticular meshwork that occupies the pulp spaces *between* the sinusoids of the red pulp (Fig. 10-14). Because this blood is not delivered directly into the sinusoids, such a path of circulation is described as *open* to distinguish it from the usual closed path of circulation found elsewhere in the body.

Observations of splenic blood flow carried out *in vivo* nevertheless suggest that blood arriving from arterioles may also be able to reach the venous circulation by a more direct route. Direct observation of the splenic circulation by Knisley led him to conclude that some of the capillaries leading from the arterioles discharged their blood directly into sinusoids, as depicted in a simplified manner on the right in Figure 10-14. Hence there may be alternative routes whereby blood cells passing through the spleen are either delivered to the reticular meshwork of the red pulp or permitted to bypass it, depending on prevailing physiological conditions. The issue of whether the splenic circulation is totally and consistently open or whether it can become partly or temporarily closed is still unresolved. A currently favored hypothesis is that the splenic circulation is structurally open but, from a functional point of view, behaves as if it were partly closed. The most likely explanation is that there are relatively wide conduits through the reticular meshwork occupying the intersinusoidal spaces of the red pulp. Strictly speaking, however, such rapidly conducting conduits would not be part of a closed circulation because they would be lined by a discontinuous layer of reticular cells instead of a continuous lining of endothelial cells. For further discussion about the splenic circulation, see Blue and Weiss.

Some of the capillaries that lead from the arteriolar branches of the penicillar arteries are surrounded near their

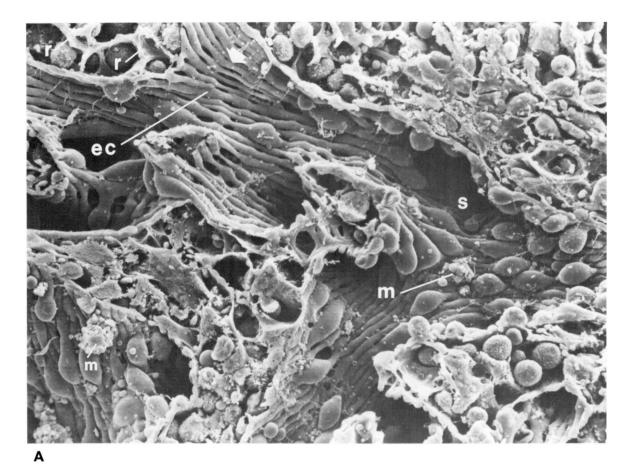

A

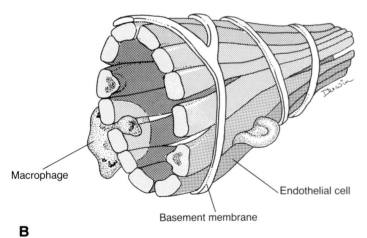

Macrophage

Basement membrane

Endothelial cell

B

Fig. 10-18. (*A*) Scanning electron micrograph (×900) of red pulp of human spleen, showing the luminal surface of the long narrow endothelial cells (*ec*) that line its sinusoids (*s*). Below the arrowhead at top left, it is possible to discern some of the slit-shaped intercellular gaps through which blood cells pass. Sinusoid-associated macrophages (*m*) and reticular cells (*r*) are also discernible in this micrograph. (*B*) Diagrammatic representation of a sinusoid in the red pulp of the spleen. Its narrow endothelial cells are held together by anastomosing hoops of basement membrane. Between these cells there are slitlike spaces that admit blood cells to the lumen. Macrophages are also closely associated with these lining cells. (*A*, Fujita, T, Kashimura M, Adachi K: Scanning Electron Microscopy/1982/I, p 435, 1982)

terminations by a reticular sheath that contains many macrophages, generally in combination with other kinds of blood cells. Such accumulations commonly have the shape of an ellipsoid; hence the term *ellipsoid* is used for these localized arrangements of macrophages.

Blood leaves the red pulp by way of its extensive system of sinusoids, which empty into the trabecular veins (Fig.

10-14). The sinusoids are lined by long thin endothelial cells that are unusually narrow and that have relatively wide, slit-shaped gaps between their lateral borders (see Fig. 10-18). Supporting these lining cells, there are anastomosing circumferential rings of basement membrane (Figs. 10-17 and 10-18) that surround the walls of the sinusoid like the hoops of a barrel, but a very leaky barrel because of the open slits between the endothelial cells (Fig. 10-18). This sievelike arrangement constitutes an effective coarse filter through which blood cells that have been discharged into the reticular meshwork of the intersinusoidal spaces are obliged to pass in order to collect within sinusoids and leave the spleen by way of the trabecular and splenic veins.

Occupying the interstices of the reticular meshwork between the sinusoids of the red pulp, there are reticular cells and numerous macrophages, erythrocytes, leukocytes, platelets, and plasma cells. In the process of negotiating the narrow slits between the lining cells of sinusoids, insufficiently deformable senescent erythrocytes and excessively fragile imperfect erythrocytes become severely damaged. Together with dead leukocytes, worn-out platelets, and superfluous particulate matter, such damaged erythrocytes are rapidly engulfed by the actively phagocytic macrophages of the red pulp, some of which extend cytoplasmic processes into the sinusoidal lumen (Fig. 10-18*B*).

Pitting. The sievelike texture of the sinusoidal walls also enables the spleen to carry out a *pitting function.* This means that it can cause deformable erythrocytes to extrude any undeformable particulate inclusions that they may contain without harming these cells in the process. Thus aggregates of denatured hemoglobin, iron-containing granules (*siderosomes*), nuclear remnants (*Howell–Jolly bodies*), and even red cell parasites can become extruded from erythrocytes as these cells squeeze through the narrow intercellular slits between the endothelial lining cells of sinusoids (Fig. 10-18*B*). Once extruded, such particles are rapidly phagocytosed by the sinusoid-associated macrophages.

In summary, then, the main roles of the red pulp are (1) to produce immunoglobulins directed against any antigens that may be circulating in the bloodstream, and (2) to filter out and dispose of worn-out blood cells, platelets, and suspended particles that might clutter up the bloodstream. The first function is achieved through the production of plasma cells that become situated in the red pulp after differentiating from B-cells activated in the white pulp. The second function of the spleen is carried out by the large population of resident macrophages situated in its red pulp. Finally, its red pulp also serves as a temporary reservoir for blood cells or platelets that are not circulating.

SELECTED REFERENCES

General

ALBERTS B, BRAY D, LEWIS J ET AL: The immune system. In Molecular Biology of the Cell, pp 951–1012, New York, Garland Publishing, 1983

BARRETT JT: Textbook of Immunology. An Introduction to Immunochemistry and Immunobiology, 4th ed. St. Louis, CV Mosby, 1983

BENACERRAF B, UNANUE ER: Textbook of Immunology. Baltimore, Williams & Wilkins, 1979

CUNNINGHAM AJ: Understanding Immunology. New York, Academic Press, 1978

FUDENBERG HH, STITES DP, CALDWELL JL, WELLS JV (eds): Basic and Clinical Immunology, 2nd ed. Los Altos, CA, Lange Medical Publications, 1978

GOLUB E: The Cellular Basis of the Immune Response: An Approach to Immunobiology, 2nd ed. Sunderland MA, Sinauer, 1981

KLEIN J: Immunology. The Science of Self–Nonself Discrimination. New York, John Wiley & Sons, 1982

PLAYFAIR JHL: Immunology at a Glance, 3rd ed. Oxford, Blackwell Scientific Publications, 1984

ROITT IM: Essential Immunology, 5th ed. Oxford, Blackwell Scientific Publications, 1984

WEISSMAN IL, HOOD LE, WOOD WB: Essential Concepts in Immunology. Menlo Park, CA, Benjamin/Cummings, 1978

B- and T-Lymphocytes: Their Development and Their Involvement in Immune Responses

ANDERSON AO, ANDERSON ND, WHITE JD: Lymphocyte locomotion, lymphatic tissues, and lymphocyte circulation in the rat. In Hay JB (ed): Animal Models of Immunological Processes, p 25. London, Academic Press, 1982

ANDERSSON J, MELCHERS F: T cell–dependent activation of resting B cells: Requirement for both nonspecific unrestricted and antigen-specific Ia-restricted soluble factors. Proc Natl Acad Sci USA 78:2497, 1981

ANDERSSON J, SCHREIER MH, MELCHERS F: T-cell–dependent B-cell stimulation is H-2 restricted and antigen dependent only at the resting B-cell level. Proc Natl Acad Sci USA 77:1612, 1980

BENACERRAF B: Regulatory T lymphocytes and their antigen receptors. In Pernis B, Vogel HJ (eds): Regulatory T Lymphocytes, p 3. New York, Academic Press, 1980

DE BRUYN PPH, FARR AG: Lymphocyte–RES interactions and their fine-structural correlates. In Carr I, Daems WT (eds): The Reticuloendothelial System, Vol I, p 499. New York, Plenum, 1980

CHEN P, TRUMMEL C, HORTON J ET AL: Production of osteoclast activating factor by normal human peripheral blood rosetting and nonrosetting lymphocytes. Eur J Immunol 6:732, 1976

CLAMAN HN, MOSIER DE: Cell-cell interactions in antibody production. Prog Allergy 16:40, 1972

COOPER MD: Pre–B cells: Normal and abnormal development. J Clin Immunol 1:81, 1981

DIAMOND BA, YELTON DE, SCHARFF MD: Monoclonal antibodies. A new technology for producing serologic reagents. N Engl J Med 304:1344, 1981

FELDMANN M, NOSSAL GVV: Cellular basis of antibody production. Q Rev Biol 47:269, 1972

GOLDSCHNEIDER I, MCGREGOR DD: Anatomical distribution of T and B lymphocytes in the rat. J Exp Med 138:1443, 1973

GUTMAN GA, WEISSMAN IL: Lymphoid tissue architecture: Experimental analysis of the origin and distribution of T-cells and B-cells. Immunology 23:465, 1972

HEDRICK SM, NIELSEN EA, KAVALER J ET AL: Sequence relationships between putative T-cell receptor polypeptides and immunoglobulins. Nature 308:153, 1984

HERBERMAN RB (ed): NK Cells and Other Natural Effector Cells. New York, Academic Press, 1982

HERBERMAN RB, ORTALDO JR: Natural killer cells: Their role in defenses against disease. Science 214:24, 1981

HORIBE K, NADLER LM: Human B cell associated antigens defined by monoclonal antibodies. In Lymphocyte Surface Antigens 1984. Perspectives in Immunogenetics and Histocompatibility, Vol 6, p 309. New York, American Society for Histocompatibility and Immunogenetics, 1984

HORTON JE, RAISZ LG, SIMMONS HA ET AL: Bone resorbing activity in supernatant fluid from cultured peripheral blood leukocytes. Science 177:793, 1972

KUPFER A, SWAIN SL, JANEWAY CA, SINGER SJ: The specific direct interaction of helper T cells and antigen-presenting cells. Proc Natl Acad Sci USA 83:6080, 1986

LEDBETTER JA, TSU TT, DRAVES K, CLARK EA: Differential expression of pan T cell antigens on human T cell subsets. In Lymphocyte Surface Antigens 1984. Perspectives in Immunogenetics and Histocompatibility, Vol 6, p 325. New York, American Society for Histocompatibility and Immunogenetics, 1984

LEVITT D, COOPER MD: Expression and function of B-lymphocyte receptors. In Bearn AG, Choppin RW (eds): Receptors and Human Diseases, p 98. New York, Josiah Macy, Jr Foundation, 1979

MELCHERS F, ANDERSSON J: B cell activation: Three steps and their variations. Cell 37:715, 1984

MILSTEIN C: Monoclonal antibodies. Sci Am 243 No 4:66, 1980

MÖLLER G (ed): Lymphocyte immunoglobulin: Synthesis and surface representation. Transplant Rev 14, 1973

NELSON DS (ed): Immunobiology of the Macrophage. New York, Academic Press, 1976

PAUL WE, BENACERRAF B: Functional specificity of thymus-dependent lymphocytes. Science 195:1293, 1977

PODACK ER: The molecular mechanism of lymphocyte-mediated tumor cell lysis. Immunology Today 6:21, 1985

RAFF MC: T and B lymphocytes and immune responses. Nature 242:19, 1973

REINHERZ EL, SCHLOSSMAN SF: The characterization and function of human immunoregulatory T lymphocyte subsets. Immunology Today April:69, 1981

REINHERZ EL, SCHLOSSMAN SF: The differentiation and function of human T lymphocytes. Cell 19:821, 1980

REINHERZ EL, SCHLOSSMAN SF: Regulation of the immune response—inducer and suppressor T-lymphocyte subsets in human beings. N Engl J Med 303:370, 1980

SCOLLAY R: Intrathymic events in the differentiation of T lymphocytes: A continuing enigma. Immunology Today 4:282, 1983

SKELLY RR, POTTER TA, AHMED A: Lymphocyte antigens and receptors. In Atassi MZ, van Oss CJ, Absolom DR (eds): Molecular Immunology. A Textbook, p 597. New York, Marcel Dekker, 1984

TONEGAWA S: The molecules of the immune system. Sci Am 253 No 4:122, 1985

TONEGAWA S: Somatic generation of antibody diversity. Nature 302:575, 1983

VOGLER LB, GROSSI CE, COOPER MD: Human lymphocyte subpopulations. In Brown EB (ed): Progress in Hematology, Vol XI, p 1. New York, Grune & Stratton, 1979

WAKSMAN BH: Tolerance, the thymus, and suppressor T cells. Clin Exp Immunol 28:363, 1977

WILLIAMS AF: The T-lymphocyte antigen receptor—elusive no more. Nature 308:108, 1984

YANAGI Y, YOSHIKAI Y, LEGGETT K ET AL: A human T cell–specific cDNA clone encodes a protein having extensive homology to immunoglobulin chains. Nature 308:145, 1984

YOSHIDA T: Lymphokines. In Atassi MZ, van Oss CJ, Absolom DR (eds): Molecular Immunology. A Textbook, p 645. New York, Marcel Dekker, 1984

YOUNG JD, COHN ZA: Cell-mediated killing: A common mechanism? Cell 46:641, 1986

Transplantation, Tolerance, and Autoimmunity

BILLINGHAM R, SILVERS W: The Immunology of Transplantation. Englewood Cliffs, NJ, Prentice-Hall, 1971

BURNET SIR MACFARLANE: The Clonal Selection Theory of Acquired Immunity. Nashville, TN. Vanderbilt University Press, and Cambridge, England, University Press, 1959

CARPENTER CB: The cellular basis of allograft rejection. Immunology Today, p 50, March 1981

ROSE NR: Autoimmune diseases. Sci Am 244 No 2:80, 1981

The Thymus

GORGOLLÓN P, OTTONE–ANAYA M: Fine structure of canine thymus. Acta Anat 100:136, 1978

HWANG WS, HO TY, LUK SC, SIMON GT: Ultrastructure of the rat thymus: A transmission, scanning electron microscope, and morphometric study. Lab Invest 31:473, 1974

RAVIOLA E, KARNOVSKY MJ: Evidence for a blood–thymus barrier using electron-opaque tracers. J Exp Med 136:466, 1972

SMITH C: Studies on the thymus of the mammal. VIII. Intrathymic lymphatic vessels. Anat Rec 122:173, 1955

Lymphatic Nodules, Lymph Nodes, and Mucosal Immunity

ANDERSON AO, ANDERSON ND: Lymphocyte emigration from high endothelial venules in rat lymph nodes. Immunology 31:731, 1976

ANDERSON AO, ANDERSON ND: Studies on the structure and permeability of the microvasculature in normal rat lymph nodes. Am J Pathol 80:387, 1975

BAILEY RP, WEISS L: Light and electron microscopic studies of postcapillary venules in developing human fetal lymph nodes. Am J Anat 143:43, 1975

BEFUS AD, BIENENSTOCK J: The mucosa-associated immune system of the rabbit. In Hay JB (ed): Animal Models of Immunological Processes, p 167. London, Academic Press, 1982

BIENENSTOCK J (ed): Immunology of the Lung and Upper Respiratory Tract. New York, McGraw-Hill, 1984

BRANDTZAEG P: Immune functions of human nasal mucosa and tonsils in health and disease. In Bienenstock J (ed): Immunology of the Lung and Upper Respiratory Tract, p 28. New York, McGraw-Hill, 1984

LUK SC, NOPAJAROONSRI C, SIMON GT: The architecture of the normal lymph node and hemolymph node. A scanning and transmission electron microscopic study. Lab Invest 29:258, 1973

NOPAJAROONSRI C, LUK SC, SIMON GT: Ultrastructure of the normal lymph node. Am J Pathol 65:1, 1971

OWEN RL: Sequential uptake of horseradish peroxidase by lymphoid follicle epithelium of Peyer's patches in the normal unobstructed mouse intestine: An ultrastructural study. Gastroenterology 72: 440, 1977

OWEN RL, BHALLA DK: Lympho-epithelial organs and lymph nodes. In Hodges GM, Carr KE (eds): Biomedical Research Applications of Scanning Electron Microscopy, Vol 3. New York, Academic Press, 1983

SYRJÄNEN KJ: The Lymph Nodes: Reactions to Experimental and Human Tumors. Exp Pathol (Suppl 8) New York, Gustav Fischer, 1982

The Spleen

BARNHART MI, LUSHER JM: The human spleen as revealed by scanning electron microscopy. Am J Hematol 1:243, 1976

BLUE J, WEISS L: Species variations in the structure and function of the marginal zone: An electron microscopic study of the cat spleen. Am J Anat 161:169, 1981

BLUE J, WEISS L: Vascular pathways in non-sinusal red pulp: An electron microscope study of cat spleen. Am J Anat 161:135, 1981

BURKE JS, SIMON GT: Electron microscopy of the spleen. I. Anatomy and microcirculation. Am J Pathol 58:127, 1970

CHEN L-T, WEISS L: Electron microscopy of the red pulp of human spleen. Am J Anat 134:425, 1972

CHEN L-T, WEISS L: The role of the sinus wall in the passage of erythrocytes through the spleen. Blood 41:529, 1973

FUJITA T, KASHIMURA M, ADACHI K: Scanning electron microscopy (SEM) studies of the spleen—normal and pathological. Scanning Electron Microscopy/1982/I, p 435. AMF O'Hare (Chicago), SEM Inc, 1982

KNISLEY MH: Spleen studies: I. Microscopic observations of the circulatory system of living unstimulated mammalian spleens. Anat Rec 65:23, 1936

ROBINSON WL: Some points on the mechanism of filtration by the spleen. Am J Pathol 4:309, 1928

SOLNITZKY O: The Schweigger–Seidel sheath (ellipsoid) of the spleen. Anat Rec 69:55, 1937

SONG SH, GROOM AC: Scanning electron microscope study of the splenic pulp in relation to the sequestration of immature and abnormal red cells. J Morphol 144:439, 1974

WEISS L: A scanning electron microscopic study of the spleen. Blood 43:665, 1974

11

Tendons, Ligaments, and Cartilage

DENSE ORDINARY CONNECTIVE TISSUE

TENDONS

LIGAMENTS

CARTILAGE

HYALINE CARTILAGE
Cartilage Matrix
FIBROCARTILAGE
ELASTIC CARTILAGE

With tendons, ligaments, and cartilage, we now begin a histological survey of the various types of skeletal tissues. A thorough knowledge of these tissues is essential preparation for important branches of surgery, medicine, and dentistry. Furthermore, although many diseases have now been brought under control in civilized societies, the incidence of accidents involving damage to the skeleton has increased because of widespread use of the automobile. In addition to contributing in large measure to the literature on *orthopedics* (Gr. *orthos*, straight; *pais*, child) (*i.e.*, the surgical specialty concerned with the preservation and restoration of the normal structure and function of bones and joints), this unfortunate consequence of having to share the road with others has provided added incentive for basic research on cartilage and bone. Moreover, because calcium metabolism is hormonally regulated and bones represent the main *calcium reservoir* in the body, skeletal manifestations of metabolic diseases constitute another very active field of investigative medicine. *Arthritis* (inflammation of the joints) and *periodontal disease* (deterioration of tooth attachments in alveolar bone) are also areas of current intensive investigation.

   In this chapter, we shall first consider *dense ordinary connective tissue*, the tissue of which tendons and ligaments are composed. A similar kind of tissue constitutes the fibrous wrappings of other parts of the body, but there it is less regularly arranged.

DENSE ORDINARY CONNECTIVE TISSUE

Dense ordinary connective tissue can be *regularly* or *irregularly* arranged. In the type that is regularly arranged, all the collagen fibers run in the same direction. Structures composed of this type of connective tissue are adapted to withstand unidirectional pull transmitted along these fibers. The regular type of dense ordinary connective tissue is found in tendons and aponeuroses (which are flat tendons expanded into a wide fibrous sheet), which are both structures that are required to transmit the full force of muscular contractions to bones or cartilages without stretching. The same type of connective tissue constitutes ligaments, which are strong bands of fibrous connective tissue that hold bones together at joints.

In the irregular type of dense ordinary connective tissue, the collagen fibers can run in a variety of different directions. Where sheets of this tissue comprise sheaths of various sorts, the fibers lie more or less in a single plane but run in different directions. Such sheets can withstand stretching in any of the directions in which their fibers run. In the reticular (deep) layer of the dermis, for example, the collagen fibers run in different directions and also in different planes, enabling the dermis to withstand stretch in any direction. In addition, the irregular type of dense ordinary connective tissue constitutes the fibrous capsule and septa or trabeculae of glands and organs; the fibrous wrappings of the heart, nervous system, bones, cartilages, and muscles; and the valves of the heart and blood vessels.

In this chapter, we shall be dealing primarily with dense ordinary connective tissue that is regularly arranged.

TENDONS

Tendons are composed of closely packed parallel bundles of collagen fibers (Fig. 11-1), with intervening rows of highly compressed fibrocyte nuclei representing the cells that produced this collagen. Blood capillaries are also present between these bundles but they are seldom evident. Some tendons are enclosed within sheaths at sites where they would otherwise rub against bone or some other friction-generating surface. Actually, a tendon sheath is made up of two sheaths. The outer sheath is a connective tissue tube attached to the surrounding tissues. The inner sheath directly encloses the tendon and is firmly attached to it. Between the inner and the outer sheath, there is a narrow fluid-filled space containing friction-reducing *synovial fluid,* which will be described in connection with synovial joints in Chapter 13. Both the outer surface of the inner sheath and the inner surface of the outer sheath lack continuous cellular linings, so the smooth surfaces that glide past each other are composed mostly of collagen. Among the collagen fibers, however, scattered cells are present as in the synovial membrane of a synovial joint (which will be described in Chap. 13).

Severed Tendons Can Be Rejoined Surgically. Tendons can become severed in accidents. However, with proper surgical management, they can heal effectively, and with time, they may become as strong as before. The preexisting fibrocytes in the tendon contribute very little to the repair process. Instead, repair is effected by fibroblasts that are derived from the inner tendon sheath or, if the tendon has no distinct sheath, from the loose connective tissue around its periphery. These cells proliferate, and their progeny grow into the site where the severed ends are apposed. As soon as the new fibroblasts become oriented along the tendon axis, they reenact the stages of collagen production that occur during tendon development. In the early stages of

repair, when there is a rich capillary supply, these cells deposit much collagen in the form of bundles that extend along the tendon axis. Furthermore, some of these cells grow into the severed ends of the tendon, enabling the new collagen being formed to unite with the old. With increasing collagen deposition, the capillary blood supply diminishes to its former level. If tendon grafts are employed, these become incorporated into rejoined tendons in a similar manner.

A common complication of tendon surgery is the development of fibrous adhesions between the tendon and its neighboring tissues. Adhesions to bone, for example, can immobilize the tendon and prevent the return of satisfactory function. Yet successful repair of a rejoined tendon depends on the very same factors that lead to the development of adhesions. Because the healing process is a result of ingrowth of fibroblasts and capillaries from outside the tendon, any attempt to prevent the development of adhesions between the healing tendon and its neighboring connective tissue by isolating the sutured ends of the severed tendon from this tissue also prevents the tendon ends from becoming united.

LIGAMENTS

Ligaments are also largely composed of closely packed parallel bundles of intercellular fibers with intervening rows of compressed fibrocyte nuclei. The longitudinal fibers in most ligaments are collagen fibers. However, closely interwoven with these main fibers, there are finer collagen fibers and a variable number of elastic fibers. Such a weblike construction confers a degree of inextensibility on ligaments sufficient for them to provide the strong support needed at articulating (synovial) joints. Here they serve to limit excessive or inappropriate joint movement. Due to their special construction, they are nevertheless flexible enough not to hinder appropriate joint movement. At a few joints, the ligaments are more extensible. Thus in the ligamenta flava, which hold together the laminae of the contiguous vertebral arches in the vertebral column, the parallel fibers that take the strain are elastic fibers and the fibers that weave them together are made of collagen. Ligaments of this type are known as *elastic ligaments.*

Torn Ligaments Can Also Heal Satisfactorily. A joint injury can impose excessive strain on a ligament, causing it to tear. Fortunately, however, effective repair ensues when the injury is properly managed. Most torn ligaments will heal satisfactorily provided their torn ends are promptly apposed, for example, by taping the joint in the right position to hold these ends together. However, suturing is occasionally necessary to bring the torn ends close enough together for adequate repair. As in the case of tendon repair, restoration of former strength to the torn ligament depends on collagen deposition, but the source of the cells that produce this new collagen has not been elucidated.

How Are Tendons and Ligaments Attached? Tendons connect muscles to bone or cartilage and enable muscular contractions to pull on the bone or cartilage into which the

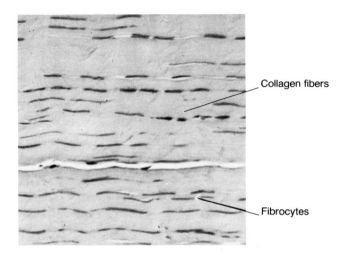

Collagen fibers

Fibrocytes

Fig. 11-1. Photomicrograph of a tendon cut in longitudinal section.

tendon is said to be *inserted.* Tendon attachments to muscles will be described in Chapter 15.

It is perhaps misleading to say that one end of the tendon is inserted into bone or cartilage because it makes it sound as if this end were somehow poked in so as to gain some sort of firm attachment. Actually, what happens is that the cells forming the collagen fibers at this end of the tendon are not ordinary fibroblasts; they are of the type found in the coverings of bones or cartilages, and such cells can produce the intercellular substances of bone or cartilage. Because these tissues both contain much collagen, cartilage- or bone-forming cells are capable of producing the collagen of the tendon at the site where it is inserted. But they also produce the amorphous intercellular substances characteristic of bone or cartilage. So where tendon insertions are forming at the surface of a bony or cartilaginous structure, the cells produce a mixture of (1) the intercellular substances of tendon and (2) the intercellular substances of bone or cartilage. Accordingly, there is a gradual transition along the tendon near its insertion from being pure dense connective tissue to being a mixture of dense connective tissue and either bone or cartilage. When this is cartilage, the tissue is said to be *fibrocartilage,* soon to be described.

Furthermore, during growth, the bones to which tendons are inserted grow when bone is added to their surface. Thus a tendon insertion into what began as a small bone eventually becomes an insertion into a large bone. This requires constant rebuilding of the tendon insertion during the growth of the bone. Hence as a result of the growth of the bone, the early attachment of the tendon becomes buried deeper and deeper within its substance. When the collagen bundles of the tendon insertion lie buried in the new bone, they are termed *Sharpey's fibers.*

In all major respects, *ligament attachments* are closely similar to *tendon insertions.*

Next, we shall consider the skeletal tissues, beginning with cartilage.

CARTILAGE

Cartilage (L. *cartilago,* gristle) is a relatively solid weight-bearing connective tissue that lacks the strength of bone. It is found in only two kinds of sites after growth is over in postnatal life. First, some extraskeletal cartilaginous structures exist in the body. For example, there are horseshoe-shaped rings of cartilage in the wall of the trachea. The role of these rings is to prevent the wall of the trachea, which otherwise consists chiefly of ordinary connective tissue, from collapsing when air is drawn into the lungs. Irregular cartilaginous structures are also present in the walls of the larger air tubes leading into the lungs. Moreover, plates of cartilage are found in the larynx, nose, and in the wall of the medial portion of the auditory tube (which connects the middle ear with the nasopharynx and permits air pressure to be equalized between the two cavities). Cartilage also remains in the costal cartilages (which connect the anterior ends of the ribs to the sternum), where it provides a connection between the ribs and the sternum that is firm yet flexible enough to permit the rib cage to expand in respiratory movements.

The second kind of site where cartilage remains throughout life is in articulating joints. In freely movable joints, the ends of bones are capped with cartilage. In this instance, the cartilage is termed *articular cartilage,* and its intercellular component (which is known as its *matrix*) provides the smooth gliding surfaces that are seen on the articulating ends of bones. Articular cartilage will be dealt with in some detail in Chapter 13. Cartilage also persists in some joints that are not freely movable.

Much of the cartilage that develops in prenatal life has only a temporary existence because it is replaced by bone. Its formation is nevertheless a key stage in the development of long bones. Furthermore, some of this cartilage persists until postnatal growth is over, providing a mechanism

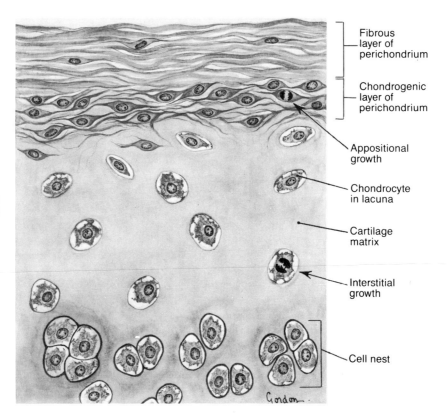

Fibrous
layer of
perichondrium

Chondrogenic
layer of
perichondrium

Appositional
growth

Chondrocyte
in lacuna

Cartilage
matrix

Interstitial
growth

Cell nest

Fig. 11-2. Diagram of growing hyaline cartilage with its perichondrium, depicting its appositional and interstitial growth.

whereby such bones grow in length. The fate of this cartilage will be discussed in Chapter 12.

Ordinary cartilage is described as *hyaline* (Gr. *hyalos*) because its matrix is bluish–pearly-white and is somewhat translucent in the fresh state. In a few sites, however, cartilage is described as *elastic* because it also contains elastic fibers, and at other sites, it contains a number of substantial collagen fibers sufficient to warrant its being called *fibrocartilage*. These two special forms of cartilage will be described at the end of the chapter.

HYALINE CARTILAGE

Embedded in the *intercellular matrix* of hyaline cartilage there is a population of cells known as *chondrocytes* (Fig. 11-2). These cells occupy such a position for the following reason. At the site where a cartilage will develop in the embryo, the mesenchymal cells undergo condensation and differentiate into cells called *chondroblasts* that then begin to secrete the macromolecular constituents of cartilage matrix. At the same time, the cells at the periphery of the site start to form a fibrous covering termed the *perichondrium* (Gr. *peri*, around). The cells in the innermost layer of the perichondrium repeatedly generate new chondroblasts that deposit new cartilage matrix over the surface of that already formed, so this innermost layer of the perichondrium is

called its *chondrogenic layer* (Fig. 11-2). The cells in the outer layer of the perichondrium, on the other hand, differentiate into *fibroblasts* that produce collagen, and as a result, the cartilage acquires an investment of irregular dense ordinary connective tissue that is known as the *fibrous layer* of the perichondrium (Fig. 11-2). In certain instances, the fibrous part of the perichondrium persists into adult life, but in other instances, both layers disappear, leaving the cartilage uncovered. Articular cartilage is an example of the type of cartilage that is *not* covered by a perichondrium.

After chondroblasts have become deeply buried in cartilage matrix, they are described as *chondrocytes*. Thereafter they live in tiny matrix spaces known as *lacunae* (L. for small pits or cavities) in the matrix they have secreted. However, the prominence of these lacunae in light microscope (LM) sections is due to a *shrinkage artifact* that creates an artificial space between the chondrocyte and the walls of its lacuna. When a chondrocyte has finished secreting intercellular substance around itself, the lacuna in which it resides is termed a *primary lacuna*. However, such a chondrocyte may still be able to divide a few times more (mitotic figure, labeled *interstitial growth* in Fig. 11-2), and, if so, the tendency is for daughter cells to reside in the same lacuna, with only a thin partition of intercellular substance being formed between them. Sometimes each of these daughter cells divides again so that there may now be four cells in the primary lacuna (labeled *cell nest* in Fig. 11-2). Because each chondrocyte secretes enough intercellular substance to form a thin wall between itself and its sister cell, it lives in what is termed a *secondary lacuna* and the secondary lacunae of a *cell nest* are therefore all within the original primary lacuna. Cartilage cells seen in a cell nest represent a clone (*i.e.*, the progeny of the original cell occupying the primary lacuna). Typically, chondrocytes have a rounded nucleus with one or more nucleoli. Glycogen and fat may be present in the cytoplasm of large chondrocytes. Chondrocytes vary in size and shape; generally this reflects their degree of maturation. Young chondrocytes are commonly flattened (Fig. 11-2). Mature chondrocytes tend to be large and rounded (Fig. 11-2). Size, then, is an important indication of the extent to which chondrocytes have matured.

With improved methods of electron microscopic preparation, it is now clear that living chondrocytes fill their lacunae completely (Fig. 11-3). Scattered throughout the extended chromatin in their round-to-ovoid nucleus, there are small clumps of condensed chromatin, which is also seen at the periphery of the nucleus (Fig. 11-3). Their cytoplasm is replete with secretory organelles that are arranged in an essentially unpolarized manner. Cisternae of rough-surfaced endoplasmic reticulum are prominent and commonly dilated with secretory product (Fig. 11-3). Substantial glycogen deposits may also be present in the cytoplasm (Fig. 11-3*B*).

Cartilage Grows in Two Different Ways. A point to establish here that will become relevant when we consider how a long bone develops and lengthens is that one of the ways in which cartilage grows is by *interstitial growth*. In other words, even after young chondrocytes have become embedded in cartilage matrix, they are still able to divide, whereupon matrix production by each daughter cell causes the cartilage matrix as a whole to expand from within (Fig. 11-2, *interstitial growth*). The other way in which cartilage grows is by having more matrix deposited on its surface. This growth mechanism is described as *appositional growth* (Fig. 11-2). This second mechanism of growth depends on the formation of new matrix-secreting chondroblasts at the cartilage surface.

Cartilage Matrix

Cartilage matrix is basically a resilient *amorphous gel* with a special kind of macromolecular organization. This gel consists mainly of proteoglycan, but some proteins and glycoproteins are also present. Distributed throughout the gel, there are fine *collagen fibrils* made of *type II collagen*. These fine reinforcing fibrils are strong enough to withstand tensile forces but are too narrow to be resolved in the LM because they are only 10 nm to 100 nm in diameter. Minimal and maximal estimates of the collagen content of cartilage matrix are 40% and 70% of its dry weight, but these estimates appear to vary with the source. Approximately half the organic matrix is a gel consisting mainly of viscous hydrophilic *cartilage proteoglycan*.

Like type II collagen, cartilage proteoglycan is synthesized locally by chondrocytes. The general nature of proteoglycans has already been discussed in connection with Amorphous Ground Substance in Chapter 7. An added distinctive feature of cartilage matrix is the presence of huge supramolecular *proteoglycan aggregates*, the proteoglycan content of which provides the molecular basis for its remarkable resilience.

Most Cartilage Proteoglycan Is Present as Proteoglycan Aggregates. Up to approximately 100 proteoglycan molecules, each with a configuration corresponding to the centipedelike representation of heparan sulfate proteoglycan shown in the inset of Figure 7-9, can become laterally arranged along the length of a hyaluronic acid molecule. The resulting *proteoglycan aggregate* resembles a bottle brush with an equivalent number of bristles. However, each bristle would have a distinctive centipedelike configuration (as represented in two dimensions in the *inset* of Fig. 7-9) because of its own laterally projecting glycosaminoglycan chains. The detailed molecular arrangement will now be described.

The long axis of the bottle brush in this analogy is a stretched-out linear molecule of *hyaluronic acid*. Each of the proteoglycan molecules that extends laterally like a bristle from this axis is itself made up of (1) a long central axial molecule of *core protein* with (2) a number of proximal side chains of *keratan sulfate* and (3) an even greater number of distal side chains of *chondroitin sulfate*. The two kinds of side chains extend radially from the molecule of core protein. *Link proteins* anchor the core protein molecules to the hyaluronic acid molecule. For further information about the structure of proteoglycan aggregates, see Rosenberg, and Caplan.

Cartilage proteoglycan and proteoglycan aggregates evidently intermesh to form the kind of network that is discernible in Figure 11-3. This type of organization can only be seen if adequate precautions are taken to maintain its integrity (*e.g.*, through the use of a mild and carefully controlled fixation process carried out in the frozen state [freeze-substitution]). This network is believed to be anchored to a supporting framework of inextensible type II collagen fibrils, probably through interaction between its proteoglycan aggregates and this collagen.

Cartilage Proteoglycan Binds Water and Provides Resilience. The entire length of each glycosaminoglycan chain of a proteoglycan molecule is richly endowed with negatively charged carboxyl and sulfate groups. Mutual electrostatic repulsion between such like charges expands proteoglycan molecules to their maximal volume and provides innumerable interstices to harbor interstitial water molecules and ions. Some of the interstitial water molecules even undergo hydrogen bonding to the negatively charged groups in the glycosaminoglycan chains. This arrangement serves two useful purposes. Not only does it ensure that the proteoglycan network will trap and retain a substantial volume of interstitial fluid, but it also provides cartilage matrix with an intrinsic mechanism of resilience. This is because an applied compressive force sufficient to displace interstitial hydrogen-bonded water molecules from the negatively charged domains on the glycosaminoglycan chains brings these domains into closer apposition, whereupon their in-

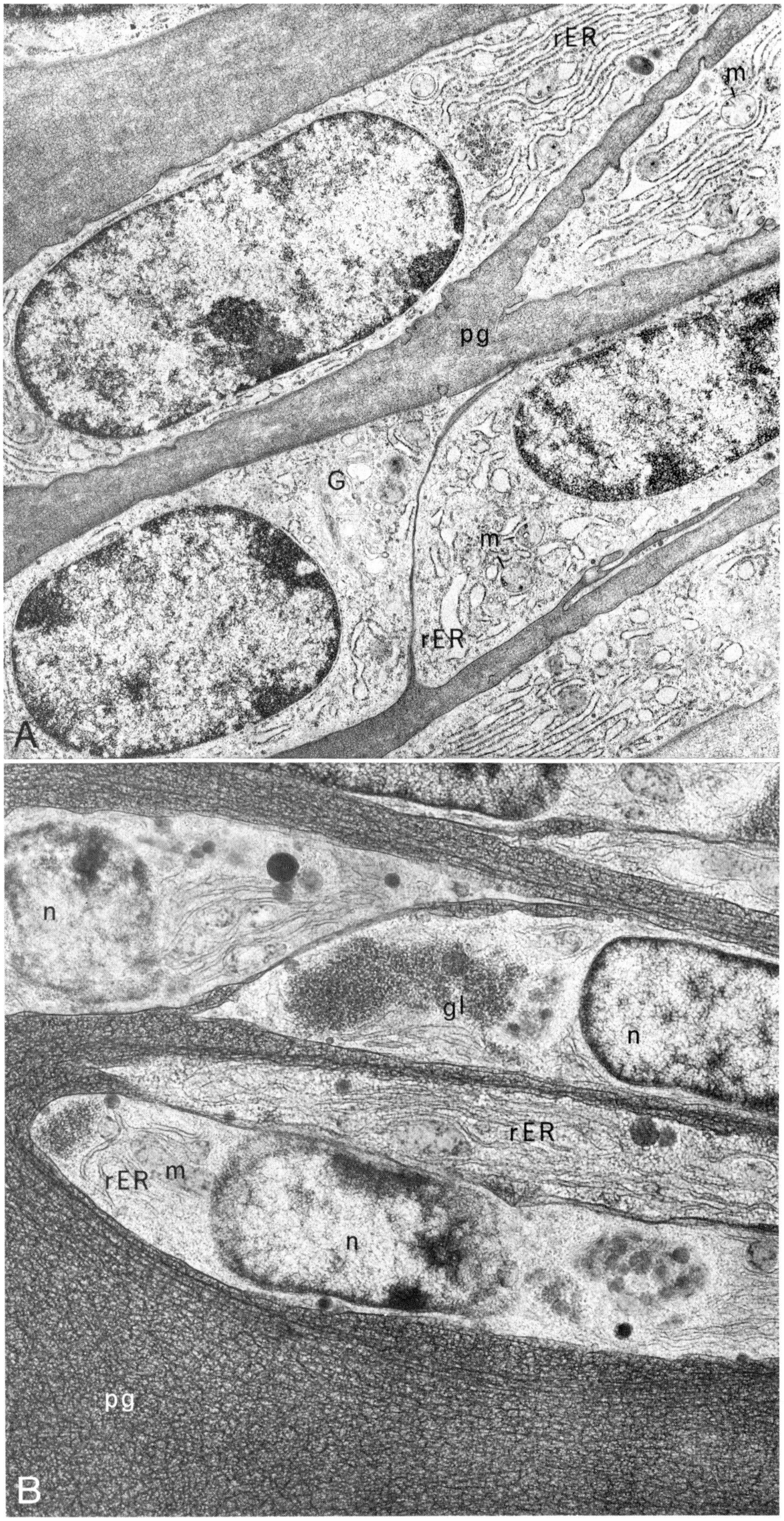

Fig. 11-3. (*A*) Electron micrograph (×8000) of chondrocytes (zone of proliferating cartilage in epiphyseal plate of mouse) prepared by freeze-substitution, which preserves their fine structure and discloses the macromolecular organization of cartilage matrix. Mitochondria (*m*) and cisternae of rough ER (*rER*) distended with secretory product are readily recognized in their cytoplasm. A Golgi region (*G*) can also be distinguished. At this magnification, it is just possible to see that the proteoglycan (*pg*) in the extracellular matrix is arranged in the form of a network. (*B*) Electron micrograph (×7000) of chondrocytes from the same source, prepared by freeze-substitution and observed under the high-voltage EM in a 1-μm section. The increased thickness of section reveals to advantage the glycogen deposits (*gl*) that are now beginning to accumulate in these cells. Mitochondria (*m*) and other organelles, together with nuclei (*n*), can also be discerned. Both micrographs show that the proteoglycan network (*pg*) of cartilage matrix lies in intimate contact with the cell membrane. (Courtesy of L. Arsenault)

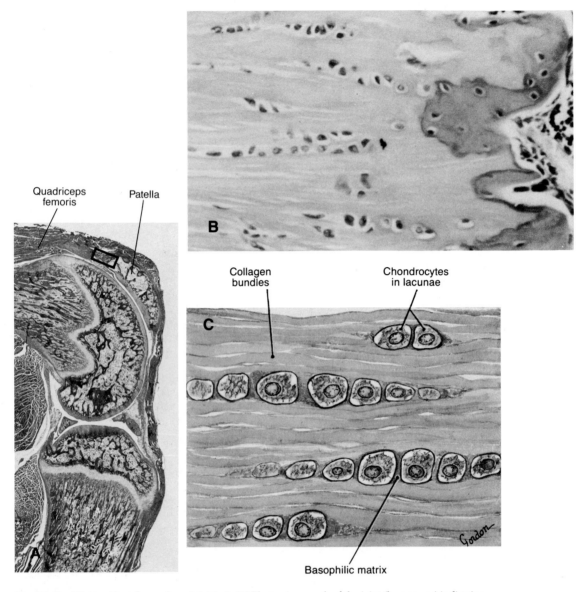

Fig. 11-4. Fibrocartilage from a knee joint (rat). (*A*) Photomicrograph of the joint (low power) indicating the site of part of the attachment of the tendon of the quadriceps femoris muscle to the patella (*box*). (*B*) Photomicrograph of fibrocartilage of the tendon attachment (high power). (*C*) Interpretive drawing of the fibrocartilage seen on the left in *B*.

creased mutual repulsion opposes the compressive force that is responsible for such displacement.

The main proteins in cartilage matrix are *type II collagen* and the *link proteins* mentioned above. *Chondronectin* is a glycoprotein that is secreted by chondroblasts and that promotes the adherence of these cells and chondrocytes to cartilage collagen. Another matrix protein called *chondrocalcin* is believed to play a role in the calcification of hyaline cartilage, as will be explained when we consider calcification in the following chapter.

In hematoxylin and eosin sections, the matrix of hyaline

cartilage either stains a pale blue or it remains almost colorless; it nevertheless tends to stain a little more intensely around cell nests (Fig. 11-2). Such staining is largely due to the sulfated glycosaminoglycan content of cartilage proteoglycan, which is the main constituent of the matrix surrounding chondrocytes (Fig. 11-3). Known as *territorial (capsular) matrix*, this surrounding zone of matrix also stains metachromatically because of the abundance of glycosaminoglycans, and it is stained positively by the PAS reaction because of its glycoprotein content. In its outermost region, many of the collagen fibrils have a circumferential orientation with respect to the chondrocytes or cell nest that they surround. Between the territorial matrix of a given chondrocyte or cell nest and that of its neighbors, there is an intervening region of uniformly staining *interterritorial matrix*.

Finally, 65% to 80% of the wet weight of cartilage matrix represents *tissue fluid* that is partly trapped and partly bound within the complex internal structure of the matrix. Viability of the embedded chondrocytes ultimately depends on adequate diffusion through this essential component of the matrix. Moreover, cartilage is an *avascular* tissue, meaning that is not provided with a capillary blood supply even though larger vessels can course through it without providing nourishment; lymphatics, too, are absent in this tissue. However, the large volume of tissue fluid held in the interstices of its proteoglycan network enables nutrients and oxygen to reach its chondrocytes by long-range diffusion from capillaries that lie *outside the cartilage itself.* Waste products are able to diffuse in the reverse direction to enter such vessels. Total dependence on this very long diffusion path nevertheless presents some problems, especially if insoluble calcium salts have been deposited in the matrix. In most situations in which cartilage matrix becomes heavily impregnated with such salts, the embedded chondrocytes become replaced by bone tissue. As we shall see, bone tissue has a unique canalicular organization that allows its matrix to become heavily calcified without jeopardizing the nourishment of its embedded cells.

Allografts of Hyaline Cartilage Are Suitable for Reconstructive Surgery. A basic difficulty in reconstructive surgery is that there is very little extraskeletal cartilage from which to obtain an autograft. Hence if the nose or an ear requires major reconstructive surgery there is not very much autologous cartilage that can be spared. Fortunately, however, allografts of hyaline cartilage that is removed from accident victims who do not survive have been fairly successful.

Before considering why such grafts survive, we should point out that for a cartilage graft to persist, its chondrocytes must remain viable and capable of producing cartilage proteoglycan. Grafts of dead cartilage become invaded by capillaries and fibroblasts and eventually undergo resorption, but the matrix of living cartilage has the capacity to resist such invasion. As long as its graft bed yields adequate amounts of nutrients and oxygen, a cartilage allograft is able to survive for years. This is because its chondrocytes are embedded in a matrix that limits the diffusion of substances of high molecular weight and therefore tends to shield the foreign antigens of the chondrocytes in the allograft from the immune system of the host. As a result, cartilage allografts are not particularly immunogenic. However, an even more important factor is that the matrix constitutes a physical barrier between the grafted chondrocytes and the surrounding host tissues. Hence even if cytotoxic T-cells are generated, they are prevented from coming into direct contact with their target cells, and with-

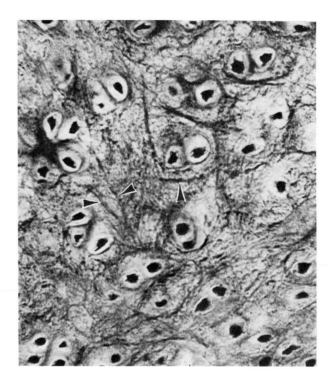

Fig. 11-5. Photomicrograph of elastic cartilage (external ear). Arrowheads indicate elastic fibers in the matrix.

out this contact, they are unable to kill such cells. Finally, the matrix of a viable cartilage graft has the capacity to resist ingrowth of blood vessels from the graft bed, and it remains largely impervious to any antibody molecules that may be formed.

FIBROCARTILAGE

Fibrocartilage is conveniently studied at sites where a tendon is inserted into cartilage. On approaching such an insertion, the tendon takes on a different appearance, as shown in Figure 11-4. Earlier in this chapter, we noted that where a tendon becomes inserted into cartilage, the collagen is formed by chondroblasts instead of fibroblasts. At such insertions, the cells are larger and more rounded than fibroblasts and they lie in rows or layers between parallel bundles of collagen fibers (Fig. 11-4). Between these cells, there is a basophilic amorphous matrix (Fig. 11-4) that resembles the territorial matrix of hyaline cartilage (the darker staining matrix seen around the cell nests at the bottom of Fig. 11-2). Similarly, its basophilia is due to sulfated glycosaminoglycans. Fibrocartilage is avascular, and in adult life, it lacks a perichondrium. In addition to constituting tendon insertions, fibrocartilage is present in the symphysis pubis and intervertebral disks, which will be described in Chapter 13.

ELASTIC CARTILAGE

Elastic cartilage is a highly resilient form of cartilage that is specially adapted to withstand repeated bending. This type of cartilage supports the external ear and the epiglottis, both of which need to be resilient enough to spring back into shape when bent. Elastic cartilage resembles hyaline cartilage except that in addition to widely dispersed type II collagen fibrils, its matrix contains *elastic fibers* (Fig. 11-5). Chondroblasts produce all the components of the matrix and then become embedded as chondrocytes in the matrix that they produce. As in the case of hyaline cartilage, the chondrocytes reside in lacunae and some are present in the form of cell nests (Fig. 11-5). Furthermore, this type of cartilage retains its fibrous layer of perichondrium in adult life.

SELECTED REFERENCES

Tendons and Ligaments

PEACOCK RC, VAN WINKLE W: Surgery and Biology of Wound Repair. Philadelphia, WB Saunders, 1970

POTENZA AD: The healing process in wounds of the digital flexor tendons and tendon grafts: An experimental study. In Verdan C (ed): Tendon Surgery of the Hand, GEM Monograph 4, p 40. Edinburgh, Churchill Livingstone, 1979

Cartilage*

ALBRIGHT JA, MISRA RP: Mechanisms of resorption and remodeling of cartilage. In Hall BK (ed): Cartilage, Vol 3, p 49. New York, Academic Press, 1983

CAPLAN AI: Cartilage. Sci Am 251 No 4:84, 1984

HALL BK (ed): Cartilage, Vols 1 to 3. New York, Academic Press, 1983

HAY ED (ed): Cell Biology of the Extracellular Matrix. New York, Plenum Press, 1981

HEINEGÅRD D, PAULSSON M: Structure and metabolism of proteoglycans. In Piez KA, Reddi AH (eds): Extracellular Matrix Biochemistry, p 277. New York, Elsevier, 1984

HUNZIKER EB, HERRMANN W, SCHENK RK ET AL: Cartilage ultrastructure after high pressure freezing, freeze substitution, and low temperature embedding. I. Chondrocyte ultrastructure—Implications for the theories of mineralization and vascular invasion. J Cell Biol 98:267, 1984

REDDI AH (ed): Extracellular Matrix Structure and Function. UCLA Symposia on Molecular and Cellular Biology, New Series, Vol 25. New York, Alan R Liss, 1985

ROSENBERG L: Structure of cartilage proteoglycans. In Burleigh PMC, Poole AR (eds): Dynamics of Connective Tissue Macromolecules, p 105. Amsterdam, North-Holland, 1975

* See also references on Calcification under Selected References, Chapter 12, and Articular Cartilage under Selected References, Chapter 13.

12

Bone

Bone represents the chief supporting tissue of the body. In this second chapter on the skeletal tissues, we shall consider the nature of bone matrix and also the several different types and arrangements of cells that are found in flat bones and long bones. Among the clinically relevant aspects of bone histology that will be discussed in this chapter and in Chapter 13 are the cellular mechanisms that bring about bone growth and remodeling, the pathways that are involved in the nourishment of different parts of a bone, and the nature of the repair processes that lead to the effective healing of a bone that has broken.

A logical way to begin a histological study of bone is to note some basic similarities between bone and cartilage. Thus both of these tissues contain populations of living cells that become embedded in the intercellular matrix they produce, and in both tissues, the matrix is made up of an amorphous component that is reinforced by collagen fibrils. However, bone matrix possesses more collagen and a smaller proportion of amorphous component, and it is heavily mineralized. Bone tissue is accordingly much harder and less supple than cartilage. The embedded cells of bone are called *osteocytes* (Gr. *osteon*, bone), and like chondrocytes, they occupy matrix spaces termed *lacunae*. Furthermore, bone possesses a fibrous connective tissue counterpart of the perichondrium; this is called the *periosteum*. A final similarity between bone and cartilage is that osteoblasts and chondroblasts both arise directly from mesenchyme. Yet a fundamental difference is that osteoblasts differentiate in the vicinity of blood capillaries whereas chondroblasts differentiate in regions of mesenchyme that are devoid of such vessels.

The stony consistency of bone matrix, which is so heavily calcified that it can resist bending and hence can bear weight, makes it impossible to cut sections of bone using ordinary methods. To cut histological sections of bone, it must first be treated with a suitable decalcifying agent (*e.g.,* EDTA [ethylenediaminetetra-acetic acid]), which is a chelating agent that has a high affinity for Ca^{2+}. The decalcified organic matrix is left comparatively soft; indeed, it is so supple that a decalcified bone can be tied into a knot (Fig. 12-1). Hence the common type of hematoxylin and eosin (H & E) section studied in the laboratory is prepared from *decalcified bone.* Although decalcification makes it possible to cut bone into sections, it unfortunately also ruins the histological appearance of osteocytes, leaving only their nucleus and a remnant of shriveled cytoplasm to be studied (Fig. 12-2A). In the living state, each of these cells would occupy its entire lacuna. Bone that has not been treated with a decalcifying agent is often described as *undecalcified bone.* It, too, can be studied in the light microscope (LM), as explained in the next section.

Capillaries and Canaliculi in Bone Tissue Facilitate Nourishment of Its Osteocytes. Several of the principal differences that exist between bone and cartilage are related to the distinctive manner in which osteocytes are nourished. To observe how this is achieved, it is best to study *ground bone sections,* which are paper-thin slices of bone that are prepared by laboriously grinding down thin sawn-off slices of undecalcified bone until they become translucent enough to study under a microscope.

In contrast to cartilage, the matrix composition of which facilitates long-range diffusion of nutrients and oxygen from sources outside the tissue, bone has a high mineral content that renders long-range diffusion inefficient. A different kind of organization is needed to keep its cells alive. Unlike the arrangement found in cartilage, all the osteocytes of bone tissue lie within a 0.2-mm radius of a blood capillary. This is because capillaries become incorporated into bone tissue as a consequence of the way it develops. In this respect, *highly vascular bone tissue* differs markedly from *avascular cartilage.*

In addition, it can be seen from ground bone sections that bone matrix is traversed by numerous fine canals (Fig. 12-2B). Known as *canaliculi,* these are narrow fluid-filled channels that interconnect osteocyte lacunae and directly or indirectly link them with bone surfaces that are continuously bathed with fresh tissue fluid from capillaries. Within each canaliculus, there is a long thin osteocyte process that is surrounded by tissue fluid (see Fig. 12-3C). The functional significance of these channels is that they serve as miniature lifelines that permit the diffusion of nutrients and oxygen to all the osteocytes in bone tissue, enabling these cells to remain viable in an environment that is very heavily mineralized.

Bone Grows Only by Apposition. In contrast to cartilage, which grows both interstitially and by apposition,

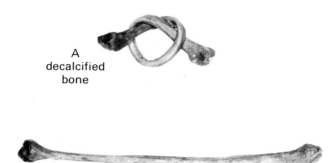

A
decalcified
bone

Fig. 12-1. A simple demonstration of the remarkable flexibility of a decalcified bone as compared with a rigid undecalcified bone.

bones grow entirely by apposition. This is because, unlike chondrocytes, osteocytes do not divide. Furthermore, bone matrix calcifies soon after being produced, and this does not allow the tissue to undergo any further expansion from within. All bone growth is therefore the result of bone deposition on some *preexisting surface.*

The preceding section comparing bone with cartilage constitutes a useful introduction for our next consideration, the prenatal development of bone.

There Are Two Distinct Mechanisms of Osteogenesis. Bone development is called *osteogenesis* (Gr. *gennan,* to produce) or *ossification.* It occurs in two general sites: (1) directly in vascularized mesenchyme and (2) in the central ossifying regions of cartilaginous forerunners of future bones.

The cranial and facial flat bones and the mandible and clavicles develop *directly* in areas of vascularized mesenchyme through a process called *intramembranous ossification,* which is so named because the layer of mesenchyme in which such bones develop can be considered an *embryonic connective tissue membrane.* Although the other bones of the axial and appendicular skeleton are also derivatives of mesenchyme, their development is largely *indirect,* involving a considerably more complex process called *endochondral ossification.* In this case, the bone is preceded by a cartilaginous forerunner termed its *cartilage model,* the skeletal role of which is subsequently assumed by bone tissue when this replaces most of the cartilage in the model during fetal life. Such bones therefore develop and grow as a result of progressive replacement of preexisting cartilage. It should nevertheless be pointed out that the only difference between these two distinct mechanisms of osteogenesis is the *environment* in which ossification occurs. There are no differences in ossification itself or in the kind of bone that it produces, which is always the same.

Because endochondral ossification is a somewhat involved process, it is best dealt with in connection with bone growth. At this point, it is nevertheless helpful to consider the process of intramembranous ossification because it explains the presence of several characteristic features of bone tissue.

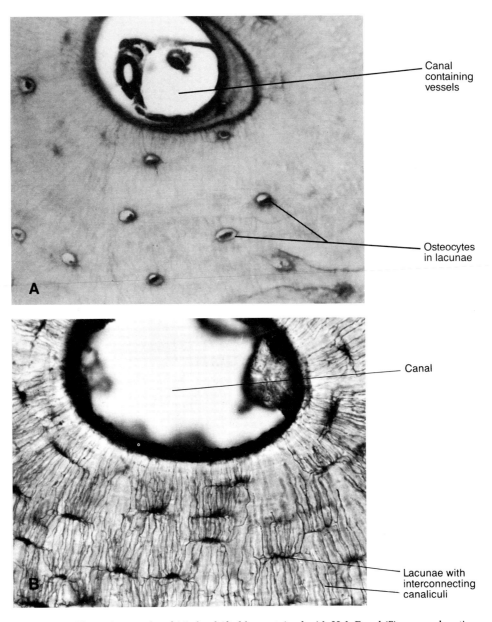

Fig. 12-2. Photomicrographs of (*A*) decalcified bone stained with H & E and (*B*) a ground section of undecalcified bone. Canaliculi are much more distinct in *B,* but osteocytes and the contents of the canal are not preserved.

INTRAMEMBRANOUS OSSIFICATION

Intramembranous ossification begins toward the end of the second month of gestation. The process is conveniently studied in the developing cranium, so we shall use the formation of a parietal bone for our example. At the site where a parietal bone will develop, there is initially a layer of loose mesenchyme. Prior to ossification, this mesenchyme appears as widely separated, pale-staining stellate cells with interconnecting cytoplasmic processes (seen at periphery in Fig. 12-3A). Then, at the site where a parietal

bone will form, a *center of osteogenesis* begins to develop in association with capillaries that grow into the mesenchyme (Fig. 12-3A).

The mesenchymal cells in such a center take on a rounded basophilic appearance and also exhibit slightly thicker interconnecting processes (Fig. 12-3A, *middle*). Such cells have passed imperceptibly through the *osteogenic cell* stage (which will be described later in this chapter) and then differentiated into *osteoblasts* (Gr. *blastos,* germ), the cells that generate the organic matrix of bone. Once surrounded with bone matrix, they are called *osteocytes* (Fig. 12-3B).

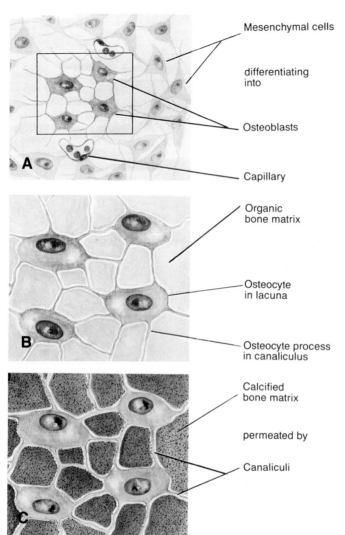

Mesenchymal cells

differentiating
into

Osteoblasts

Capillary

Organic
bone matrix

Osteocyte
in lacuna

Osteocyte process
in canaliculus

Calcified
bone matrix

permeated by

Canaliculi

Fig. 12-3. Schematic diagram showing three stages of intramembranous ossification. For details, see text.

This matrix soon begins to calcify (Fig. 12-3C), but the osteocytes can still obtain their nutrients and oxygen by diffusion along bone canaliculi (Fig. 12-3C). These tiny channels are formed in the following way.

The organic matrix produced by osteoblasts is also formed around their interconnecting processes (Fig. 12-3B). After it is impregnated with mineral, this matrix therefore remains riddled with canaliculi (Fig. 12-3C). The narrow spaces between the osteocyte processes and the walls of their surrounding canaliculi are filled with tissue fluid that is derived from capillaries situated just outside the islands of forming bone. Tissue fluid also occupies the narrow space between each osteocyte and the walls of its surrounding lacuna.

The first small mass of newly formed bone matrix takes the form of a tiny, irregularly shaped *spicule* (Fig. 12-4) that gradually lengthens into a longer anastomosing structure that is described as a *trabecula* (L. for small beam). Spicules and trabeculae of bone are easy to recognize in

H & E sections because their matrix stains a bright pink color and because they are covered with large rounded osteoblasts that have an intensely basophilic cytoplasm (Fig. 12-4). Canaliculi are not usually discernible in H & E sections.

The further growth of a developing parietal bone is a result of trabeculae extending from it in a radial pattern. Continued growth leads to the formation of an anastomosing network of trabeculae that is characteristic of a form of bone known as *spongy* or *cancellous bone* (L. *cancellus*, lattice). The latticelike structure of this form of bone is illustrated in Figure 12-5B. By the time cancellous bone has formed, there are few mesenchyme-derived cells in the area that remain undifferentiated. However, before these cells entirely disappear, they leave a heritage of thin, flattened cells known as *osteogenic cells* on the parts of trabecular surfaces that are not occupied by osteoblasts. In richly vascularized regions, these osteogenic cells give rise to osteoblasts that then form bone tissue, but if no local

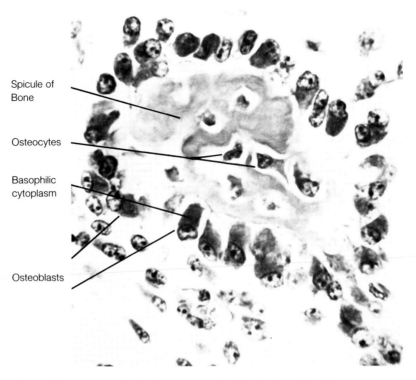

Spicule of
Bone

Osteocytes

Basophilic
cytoplasm

Osteoblasts

Fig. 12-4. Photomicrograph of a bone spicule that is being formed by intramembranous ossification (skull of pig embryo).

capillary blood supply has been established, they give rise to chondroblasts and hence cartilage instead. Osteogenic cells are not only *bipotential* but also *self-renewing;* they therefore represent a *stem cell* population that is capable of giving rise to either bone or cartilage. Because they persist in adult life, they constitute a potential source of new skeletal tissue for the repair of broken bones.

Appositional Growth of Cancellous Bone Can Result in Its Conversion into Compact Bone. The bone cell population that covers the surfaces of spicules and trabeculae of developing bone includes both osteoblasts and osteogenic cells. Because these osteogenic cells are proliferating in an environment that is richly vascularized, they give rise to osteoblasts that thereupon deposit new layers of bone matrix on the preexisting bone surfaces. Moreover, this process does not alter the relative position of the osteogenic cells, so they remain in a superficial position, ready to repeat this process over and over again. Such an *appositional growth mechanism* results in the buildup of bone tissue one layer at a time. Each new generation of osteoblasts produces their own additional canaliculi, with the result that all the new osteocytes remain linked, by their canaliculi, both to the bone surface above and to the osteocytes below (Fig. 12-5*A*, stage 3). Furthermore, as the trabeculae increase in width as a result of appositional growth, they incorporate neighboring capillaries that then are able to deliver nutrients to their most deeply situated osteocytes. Such small vessels become incorporated into bone tissue because the tissue

envelops and encloses them during the course of becoming built up layer upon layer. Such an arrangement ensures that no osteocytes are required to live more than 0.2 mm from a source of fresh tissue fluid.

Whereas new bone is being deposited on some bone surfaces, a certain amount of preexisting bone is being removed from surfaces where it is no longer needed. This progressive removal of excess bone tissue starts as soon as bone deposition begins, and it avoids any unnecessary buildup of the tissue. The cells responsible for bone removal, which is more often described as *bone resorption,* are specialized multinucleated cells called *osteoclasts* (Gr. *klan,* to break) that have the capacity to erode bone surfaces. The net result of bone deposition at some sites and bone resorption at others is that bony trabeculae become *remodeled.* These two opposing processes (*i.e.,* appositional growth and bone resorption) enable bones to maintain or change their shape and size as necessary throughout pre- and postnatal life.

Continuing appositional growth and remodeling of the bony trabeculae of a parietal bone eventually convert its cancellous bone into a more solid form of bone known as *dense* or *compact bone.*

The Development of Compact Bone

The most striking difference between *cancellous* and *compact* bone is the dissimilarity between their respective pro-

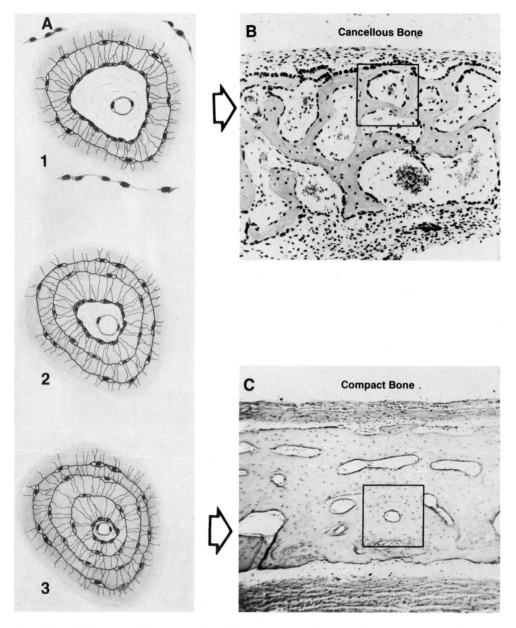

Fig. 12-5. (A) Diagrammatic representation of the process by which a soft tissue space in cancellous bone of the developing skull becomes filled in with concentric lamellae to form an osteon of compact bone. The space becomes reduced to a narrow canal that retains a lining of osteogenic cells. (B) Photomicrograph of a plate of cancellous bone of the developing cranial vault at the stage illustrated in part 1 of A. The large basophilic cells present on the periosteal and endosteal surfaces are osteoblasts. (C) Photomicrograph of a plate of compact bone (cranial vault of a child) at the stage illustrated in part 3 of A.

portions of soft tissue spaces and bone matrix. Thus cancellous bone has such large soft tissue spaces (which are initially filled with vascular loose connective tissue but later contain myeloid tissue) that their total volume exceeds that of the bone matrix itself (Fig. 12-5B). *Compact bone*, on the other hand, is characterized by having a higher proportion

of bone matrix than of soft tissue spaces (Fig. 12-5C). Throughout the gradual transition from cancellous to compact bone, the trabecular surfaces—including the lining surfaces of soft tissue spaces—retain their population of associated osteogenic cells. As consecutive layers of bone tissue build up by apposition on these surfaces, the trabeculae thicken and the soft tissue spaces that they enclose become progressively narrower, as illustrated in Figure 12-5A. This process can convert cancellous bone with large soft tissue spaces (Fig. 12-5B) into compact bone with only small soft tissue spaces (Fig. 12-5C). A certain amount of cancellous bone is nevertheless retained in the central parts of most bones.

Osteons (Haversian Systems) Are Formed by the Filling in of Soft Tissue Spaces. The gradual filling-in process that converts cancellous bone into compact bone creates a number of narrow canals that are lined with osteogenic cells. Such canals enclose the vessels that were formerly present in the soft tissue spaces of the cancellous network. Each multilayered arrangement that is built up as consecutive *lamellae* (layers) of bone become added to the bony walls of the spaces in cancellous bone (stages 1 to 3 in Fig. 12-5A) is called an *osteon* or a *haversian system* (named after Havers, who first described it). When cut in transverse section, these lamellae appear as a series of concentric rings situated around a small central *haversian canal* that contains one or two small blood vessels and a lining of osteogenic cells (stage 3 in Fig. 12-5A). Osteons have an average diameter of 0.3 mm, and they represent the basic structural unit of compact bone. Because osteons that develop in flat bones are short in comparison to the osteons that are present in long bones, they are commonly referred to as *primitive osteons*.

After the spaces in the network of cancellous bone have become filled in with osteons, a parietal bone becomes a simple plate of compact bone (Fig. 12-5C). Yet to accommodate the growing brain, it still has to enlarge and adjust its curvature, processes that have to continue until the head attains its adult size.

The Growing Plate of Compact Bone Undergoes Remodeling. Throughout the period of growth of the cranial vault, the margins of the flat bones of which it is composed remain separated from one another by special joints that are described as *sutures* (L. *sutura*, seam). During the growing period, these sutures contain loose connective tissue, blood vessels, and osteogenic cells (*i.e.*, everything necessary to facilitate appositional growth of the bone margins that meet at the suture). Enlargement of the cranial vault is believed to be brought about by a combination of (1) peripheral growth of these bones into the sutures that join them (Fig. 12-6A and B); and (2) bone deposition on their broad convex surfaces, accompanied by compensatory bone resorption from their concave surfaces (Fig. 12-6B) to avoid undue thickness and to match their curvature to the contours of the growing brain.

By the time of birth, the flat bones of the cranium are separated only by narrow sutures. However, at the sites where *more* than two bones meet, the suture space remains larger and such areas are termed *fontanelles* (soft spots). There are six of these soft areas that are not yet filled with bone in the skull of the newborn infant. The most prominent, the *anterior* or *frontal* fontanelle, is situated at the

point where the two parietal bones and the bone advancing from dual centers of ossification of the frontal bone meet. Palpation of this fontanelle can give the physician valuable information about whether ossification is proceeding normally in an infant.

As they grow, the parietal bones are, for some time after birth, composed of only a single plate of bone. However, the plate of bone contains some spaces filled with loose connective tissue and thin-walled veins (Fig. 12-5C). As growth of the skull continues, the remodeling process (appositional growth in some sites and resorption in others) gradually converts these single plates of bone over most of the skull into double plates of compact bone, between which there is some cancellous bone and a considerable amount of marrow.

Because cancellous bone and the bone marrow it contains in its spaces separate two plates of compact bone at this stage, this arrangement of two plates of bone is termed the *diploë* (Gr. meaning double) and the many large, thin-walled veins present in the marrow between the two plates are correspondingly called the *diploetic veins*. The double-plate arrangement of the diploë is attained at approximately 8 years of age. In adult life, the bones meeting at the various sutures fuse and it becomes possible for diploetic veins to pass from one skull bone to another.

IMMATURE AND MATURE BONE

It has already been emphasized that bone forming as a result of intramembranous ossification is no different from that forming by endochondral ossification. Hence if the terms *membrane bone* and *cartilage bone* are ever used, they do not signify different kinds of bone but only that the bone was, in these two instances, formed in different tissue environments in the embryo. However, as described above, there are two kinds of bone that are characterized by whether they consist chiefly of trabeculae, with relatively large spaces between them (*cancellous bone*), or primarily of bone substance, with small spaces (*compact* or *dense bone*). We shall now describe how in addition to being classified as cancellous or compact, bone can be classified as either *immature* or *mature*. These two types of bone are distinguished from each other by the arrangement and relative amounts of the various components of their intercellular substance and also by the relative numbers of osteocytes they possess in relation to their content of intercellular substance. Such morphological criteria also permit bone to be classified as (1) *bundle bone*, (2) *woven bone*, or (3) *fine-fibered bone* (Pritchard).

The basis for distinguishing between *immature* and *mature* bone is that bundle bone and woven bone are generally the first types of bone to develop in prenatal life. Fine-fibered bone is formed later, so it is often referred to as *mature* bone to distinguish it from the *immature* bone that is formed earlier. Most immature bone has only a temporary

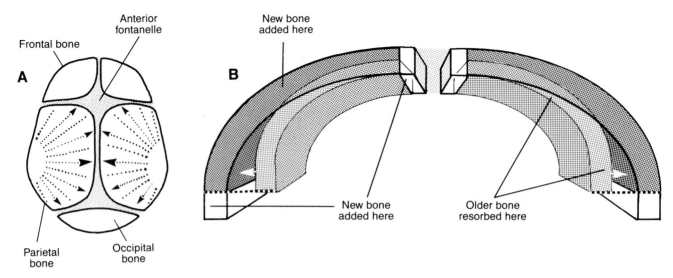

Fig. 12-6. Diagrams illustrating growth of the cranial vault. (*A*) Superior view of fetal skull. The sutures and fontanelles are indicated in gray. (*B*) Schematic representation of growth and change of curvature of the bones of the cranial vault (coronal section). For details, see text.

existence; it is replaced with mature bone as growth continues.

Immature Bone.   A distinctive feature of immature bone is that it contains a relatively higher proportion of osteocytes than mature bone (Fig. 12-7). Its two subtypes are known as *woven bone* and *coarsely bundled bone.* In the former subtype, bundles of collagen fibers run in various directions through the matrix; this accounts for the name *woven.* Also, the matrix of woven bone tends to be tinged with blue in H & E sections, possibly indicating that it has a higher proteoglycan content than mature bone. Bundle bone differs from woven bone in that it contains thick collagen bundles, most of which are arranged parallel to one another with osteocytes between them.

Although the matrix of immature bone stains unevenly, it so commonly demonstrates basophilia that areas of immature bone that have become surrounded by mature bone may be spotted easily on low-power examination (Fig. 12-7). Unless it is appreciated that regions of immature bone can become surrounded by mature bone, as seen in Figure 12-7, its presence can be *mistakenly interpreted as being due to some degenerative change* that occurred in mature bone.

As already noted, almost all the immature bone that forms during prenatal life is subsequently replaced by mature bone. According to Pritchard, some immature bone persists in tooth sockets, near cranial sutures, in the osseous labyrinth, and near tendon and ligament attachments; in these sites, however, it is usually mixed with mature bone. It should also be mentioned that immature bone can be formed in postnatal life in the repair of fractures and in rapidly growing tumors of bone that arise from osteogenic cells.

Mature Bone.   Alternatively described as *lamellar bone,* mature bone is characterized by a distinctive orderly ar-

rangement that is the result of the repeated addition of uniform lamellae to bony surfaces during appositional growth. These lamellae are from 4 μm to 12 μm thick. The osteoblasts that produce them become incorporated as osteocytes in the layers of bone matrix that they form. In general, the direction of the collagen fibrils in any given lamella lies at right angles to that of the fibrils in the adjacent lamellae. Because of this difference in the orientation of the collagen, optical differences can be detected between adjacent lamellae if they are viewed under polarized light.

Some microscopic features of mature bone that may be helpful in distinguishing mature bone from immature bone are (1) the comparatively even acidophilic staining of its matrix, (2) the comparatively regular arrangement of its lamellae, and (3) the fact that its osteocytes are fewer, more evenly arranged, and present in flatter lacunae (Fig. 12-7).

Secondary Cartilage.   Another term that is sometimes encountered in descriptions of the development and growth of the skull is *secondary cartilage.* This type of cartilage develops in association with bones that are formed by intramembranous ossification. If it were not for the development of secondary cartilage, all bones that formed intramembranously would lack articular cartilages. Hence secondary cartilage develops *after* the bone with which it is associated.

We shall now provide some more details about the cell types that are associated with bone tissue and then elaborate further on the nature of bone matrix itself.

OSTEOGENIC CELLS

Osteogenic cells, which are also sometimes referred to as *osteoprogenitor cells,* are small, pale-staining, spindle-

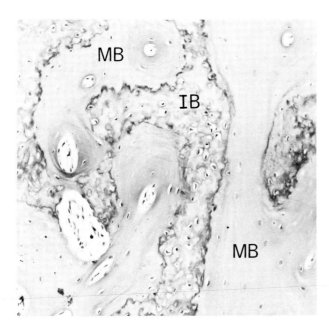

Fig. 12-7. Low-power photomicrograph showing immature bone (*IB*) and mature bone (*MB*) in an H & E section of decalcified bone. Regions of immature bone have been replaced by mature bone.

shaped cells that are present on all nonresorbing surfaces of living bone as constituents of two membranes: (1) as the deepest layer of the *periosteum* (Gr. *peri,* around), the membrane that *covers the outer surface* of any given bone; and (2) the *endosteum* (Gr. *endon,* within) that *lines the internal surfaces* of all cavities within bones. The bony walls of bone cavities are said to be lined with endosteum (these cavities include the marrow cavities, all the haversian canals of compact bone, and all the spaces in cancellous bone). But because some trabeculae of cancellous bone in a given section may appear not to be continuous with one another, and hence may seem not to surround cavities, such trabeculae should be said to be *covered* with endosteum, not *lined* with it.

Osteogenic cells are also a stromal component of the bone marrow that fills the cavities of bones.

The *periosteum* is a substantial and vascular connective tissue membrane that covers the outer surface of the bone except for its articular surfaces. Its comparatively thick outer region is called its *fibrous layer* because it is composed of dense ordinary connective tissue (irregularly arranged). Its less well-defined inner region is called its *osteogenic layer* because it is made up of osteogenic cells. When neither appositional growth nor bone resorption is occurring, this membrane is described as *resting periosteum* and its outer region, which consists primarily of collagen fibers, elastic fibers, and a few fibroblasts, is thicker than its inner region.

The *endosteum* consists only of a layer of flat osteogenic cells without a fibrous component. Its osteogenic cells are

nevertheless able to participate with those of the periosteum in the repair of broken bones. They also serve as a source of the osteoblasts that are needed to form new haversian systems when old ones are resorbed, as will be described later in this chapter.

Because the osteogenic cells in resting periosteum are poorly differentiated, it is not possible to identify them by their microscopic appearance alone. However, their relative position in this membrane is well established, and evidence of their proliferation and differentiation in response to an activating stimulus (*e.g.,* a fracture) can easily be recognized in a bone section (Fig. 12-8).

When circumstances cause osteogenic cells of the periosteum or endosteum to proliferate, these cells give rise to *osteoblasts* in regions that are well vascularized (Fig. 12-8) and to *chondroblasts* in regions that are avascular. Moreover, some of their descendants self-renew without differentiating any further, and this ensures that a pool of osteogenic cells will remain for future use. Osteogenic cells therefore constitute a population of *bipotential stem cells* that can give rise to either bone or cartilage, whichever is required. Furthermore, the different expression of these two potentialities in vascular and avascular environments explains why cartilage forms during the development, growth, and repair of long bones.

Osteogenesis Does Not Occur Without Prior Vascularization. Ham's early studies on the contribution made by the periosteum to fracture repair led him to observe that the only osteogenic cells that give rise to bone tissue are those that are situated near blood capillaries. The conclusion that vascularization is required before osteogenesis will occur *in vivo* is now borne out by many observations. Yet the reasons for this dependence have not been fully elucidated. Because the capillary blood supply of a region serves as its principal source of oxygen, it was at first believed that the primary determinant inducing differentiation into osteoblasts was a high local oxygen tension, and that a low local oxygen tension would result in differentiation into chondroblasts. However, it subsequently became evident that other factors such as compression are also involved. Thus a combination of compression forces and adequate oxygen tension has been found to promote bone formation whereas compression forces in combination with a reduced oxygen tension promote cartilage formation (Bassett and Herrmann). Furthermore, one of the factors that determines how much cartilage is produced at a fracture site is the amount of free movement that is allowed to occur at the site. Lastly, oxygen is certainly not the only constituent that comes from capillaries. There is every reason to suppose that capillaries could also provide a continuous supply of fresh tissue fluid, nutrients, and any differentiation or growth factors that might also be needed for osteogenesis to occur.

A Protein Present in Bone Matrix Can Induce the Formation of Osteogenic Cells. Bone tissue is not only called upon to repair itself if fractured. It is also submitted to a lifelong process of remodeling. The total number of osteogenic cells required for such purposes is so great that unless new cells could be recruited, the population of osteogenic cells might become depleted. Two lines of evidence suggest that new osteogenic cells can arise from more primitive mesenchymal progenitors during postnatal life.

First, under certain circumstances soft tissue sites can become

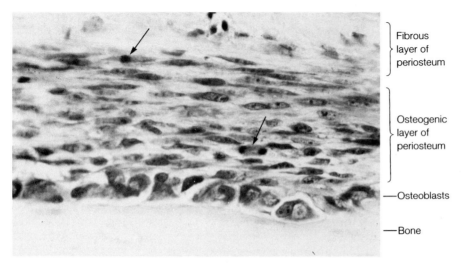

Fig. 12-8. Photomicrograph of periosteum near a fracture. The fibrous layer has become lifted away from the bone by the thickened osteogenic layer in which osteogenic cells are proliferating. Mitotic figures are indicated by arrows. At the bone surface, osteogenic cells have differentiated into osteoblasts that will form a new layer of bone. (Ham AW, Harris WR: In Bourne GH (ed): The Biochemistry and Physiology of Bone, 2nd ed, Vol 3. New York, Academic Press, 1971)

sites of ossification. Such misplaced bone formation is called *het-erotopic* (Gr. *heteros*, other) or *ectopic* (Gr. *ektopos*, displaced) *osteogenesis*. For example, as a result of aging, trauma, or disease, osteogenesis can occur in the walls of arteries, tendon attachments to bone, damaged muscles, diseased kidneys, or old incisional scars. Heterotopic osteogenesis has aroused much curiosity on the part of investigators about which type of cell is involved and which factors would induce bone formation in such strange places. Clearly, osteogenic cells could hardly be expected to exist at such atypical sites, so a more likely explanation would be that they are generated locally from more primitive mesenchymal cells.

The second line of evidence comes primarily from investigations by Urist and his associates and also by Reddi et al. Studies by the latter group showed that demineralized bone powders have the capacity to induce new bone formation *in vivo* (Reddi et al). Urist's group has succeeded in identifying and partly characterizing a noncollagen protein or glycopolypeptide that is associated in low concentration with the collagen of bone matrix and dentin, and that is released during bone resorption. They call this protein *bone morphogenetic protein* (BMP); the word morphogenetic means that it induces the formation of entirely new bone. Implied in its name is the fact that this protein has the capacity to initiate what is termed the *morphogenetic phase* of bone development, which includes the migration, aggregation, and proliferation of mesenchymal-type cells and their ensuing differentiation into osteogenic cells. One of the places where such primitive mesenchymelike cells are known to persist is the perivascular loose connective tissue that is associated with capillaries and other kinds of small blood vessels. It is also of interest that the content of BMP in bone matrix declines with age and that this decline follows a time course similar to that of age-related loss of bone density. There is also some evidence to suggest that in certain forms of osteoporosis (reduction of total bone mass), autoimmunity to BMP may be responsible for reducing bone formation (Urist et al).

OSTEOBLASTS

The primary role of osteoblasts is to synthesize and secrete the macromolecular organic constituents of bone matrix. This matrix is deposited not only around their cell bodies but also around their cytoplasmic processes, resulting in the formation of canaliculi. A further function of osteoblasts is to participate in the nucleation of crystalline bone mineral, which is considered below.

Osteoblasts are relatively large nondividing cells with a shape that is generally rounded to polygonal (Fig. 12-8). Their nucleus is commonly situated eccentrically in the part of the cell that is farthest away from the adjacent bone surface. Their cytoplasm is deeply basophilic, and commonly it exhibits a distinct negative Golgi image (see Fig. 4-15). The cytoplasmic processes of osteoblasts (see Fig. 12-9, labeled *cp*) are not visible in H & E sections, but from other types of preparations, it is known that they are in contact with one another and also with the processes of osteocytes in the lacunae beneath them.

The fine structure of osteoblasts is typical of secretory cells in general. Thus their intense cytoplasmic basophilia is due to an abundance of rough-surfaced endoplasmic reticulum (rER; Fig. 12-9). The procollagen and other organic constituents of bone matrix synthesized by this organelle enter its lumen and are carried by transfer vesicles to the prominent Golgi complex, where they become packaged into secretory vesicles. Exocytosis of these secretory products occurs from all parts of the cell surface as it does in fibroblasts. The composition of the organic matrix that osteoblasts produce in this way is described in the following section.

BONE MATRIX AND CALCIFICATION

There are differences in matrix composition between bone and cartilage that are closely related to the respective functions of these two tissues. For example, whereas cartilage matrix has a substantial proteoglycan content and can hold enough interstitial water to support long-range diffusion, bone matrix has only a low proteoglycan content and cannot hold as much water. Its water content is, in fact, only approximately 25% as compared with 65% to 80% for cartilage. Nevertheless, because bone tissue is provided with canaliculi, it does not have to depend on diffusion through its matrix to keep its cells alive.

Bone matrix, on the other hand, is often called upon to provide great tensile strength, for which it requires a greater collagen content than cartilage. Approximately 90% of the organic content of bone matrix is therefore collagen, as compared with only 40% to 70% of the dry weight of cartilage matrix. Most of the collagen in bone matrix is type I collagen, but small quantities of type V collagen have also been reported. The pink to red color of bone matrix that can be seen in H & E sections is due to this substantial collagen content.

The remaining 10% or so of the organic content of bone matrix represents an amorphous component containing chondroitin sulfate and hyaluronic acid (which are initially associated with protein as proteoglycan aggregates) together with some noncollagen proteins and glycoproteins. *Osteonectin* is a bone-specific protein that serves to anchor the collagen of bone matrix to bone mineral. *Osteocalcin* is a calcium-binding protein that is believed to be involved in bone calcification. During bone formation, bone matrix also takes up detectable amounts of albumin from tissue fluid. For further details about the composition of bone matrix, see Triffitt.

Our next consideration will be how bone matrix acquires its high mineral content, which requires an initial explanation of some of the terms that are used. The following section will also provide a certain amount of necessary clinical perspective regarding the process of calcification.

Calcification Has Broad Clinical Significance. Medical students are probably already well aware that the terms *ossification* and *osteogenesis* (both of which are used to denote the process of bone formation) do not mean the same thing as *calcification* (the deposition of insoluble calcium salts in a tissue). The process of ossification would normally include both the production of organic bone matrix and its ensuing calcification. However, the terms ossification and osteogenesis can also be used in a more restricted sense to denote the production of bone-forming cells and the following deposition of organic bone matrix. Furthermore, under certain conditions, even soft tissues will undergo ectopic (misplaced) calcification. Hence it is possible for calcification to occur in the absence of ossification, and ossification can proceed without reaching the stage of calcification. Bone tissue that is still uncalcified is called *osteoid tissue* (*osteoid* denoting bonelike) or *prebone*. Thus if the combined ion product of the calcium and phosphate ions in tissue fluid is too low, ossification proceeds without calcification, leading to the production of osteoid tissue but not bone. Two dietary-deficiency diseases that are characterized by such failure to calcify are *rickets* in infants and *osteomalacia* in adults. Both are bone conditions that will be described later in this chapter. Also of relevance to medicine and dentistry is the fact that it is difficult to recognize osteoid tissue in radiographs because only bone that is calcified shows up clearly on x-ray examination. Nor can the healing of a fracture be counted on to show up radiographically until the fracture repair tissue (termed *callus*) has begun to calcify.

A zone of osteoid tissue persists around each osteoblast (Fig. 12-9) and osteocyte during normal calcification. In the electron microscope (EM), this zone appears as a pale region containing collagen fibrils that are widely dispersed in a lightly stained amorphous matrix (see Fig. 12-12). An irregular *calcification front* extending along the interface between the osteoid tissue and the surrounding calcified bone indicates where calcification is taking place. The sharp but irregular border between these two tissues can just be discerned where it is labeled *b* in Figure 12-12.

Bone matrix owes a great deal of its intrinsic strength to its abundant collagen (approximately 90% of its organic content) and bone mineral (almost 70% of its wet weight). Why skeletal and dental tissues should be the only tissues that, under normal conditions, acquire such a high mineral content is an issue that has intrigued many investigators. The absolute physiological necessity for precise regulation of Ca^{2+} levels in all parts of the body makes strict local control of the onset of mineralization essential. One need only consider the clinical complications of calcification occurring in atherosclerotic plaques on the walls of essential arteries, or the kidney damage inflicted by the continuing growth of kidney stones, to appreciate the full importance of such regulation. Moreover, if the process of mineralization were initiated but then allowed to proceed unabated, it could cause potentially dangerous hardening of clinically important tissues such as heart valves and arterial walls. Also, Ca^{2+} ions might become locked too stably in crystalline arrays to be freely available to mediate essential cellular and physiological processes. Because ectopic calcification can have such devastating clinical consequences, investigators have now widened their attention to include mechanisms by which the soft tissues normally protect themselves from such calcification, which is a matter that we shall come back to consider later in this chapter.

Calcification Is Essentially the Extracellular Deposition of Hydroxyapatite. A good deal of the early work on calcification appears to have been based on the assumption

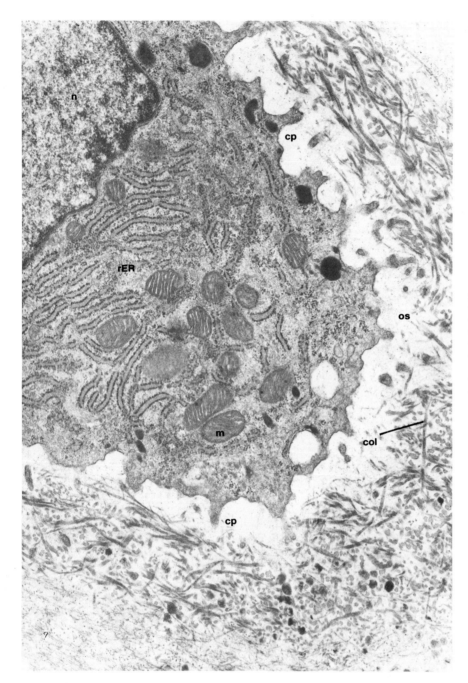

Fig. 12-9. Electron micrograph of part of an osteoblast, the nucleus (*n*) of which is seen in the top left-hand corner. This cell possesses numerous mitochondria (*m*) and a highly developed rough ER (*rER*), and it has many cytoplasmic processes (*cp*) extending from it. The pale zone of osteoid tissue (*os*) surrounding the cell contains an abundance of newly formed collagen fibrils (*col*). (Courtesy of L. Arsenault)

that a single universal mechanism underlies the mineralization of bone and cartilage and perhaps accounts for the calcification of degenerating soft tissues as well. However, there has been very little agreement about what constitutes the *primary cause* of such mineralization. It now seems likely that instead of only a single set of conditions that pertains in every situation, a number of different factors may operate synergistically or interchangeably to initiate mineral deposition. Also, it is still not entirely clear whether the first-formed solid phase is amorphous or crystalline, even though it is widely conceded that amorphous calcium phosphate ($Ca_9(PO_4)_6$) that is present early in mineralization undergoes progressive transformation into the crystalline state. It is nevertheless firmly established that the final mineral deposit in bone is crystalline *hydroxyapatite* ($Ca_5(PO_4)_3OH$).

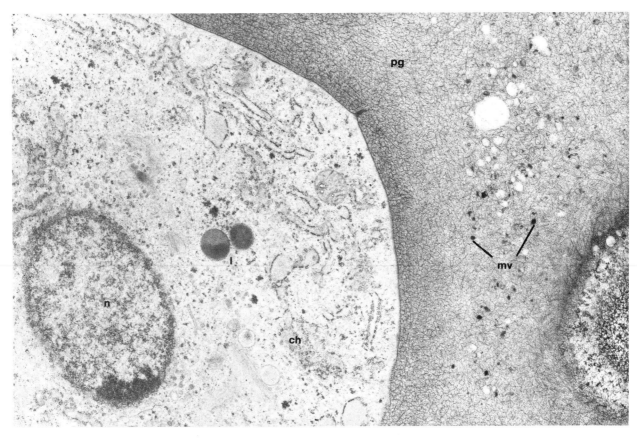

Fig. 12-10. Electron micrograph (×11,000) of a hypertrophied chondrocyte (*ch*) in the zone of maturing cartilage of an epiphyseal plate, prepared by freeze-substitution. The matrix vesicles (*mv*) produced by these cells appear as small electron-dense vesicles in the proteoglycan network (*pg*) of cartilage matrix. The cell nucleus (*n*) and two lysosomes (*l*) can also be recognized in this section. (Courtesy of L. Arsenault)

Under normal conditions, there seem to be insufficient concentrations of available Ca^{2+} and *phosphate* ions in blood and tissue fluid for calcium phosphate to crystallize or precipitate spontaneously. The critical factor is the local $[Ca^{2+}] \times [P_i]$ ion product, commonly referred to as the $Ca^{2+} \cdot P_i$ *product*, where P_i denotes total free inorganic orthophosphate (*i.e.*, HPO_4^{2-} and $H_2PO_4^-$ as well as PO_4^{3-}). When factors operate locally to raise this ion product, calcium phosphate separates out in the solid phase and then undergoes solid phase transition and interconversion into a number of alternative crystalline arrangements of varying degrees of complexity. Once microcrystals of *hydroxyapatite* have begun to form, they will then (1) continue to grow and (2) catalyze further crystallization of calcium phosphate even at sites where the local $Ca^{2+} \cdot P_i$ product does not exceed the plasma level. This, of course, explains why it is so important to keep crystal nucleation under strict control.

The two most widely accepted theories of how such a local increase in the $Ca^{2+} \cdot P_i$ product is brought about are not really mutually exclusive; hence either or both might apply depending on prevailing circumstances. Both theories invoke the trapping of Ca^{2+} and P_i in concentrations that would initiate deposition of calcium phosphate in the solid phase, followed by its conversion to crystalline hydroxyapatite. However, one theory holds some cellular component directly responsible for nucleation, whereas the other hypothesis is based on the idea that nucleation depends on specific properties of some cell-derived macromolecular constituent of mature organic matrix.

Crystals of Hydroxyapatite Can Form in Association with Matrix Vesicles. Until fairly recently, attention was focused almost exclusively on cell-derived structures termed *matrix vesicles* (Figs. 12-10 and 12-11). These are small membrane-bounded structures, 25 nm to 250 nm in diameter, that have been observed lying free in the matrix at many different sites where calcification is known to be underway, including calcifying cartilage, osteoid tissue, and dentin. They seem to arise as rounded outgrowths of the cell membrane that bud from chondrocytes, osteoblasts, and odontoblasts into the extracellular matrix. The current view that they are independent structures that are derived from the cell surface is partly based on the qualitative similarity found between their enzyme complement and the enzymes known to be associated with the cell membrane of such cells. A detailed characterization of these enzymes has disclosed several reasons for believing that matrix ves-

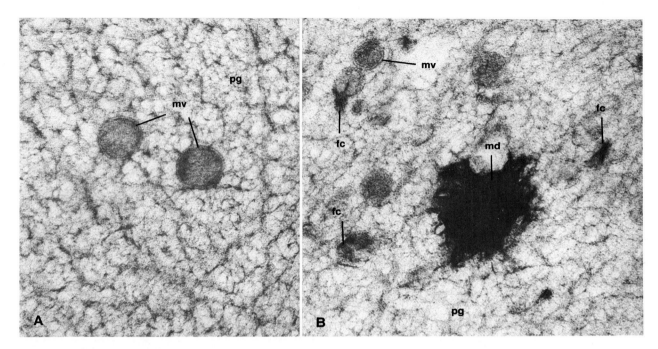

Fig. 12-11. Electron micrographs (×90,000) of matrix vesicles (*mv*) prepared by freeze-substitution, which preserves their unit-membrane appearance. (*A*) Seen prior to calcification in the zone of proliferating cartilage of an epiphyseal plate. (*B*) Seen acting as early foci of calcification (*fc*) in the zone of maturing cartilage of the plate. The larger electron-dense mass is a mineral deposit (*md*) seeded by matrix vesicles. The proteoglycan network (*pg*) in cartilage matrix is well preserved in these preparations. (Courtesy of L. Arsenault)

icles could act as *calcification initiators.* Such a role would explain the close association often found between matrix vesicles and some of the first-formed crystals of hydroxyapatite, which seem to form either within or in the immediate vicinity of such vesicles. This close association suggests that matrix vesicles may furnish a suitable microenvironment for the nucleation of hydroxyapatite.

The enzyme first suspected of participation in the process of calcification was *alkaline phosphatase* because its presence is demonstrable at virtually every site where calcification is in progress. It is now established that this enzyme is able to hydrolyze a broad range of organic phosphate-containing substrates, and also that it mostly resides in matrix vesicles (Ali). It has even been shown that this enzyme can release Ca^{2+} as well as P_i from calcium β-glycerophosphate at pH 7.4. Through its broad-based capacity for elevating local Ca^{2+} and P_i concentrations, the alkaline phosphatase in matrix vesicles could be instrumental in bringing about a $Ca^{2+} \cdot P_i$ product that is high enough to facilitate mineral deposition. Furthermore, it has now been established that this enzyme also hydrolyzes pyrophosphate and other naturally occurring polyphosphates that are capable of inhibiting calcification. Hence it is believed that alkaline phosphatase is not only a putative *promoter* of calcification but also an important *anti-inhibitor* as well. This role of maintaining an inhibitor-free microenvironment within the lumen of matrix vesicles is considered to be critical for crystal nucleation.

Matrix vesicles are also able to accumulate Ca^{2+}, and there is a possibility that their membrane could furnish appropriate binding sites for the nucleation of hydroxyapatite crystals. It has been sug-

gested that the basis of such nucleation might be the unique spacing of Ca^{2+}-binding and P_i-binding sites on acidic phospholipid or proteolipid molecules in the vesicle membrane.

Mitochondria Can Also Store Calcium and Phosphate. The mitochondria of chondrocytes and osteoblasts may also play an indirect role in the calcification process, but the nature of their involvement is less clear than that of matrix vesicles. In the upper region of the zone of maturing (hypertrophying) cartilage of an epiphyseal plate, the mitochondria of chondrocytes not only accumulate calcium but also contain amorphous calcium phosphate. Yet in the lower part of this zone, calcium is primarily associated with matrix vesicles in the form of crystalline hydroxyapatite. This shift in position of the calcium led to the proposal that mitochondria might be the earliest storage site of calcium and phosphate in the form of amorphous calcium phosphate. It was also suggested that this stored mineral might then be made available extracellularly (either by being liberated directly due to cell destruction or by being released indirectly in the form of constituent ions), and that it would thereupon support the growth of hydroxyapatite crystals forming extracellularly in association with matrix vesicles. This still hypothetical participation by mitochondria could lead to an accumulation of ions for mineralization but would be unlikely to achieve any nucleation of crystalline hydroxyapatite. The critical step, namely *initiation* of calcification as a result of such nucleation, would then follow extracellularly, generally in the vicinity of matrix vesicles.

Macromolecular Constituents of Bone and Cartilage Matrix Are Also Directly Implicated in Calcification. Cartilage, and to a lesser extent osteoid tissue, have a relatively substantial content of *proteoglycan,* a macromolec-ular matrix constituent for which several relevant roles have been proposed. These are described in the following section.

Initially, the proteoglycan is thought to bind extracellular Ca^{2+} and thereby *facilitate* calcification. However, there is evidence that certain matrix proteoglycans and proteoglycan aggregates can actually *inhibit* the crystallization of bone mineral. Hence it is widely believed that calcification will not occur unless the matrix proteo-glycans and proteoglycan aggregates have undergone some mod-ification. Such processing is presumed to release their bound Ca^{2+} and perhaps also to relinquish sufficient space to accommodate bone mineral deposited following partial degradation of the inhibiting proteoglycan. Consistent with this hypothesis, the inhibitory pro-teoglycan does seem to lose its inhibitory activity once its protein moiety has been enzymatically removed. However, it now seems that even if proteoglycans are partly degraded or otherwise mod-ified, the liberated constituent sulfated glycosaminoglycans may play a further role in *promoting* mineral deposition, as described below. The relatively high sulfur content of so-called crystal ghosts (the spaces occupied by mineral crystals before a tissue is decal-cified) has also been cited as evidence that sulfated glycosami-noglycans play a direct role in mineral deposition.

A protein called *osteocalcin,* which can be isolated from bone matrix, and a protein named *chondrocalcin,* which builds up as a constituent of cartilage matrix just prior to its calcification, have also been shown to bind extracellular Ca^{2+} with high affinity. Im-munofluorescent staining discloses that chondrocalcin is diffusely distributed throughout the matrix and is not specifically associated with matrix vesicles. By augmenting the extracellular Ca^{2+} con-centration of cartilage matrix, this protein could substantially sup-plement the calcification-promoting effects of matrix vesicles. It is even possible that the deposition of mineral in cartilage may actually be nucleated when chondrocalcin becomes associated with pro-teoglycan-containing foci (Poole et al).

Until recently, it was widely believed that matrix pro-teoglycans would only contribute Ca^{2+} for the growth of crystals that had already been seeded. However, totally new evidence has now come to light that cartilage proteo-glycans, or sulfated glycosaminoglycans that are liberated as a result of their degradation, could, in fact, play a central role in bringing about mineral deposition.

Electron Spectroscopic Imaging Confirms That Intermediate Stages Exist in the Association Between Calcium and Phosphorus. A powerful new analytical technique called *electron spectroscopic imaging,* recently developed by Ottensmeyer et al, has the advan-tage of being able to reveal the chemical nature of the structures seen in the transmission EM (TEM) in terms of elements that are present. Elements such as calcium (Ca), phosphorus (P), and sulfur (S) each can be directly visualized and independently quantitated, and their distributions can be resolved in considerable detail be-cause of the remarkable resolving power of the instrument.

The basis of the technique is as follows. When electrons bombard the specimen, they interact in a characteristic manner with atoms of the various elements. An energy analyzer is used to separate the electrons leaving the specimen into distinct energy bands, each characteristic of a specific element. The information obtained from the instrument is then computerized and viewed on a video display system that reveals the distribution of the element in question su-perimposed over a TEM image of the specimen. When applied to calcifying cartilage and bone, this novel way of looking at a min-eralized matrix produced results that quite surprised those who had assumed direct initial interaction between Ca^{2+} and P_i. The Ca of calcifying cartilage, instead of codistributing with P, was undeniably first associated with S (Arsenault and Ottensmeyer). Among the most abundant S-containing macromolecular compo-nents of cartilage matrix are the sulfated glycosaminoglycans, major constituents of proteoglycan subunits and aggregates. This finding is therefore consistent with the hypothesis that cartilage proteo-glycans or their S-containing degradation products (sulfated gly-cosaminoglycans) perform a key role in the mineralization process. At a later time, as might be expected, the distribution of P super-imposes with that of both Ca and S, further suggesting that an S-containing matrix constituent mediates the eventual deposition of crystalline calcium phosphate during endochondral ossification. Furthermore, whereas Ca and S are both diffusely distributed, P manifests a punctate (dotted) as well as a diffuse distribution.

In contrast, when bone is undergoing intramembranous devel-opment, these three elements associate in a different sequence. The initial association seems to be between S and P, later followed by Ca as well. A widely distributed S-containing matrix component such as sulfated glycosaminoglycan is thought to acquire diffuse and punctate accumulations of P_i that might both then proceed to take up Ca^{2+}. Again, S persists in the mineral deposit and hence appears to be of central importance for nucleation. Nucleation sites, but not matrix vesicles, are found in close proximity to osteoblast processes, suggesting that matrix vesicles may not be an absolute requirement for calcification when bone matrix is forming in an intramembranous environment (Arsenault and Ottensmeyer).

Calcification Inhibitors Protect Noncalcifying Tissues from Mineralization. Pyrophosphate, nucleotides, citrate, and Mg^{2+} are among the naturally occurring substances of low molecular weight that are known to inhibit the nucle-ation and growth of crystals of bone mineral. Synthetic diphosphonates (already shown to have clinical potential for combating excessive bone turnover) and a few mac-romolecular skeletal matrix constituents (including certain proteoglycans of high molecular weight and noncollagen bone proteins) can also inhibit the mineralization process. It is believed that all nonmineralizing tissues normally contain sufficient levels of naturally occurring calcification inhibitors to preclude them from undergoing inappropriate calcification, and that mineralization can only proceed at a site of potential calcification when such inhibitors are enzymatically destroyed or otherwise removed. However, conditions such as necrosis, inflammation, and local ele-vation of alkaline phosphatase levels can reduce or over-come such inherent resistance to calcification, and this can lead to inappropriate ectopic calcification at extraskeletal sites.

OSTEOCYTES

Osteocytes are somewhat smaller and less basophilic than osteoblasts, but this is seldom appreciated from routine LM sections because osteocytes become excessively dis-torted during the decalcification stage of bone section preparation. Their numerous interconnecting cytoplasmic processes (Fig. 12-3*B*) are not evident in H & E sections

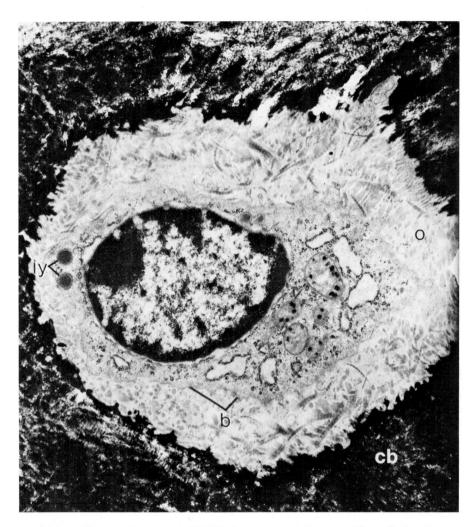

Fig. 12-12. Electron micrograph (×25,000) of an osteocyte in its lacuna. The wall of the lacuna consists of uncalcified osteoid tissue (prebone), labeled o, containing abundant collagen fibrils; peripheral to this is calcified bone (*cb*). The border (*b*) between the osteocyte and the osteoid tissue is not easy to discern. Two dense bodies representing lysosomes (*ly*) are seen at center left. (Holtrop ME, Weinger JM: Ultrastructural evidence for a transport system in bone. Proc 4th Parathyroid Conference. Amsterdam, Excerpta Medica, 1971)

(Fig. 12-2*A*), but in ground bone sections it is possible to discern the canaliculi along which such processes extend (Fig. 12-2*B*). In the EM, it can also be seen that osteocytes encased in calcified bone matrix generally retain a thin layer of uncalcified osteoid tissue as a lining to their lacuna (Fig. 12-12). Osteocyte lacunae can appear ovoid (Fig. 12-12) or flattened (Fig. 12-13). Futhermore, whereas a primary lacuna in cartilage may contain more than one chondrocyte, it is very rare for a lacuna in bone to contain more than a single osteocyte. Hence there is no histological evidence to suggest that osteocytes proliferate *in vivo.*

The cytoplasm of most osteocytes retains sufficient rER and a large enough Golgi region (Figs. 12-12 and 12-13) to suggest that these cells would be capable of keeping

bone matrix in a state of good repair. Furthermore, gap junctions are present in the extensive areas of contact between the processes of neighboring osteocytes. Because ions and small molecules can pass directly from one osteocyte to another by way of such junctions, it has been suggested that there may be some sort of intracellular transport mechanism between osteocytes and bone surfaces supplied with capillaries (Holtrop and Weinger). Various kinds of dense bodies such as the two lysosomes seen in Figure 12-12 have also been described, particularly in older osteocytes. Their possible significance in these cells will be discussed later in this chapter.

Two popular beliefs about osteocyte function are that they (1) maintain bone matrix and (2) release calcium ions

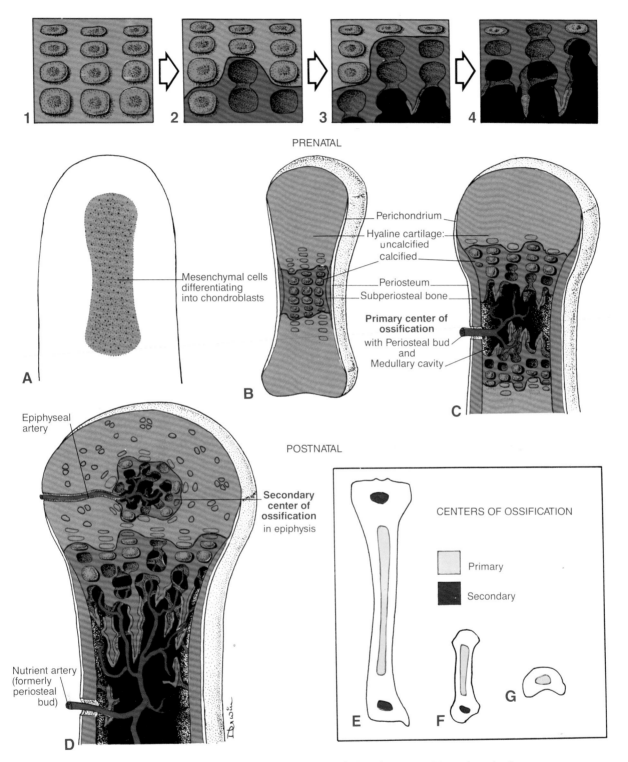

PLATE 12-1. Diagrammatic representation of endochondral ossification. (A) Mesenchymal cells condense and differentiate into chondroblasts. (B) Cartilage in midregion of model calcifies, and a collar of bone forms under the periosteum. (C) Calcified cartilage begins to break down, and periosteal bud (periosteal capillaries with osteogenic cells) grows in and establishes primary (diaphyseal) center of ossification. Medullary cavity begins to form. (D) Secondary (epiphyseal) centers of ossification develop postnatally by the same process. The top series of drawings depicts the formation of trabeculae with cores of calcified cartilage. (*Inset*) The arrangement of primary and secondary centers of ossification in long and short bones. (E) Typical long bone with primary center and a secondary center at both ends (tibia). (F) A long bone with primary center and only a proximal secondary center (phalanx). (G) Typical short bone with primary center but no secondary centers (lunate bone of wrist).

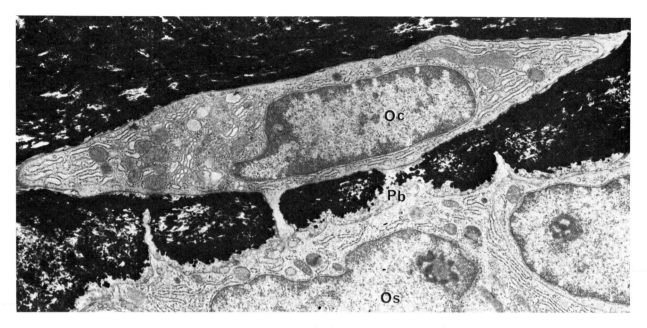

Fig. 12-13. Electron micrograph of a young and relatively flat osteocyte (*Oc*) in its lacuna in calcified bone. The cells below it are osteoblasts (*Os*). A process from the osteocyte connects with an osteoblast in the plane of section. Parts of processes of osteoblasts are also seen. Some osteoid tissue (prebone), labeled *Pb,* is present between the osteoblasts and the calcified bone, but very little of it can be discerned between the osteocyte and the walls of its lacuna. (Courtesy of M. Weinstock)

from bone matrix when calcium demands increase. The first hypothesis is based on the observation that osteocytes possess an appropriate complement of organelles for them to continue producing relatively small amounts of matrix constituents throughout life. Before discussing the second theory, which is that osteocytes have the capacity to transfer calcium ions from bone mineral to the blood plasma, it is necessary to describe the cells that are specially adapted for bone resorption.

OSTEOCLASTS

Osteoclasts are multinucleated nondividing cells that move around on bone surfaces, resorbing bone matrix from sites where it is either deteriorating or not needed. Large and variable in shape due to their motility, osteoclasts are characteristically found on *resorbing surfaces.* Such surfaces can be readily recognized because instead of appearing smooth and evenly covered with a uniform layer of cells, they are etched or scalloped and exhibit scattered osteoclasts rather than osteoblasts or osteogenic cells along their free margin (see Fig. 12-34). Some osteoclasts lie in recesses termed *Howship's lacunae* or *resorption bays* that they have eroded on these surfaces. Examples of osteoclasts that are situated on such surfaces can generally be found in the resorption sites present near the ends of a growing long bone, for example, those indicated by the arrows marked *1* and *3* in Figure 12-26. Osteoclasts are generally distinguishable by

their large size, multiple nuclei (several are usually seen in an LM section), and their close proximity to a bone surface (Fig. 12-14). However, where they are peeled off from an endosteal surface by shrinkage artifact, detached osteoclasts may superficially resemble megakaryocytes of myeloid tissue, even though megakaryocytes possess a single multi-lobed nucleus and not multiple nuclei. The side of the cell adjacent to the bone generally contains fewer nuclei than the opposite side. In LM sections, shrinkage artifact occasionally discloses a frayed border on surfaces where bone matrix is undergoing resorption. Because the projecting free collagen fibrils can look like the bristles of a brush, such edges were originally called *brush* (or *striated*) *borders,* but this term is now generally reserved for cell borders that are made up of large numbers of microvilli (*e.g.,* the apical border of an absorptive intestinal epithelial cell).

Fine Structure of Osteoclasts. The part of an osteoclast that is directly responsible for carrying out bone resorption is a transitory and highly motile structure called its *ruffled border* (Figs. 12-15, 12-16, and 12-17). This border of the cell is made up of branching fingerlike processes that poke down into the bone surface on which it is situated. Whereas the brush border seen in the LM corresponds to collagen fibrils exposed through erosion and extracellular digestion of bone matrix components, the ruffled border visible in the EM represents an integral part of the osteoclast's surface. Encircling the periphery of the ruffled border is the *clear zone,* a ring-shaped region seen on both sides of the

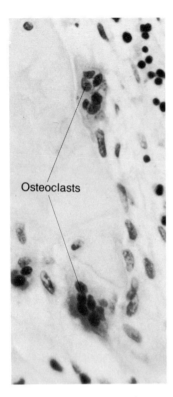

Osteoclasts

Fig. 12-14.   Photomicrograph of two large multinucleated osteoclasts in shallow cavities (Howship's lacunae) that they have eroded in bone. (Ham AW: In Cowdry's Special Cytology, 2nd ed, Vol 2. New York, Hoeber, 1932)

ruffled border in cross sections (Fig. 12-16). This zone is described as clear because it lacks large organelles but contains abundant microfilaments that give it a characteristic mottled appearance (Fig. 12-16). Deep to the ruffled border there is a *vesicular region* containing vesicles of various shapes and dimensions (Figs. 12-15 and 12-16), but almost all of these so-called vesicles probably represent cross or oblique sections through clefts that extend down into the cytoplasm, between the branching fingerlike processes of the ruffled border. Farthest away from the bone lies the *basal region* of the cell (Figs. 12-15 and 12-16), which contains multiple nuclei surrounded by stacks of Golgi saccules together with numerous mitochondria, some secretory vesicles and lysosomes, and a small amount of rER.

Local Conditions at the Ruffled Border Bring About Bone Resorption.   The fine structure of the osteoclast suggests that it is a secretory cell that is capable of active ion transport. The highly motile ruffled border presents an extensive area of cell membrane to the bone surface, and the ringlike clear zone is probably able to seal off the working area to some extent. Furthermore, the presence of numerous actin-containing microfilaments in the clear zone suggests substantial contractile activity, and perhaps even the capacity to (1) maintain limpetlike attachment of the

cell to bone surfaces and (2) agitate the ruffled border and thereby facilitate resorption. Consistent with such a hypothesis are the observations that the clear zone and ruffled border both adhere tightly to bone surfaces and that osteoclasts lose their ruffled borders and clear zones after they have left a bone surface. The basal region of the cell contains an abundance of energy-providing mitochondria (Figs. 12-15 and 12-17) as well as perinuclear stacks of Golgi saccules that package hydrolytic enzymes into vesicles. Some of these vesicles are thought to be secretory vesicles that are destined to empty their contents into the bottoms of the clefts between the cytoplasmic processes of the ruffled border.

Once liberated by exocytosis into the tiny extracellular compartment between the ruffled border and an apposed bone surface, such hydrolytic enzymes are in an appropriate position to degrade amorphous organic constituents of bone matrix. This, in turn, can liberate and expose enough of the collagen component for this to become visible as a striated border. However, it is doubtful whether such an action would have any effect without concomitant demineralization of the bone matrix, which is one of the principal functions ascribed to osteoclasts. It has been proposed that the large expanse of cell membrane exposed at the ruffled border could excrete sufficient quantities of organic acids (metabolic by-products such as carbonic, citric, and lactic acid) into the tiny tissue fluid–containing compartment circumscribed by the clear zone to generate a local acidic environment that is capable of bringing about focal decalcification of bone matrix. Carbonic anhydrase, an enzyme known to augment carbonic acid production, is detectable in the vicinity of the ruffled border, and there is some evidence that the extracellular *p*H is lower in the general neighborhood of this compartment. It seems likely that in acting to buffer the local acidity, the relatively insoluble calcium salts in bone mineral become converted into acid salts that steadily pass into solution because they are more soluble. Thus the degradation of mineralized bone matrix by osteoclasts is considered to be primarily due to a combination of (1) *focal decalcification* by organic acids building up under the ruffled borders of osteoclasts and (2) *extracellular digestion* by acid hydrolases liberated by exocytosis at such borders. Although there is no evidence that osteoclasts are intensely phagocytic, an abundance of coated vesicles and coated pits in these cells suggests active uptake of the products of extracellular digestion (and also membrane retrieval) through receptor-mediated endocytosis. Hence as well as constituting the principal site of release of digestive enzymes, the ruffled border and its associated vesicular region are considered to be a major site of endocytosis and absorption.

Other types of cells may participate in disposing of the collagen released from bone matrix. For example, fibroblasts produce collagenase, and there is evidence that they phagocytose and degrade collagen within secondary lysosomes at sites where collagen turnover and bone re-

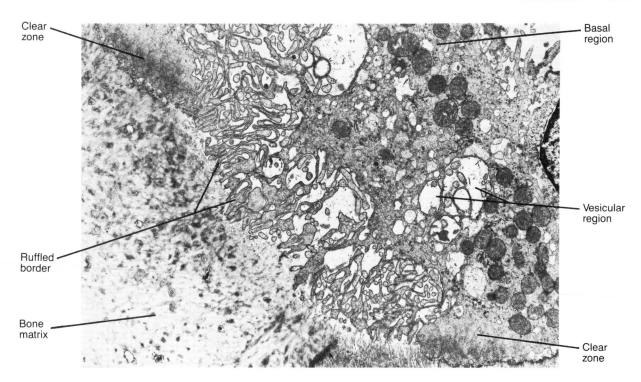

Clear zone

Basal region

Ruffled border

Vesicular region

Bone matrix

Clear zone

Fig. 12-15. Electron micrograph (×8500) of the ruffled border of an osteoclast, also showing the clear zone. The bone matrix that this cell is eroding is seen at lower left. The basal part of the cell contains numerous mitochondria. The vesicular region lies between the ruffled border and the basal region. (Holtrop ME, King GJ: Clin Orthop 123:177, 1977)

modeling are both very active (Ten Cate et al). Collagenase is also produced by monocytes and macrophages, and it is known to be released from explants of bone tissue.

Osteoclasts Are Derived from Monocytic Precursors. Until recently, it was widely thought that osteoclasts were derived from osteogenic cells or osteoblasts, but a number of different lines of investigation now indicate that they come from *mononuclear precursors*, in all probability from *blood monocytes*. In favor of such a hypothesis is evidence that in addition to being chemotactically attracted to dead bone by some organic constituent of bone matrix, monocytes manifest a certain capacity for bone resorption *in vitro*. There are also indications that such cells can form osteoclasts by fusing with one another or by fusing with preexisting macrophage- or osteoclastlike cells. For example, such precursor cells seem able to fuse with perivascular macrophages that are associated with the thin-walled blood vessels of calcifying cartilage. Recently reported for ossifying deer antlers, such a mechanism of formation is consistent with an earlier finding that in each metaphysis of a growing long bone, the first-formed osteoclasts on the diaphyseal side of the epiphyseal plate are found close to the zone of calcifying cartilage. Thus instead of representing an extension of the bone cell lineage, osteoclasts appear to be a part of the monocyte–macrophage–multinucleated giant cell line of differentiation.

The ingenious means by which osteoclasts were shown to be derived from cells of the monocytic series constitute a fascinating story. In addition, they illustrate that existing knowledge is not always the truth. Had it not been for critical reevaluation of the earlier evidence for the osteogenic origin of osteoclasts, everyone might have continued to believe in it forever.

The Extraskeletal Origin of Osteoclasts: Historical Perspective. From the evident intimate association of osteoclasts with bone tissue, it was at first surmised that they were derived from the same progenitor cells as other types of bone cells. However, the microscopic resemblance between osteoclasts and multinucleated foreign-body giant cells generated some speculation that they might instead arise from macrophages or monocytes. Early *in vivo* studies using tritiated thymidine did not enable any distinction to be made between an origin from (1) labeled osteogenic cells or (2) myeloid progenitors that may have become labeled at the same time. A virtual breakthrough came when Walker began a series of studies in experimental animals with congenital *osteopetrosis* (Gr. *petros*, stone), a bone condition in which defective resorption by osteoclasts leads to the production of abnormally dense bone tissue. Through the expedient of crossing the blood circulation of osteopetrotic animals with that of their normal littermates (parabiosis), he was able to demonstrate that ensuing normal bone resorption in the osteopetrotic animals resulted from the transfer of some type of circulating cell. It was later found that when osteopetrotic mice were given bone marrow or spleen cells from nonosteopetrotic *beige* mice, a mutant strain characterized by the presence of exceptionally large lysosomal granules in its

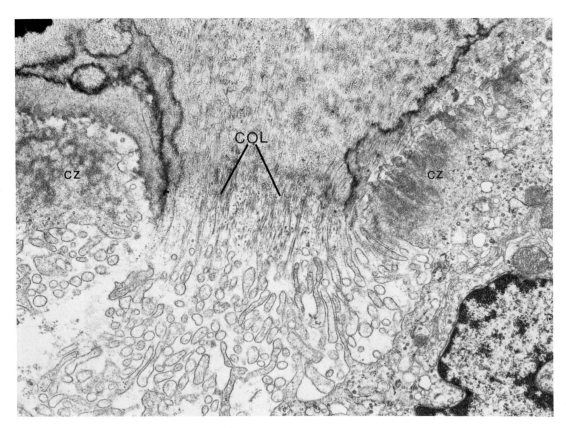

Fig. 12-16.   Electron micrograph (×11,000) of part of the ruffled border of an osteoclast (which lies *below*) wrapped around the bottom of the tip of a trabecula of partly calcified cartilage (which is seen at *top*). This trabecula extends down from an epiphyseal plate into the shaft of a developing bone. At such sites, resorption of cartilaginous trabeculae proceeds at their free ends, as will be explained later in this chapter. At center the osteoclast is removing the calcified amorphous component of the cartilage more rapidly than the collagen fibrils (*COL*) of the cartilage matrix. The clear zone (*cz*) is seen on each side of the ruffled border, which occupies most of the lower part of the micrograph. A nucleus is seen at lower right. (Courtesy of M. Holtrop)

leukocytes, mast cells, and osteoclasts, effective bone resorption ensued in the recipient mutant mice. Moreover, their osteoclasts exhibited the same characteristic granules in their cytoplasm, indicating donor origin from some type of *myeloid* progenitor or stem cell. Subsequent work, in which suspensions of normal myeloid cells or normal spleen cells (the latter being entirely free of osteogenic cells) were injected into irradiated osteopetrotic mice, indicated the likelihood that the osteoclast-producing cells were circulating progenitors belonging to the *monocytic* series. The permanent cure effected by infusing normal myeloid or spleen cells into irradiated osteopetrotic mice is due to seeding of their bone marrow and spleen (which, in mice, is a hematopoietic organ) with normal multipotential hematopoietic stem cells that are capable of producing normal descendants of the monocytic series. A tangible result of this important line of research is that it has now become possible to cure debilitating human *infantile* and *juvenile osteopetrosis* by means of histocompatible bone marrow transplants (Coccia et al; Sorell et al).

Convincing evidence of an extraskeletal source of osteoclasts also came from studies of chick-quail chimeras. Following the vascularization of transplanted quail bone rudiments by chick blood vessels, the bone cells remained representative of quail cells but the majority of osteoclasts were chick-derived (Kahn and Simmons). For more detailed discussion of the origin of osteoclasts, see Marks. Finally, it should be noted that in view of the substantial evidence that osteoclasts are not derived from the same skeletal tissue stem cell as osteoblasts and osteocytes are, it is necessary to abandon the old mistaken notion, still sometimes heard in clinical circles, that osteoclasts can serve as a source of new osteoblasts for continued bone growth.

Our next major concern will be the problem of whether osteocytes liberate calcium from bone matrix. We shall begin discussion of this topic by considering some of the main ways in which the body regulates its blood calcium level.

The Systemic Regulation of Blood Calcium Levels

Two hormones, *parathyroid hormone* (PTH) and *calcitonin* (CT), are involved in regulating the calcium ion concen-

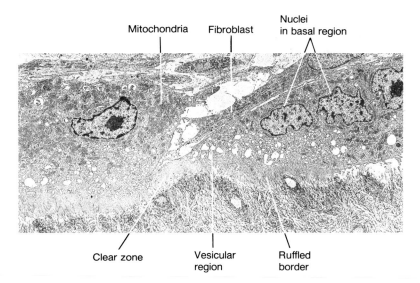

Fig. 12-17.   Electron micrograph (×7150) of parts of two osteoclasts resorbing dentin of a tooth. A fibroblast process (labeled) is also seen extending down from top right. The tissue extending across the bottom of the micrograph is dentin. (Courtesy of A. R. Ten Cate)

tration of blood plasma. Also, at least one *vitamin D metabolite* is known to play an important role in the regulatory process. PTH elicits a combination of physiological responses that *raise* the blood calcium level, and CT can elicit responses that counterbalance this action, *lowering* the blood calcium level. Normally, the two opposing actions maintain the calcium ion concentration of plasma and tissue fluid between precise limits. If the blood calcium level stays above or below these normal limits for any length of time, clinical manifestations will occur.

Thus *hypercalcemia*, the term used for an *elevated blood calcium level*, can lead to ectopic calcification in soft tissues and to the development of kidney stones, and it may also result in neuromuscular and behavioral symptoms. Persistent hypercalcemia can result from diffuse parathyroid hyperplasia, or it can reflect the continuous and autonomous production of PTH by a parathyroid adenoma or the continuous secretion of a PTH-mimicking product by a nonparathyroid malignancy.

Hypocalcemia, which means an abnormally *low blood calcium level*, can have clinical consequences that are potentially even more serious. This is because the calcium ion concentration of tissue fluid, related to the calcium ion concentration of plasma, profoundly affects the electrical excitability of the cell membrane of nerve and muscle cells. The permeability of their cell membrane to sodium ions is lowered by the presence of a normal concentration of calcium ions. In the hypocalcemic patient, an evident manifestation of the heightened neural excitability resulting from an insufficiency of calcium ions is the generation of inappropriate motor impulses in response to stimuli that, under normal conditions, would remain subliminal. Such impulses

may then bring about unwanted and prolonged contraction in skeletal muscles and result in the clinical condition *tetany*.

In addition to experiencing recurrent cramps, hypocalcemic individuals are subject to *carpopedal spasms* with characteristic flexion of the wrist and metacarpophalangeal joints, extension of the fingers, and plantar flexion of the toes. They are also at risk of developing prolonged laryngeal muscle spasms that are capable of closing off all movement of air through the glottis, which can result in fatal *asphyxiation* (suffocation) unless the muscular spasm subsides. Because hypocalcemia raises the general level of excitability of the whole nervous system, it occasionally also results in generalized convulsions. In many instances, the cause of hypocalcemia can be traced to unintentional extirpation of the parathyroid glands or their accidental mutilation during surgery (*e.g.*, thyroidectomy or the resection of extensive laryngeal or esophageal tumors).

In broad terms, the basis of systemic regulation of the blood calcium level is as follows. The PTH-secreting (chief) cells of the parathyroid glands monitor the plasma concentration of calcium ions, and when this drops below normal, they release more PTH, which then raises the blood calcium level. Whenever the calcium level rises above normal, they stop releasing PTH, and the CT-secreting (C) cells of the thyroid release the antagonistic hormone CT, which temporarily lowers the blood calcium level. The intriguing hypothesis has recently been proposed that this antihypercalcemic action of CT may, in fact, be a secondary effect; the primary effect of CT is to regulate plasma levels of inorganic phosphate. Furthermore, the overall importance of CT in human calcium homeostasis remains difficult to evaluate (Talmage et al). PTH promotes (1) the resorption of calcium from glomerular filtrate produced in the kidneys and (2) the synthesis of a hydroxylated vitamin D_3 derivative called 1,25-*dihydroxycholecalciferol,* an important action of which is to enhance calcium absorption from the intestine (see also Chap. 22). Of particular interest in this discussion is the third major action of PTH, which is to bring about the release of calcium from mineralized bone matrix. We shall now consider some of the ideas about how this is achieved.

Which Cells Liberate Calcium Ions from Bone Mineral: Osteocytes or Osteoclasts? Evidence is rapidly accumulating that *osteoclasts* equipped with ruffled borders demineralize bone as part of the resorption process. The calcium ions they liberate enter the tissue fluid and lymph and thereby contribute to the blood calcium level. Not quite as widely accepted is an alternative hypothesis that is based on the vast number and huge surface area of *osteocytes* and their cytoplasmic processes, proposed by Bélanger and others. Irregularities in the shape and size of osteocytic lacunae suggested to these investigators that the lacunar walls were being eroded. They postulated that such resorption was brought about by the liberation of lysosomal enzymes and organic acids from the osteocytes. Although the theory that the cells liberating bone calcium under the stimulus of PTH are *osteocytes* was initially upheld, it is now less universally accepted for reasons that will be discussed in the following paragraph. The term *osteocytic osteolysis* is widely used in the literature to mean the induced retrieval of calcium from bone matrix by osteocytes.

However, it has since been pointed out that, in many cases, instead of indicating perilacunar decalcification, enlarged and irregular osteocytic lacunae might reflect the persistence of a substantial zone of pericellular osteoid tissue that has never become uniformly calcified (Fig. 12-12). Furthermore, osteocytes do not develop ruffled borders or clear zones, specializations that clearly are manifestations of marked resorptive activity in osteoclasts. Thus the histological evidence for osteocytic osteolysis remains meager and far from conclusive. Also, it is somewhat doubtful whether PTH-stimulated osteocytes could liberate as much bone calcium as can osteoclasts that are engaged in acid-mediated demineralization as part of a prolonged episode of PTH-induced bone resorption.

Thus osteoclasts could be the cells that play the major role in massive liberation of calcium from bone matrix under the stimulus of PTH. Supporting such a view are the observations that PTH increases (1) the number of osteoclasts present on resorbing surfaces and (2) the size of the ruffled borders on osteoclasts. There is also electron microscopic evidence that the resorptive activity of osteoclasts increases following administration of PTH. Furthermore, CT administration has the reverse effect, reducing the dimensions of any ruffled borders that may have enlarged in response to PTH, with the result that some of these borders become restored to their former size and others vanish entirely. CT also brings about the dissociation of carbonic anhydrase from ruffled borders. Because the role of this enzyme is to facilitate H^+ production (as carbonic

acid), such dissociation could be expected to decrease the amount of acid being generated by ruffled borders. In addition to inhibiting the resorptive activity of existing osteoclasts, CT is believed to reduce the rate at which new osteoclasts (or their precursors) become recruited.

This is not to say, however, that osteocytes and osteoblasts do not respond to PTH. Indeed, there is immunohistochemical evidence that PTH can become bound to osteoblasts and osteocytes as well as to osteoclasts, and certain osteocytes and osteoblasts also seem able to bind CT much as osteoclasts do (Rao et al). Furthermore, it has never been unequivocally demonstrated that osteoclasts possess specific PTH receptors on their cell membrane, and it is becoming increasingly apparent that their response to PTH may depend on mediation by some other type of bone cell.

Whereas osteocytes show little ultrastructural evidence of secreting hydrolytic enzymes, they do, in fact, reach a stage at which lysosomes become more prominent in their cytoplasm, and there are reports that PTH increases the proportion of osteocytes entering this postulated resorptive stage. It nevertheless seems unreasonable to expect that their lysosomal enzymes, even if freely liberated as a result of exocytosis, could exert an almost instantaneous resorptive effect that, in the absence of vast expanses of ruffled membrane, would generate sufficient acidity to decalcify the matrix. It is possible, of course, that local breakdown of matrix and decalcification might result from death of osteocytes, and this could be expected to enlarge their lacunae. Indeed, dead bone is characterized by the presence of empty lacunae that almost always do appear enlarged. It is also conceivable that when stimulated by PTH, osteocytes might enter their terminal stage of maturation, after which there would be an increased probability of their dying, creating an impression that the normal physiological response to this hormone is osteocytic osteolysis.

On the issue of whether osteocytes are primarily responsible for the retrieval of calcium from bone mineral, opinion is now sharply divided. There are those who contend that even allowing for rapid calcium-retrieving responses in the kidneys and gut, without a very substantial contribution by osteocytes and osteoblasts, PTH-stimulated osteoclastic resorption would be insufficient to raise the plasma calcium level with the degree of rapidity that is observed. An alternative theory to the belief that lysis is required for the liberation of calcium from bone mineral is that PTH augments the activity of calcium pumps in the cell membrane of the osteocytes and osteoblasts that constitute the interconnecting system of cells present at the interface between the matrix of living bone and the remainder of the body. This theory, based solely on indirect physiological evidence, proposes that such cells are capable of (1) withdrawing calcium ions from so-called *bone fluid* (the tissue fluid present in bone canaliculi, for example) and (2) redistributing these ions in such a way that they enter the tissue fluid compartment outside the bone tissue and enter the blood plasma. According to such a hypothesis, PTH would accelerate calcium withdrawal and deplete the calcium ion concentration of bone fluid to an extent that would favor the dissociation of calcium from phosphate in bone mineral. A more recent proposal that has gained acceptance is that in response to PTH, *osteoblasts* selectively uncover bone surfaces that are ready for resorption and liberate some mediator that effectively recruits resorptive cells such as osteoclasts and their precursors to the resorption site (Rodan and Martin).

Hence PTH may be able to facilitate the withdrawal of calcium from bone mineral by more than one mechanism, and calcium retrieval from this source may involve osteo-blasts or osteocytes as well as osteoclasts. At present, it would seem that whereas CT is able to inhibit the resorptive activity and motility of osteoclasts directly by interacting with their cell-surface receptors, PTH acts primarily on osteoblasts that respond by liberating a mediator that is capable of reversing such inhibition and stimulating the resorptive activity and motility of osteoclasts. When considered in the context of the direct coupling that is now known to exist between new bone deposition and prior bone resorption (such coupling will be explained later in this chapter), it is clear that this putative role of osteoblasts in mediating PTH-induced osteoclastic resorption represents yet another example of the very close integration that must be maintained between osteoblastic and osteoclastic activity. Finally, there seems to be little reason to suppose that extracellular calcium levels would be adequately regulated if this regulation occurred only at a systemic level. Hence there may be additional mechanisms operating at the local tissue level that are still being overlooked.

The various roles of the hydroxylated derivative of vitamin D_3 remain incompletely explored, but a general effect is that it facilitates the calcification of newly formed bone matrix by increasing the plasma concentrations of both calcium and inorganic phosphate. Its well-established effects include (1) enhancement of intestinal absorption of calcium and phosphate, and (2) augmentation of bone resorption by osteoclasts. Accordingly, this active metabolite of vitamin D and the hormone PTH *potentiate each other's effects* with respect to raising the blood calcium level.

Returning now to our consideration of osteogenesis, we noted earlier in this chapter that bones develop in two different kinds of environments. In contrast to flat bones, which form directly in vascularized mesenchyme, long or short tubular bones form indirectly by *endochondral ossification,* that is, through the development and ossification of a temporary cartilage model. Students will find a general knowledge of the stages of formation of a long bone very helpful in understanding the processes by which a long bone grows and repairs itself if it is broken.

ENDOCHONDRAL OSSIFICATION

At each site where a limb will later emerge, a small structure known as a *limb bud* grows out from the embryo. This limb rudiment is basically a mesodermal outgrowth covered by ectoderm. The earliest signs of long bone development within such a bud are seen in the mesenchyme at the site where the bone is going to form.

Endochondral Ossification Starts with the Development of a Cartilaginous Model.   The mesenchymal cells at the site condense and delineate the shape of the future bone (Plate 12-1A). They then differentiate into *chondroblasts* that produce cartilage matrix, resulting in the development of a model that consists of hyaline cartilage (Plate 12-1B

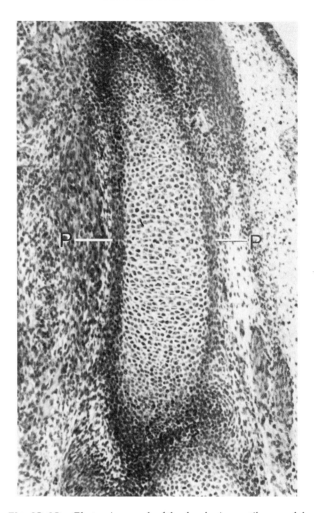

Fig. 12-18.   Photomicrograph of the developing cartilage model of a metatarsal. The middle region of developing cartilage is distinguishable from the surrounding perichondrium (*P*).

and Fig. 12-18). Also, a *perichondrium* made up of an inner chondrogenic layer and an outer fibrous layer develops at its periphery (Plate 12-1B and Fig. 12-18). At this stage, no osteoblasts are produced by the cells in the chondrogenic layer because differentiation is taking place in an avascular environment. Fibroblasts differentiate in the fibrous layer and begin producing collagen, with the result that this layer becomes a dense fibrous covering.

The Cartilage Model Grows Interstitially and by Apposition.   Ensuing growth of the cartilage model is a combined result of interstitial and appositional growth. Its increase in length is mostly due to repeated division of its chondrocytes, accompanied by the production of additional matrix by the daughter cells (as depicted in Fig. 11-2, *interstitial growth*), whereas widening of the model is primarily due to the further addition of matrix to its periphery by new chondroblasts that are derived from the chondrogenic layer of its perichondrium (as depicted in Fig. 11-2,

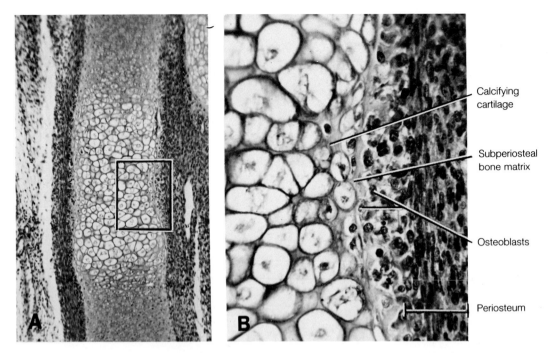

Fig. 12-19. (A) Photomicrograph of a developing cartilage model of a long bone. The chondrocytes in the middle part of the model have hypertrophied, and the matrix around them has calcified. (B) High-power photomicrograph of the area indicated in A. The osteogenic cells of the former perichondrium (now the periosteum) have differentiated into osteoblasts, and these have laid down a thin shell of subperiosteal bone matrix around the midsection of the model.

appositional growth). Most of the cellular proliferation responsible for the increase in the length of the model occurs near its ends rather than in its midsection.

As the model continues to grow, the chondrocytes in its midsection undergo hypertrophy (enlarge) and mature. However, this stage is associated with the deposition of insoluble calcium salts in the thin partitions of matrix that separate their lacunae (Plate 12-1B and Fig. 12-19). It will be recalled that the viability of chondrocytes depends on the maintenance of a free diffusion of nutrients and oxygen through cartilage matrix, and it is widely believed that heavy mineralization of cartilage matrix eventually impedes this diffusion process. However, it is now becoming evident that the main basis for this belief—the degenerating appearance of hypertrophied chondrocytes as seen in LM sections of calcified cartilage (Fig. 12-19)—can result from fixation artifact, and this raises the question of whether the ensuing changes in the midsection of the model are a result of cell death and passive disintegration of the cartilage, active erosion of the cartilage, or some combination of both these processes. We shall encounter the same problem of interpretation when we consider the zone of calcifying cartilage in the epiphyseal plates. It is nevertheless safe to say that after the midsection of the cartilage model has become heavily calcified, it begins to become replaced by bone. In LM sections, many of the lacunae in the mid-

section of the model now appear empty, and the thin partitions that separate them show signs of breaking down to form little cavities, as may be seen at a more advanced stage in Figure 12-20.

In the meantime, capillaries grow into the part of the perichondrium that ensheaths the midsection of the model. The cells produced by the inner layer of the perichondrium then begin to differentiate in a vascular environment, with the result that they become osteoblasts that start to lay down a thin collar of bone matrix around the midregion of the model (Plate 12-1B and Fig. 12-20). Now that differentiation of the cells arising from the inner layer of the perichondrium leads to bone production, this membrane is referred to as a *periosteum*. The bony collar that forms below the periosteum and that strengthens the midregion of the model where it has become weakened through loss of calcified cartilage is described as *subperiosteal bone*, but it is the same kind of bone that is formed at other sites. With increasing vascularity of the periosteum (a change that is necessary for continuing bone formation), the osteogenic and fibrous layers of this membrane become more distinct.

A Primary Center of Ossification Becomes Established. Periosteal capillaries, accompanied by osteogenic cells, invade the calcified cartilage near the middle of the model and thereafter supply its interior (Fig. 12-20, *arrow,*

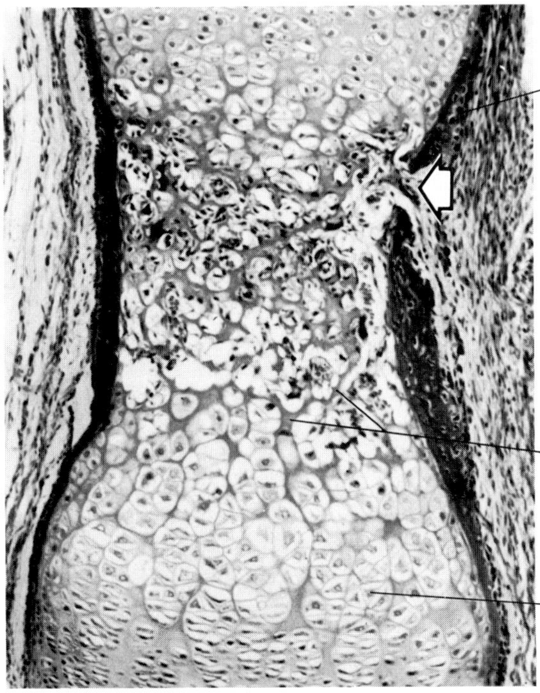

Fig. 12-20. Photomicrograph of a developing cartilage model of a long bone at the stage where its calcified cartilage is being invaded by periosteal capillaries and associated osteogenic cells. The site where these components grew in as the periosteal bud is indicated by an arrow. This is the stage of endochondral ossification depicted in Plate 12-1C, and it represents the beginning of development of the primary center of ossification.

Subperiosteal bone traversed by periosteal bud (*arrow*)

Disintegrating calcified cartilage

Hypertrophied chondrocytes

and Plate 12-1C). Together with their associated osteogenic cells, these vessels comprise a structure called the *periosteal bud;* however, some bones develop more than one periosteal bud. These periosteal capillaries grow into the cartilage model and initiate development of a *primary center of ossification* that is so called because the bone tissue it produces eventually replaces most of the cartilage in the model. The majority of long bones develop such an ossification center toward the end of the second month of gestation. In this newly vascularized environment, the osteogenic cells brought in by the periosteal bud give rise to osteoblasts that begin to deposit bone matrix over the residual calcified cartilage, as shown in boxes 3 and 4 at the top of Plate 12-1. This process results in the formation of *cancellous bone* that has small remnants of calcified cartilage in its trabeculae. The presence of calcified cartilage in the cores of these trabeculae can generally be recognized in H & E sections because they stain pale blue to mauve in contrast to the bright pink to red color of the bone matrix that covers their surfaces (Plate 12-1C and D). Eventually, the central portion of the cancellous bone in the midsection of the model undergoes resorption, and this leaves a central *medullary cavity* (Plate 12-1C) surrounded by cortical bone (*bone cortex*). After the medullary cavity has begun to form, it becomes seeded by circulating multipotential hematopoietic stem cells that give rise to *myeloid tissue* (Fig. 12-21).

The Bone Acquires Epiphyses and a Diaphysis. Developing bone tissue has now replaced the middle third or so of what was formerly a solid mass of cartilage, and

a medullary cavity filled with myeloid tissue has developed in its central region. The two ends of the developing bone are nevertheless still composed entirely of cartilage. Hence at this stage, the forming bone tissue consists of (1) an elongating collar of subperiosteal bone that extends along the midsection of the bone and (2) a decreasing amount of cancellous bone that borders on an enlarging central medullary cavity (Fig. 12-21). The midsection of the bone becomes its shaft or *diaphysis* whereas the cartilaginous ends of the bone become its *epiphyses* (Fig. 12-21). Its primary center of ossification is accordingly often referred to as its *diaphyseal center of ossification.*

Interstitial growth occurs in the cartilaginous epiphyses, causing the bone to lengthen. Yet the epiphyses themselves do not lengthen because the cartilage on either side of the diaphyseal center of ossification undergoes progressive maturation, calcification, and replacement by bone. Because elongation of the diaphyseal center of ossification keeps pace with interstitial growth of the cartilaginous epiphyses, the epiphyses remain approximately the same size while the bony diaphysis between them lengthens.

Cartilage models of the developing short bones (*e.g.,* carpals of the wrists and most of the tarsals of the feet) lengthen as a result of interstitial growth. After they have finished growing, their cartilaginous epiphyses become almost entirely replaced by bone from the diaphysis; only a thin rim persists as each articular cartilage. Immediately beneath the articular cartilage, bony trabeculae form a supporting platelike structure.

Secondary (Epiphyseal) Centers of Ossification Become

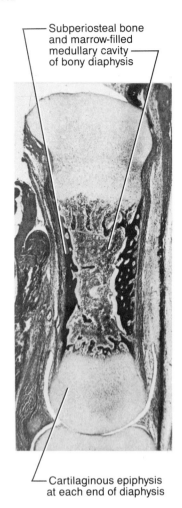

Subperiosteal bone
and marrow-filled
medullary cavity
of bony diaphysis

Cartilaginous epiphysis
at each end of diaphysis

Fig. 12-21. Low-power photomicrograph of a developing long bone. At this stage there is a substantial layer of subperiosteal bone around its midsection, and cartilage has disappeared from this central part of the model, which now contains myeloid tissue. Bone formation is advancing toward the ends of the bone, but the epiphyses are still wholly cartilaginous. They will eventually develop epiphyseal centers of ossification and become almost entirely replaced by bone except for their tips, which will remain as articular cartilages.

Established. The formation of long bones is slightly more complex because these bones develop *secondary (epiphyseal) centers of ossification.* The majority of secondary centers are formed postnatally, but those in the lower end of the femur and the upper end of the tibia begin to appear just prior to birth. In the simplest kind of long bone, a secondary center of ossification develops in each cartilaginous epiphysis. In due course the cartilaginous epiphysis gives rise to a bony epiphysis that retains a covering of articular cartilage. Each secondary center is formed as described in the following paragraph.

The chondrocytes in the middle of an epiphysis hypertrophy and mature, whereupon the matrix partitions between their lacunae calcify. Capillaries with associated os-

teogenic cells then invade cavities in the calcified cartilage (Plate 12-1D), much as the periosteal bud grew into the diaphysis, and in this newly vascularized environment, the osteogenic cells give rise to osteoblasts that deposit bone matrix on the remnants of calcified cartilage. Meanwhile, the chondrocytes that are situated at the periphery of this region also start to hypertrophy, whereupon their surrounding matrix becomes calcified and then becomes replaced by bone. The resulting wave of ossification spreads from the secondary center in all directions. In this manner, the cartilage in the middle of the epiphysis gradually becomes replaced by a mass of cancellous bone with its associated marrow spaces (Fig. 12-22). Cartilage nevertheless remains as (1) the *articular cartilage* that covers the articular surface (Fig. 12-22A) and (2) a transverse disk of hyaline cartilage called the *epiphyseal plate* that borders on the diaphysis (Fig. 12-22A). The functional significance of the epiphyseal plate is that it enables the bone to grow until full adult stature is attained, at which time it becomes entirely replaced by bone tissue. The site of entry of the periosteal bud is marked by the foramen of the nutrient artery, and the places where capillaries grew in to initiate development of the secondary centers of ossification are indicated by the foramina of the epiphyseal arteries (compare Plate 12-1D with Fig. 12-39).

The majority of long bones develop two secondary centers in addition to a primary center of ossification (Plate 12-1E). However, a few long bones develop a secondary center at one end only (Plate 12-1F). Typical short bones ossify entirely from their primary center (Plate 12-1G).

POSTNATAL GROWTH OF LONG BONES

Until skeletal growth is completed, a long bone continues to lengthen as a result of interstitial growth of the cartilage that is retained as its epiphyseal growth plates. However, the production of new cartilage matrix does not increase the thickness of such a plate because cartilage formation within the plate is only sufficient to keep pace with its replacement by bone tissue on the diaphyseal aspect of the plate. Because the epiphyseal plates grow on one side and become replaced by bone on the other, they are gradually shifted farther apart, lengthening the bony diaphysis that lies between them. Bony replacement eventually catches up with cartilage production, at which time the bone attains its adult size and its cartilaginous growth plates disappear.

The structure of the cartilaginous plates on which longitudinal growth of all long bones depends is described in the following section.

Epiphyseal Plates Are Subdivided into Four Zones

An epiphyseal plate exhibits a highly distinctive microscopic appearance when observed in longitudinal section. It consists of four successive zones that merge imperceptibly with

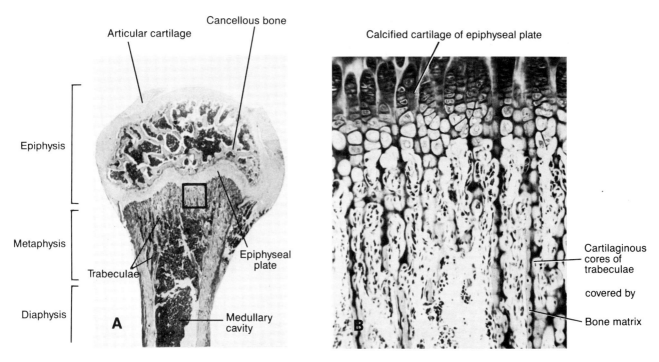

Fig. 12-22. (*A*) Low-power photomicrograph of end of growing long bone. Osteogenesis has now spread from the epiphyseal center of ossification so that only the articular cartilages and the epiphyseal plates remain cartilaginous. On the diaphyseal side of the epiphyseal plate, bony trabeculae extend down into the diaphysis. (*B*) Medium-power photomicrograph of the area indicated in *A*, showing trabeculae on the diaphyseal side of the epiphyseal plate. They have cores of darker stained calcified cartilage on which lighter stained bone has been deposited.

one another. From epiphysis to diaphysis, these are termed the *zones* of (1) *resting cartilage,* (2) *proliferating cartilage,* (3) *maturing cartilage,* and (4) *calcifying cartilage.* Extending from the fourth zone into the diaphysis, there are remnants of calcified cartilage (shown in a dark tone in Fig. 12-22*B*) with a thin layer of bone matrix (light in Fig. 12-22*B*) on their surface.

1. *Zone of Resting Cartilage.* The cartilage zone nearest to the bone tissue in the epiphysis (Fig. 12-23) is described as *resting* because its chondrocytes do not actively contribute to bone growth. The main function of this zone is to anchor the other zones of the epiphyseal plate to the bony epiphysis. Capillaries are present between it and the adjacent bony epiphysis (Fig. 12-23, marked with *arrows*). These vessels are important because in addition to providing nutrients and oxygen for the bone tissue in the epiphysis, they nourish all the chondrocytes in the epiphyseal plate down as far as its zone of calcifying cartilage.

2. *Zone of Proliferating Cartilage.* This zone, which would be better described as the zone of proliferating *chondrocytes,* contains chondrocytes that repeatedly divide and supply new chondrocytes to replace those that disappear from the diaphyseal side of the plate. As the plate's chondrocytes proliferate, they form char-

acteristic longitudinal columns that look like stacks of coins (Fig. 12-23). Furthermore, mitotic figures can sometimes be found in this zone. Figure 12-24 shows the electron microscopic appearance of the chondrocytes and the matrix of this zone.

3. *Zone of Maturing Cartilage.* In this zone, which is also known as the *zone of hypertrophying cartilage,* the chondrocytes are still arranged in longitudinal columns, but they undergo hypertrophy and accumulate glycogen and lipid. As a result, they appear large and pale staining (Fig. 12-23). Furthermore, they produce large amounts of alkaline phosphatase, an enzyme that, as noted earlier in this chapter, is believed to facilitate the calcification of extracellular matrix. At the EM level, the cells and matrix of this zone appear as illustrated in Figure 12-25.

4. *Zone of Calcifying Cartilage.* Also termed the *zone of provisional calcification,* this is the zone where the cartilage matrix becomes heavily impregnated with bone mineral. Yet careful measures to preserve its cells, through the use of rapid high-pressure freezing followed by freeze substitution of the frozen water by methanol and embedding at a low temperature (−35°C), have shown that the chondrocytes in this zone are still structurally intact, not degenerating as was previously believed (Hunziker et al). This finding

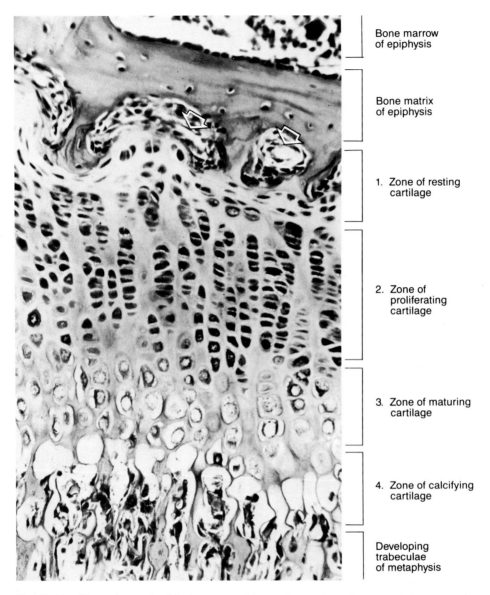

Bone marrow
of epiphysis

Bone matrix
of epiphysis

1. Zone of resting
   cartilage

2. Zone of
   proliferating
   cartilage

3. Zone of maturing
   cartilage

4. Zone of calcifying
   cartilage

Developing
trabeculae
of metaphysis

Fig. 12-23. Photomicrograph of the four zones of the epiphyseal plate. The position of the capillaries that nourish its chondrocytes is indicated by arrows.

makes it necessary to reevaluate the earlier hypothesis, which was based on morphological observations made when only standard methods of chemical fixation were available, that calcification of this zone results in its disintegration because it causes death of its chondrocytes. As in the case of development of primary and secondary centers of ossification in a cartilage model, it is unclear whether osteogenesis is preceded by disintegration or erosion of calcified cartilage. It is nevertheless evident that bone deposition occurs only after the cartilage has calcified. In LM sections, the transverse partitions of matrix between the lowermost lacunae in this zone can show signs of breaking down

(Fig. 12-23). Capillaries with associated osteogenic cells invade this zone from the medullary cavity below and provide a vascular environment that promotes the differentiation of osteoblasts and the deposition of bone matrix on the remnants of calcified cartilage, as described in the following section.

New Bone Forms on the Diaphyseal Side of the Epiphyseal Plate

The longitudinal partitions of calcified cartilage matrix that are present between neighboring columns of chondrocytes remain intact longer than the flimsier transverse partitions

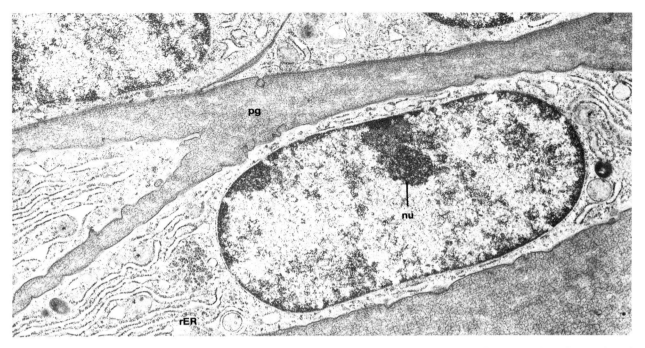

Fig. 12-24. Electron micrograph of a chondrocyte in the zone of proliferating cartilage of an epiphyseal plate, prepared by freeze-substitution. Dilated cisternae of rough ER (*rER*) and ER-associated polysomes can be recognized in the cytoplasm. A prominent nucleolus (*nu*) is seen in the nucleus. The proteoglycan network (*pg*) of cartilage matrix also shows to advantage in this section. (Courtesy of L. Arsenault)

that separate the chondrocytes in each longitudinal column (Fig. 12-22*B* and box 4 in Plate 12-1). Capillary sprouts (see Fig. 12-29*A*) invade the spaces vacated by the columns of chondrocytes on the diaphyseal side of the plate (Figs. 12-22*B* and 12-23).

In the process of growing into vacated lacunae, it would appear that some of these capillary sprouts are susceptible to damage, whereupon small amounts of blood leak into the lacunae. Although such extravasation is relatively minor, it may well explain why the juvenile type of *osteomyelitis* (Gr. *osteon*, bone; and *myelos*, marrow, meaning inflammation of bone marrow) commonly begins at this particular site. This inflammatory condition can develop in children who have a bacterial infection in some other part of the body that permits bacterial access to the bloodstream. Even such minor capillary bleeding into the marrow cavity could enable circulating bacteria to set up new foci of infection at the sites of blood leakage.

The longitudinal remnants of calcified cartilage on the diaphyseal border of the epiphyseal plate serve as a scaffolding on which diaphyseal osteoblasts lay down bone matrix. When seen in longitudinal section, long tapering spikes of bone described as *trabeculae* project down from the diaphyseal side of the epiphyseal plate like stalactites from the roof of a cave (Plate 12-1*D* and Fig. 12-22). The residual calcified cartilage in the cores of these structures stains a pale blue to mauve color in H & E sections whereas the bone matrix that covers them generally stains a bright pink (Plate 12-1*D*).

Thus as soon as the new cartilage that is produced in the epiphyseal plate undergoes calcification, it becomes replaced by bone. Resulting progressive replacement of the cartilage that calcifies on the diaphyseal side of both epiphyseal plates gradually increases the length of the bony diaphysis. Furthermore, as quickly as new bone is formed at the advancing end of the tapering trabeculae (described as their base), a comparable amount of slightly older bone is resorbed from the trailing tips of these structures (Fig. 12-26). Osteoclasts are particularly plentiful at the trailing ends of diaphyseal trabeculae; Figure 12-16 shows such an osteoclast wrapped around the tip of a trabecula. Hence the process of elongation of the diaphysis and its medullary cavity does not require comparable changes in the length of the diaphyseal trabeculae.

Whereas the diaphyseal trabeculae that lie below the central region of the epiphyseal plate contain bone that is undergoing the continuous turnover described above, the trabeculae that form at the *periphery* of the plate are progressively *incorporated into the shaft* (Fig. 12-26). Their fate can be followed by the use of radioautography after the injection of experimental animals with radioactively labeled phosphorus. If a single dose of radioactive phosphorus is injected so as to mark the newly formed bone tissue that is becoming calcified at the time of injection, radioactivity can first be detected at the base of the diaphyseal trabeculae (Fig. 12-27*A*). It is then found in the tips of these structures

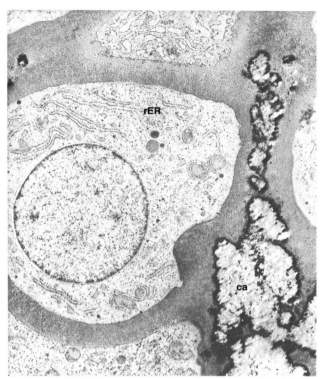

Fig. 12-25. Electron micrograph of a hypertrophied chondrocyte in the zone of maturing cartilage of an epiphyseal plate. Its rough ER (*rER*) is still fairly prominent. Calcification (*ca*) has already started in the longitudinal partition of matrix extending from top to bottom on the right. The pale middle in the site of calcification is due to a loss of mineral during staining. (Courtesy of L. Arsenault)

and also in the walls of the flared region of the shaft (Fig. 12-27B). Finally, it is incorporated into the bone cortex at the base of this region (Fig. 12-27C).

The Metaphyses Undergo Active Remodeling. The *metaphyses* are the flared regions near the ends of a long bone where the diameter of the diaphysis increases and becomes equal to that of the epiphyses (Fig. 12-22A). In these regions, the bony trabeculae that form at the periphery of the epiphyseal plates are gradually becoming incorporated into the diaphysis; the cartilaginous growth plates themselves are regarded as parts of the epiphyses (Fig. 12-22A). The metaphyses of a lengthening bone retain the same general shape because of the resorptive activity of numerous osteoclasts that remove bone from the flared periphery of the metaphyses, which, as a result, become reduced in diameter to match the width of the shaft. The effect of such bone removal can be appreciated by comparing the left and right sides of Figure 12-26, where active bone resorption at the site labeled 1 has markedly changed the previous epiphyseal contour (indicated by a *dotted line*). At the same time, new bone is being built up on the inner aspect of the bony walls of the metaphyses to compensate for bone lost through resorption from their periphery (Figs.

12-22A and 12-26). Such adjustment of the general shape of a bone while it is growing is described as *bone remodeling.*

Next the stages of ossification that take place in the metaphyses will be considered in three dimensions.

Trabeculae Represent the Walls of Tunnels. A longitudinal section through a metaphysis of a growing long bone tends to give the impression that the diaphyseal trabeculae hang down from the diaphyseal border of the epiphyseal plate like stalactites from the roof of a cave (Plate 12-1D). In fact, it is only the free ends of such trabeculae that do this. Closer to the epiphyseal plate from which they extend, the trabeculae remain interconnected in a honeycomblike arrangement that is riddled with tunnel-like spaces (Fig. 12-28B). Such spaces are formed as described in the following paragraph.

As may be seen from boxes 1 to 4 in Plate 12-1 and also from Figure 12-28B, the chondrocytes in the lower part of the epiphyseal plate are arranged in parallel longitudinal columns. Breakdown of the thin transverse partitions between their lacunae therefore creates an arrangement of tubular spaces separated by longitudinal partitions of calcified cartilage matrix (*purple* in Plate 12-1) that constitute the walls of longitudinal tunnels. These tunnels can be viewed directly in the scanning electron microscope following removal of the other tissues by enzymatic digestion. Figure 12-29B shows the honeycomblike texture of the zone of calcifying cartilage as seen by this means. The cartilaginous tunnels become invaded by branching terminal capillary sprouts with characteristic bulbous tips (Fig. 12-29A) that penetrate the vacated lacunae. Such capillaries are accompanied by osteogenic cells and osteoblasts that begin to line the tunnels with a layer of bone matrix (Fig. 12-26, site labeled 4).

Each longitudinal partition between neighboring tunnels appears in longitudinal section as a more or less isolated trabecula with calcified cartilage in its core and bone tissue on its lateral surfaces (Fig. 12-28A and B). Hence the bone tissue that apparently *covers* the cartilaginous cores of trabeculae is, in fact, *lining* the cartilaginous tunnels (Fig. 12-28B), and the osteoblasts, osteogenic cells, and capillaries that seem to lie in the spaces between the trabeculae constitute the contents of such tunnels.

Haversian Systems Are Formed by the Filling In of Tunnels with Concentric Bone Lamellae. The relatively wide cartilaginous tunnels that form under the periphery of an epiphyseal plate begin to fill in with consecutive lamellae of bone matrix (Fig. 12-26, site labeled 4). These lamellae gradually decrease the diameter of the tunnel until it is no more than a narrow canal that encloses some osteogenic cells, osteoblasts, and one or two small blood vessels. The characteristic arrangement of concentric lamellae that surrounds each central canal constitutes an *osteon* or *haversian system,* the basic structural unit of compact bone (see Figs. 12-32 and 12-33). Indeed, the only way an osteon can develop is through the progressive filling in of a tunnel of some kind with successive lamellae of bone. The total

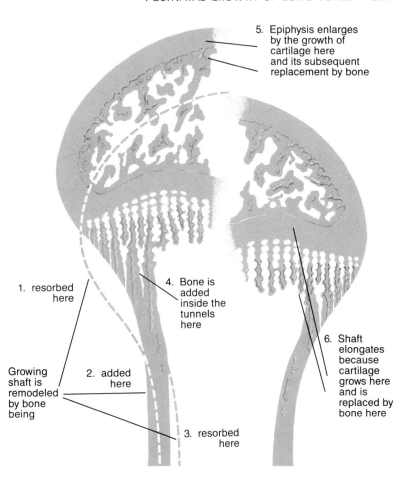

5. Epiphysis enlarges by the growth of cartilage here and its subsequent replacement by bone

4. Bone is added inside the tunnels here

6. Shaft elongates because cartilage grows here and is replaced by bone here

1. resorbed here

Growing shaft is remodeled by bone being

2. added here

3. resorbed here

Fig. 12-26. Schematic diagram indicating the surfaces where bone is deposited or resorbed during remodeling at the ends of a growing long bone with flared extremities. Bone is shown in black and cartilage is shown in blue. (Ham AW: J Bone Joint Surg 34-A:701, 1952)

diameter of an osteon is limited by the diameter of the preexisting tunnel and also by the farthest distance over which osteocytes can be nourished through their canalicular system. A typical osteon is generally 3 mm to 5 mm long with an average diameter of 0.3 mm, and it is made up of up to approximately six lamellae (see Fig. 12-32). In general, it is only the osteons that are laid down under the periphery of the epiphyseal plate that become incorporated into compact bone of the diaphysis. Any osteons that are starting to form under the central region of the plate are resorbed long before completion because of extension of the medullary cavity.

We shall now consider how a bone grows in width.

Increase in Diameter Is Due to Appositional Growth at the Periphery of the Diaphysis

Successive generations of osteoblasts arise from osteogenic cells of the periosteum and contribute successive lamellae of bone matrix to the outer surface of the diaphysis (Fig. 12-26, site labeled 2). Such appositional growth results in an increase in the diameter of the shaft, which then requires compensatory widening of the medullary cavity (Fig. 12-26, site labeled 3) to prevent the bone cortex from becoming too thick and heavy. Some osteoclasts that are helping to widen the medullary cavity can be seen in Figure 12-30. At this stage, new bony trabeculae are being formed as a result of subperiosteal appositional growth and are becoming incorporated into the periphery of the diaphysis. At the same time, older bone is being resorbed from the inner aspect of the cortex so as to widen the medullary cavity. In the inner region of the bone cortex, the soft tissue spaces that were present in the preexisting cancellous bone are becoming filled in, with the result that the cancellous bone is becoming converted into compact bone (Fig. 12-30).

At a later stage, bone is added to the periphery of the diaphysis primarily in the form of new osteons that develop

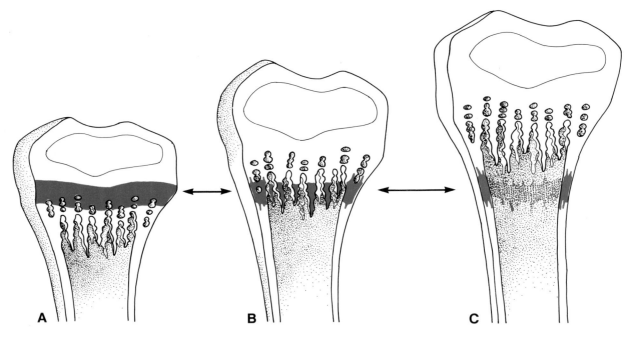

Fig. 12-27. Diagram indicating the relative position of newly formed bone tissue in the end of a tibia over an 8-day period. Its position has been followed by radioautography following the injection of radiophosphorus into a rat. (*A*) Five minutes after injection. (*B*) Two days after injection. (*C*) Eight days after injection. See text for description. (Based on studies by Leblond CP, Wilkinson P, Bélanger GW, Robichon J: Am J Anat 86:289, 1950)

under the periosteum in the following manner. The first stage is the formation of a longitudinal groove between ridges along the diaphysis (Fig. 12-31*A*). Bone matrix is then deposited in a way that extends the two longitudinal ridges toward each other (Fig. 12-31*B*) until they meet and fuse (Fig. 12-31*C*), and as a result the groove becomes

transformed into a bony tunnel. The former groove is still lined by periosteum, and eventually, it encloses one or two small periosteal vessels (Fig. 12-31*B*). Hence the resulting tunnel is lined by osteogenic cells, and it has one or two small blood vessels extending along it (Fig. 12-31*D*). The deposition of successive lamellae of bone on the walls of

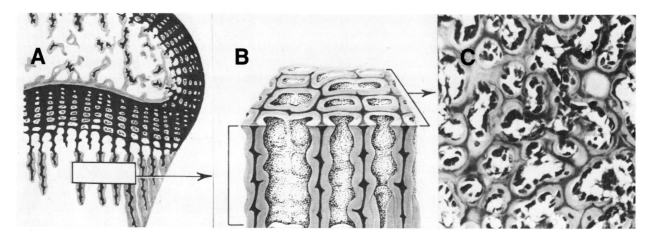

Fig. 12-28. (*A*) Schematic diagram of metaphyseal trabeculae just below the epiphyseal plate, as seen in longitudinal section. (*B*) Interpretive drawing showing that in boxed-in area in *A*, the so-called trabeculae are tunnel walls. Cartilage is depicted in black; bone is shown in gray. (*C*) Photomicrograph showing boxed-in area in *A*, as seen in transverse section.

the tunnel culminates in the formation of an osteon (Fig. 12-31*D* to *F*).

Volkmann's Canals Are Also Formed. The osteons that form under the periosteum become built up (in the manner just described) around their central periosteally derived vessels that are then referred to as *haversian vessels* (Fig. 12-31). Now incorporated into compact bone, such vessels may continue to receive blood by way of small periosteally derived vessels that reach them by way of other canals known as Volkmann's canals (Fig. 12-32; see also Fig. 12-39, *lower right*). Vessels in Volkmann's canals can also connect haversian vessels with blood vessels in the medullary cavity (Fig. 12-32; see also Fig. 12-39). Volkmann's canals can be recognized by the fact that they run obliquely or transversely *in a radial direction* through the shaft, not in a longitudinal direction as in the case of the haversian canals they interconnect (Fig. 12-32). Hence unlike haversian canals, Volkmann's canals are *not* surrounded by a concentric pattern of lamellae.

Compact Bone May Also Contain Circumferential and Interstitial Lamellae. In a long bone that is nearing its adult size, the outer and inner circumferential surfaces of the diaphysis, which are initially rough (Fig. 12-30), become smoothed off through the addition of a few *outer* and *inner circumferential lamellae* (Figs. 12-32 and 12-33). The remainder of the cortex is made up primarily of osteons (Figs. 12-32 and 12-33), but in the crevices between these osteons, there are small remnants of either preexisting osteons or preexisting circumferential lamellae that have been almost entirely replaced by new osteons as a result of remodeling. These remnants are described as *interstitial lamellae* (Fig. 12-32).

It might be thought that the laying down of outer circumferential lamellae at the periphery of the diaphysis would terminate its further growth in width. However, this is not so because osteoclasts can still erode grooves in its external surface, and these grooves can then become filled in with successive lamellae of bone derived from osteogenic cells of the periosteum. As a result, new osteons can be added to the periphery of the diaphysis by a process that is essentially similar to that illustrated in Figure 12-31.

Bone Undergoes Lifelong Remodeling

In addition to the process of *structural remodeling* that occurs as bones grow, bones continually adapt to prevailing stresses through remodeling of their internal structure. Marked changes in such stresses can lead to compensatory deposition or resorption of compact bone and changes in alignment of the bony trabeculae in their cancellous regions. Furthermore, if a limb remains unused for a prolonged period, its bones are not subjected to the usual stresses and a process of remodeling ensues that can result in excessive bone resorption with consequent weakening of the bones.

This degenerative change in bones is often referred to as *atrophy of disuse.*

Bones also have to undergo a lifelong process of constitutive *internal remodeling*, which is required because bone tissue can weaken and some of its osteocytes may die, making a certain amount of daily bone replacement necessary. Compact bone is always being resorbed to some extent by osteoclasts, and the resorbed bone is then replaced with new compact bone. This new bone is laid down as osteons that form within *resorption tunnels* (*resorption cavities*) made by osteoclasts. Such tunnels can generally be distinguished from haversian canals or Volkmann's canals by (1) their *irregularly etched outlines* and (2) the presence of *osteoclasts* (instead of osteoblasts and osteogenic cells) along their borders (Fig. 12-34). Resorption cavities are nevertheless rapidly invaded by osteogenic cells and osteoblasts that fill them in with new osteons. The microscopic appearance of a resorption tunnel that is becoming filled in with bone is illustrated in Figure 12-35. The border between the edge of the tunnel and the new bone that has been deposited is marked by a *cementing line* (Fig. 12-35). The *calcification front* is represented by the indistinct border between the inner lamella of *prebone* (*osteoid tissue*) and the surrounding lamellae of *calcified bone* (Fig. 12-35).

Bone Formation Is Normally Coupled Directly to Previous Bone Resorption. It is well established that bone resorption continues throughout life as an intrinsic part of the remodeling process. Yet under most circumstances adult bones show little day-to-day variation in their total bone mass, suggesting that under most circumstances, a local regulatory mechanism gears the amount of new bone formed during remodeling to the quantity of older bone lost through resorption. It has recently been established that resorbing bone does indeed liberate a macromolecular *coupling factor*, probably a protein, that is capable of eliciting the compensatory deposition of new bone matrix by osteoblasts. Hence there is reason to believe that signaling molecules produced by bone-forming (or even bone-resorbing) cells and liberated during degradation of bone matrix have the capacity to couple compensatory bone formation directly to bone resorption, thereby bringing about site-specific replacement of bone that is being resorbed.

The existence of a direct coupling mechanism could help to explain the well-substantiated observation that PTH acts as a stimulus for bone formation as well as bone resorption. It now seems that one of the primary effects of PTH is to stimulate osteoclastic activity, and that an outcome of this activity would be the release of coupling factor from foci of bone resorption. The liberated coupling factor could then elicit compensatory bone deposition at such foci. However, there is evidence that PTH can also elicit bone deposition by a mechanism that does not depend solely on increased bone resorption (Tam et al).

The nature of the cellular response to coupling factor is not yet established. It is conceivable that preexisting osteogenic cells may become supplemented by subsequent generations of osteogenic cells that are induced to differentiate from more primitive perivascular mesenchymal progenitors by bone morphogenetic protein

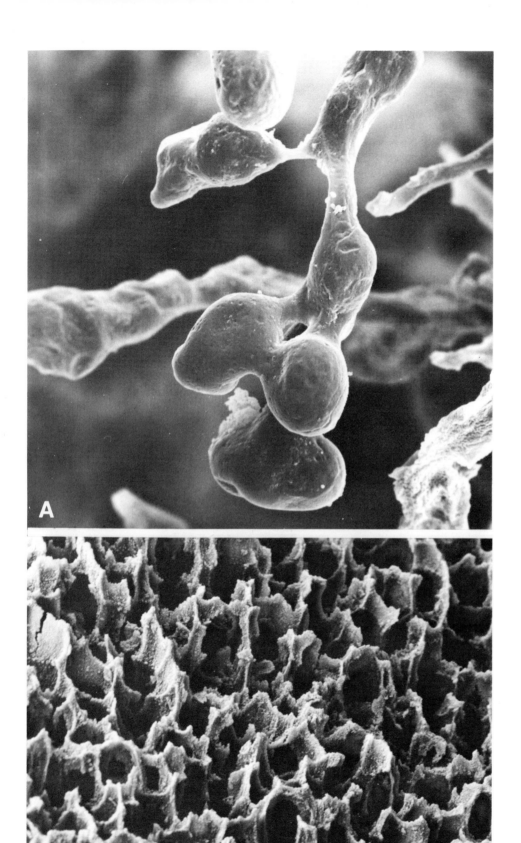

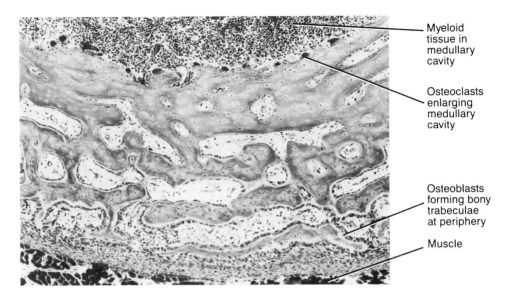

Myeloid
tissue in
medullary
cavity

Osteoclasts
enlarging
medullary
cavity

Osteoblasts
forming bony
trabeculae
at periphery

Muscle

Fig. 12-30. Photomicrograph of a growing long bone (femur of kitten, cross section). Trabeculae of cancellous bone are being formed at its periphery, and its medullary cavity is being widened by the resorptive activity of numerous osteoclasts. (Courtesy of M. Weinstock)

(BMP). The cellular response would then include the further recruitment of osteogenic cells accompanied by their proliferation under the stimulus of coupling factor and other putative bone-derived growth factors (Urist et al).

Thus under normal conditions, resorptive stimuli bring about a *coupled increase in bone deposition,* augmenting bone *turnover* rather than eliciting bone *loss.* In clinical conditions in which there is a net loss of bone, this coupling mechanism presumably fails to operate adequately. Indeed, it has been suggested that *osteoporosis,* a fairly common bone condition in the elderly that is characterized by an overall reduction in the total bone mass, commonly represents the outcome of generalized uncoupling. This condition is a major factor that predisposes the elderly to bone fractures, particularly fractures of the hip, wrist, and vertebrae.

Next we shall discuss some clinically relevant nutritional and metabolic factors that are known to exert a profound effect on bones and their formation.

NUTRITIONAL AND METABOLIC FACTORS THAT INFLUENCE BONE GROWTH

The ossification that takes place in the metaphyses is markedly affected by factors that can interfere with either

(1) *secretion* of the organic constituents of bone matrix or (2) *calcification* of intercellular organic matrix. Normally, these two processes are kept strictly in balance, but under certain circumstances, an imbalance develops in growing bones that profoundly changes the histological appearance of their metaphyses. Two examples of such an imbalance are described in the following sections.

Scurvy. A particularly striking consequence of impaired synthesis of the main organic constituent of bone matrix is seen in *scurvy.* This disease stems from inadequate hydroxylation of proline, as described under Collagen in Chapter 7. In the absence of sufficient dietary *vitamin C (ascorbic acid)* to act as a cofactor in the hydroxylation of proline and lysine, collagen is unable to assume its normal triple-helix configuration. Such inability results in the accumulation of procollagen within osteoblasts and various other cells that secrete it, leading to inhibition of procollagen synthesis in these cells.

The main skeletal manifestations of inadequate levels of vitamin C are that the formation of osteoid tissue is greatly reduced and that the thickness of the bone cortex is accordingly decreased. This, in turn, leads to increased fragility of long bones and increased risk of fracture. During the period of bone growth, the epiphyseal growth plates

Fig. 12-29. Scanning electron micrographs of the zone of calcifying cartilage of an epiphyseal plate and of the diaphyseal capillaries that invade this zone (proximal epiphysis of rat humerus). These capillaries are outgrowths of capillary loops in the adjacent metaphysis. (*A*) Plastic corrosion cast of invading capillaries. All the surrounding tissues have been removed by enzymatic digestion. (*B*) Mineralized portion of the growth plate (epiphyseal aspect of calcified zone), prepared by enzymatic removal of the other tissues. The diaphyseal capillaries invade tunnels and chondrocyte lacunae on the diaphyseal side of this zone of calcifying cartilage. (Courtesy of L. Arsenault)

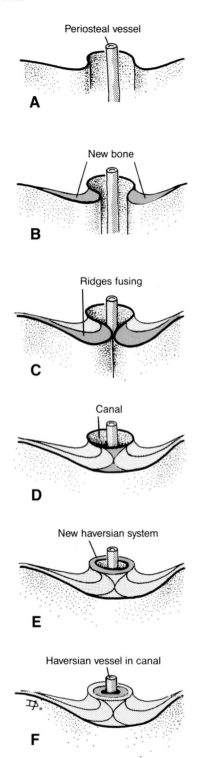

Periosteal vessel

A

New bone

B

Ridges fusing

C

Canal

D

New haversian system

E

Haversian vessel in canal

F

Fig. 12-31. Diagrammatic representation of the addition of a new haversian system to the periphery of the diaphysis of a growing long bone. (See text for details.) Note how a periosteal vessel can end up within a haversian canal.

remain unduly thin (Fig. 12-36). Other consequences of this slow rate of production of organic bone matrix are that the bony walls of the metaphyses also remain very thin and that only minimal amounts of bone are formed to support the epiphyseal plate (Fig. 12-36). The adult form of scurvy, which affects the maintenance of bones rather than their growth, plagued the life and welfare of many sailors until it was realized that liberal supplies of leafy green vegetables and fresh citrus fruits needed to be taken on board for long voyages. The possibility of an outbreak of scurvy also hung heavily over the heads of those engaged in polar explorations, and scurvy was so widespread among early settlers of the northern regions of the American continent that it is a wonder anyone remained here unless compelled to do so through force of circumstance.

However, scurvy is not associated with any impairment of calcification. The little organic matrix that is formed becomes heavily calcified.

Rickets. Calcification is dependent on the presence of a sufficient local $Ca^{2+} \cdot P_i$ product for it to proceed. Inadequate dietary levels of either calcium or phosphorus do not necessarily impede calcification; it is the local product of these two concentrations (and the effective removal of calcification inhibitors) that determines whether calcification will take place. Adequate levels of *vitamin D* are also required because, as noted earlier in this chapter, a hydroxylated derivative of this vitamin promotes calcium and phosphate absorption from the gut. If infants are deprived of this vitamin as well as sunshine (because long-wave ultraviolet light reaching their skin will convert the provitamin 7-dehydrocholesterol into vitamin D_3), they run the risk of developing *rickets*, a bone disease that can lead to permanent skeletal deformities. Their weight-bearing bones are poorly calcified and bend under the strain of supporting the weight of the body, and this typically results in the development of bowed legs or knock-knees. The low $Ca^{2+} \cdot P_i$ product impedes calcification in their epiphyseal plates, the cartilage of which continues to grow until it becomes markedly and irregularly thickened (Fig. 12-37). Calcification is also impaired in the organic bone matrix that is being laid down on the diaphyseal side of these plates, with the result that comparatively weak osteoid tissue, rather than properly mineralized bone, accumulates in the metaphyses. Large amounts of subperiosteal osteoid tissue are also produced by osteoblasts arising from the periosteum (Fig. 12-37). This makes the metaphyseal regions of long bones knobby. The knobs thus produced at the growing ends of the ribs are responsible for what is termed the "rachitic rosary" typical of a rachitic child's chest.

Hence in rickets, the changes that occur in the metaphyseal growth zones of a long bone are the result of bone growth proceeding while calcification fails.

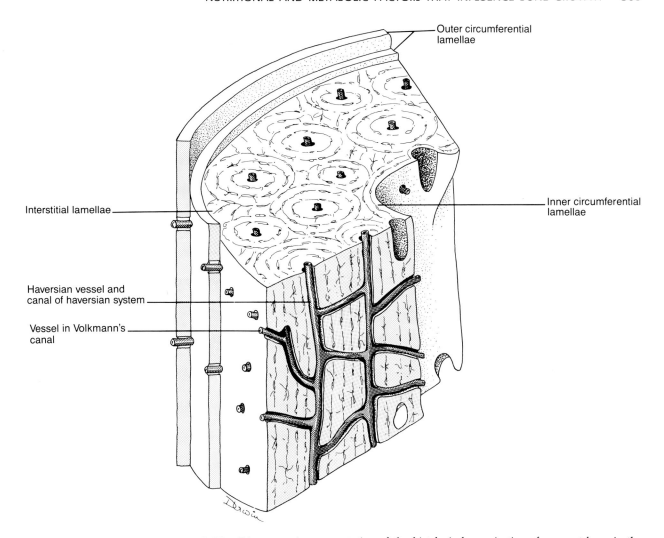

Fig. 12-32. Diagrammatic representation of the histological organization of compact bone in the diaphysis of an adult long bone. The number of osteons has been reduced for simplicity (compare with Fig. 12-33).

Nutritional and metabolic bone defects take longer to be manifested in the bones of adults than in the metaphyses of children's bones. However, adult bones still have to be maintained, and this requires a steady turnover of bone tissue throughout life. Two examples of conditions in which bone maintenance becomes inadequate will now be mentioned.

Osteomalacia. This condition is also sometimes referred to as *adult rickets* because it affects the bones of adults. In this case, the new bone tissue being formed to maintain the skeleton does not become properly calcified. Osteomalacia can develop in adults who are obliged to exist on a poor diet that is deficient in calcium or vitamin D. However, it is more often the result of (1) some metabolic dis-order that interferes with the absorption or excretion of minerals, or (2) loss of vitamin D from the gut or failure to convert it into its active form within the body.

Osteoporosis. Already mentioned in connection with bone morphogenetic protein (BMP) and also coupling, osteoporosis is a skeletal disorder that commonly develops in elderly people. In this instance, the defect is not failure of the newly formed bone tissue to become adequately calcified. It results primarily because the amount of new bone matrix produced is insufficient to keep pace with bone resorption. As a result, the body's total bone mass becomes progressively diminished.

A useful histological method that can be used to investigate both these conditions is microradiography, the basis of which is described in the following section.

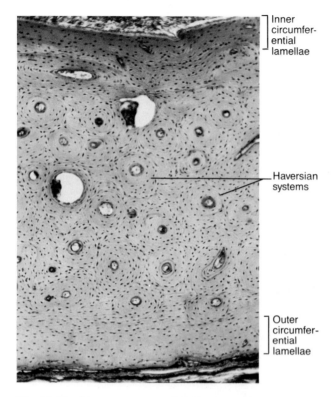

Inner circumferential lamellae

Haversian systems

Outer circumferential lamellae

Fig. 12-33. Transverse section of the diaphysis of a mature long bone. Both the inner and the outer surfaces of the bone are now smoothed off by circumferential lamellae. Part of the periosteum is seen external to the outer circumferential lamellae. The interstices between neighboring haversian systems are filled by interstitial lamellae. (Courtesy of M. Weinstock)

Microradiography. An undecalcified section of the bone sample to be investigated is placed in contact with a photographic emulsion and then is exposed to soft x-rays. The extent to which the x-rays penetrate the different parts of the section is indicative of the amount of calcium present. Hence the resulting developed *microradiograph* reveals not only the numbers and relative sizes of the osteons in the section but also the extent to which their component lamellae are calcified. Three microradiographs of representative cortical bone samples obtained from individuals of different ages are illustrated in Figure 12-38, and the findings are discussed in its caption.

From Figure 12-38 it will be appreciated that young adults have a slower rate of bone turnover than children and that in old age the rate of bone resorption exceeds that of bone replacement.

THE BLOOD SUPPLY OF A LONG BONE

The main blood supply to the diaphysis, metaphyses, and bone marrow of a long bone comes from its *nutrient artery* or *arteries* (Fig. 12-39). The metaphyses receive a supplementary blood supply from their *metaphyseal arteries,* and

the epiphyses are supplied by their *epiphyseal arteries* (Fig. 12-39). In addition, the osteocytes in the outermost lamellae of the bone cortex obtain nourishment by diffusion through their canalicular system from periosteal capillaries that are supplied by *periosteal arteries* (Fig. 12-39).

For the most part, blood enters haversian vessels of the cortex from the nutrient arterial branches in the medullary cavity and it leaves the periphery of the cortex by way of periosteal vessels. Under normal conditions, periosteal arteries supply very little blood to the cortex; the nutrient arteries supply at least its inner two thirds. For further information, see Brookes.

The various arteries supplying the bone become incorporated as follows. Each nutrient artery represents the principal vessel of a periosteal bud from which the primary center of ossification developed. Similarly, the epiphyseal arteries are derivatives of the vessels that initiated development of the secondary centers of ossification. The metaphyseal arteries represent periosteal arteries that became incorporated into the metaphyses as these grew in width.

By the time a long bone is fully grown (*i.e.,* its epiphyseal plates have become entirely replaced by bone tissue), numerous anastomoses have been established between terminal branches of the nutrient, metaphyseal, and epiphyseal arteries (Fig. 12-39). A distinct advantage of receiving nourishment from so many anastomosing arteries is that in the event of failure of the main blood supply by way of the nutrient artery, enough blood is provided by the other arteries to keep most parts of the bone viable.

The Epiphyseal Plates Are Nourished by Epiphyseal Capillaries. The growth plates of a growing bone are made of cartilage and hence are not supplied with any capillaries of their own. On the other hand, the bony trabeculae present on the diaphyseal border of each epiphyseal plate are richly provided with capillaries. Yet the zone of

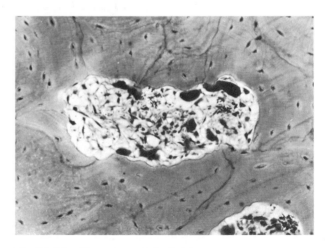

Fig. 12-34. Photomicrograph of a bone resorption cavity, probably in oblique section. The large dark cells are osteoclasts; their activity explains the etched-out borders of the cavity. (Courtesy of C. P. Leblond)

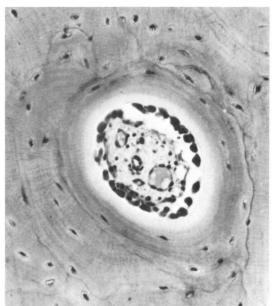

Fig. 12-35. (*A*) Photomicrograph of a former resorption cavity being filled in to form a new osteon. The dark cells encircling the cavity are osteoblasts. (*B*) Interpretative diagram showing that the ring of osteoblasts lining the cavity in *A* is separated from bone by a layer of pale-staining osteoid tissue (prebone), the matrix of which has not yet calcified. Cementing lines indicate where new layers of bone began to be laid down on the older bone. A fully formed osteon is shown at left. (Courtesy of C. P. Leblond)

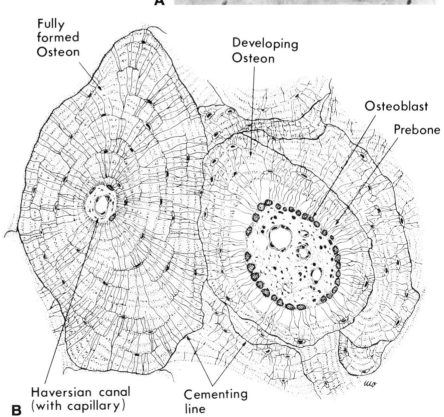

calcifying cartilage on the diaphyseal side of each plate is so heavily mineralized that the amount of nourishment that would reach the chondrocytes by diffusion from these vessels would be insufficient for the chondrocytes to remain viable. Throughout the period of bone growth, the primary source of nourishment of these chondrocytes is another important set of capillaries that are situated along the *epiphyseal border* of the plate, adjacent to its zone of resting cartilage. Marked with arrows in Figure 12-23, these capillaries receive blood from the *epiphyseal arteries.* Some nourishment may also reach the chondrocytes by diffusion from the perimeter of the plate.

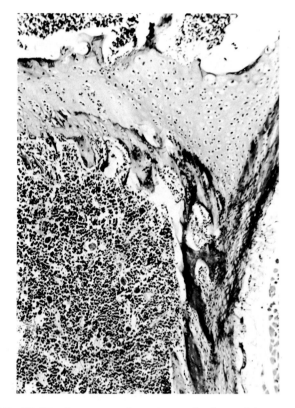

Fig. 12-36. Low-power photomicrograph of part of the upper end of a tibia (guinea pig), from an animal maintained for several weeks on a diet deficient in vitamin C so that it would develop scurvy. Note the inadequate formation of trabeculae on the diaphyseal side of the epiphyseal plate (just above *middle*). As a result, the plate is not supported by the proper number of trabeculae. Bone building for the shaft has almost ceased at the metaphysis so that it is very thin (*lower right*) and breaks easily. (Ham AW, Elliott HC: Am J Pathol 14:323, 1938)

A thorough knowledge of the vessels that supply the different parts of a long bone and of changes in blood supply that can result from bone injuries or surgical procedures is of prime importance to those engaged in orthopedic or reconstructive surgery.

Epiphyseal Displacement Can Rupture Epiphyseal Blood Vessels. Two basically different types of arrangement are found in the epiphyses of growing long bones (Dale and Harris). In the head of the femur, for example, the epiphyseal plate is continuous with the articular cartilage (Fig. 12-40*A*), whereas in many other cases it is not (Fig. 12-40*B*). In the former type of arrangement, the epiphyseal arteries penetrate the zone of cartilaginous continuity between the epiphyseal plate and the articular cartilage (Fig. 12-40*A*), whereas in the latter type of arrangement they penetrate the perichondriumlike tissue covering the sides of the epiphysis without having to pass through either the epiphyseal plate or the articular cartilage (Fig. 12-40*B*). The clinical significance of these two somewhat different arrangements will now be discussed.

In children, *epiphyseal separation* can occur as a result of an accident. Such separation generally involves the weakest zone of the epiphyseal plate, which is its zone of maturing (hypertrophying)

cartilage. If this happens to an epiphysis of the type shown in Figure 12-40*A*, the blood vessels entering the cartilage at the perimeter of the plate are likely to be ruptured. Separation of this type of epiphysis leads to death of the detached fragment. However, separation of the other type of epiphysis (Fig. 12-40*B*) does not cut it off from its blood supply and therefore does not cause death of the chondrocytes in its epiphyseal plate.

Haversian Vessels. The small blood vessels within haversian canals constitute an anastomosing network that is connected to vessels of the medulla and also to vessels of the periosteum. Some haversian canals contain an arteriole and a venule (Fig. 12-41), but others contain only a single capillary. Small nerve fibers can also be present in haversian canals but lymphatics are absent. Indeed, the only part of a bone that is known to be provided with a lymphatic drainage is its periosteum.

The remainder of this chapter and much of Chapter 13 will be of particular interest to medical students who intend to specialize in orthopedics.

MECHANISM OF HEALING OF A SIMPLE FRACTURE OF A LONG BONE

A *simple fracture* breaks a bone into two parts that are referred to clinically as *fragments*. It usually also results in some tearing of the periosteum and can cause displacement of the fragments relative to each other that is sufficient to warrant some *reduction* of the fracture. The standard procedure is to manipulate the broken ends of the bone back into apposition in a manner that realigns the fragments and restores the former line of the bone. To maintain the appropriate position for proper healing, the bone is then usually stabilized externally by applying a plaster cast. In some cases, however, fractures require reduction at open operation followed by internal stabilization through the use of a suitable rigid fixation device. Under such circumstances, healing takes place in a somewhat different manner, as will be discussed later in this chapter.

Fracturing a Bone Has Some Immediate Consequences. Because blood vessels in the bone itself and in its adjacent soft tissues are torn, the bone tissue manifests signs of indirect as well as direct damage. In general, the amount of bleeding that results from the injury depends on the size of the bone and on the extent to which its fragments become displaced. Major fractures can result in severe hemorrhage; in a fracture of the femoral shaft, for example, more than 1 liter of blood may be lost from the circulation. The extravasated blood coagulates into a clot (Fig. 12-42) that, if substantial, may persist at the fracture site for a week or two.

In addition to such direct injury, indirect damage is sustained because of tearing of the haversian vessels that cross the fracture line. Blood circulation ceases in these vessels back to sites where they anastomose with other haversian vessels (or vessels of other kinds), and a consequence of

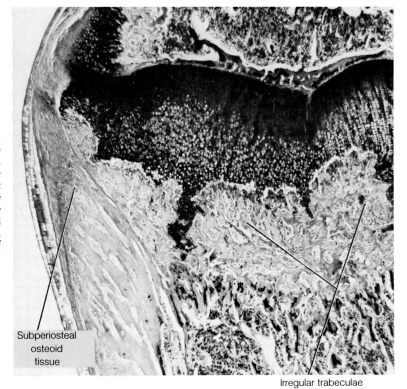

Fig. 12-37. Low-power photomicrograph of part of the upper end of a tibia (rat), from an animal maintained on a diet with low $Ca^{2+} \cdot P_i$ product so that it would develop rickets. Because calcification cannot proceed properly, the chondrocytes in the epiphyseal plate live longer, with the result that the plate becomes thick (darkly stained, just above *middle*). Irregular trabeculae of osteoid tissue are evident below the cartilage (under the epiphyseal plate), and much subperiosteal osteoid tissue is seen in the metaphysis, at left. (This is an example of severe low-phosphorus rickets.)

Subperiosteal
osteoid
tissue

Irregular trabeculae
of osteoid tissue

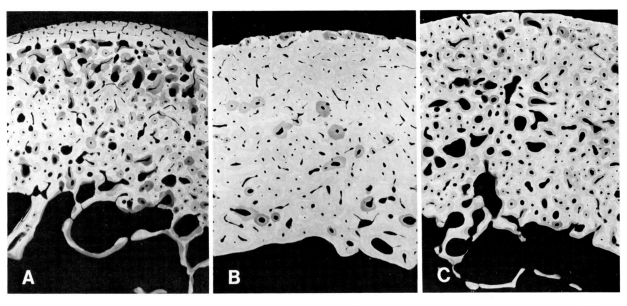

Fig. 12-38. Microradiographs of undecalcified sections of midshaft of a femur from people of different ages. (*A*) A 7-year-old. This indicates the relatively rapid turnover of bone that is normal for this age. It shows many resorption tunnels and newly formed osteons that are not yet as heavily calcified as the older bone and that therefore appear darker in comparison. (*B*) A 25-year-old. There is little indication here of turnover of haversian systems. There are almost no resorption tunnels, and most of the systems are well calcified and of similar density. (*C*) An 85-year-old. This shows two features that are characteristic of bone of people this age: (*1*) there are many resorption tunnels, which indicates increased resorption, and (*2*) the new layers of bone beginning to fill in some of the tunnels are poorly calcified (darker than well-calcified bone). Hence bones of the old have a higher content of bone of low density than bones of young adults. (Courtesy of J. Jowsey)

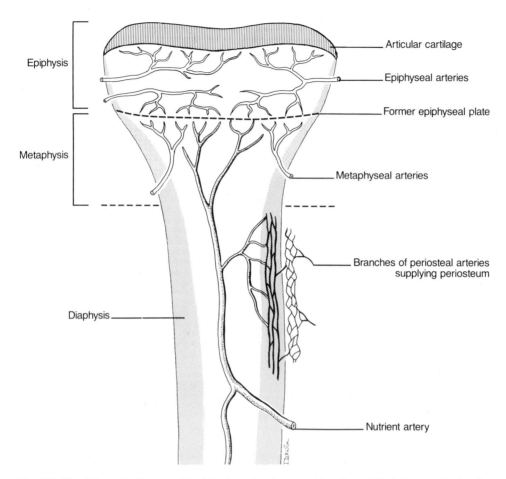

Epiphysis

Metaphysis

Diaphysis

Articular cartilage

Epiphyseal arteries

Former epiphyseal plate

Metaphyseal arteries

Branches of periosteal arteries
supplying periosteum

Nutrient artery

Fig. 12-39. Schematic diagram of the blood supply of a mature long bone (tibia). See text for details.

such interruption of the blood flow is that the bone tissue on either side of the fracture line becomes deprived of oxygen and nutrients. This, in turn, leads to death of osteocytes for some distance on each side of the fracture line. The *dead bone tissue* can be recognized by its characteristic *empty lacunae* (Fig. 12-42). The associated necrotic regions

of bone marrow and periosteum do not extend quite as far on either side of the fracture line (Fig. 12-42) because these tissues have an even richer blood supply than bone tissue.

Early Stages of Repair.   In bone sections obtained one or two days post fracture, there is histological evidence that

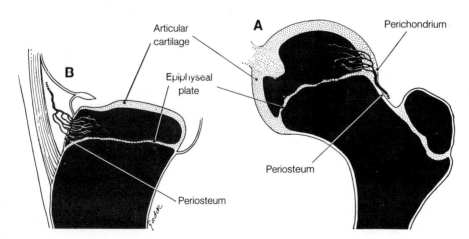

Articular
cartilage

A

Perichondrium

B

Epiphyseal
plate

Periosteum

Periosteum

Fig. 12-40. Diagram illustrating that where an epiphysis is entirely covered by articular cartilage (*A, right side*), its blood vessels must enter it by traversing the perichondrium at the periphery of the epiphyseal plate. This makes them vulnerable to rupture on epiphyseal displacement. In contrast, where an epiphysis is only partly covered by articular cartilage (*B, left side*), its blood vessels enter in such a way that separation could occur without serious damage to them. (Dale GG, Harris WR: J Bone Joint Surg 40-B:116, 1958)

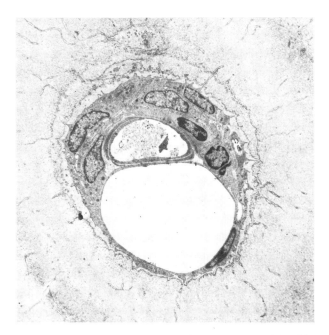

Fig. 12-41. Electron micrograph of a haversian canal lined by cells of the bone cell series. Some of these are osteogenic cells; others are differentiating into osteoblasts (note their cytoplasmic processes extending into canaliculi). An arteriole (*upper center*) and a venule (*center*) are also evident in the canal. (Courtesy of S. C. Luk and G. T. Simon)

an *acute inflammatory reaction* is underway. Early on, polymorphs appear in abundance. Later, macrophages are seen as well; their role is to complete the task of scavenging the extravasated blood cells, fibrin, and necrotic tissue. The blood clot is still recognizable (1) between the medullary cavities of the fragments and (2) between the broken ends of the bone (see Fig. 12-44). If the blood clot is extensive, it may manifest some degree of cellular invasion and vascularization, early signs that osteogenesis is about to commence at these two sites. Transition of the initial inflammatory phase of fracture repair into the ensuing reparative phase of this process is nevertheless generally heralded by *progressive removal* of the blood clot through phagocytosis. The events that follow are influenced both by the degree of vascularity at the fracture site and by the amount of free movement permitted there during healing. Much of the new bone tissue forms directly, but a variable amount can form indirectly through the process of endochondral ossification, as we shall now explain.

Fracture Repair Tissue Is Termed Callus.   Strong collars of repair tissue form both around and between the ends of the fragments. It is this repair tissue, termed *callus*, that first bridges the gap between the fragments and brings about their union. The callus that forms *around* the broken ends of the bone is variously known as the *external, periosteal*, or *anchoring callus*, whereas that forming *between* the bone fragments and constituting the bridge between

their respective medullary surfaces is called *internal callus* (see Fig. 12-46), sometimes also referred to as *medullary, endosteal*, or *bridging callus*.

The cellular origin of callus is well documented for rib fractures in experimental animals. Because such fractures are subjected repeatedly to respiratory movements, they develop larger quantities of callus than better stabilized fractures do. A short distance from each side of the fracture gap, the periosteum thickens markedly as a result of active proliferation of its osteogenic cells (Figs. 12-8 and 12-42), and endosteal cells also start showing signs of mitotic activity. Continued thickening of the periosteum leads to the formation of a cuff of osteogenic cells around each fragment (Figs. 12-43 and 12-44). Because the rate of proliferation of periosteal osteogenic cells exceeds the rate of accompanying growth of periosteal capillaries, only the cells in the deepest part of the external callus (*i.e.* nearest to the original outer surface of the bone fragment) are richly supplied with capillaries. Such osteogenic cells differentiate into osteoblasts that start laying down bone matrix on the outer surface of the fragment (Fig. 12-45). The new bony trabeculae they produce are firmly cemented to the matrix of the fragment, including sites where the preexisting bone tissue has died (Figs. 12-43 and 12-44). In the more superficial parts of the growing collar of callus tissue, however, osteogenic cells may differentiate in a virtually avascular environment, in which case they become chondroblasts that produce cartilage.

Thus cartilage can be present in the outer region of the collar (Fig. 12-43), particularly if callus is growing rapidly. Such cartilage formation is markedly increased when excessive local mobility occurs at the fracture site during healing. Indeed, the development of a great deal of external callus that contains a relatively high proportion of cartilage is considered to be the hallmark of instability at the fracture site. Provided that the damage done to the local blood supply and to the periosteum is not excessive, and provided that adequate stability is maintained throughout the healing period, a properly set fractured major long bone will not develop as much cartilage in its callus as a broken rib will.

At this stage, the external callus of a fractured rib exhibits the three zones depicted in Figures 12-43 and 12-44. Closest to each fragment lies a zone of new *bony trabeculae* that are cemented to the bone tissue. Then comes an intermediate *cartilaginous region* that merges superficially with a third and outermost zone that is made up of *proliferating osteogenic cells*. The three zones merge with one another, as can be seen in Figure 12-45. Proliferation and differentiation of the osteogenic cells and subsequent interstitial growth of the cartilage cause the two collars to enlarge and to grow toward each other so that they fuse (Figs. 12-43 and 12-44). Because the callus tissue that is responsible for external union of the fragments is peripheral in position, its strength is sufficient to stabilize an otherwise unstable fracture. Meanwhile, weaker internal union is effected within the medullary cavity through bridging of the fracture gap by newly formed bony trabeculae (Fig. 12-43). The healing fracture then appears as in Figure 12-46.

Whenever a surgical procedure becomes necessary to facilitate fracture repair, it is essential to keep as much of the periosteum as intact as possible to preserve its vascular connections with the bone tissue. Also, sufficient numbers of periosteal osteogenic cells should be conserved to ensure that adequate amounts of external

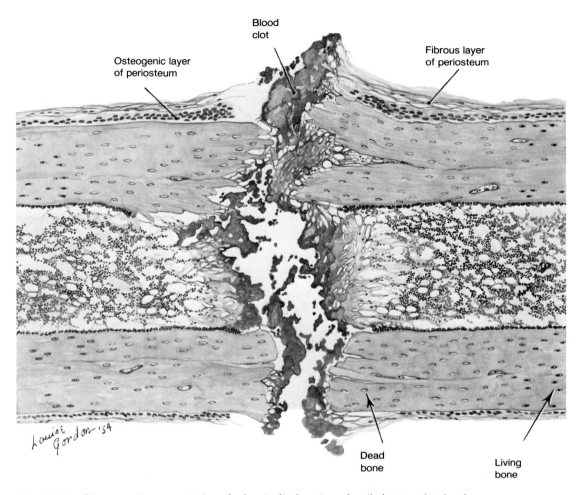

Blood
clot

Osteogenic layer
of periosteum

Fibrous layer
of periosteum

Dead
bone

Living
bone

Fig. 12-42. Diagrammatic representation of a longitudinal section of a rib fracture that has been healing for 2 days (rabbit). See text for explanation. (Ham AW, Harris WR: In Bourne GH (ed): The Biochemistry and Physiology of Bone, 2nd ed, Vol 3, p 338. New York, Academic Press, 1971)

callus will form. The contribution made by the external callus is particularly important in cases in which it becomes necessary to ream the medullary cavity and insert a tight-fitting intramedullary rod to maintain sufficient stability at the fracture site. Because such a procedure damages the endosteum and the osteogenic cells on trabecular surfaces, it hinders the formation of internal callus.

The Cartilage in Callus Becomes Replaced with Bone. As in the case of prenatal development of a long bone, cartilage formation in the external or internal callus is of only temporary significance because it all becomes replaced by bone through the process of endochondral ossification. The chondrocytes adjacent to the newly formed bone tissue hypertrophy and mature, resulting in calcification of the cartilage matrix in this region and its progressive replacement by bone. In a longitudinal section of a fracture site, the ossification fronts appear as a V-shaped line (Fig. 12-46). The advancing ossification fronts encroach on the wedge-shaped mass of cartilage, reducing the angle be-

tween them and culminating in total replacement of the cartilage with newly formed trabeculae of cancellous bone. Like the bony trabeculae on the diaphyseal border of an epiphyseal plate, these trabeculae exhibit occasional remnants of calcified cartilage in their cores. In due course, myeloid hematopoiesis begins in the spaces between the trabeculae as a result of seeding by circulating multipotential hematopoietic stem cells.

Bony Callus Is Remodeled. The first-formed bony trabeculae that bridge the fracture gap are cemented to dead bone tissue as well as to living bone (Fig. 12-43). However, this dead bone tissue is subsequently resorbed by osteoclasts that gain access to it from the soft tissue spaces between trabeculae. Due to coupling (which was described earlier in this chapter), removal of dead bone then paves the way for osteoblasts to move in and to replace almost all the dead bone with living bone.

At this stage, the callus is a spindle-shaped mass of cancellous bone that is made up of internal as well as external

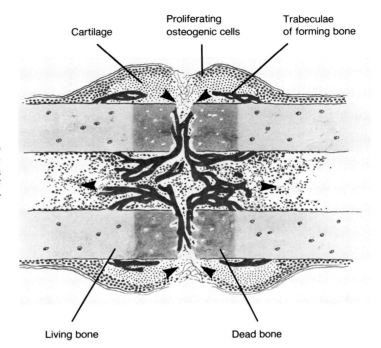

Cartilage — Proliferating osteogenic cells — Trabeculae of forming bone

Living bone — Dead bone

Fig. 12-43. Summary diagram of healing rib fracture. New cancellous bone is shown in black; cartilage is indicated in light stipple. Arrowheads indicate the direction of growth of trabeculae of new bone in the external and internal callus. For details, see text.

callus (Fig. 12-43). Due to its central position, the *internal callus* does not contribute much strength to the union, but it can participate substantially in the healing process. This callus arises from two sources. First, new bony trabeculae arise in the medullary cavity of each fragment from osteogenic cells of the endosteum and bone marrow. The trabeculae growing from each fragment interconnect with those growing from the other (Fig. 12-43). The second contribution to the internal callus is a similar group of new bony trabeculae that form between the broken ends of the bone (Fig. 12-43). A sufficient number of trabeculae of cancellous bone is formed in the internal callus to constitute a secure bridge between the apposed fragments. A substantial amount of internal bony callus is formed only if the medullary blood supply remains virtually intact. If relative displacement of the fragments disrupts this main blood supply, the formation of internal bony callus is delayed and the contribution made by the external callus becomes of major importance to the mechanics of repair.

Subsequent remodeling converts the newly formed cancellous bone tissue into dense cortical bone and thereby increases the strength of the bony union between the fragments. When the supplementary supporting trabeculae in the periphery of the callus are no longer required, they undergo resorption, and this reestablishes the original contours of the bone and renders the fracture site radiographically indistinguishable from the remainder of the bone.

Fracture Healing Is Slightly Different in Bones with a Thick Cortex. A bone that has a relatively thick cortex possesses so many osteons that the osteogenic cells lining its haversian canals (Fig. 12-41) can also contribute sub-

stantially to the healing process. If a fractured major long bone is treated without operation by means of a cast, external callus develops and the healing process commences in the manner described previously. The degree of development of this external callus increases with the amount of relative movement that is permitted between the fragments during healing. Capillaries and accompanying osteogenic cells subsequently grow out of the existing haversian canals and into the gap between the apposed fragments, where they then participate in forming the part of the internal callus that develops between the cortical regions of both fragments. The resulting stability of the fracture site increases with the width of the bone that was fractured.

When it becomes necessary to manage such a fracture by stable internal fixation, haversian canals constitute an even more important source of the repair tissue, as will be explained in the following section.

Fractures Also Exhibit the Capacity to Heal Directly Under Conditions of Stable Internal Fixation. In addition to being able to heal *indirectly* through the production of callus, bone fractures can undergo *direct* repair provided their fragments are accurately aligned and impacted on each other by means of a lag screw, an axial compression plate, or some other type of rigid internal fixation device. Following stable internal fixation, the fragments become united, with the formation of little or no external stabilizing callus. This direct type of union is promoted by stable fixation, not by compression itself. Its basis is described in the following paragraphs.

Interruption of the capillary circulation at the fracture site results in the death of osteocytes; hence initially, only dead bone is found

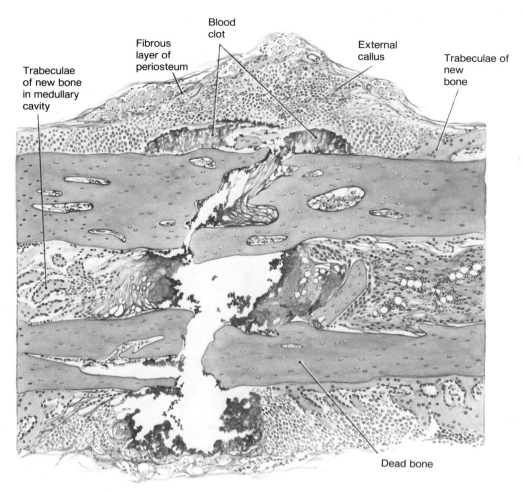

Fibrous layer of periosteum

Blood clot

External callus

Trabeculae of new bone

Trabeculae of new bone in medullary cavity

Dead bone

Fig. 12-44. Diagrammatic representation of a longitudinal section of a rib fracture that has been healing for 1 week (rabbit). For details, see text. (Ham AW, Harris WR: In Bourne GH (ed): The Biochemistry and Physiology of Bone, 2nd ed, Vol 3, p 338. New York, Academic Press, 1971)

on either side of the fracture line. However, capillary buds and accompanying osteogenic cells then begin to invade this dead bone from haversian canals of adjacent bone tissue that is still viable. Associated with the invading capillaries are osteoclasts that ream new *resorption tunnels* in the dead bone tissue, and following immediately behind the osteoclasts are osteoblasts that start building up *new osteons* within these tunnels. As a consequence of coupling, the dead bone becomes replaced by new bone as soon as it is resorbed; hence loss of cortical bone is minimal and compression between the fragments is maintained. The coupled processes of bone resorption and bone deposition advance slowly toward the fracture line, where, under favorable experimental conditions (*e.g.,* in the case of a straight saw cut), some of the newly forming osteons in each fragment begin to cross the fracture line and then extend into the other fragment, much as dowel pins can be used to join adjacent parts of a piece of wooden furniture. This is a relatively slow process that is essentially similar to ordinary remodeling of the shaft (*i.e.,* ongoing replacement of preexisting osteons by new ones). The only substantial differences are that (1) it is not quite so slow and (2) the tunneling is more directed toward the fracture line.

Yet with accidental fractures it is usually impossible to fit the broken ends of bones together with total accuracy. The closest possible apposition still leaves minute spaces between the fragments. Furthermore, new gaps continue to develop as the dead bone becomes resorbed. Capillaries and accompanying osteogenic cells continue to grow along resorption tunnels toward the fracture line, but before the fracture gap becomes effectively bridged by new osteons, each empty space fills in with bone, generally bone of the immature type. Hence the earliest bony union between the fragments, and in particular the bony union that occurs on the opposite side of the bone to an axial compression plate, is largely dependent on the deposition of *immature bone* that is relatively weak. Only after a month or so has elapsed do strong new osteons begin to peg the fragments securely together. Solid union is not achieved until the entire region of bone encompassing the fracture site has had an opportunity to become remodeled and multiple pegging has been accomplished across the dead bone tissue that borders on the fracture line. Compared with the indirect mechanism of healing, this is a slow process, taking at least a year to complete.

Much of the delay in such union is probably attributable to the relatively slow rate at which dead bone obtains a new blood supply

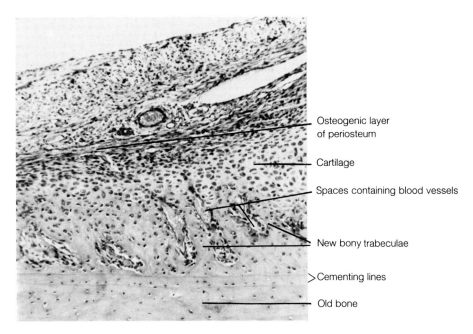

Fig. 12-45. Photomicrograph of the surface of a rib near a fracture that has been healing for 5 days (rabbit). Osteogenic cells have differentiated into osteoblasts that have formed bony trabeculae cemented to the bone. This region is vascular. Toward the right, the osteogenic cells have differentiated into chondroblasts that have formed a mass of avascular cartilage. (Ham AW, Harris WR: In Bourne GH (ed): The Biochemistry and Physiology of Bone, 2nd ed, Vol 3. New York, Academic Press, 1971)

under conditions of stable internal fixation. Furthermore, rigid plating may deprive the bone tissue in the immediate vicinity of the fracture of certain stresses and strains to which it is ordinarily subjected. Such bone exhibits an increased porosity because of rapid remodeling and resulting acquisition of many new haversian canals. However, it is not clear whether this extra porosity develops as a result of stress protection or whether it reflects a change in the local blood supply brought about by implantation of the fixation device. Although increased porosity might be expected to weaken the cortical bone in the vicinity of a stably fixed fracture, the incidence of refracture at such sites is low, provided the compression device is left in place until the fragments have become soundly united. Nevertheless, a substantial period must elapse before the *direct* (*primary*) type of cortical union obtained using stable internal fixation becomes as strong as the *indirect* (*secondary*) type of union achieved through callus formation.

BONE TRANSPLANTATION

Bone *grafts* (which are more often called *transplants*) are routinely employed in orthopedic procedures for two main purposes: (1) repairing fracture defects that otherwise would probably not heal properly and (2) filling in extensive regions of bone that have been destroyed through injury or disease. In addition, they can be used in reconstructive procedures and to bring about the bony fusion (*arthrodesis*) of a joint in the event that such a drastic measure becomes necessary. A bone transplant is described as *autogeneic* if

it is made to a different site on the *same* individual, and as *allogeneic* if it is made from one individual to *another*.

Autogeneic Bone Transplants (Autografts). Even though relatively few of the osteocytes in an *autogeneic* transplant of *compact bone* are able to survive the trauma of transplantation, the resulting dead bone tissue still serves a useful purpose because it gradually becomes *replaced by new bone.*

Cell death in an autogeneic transplant generally reflects inadequacy of the blood supply at its new site. However, in certain situations, it is now becoming possible to enhance the cellular viability of massive bone transplants by attaching the vessels that supply the transplant to vessels that supply the graft bed. Osteogenic cells of transplanted endosteum or periosteum have a better chance of survival than osteocytes do because of their close proximity to tissue fluid. Even so, the trabeculae of new bone that form are derived mainly from any periosteal, endosteal, or myeloid osteogenic cells of the *host bone* that are present at the graft site. Together with their associated capillaries, these linking trabeculae grow in toward the transplant and unite with it, thereby incorporating it into the graft bed. Initial incorporation of the transplant into the host bone is therefore due to these trabeculae of new bone becoming firmly cemented to the dead bone of the transplant. During the course of subsequent remodeling, the dead bone then becomes almost entirely replaced by new bone.

Fragments of *cancellous bone* that are suitable for autogeneic transplants are conveniently obtained from the crest of the ilium. Here again, only a few of the original osteo-

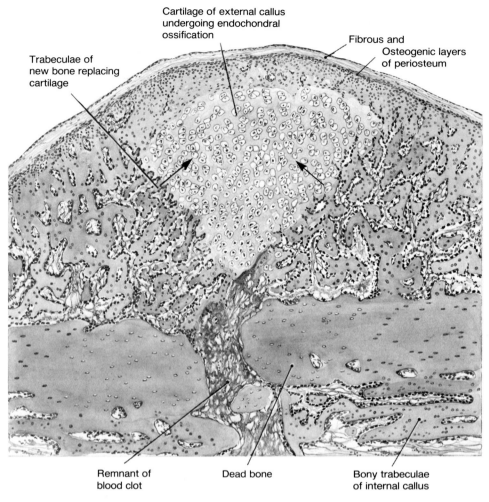

Cartilage of external callus
undergoing endochondral
ossification

Fibrous and
Osteogenic layers
of periosteum

Trabeculae of
new bone replacing
cartilage

Remnant of
blood clot

Dead bone

Bony trabeculae
of internal callus

Fig. 12-46. Diagrammatic representation of a longitudinal section of a rib fracture that has been healing for 2 weeks (rabbit). For explanation, see text. (Ham AW, Harris WR: In Bourne GH (ed): The Biochemistry and Physiology of Bone, 2nd ed, Vol 3, p 338. New York, Academic Press, 1971)

cytes in such transplants survive, but there are enough osteogenic cells on the extensive surfaces of cancellous bone to ensure the rapid deposition of new bone tissue in a vascular environment. Hence autogeneic cancellous bone fragments are routinely employed whenever there is a need to set up new foci of osteogenesis.

Allogenic Bone Transplants (Allografts). The long-term value of an *allogeneic* transplant of *compact bone* is its intrinsic ability to *elicit new bone formation* at the site of transplantation. In other words, it possesses the latent capacity to induce a *bone morphogenetic response* on the part of the host at the site of the transplant. Such *induced osteogenesis* is believed to be elicited by the content of bone morphogenetic protein (BMP) in the matrix of the transplant. In due course, the transplanted piece of foreign bone tissue becomes entirely replaced with new bone tissue that is produced by the host.

Allografts of compact bone are less frequently used than autografts because they can elicit a cell-mediated immune response, but the success rate is still high. To minimize the immune response, the transplant can be pretreated to remove the donor cells and their remains. Even so, it still seems to elicit graft rejection responses that can block the valuable osteoinductive potential of the bone transplant. Hence in situations in which a bone defect is not too extensive, an autograft is considered preferable whenever technically feasible.

If fragments of allogeneic *cancellous bone* are used as transplants, the osteogenic cells on their extensive surfaces proliferate and give rise to progeny that differentiate and that may even start to deposit some new bone matrix. Nevertheless, the ensuing immune response elicited by the foreign histocompatibility antigens on the donor's cells then destroys all the cells in the transplant, and host-derived osteoclasts invade the transplant and eventually dispose of it entirely. Because this procedure results in nothing that is of any value, the earlier practice of employing allogeneic cancellous bone fragments for bone transplantation has largely been discontinued.

SELECTED REFERENCES

Prenatal Bone Development

BERNARD GW, PEASE DC: An electron microscope study of initial intramembranous osteogenesis. Am J Anat 125:271, 1969

GARDNER E: Osteogenesis in the human embryo and fetus. In Bourne GH (ed): The Biochemistry and Physiology of Bone, 2nd ed, Vol 3, p 77. New York, Academic Press, 1971

HALL BK: Cellular differentiation in skeletal tissues. Biol Rev 45: 455, 1970

HALL BK: Histogenesis and morphogenesis of bone. Clin Orthop 71:249, 1971

HUNTER SJ, CAPLAN AI: Control of cartilage differentiation. In Hall BK (ed): Cartilage, Vol 2, p 87. New York, Academic Press, 1983

OGDEN JA: Chondro-osseous development and growth. In Urist MR (ed): Fundamental and Clinical Bone Physiology, p 108. Philadelphia, JB Lippincott, 1980

Osteogenic (Osteoprogenitor) Cells, Bone Induction, Osteoblasts, and Osteocytes

BASSETT CAL, HERRMANN I: Influence of oxygen concentration and mechanical factors on differentiation of connective tissues in vitro. Nature 190:460, 1961

BÜRING K: On the origin of cells in heterotopic bone formation. Clin Orthop 110:293, 1975

HALL BK: Cellular differentiation in skeletal tissues. Biol Rev 45: 455, 1970

HOLTROP ME: The ultrastructure of bone. Ann Clin Lab Sci 5:264, 1975

HOLTROP ME, WEINGER JM: Ultrastructural evidence for a transport system in bone. In Talmage RV, Munson PL (eds): Calcium, Parathyroid Hormone and the Calcitonins, p 365. Amsterdam, Excerpta Medica, 1970

MATTHEWS JL: Bone structure and ultrastructure. In Urist MR (ed): Fundamental and Clinical Bone Physiology, p 4. Philadelphia, JB Lippincott, 1980

OWEN M: Cellular dynamics of bone. In Bourne GH (ed): The Biochemistry and Physiology of Bone, 2nd ed, Vol 3, p 271. New York, Academic Press, 1971

OWEN M: The origin of bone cells. Int Rev Cytol 28:213, 1970

PRITCHARD JJ: The osteoblast. In Bourne GH (ed): The Biochemistry and Physiology of Bone, 2nd ed, Vol 1, p 21. New York, Academic Press, 1972

REDDI AH, ANDERSON WA: Collagenous bone matrix induced endochondral ossification and hemopoiesis. J Cell Biol 69:557, 1976

TONNA EA, PENTEL LP: Chondrogenic cell formation via osteogenic cell progeny transformation. Lab Invest 27:418, 1972

URIST MR: Heterotopic bone formation. In Urist MR (ed): Fundamental and Clinical Bone Physiology, p 369. Philadelphia, JB Lippincott, 1980

URIST MR, HUDAK RT, HUO YK, RASMUSSEN JK: Osteoporosis: A bone morphogenetic protein autoimmune disorder. In Dixon AD, Sarnat BG (eds): Normal and Abnormal Bone Growth: Basic and Clinical Research. p 77. New York, Alan R Liss, 1985

Bone Matrix and Calcification

ALI SY: Calcification of cartilage. In Hall BK (ed): Cartilage, Vol 1, p 343. New York, Academic Press, 1983

ANDERSON HC: Matrix vesicles of cartilage and bone. In Bourne GH (ed): The Biochemistry and Physiology of Bone, 2nd ed, Vol 4, p 135. New York, Academic Press, 1976

ARSENAULT AL, OTTENSMEYER FP: Quantitative spatial distributions of calcium, phosphorus, and sulfur in calcifying epiphysis by high resolution electron spectroscopic imaging. Proc Natl Acad Sci USA 80:1322, 1983

ARSENAULT AL, OTTENSMEYER FP: Visualization of early intramembranous ossification by electron microscopic and spectroscopic imaging. J Cell Biol 98:911, 1984

BONUCCI E: The origin of matrix vesicles and their role in the calcification of cartilage and bone. In Schweiger HG (ed): International Cell Biology 1980–1981, p 993. Berlin, Springer-Verlag, 1981

BONUCCI E: The structural basis of calcification. In Ruggeri A, Motta PM (eds): Ultrastructure of the Connective Tissue Matrix, p 165. Boston, Martinus Nijhoff, 1984

HUNTER GK, HEERSCHE JNM, AUBIN JE: Proteoglycan synthesis and deposition in fetal rat bone. Biochemistry 23:1572, 1984

LEBLOND CP, WEINSTOCK M: Radioautographic studies of bone formation. In Bourne GH (ed): The Biochemistry and Physiology of Bone, 2nd ed, Vol 3, p 181. New York, Academic Press, 1971

OWEN M, TRIFFITT JT: Extravascular albumin in bone tissue. J Physiol 257:293, 1976

POOLE AR, PIDOUX I, REINER A ET AL: Association of an extracellular protein (chondrocalcin) with the calcification of cartilage in endochondral bone formation. J Cell Biol 98:54, 1984

RUSSELL RGG, FLEISCH H: Pyrophosphate and diphosphonates. In Bourne GH (ed): The Biochemistry and Physiology of Bone, 2nd ed, Vol 4, p 61. New York, Academic Press, 1976

TRIFFITT JT: The organic matrix of bone tissue. In Urist MR (eds): Fundamental and Clinical Bone Physiology, p 45. Philadelphia, JB Lippincott, 1980

VEIS A: Bones and teeth. In Piez KA, Reddi AH (eds): Extracellular Matrix Biochemistry, p 329. New York, Elsevier, 1984

Osteoclasts and Bone Resorption

ANDERSON RE, SCHRAER H, GAY CV: Ultrastructural immunocytochemical localization of carbonic anhydrase in normal and calcitonin-treated chick osteoclasts. Anat Rec 204:9, 1982

BONUCCI E: New knowledge on the origin, function and fate of osteoclasts. Clin Orthop 158:252, 1981

CHAMBERS TJ: The cellular basis of bone resorption. Clin Orthop 151:283, 1980

COCCIA PF, KRIVIT W, CERVENKA J ET AL: Successful bone-marrow transplantation for infantile malignant osteopetrosis. N Engl J Med 302:701, 1980

DOTY SB, SCHOFIELD BH: Electron microscopic localization of hydrolytic enzymes in osteoclasts. Histochem J 4:245, 1972

GAY CV, ITO MB, SCHRAER H: Carbonic anhydrase activity in isolated osteoclasts. Metab Bone Dis Relat Res 5:33, 1983

GÖTHLIN G, ERICSSON JLE: The osteoclast. Clin Orthop 120:201, 1976

HEERSCHE JNM: Mechanism of osteoclastic bone resorption: A new hypothesis. Calcif Tissue Int 26:81, 1978

HOLTROP ME, KING GJ: The ultrastructure of the osteoclast and its functional implications. Clin Orthop 123:177, 1977

HOLTROP ME, KING GJ, COX KA, REIT B: Time-related changes in the ultrastructure of osteoclasts after injection of parathyroid hormone in young rats. Calcif Tissue Int 27:129, 1979

IBBOTSON KJ, D'SOUZA SM, KANIS JA ET AL: Physiological and pharmacological regulation of bone resorption. Metab Bone Dis Relat Res 2:177, 1980

JOTEREAU FV, LE DOUARIN NM: The developmental relationship between osteocytes and osteoclasts: A study using the quail-chick nuclear marker in endochondral ossification. Dev Biol 63:253, 1978

KAHN AJ, SIMMONS DJ: Investigation of cell lineages in bone using a chimaera of chick and quail embryonic tissue. Nature 258:325, 1975

KALLIO DM, GARANT PR, MINKIN C: Evidence of coated membranes in the ruffled border of the osteoclast. J Ultrastruct Res 37:169, 1971

KALLIO DM, GARANT PR, MINKIN C: Ultrastructural effects of calcitonin on osteoclasts in tissue culture. J Ultrastruct Res 39:305, 1972

KING GJ, HOLTROP ME, RAISZ LG: The relation of ultrastructural changes in osteoclasts to resorption in bone cultures stimulated with parathyroid hormone. Metab Bone Dis Relat Res 1:67, 1978

MARKS SC: The origin of osteoclasts: Evidence, clinical implications and investigative challenges of an extra-skeletal source. J Pathol 12:226, 1983

NEWBREY J, TRUITT S: Osteoclast formation in deer antler. Anat Rec 208:126A, 1984

SORELL M, KAPOOR N, KIRKPATRICK D ET AL: Marrow transplantation for juvenile osteopetrosis. Am J Med 70:1280, 1981

TEN CATE AR, DEPORTER DA, FEEEMAN E: The role of fibroblasts in the remodeling of periodontal ligament during physiologic tooth movement. Am J Orthodont 69:155, 1976

WALKER DG: Bone resorption restored in osteopetrotic mice by transplants of normal bone marrow and spleen cells. Science 190:784, 1975

WALKER DG: Experimental osteopetrosis. Clin Orthop 97:158, 1973

WALKER DG: Spleen cells transmit osteopetrosis in mice. Science 190:785, 1975

Systemic Regulation of Blood Calcium Levels

BÉLANGER LF: Osteocytic osteolysis. Calcif Tissue Res 4:1, 1969

BÉLANGER LF: Osteocytic resorption. In Bourne GH (ed): The Biochemistry and Physiology of Bone, 2nd ed, Vol 3, p 240. New York, Academic Press, 1971

DELUCA HF: Metabolism of actions of vitamin D—1982. In Peck WA (ed): Bone and Mineral Research Annual, 1, p 7. Amsterdam, Excerpta Medica, 1983

JANDE SS, BÉLANGER JF: The life-cycle of the osteocyte. Clin Orthop 94:281, 1973

RAO LG, HEERSCHE JNM, MARCHUK LL, STURTRIDGE W: Immunohistochemical demonstration of calcitonin binding to specific cell types in fixed rat bone tissue. Endocrinology 108:1972, 1981

RAO LG, MURRAY TM, HEERSCHE JNM: Immunohistochemical demonstration of parathyroid hormone binding to specific cell types in fixed rat bone tissue. Endocrinology 113:805, 1983

RODAN GA, MARTIN TJ: Role of osteoblasts in hormonal control of bone resorption—a hypothesis. Calcif Tissue Int 33:349, 1981

TALMAGE RE: The physiological significance of calcitonin. In Peck WA (ed): Bone and Mineral Research Annual, 1, p 74. Amsterdam, Excerpta Medica, 1983

Nutritional, Metabolic, and Coupling Factors in Bone Growth and Remodeling

BAYLINK FJ, LIU CC: The regulation of endosteal bone volume. J Periodontol 50(special issue):43, 1979

DIXON AD, SARNAT BG (eds): Factors and Mechanisms Influencing Bone Growth. Progress in Clinical and Biological Research, Vol 101. New York, Alan R Liss, 1982

DRIVDAHL RH, HOWARD GA, BAYLINK DJ: Extracts of bone contain a potent regulator of bone formation. Biochim Biophys Acta 714:26, 1982

FROST HM: Tetracycline-based histological analysis of bone remodelling. Calcif Tissue Res 3:211, 1969

HARRIS WR, HAM AW: The mechanism of nutrition in bone and how it affects its structure, repair and transplantation. In Ciba Foundation Symposium on Bone Structure and Metabolism, p 135. London, J & A Churchill, 1956

HARRIS WH, HEANEY RP: Skeletal renewal and metabolic bone disease. N Engl J Med 280:193, 303; 1969

HOWARD GA, BOTTEMILLER BL, TURNER RT ET AL: Parathyroid hormone stimulates bone formation and resorption in organ culture: Evidence for a coupling mechanism. Proc Natl Acad Sci USA 78:3204, 1981

HUNZIKER EB, HERRMANN W, SCHENK RK ET AL: Cartilage ultrastructure after high pressure freezing, freeze substitution, and low temperature embedding. I. Chondrocyte ultrastructure—Implications for the theories of mineralization and vascular invasion. J Cell Biol 98:267, 1984

JOWSEY J, GORDAN G: Bone turnover and osteoporosis. In Bourne GH (ed): The Biochemistry and Physiology of Bone, 2nd ed, Vol 3, p 202. New York, Academic Press, 1971

JOWSEY J, RIGGS BL: Assessment of bone turnover by microradiography and autoradiography. Semin Nucl Med 2:3, 1972

RASMUSSEN H, BORDIER P: The cellular basis of metabolic bone disease. N Engl J Med 289:25, 1973

RASMUSSEN H, BORDIER P: The Physiological and Cellular Basis of Metabolic Bone Disease, Baltimore, Williams & Wilkins, 1974

TAM CS, HEERSCHE JNM, MURRAY TM, PARSONS JA: Parathyroid hormone stimulates the bone apposition rate independently of its resorptive action: Differential effects of intermittent and continuous administration. Endocrinology 110:506, 1982

URIST MR, DELANGE RJ, FINERMAN GAM: Bone cell differentiation and growth factors. Science 220:680, 1983

Blood Supply of Bones

BROOKES M: The Blood Supply of Bone. An Approach to Bone Biology. London, Butterworths, 1971

COHEN J, HARRIS WH: The three-dimensional anatomy of haversian systems. J Bone Joint Surg 49-A:419, 1958

DALE GG, HARRIS WR: Prognosis of epiphyseal separation. J Bone Joint Surg 40-B:116, 1958

IRVING MH: The blood supply of the growth cartilage in young rats. J Anat 98:631, 1964

RHINELANDER FW: Circulation of Bone. In Bourne GH (ed): The

Biochemistry and Physiology of Bone, 2nd ed, Vol 2, p 1. New York, Academic Press, 1972

SALTER RB, HARRIS WR: Injuries involving the epiphyseal plate. J Bone Joint Surg 45-A:587, 1963

Repair and Transplantation of Bone

BYERS PD, GRAY JC, MOSTAFA AGSA, ALI SY: The healing of bone and articular cartilage. In Glynn LE (ed): Tissue Repair and Regeneration. Handbook of Inflammation, Vol 3, p 343. Amsterdam, Elsevier North-Holland, 1981

CHALMERS J: Bone transplantation. Symp on Tissue and Organ Transplantation. J Clin Pathol (Suppl) 20:540, 1967

CRELIN ES, WHITE AA, PANJABI MM, SOUTHWICK W: Microscopic changes in fractured rabbit tibias. Conn Med 42:561, 1978

HAM AW: An histologic study of the early phases of bone repair. J Bone Joint Surg 12:827, 1930

HAM AW, HARRIS WR: Repair and transplantation of bone. In Bourne GH (ed): The Biochemistry and Physiology of Bone, 2nd ed, Vol 3, pp 338 and 379. New York, Academic Press, 1971

OWEN R, GOODFELLOW J, BULLOUGH P (eds): Scientific Foundations of Orthopaedics and Traumatology. London, William Heinemann Medical Books, 1980

SEVITT S: Bone Repair and Fracture Healing in Man. Edinburgh. Churchill Livingstone, 1981

SEVITT S: Healing of fractures in man. In Owen R, Goodfellow J, Bullough P (eds): Scientific Foundations of Orthopaedics and Traumatology, p 258. London, William Heinemann Medical Books, 1980

SIMMONS DJ: Fracture healing. In Urist MR (ed): Fundamental and Clinical Bone Physiology, p 283. Philadelphia, JB Lippincott, 1980

URIST MR: Bone transplants and implants. In Urist MR (ed): Fundamental and Clinical Bone Physiology, p 331. Philadelphia, JB Lippincott, 1980

13

Joints

Because joint afflictions probably represent the single most common cause of disability seen by physicians, medical students should make every effort to become thoroughly familiar with all relevant aspects of joint structure and function.

The words *articulation* (L. *articulatio,* junction between bones) and *joint* (L. *junctio,* joining or connection) are used as synonyms to describe a structural arrangement that connects two or more bones to each other at their sites of contact. Whereas many joints permit free *movement* between the bones they connect, such movement is not essential for a connecting structure to be termed a *joint;* indeed, some joints become as solid as the bones that they connect. Another important function of certain joints is that they facilitate *growth* of the bones that they interconnect.

Because the most common joint problems encountered in medical practice involve either synovial joints or symphyses, these two types of joints will be dealt with first.

SYNOVIAL JOINTS

Free movement between the bones that meet at a *synovial joint* is facilitated because the gliding surfaces are efficiently lubricated. Because the lubricant in such a joint (represented in *black* in Fig. 13-1) is viscous and clear like the white of an egg, it is called *synovial fluid* (Gr. *syn,* together; L. *ovum,* egg), hence the term *synovial joint.* Furthermore, to minimize friction, the gliding surfaces are quite smooth and shiny because the articulating ends of the bones are capped with hyaline cartilage. This cartilage *is not covered by a perichondrium.* Hence the surfaces that glide over each other consist of naked uncalcified matrix of *articular cartilage* (cross-striped in Fig. 13-1).

At the boundary of the joint, there is a tough *joint capsule* that merges with the periosteum of the bones meeting at the joint (Fig. 13-1). The capsule is lined by a more delicate connective tissue layer called the *synovial membrane* (Fig. 13-1) that produces and resorbs synovial fluid, as will be described later in this chapter.

Synovial Joint Development. From Chapter 12 it will be recalled that during the early stages of development of a long bone, embryonic mesenchymal cells at the site where the bone is about to form begin to condense and differentiate into chondroblasts that produce a cartilage model of the bone (see Endochondral Ossification in Chap. 12). Between the apposed ends of such developing cartilage models, the mesenchyme condenses and forms an *articular disk* (*primitive joint plate*). Meanwhile, the mesenchyme forming the side walls of the developing joint progressively delineates the future joint capsule. This lateral layer of mesenchyme gives rise to a connective tissue sleeve that surrounds the articulating ends of the cartilage models, initially merging with

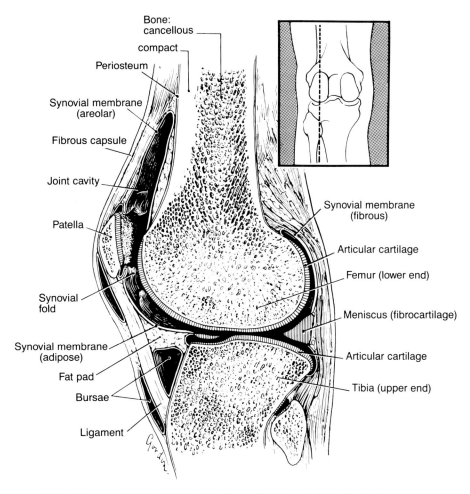

Fig. 13-1. Diagram of a knee joint, cut in the sagittal plane indicated in the inset.

their perichondrium but then becoming attached to periosteum after the models ossify.

As development proceeds, fluid-filled spaces form between the cells of the articular disk. These spaces then coalesce and a continuous *synovial cavity* is established in the central part of the disk. The formation of this cavity enables the ends of the two cartilage models to come into contact and to articulate with each other. Differentiation also continues in the developing joint capsule. Its outer layer gives rise to dense fibrous tissue that becomes the stronger and thicker part of the joint capsule, and its thin inner layer becomes the synovial membrane.

Articular Cartilages

Articular cartilages are unique in that they present a smooth and almost perfectly even (matte) surface of *naked cartilage matrix*. Their cells represent descendants of the chondrocytes that were present in the cartilage model of the bone. In postnatal life these cartilages are required to keep on growing until the epiphyses reach their adult size. However, they cannot grow by apposition because they lack a peri-

chondrium; hence all their growth is interstitial. It depends on proliferation of the chondrocytes that lie just under the articular surface.

Deeper down in the cartilage, the chondrocytes are arranged in longitudinal columns that are oriented perpendicular to the surface, and for the most part, they are longitudinally disposed in cell nests (Fig. 13-2). They assume this arrangement because the majority of the collagen fibrils in the deeper part of articular cartilage matrix have a perpendicular orientation with respect to the articular surface. Near to this surface, however, the fibrils arch over and run parallel with the surface. Hence the arrangement of cell nests in an articular cartilage is determined by the predominant orientation of its collagen fibrils, as in an epiphyseal plate where the chondrocytes become similarly arranged in longitudinal columns. Furthermore, the proliferation that is responsible for generating such cell nests during growth of this cartilage is limited to the superficial zone near the articular surface. Farther down the columns, the chondrocytes undergo hypertrophy.

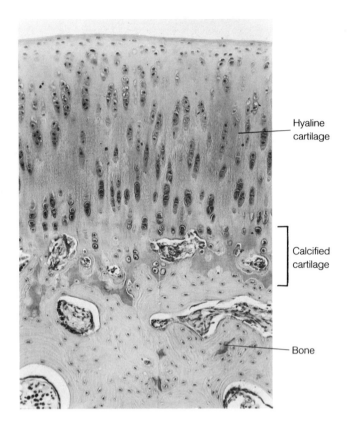

Hyaline
cartilage

Calcified
cartilage

Bone

Fig. 13-2. Photomicrograph of articular cartilage and subchondral bone (knee joint of rabbit). The articular cartilage consists of three ill-defined zones. In the superficial zone, the chondrocytes are small and flattened. In the middle zone, the cells are arranged in columns lying perpendicular to the surface. Both the superficial and the middle zones are typical hyaline cartilage. The deep zone consists of calcified cartilage and contains small chondrocytes. (Courtesy of R. Salter and E. Bogoch)

The deepest part of an articular cartilage is darker staining and *calcified* (Fig. 13-2). During postnatal growth, this part of the cartilage becomes progressively replaced by bone as the diaphyseal side of an epiphyseal plate does. However, in this case, replacement is less regular. Compared with the calcified cartilage to which it is attached, the underlying bone tissue is somewhat lighter staining (Fig. 13-2). Interlocking with the undersurface of the calcified cartilage, it constitutes a plate of *subchondral bone* that supports the articular cartilage. The superficial zone of the subchondral bone is fairly compact, but some of the canals and soft tissue spaces remain rather wide (Fig. 13-2).

The chondrocytes of articular cartilage remain capable of secreting further quantities of matrix constituents throughout life, but they do not normally divide. Hence renewed matrix production seems to be the only mechanism by which articular cartilage can compensate for everyday wear and tear. This limitation is borne out by estimates of the proportion of chondrocytes to matrix, which indicate that the relative number of cells in articular cartilage diminishes with age. More will be said about factors that influence matrix deposition later in this chapter.

The Chondrocytes in Articular Cartilage Obtain Nourishment from Synovial Fluid. As already emphasized in the preceding chapters, cartilage is an avascular tissue; hence nutrients and oxygen have to reach the chondrocytes in articular cartilages by diffusion from outside sources.

Furthermore, the deepest part of an articular cartilage is so heavily calcified that it is doubtful whether much nourishment or oxygen could reach its chondrocytes by diffusion from the vessels in subchondral bone tissue. The *main source of nourishment* for its cells is therefore the *film of synovial fluid* that covers its free surface. Nutrients and oxygen pass into this fluid by diffusion from capillaries that are situated near the inner surface of the synovial membrane. Additional nourishment may also reach the chondrocytes in the periphery of the articular cartilage by direct diffusion from capillaries in the synovial membrane.

Two lines of evidence support the conclusion that synovial fluid serves as the primary source of nourishment for the articular cartilages. First, detached fragments of articular cartilage that are floating as nonvascularized loose bodies in the synovial cavity remain viable and sometimes show evidence of growth. Second, an epiphyseal separation that disrupts all blood supply to an epiphysis does not result in death of the chondrocytes in its articular cartilage. Until the epiphysis becomes revascularized following its surgical reattachment to the diaphysis, the chondrocytes are obliged to obtain all the nourishment they need from the synovial fluid.

Articular Cartilage Matrix. The organic composition of this matrix has already been described under Cartilage Matrix in Chapter 11. The diameter of its type II collagen fibrils varies according to where they lie in relation to the chondrocytes that produced them. Thus the narrow zone of matrix that lines the lacunae, described as a *pericellular*

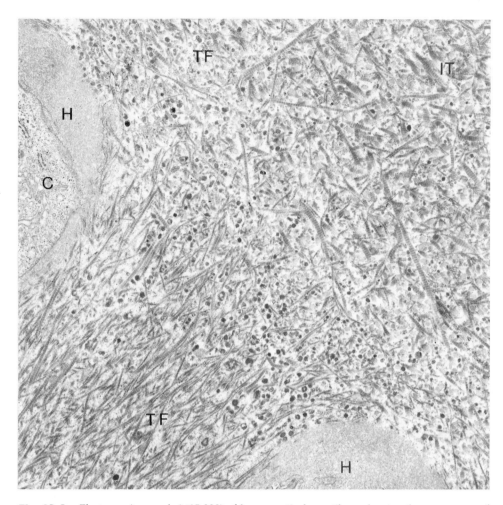

Fig. 13-3. Electron micrograph (×15,000) of human articular cartilage, showing the appearance of collagen fibrils in its matrix. At upper left, part of a chondrocyte (C) can be seen in its lacuna. Surrounding each chondrocyte is a relatively homogeneous-looking region termed a pericellular halo (*H*) containing extremely fine collagen fibrils (only 4 nm to 10 nm in diameter). External to this (*lower left*), fibrils of the territorial zone are seen; these are labeled TF. They are oriented circumferentially around the lacunae. At upper right, the wide mature fibrils (30 nm to 200 nm in diameter) characteristic of the interterritorial matrix (*IT*) have a random arrangement. (Lane JM, Weiss C: Review of articular cartilage collagen research. Arthritis Rheum 18:553, 1975)

halo (labeled *H* in Fig. 13-3) because it appears so pale in the electron microscope (EM), contains collagen fibrils that are extremely fine. A little farther away from the cell, the collagen fibrils are slightly wider and they are arranged circumferentially around the lacuna. These fibrils (labeled *TF* in Fig. 13-3) characterize the so-called *territorial matrix*. The regions of matrix that lie between the zones of territorial matrix constitute the *interterritorial matrix* (labeled *IT* in Fig. 13-3). Here the collagen fibrils are randomly arranged, and they are substantial enough for their cross-banding to be seen (Fig. 13-3).

The main reason why articular cartilage has been studied in considerable detail is that sooner or later it begins to show signs of degeneration, as will now be described.

Aging or Injury Can Lead to the Development of Degenerative Changes in Articular Cartilage. Also described as *degenerative arthritis*, the condition *osteoarthritis* generally affects the weight-bearing synovial joints of most people by the time they reach old age. It is considered pathological when it is premature in onset or clinically severe. This condition is characterized by a unique combination of degenerative and proliferative changes in the articular cartilage. For example, in the central part of the articular surface, collagen fibrils of the cartilage matrix may become exposed in such a way that they resemble the pile of a carpet. Such microscopic signs of degeneration are described as the *fibrillation* of articular cartilage. The proliferative changes that are also characteristic of osteoarthritis are manifested around the periphery of the cartilage, in particular at attachment sites of tendons, ligaments, or the synovial membrane. Here the cartilage develops to excess and subsequently becomes replaced by bone, with the result that bony spurs known as *osteophytes* form a rim at the periphery of the cartilage and protrude from the joint margins. It has been suggested that such formation of bony outgrowths may be a compensatory measure that progressively "stabilizes" the joint by limiting its mobility.

Degenerative arthritis can also develop in younger patients (1) when the stress applied to part of a joint surface has increased because of altered joint alignment resulting from trauma, or (2) when there is a marked degree of congenital malalignment in the joint. Furthermore, it can develop as a complication of the management of intra-articular fractures or other types of joint injuries. Clinically, this can present quite a problem because under ordinary circumstances, articular cartilage manifests a disappointingly poor capacity for effective healing and regeneration. Hence it has become somewhat of a challenge to find a suitable way of managing intra-articular fractures or damaged articular cartilages that will promote their effective repair and at the same time reduce the associated risk of developing degenerative arthritis. An innovative way of dealing with this problem is described in the following section.

How Can Effective Repair of Damaged Articular Cartilage Be Promoted?

Until fairly recently, prospects for the satisfactory repair of damaged articular cartilages were not very encouraging. Their remarkably poor capacity for effective restoration seemed to be attributable to a general disinclination on the part of their chondrocytes to undergo mitosis in adult life. The most that could be hoped for was an ineffective and barely detectable mitotic response in chondrocytes situated close to the defect, a response that was too minimal to result in significant deposition of new matrix and resulting repair. Yet it was found that if an intra-articular fracture involved the underlying subchondral bone tissue as well as the articular cartilage, a defect of this nature would fill in with loose connective tissue or a mixture of poorly differentiated cartilage and loose connective tissue. However, the repair process that ensues under such circumstances is an outcome of the damage sustained by the subchondral bone tissue; it is not achieved through proliferation of the preexisting chondrocytes. Under ordinary conditions of healing, the callus tissue that develops at the site of a healing intra-articular fracture extends along the fracture gap and then proceeds to fill in any defect in the articular cartilage. As a result, the cartilage defect generally becomes filled in with a mixture of poorly differentiated cartilage (sometimes regrettably referred to in the literature as "fibrocartilage"), regenerating subchondral bone, and loose connective or fibrous tissue. The callus tissue (cartilage and bone) is generated by osteogenic cells as described in connection with fracture healing in Chapter 12, and the accompanying fibrous tissue arises from pericytes and fibroblasts. Such a heterogeneous and disorganized mass of repair tissues fails to provide the smooth gliding surfaces needed for articular cartilage. Furthermore, it is poorly adapted to withstand the stresses that result from normal joint function, so this type of repair tissue degenerates prematurely, leading to the development of an arthritic joint.

We have already pointed out some features of synovial joints that facilitate their movement. A keen awareness of the importance of joint movement in facilitating the nutrition of articular cartilage has led to the proposal that healing of damaged articular cartilage would be enhanced by gentle passive motion of the joint during healing, as opposed to keeping the joint at rest in order for it to heal (Salter). It is well established that local mobility at the site of a fracture will promote the formation of cartilage during repair. When excessive, such local mobility can even lead to the development of a *pseudarthrosis*, a false joint in which so much cartilage is formed between the broken ends of the bone that it allows free movement to occur between them. Moreover, it seems likely that a certain amount of joint movement would be necessary to ensure continual replenishment of the film of synovial fluid, the main source from which the articular cartilages obtain their nutrients and oxygen.

Continuous Passive Motion Promotes the Regeneration of Articular Cartilage. Nearly 20 years ago, a strong conviction that gentle continuous passive motion would enhance the effective healing of damaged articular cartilage led Salter to abandon the hitherto long-accepted practice of total joint immobilization following joint injury. Instead, he and his research associates decided to administer a course of *continuous passive motion* to promote healing and regeneration of the damaged articular tissues. Encouraged by the results they obtained over the years using experimental rabbits, they are now applying this new approach to the clinical management of certain disorders and injuries of synovial joints in man (Salter et al).

Unlike *active* joint motion, which is intermittent and voluntary, continuous *passive* motion is uninterrupted and does not require any voluntary effort. A mechanical device does the work of skeletal muscles that would otherwise fatigue, and it also enables the individual to get a customary amount of sleep. When continuous passive motion is applied to rabbits with an experimentally induced intra-articular fracture or a small drill-hole extending down into the subchondral bone tissue of a knee joint, it encourages healing of the cartilage defect by repair tissue that is virtually indistinguishable from hyaline cartilage (Figs. 13-4*B* and *C*, and 13-5*B*).

If instead of having their joints submitted to continuous *passive* motion, the animals are simply allowed to resume normal cage activity (intermittent *active* motion), there are noticeably fewer instances in which hyaline cartilage develops as the repair tissue and a substantially higher incidence of degenerative arthritis ensuing as a complication. A complete absence of joint motion (*Immobilization*) predisposes the animals to the development of joint adhesions as well as fibrous scarring of the defect (Figs. 13-4*A* and 13-5*A*) and degenerative arthritis in the joint.

The cells most likely to give rise to the reparative cartilage filling in the drill hole seen on the right of Figure 13-4*C* are uncommitted mesenchyme-derived cells from the bone marrow spaces in the subchondral bone tissue (visible under the articular cartilage in this illustration). The combination of continuous passive motion and a relatively avascular environment is evidently conducive to the differentiation of such cells into chondrocytes. Furthermore, the

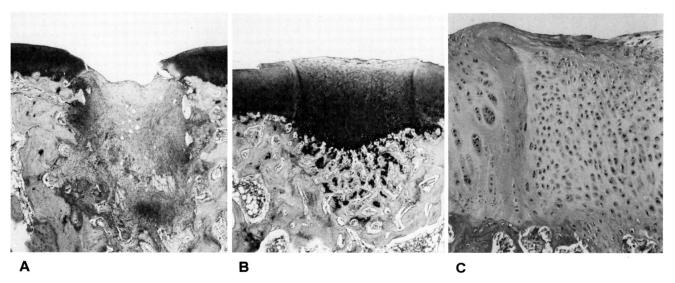

A   B   C

Fig. 13-4. Low-power photomicrographs (*A* and *B* stained with toluidine blue; *C,* H & E), showing articular cartilage in a rabbit knee joint healing under different conditions. The defect was created by drilling a hole through the cartilage into the subchondral bone. (*A*) Healing obtained after 3 weeks if the joint is immobilized. Note inadequate healing of the defect with loose connective tissue. (*B*) Healing obtained after 3 weeks of continuous passive motion. The defect has become filled with newly formed hyaline cartilage. (*C*) Cartilaginous repair after 3 weeks of continuous passive motion. The reparative tissue is entirely cartilaginous. (*A* and *B,* courtesy of R. Salter and E. Bogoch; *C,* courtesy of R. Salter, D. Simmonds, B. Malcolm, and E. Rumble)

chondrocytes synthesize cartilage matrix constituents in amounts that are sufficient to repair small defects that are approximately 1 mm in diameter. Thus it would seem that reparative cartilage can arise from uncommitted pluripotential mesenchyme-derived cells that are derived from the underlying subchondral bone tissue and its associated marrow. Another reason for believing that repair depends on such uncommitted mesenchymal progenitor cells coming from the subchondral bone tissue is that even under conditions of continuous passive motion, partial-thickness cartilage defects situated above subchondral bone tissue that remains intact show little or no evidence of repair. It also seems safe to conclude that preexisting chondrocytes of mature articular cartilage do not make any significant contribution to the repair process.

When an experimentally-induced intra-articular fracture is managed by open reduction and stable internal fixation (by means of a screwnail) and this procedure is followed by a course of continuous passive motion, healing of the fracture within the cartilage is remarkably good (Fig. 13-5*B*). On the other hand, if the joint is immobilized, loose connective tissue grows into the fracture gap from below and fills it with fibrous tissue (Fig. 13-5*A*). These findings have been interpreted as indicating that in the case of stably fixed intra-articular fractures, continuous passive motion promotes effective healing of articular cartilage by augmenting the secretion of organic matrix constituents such as proteoglycan, and furthermore that such additional matrix production can result in sufficient interstitial growth of cartilage on both sides of the fracture line to close up the fracture gap. Another possibility is that under the influence of continuous passive motion, new chondroblasts might also arise from uncommitted mesenchymal cells that are associated with the subchondral bone tissue.

The results of these experimental studies indicate that during

early postfracture healing, continuous passive motion is able to exert beneficial effects that promote the satisfactory restoration of articular cartilage. Perhaps the most useful attribute of continuous passive motion is that it increases the chances that a full-thickness articular cartilage defect will become replaced with *hyaline cartilage.* An encouraging finding is that in rabbits, the resulting cartilaginous repair tissue stands up to at least a year of routine weight-bearing and normal cage activity without manifesting signs of deterioration. Furthermore, postoperative continuous passive motion considerably reduces the risk of developing postoperative degenerative arthritis.

Strategies Are Now Being Developed to Repair Major Osteochondral Defects. Provided a full-thickness defect in articular cartilage is not very large, sufficient ingrowth of uncommitted mesenchymal cells from the subchondral bone tissue occurs to enable the defect to heal satisfactorily under the stimulus of continuous passive motion. However, the healing of an extensive defect is both qualitatively and quantitatively inferior. In most clinical situations, the entire joint has to be replaced with a suitable prosthesis—an "artificial joint replacement." Joint prostheses nevertheless have a regrettable tendency to become loose and to cause pain, particularly in young patients. A better alternative would be a surgical approach that takes full advantage of the chondrogenic properties of the bipotential "osteochondrogenic" cells in the osteogenic layer of the periosteum. We should explain that the stem cells of bone (*osteogenic* or *osteoprogenitor cells*) are often described as "osteochondrogenic" cells to emphasize the fact that they also possess *chondrogenic,* and not just *osteogenic,* potential. At this point, we also need to introduce the term *cambium layer,* which means the *osteogenic layer* of the periosteum.

Whereas in a vascular environment the cambium layer of the

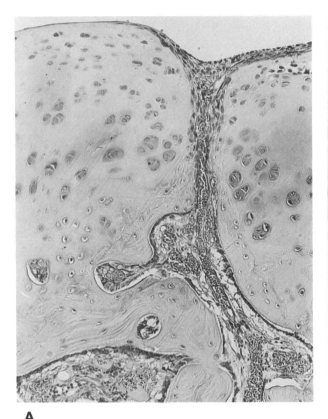
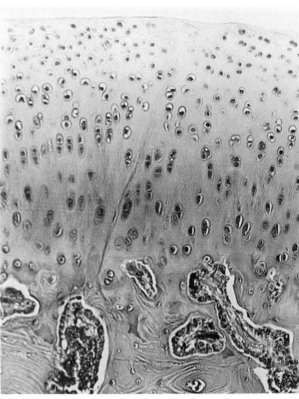

A   **B**

Fig. 13-5. Photomicrographs (safranin O stain) showing experimentally induced fracture site of lateral condyle of a rabbit femur healing under different conditions. (*A*) Healing obtained after 4 weeks of immobilization. The gap in the cartilage has become invaded from below by loose connective tissue. (*B*) Healing obtained after 4 weeks of continuous passive motion. The gap in the cartilage has closed, apparently without any new tissue invading it from below. (Courtesy of R. Salter and D. Harris)

periosteum gives rise to bone, in an avascular environment, it tends to produce cartilage. Such new cartilage formation is termed *periosteal neochondrogenesis* (Gr. *neos,* new). Experimental studies by O'Driscoll and Salter have revealed that it may be feasible to resurface relatively large osteochondral defects by using (1) free periosteal autografts or (2) osteoperiosteal autografts that are made up of bone and periosteum, provided that the joint is also managed postoperatively with a course of continuous passive motion. Nonvascularized autografts of periosteum alone, transplanted as loose bodies into knee joints of rabbits, have been found to manifest a capacity for neochondrogenesis. To investigate the suitability of osteoperiosteal grafts (disks of cortical bone covered with periosteum and transplanted as a combined graft), full-thickness defects, 3.5 mm in diameter, were created in the articular cartilage of rabbit knee joints (Fig. 13-6*A*). A disk of cortical bone, enclosed in a piece of periosteum that was oriented with its deep (cambium) layer facing outward, was then pressed into the defect (Fig. 13-6*B*). This procedure brought the cambium layer of the periosteum into direct contact with the edges of the defect and also exposed the cambium layer on the free (articulating) surface of the joint (Fig. 13-6*B*). In almost every case, the bipotential "osteochondrogenic" cells in the covering layer of the graft produced enough cartilage under the stimulus of continuous passive motion to bond the graft edges to the graft bed (Fig. 13-7*A*). Meanwhile,

on the articulating surface, "osteochondrogenic" cells produced pearly white tissue that was histologically indistinguishable from hyaline cartilage (Fig. 13-7*B*). Furthermore, as the bony component of the graft gradually became incorporated into the subchondral bone, it secured the graft in its graft bed and helped to restore the lost bone tissue (Fig. 13-7*A*).

Recent additional experimental studies by O'Driscoll and Salter indicate that it is also feasible to resurface an extensively denuded joint surface with cartilage by covering it with a large free periosteal autograft, oriented with its cambium layer next to the denuded surface, and then submitting the joint to postoperative continuous passive motion. This procedure leads to successful restoration of the surface with biochemically and histologically normal articular cartilage.

Now that we have discussed articular cartilage and some interesting new developments regarding its repair, we shall briefly consider the remaining parts of a synovial joint.

Joint Capsule, and Ligament and Tendon Insertions

The *joint capsule* consists of an outer fibrous layer called the *fibrous capsule* and an inner layer called the *synovial*

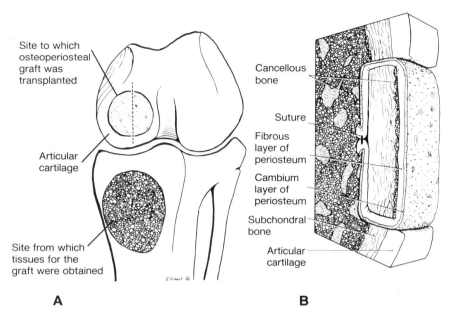

Fig. 13-6. Diagrams illustrating the experimental procedure adopted for osteoperiosteal grafting into a full-thickness articular cartilage defect. (*A*) Knee joint of a rabbit, showing the site where a full-thickness defect was created in the articular cartilage and also the tibial site from which bone tissue and periosteum were obtained to construct an osteoperiosteal graft. (*B*) Osteoperiosteal graft positioned within this defect, showing the orientation of its components. (O'Driscoll SW, Salter RB: Clin Orthop 208:131, 1986)

membrane (Fig. 13-1). The *fibrous capsule* is continuous with the fibrous layer of periosteum of the bones meeting at the joint (Fig. 13-1). It is composed of sheets of collagen fibers that extend from the periosteum of one bone to the periosteum of the other. Because it is inelastic, it contributes to the stability of the joint. When gaps are present in the fibrous capsule, the synovial membrane adheres to other tissues bordering on the joint.

The *ligaments* of the joint are cordlike thickenings of the fibrous capsule. Some of them are incorporated into the capsule whereas others are separated from it by *bursae* formed by outpouchings of the synovial membrane (Fig. 13-1). Near their attachments to cartilage, both ligaments and tendons generally undergo a transition into *fibrocartilage* (Fig. 13-8*A*). Where their bundles of collagen fibers are attached to bone, these are anchored in the bone tissue as typical *Sharpey's fibers* (Fig. 13-8*B*).

Synovium, Menisci, Blood Supply, and Afferent Innervation

The *synovial membrane* (*synovium*) lines the joint cavity everywhere except for the articular cartilages (Fig. 13-1). Its smooth and glistening inner surface is raised into *synovial folds* and *villi* (Fig. 13-1). It is abundantly provided with blood vessels, nerves, and lymphatics. The *synovial cells* (*synovocytes*) in this membrane tend to be concentrated along its inner border, often giving the impression of a

continuous cellular membrane. However, careful observation shows that along its inner border, these cells lie *among* rather than *on* collagen fibers; hence these fibers are also present on the inner surface of the membrane. For this reason, the synovial membrane is classified as a connective tissue membrane but not as an epithelial membrane.

The lining layer that contains these synovial cells can lie directly on the fibrous capsule, or it can be attached to it by a layer of loose connective tissue (areolar tissue) or adipose tissue (Fig. 13-1). Accordingly, three morphological subtypes of synovial membrane can be distinguished: *fibrous, areolar,* and *adipose.*

The *fibrous* type of synovial membrane is present over ligaments and tendons and in other regions in which the synovial membrane is subjected to pressure (Fig. 13-1). As illustrated in parts 1 and A of Figure 13-9, some of the surface cells are widely separated from one another, and in the light microscope, they look like underlying fibroblasts. The *areolar* type of synovial membrane is present at sites where the membrane has to move freely with respect to the fibrous capsule as it does, for example, in the suprapatellar pouch of the knee joint (Fig. 13-1). Here the synovial cells are arranged in three or four layers (parts 2 and B of Fig. 13-9), enmeshed in collagen fibers of the underlying areolar tissue. Elastic fibers are also present in this type of lining to keep its various projections from becoming pinched between the articular cartilages. The *adipose* type of synovial membrane covers the intra-articular fat pads (Fig. 13-1). Its synovial cells are generally arranged

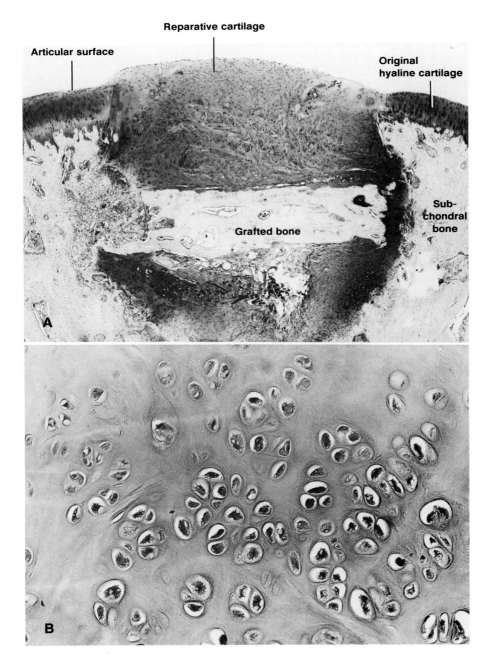

Reparative cartilage

Articular surface

Original hyaline cartilage

Grafted bone

Sub-chondral bone

A

B

Fig. 13-7. (*A*) Photomicrograph showing the type of repair tissue that was obtained during healing of a full-thickness articular cartilage defect in a rabbit's knee joint (safranin O). The defect was filled with an osteoperiosteal graft as depicted in Figure 13-6, after which the joint was submitted to a course of continuous passive motion. (*B*) High-power photomicrograph of the type of reparative tissue seen in *A* in the region superficial to the grafted bone tissue (safranin O). The chondrocytes present in cell nests and their surrounding hyaline matrix closely resemble those of articular cartilage. For further details, see text. (O'Driscoll SW, Salter RB: Clin Orthop 208:131, 1986)

as a single layer that appears to cover the adipose tissue (parts 3 and C of Fig. 13-9), but they are, in fact, enmeshed in collagen fibers as they are in the other types of synovial membrane.

In the EM, synovial cells exhibit two distinct appearances. Most of them (*type A cells*) resemble macrophages in that they possess a prominent Golgi complex and many lysosomes and show evidence of endocytosis. Other cells (*type B cells*) are more like fibroblasts because they have a very prominent rough-surfaced endoplasmic reticulum; these cells are believed to be the source of the hyaluronic acid and glycoprotein lubricant in synovial fluid. Intermediate

Fibrocartilage of
tendon insertion

Ligament insertion

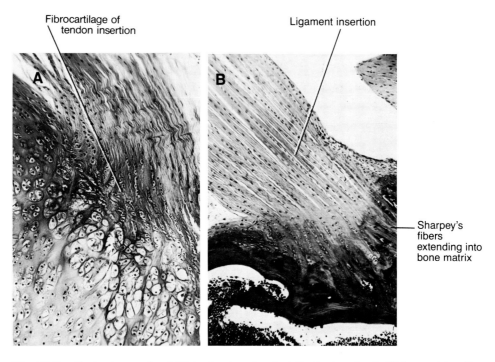

Sharpey's
fibers
extending into
bone matrix

Fig. 13-8. Photomicrographs of (*A*) tendon insertion (patellar tendon of rat), (*B*) ligament insertion (anterior cruciate ligament of rat).

cells (*type C cells*) have also been described, so it is possible that A and B cells are not really different cell types.

In contrast to the articular cartilages, the synovial membrane is capable of rapid and complete regeneration, which is helpful to know because synovial tissue must sometimes be removed during joint surgery.

Synovial Fluid. The slightly yellowish viscous fluid in the synovial cavity is essentially a plasma dialysate that contains hyaluronic acid and a lubricating glycoprotein that seems to be either attached to hyaluronic acid molecules or held in place by them. The plasma dialysate is produced by an extensive capillary plexus that is situated close to the inner surface of the synovial membrane, and the constituents concerned with lubrication are produced by the type B synovial cells. Under normal conditions, synovial fluid contains only a small number of suspended cells (less than 100 cells per cubic millimeter) over half of which are monocytes. The remainder include lymphocytes, macrophages, and a small proportion (less than 10%) of neutrophils.

Macromolecular constituents are able to leave the synovial cavity by way of lymphatic capillaries in the synovial membrane. Any particulate matter that enters the synovial fluid is engulfed by its macrophages.

Intra-articular Menisci. These cushions of fibrocartilage (Fig. 13-1) can have a free inner border (as in the knee joint), or they can traverse the joint, thereby dividing it into two separate synovial cavities (as in the sternoclavicular joint). Menisci of the knee joint sometimes tear as a result of an injury and may require surgical removal. Following such excision of a meniscus, a new one may grow in from the fibrous capsule. This is an almost exact replica of a meniscus except that it is made of dense fibrous tissue instead of fibrocartilage.

Blood Supply. Synovial joints have a relatively rich blood supply. The arterial branches approaching a joint commonly supply three structures: one branch goes to the epiphysis, another to the joint capsule, and the third to the synovial membrane. Arteriovenous anastomoses are also present in joints, but their significance is uncertain.

The synovial membrane has an abundance of capillaries that approach its inner surface very closely. As a consequence, extravasated blood can enter the synovial fluid from a relatively minor joint injury.

Afferent Innervation. Although the articular cartilages contain no nerve endings, the joint capsule and its associated structures are provided with several different types of afferent (sensory) endings. Those of the joint capsule itself are mostly of the Ruffini type, which will be described in Chapter 17. The afferent endings in tendons will be described in Chapter 15. Small myelinated afferent fibers also terminate in free endings in the joint capsule and ligaments; these fibers are involved in the sense of pain. The synovial membrane contains relatively few free afferent

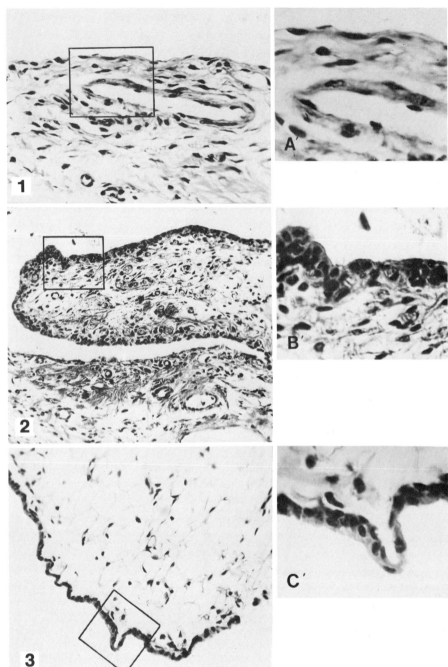

Fig. 13-9. Photomicrographs of the three subtypes of synovial membrane (rat). (*1*) Low-power and (*A*) high-power view of fibrous type. (*2* and *B*) Similar views of areolar type. (*3* and *C*) Similar views of adipose type.

endings and is correspondingly less sensitive to pain. Most kinds of joint pain are poorly localized.

SYMPHYSES

A *symphysis* is a slightly moveable type of joint in which bones are connected by a combination of hyaline cartilage and fibrocartilage. At the beginning of this chapter, we noted that there are two types of joints that commonly require medical attention. The second type is the *anterior intervertebral joint*, which represents a modified type of symphysis. Here the bodies of adjacent vertebrae are held together by structures known as intervertebral disks that have a regrettable tendency to degenerate, and problems resulting from their degeneration are a common cause of recurrent low back pain, as we shall now explain.

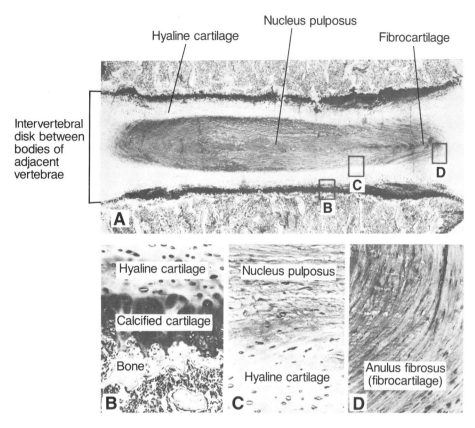

Fig. 13-10. Photomicrographs of representative regions of an intervertebral disk (young child). (*A*) Low power; (*B, C,* and *D*) medium-power views of the areas indicated in *A*.

Intervertebral Disks

In the course of vertebrate evolution, the notochord became replaced by bony vertebrae, the bodies of which are joined together by *intervertebral disks*. The structure of these joints is illustrated in Figures 13-10 and 13-11. Parts A and B of Figure 13-10 show the covering of *hyaline cartilage* on the body of each vertebra (part of one vertebra is seen at the *top* and part of another vertebra is seen at the *bottom* of Fig. 13-10*A*). The side of the cartilage that borders on the bone tissue is calcified (Fig. 13-10*B*). Interconnecting the cartilaginous coverings of the vertebrae are the *intervertebral disks.* In Figure 13-10*A*, a darkly stained, flattened oval region can be distinguished in the middle of such a disk. This region is filled with a soft gelatinous matrix described as the *nucleus pulposus* (Figs. 13-10*C* and 13-11*A*). The periphery of the disk, on the other hand, is a strong ringlike collar of fibrocartilage termed the *anulus fibrosus* (Figs. 13-10*D* and 13-11*A*). The nucleus pulposus is believed to be the evolutionary heritage of the notochord, which is the primitive axial supporting structure of vertebrates. The organic constituents of this matrix are essentially similar to those of hyaline cartilage. Like cartilage, the central part of the nucleus pulposus and the innermost layers of the

anulus fibrosus (both of which are loaded in compression) contain mainly type II collagen. However, the peripheral part of the nucleus pulposus and the bulk of the anulus fibrosus (both of which are loaded in tension) contain mainly type I collagen, the type found in tendons and bone.

This unique combination of the incompressible gelatinous nucleus pulposus and the inextensible anulus fibrosus at its periphery provides a cushion between adjacent vertebral bodies that permits slight movement between them.

Under Undue Strain, Intervertebral Disks Are Inclined to Rupture. Intervertebral disks, like articular cartilages, are susceptible to degenerative changes as part of the aging process. For example, tiny fissures can develop between the collagen fibers in the anulus fibrosus. Such fissures constitute weak spots through which the soft nucleus pulposus is inclined to rupture (*herniate*). Herniation generally occurs posterolaterally or posteriorly, and it is quite common in the lumbar region where the anulus fibrosus is thinnest. Any extruded matrix trapped in the vicinity of the spinal nerve roots can imbibe sufficient tissue fluid for the matrix to swell and compress the spinal nerve roots. Moreover, the herniation commonly elicits an acute inflammatory reaction and the resulting edema can also

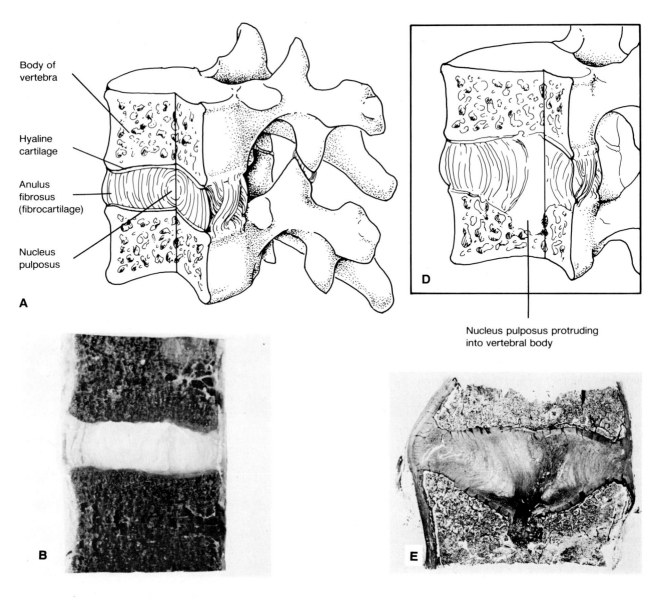

Body of
vertebra

Hyaline
cartilage

Anulus
fibrosus
(fibrocartilage)

Nucleus
pulposus

A

D

Nucleus pulposus protruding
into vertebral body

B

E

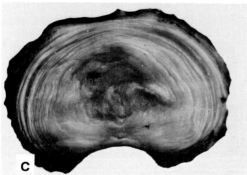

C

Fig. 13-11. (*A*) Diagrammatic representation of an intervertebral disk. (*B*) Photomicrograph of a vertical section through the bodies of two vertebrae and the intervertebral disk between them (very low power). The fibers of the anulus fibrosus can just be discerned near the periphery of the disk; the pale middle is the nucleus pulposus. (*C*) Photomicrograph of a horizontal section of an intervertebral disk (very low power). Concentrically arranged fibers of the anulus fibrosus can be seen in the periphery; the darker central region is the nucleus pulposus. (*D*) Diagrammatic representation of an intervertebral disk that has herniated into the marrow of the vertebral body below. (*E*) Photomicrograph of a vertical section of an intervertebral disk that has herniated into the marrow of the vertebral body below (very low power). (*B, C,* and *E,* courtesy of W. Donohue).

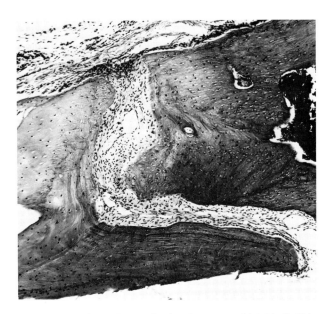

Fig. 13-12. Photomicrograph of parietotemporal joint (rat). This is an example of a suture (syndesmosis).

compress these nerves, causing pain. This condition is known as a *ruptured* or *prolapsed disk*, a misnomer for which is "slipped disk."

If, on the other hand, an intervertebral disk herniates axially through the cartilage that borders on it, the extruded matrix enters the marrow of a vertebral body instead (Fig. 13-11*D* and *E*). Such a protrusion is called a *Schmorl's node*, and it seldom presents any problem.

Degenerative changes, primarily proteoglycan degradation, also occur in the nucleus pulposus. Such degeneration is accompanied by a gradual decline in the fluid content of the nucleus pulposus that is manifested as a decrease in the turgor and thickness of the intervertebral disks and a correspondingly reduced risk of disk herniation in the elderly.

SYNDESMOSES

Syndesmoses are joints in which bones are held together by bands of dense fibrous tissue (Gr. *syn*, together; *desmos*, band or bond). Joints of this type facilitate growth of the flat bones that constitute the vault of the skull. As explained under Intramembranous Ossification in Chapter 12, the persistence of *cranial sutures* between these bones enables their margins to grow by apposition (see Fig. 12-6). Such growth results in reduction in width of the connective tissue between the edges of adjacent bones until it is only a narrow band that holds the bones together (Fig. 13-12). Hence a cranial suture is a syndesmosis. Osteogenic cells capable of proliferating and differentiating into osteoblasts nevertheless persist within the suture, and new bone continues

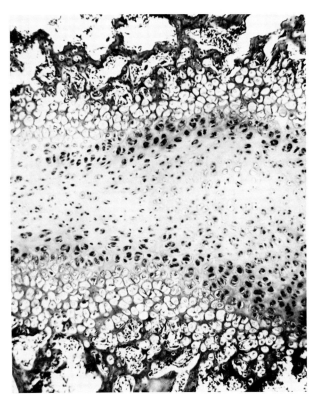

Fig. 13-13. Photomicrograph of basisphenoid joint (rat). The cartilage is being replaced by bone on both sides.

to be added to the margins of these bones by apposition. At the end of skeletal growth, the flexible fibrous joints become replaced by rigid bony joints called *synostoses*, and the individual cranial bones thereby become cemented together into a single caselike structure.

Suture lines generally present an irregularly serrated or interlocking toothlike appearance, and in cross section, the course that many of them take appears irregular or oblique (Fig. 13-12). An isolated ossicle called a *Wormian bone* is occasionally formed in a suture if a small group of osteoblasts or bone spicule becomes detached during bone growth.

SYNCHONDROSES

During skeletal growth, the cartilaginous growth plates of a long bone represent *synchondroses* (*i.e.*, joints in which bones are interconnected by *cartilage*), because they connect the bony epiphyses derived from the secondary centers of ossification to the bony diaphysis derived from the primary center of ossification. In these epiphyseal plates, bone growth occurs on the diaphyseal side of the plate. However, the synchondrosis between the basioccipital and basisphenoid bones facilitates growth of both these bones; hence it has the cross-sectional appearance of a "double-sided" epiphyseal plate (Fig. 13-13).

SYNOSTOSES

When skeletal growth is over, most syndesmoses and synchondroses become *synostoses* (*i.e.*, joints in which bones have become cemented to each other). Hence the main role of syndesmoses and synchondroses is to facilitate bone *growth* rather than *movement*. When pathological conditions make the movement of a synovial joint undesirable, it sometimes becomes necessary to convert it into a synostosis surgically.

SELECTED REFERENCES*

Joint Structure

ADAMS P, EYRE DR, MUIR H: Biochemical aspects of development and ageing of human lumbar intervertebral disc. Rheumatol Rehab 16:22, 1977

BARNETT CH, DAVIES DV, MACCONAILL MA: Synovial Joints. London, Longman, Green & Co, 1961

BRADFORD FK, SPURLING RG: The Intervertebral Disc. Springfield, IL, Charles C Thomas, 1941

GARDNER E: The anatomy of the joints. Instruc Lect Am Acad Orthop Surg Vol 9. Ann Arbor, Edwards, 1952

GARDNER E: Blood and nerve supply of joints. Stanford Med Bull 11:203, 1953

MCDEVITT CA: The proteoglycans of cartilage and the intervertebral disk in ageing and osteoarthritis. In Glynn LE (ed): Tissue Repair and Regeneration. Handbook of Inflammation, Vol 3, p 111. Amsterdam, Elsevier/North-Holland Biomedical Press, 1981

SOKOLOFF L (ed): The Joints and Synovial Fluid. New York, Academic Press, 1978

Articular Cartilage

ALBRIGHT JA, MISRA RP: Mechanisms of resorption and remodeling of cartilage. In Hall BK (ed): Cartilage, Vol 3, p 49. New York, Academic Press, 1983

BYERS PD, GRAY JC, MOSTAFA AGSA, ALI SY: The healing of bone and articular cartilage. In Glynn LE (ed): Tissue Repair and Regeneration. Handbook of Inflammation, Vol 3, p 343. Amsterdam, Elsevier/North-Holland Biomedical Press, 1981

CONVERY FR, AKESON WH, KEOWN GH: The repair of large osteochondral defects. Clin Orthop 82:253, 1982

GREENWALD AS: A pathway for nutrients from the medullary cavity to the articular cartilage of the human femoral head. J Bone Joint Surg 51-B:797, 1969

---

* For additional references on Cartilage, see Selected References, Chapter 11.

HJERTQUIST S, LEMPERG R: Histological, autoradiographic and microchemical studies of spontaneously healing osteochondral articular defects in adult rabbits. Calcif Tissue Int 8:54, 1971

HONNER R, THOMPSON RC: The nutritional pathways of articular cartilage. J Bone Joint Surg 53-A:4, 1971

LANE JM, WEISS C: Review of articular cartilage collagen research. Arthritis Rheum 18:553, 1975

MANKIN HJ: The reaction of articular cartilage to injury and osteoarthritis. Part I. N Engl J Med 291:1285, 1974; and Part II, 291:1355, 1974

O'DRISCOLL SW, SALTER RB: The induction of neochondrogenesis in free intra-articular periosteal autografts under the influence of continuous passive motion. An experimental investigation in the rabbit. J Bone Joint Surg 66-A:1248, 1984

O'DRISCOLL SW, SALTER RB: The repair of major osteochondral defects in joint surfaces by neochondrogenesis with autogenous osteoperiosteal grafts stimulated by continuous passive motion: An experimental investigation in the rabbit. Clin Orthop 208:131, 1986

RODNAN GP, SCHUMACHER HR, ZVAIFLER NJ (eds): Primer on the Rheumatic Diseases, 8th ed, p 16. Atlanta Arthritis Foundation, 1983

ROSENBERG L: Structure of cartilage proteoglycans. In Burleigh PMC, Poole AR (eds): Dynamics of Connective Tissue Macromolecules, p 105. Amsterdam, North-Holland, 1975

SALTER RB: Motion vs. rest: Why immobilize joints?—Presidential Address. Can Orthop Assoc, Halifax, June 1981. J Bone Joint Surg 64B:251, 1982

SALTER RB, HAMILTON HW, WEDGE JH ET AL: The clinical application of basic research on continuous passive motion (CPM) for disorders and injuries of synovial joints: A preliminary reporty. J Orthop Res 1:325, 1983

SALTER RB, HARRIS DJ, CLEMENTS ND: The healing of bone and cartilage in transarticular fractures with continuous passive motion. Orthop Trans 2:77, 1978

SALTER RB, OGILVIE–HARRIS DJ: Healing of intra-articular fractures with continuous passive motion. In American Academy of Orthopaedic Surgeons Instructional Course Lectures, Vol 28, p 102, St Louis, CV Mosby, 1979

SALTER RB, SIMMONDS DF, MALCOLM BW ET AL: The biological effect of continuous passive motion on the healing of full-thickness defects in articular cartilage. J Bone Joint Surg 62-A:1232, 1980

SERAFINI–FRACASSINI A, SMITH JW: The Structure and Biochemistry of Cartilage. Edinburgh, Churchill-Livingstone, 1974

SHEPARD N, MITCHELL N: The localization of articular cartilage proteoglycan by electron microscopy. Anat Rec 187:463, 1977

SKOOG T, JOHANSSON SH: The formation of articular cartilage from free periochondrial grafts. Plast Reconstr Surg 57:1, 1976

SKOOG T, OHLSEN L, SOHN A: Perichondrial potential for cartilaginous regeneration. Scand J Plast Reconstr Surg 6:123, 1972

SOKOLOFF L: Aging and degenerative diseases affecting cartilage. In Hall BK (ed): Cartilage, Vol 3, p 109. New York, Academic Press, 1983

14

Nervous Tissue and the Nervous System

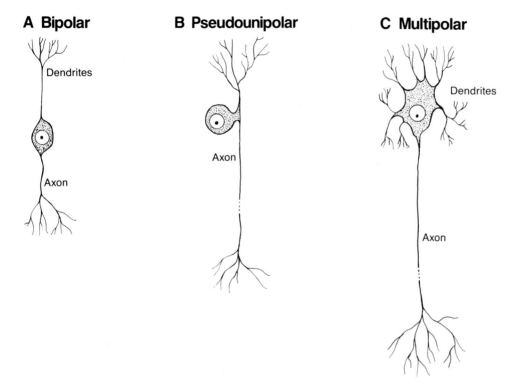

A Bipolar   **B Pseudounipolar**   **C Multipolar**

Fig. 14-1. Diagram showing the three main classes of neurons classified on the basis of their cell shape.

The general organization and distribution of *nervous tissue,* the third basic tissue, are to a large extent determined by its course of evolution. It therefore makes sense to consider the organization of nervous tissue in relation to the evolution of the *nervous system.* We shall begin with a brief description of the two major subdivisions of the nervous system.

THE ORGANIZATION OF NERVOUS TISSUE

The axial part of the nervous system, called the *central nervous system* (CNS), lies deep inside the body, surrounded and protected by bone. It consists of the *brain,* which is encased by the skull, and the *spinal cord,* which extends down the vertebral canal to a position between the first and second lumbar vertebrae.

The other broad division of the nervous system, the *peripheral nervous system* (PNS), is represented primarily by cordlike *nerves* that emerge bilaterally from the brain and spinal cord. Those that emerge from the brain pass through small canals (*foramina*) in the skull; they are termed the *cranial nerves.* Those that emerge from the spinal cord do so by way of the intervertebral foramina and are called the *spinal nerves.*

Parts of the Neuron.   The structural and functional unit of the nervous system is, of course, the nerve cell or *neuron* (Gr. for nerve). A unique feature of neurons is that they possess delicate cytoplasmic processes called *nerve fibers,* some of which approach approximately 1 m in length. The number of nerve fibers that neurons possess provides a structural basis for their classification. Those with only one process are termed *unipolar* neurons, those with two, *bipolar* neurons (Fig. 14-1A), and those with more than two, *multipolar* neurons (Fig. 14-1C). Unipolar neurons are relatively rare, and multipolar ones are very common in nervous tissue.

A neuron thus has two characteristic features. First, it has a *cell body.* This consists of its nucleus and generally a large amount of cytoplasm that encloses the nucleus and is therefore sometimes called the *perikaryon* (Gr. *peri,* around; *karyon,* nut or nucleus). It houses most of the organelles that maintain the structural and functional integrity of the *nerve fibers* extending from it; the latter constitute the second characteristic feature of a neuron.

It is important to realize that neurons do not divide. Furthermore, from shortly after birth, new ones do not develop from precursor cells.

Neurons have one (and only one) process known as an *axon* (Gr. for axle or axis), probably so called because the axon tends to be straight. Thus only one of the two fibers of a bipolar neuron and one of the many fibers of a mul-

Posterior

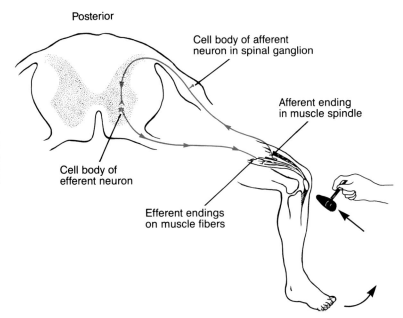

Cell body of afferent
neuron in spinal ganglion

Afferent ending
in muscle spindle

Cell body of
efferent neuron

Efferent endings
on muscle fibers

Fig. 14-2. Schematic diagram of the stretch reflex, a simple monosynaptic reflex requiring only two neurons. The first, which is afferent, has its cell body in a spinal ganglion. The second, which is efferent, is an anterior horn cell of the spinal cord (lower motor neuron).

tipolar neuron is an axon (Fig. 14-1). The other fiber of a bipolar neuron and all the remaining ones of a multipolar neuron are called *dendrites* (Gr. *dendron,* tree) because they branch like trees (Fig. 14-1).

Nerve impulses are propagated by a neuron along the axon to its destination, whereas impulses received by dendrites are transmitted toward the cell body. So in general, the axon propagates impulses away from the cell body and dendrites transmit impulses toward it. (There are, however, exceptions to this general rule in that certain fibers that are considered to be axons because of their structural and functional characteristics transmit impulses toward the cell body. Nevertheless the general rule is useful.) Axons and dendrites will be considered in detail later in this chapter.

Neurons are functionally linked by their fibers. The connections that enable impulses to pass from one neuron to another are called *synapses* (Gr. *synapsis,* a conjunction, connection) and are commonly positioned at sites where the axon of one neuron ends in a special structural arrangement on part of another neuron. When impulses arrive at a synapse, they either trigger or inhibit initiation of impulses in the second neuron.

Broadly speaking, all the neuronal linkages within the nervous system conform to the basic functional pattern described in the following section.

Functional Organization of Nervous Tissue

During the course of evolution, it would seem that muscle cells (in which the fundamental properties of irritability, conductivity, and contractility were all highly developed) evolved prior to nerve cells. Contraction of these first-formed muscle cells was probably elicited directly by environmental stimuli. Attainment of a more complex body

organization brought with it the requirement for surface *nerve cells* that were sensitive to external stimuli. By transmitting nerve impulses along a nerve fiber, such sensory cells on the body surface could stimulate the contraction of muscle cells that were situated more deeply in the body.

Neural pathways then evolved in which the impulses originating in such a neuron were able to reach another neuron by way of a synapse. Here the impulses from the first neuron could either stimulate or inhibit the firing of new impulses by the second neuron. In the simplest kind of neural pathway, which is made up of only two neurons, impulses generated as a response to external stimuli elicit the contraction of muscle cells that are situated deep in the body. The first neuron in such a pathway is described as *afferent* (L. *ad,* to; *ferre,* to carry) because it carries *afferent (sensory) impulses* deep into the body. The second neuron is described as *efferent* (L. *ex,* out of) because it carries *efferent (motor) impulses* outward to a muscle fiber. These two neurons comprise the simplest type of *reflex arc* (Fig. 14-2).

The basic body plan of multicellular animals such as man is made up of body segments, each with its own afferent and efferent neurons that are capable of carrying out reflex activities that are segmentally based. However, the need also arose for *interneurons (association neurons)* to coordinate autonomous neural activities of the individual body segments. Furthermore, as evolution progressed, the population size of interneurons in the axial part of the nervous system expanded considerably, and in the vertebrates, these cells are well protected by the skull and the vertebral column. Interneurons became particularly abundant in the head region and comprise almost all of the brain. In man and the other vertebrates, the body segments are represented by the adjacent halves of contiguous vertebrae; the spinal nerves of each body segment emerge bilaterally by way of the intervertebral foramina and innervate the tissues of that segment.

From the foregoing discussion, it will be appreciated that *interneurons all lie within the CNS.* Furthermore, *portions of afferent and efferent neurons* of each body segment also *lie within the CNS.* As we shall see, the other parts of the afferent and efferent neurons, because they lie outside the CNS, constitute the PNS. To explain this, we must now describe how the position of the cell bodies of afferent neurons changed as evolution proceeded.

Posterior Root Ganglia and Cranial Ganglia. The first afferent neurons to evolve, as noted, had their cell bodies at the surface of the animal. However, the body surface was not a suitable place because the cell bodies of these neurons were far too easily injured there. Damage to the cell body of a neuron is particularly serious because nerve cells are not replaced. Nevertheless, the cell body of a viable nerve cell can, under suitable circumstances, *regenerate new fibers* if its fibers are damaged. It is therefore better to have cell bodies of afferent neurons located more deeply, with a long fiber reaching to the surface from each to pick up stimuli; then if this fiber is damaged, it can be regenerated by the protected cell body. This arrangement is general in the sensory neurons of higher animals.

In man, the nerve cell bodies of almost all afferent neurons lie extremely close to the CNS without becoming part of it. As shown in Figure 14-2, the cell bodies of such neurons are housed in small rounded nodules termed *ganglia* (meaning a lump). The ganglia housing cell bodies of afferent neurons of body segments are called *spinal* or *posterior* (*dorsal*) *root ganglia.* There are two ganglia for each segment, one lying on each side of the vertebral column. However, it should be borne in mind that although segmentation of the body is indicated by vertebrae of the vertebral column, each segment corresponds to adjacent halves of vertebrae. Figure 14-25 shows the cross-sectional appearance of the vertebral column at a level where two intervertebral foramina extend from the vertebral canal, one on each side; such foramina lie between contiguous vertebrae and mark the middle of a segment. As can be seen at left in Figure 14-25, spinal ganglia lie protected within these intervertebral foramina.

Other afferent fibers enter the brain by way of certain cranial nerves. The cell bodies of these afferent neurons are also situated in ganglia (termed *cranial ganglia*) that are close to the brain but not actually inside it. All the *cell bodies of the afferent neurons* entering the CNS from body segments are therefore *housed in either spinal or cranial ganglia.*

Afferent Neurons. The afferent neurons are essentially bipolar cells. In evolution they began by having one fiber that reached to the surface and brought impulses toward the cell body and another that passed inward, conducting

impulses toward the spinal cord. This type of bipolar afferent neuron is shown in Figure 14-1A. During evolution the two fibers moved, as it were, toward one another like the hands of a clock until they fused, so that except in a few places, such bipolar cells *appear to have only one pole and are therefore often called pseudounipolar* (Fig. 14-1B) and occasionally even *unipolar.* It is interesting that the two fibers also move together and fuse to form a common proximal segment during embryonic development of afferent neurons in the posterior root ganglia. As can be seen in Figure 14-1B, the common proximal process branches at a position that is close to the cell body to form a T-shaped junction with two fibers extending in opposite directions from it. The longer of the two branches (the *peripheral fiber*) extends to a sensory ending whereas the shorter one (the *central fiber*) enters the spinal cord. Except for the termination of the peripheral fiber at the sensory ending, which receives impulses locally and is therefore dendritic, both the central and the peripheral fibers have the structure of an axon. Furthermore, they both actively propagate impulses toward the spinal cord. So in this special instance, both fibers are generally regarded as constituting the axon, with the cell body being attached, as it were, to one side of the axon. Alternatively, these fibers may be referred to as the central and peripheral branches, respectively, of an afferent fiber.

The fibers of afferent neurons enter the spinal cord posterolaterally and within the cord may synapse directly with efferent neurons of the same segment (as in Fig. 14-2) or with intersegmental interneurons. However, some also pass for short distances down the cord, or for longer distances up the cord, to synapse with efferent neurons of other segments or other interneurons.

Efferent Neurons. The cell bodies of efferent neurons are multipolar and, except for certain autonomic neurons (which will be described later in this chapter), all lie *within the CNS.* The axons of spinal efferent neurons in general leave the spinal cord by way of the anterior roots of spinal nerves of the same segment as that in which the cell bodies lie (as in Fig. 14-2). They terminate at efferent endings in the muscles. Muscle cells of viscera, however, are innervated by efferent fibers from autonomic neurons that lie outside the CNS. We shall describe the efferent endings on muscle cells in Chapter 15.

The Knee Jerk Is an Example of a Monosynaptic Reflex. Medical students will soon be testing reflexes to learn whether various parts of the nervous system are functioning properly. One reflex that is frequently tested is the *knee jerk.* A patient crosses his knees and relaxes his leg muscles, and the dangling knee is given a sharp tap just below the patella (Fig. 14-2). The stretch on the tendon pulls on the quadriceps femoris muscle, stimulating stretch receptors (described in Chap. 15) in the muscle. This causes impulses to be generated in afferent neurons that conduct them toward the spinal cord. Here these afferent neurons synapse with efferent neurons, the axons of which extend to muscle fibers in the same muscle (Fig. 14-2). It is common for both afferent and efferent fibers of a given segment to travel in the same peripheral nerve. The contraction elicited in the muscle by the efferent impulses causes the foot to kick forward. The knee jerk is an example of the simplest kind of reflex found in the body, involving a monosynaptic pathway between only two neurons. Most other reflexes are polysynaptic, involving more than two neurons.

Reflexes, of course, are basic to human behavior. Nevertheless, reflex behavior can undergo modification by conditioning. Although synapses between afferent and efferent neurons exist in the spinal cord, afferent impulses commonly pass to the brain before they activate an efferent response. Because the brain contains countless alternative circuits, afferent impulses reaching the brain can elicit a variety of alternative efferent responses, depending on the circuit employed. Conditioning procedures influence which of these circuits s preferred and extend the range of possible responses to given stimuli. All in all, it is understandable why a particular stimulus does not evoke the same response in everyone; indeed, what is distinctly enjoyable for one individual may be quite unpleasant for another.

Innervation Has a Segmental Basis. To understand the nerve supply and reflexes of the various parts of the body, it is important to appreciate that the organization of the nervous system reflects the *basic segmental plan* of the body. Spinal nerves, for instance, contain the afferent and efferent fibers of an individual body segment and supply only tissues that develop from that segment. However, muscle fibers in any given segment commonly blend with those of other segments to form muscles that traverse many segments. Muscle fibers arising from a given segment nevertheless retain their efferent innervation from that segment, so that large muscles may have efferent innervation from several segments.

The clinical relevance of segmental innervation becomes evident when a site of injury of the spinal cord is being investigated, because if the injury destroys afferent or efferent neurons (or their fibers) in a segment, the site of the lesion may be determined by locating the region from which sensation has been lost or by investigating which particular muscles have lost their function.

In summary, then, the cell bodies of afferent neurons lie within spinal or cranial ganglia just outside the CNS. However, the cell bodies of (1) all interneurons and (2) all somatic efferent neurons (but not all autonomic efferent neurons) lie within the CNS. The skin and muscles that develop from a given body segment are innervated by nerves of that segment.

THE CENTRAL NERVOUS SYSTEM

The *central nervous system* (CNS) is derived from the *neural plate* that develops in the mid-dorsal axial ectoderm of the embryo as described in Chapter 5 and illustrated in Figures 5-1 and 5-3. Tiny traces of delicate loose connective tissue are associated with its many capillaries, but other than this,

the CNS is virtually unsupported by connective tissue. As a consequence, the brain and spinal cord have a characteristic consistency that is rather soft and mushy. Instead of being supported by connective tissue, their neuronal cell bodies and processes obtain support from other kinds of cells that are similarly derived from neuroectodermal cells of the neural tube. These non-neuronal constituents of the CNS are called *neuroglia* or *glial cells* (Gr. *glia,* glue) to reflect their evident role of holding neuronal cell bodies and nerve fibers in position, but they have other important functions as well. Thus oligodendrocytes produce myelin, the fatty material that insulates myelinated axons and enables them to transmit impulses with great rapidity. Astrocytes constitute the main supporting element in the CNS. Ependymal cells constitute an epithelium that lines the brain ventricles and the central canal of the spinal cord. Microglia, also classified as glial cells, can become active phagocytes and can dispose of cellular debris, but they do not really support the CNS in any physical sense. These various types of neuroglia will be described later in this chapter.

We shall now discuss how nervous tissue is arranged within the CNS and to point out where neuronal cell bodies can be found in sections of the spinal cord.

SPINAL CORD

Two main components of central nervous tissue can be recognized in slices of the spinal cord or brain even without a microscope. These two components are known as *gray matter* and *white matter.*

Gray Matter. As a result of proliferation in the inner part of the wall of the neural tube, cells are pushed into the middle layers of the wall. Most of these cells differentiate into neurons, but some differentiate into *neuroglia.* The *cell bodies of neurons* and their various associated glial cells (the nuclei of which are labeled *NN* in parts 2 and 3 of Fig. 14-4) are the principal components of *gray matter.* The cell bodies of neurons lie surrounded by tangled masses of fibers that represent the beginnings and endings of nerve fibers. Due to its matted appearance in the light microscope (LM), this component of gray matter is called *neuropil* (Gr. *pilos,* felt). Its appearance is illustrated in part *B* of Figure 14-3 and parts 2 and 3 of Figure 14-4. The axons in the neuropil are not heavily myelinated, and the dendrites lack myelin.

In the spinal cord, the gray matter roughly resembles an ''H'' when seen in cross section (Fig. 14-3*A* and part 1 of Fig. 14-4). Hence the gray matter is said to have two *posterior horns* and two *anterior horns.* Actually, the horns are continuous columns that extend up and down the cord. In some parts of the cord, there is a lateral column on each side as well. Cell bodies of neurons are seen to advantage in the anterior horns (Fig. 14-3*B* and parts 2 and 3 of Fig.

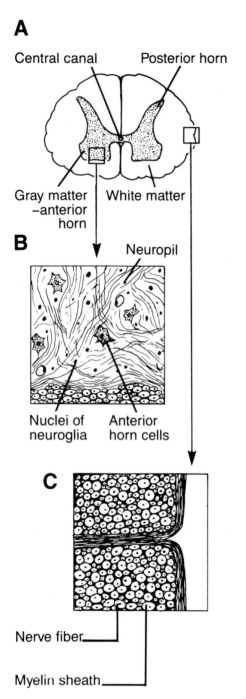

A

Central canal   Posterior horn

Gray matter
–anterior   White matter
horn

B

Neuropil

Nuclei of   Anterior
neuroglia   horn cells

C

Nerve fiber

Myelin sheath

Fig. 14-3. Diagrammatic representation of the basic organization of the spinal cord. (*A*) Transverse section. (*B*) Gray matter. (*C*) White matter.

14-4). Gray matter is gray because it contains many cells but not much myelin.

White Matter.   In the spinal cord, the white matter, which surrounds the H-shaped region of gray matter (Fig. 14-3*A*),

contains a vast number of nerve fibers extending up and down the cord. It is white because the majority of fibers are ensheathed with the white fatty material *myelin.* Hence myelin makes up most of the substance of white matter.

White matter *does not contain any cell bodies of neurons.* The fibers it contains originate from cell bodies lying either in the gray matter of the brain or spinal cord or in the spinal ganglia. The fibers are organized into tracts, each of which contains fibers from neurons with similar roles, so there are separate motor and sensory tracts.

Although white matter contains no cell bodies of neurons, it does contain many glial cells. In the developing spinal cord, cells called spongioblasts from the developing middle layer differentiate into astrocytes and oligodendrocytes. These two types of glial cells (chiefly oligodendrocytes) fit into the crevices between the axons. Oligodendrocytes are commonly arranged in rows between myelinated axons and, as noted, are responsible for laying down myelin in the CNS. Because myelin is a lipid–protein complex containing cholesterol, phospholipids, and glycolipids in addition to a few proteins, it is mostly dissolved by fat solvents. Hence when ordinary paraffin sections of nervous tissue are prepared, the lipid component of the myelin is extracted. When such sections are then stained with hematoxylin and eosin (H & E), each site where myelin was present appears as a round space that seems empty except for a little round dot representing a cross section of the axon that, in life, was surrounded by the myelin (Fig. 14-3*C*). Occasional nuclei are seen in white matter between the empty round spaces; these belong to glial cells.

By utilizing fixatives that render myelin insoluble, it is possible to demonstrate myelin with suitable special stains, even in paraffin sections. Osmic acid fixes myelin so that it is not extracted in paraffin sections and moreover stains myelin black, so that in sections of spinal cord fixed in osmic acid, the white matter of the cord appears black.

Myelination in the CNS.   In the CNS, myelin is formed by *oligodendrocytes,* chiefly those lying between nerve fibers of white matter. However, some myelin is also formed (although to a much lesser extent) by oligodendrocytes in the gray matter. Each oligodendrocyte participates in forming a myelin sheath by wrapping a segment of a nerve fiber in spiral fashion with successive layers of one of its processes (see Fig. 14-18). The cytoplasm of the process becomes squeezed back into the cell body so that the wrapping material consists of little more than double layers of cell membrane, which supply the lipids, phospholipids, and cholesterol for the myelin. The process of myelination here is, in some ways, similar to that occurring in the PNS in the myelination of peripheral nerve fibers, but in other ways, it is more complicated. After myelination in the PNS has been described later in this chapter, myelination in the CNS will be easier to visualize.

The process of myelination in the CNS begins in the gray matter, close to the cell body of a neuron, and advances along the axon into the white matter. This process begins early in the fourth month of fetal life, and it is incomplete at birth, so that some fibers become myelinated only during the first year of life. The total amount of myelin in the CNS increases from birth to maturity, and individual fibers become more heavily myelinated during the growth period. In both the CNS and PNS, the myelin sheath is interrupted at *nodes of Ranvier* (see Fig. 14-18). The structure and significance of these nodes will be explained when we discuss the conduction of nerve impulses. The segments of a nerve fiber between consecutive nodes are called *internodes.*

In the Brain, the Relative Positions of Gray and White Matter Are Reversed. In the brain, the formation of gray and white matter initially follows a pattern similar to that in the spinal cord, where gray matter forms from the middle layers and white matter forms from the outer layer of the neural tube. In the medulla, pons, midbrain, and parts of the forebrain, gray matter develops in positions corresponding roughly to those in the spinal cord, and the gray matter becomes covered by white matter, as in the spinal cord. In certain other parts of the brain, however, neuroblasts from the middle layers of the neural tube migrate out through the outer layer of the wall (where white matter will develop) and assume a position on the outside of the tube. Because of this, the cerebral hemispheres and the cerebellum acquire a covering (*cortex*) of *gray matter.* Hence in these two parts of the brain, the gray matter exists not only deep to the white matter but also superficial to it. This explains why the outer region of the spinal cord consists of white matter whereas that of the cerebrum and cerebellum is gray matter.

We shall now describe how nerve cells are arranged in the brain cortex.

CEREBRAL CORTEX

In the *cerebral cortex* that constitutes the covering of the two cerebral hemispheres, sensory information is integrated and voluntary motor responses are initiated and coordinated. Furthermore, this is the part of the brain where complex and generally useful thought processes such as acquisition and the use of language, learning, and memorization occur. For such purposes, the cerebral cortex needs to be very extensive; hence the outer surface of the cerebral hemispheres is deeply convoluted; the deeper grooves are known as *fissures* and the shallower ones as *sulci.* The latter lie between ridges of cortex called *gyri.*

The cerebral cortex is composed of gray matter. It constitutes a covering, approximately 1.5 mm to 4 mm thick, over the white matter of the cerebral hemispheres (Fig. 14-5). Different regions of the hemispheres show the same general plan of microscopic organization, but this plan is modified in the different areas of the cerebral cortex that perform different functions. In general, the cell bodies of the neurons in the cerebral cortex are arranged in six some-

what indistinct layers (Fig. 14-5, *left*); however, the extent to which each layer is developed depends on the area involved.

The most superficial layer is called the *molecular layer* (Fig. 14-5, *left*). It contains relatively few cell bodies and consists chiefly of fibers of underlying cells, the fibers of which run in many directions but generally parallel with the surface (Fig. 14-5, *right*). The second layer is called the *outer granular layer* because it contains the cell bodies of many small nerve cells, which gives it a granular appearance when examined under low power (Fig. 14-5, *left*). The third layer is called the *pyramidal cell layer* because of its content of pyramid-shaped cell bodies of neurons (Fig. 14-5, *left*). The fourth layer is termed the *inner granular layer* because it is "granulated" with small nerve cell bodies (Fig. 14-5, *left*). The fifth layer is termed the *internal pyramidal layer* because its most prominent feature is its content of pyramidal cell bodies. In one part of the cortex, the *motor area*, the pyramidal cells of this layer are huge; they are called *Betz cells.* The sixth and final layer is named the layer of *polymorphic cells* because the cells of this layer have many shapes. It can be seen from Figures 14-5 and 14-6A that the cell bodies of the neurons in the deeper parts of the cerebral cortex are larger than those in its more superficial parts.

In an H & E section of the cerebral cortex (such as that illustrated in Fig. 14-6), it is possible to distinguish the following componets: (1) the cell bodies of pyramidal cells and other cortical neurons; (2) cell nuclei belonging to neurons or glial cells; (3) the many capillaries that provide the cortex with nutrients and oxygen; and (4) the neuropil, which is seen as a pale-staining fibrillar mass in which these other components are embedded.

It has been estimated that there are close to 10 billion neurons in the cerebral cortex, and because one neuron can establish synaptic connections with as many as 100,000 others, the possibilities with regard to the number of available pathways are overwhelming.

CEREBELLAR CORTEX

The gray matter in the *cerebellar cortex* is arranged somewhat differently and forms only three layers. The superficial one is termed the *molecular layer* because it contains relatively few small neurons, together with numerous unmyelinated fibers. Deep to this, there is a layer of huge flask-shaped cells named *Purkinje cells* after the Czech physiologist Johannes Purkinje, who first described them. The remainder of the gray matter of the cerebellar cortex consists of an inner *granular layer* containing abundant small neurons. The three layers are illustrated in Figure 14-7.

The several kinds of neurons and their fibers are arranged in a somewhat complex manner, with the Purkinje cells receiving both excitatory and inhibitory impulses. Their

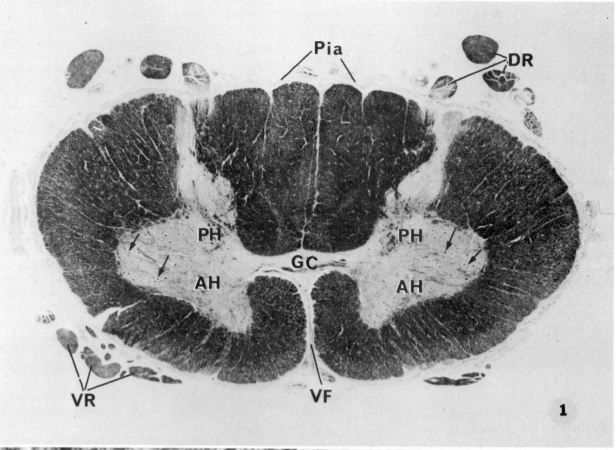

Pia DR

PH PH

GC

AH AH

VR VF

1

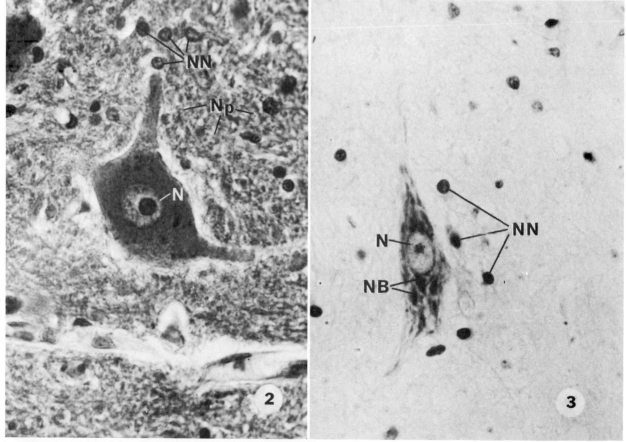

NN

Np

N

2

N

NN

NB

3

Layers:

1. Molecular

2. Outer granular

3. Pyramidal cell

4. Inner granular

5. Inner pyramidal cell

6. Polymorphic cell

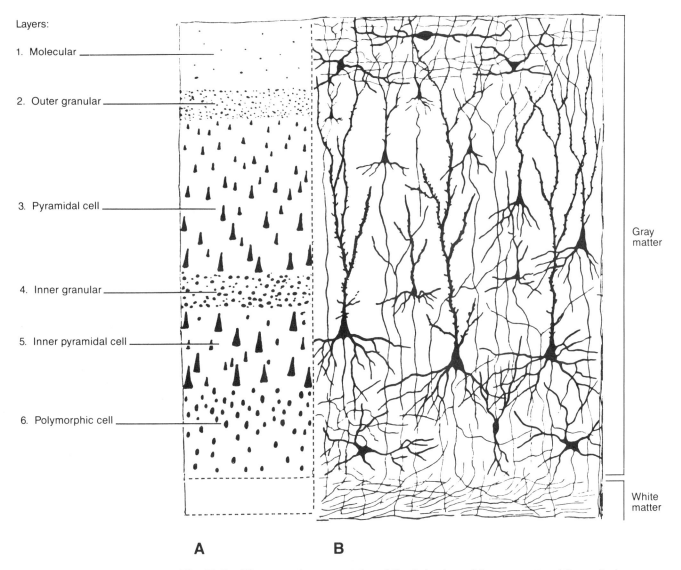

Gray matter

White matter

A   B

Fig. 14-5.   Diagrammatic representation of the six laminae of the gray matter of the cerebral cortex, as seen (*A*) with H & E staining and (*B*) with Golgi staining. (After Villiger E: Brain and Spinal Cord. Philadelphia, JB Lippincott, 1925)

huge dendritic arborizations extend up into the molecular layer, as shown in Figure 14-8, where they collect excitatory impulses arriving primarily from the motor area of the cerebral cortex. The cerebellum modulates and organizes the motor impulses so as to regulate and coordinate movements involving groups of muscles. For details of the neuronal and functional organization of the cerebellum, see Llinás.

Now that we have dealt with the distribution and arrangement of neurons in the CNS, we shall consider them in more detail.

Fig. 14-4.   Photomicrographs of the spinal cord. (*1*) Cross section of spinal cord (cervical region). The myelin of the white matter is darkly stained. The pale-stained gray matter in the central area is made up of bilateral anterior horns (*AH*) and posterior horns (*PH*) joined by the gray commissure (*GC*). The anterior (ventral) fissure (*VF*), and anterior (ventral) and posterior (dorsal) roots of spinal nerves (*VR* and *DR*) are also clearly discernible. (*2*) Anterior horn cell (*center*), neuropil (*Np*), and nuclei of neuroglia (*NN*) in an H & E section. The anterior horn cell has a prominent nucleolus in its nucleus (*N*). (*3*) Anterior horn cell, stained with toluidine blue to demonstrate its Nissl bodies (*NB*). Other labels as in *2*. (Ross MH, Reith EJ: Histology: A Text and Atlas. New York, Harper & Row/JB Lippincott, 1985)

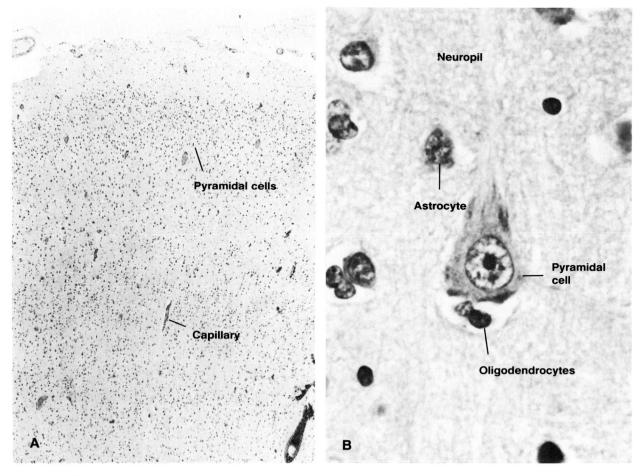

Fig. 14-6. Photomicrographs of cerebral cortex (motor area). (*A*) Seen at very low power, the laminar organization depicted in Figure 14-5 is just discernible. The gray background is neuropil. (*B*) Representative pyramidal and glial cells (high power). The pyramidal cell exhibits Nissl bodies in its cytoplasm and a prominent central nucleolus in its nucleus. Individual nerve fibers are discernible in the neuropil.

NEURONS

Most neurons of the CNS are multipolar and have many dendrites (Fig. 14-1C). In most cases, their cell bodies are relatively large (up to 135 μm in diameter), but a few are small (only 4 μm in diameter). Their cell bodies can be spherical, flattened, ovoid, or pyramidal, and, as noted, in the CNS they are all located in gray matter.

In most neurons the nucleus lies centrally in the cell body, but in autonomic neurons of the PNS it more commonly has an eccentric position. It is typically large and spherical (Figs. 14-9 and 14-10), and most of its chromatin is of the extended type; hence in the LM, its chromatin granules appear very small or are not seen at all. As a result, the large central nucleolus is very prominent. Its characteristic LM appearance (see part 2 of Fig. 14-4 and Fig. 14-9) has been likened to an owl's eye, possibly by a student who was accustomed to doing most of his studying

by night. In the electron microscope (EM), a small amount of peripheral chromatin can be seen on the inner aspect of the nuclear envelope (Fig. 14-10).

Localized regions of basophilia are common in the cell body and also in the larger dendrites of neurons (see part 3 of Fig. 14-4 and Fig. 14-9). These regions are termed *Nissl bodies* after the German neurologist who first described them. Seen in the EM, Nissl bodies are regions of the cytoplasm where there are many cisternae of rough-surfaced endoplasmic reticulum (rER) and also many free ribosomes and polysomes in the spaces between the cisternae (Fig. 14-10). The abundant ribosomal RNA of the free and attached ribosomes in Nissl bodies is what causes their intense basophilia. The great abundance of free ribosomes in the cell body (Fig. 14-10) is required to synthesize cytoplasmic proteins that continuously flow along the axon (and the dendrites, too) to replace the proteins used up in metabolism.

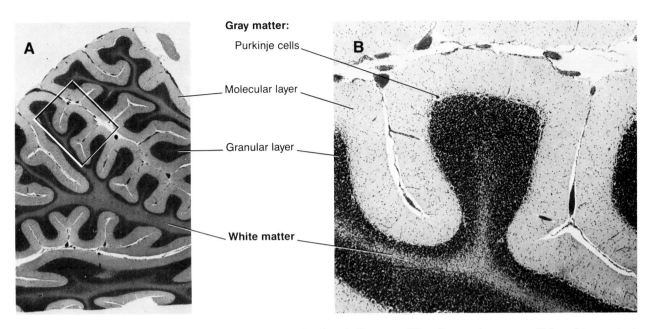

Gray matter:

Purkinje cells

Molecular layer

Granular layer

White matter

Fig. 14-7. Photomicrographs of cerebellar cortex (*A*) under very low power; (*B*) boxed-in area in *A* under higher magnification, showing its three layers.

If, as a result of an accident, the axon of a neuron becomes severed, a change known as the *axon reaction* ensues. The Nissl bodies temporarily disappear from the cell body (a change termed *chromatolysis*), and the nucleus moves to one side. In the event that the axon regenerates, the Nissl bodies reappear.

In addition to having prominent organelles for protein synthesis, the cell body possesses a relatively large number of energy-providing mitochondria (Figs. 14-10 and 14-11). Its characteristic shape is maintained by numerous microtubules (Fig. 14-11) that also furnish the neuron with a mechanism of intracellular transport. In addition, the cell body contains many intermediate filaments (Fig. 14-11). Usually referred to as *neurofilaments*, these filaments provide added internal support for the nerve cell, particularly

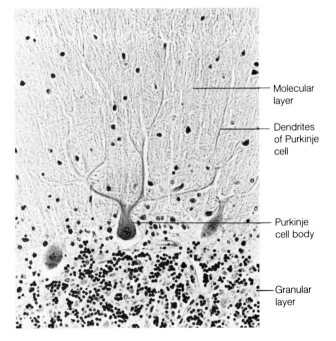

Molecular layer

Dendrites of Purkinje cell

Purkinje cell body

Granular layer

Fig. 14-8. Photomicrograph of a Purkinje cell of the cerebellar cortex, showing its extensive dendritic tree extending up into the molecular layer. (Courtesy of C. P. Leblond)

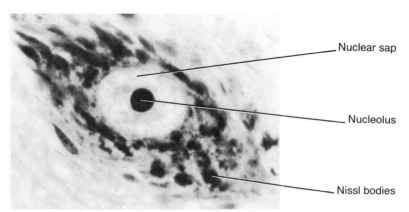

Nuclear sap

Nucleolus

Nissl bodies

Fig. 14-9. Photomicrograph of the cell body of a multipolar neuron (anterior horn cell of cat spinal cord), stained with cresyl violet. Note its prominent rounded nucleolus and large basophilic Nissl bodies. (Barr ML, Bertram LF, Lindsay HA: Anat Rec 107:283, 1950)

for its long fragile extensions. Furthermore, neurofilaments of the axon are associated with a system of crosslinkers (see Fig. 4-28B) that interconnects them with microtubules, the axolemma, and other membranous organelles. Lastly, the cell body contains an elaborate Golgi complex (Figs. 14-10 and 14-11) and some lysosomes. Pigments, too, may be present. Thus ganglion cells of the PNS (see Fig. 4-42) and neurons of the CNS may accumulate the wear-and-tear pigment lipofuscin, and in the substantia nigra of the midbrain, the neurons even contain melanin.

The Axon. The *axon* is generally the neuron's longest nerve fiber. Its diameter remains constant along its length, ranging from 0.2 μm to 20 μm, depending on the type of neuron. An axon that has a large diameter conducts impulses more rapidly than an axon of narrower diameter. *Collateral* branches, where they exist, leave the axon more or less perpendicularly (Fig. 14-12) and then make another more or less right-angled turn and either (1) continue in the same direction, or (2) extend back alongside the axon from which they branched, in which case they are termed *recurrent collaterals* (Fig. 14-12). The part of the cell body from which the axon emerges is called the *axon hillock* (Fig. 14-11). Although relatively free of rER, it contains many microtubules and neurofilaments.

Both efferent and afferent nerve fibers situated in the white matter of the spinal cord and brain are myelinated. The proximal (initial) segment of the axon lies in the gray matter and remains devoid of myelin. It is covered instead by the cytoplasmic processes of oligodendrocytes and astrocytes. This initial segment of the axon is also slightly narrower than the myelinated portion. The part of the cell membrane that covers the axon is known as the *axolemma*, and the part of the cytoplasm that lies within the axon is termed the *axoplasm*. In a *myelinated axon*, the axolemma is invested by a segmented *myelin sheath* that is interrupted at regularly spaced intervals by myelin-free gaps called *nodes* (*of Ranvier*), which will be described when we consider the PNS. However, not all axons are myelinated. Figure 14-13 illustrates the fine structure of an *unmyelinated axon*. The axoplasm of both types of axons contains many

threadlike mitochondria, some elements of smooth-surfaced endoplasmic reticulum (sER) known as the *axoplasmic reticulum,* and an abundance of microtubules and uniformly spaced neurofilaments. The axon is nevertheless almost devoid of ribosomes, so it depends on the cell body for its maintenance. Proteins and many of the other macromolecular constituents required for the neuron's metabolic and synaptic activities are synthesized solely in its cell body. Together with certain types of organelles, such constituents must be conveyed along the entire length of the axon to its terminals by a distinctive process known as *axonal (axoplasmic) transport.*

Axonal (Axoplasmic) Transport Represents a Combination of Slow, Intermediate, and Fast Components. Due to the considerable length of the axon, it is not unusual for the volume of this part of the cell to be several hundred times greater than that of the cell body. However, the amount of protein synthesis occurring in the axon itself is insignificant; hence required proteins and glycoproteins, together with mitochondria and vesicular or tubulovesicular structures called *axoplasmic vesicles* that serve as a source of ready-made membrane, must be continually transported along the axon, away from the cell body. Radioautographic studies have shown that within minutes of becoming incorporated into newly synthesized proteins, labeled amino acids start moving along the axon. Cytoplasmic proteins and organelles migrate in two main streams that travel along the axon at different speeds.

First, there is a unidirectional *slow stream* of axoplasmic matrix that is sometimes described as *axoplasmic flow.* This stream moves along the axon in an anterograde direction (*i.e.,* away from the cell body) at a speed of about 1 mm to 4 mm per day. It carries cytosolic enzymes (*e.g.,* tyrosine hydroxylase, an enzyme involved in the synthesis of norepinephrine), actin (in soluble form and in the form of microfilaments), myosin, and clathrin (the protein that becomes associated with coated vesicles). The microtubule and neurofilament proteins move at a slightly slower rate, probably in the form of a slowly advancing, crosslinked microtrabecular lattice or scaffolding (see Fig. 4-28B) that carries tiny pockets of axoplasmic matrix along with it in

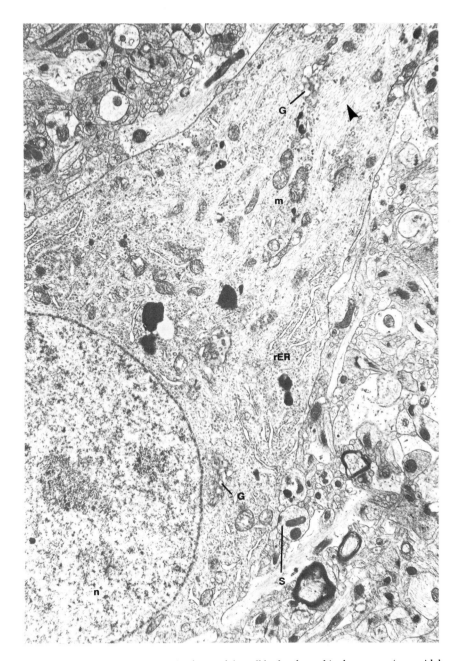

Fig. 14-10. Electron micrograph of part of the cell body of a multipolar neuron (pyramidal cell of human cerebral cortex). A portion of the spherical nucleus (*n*) is seen at lower left; it is characterized by its considerable content of extended chromatin. Mitochondria (*m*), Golgi stacks (*G*), and patches of rough-surfaced endoplasmic reticulum (*rER*) are discernible in the cytoplasm. A synapse (*s*) is readily identifiable near the nucleus. At this magnification, microtubules and neurofilaments are also just discernible at upper right in the region above the arrowhead. (Courtesy of J. Bilbao and S. Briggs)

its interstices. This slow stream is thought to be necessary for axon growth and general maintenance of the axoplasm.

Secondly, a *fast stream* travels along the axon in an anterograde direction at a rate of 50 mm to 400 mm per day, which is approximately 100 times faster than the slow stream described above. This fast-moving stream transports neurotransmitter-filled vesicles and membrane-associated and membrane-bounded constituents that are involved in synaptic transmission. An example of such a constituent is dopamine-β-hydroxylase, another enzyme that is involved in the local synthesis of norepinephrine at nerve terminals. The extra glycoproteins, proteins, and phospholipids

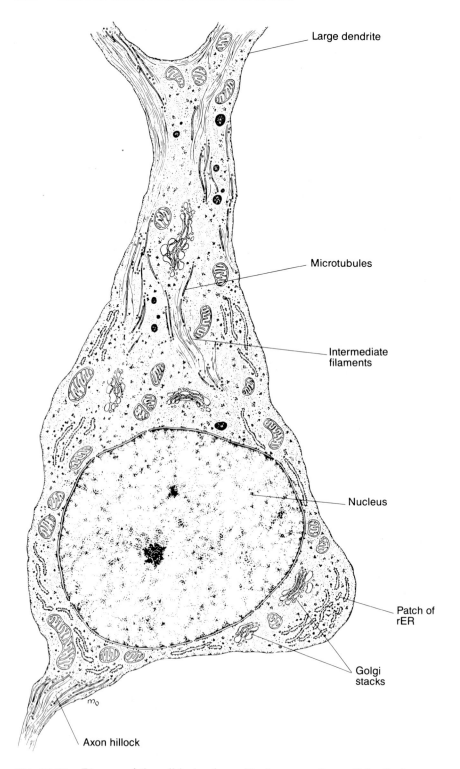

Large dendrite

Microtubules

Intermediate
filaments

Nucleus

Patch of
rER

Golgi
stacks

Axon hillock

Fig. 14-11. Diagram of the cell body of a multipolar neuron (pyramidal cell of motor cortex), showing its features as seen in the EM. (Courtesy of C. P. Leblond)

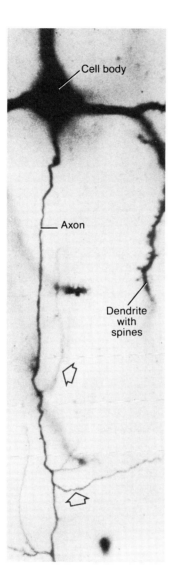

Fig. 14-12. Photomicrograph of a multipolar neuron (pyramidal cell of cat, modified Golgi stain) showing a dendrite with spines and the axon with collaterals. Arrows indicate axon collaterals. (Courtesy of E. G. Bertram)

role. It has also been established that such transport depends on the presence of calcium ions and the expenditure of metabolic energy from adenosine triphosphate (ATP). A currently favored hypothesis is that membranous organelles and vesicles are somehow moved along the microtubules by becoming attached to crosslinkers that can interact with microtubules of the axonal microtrabecular scaffolding. One idea is that such crosslinkers possess adenosinetriphosphatase (ATPase) activity and that when bound to a membranous structure, they utilize energy liberated from ATP to pull this structure along a microtubule (Miller and Lasek). An extensive crosslinker system that interconnects axonal microtubules, neurofilaments, and the axolemma with membranous organelles has indeed been demonstrated (Hirokawa; see Fig. 4-28*B*). However, in this

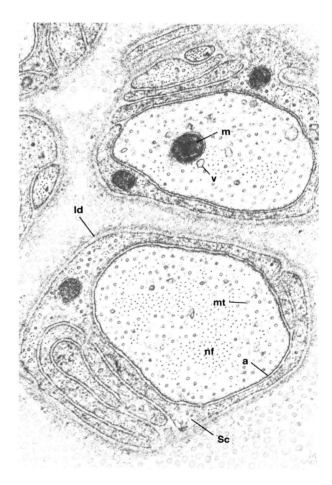

Fig. 14-13. Electron micrograph (×45,000) of unmyelinated axons in transverse section (biopsy of human peripheral nerve). Each axon is invested by a Schwann cell (*Sc*), the cytoplasm of which closely surrounds its axolemma (*a*). Within the axoplasm, a mitochondrion (*m*), smooth-surfaced vesicles (*v*), microtubules (*mt*), and neurofilaments (*nf*) are readily distinguished. The lamina densa (*ld*) of the Schwann cell basement membrane and interstitial collagen fibrils cut in transverse section also can be seen. (Courtesy of J. Bilbao and S. Briggs)

needed for the local formation of synaptic vesicles in the axon terminals are transported to these terminals in the fast stream. All such membrane constituents of synaptic vesicles are nevertheless obliged to pass through the Golgi complex on their way to the axon.

Other axon components, notably mitochondria, have been found to travel at a speed that is intermediate between those of the slow and fast streams. Such transport represents a combination of fast anterograde transport and intermittent stopping or backward (retrograde) movement.

It is not yet clear how axonal transport is brought about, but because both colchicine and vinblastine inhibit this process, it is widely accepted that microtubules play a key

type of preparation, it is not clear whether these organelles are actually being transported or not. Recent evidence indicates that the crosslinkers responsible for mediating axonal transport may be of a special type that interacts only with membranous organelles and microtubules (Miller and Lasek). Others have suggested that microfilaments and associated myosin might somehow be involved, but the nature of their involvement remains a matter of speculation.

In summary, then, slow axonal transport (axoplasmic flow) conveys the cytoskeletal, cytoskeleton-associated, and cytosolic constituents of the axoplasm, whereas fast axonal transport conveys the membranous organelles and membranous and membrane-associated constituents of the axon.

Dendrites. Dendrites are branched, tapering processes that seldom exceed 1 mm in length. In most kinds of multipolar neurons, they extend in all directions from the cell body (Fig. 14-1C). In contrast to the axon, the dendrites branch dichotomously and at an acute angle. Several orders of branching give rise to dendritic branches of progressively diminishing diameter that greatly increase the surface area available for receiving nerve impulses. The major dendritic processes differ from the axon in that they contain Nissl bodies (rER and ribosomes) as well as abundant microtubules, neurofilaments, and mitochondria (Fig. 14-11).

Dendritic Transport. Certain proteins (*e.g.,* acetylcholinesterase, an enzyme that can be conveyed by fast axonal transport and that degrades acetylcholine released at synapses) can also be transported to the dendritic terminals (away from the cell body) at a speed of approximately 3 mm per hour, which is close to that of fast axonal transport. Much less is known about the mechanism of dendritic transport, but it is believed to have a similar basis to axonal transport.

Retrograde Flow. Cytoplasmic components do not only migrate away from the cell body of the neuron toward the tips of its processes. Some components are transported in the reverse direction, that is, away from the pre- and postsynaptic terminals and toward the cell body. This movement is termed *retrograde flow*. Such retrograde streams can transport cytoplasmic components from the axon and dendrites to the cell body at approximately half the speed of the anterograde fast axonal stream. This reverse flow avoids accumulation of such components at the nerve fiber terminals, and it enables the neuron to recycle the membranous component of its pre- and postsynaptic terminals so as to maintain them in good condition. Furthermore, in situations in which the axon has become damaged, retrograde flow of substances that, under normal circumstances, would not enter the axoplasm is believed to signal to the cell body the need for axon regeneration. As in the case of anterograde axonal transport, retrograde axonal transport of membranous organelles appears to be mediated by

crosslinkers that become attached to these organelles and thereupon interact with microtubules (Miller and Lasek).

Among the organelles that return to the cell body in the retrograde stream from axon terminals are phagosomes and other types of vesicles that result from receptor-mediated and nonspecific endocytosis. It so happens that EM markers (*e.g.,* horseradish peroxidase) can be taken up by endocytosis at axon terminals as a consequence of the local recycling mechanism that retrieves synaptic vesicle membrane constituents from the presynaptic membrane. Such uptake of a recognizable marker can be utilized to follow the axonal pathway by which endocytotic vesicles return to the cell body to submit their contents to lysosomal degradation. This experimental approach has enabled investigators to trace the course of axons back to the cell bodies from which they originated, and this has revealed the presence of hitherto undiscovered connections between the various nuclei (groups of neuronal cell bodies) of the brain. Of clinical importance is the fact that retrograde axonal transport can also carry infective viruses (*e.g.,* rabies virus and herpes virus) or infection-derived toxins (*e.g.,* tetanus toxin) from the peripheral tissues into the CNS, and this can result in a viral encephalitis that, in the case of rabies, may prove fatal.

In the next part of this chapter, we shall consider how myelin facilitates saltatory conduction and how nerve impulses become transmitted at synapses. Students who are already familiar with the general nature of nerve impulses will have little difficulty understanding the structural basis of impulse conduction, but those with no background in physiology may find it useful to peruse the following introductory account of how nerve impulses are transmitted along nerve fibers.

NERVE IMPULSES

When a Neuron Is Not Being Stimulated, Its Cell Membrane Carries a Resting Potential. In this particular context, the word *potential* refers to the *transmembrane potential,* that is, the difference between the electrical charges that are present internal and external to the cell membrane. In a neuron that is firing no impulses, there is a difference of -70 mv that is known as its *resting potential.* Hence the *inner side* of the cell membrane of a neuron is *negatively charged* with respect to its outer side. Such a membrane is described as being electrically *polarized.*

The reason for this resting potential is that the total concentrations of positively and negatively charged ions on either side of the cell membrane are unequal. There is a higher concentration of positive ions in the intercellular fluid and a higher concentration of negative ions in the cell cytoplasm. The basis for this difference will now be described.

First, it will be recalled that the cell membrane actively transports certain cations against their respective concentration gradients. Using ATP as its energy source, the *sodium–potassium pump* (Na$^+$–K$^+$ ATPase) pumps sodium ions out of the cytoplasm at the same time that it pumps potassium ions into the cytoplasm from the intercellular fluid. Next, whether these ions stay where they have been pumped depends on the selective permeability of the cell membrane. The selectivity of the cell membrane determines which ions subsequently diffuse back along their respective concentration gradients into the compartments from which they were pumped. The nerve cell membrane is fairly permeable to potassium ions, so these are able to leave the cytoplasm after being pumped into it. This raises the concentration of positive ions outside the cell membrane. However, permeability of the membrane to sodium ions is low, so these do not reenter the cytoplasm after being pumped into the intercellular fluid. Because the potassium ions leaking from the cytoplasm and the excluded sodium ions are both positively charged, the total concentration of positive ions is greater in the intercellular fluid than in the cytoplasm. This is the chief reason why the inner aspect of the cell membrane is negative with respect to its outer aspect in a resting neuron.

Another factor that contributes to negativity on the cytoplasmic side of the cell membrane is the presence of relatively large numbers of negatively charged organic macromolecules in the cytoplasm. Because the cell membrane is impermeable to such molecules, their presence adds negativity only to its cytoplasmic side.

Nerve Impulses Are Essentially Waves of Transient Membrane Depolarization. A nerve impulse originates in response to a *stimulus* of electrical, chemical, thermal, or mechanical nature that has been received by the cell membrane of a neuron. Later we shall consider how impulses are generated at afferent endings and describe how they are transmitted so that a second neuron can be stimulated by such impulses. But first it is necessary to consider what would happen at the site of a stimulus applied to the cell membrane of an unmyelinated axon at some point along its course—with the realization, of course, that this would not be the usual part of a neuron to receive stimuli. When we have described how impulses are propagated along an unmyelinated axon, we shall explain how they travel along a myelinated axon.

The first detectable change at the site on an *unmyelinated axon* that receives an effective stimulus is a sudden influx of sodium ions from outside the axolemma into the axoplasm. Prior to this, the sodium–potassium pump in the axolemma maintains an excess of sodium ions outside the axolemma against their concentration gradient. The immediate influx of sodium ions is due to a sudden increase in the permeability of the axolemma that allows sodium ions to pass inward along their concentration gradient.

Because sodium ions carry a positive charge, their influx into the cytoplasm reduces the total positive charge on the outer aspect of the axolemma and adds to the content of positive ions within the axoplasm. As a result, the *resting potential disappears* from the site where the stimulus was received. Indeed, the influx is so great that the inner side of the axolemma temporarily becomes slightly positively charged relative to its exterior. Because the sodium ions enter as a result of their concentration gradient, their influx stops as soon as the sodium ion concentration of the axoplasm equilibrates with that of the intercellular fluid. However, just as their influx is arrested, the axolemma becomes freely permeable to potassium ions. Because these ions were previously in excess in the axoplasm (due to the action of the sodium–potassium pump)

and because the axolemma now permits their free movement, they flow outward into the intercellular fluid. This has two effects. First, it reduces the total positive charge in the axoplasm, and secondly it increases the total positive charge outside the axolemma. This combined effect *restores the resting potential* to the site of depolarization.

In this manner, the application of a stimulus to some site along the axolemma elicits a rapid *depolarization* that is almost immediately followed by a *repolarization*. This is manifested as a wave of depolarization and ensuing repolarization that spreads along the axolemma, away from the site where the stimulus was received. Hence the transmission of a nerve impulse amounts to the sweeping of a wave of depolarization and repolarization along the cell membrane.

The depolarization and ensuing repolarization of the cell membrane of a nerve or muscle cell are commonly described as an *action potential*. Semantically, this is a puzzling term. It was probably devised to contrast with the term *resting potential* and to denote that the depolarization and repolarization are transmitted along the membrane in a wavelike manner, with the result that the stimulus causes action.

If a stimulus were applied to an unmyelinated nerve fiber at some point along its course, a wave of depolarization and repolarization would spread away from the site of stimulation in both directions (*i.e.,* toward both ends of the nerve fiber). In life, however, afferent or efferent fibers are stimulated only at one end, and hence the wave of depolarization and repolarization travels in one direction only. Because a site on a nerve fiber becomes repolarized within a few milliseconds of becoming depolarized, it might be thought that a wave of depolarization traveling along the fiber in one direction might also spread backward to depolarize the repolarized site immediately behind it—which, of course, would initiate a retrograde wave of depolarization. However, this does not happen because, as explained below, the repolarizing site immediately behind the wave of depolarization remains *temporarily refractive to further stimulation.*

In Unmyelinated Axons, Impulse Propagation Involves the Entire Axolemma. The influx of positively charged sodium ions at the site of a stimulus is sufficient to render the axoplasm at that site transiently positive. A local circuit is established that enables electrical current to flow between the depolarized site and the surrounding region of polarized axolemma by way of the axoplasm and the intercellular fluid. Positively charged ions entering the axoplasm at this site flow toward the surrounding region of negatively charged axoplasm, and on the outer aspect of the axolemma, the site of depolarization attracts positive charges to it from the surrounding region of polarized membrane. As a result, there is an inward flow of positive current at the site of depolarization and an outward flow of such current through the surrounding region of polarized membrane. This outward flow of current then triggers depolarization of the region of membrane that is still polarized.

Under normal circumstances, the wave of depolarization originates at one end of the fiber and proceeds in one direction only. Propagation in the same direction is ensured because depolarization of the axolemma is followed by a short period during which its sodium channels become temporarily inactivated (*i.e.,* unresponsive to further excitation). Such inactivation permits the wave of depolarization to elicit depolarization of the region of axolemma just ahead of it but prevents the wave of depolarization from being propagated backward.

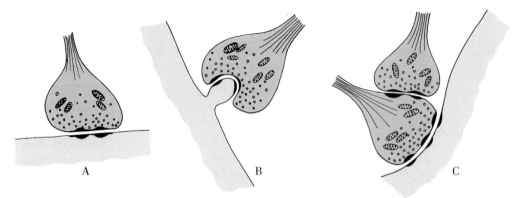

Fig. 14-14. Diagram illustrating some common kinds of synapses. (*A*) Axodendritic or axosomatic synapse. (*B*) Axodendritic synapse in which an end bulb synapses with a dendritic spine. (C) Axoaxonic synapse of the end bulb to end bulb type. (Barr ML: The Human Nervous System. New York, Harper & Row, 1972)

Myelin Plays a Key Role in Saltatory Conduction. The myelin sheath that surrounds myelinated nerve fibers is interrupted at regular intervals along its length by *nodes* (*of Ranvier*). These nodes are present along myelinated fibers of both the CNS and the PNS. The distance between consecutive nodes varies; it is at least 0.2 mm but can be more than 1 mm in large fibers. In myelinated fibers, each region of the fiber between nodes is invested with a thick coat of *myelin* that acts as an electrical insulator. However, at the nodes, the axolemma is *freely exposed to tissue (intercellular) fluid.* Because the internodal segments of the fiber are so well insulated, almost no current flows through the internodal parts of the axolemma. Current is nevertheless able to flow very readily through the nodal parts of the axolemma that lack a covering of myelin. Hence in myelinated fibers, it is only the *nodal parts* of the axolemma that undergo depolarization. Temporary flow of current (*i.e.,* net movement of ions) through a circuit that is made up of the axoplasm and the surrounding tissue fluid enables each depolarized node to initiate depolarization of the next. This process is known as *saltatory conduction* (L. *saltare,* to jump) because instead of proceeding in a continuous manner along the entire axolemma, the action potential jumps consecutively from node to node. Its advantages are that it substantially increases the speed of impulse conduction and that it requires less energy expenditure on the part of the neuron.

SYNAPSES

Nerve impulses are transmitted from one neuron to another at morphologically recognizable sites of contact that are known as *synapses.* Most synapses transmit impulses indirectly and in one direction only through the action of one or more chemical *neurotransmitters;* these are called *chemical synapses.* In addition, there is a much rarer type

of synapse called the *electrical synapse* that is basically a gap junction through which ions can pass freely, thereby conducting nerve impulses directly and with virtually no delay. In some sites, there are mixed *conjoint synapses* that represent a combination of the two.

The part of a neuron that delivers impulses at a synapse is referred to as a *presynaptic terminal* and the part receiving them is called a *postsynaptic terminal.* The presynaptic part of a synapse is commonly an axon terminal. Here the end of an axon branch is expanded into an *end bulb* (or *end foot*), the shape of which is shown in Figure 14-14. The end bulb is, of course, bounded by axolemma, and the region of the axolemma that closely approaches the postsynaptic neuron at a synapse forms the *presynaptic membrane.* The region of cell membrane of the postsynaptic neuron closely associated with the presynaptic membrane is referred to as the *postsynaptic membrane.* Between the pre- and postsynaptic membranes, there is an intercellular space visible only with the EM and termed the *synaptic cleft* (see Fig. 14-16).

Synapses can be classified on the basis of their position on the postsynaptic neuron. Only the common types will be mentioned here. Where axons terminate on dendrites, they form what are termed *axodendritic* synapses (Fig. 14-14*A*; see also Fig. 14-17*B*). In some of these, the dendrite possesses little protrusions called *dendritic spines,* on or around which a terminal end bulb of the axon fits (Figs. 14-14*B* and 14-17*C*). Axon endings that terminate on the cell body of a neuron form what are termed *axosomatic* synapses (Figs. 14-14*A* and 14-17*D*). About half the total surface of the cell body of a neuron and almost all the surface of its dendrites may be involved in synaptic contact with other neurons. Axons that terminate on other axons form what are termed *axoaxonic* synapses (Fig. 14-14*C*). An axon can form a synapse with a second axon only at a region of the latter that is not myelinated. This situation is encountered in the *proximal segment* of an axon, because

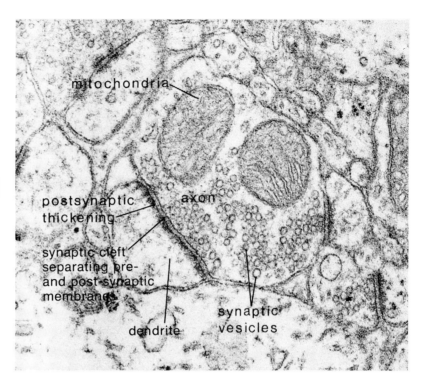

Fig. 14-15. Electron micrograph (×41,000) of asymmetrical synapses in occipital cortex of rat. (Courtesy of D. G. Jones)

here the axon remains naked since myelination does not begin right at the axon hillock but at a short distance from it. The *end bulb* regions of axons also lack myelin sheaths, so another way in which axoaxonic synapses can be formed is between terminal end bulbs of a presynaptic axon and those of a postsynaptic axon (Fig. 14-14C). There are also other anatomical sites and arrangements of synapses that will be described later in this chapter.

From electron micrographs it can be estimated that the synaptic cleft of a chemical synapse is 20 nm to 30 nm across. Presynaptic terminals that are axon end bulbs contain numerous mitochondria (an indication of their intense metabolic activity) and are characterized by a relative abundance of synaptic vesicles (Fig. 14-15). In most cases, the synaptic vesicles are spherical with a diameter of 40 nm to 50 nm. At some synapses, such vesicles appear flattened after glutaraldehyde fixation, and at others, the vesicles appear spherical with an electron-dense core. However, the shape of these vesicles is not always a reliable indication of the type of neurotransmitter that they contain.

Synapses Can Have an Asymmetrical or a Symmetrical Appearance. The type of synapse that is most often found between axon terminals and small dendrites or dendritic spines has an *asymmetrical* appearance (Gray and Guillery). Here the synaptic cleft is approximately 30 nm across, and it generally contains a plaquelike arrangement of slightly electron-dense material. Whereas only small aggregates of moderately electron-dense material are found on the cytoplasmic aspect of the presynaptic membrane, prominent aggregates of electron-dense material can be seen on the

cytoplasmic aspect of the postsynaptic membrane in this type of synapse (Fig. 14-15). This type of synapse accordingly appears asymmetrical in the EM.

Attached to the cytoplasmic aspect of the presynaptic membrane, there is a hexagonal array of conical electron-dense projections, approximately 60 nm in diameter, that extend into the axoplasm of the presynaptic terminal. Between these projections, there are spaces that are just wide enough to permit synaptic vesicles to establish contact and fuse with this membrane when nerve impulses arrive at the synapse. The synaptic cleft into which these vesicles release their content of neurotransmitter contains tissue fluid and little wisps of slightly electron-dense material (Fig. 14-16). Wispy filamentous structures can also sometimes be discerned traversing the cleft. EM markers such as horseradish peroxidase are able to penetrate the synaptic cleft, showing that it is a true intercellular space. Although there is no intervening basement membrane between the pre- and postsynaptic membranes at a neural synapse, a basement membrane is found in the equivalent position at a motor nerve ending, which represents a synapse between an axon and a skeletal muscle fiber. The prominent thickening that characterizes the postsynaptic membrane seems to represent a perforated plate of electron-dense granular material. Because the pre- and postsynaptic membranes tend to remain in intimate association with each other even after nervous tissue has been disrupted and fractionated, it appears that they are held together by some arrangement that serves the same purpose as do the desmosomes found between cells of other types.

There is a second type of synapse in which the synaptic cleft is slightly narrower (20 nm across) and the postsynaptic densities appear as more or less discrete patches that resemble the patches seen on the presynaptic membrane.

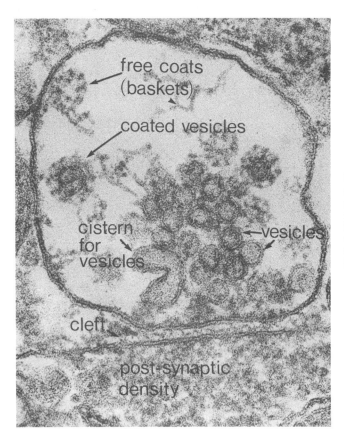

Fig. 14-16. Electron micrograph of a synapse in the cerebral cortex (rat). The synaptic vesicles fuse with the presynaptic membrane and release their contents of neurotransmitter. Coated vesicles subsequently arise from the membrane of the presynaptic terminal by endocytosis. The free coats fall off, leaving smooth vesicles that fuse with the collecting cisterna. Vesicles later bud from the cisterna and become reloaded with neurotransmitter. (Courtesy of P. Seeman)

This type of synapse is consequently described as having a *symmetrical* appearance (Gray and Guillery). Several other morphologically different types of chemical synapses have now been distinguished on the basis of the EM appearance of their synaptic vesicles, the width of their synaptic cleft, and the prominence of their synaptic densities, but their respective functional roles remain to be elucidated.

Neurotransmitter Release Can Result in Excitation or Inhibition. In the previous section on Nerve Impulses, we noted that the first phase of an action potential is the sudden influx of sodium ions from the intercellular fluid. This is because the arrival of the nerve impulse causes the *sodium channels* in the nerve cell membrane to open and then close, which is followed almost immediately by similar opening and closing of the *potassium channels*. The presynaptic membrane of synapses also possesses *calcium channels*, and these, too, open for a brief period when the action potential arrives. Prior to opening of the calcium channels, the negative charges on the inner side of the cell membrane (discussed above in connection with the resting potential) prevent the synaptic vesicles (also negatively charged on their external surface) from establishing contact with the presynaptic membrane. The local influx of calcium ions, however, reduces the negative charges to such an extent that a substantial number of these vesicles become able to make contact with the membrane, whereupon they

fuse with it and, by exocytosis, liberate their content of neurotransmitter molecules into the synaptic cleft. Exocytosis of neurosecretory granules, the contents of which are released by a similar mechanism, is illustrated in Figure 4-19.

Neurotransmitter molecules released into the synaptic cleft interact with the *neurotransmitter receptors* in the postsynaptic membrane and elicit an electrical response in this membrane also. At some synapses, the neurotransmitter acts to *depolarize* the postsynaptic membrane. These synapses are called *excitatory* because their activity promotes the firing of new impulses by the postsynaptic neuron. At other synapses, however, the neurotransmitter acts to *hyperpolarize* (*i.e.*, further polarize) the postsynaptic membrane. These synapses are called *inhibitory* because their activity reduces the chances of any new impulses being generated in the postsynaptic neuron. At any given moment, the factor that determines whether the postsynaptic neuron will generate any impulses of its own is the net balance (summation) of all the excitatory and inhibitory impulses it is receiving.

Excitatory neurotransmitters such as acetylcholine increase the ionic permeability of the postsynaptic membrane, opening up cation channels that admit *sodium ions*, whereas *inhibitory neurotransmitters* such as γ-aminobutyric acid (GABA) open up anion channels that admit *chloride* ions. At some inhibitory synapses, the postsynaptic membrane also becomes permeable to *potassium ions*, with the result that these begin to leave the postsynaptic terminal.

Synaptic Transmission Is Accompanied by Retrieval of the Excess Membranous Constituents. Synaptic activity can contribute significant amounts of extra membrane to the presynaptic terminal. Accumulation of excess synaptic membrane is avoided by a local recycling mechanism that retrieves this extra membranous component—and in the case of norepinephrine, excess neurotransmitter as well—and reutilizes such products in the formation of further synaptic vesicles. Superfluous synaptic membrane-derived constituents of the presynaptic membrane that reach its periphery by lateral diffusion are retrieved through endocytosis. The coated vesicles responsible for such endocytosis shed their basketlike polygonal frameworks and fuse with a presynaptic smooth-surfaced membranous cisterna from which new synaptic vesicles are subsequently formed (Fig. 14-16). Certain neurotransmitters (*e.g.,* acetylcholine) are synthesized locally within this presynaptic cisterna, utilizing precursors and enzymes that are synthesized in the cell body and then conveyed along the axon by axonal transport.

Synapses Can Be Chemical, Electrical, or a Mixture of the Two. Although impulses are mediated at most synapses by means of neurotransmitter substances (referred to as *neurochemical* transmission), there are some synapses at which direct electrical transmission of impulses (*neuroelectrical* transmission) occurs. Such synapses, which are called *electrical synapses,* have a symmetrical appearance and are characterized by a much narrower synaptic cleft, only 2 nm to 4 nm wide. Furthermore, because there is no delay in transmission caused by chemical mediation, neuroelectrical transmission is virtually instantaneous. In the EM, electrical synapses (which have been demonstrated in certain regions of the brain) have all the characteristics of *gap junctions* and, like them, permit free movement of ions between the pre- and postsynaptic terminals.

Certain other synapses contain some regions similar to gap junctions and other regions where there are wider synaptic clefts, together with associated synaptic vesicles on the presynaptic side and postsynaptic densities on the other. Such mixed synapses are sometimes referred to as *conjoint synapses,* and they apparently mediate impulses by both electrical and chemical means.

Other Kinds of Synaptic Arrangements Also Exist Between Neurons. The presynaptic terminal of a synapse is commonly an axonal end bulb, but this is not always the case. Other kinds of arrangements also exist, a number of which are illustrated in Figure 14-17. Thus *dendrodendritic* synapses (Fig. 14-17F) may be present between the dendrites of two neurons, as in the olfactory bulbs. These structures represent relay stations between the olfactory receptors of the nose and the olfactory area of the cerebral cortex, and they are concerned with the processing of neural information about smells. The presynaptic terminal of such synapses has synaptic vesicles associated with its synaptic membrane even though it represents part of a dendrite. In the olfactory bulbs, dendroden-

dritic synapses with opposing polarities and functions are arranged in reciprocal pairs, with an excitatory synapse positioned next to an inhibitory synapse that transmits inhibitory impulses between the same two dendrites, but in the reverse direction. Hence some of the complex neural activities that occur in the CNS involve the participation of microcircuits that incorporate reciprocal synapses between dendrites. Lastly, *dendrosomatic* synapses can exist between the dendritic spines of one neuron and the cell body of another (Fig. 14-17E), and electrical *soma-somatic* synapses can occur between the cell body of one neuron and that of another.

To What Extent Are New Synapses Formed in Adult Life? Mental activities employ neuronal circuits that are not necessarily immutable or permanent. This is known because long-established patterns of behavior can become modified in adult life. Also, cortex-based functions such as talking are sometimes regained after being lost through focal brain damage due to a *stroke* (*i.e.,* occlusion of a cerebral vessel by a thrombus). A number of neuronal circuits in the CNS are now known to be endowed with a substantial measure of functional adaptability. Such neuronal capacity for assuming other duties is described as *neuronal plasticity.*

Neuronal plasticity is believed to be a manifestation of functional substitution by components of other existing circuits. Any such major functional reorganization would almost certainly require the establishment of some new synaptic connections. Also, it has long been held (without much evidence) that some kind of structural change would occur in such connections during learning and the establishment of long-term memory. Certainly there is morphometric evidence to suggest that supernumerary synapses are formed during growth and development of the nervous system and that many unused synapses undergo subsequent degeneration. It has been suggested that any superfluous synapses that remain could contribute to new neural circuits, yet it seems unlikely that neuronal plasticity in adult life would depend on such a haphazard arrangement. The general picture that is emerging is that neuronal and synaptic loss as a result of aging or injury can, to some extent, be compensated for by the establishment of new circuits, a process that is manifested as neuronal plasticity and that probably entails the formation of appropriate new synapses.

Morphometric studies indicate that an almost constant synaptic density is maintained in the human frontal cortex throughout the greater part of adult life, with no evidence of any decline until after the age of 74 (Huttenlocher). Synaptic density becomes maximal at the age of 1 to 2 years and then gradually drops to its adult value. Similar studies of the rat parietal cortex indicate that although an almost constant synaptic density is maintained until late in life, the types of synapses that are present do not necessarily remain the same (Adams and Jones). The changes observed in their respective morphologies are considered to be further evidence of changing patterns of communication between the neurons of the CNS.

Regenerative Responses That Occur in the CNS Are Ineffective and Fail to Restore Function. If a peripheral nerve that has been severed is rejoined by means of sutures, axon sprouts grow from the proximal stump and along the rejoined nerve to the structure that was formerly innervated, whereupon they reestablish synaptic contact with the target cells. Both afferent and efferent fibers are able to do this, and the process involves specificity. The regenerating nerve fibers seem to be able to recognize appropriate target cells with which to reestablish contact.

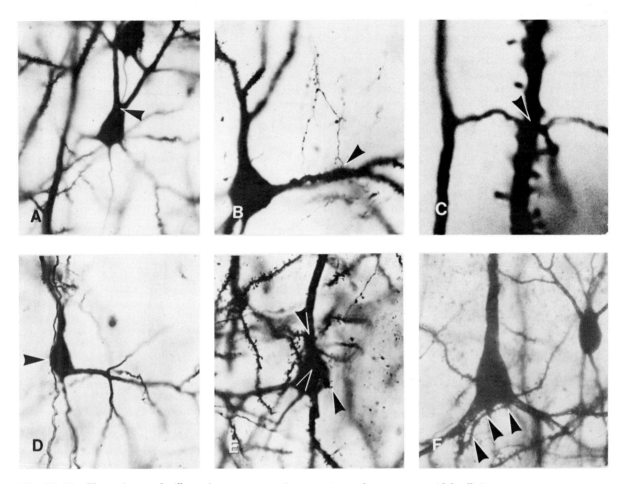

Fig. 14-17. Photomicrographs illustrating some synaptic arrangements between pyramidal cells in the cerebral cortex of a cat (modified Golgi stain). The arrows indicate (*A*) *axosomatic* synapse, between the *axon* of a neuron (cell body at *top center*) and the *cell body* of another neuron at center; (*B*) *axodendritic* synapse, between a terminal branch (*right of center*) of the *axon* of a neuron and a *dendrite* of another neuron whose cell body lies at bottom left; (*C*) *axodendritic* synapse, between a collateral branch (extending from *left* to *right* across middle of photomicrograph) of the *axon* (*left* border) of a neuron and a *dendritic spine* on a dendrite (*right of center*) of another neuron; (*D*) *axosomatic* synapse, between the *axon* (thin fiber running parallel to *left* border) of a neuron and the *cell body* of another neuron, with which it forms a *synapse en passant* (Fr., meaning in passing); (*E*) *dendrosomatic* synapses, between spines of a *dendrite* of a neuron whose cell body lies at top left and the *cell body* of the neuron at center; (*F*) *dendrodendritic* synapses between spines on a *dendrite* (which extends diagonally from *middle right* toward *bottom left*) and a major *dendritic* process that runs parallel to it and belongs to the neuron lying left of center. (Courtesy of E. G. Bertram)

Within the confines of the CNS of adult mammals, however, regeneration of nerve fibers is extremely limited and ineffective, although not nonexistent. One of the few places where it seems to occur is in the hypothalamohypophyseal tracts of neurosecretory fibers that extend into the posterior lobe of the pituitary from hypothalamic nuclei (see Fig. 22-9). Experimental studies in laboratory animals have shown that axon sprouts are able to grow for short distances across transections of the spinal cord, but such limited regeneration ceases after approximately 2 weeks and is not enough to restore lost functions. Hence the prognosis for injuries that involve the spinal cord is very poor.

A limitation of the CNS is that endoneurial sheaths lined by Schwann cells and their surrounding basement membrane, collectively believed to expedite nerve fiber regeneration in the PNS, are lacking. At present, there is a considerable amount of interest in the role played by the glial cell (or equivalent) microenvironment in promoting axonal regeneration. The importance of this influence is borne out by transplantation studies in which a segment of thoracic spinal cord was replaced by a segment of autologous sciatic nerve. These studies have shown fairly conclusively that axons in the CNS of rats and mice are capable of much more effective regeneration after they are provided with the specific microenvironment furnished by an engrafted segment of a peripheral nerve (Aguayo et al; Richardson et al). Recently, evidence has also been obtained that transplanted embryonic neurons may be able to establish functional connections in the CNS (Fine).

In many experimental studies on nerve fiber regeneration, it is difficult to distinguish nerve fiber regeneration and synaptic replacement (*i.e.*, the takeover of a former synaptic site) from collateral sprouting of intact fibers and the formation of new synapses (*i.e.*, synaptogenesis).

NEUROGLIA

Most parts of the body are supported by intercellular substances that are produced by connective tissue cells developing from mesoderm. However, the gray and the white matter of the CNS develop exclusively from ectoderm and, except for endothelial cells and pericytes of capillaries, lack connective tissue cells and fibers. The substance of the brain and spinal cord is therefore soft and mushy and requires the internal support provided by their neuroectoderm-derived *neuroglia.*

H & E sections fail to disclose that most neuroglia possess cytoplasmic processes that permeate the tissue of the CNS, binding it together and securing it to the capillaries that course through it. However, a unique way of staining nervous tissue was discovered by the Italian neurologist Camillo Golgi (who also discovered the Golgi apparatus), and this staining method has contributed a great deal to our knowledge of the form and supportive function of the neuroglial cell population in the CNS.

Forced by economic circumstances to assume the position of chief resident physician and surgeon at a hospital for incurable patients, Camillo Golgi decided to set up a rudimentary histology laboratory in his kitchen where he could work at night. There he made a useful discovery that revolutionized the study of nervous tissue. He had fixed some brain tissue in a solution of potassium bichromate and left it in this solution for a long time. He then soaked it in silver nitrate, whereupon metallic silver became deposited on some of the cells of the tissue, but not on all of them. Furthermore, the impregnated cells stood out clearly against an unstained background. By using thick sections, it became possible, with this technique, to demonstrate entire neurons (Fig. 14-17) and also the various types of neuroglia and the blood capillaries in this tissue (see Fig. 14-20).

Subsequently, the Spaniard Santiago Ramón y Cajal, who was destined to become the greatest neurohistologist of his time, saw the possibilities of Golgi's method, made some improvements in it, and systematically investigated the histology of nervous tissue.

Golgi preparations reveal that some neuroglia, of which only the nucleus can be seen in an H & E section, possess numerous processes that connect the various parts of neurons to capillaries (see Fig. 14-20). Furthermore, more refined impregnation methods and EM studies show that the neuropil is a conglomerate of cell bodies and processes of neuroglia and nerve fibers, which in the neuropil are mostly unmyelinated.

By using either silver or gold impregnation methods, Cajal and del Rio–Hortega (one of Cajal's pupils) were able to recognize the following three types of neuroglia: (1) *oligodendrocytes* (Gr. *oligos,* small; *dendron,* tree), so named because they are fairly small with treelike processes; (2) *astrocytes* (Gr. *astron,* star), which were given this name because they possess radiating processes and have a starlike appearance; and (3) cells of a third type that were called *microglia* because of their tiny size. There are also neuroglial cells of a fourth type known as *ependymal cells.* These four types of neuroglia will now be described in turn.

Oligodendrocytes

The cell bodies of oligodendrocytes are commonly found in rows between the myelinated fibers of white matter. Extending from the cell body of each cell, there is a relatively small number of fine cytoplasmic processes. The extremity of each process is spread out in the form of a thin sheet that is composed mainly of a double layer of cell membrane, and this sheet is wrapped many times around an axon in the form of a spiral. However, each process is able to wrap around a different fiber, so each oligodendrocyte wraps segments of several different fibers that lie in its vicinity (Fig. 14-18). The many double layers of cell membrane then become transformed into myelin and constitute an internodal segment of a *myelin sheath.* Thus oligodendrocytes have the same myelin-forming function as Schwann cells, which are the cells that myelinate nerve fibers in the PNS. The process of myelination will be described in further detail later in this chapter.

Three classes of oligodendrocytes are now recognized; they are described as *light, medium,* or *dark* (Mori and Leblond). Although these three kinds of cells are equally numerous in the very young, only the dark type is common in adults. It can be found both in white matter and in gray matter.

The light oligodendrocyte has abundant cytoplasm and a relatively large pale-staining nucleus with a large nucleolus (Fig. 14-19*B*). After a few weeks, it gradually transforms into a medium oligodendrocyte, which is intermediate in size and electron density between a light and a dark oligodendrocyte. A few weeks later, it transforms again into a dark oligodendrocyte, which is the last cell in the series. In the adult, dark oligodendrocytes appear as small cells that are approximately 10 μm to 20 μm in diameter with a dark-stained nucleus (Fig. 14-19*C*). The light type of oligodendrocyte is believed to play a major role in producing myelin sheaths. By the time the oligodendrocyte reaches the medium stage, these sheaths have probably already been formed. The dark type of oligodendrocyte remains connected to myelin sheaths by its processes and is probably responsible for maintaining the myelin.

Radioautographic studies indicate that even after growth is completed, light oligodendrocytes can arise from precursor or stem cells and then become medium and dark cells as just described. This process is believed to occur at a slow rate throughout life and to result in a slow turnover of the oligodendrocyte population. After oligodendrocytes start to myelinate axons, they do not divide. In the event

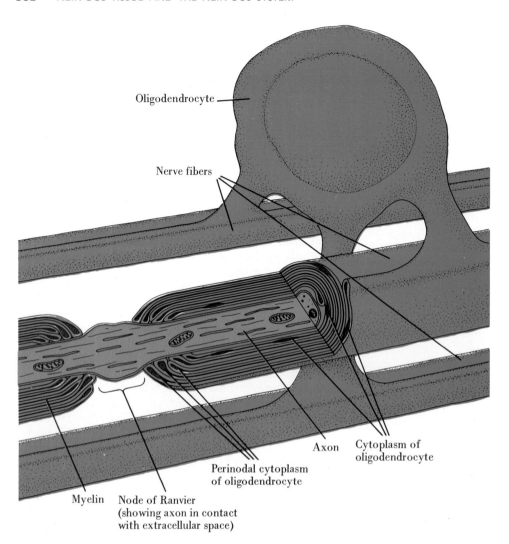

Oligodendrocyte

Nerve fibers

Axon   Cytoplasm of
oligodendrocyte

Perinodal cytoplasm
of oligodendrocyte

Myelin   Node of Ranvier
(showing axon in contact
with extracellular space)

Fig. 14-18.   Schematic diagram illustrating how oligodendrocytes are related to nerve fibers in white matter. Their wide, flattened processes wrap fibers with successive layers that become converted into myelin. Oligodendrocytes myelinate parts of more than one nerve fiber. The junction between the part of a fiber myelinated by the process of one oligodendrocyte and the part myelinated by the next oligodendrocyte is a node of Ranvier. (Bunge ML, Bunge RP, Ris H: J Biophys Biochem Cytol 10:67, 1961)

that augmented numbers of these cells are needed for re-myelination (*e.g.*, in demyelinating diseases), they have to be formed from precursors or stem cells.

Astrocytes

Astrocytes are star-shaped cells that stain fairly specifically with Cajal's gold chloride–sublimate method. On a yellow background, they then appear as dark stars due to staining of their radiating cytoplasmic processes. Some astrocytes are also stained in Golgi preparations (Fig. 14-20). A number of their processes are attached to capillaries (Fig. 14-20) whereas others adhere to neuronal cell bodies and nerve fibers. Astrocyte processes are characterized by ex-

panded tips called *astrocyte feet.* These feet comprise an almost complete sheath around capillaries (see Fig. 14-26) that is interrupted to only a minor extent by glial cells (or processes) of other kinds. Astrocyte feet are also applied to the basement membrane that lies between the CNS and its surrounding layer of loose connective tissue (pia mater).

There are two subtypes of astrocytes. *Fibrous astrocytes,* which are present mostly in white matter, have comparatively few cytoplasmic processes and these tend to be straight (Figs. 14-20 and 14-21, *inset*). *Protoplasmic astrocytes,* which are present mostly in gray matter, possess numerous processes that branch extensively and are relatively short. Astrocyte processes are supported by microtubules and are also strongly reinforced with bundles of interme-

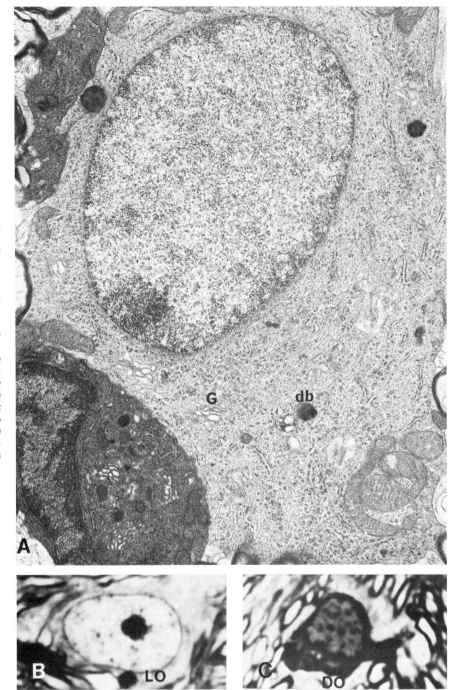

Fig. 14-19. (*A*) Electron micrograph (×15,000) of a *light oligodendrocyte* with a *dark oligodendrocyte* at lower left (rat brain). The light oligodendrocyte has cytoplasm rich in ribosomes and microtubules. A Golgi stack (*G*) and a lysosomal dense body (*db*) are indicated. The dark oligodendrocyte is small, shows densely staining cytoplasm, and has more condensed chromatin in its nucleus. Golgi saccules are prominent in its cytoplasm.

(*B* and *C*) Photomicrographs of (*B*) light oligodendrocyte and (*C*) dark oligodendrocyte (stained with toluidine blue). The light oligodendrocyte (*LO*) has a light nucleus and a prominent nucleolus; its ample cytoplasm is less pale. The dark oligodendrocyte (*DO*) shows large patches of dense chromatin in its nucleus, and its cytoplasm stains very deeply. (Courtesy of E. Ling, J. Paterson, and C. P. Leblond)

diate filaments (Fig. 14-21), the latter consisting of a distinctive protein called *glial fibrillary acidic protein* with some vimentin. Such filaments have not been found in oligodendrocytes. The microtubules and intermediate filaments that characterize astrocyte processes are believed to endow them with sufficient rigidity and tensile strength to brace the cell bodies and nerve fibers of neurons to the basement membranes that surround and support the blood vessels of the CNS.

In addition to their supportive function, it is widely believed that astrocytes play an important role in regulating the composition of the intercellular environment of the CNS. Thus there is evidence that they take up excess potassium ions when these escape from neurons during im-

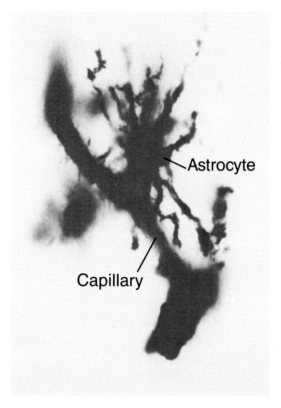

Fig. 14-20. Photomicrograph of an astrocyte adhering to a capillary (Golgi stain).

pulse conduction, and the close proximity of their processes to capillaries and to the spaces in and around the CNS that are filled with cerebrospinal fluid strongly suggests that they regulate the entry of substances into the interneuronal spaces. It is also widely believed that they take up any neurotransmitters that enter the interneuronal spaces, mediate exchanges of nutrients and metabolites between neurons and the blood, and provide metabolic intermediates for use by the neurons. Later in this chapter, we shall also mention some new findings that strongly implicate astrocytes in the induction and maintenance of the blood–brain barrier.

In the EM, the nucleus of an astrocyte appears large, ovoid, and pale staining and may exhibit surface irregularities caused by pressure from bundles of intermediate filaments. It commonly lies eccentrically in the cell. The cytoplasm contains free ribosomes and polysomes and a moderate number of threadlike mitochondria (Fig. 14-21). Besides the microtubules and intermediate filaments already mentioned, it is also generally possible to discern a few cisternae of rER, a Golgi complex, and a few lysosomes.

It is generally assumed that there is a slow renewal of the astrocyte population by new astrocytes forming from residual precursors or stem cells. Some new findings that

support this assumption are described in the following section.

Astrocytes Play a Role in Scar Formation in the CNS. When tissues and organs that have a connective tissue component recover from damage, their final stage of repair is commonly the formation of a fibrous scar; this is termed *fibrosis.* However, the CNS lacks a connective tissue component; hence when scar tissue is formed in the brain or spinal cord, it does not consist of collagen. Instead, glial cells react to the injury and proliferate to form the scar tissue, a process that is termed *gliosis.* The cells that form this scar tissue are variously described as *hypertrophied astrocytes* or *reactive astrocytes.* They are much larger than ordinary astrocytes and possess many long branched processes with prominent bundles of intermediate filaments (Fig. 14-22). They also contain more mitochondria, a more prominent sER, and more Golgi stacks than their ordinary counterparts. There is evidence that these cells also become phagocytic, so they may assist in clearing away the necrotic tissue from the space that they occupy.

Recent *in vitro* studies of cells of the mouse astrocyte lineage suggest that reactive astrocytes correspond to a type of cell that can be induced to differentiate *in vitro* from newborn mouse astroblasts (astrocyte precursors) by the addition of dibutyryl-cyclic AMP (Fedoroff et al). This, in turn, implies that astroblasts persist as a normal constituent of the CNS in postnatal life. Under normal conditions, it could be assumed that such precursors would give rise to normal astrocytes, whereas under pathological conditions, their response is evidently to give rise to reactive astrocytes.

Microglia

Microglia are small cells that are evenly distributed in gray and white matter. They are stained fairly specifically by the weak silver carbonate method of del Rio–Hortega, which stains their cell body and their relatively long angular processes (Fig. 14-23). In the EM, a small amount of rER and a fair number of lysosomes can generally be discerned in these cells.

Under normal conditions, microglia do not divide and they show little indication of motility or phagocytosis in adult life (Mato et al). Although the normal functions of such resting microglia have not been elucidated, it seems that cells of this description, sometimes referred to as *reactive microglia,* can transform into actively phagocytic *macrophages* in response to CNS damage. Such macrophages are believed to be the primary means by which necrotic tissue is cleared away prior to gliosis.

Are Microglia Related to Other Neuroglia or to Monocytes and Macrophages? The issue of how microglia originate has become a hotbed of controversy. Some investigators maintain that the first-formed microglia arise from neuroectoderm-derived progenitors of the CNS and not from cells that arrive by way of blood vessels that grow into the brain. For a discussion of the various lines of evidence on which this opinion is based, see Fujita et al. Other investigators have concluded that in postnatal life, microglia (or

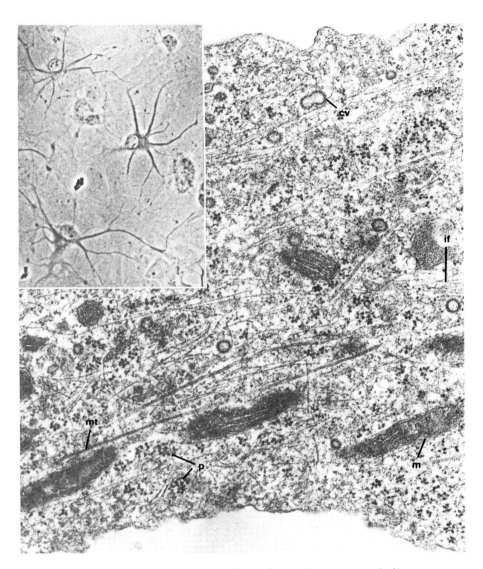

Fig. 14-21. Electron micrograph (×37,000) of part of a cytoplasmic process of a fibrous astrocyte grown *in vitro* (mouse). Mitochondria (*m*), microtubules (*mt*), intermediate filaments (*if*), and coated vesicles (*cv*) are easily recognized in its cytoplasm. Numerous polysomes (*p*) are also present. (*Inset*) Photomicrograph of three fibrous astrocytes growing in culture (mouse). (Fedoroff S, Neal J, Opas M, Kalnins VI: J Neurocytol 13:1, 1984)

reactive microglia) arise from monocytes that, in some cases, transform first into macrophages and then into microglia (Imamoto). Hence the possibility of a dual origin needs to be considered. Whichever interpretation is correct, it would appear that there is a strong morphological resemblance between (1) microglia of putative neuroectodermal origin and (2) transformed monocytes and macrophages of monocytic origin. It is not even clear whether microglia proliferating locally in response to CNS damage are monocyte-derived (Adrian and Schelper). Hence it could hardly be said that there is any general consensus at present on the origin and fate of microglia. Because there is a lack of conclusive evidence that the microglia present in adult life are derived from neuroectoderm, and they have no known supportive function, it is really only through convention that they continue be included with the neuroglia.

Ependymal Cells

The glial cells that line the ventricles of the brain and the central canal of the spinal cord are called *ependymal cells.* These cells constitute a simple lining epithelium known as the *ependyma.* They have basal processes and a cuboidal or low columnar shape, and on their free surface there are cilia and microvilli. Their intermediate filaments are of the vimentin type. Where ependymal cells cover the choroid plexuses, as described below, they constitute a specialized layer called the *choroid plexus epithelium.*

The only other parts of the CNS that remain to be described are its protective connective tissue wrappings and its distinctive central and surrounding fluid.

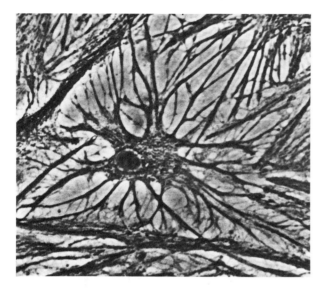

Fig. 14-22. Photomicrograph of a reactive astrocyte growing *in vitro* (mouse). This particular type of astrocyte, induced to differentiate *in vitro* by the addition of dibutyryl–cyclic AMP to the culture medium (see reference in caption for Fig. 14-21), resembles the large stellate cells seen at sites of brain trauma. Its distinctive features include its large size and its numerous long branched processes. (Courtesy of S. Fedoroff, J. Neal, M. Opas, and V. I. Kalnins)

MENINGES

The brain and spinal cord are well protected by the bony cranium and vertebral column, within which there are three connective tissue wrappings (Fig. 14-24). The innermost of these three layers, which are termed the *meninges* (Gr. pl. of *meninx*, membrane), is applied directly to the outer surface of the brain and spinal cord; it is called the *pia mater* (Figs. 14-24 and 14-25). The middle layer is known as the *arachnoid* (or *arachnoid membrane*), and the outermost layer is called the *dura mater* (Figs. 14-24 and 14-25).

Pia Mater (Pia). As indicated by its name (L. *pia*, tender; *mater*, mother), the innermost membrane is delicate. It contains interlacing bundles of collagen fibers and some fine elastic fibers, and it is covered with a continuous membrane of squamous cells that resembles the mesothelial lining of body cavities. The pia also contains a few fibroblasts and macrophages, and many blood vessels that are distributed by the pia over the surface of the brain (Fig. 14-24).

When blood vessels of the vascular pia penetrate the substance of the brain to supply its abundant capillaries, they carry with them a thin covering (*perivascular sheath*) of delicate loose connective tissue and also an investing sleeve of *pia*. Between the two, there is a narrow *perivascular space* that represents a continuation of the *subarachnoid space* and that is accordingly filled with cerebrospinal fluid.

The perivascular space disappears at the level of small arterioles and venules; hence there is no perivascular space around brain capillaries.

Arachnoid Membrane (Arachnoid). The middle layer of the meninges is termed the *arachnoid* (Gr. *arachnoeides*, cobweblike) because it is joined to the pia by a cobweblike network of delicate connective tissue trabeculae (Fig. 14-24). This layer includes a continuous roof over the pia and also a network of trabeculae that, like pillars, support this roof over the pia. The pia and arachnoid are sometimes described as a combined membrane, the *pia–arachnoid* or *leptomeninges*.

The arachnoid membrane and its trabeculae are composed chiefly of delicate collagen fibers, together with some elastic fibers. Both the outer and the inner surfaces of the membranous roof and the trabeculae are covered with a continuous lining of thin, flat lining cells similar to those covering the pia. Between the membranous roof of the arachnoid and the pia below, there is a space through which the arachnoid trabeculae extend. This space is filled with *cerebrospinal fluid* and is termed the *subarachnoid space* (Figs. 14-24 and 14-25).

The surface of the brain is extraordinarily convoluted. Whereas the pia extends down into the sulci and fissures to cover the surface of the brain intimately, the membranous part of the arachnoid (except in some larger fissures) does not. Hence over grooves, there is more accommodation for cerebrospinal fluid than at other sites. Indeed, there are sites, termed *cisternae*, where the brain surface lies at a considerable distance from the covering arachnoid so as to accommodate considerable amounts of cerebrospinal fluid.

Dura Mater (Dura). As its name suggests (L. *dura*, hard; *mater*, mother), this outermost membrane is of tough consistency and is made up of dense connective tissue. Its collagen fibers tend to run longitudinally in the spinal dura but more irregularly in the cranial dura. Some elastic fibers

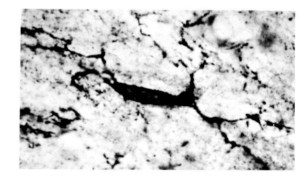

Fig. 14-23. Photomicrograph (oil immersion) of a microglial cell (stained by del Rio–Hortega's weak silver carbonate method). The nucleus and cytoplasm are deeply stained. A number of long, dark cytoplasmic processes extend out from the cell. (Courtesy of C. P. Leblond)

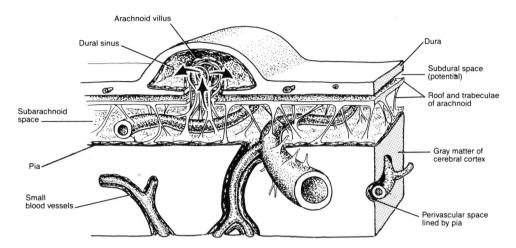

Fig. 14-24. Schematic diagram of the three connective tissue membranes (pia, arachnoid, and dura) comprising the meninges of the central nervous system. Cerebrospinal fluid is resorbed by way of the arachnoid villi projecting into the dural sinuses, as indicated by arrows. (After Weed)

are mixed with the collagen. There are certain differences between the dura of the vertebral canal and that of the cranium. In the vertebral canal, the dura consists of a relatively free dense connective tissue sheath. The potential space between its inner surface and the outer surface of the arachnoid is called the *subdural space* (Figs. 14-24 and 14-25), and it normally contains a slight amount of fluid that is *not* cerebrospinal fluid. The outer surface of the spinal dura abuts the *epidural (extradural) space* (Fig. 14-25), which is filled with loose connective tissue containing a variable amount of fat and many veins. The internal periosteum of the vertebrae, which lines the vertebral canal, forms the outer limit of the epidural space. The space between the arachnoid roof and pia, as noted, is called the *subarachnoid space* (Figs. 14-24 and 14-25).

In the cranium, there is no potential epidural space because here the dura is fused with the internal periosteum of the cranial bones.

Although the cranial dura is often described as having two layers, it is only the inner layer that forms the cranial dura that is continuous with the spinal dura in the vertebral canal. The so-called outer layer is not part of the dura but corresponds to the internal periosteum of the cranial bones. However, because these two layers adhere to each other, the cranial dura is also often described as being adherent to the skull. The dura is much less vascular than the periosteum.

Whereas the periosteum and cranial dura are adherent to each other over most of the brain surface, they are separate from each other along the lines where dural septa extend deep into brain fissures. Here there are blood-filled cavities between the origins of the dural reflections. Such cavities have a triangular cross section, bordered superficially by the cranial periosteum (the so-called outer layer of the dura) and laterally by the origins of the reflections of the cranial dura. Lined by endothelium and filled with venous blood, these spaces constitute the *venous sinuses* and *venous lacunae* of the dura mater that serve to drain blood from the brain.

BLOOD–BRAIN BARRIER

Before describing the composition of the special fluid that surrounds and protects the CNS and that occupies its various internal spaces, we shall briefly consider the composition and fate of the tissue fluid that is formed in the brain.

Cerebral Interstitial Fluid Has a Composition That Is Closely Regulated. The extent to which lipid-insoluble molecules or complexes (such as the antibiotic penicillin or albumin-bound trypan blue) gain access to brain and spinal cord tissue from the bloodstream is very limited indeed. However, this so-called *blood–brain barrier* is lacking in (1) the endocrine regions and appendages of the brain (the median eminence, pituitary, and pineal), (2) the main sites of production of cerebrospinal fluid (the choroid plexuses), and (3) the area postrema (the brain stem region where vomiting is triggered). One of the functions of the blood–brain barrier is to segregate the neurons of the CNS from blood-borne molecules that can act as neurotransmitters. Another is that it provides them with a substantial measure of protection against toxic drugs, bacterial toxins, and other harmful substances that may enter the bloodstream. Also, the presence of such a barrier helps to ensure that the composition of the interstitial fluid in the interneuronal spaces will remain virtually constant. A similar permeability barrier to polar molecules has been reported in the endoneurium of large peripheral nerves and also in the retina and iris. Wherever such a barrier exists, there are nevertheless specific transport mechanisms that ensure unrestricted access of essential metabolic substrates.

Investigations using horseradish peroxidase as an EM tracer have disclosed that in capillaries in which there is a blood–brain barrier, the entire perimeter of each endothelial cell is characterized by the presence of a highly developed *continuous tight junction* (zonula occludens) that is capable

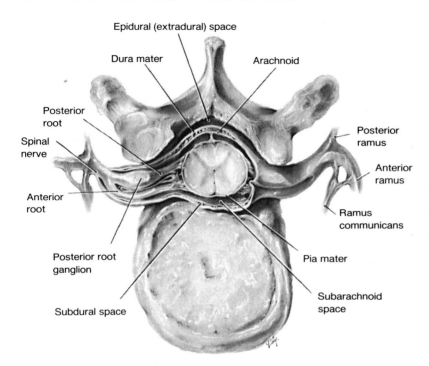

Epidural (extradural) space

Dura mater

Arachnoid

Posterior
root

Spinal
nerve

Posterior
ramus

Anterior
ramus

Anterior
root

Ramus
communicans

Posterior root
ganglion

Pia mater

Subdural space

Subarachnoid
space

Fig. 14-25. Diagrammatic drawing of a cross section of the vertebral column at the level of intervertebral foramina. It shows the anatomical relation of the meninges to the spinal cord and the way the PNS is connected to the CNS. Note the spinal (posterior or dorsal root) ganglion containing the cell bodies of afferent neurons.

of impeding passage of the marker from the lumen of the vessel into the surrounding brain tissue (Reese and Karnovsky). Complementary studies have shown that if the macromolecular tracer is injected into the cerebrospinal fluid in a brain ventricle, the tracer passes freely between the ependymal cells that line the ventricle and enters the interstitial spaces of the brain, whereupon it permeates the gaps between astrocyte feet and reaches the basement membrane around brain capillaries (Brightman and Reese). These results clearly indicate that the morphological basis of the blood–brain barrier is the continuous tight junctions that seal the clefts between contiguous endothelial cells, and not the glial sheath that invests the capillary. Any substances that leave or gain access to the capillaries in most parts of the CNS must therefore do so by passing through and not between the endothelial cells. The capillaries in regions in which there is a blood–brain barrier are further characterized by minimal transfer of substances across their endothelial cells by endocytosis. Their basement membrane is relatively thick (Fig. 14-26), and its outer surface is densely covered with glial processes, almost 90% of which are astrocyte feet.

The fact that astrocyte feet are always found in close association with the endothelial cells that maintain the permeability barrier suggests that astrocytes, too, may have a role to play in maintenance of the blood–brain barrier. The likelihood that these cells have a regulatory role in inducing the barrier characteristics of CNS capillary endothelium is substantiated by the following findings.

Transplantation studies in quail-chick chimeras have shown that

when non-neural chick mesenteric vessels are allowed to grow into transplanted fragments of unvascularized embryonic quail brain, they acquire structural and functional barrier characteristics. Conversely, when chick brain vessels are allowed to grow into transplanted fragments of non-neural unvascularized embryonic quail somite, the brain-derived vessels fail to develop their usual barrier characteristics (Stewart and Wiley). Furthermore, in the course of normal development, the time at which barrier characteristics are acquired coincides with the time at which the perivascular glial sheath first appears. Also, this sheath is either absent or slightly separated from brain capillaries at sites in the CNS where the blood–brain barrier does not exist. For further information, see Stewart and Coomber.

Interstitial Fluid Formed Within the CNS Contributes to Cerebrospinal Fluid. As in any other vascularized tissue, some tissue fluid is formed by brain capillaries. However, *the CNS is not provided with lymphatics.* Instead of draining into lymphatics, the excess tissue fluid moves through the network of intercellular channels and leaves the brain by way of the perivascular spaces that accompany its vasculature and also directly from its outer and inner surfaces, thereby entering the subarachnoid space and brain ventricles. This fluid serves as an auxiliary source of cerebrospinal fluid, contributing approximately 10% to 20% of its total volume.

CEREBROSPINAL FLUID

In addition to being protected by the skull, the vertebral column, and the meninges, the CNS is cushioned by its

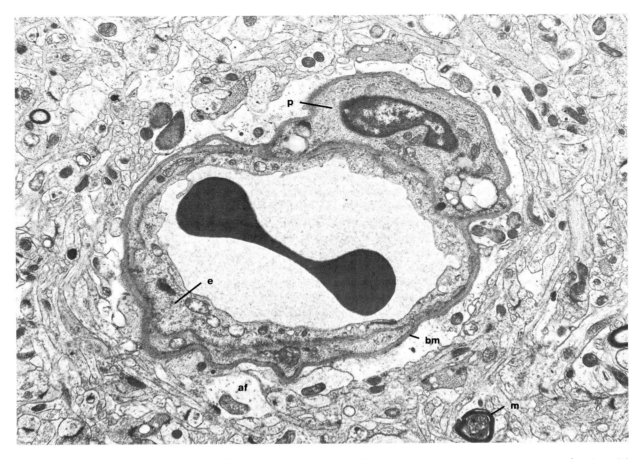

Fig. 14-26.   Electron micrograph of a capillary in human cerebral cortex. An associated pericyte (*p*) also lies enclosed within its thick basement membrane (*bm*). The pale-staining structures covering most of its external surface are astrocyte feet (*af*). Its endothelial lining (*e*) and the erythrocyte within its lumen are also easily recognized. Surrounding the capillary there is neuropil; this contains unmyelinated nerve fibers, a few myelinated axons (*m*), and glial cell processes. (Courtesy of J. Bilbao and D. McComb)

own hydraulic shock absorber. *Cerebrospinal fluid* (CSF), the cushioning fluid of the CNS, fills the brain ventricles, the subarachnoid space, and the remains of the central canal of the spinal cord. The CSF in the brain ventricles communicates with the CSF in the subarachnoid space through three openings in the roof of the fourth ventricle. These three openings allow the CSF to flow into the subarachnoid space.

CSF is a clear, colorless fluid that normally contains only a low concentration of protein (20 mg to 30 mg per 100 ml). It also contains few cells (about 5 cells per cubic millimeter), most of which are lymphocytes. Microscopic observation of CSF can be a valuable aid to diagnosis. For example, the presence of erythrocytes in CSF can confirm that there has been hemorrhage caused by a skull fracture, and an increased number of leukocytes in CSF can indicate inflammation of the brain or meninges.

Cerebrospinal Fluid Is Formed Mostly by the Choroid Plexuses.   Although some CSF exudes from the external

and internal surfaces of the brain, about 80% is formed in the brain ventricles by the *choroid plexuses,* which are little tufted vascular structures that project into the brain ventricles. The capillaries in these plexuses are fenestrated, and they lie close to the luminal surface (Fig. 14-27). The choroid plexuses are covered by a simple cuboidal epithelium known as the *choroid plexus epithelium* through which the capillary filtrate has to pass to enter a ventricle (Fig. 14-27). This epithelium possesses distinctive ion transport mechanisms (*e.g.,* for Na^+) that enable it to modify the filtrate, with the result that there are characteristic differences between the individual ion concentrations of CSF and ordinary tissue fluid.

Another function of this epithelium is to maintain a permeability barrier between CSF and the interstitial spaces of the choroid plexuses. This barrier is due to the presence of highly developed, continuous tight junctions (zonula occludens junctions) that form an intercellular seal between the epithelial cells at the luminal end of their lateral borders.

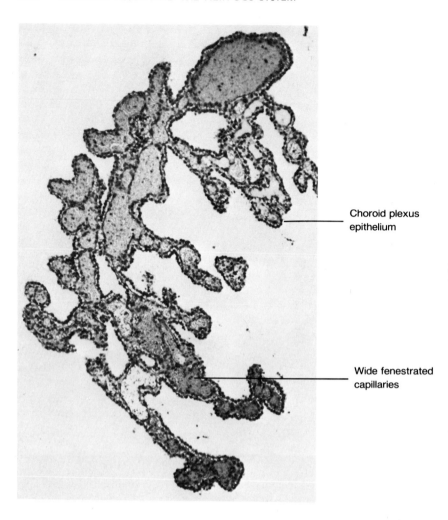

Choroid plexus
epithelium

Wide fenestrated
capillaries

Fig. 14-27. Photomicrograph of a portion of a choroid plexus. These structures elaborate cerebrospinal fluid into the brain ventricles.

It is often described as the *blood–CSF barrier* of the choroid plexuses because the fenestrations in the plexus capillaries are permeable to plasma proteins and other macromolecules, but the protein concentration of CSF is remarkably low. Hence the macromolecules leaving the blood are able to reach the interstitial spaces in the choroid plexuses, but the tight junctions between the covering epithelial cells impede the escape of such molecules into the CSF.

The best way to understand the morphology of the choroid plexuses is to consider how they develop. The part of the neural tube that forms the roof of the third and fourth ventricles becomes very thin, consisting of no more than the single layer of cuboidal cells that comprises the ependyma plus the vascular pia–arachnoid (leptomeninges) that covers it. In these sites, the pia–arachnoid, carrying the ependyma ahead of it, invaginates into the ventricles to form choroid plexuses. A similar process results in the development of choroid plexuses in the lateral ventricles. In this way, four choroid plexuses are formed: one in each lateral ventricle, one in the third, and one in the fourth.

A choroid plexus is made up of many leaflike processes, each of which is supplied by a small artery or arteriole that opens into a tortuous plexus of fenestrated capillaries. Each process is raised into small surface elevations called villi. The choroid plexus epithelium on its free surface is derived from the ependyma. In the EM, the cuboidal cells of this epithelium can be seen to have abundant microvilli on their luminal surface (Fig. 14-28). Their high content of mitochondria (Fig. 14-28) reflects their substantial energy expenditure in pumping ions across their cell membrane. Degenerative changes such as calcium deposition and cyst formation are common in the plexuses of the lateral ventricles.

Cerebrospinal Fluid Enters the Cerebral and Spinal Subarachnoid Space. The CSF produced in the lateral ventricles circulates through the interventricular foramina and, together with that produced in the third ventricle, passes through the cerebral aqueduct of the midbrain to the fourth ventricle, whereupon it leaves the brain by way of the openings in the roof of the fourth ventricle and enters the subarachnoid space. Most of the CSF surrounding the brain and spinal cord is formed within the brain, so that if outflow by way of the roof of the fourth ventricle is

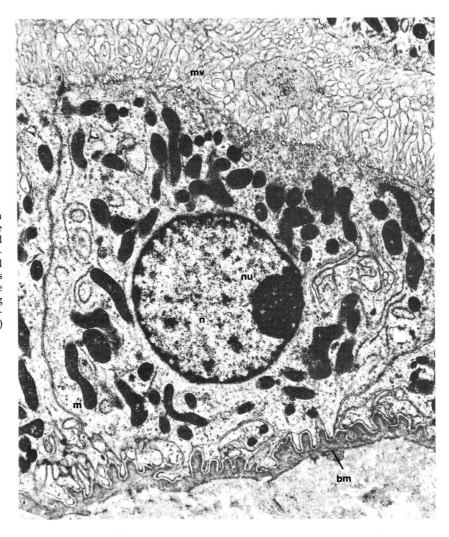

Fig. 14-28. Electron micrograph of a human choroid plexus epithelial cell. The luminal surface of this modified cuboidal epithelium is covered with abundant microvilli (*mv*). The cell possesses a spherical nucleus (*n*) with a prominent nucleolus (*nu*), and it contans a relatively large number of mitochondria. The underlying basement membrane (*bm*) is well developed. (Courtesy of J. Bilbao and S. Briggs)

blocked, CSF accumulates in the ventricles and expands them, stretching the brain from within. This can occur as a result of disease or deformity, and the condition is called *obstructive* (*noncommunicating*) *hydrocephalus*.

Cerebrospinal Fluid Is Resorbed Mostly Through Arachnoid Villi. CSF is normally resorbed into the bloodstream at the same rate at which it is being produced. Most of this resorption occurs via structures known as *arachnoid villi*, which are small villous projections of the arachnoid into venous sinuses of the dura mater, primarily the superior sagittal and lateral sinuses. The CSF present in the core of an arachnoid villus is separated from the blood in a sinus only by the thin cellular covering of the villus and the thin endothelial lining of the sinus (Fig. 14-24). Because of the lower hydrostatic pressure and higher osmotic pressure of venous blood relative to CSF, and also because of active transport mechanisms, CSF passes through the intervening cells and enters the venous blood in the sinus. As already noted, there are no lymphatics within the CNS itself to drain off excess fluid. However, some CSF is believed to be drained by way of lymphatics associated with the epidural connective tissue and the connective tissue sheaths around the cranial and spinal nerve roots. For further information, see Bradbury and Cserr.

THE PERIPHERAL NERVOUS SYSTEM

The *peripheral nervous system* (PNS) is made up of the following three types of components:

1. *Ganglia.* These are small nodules that contain the cell bodies of neurons. The ganglia of the PNS are (1) the *cranial* and *spinal ganglia*, which contain cell bodies of afferent neurons (see Figs. 14-25 and 14-31); and (2) the *autonomic ganglia*, which contain cell bodies of

efferent neurons of the autonomic nervous system (see Fig. 14-43).

2. *Nerves.* These are branching cordlike structures that extend from the brain as *cranial nerves* and from the spinal cord as *spinal nerves.* Nerves incorporate many nerve fibers, commonly both afferent and efferent. Large nerves are sometimes referred to as *nerve trunks.*

3. *Nerve Endings and Organs of Special Sense.* The various kinds of *afferent* (sensory) nerve endings, particularly those that are present in the organs of special sense, are easier to study after the organs or structures with which they are associated have been described. These endings are therefore considered in the chapters of this text that describe the parts of the body with which they are associated. All *efferent* fibers end in association with glandular cells, adipocytes, or muscle cells. The efferent nerve endings on secretory cells of exocrine glands are described at the end of this chapter; efferent and afferent nerve endings in muscle will be dealt with in Chapter 15.

This outline of the components of the PNS provides the basis for completing the classification of nervous tissue shown in Table 14-1.

DEVELOPMENT OF THE PERIPHERAL NERVOUS SYSTEM

The afferent and efferent components of the PNS develop from different sources. The afferent components will be considered first.

Afferent Neurons and Their Associated Supporting Cells. The neural plate gives rise to the neural tube and neural crest, as was outlined in Chapter 5 (see Fig. 5-3). The neural crest then gives rise to the spinal or posterior (dorsal) root ganglia of the spinal cord and also contributes to their cranial counterparts, the cranial ganglia. Each body segment develops bilateral spinal ganglia that are situated posterolaterally with respect to the spinal cord (Fig. 14-25). The neuroectodermal cells in the developing spinal ganglia follow two lines of differentiation. Some produce neurons that are initially bipolar but become pseudounipolar when their two processes fuse (Fig. 14-1B). Their single process branches at a

Table 14-1   Composition of Nervous Tissue

Part of Nervous System	Components
CNS	Gray matter White matter

PNS	Ganglia
	Nerves
	Nerve endings
	    Afferent
	    Efferent

T-shaped junction, and one of its branches grows in an axial direction into the spinal cord. Enclosed with the other nerve fibers in a nerve trunk, their other branch grows in a peripheral direction and eventually reaches a target tissue, where it terminates as afferent nerve endings (Fig. 14-29; see also Fig. 14-31).

Some of the neuroectodermal cells in the developing spinal ganglia differentiate along a second pathway that produces supporting cells. These cells represent the PNS counterparts of neuroglial cells, and they are of two main types: *capsule (satellite) cells,* which form cellular capsules around the cell bodies of the ganglion cells; and *Schwann (neurolemmal) cells,* which form cellular sheaths around the axons (see Fig. 14-30).

Efferent Neurons. These neurons arise from the middle layers of the neural tube. The axon of each efferent neuron then grows from an anterolateral aspect of the spinal cord as an efferent fiber in a peripheral nerve. The efferent fibers of the cranial nerves develop in a similar manner. Such axons leave the confines of the CNS by way of foramina (Fig. 14-25) and extend into nerve trunks (Fig. 14-29) that distribute them to the structures they innervate.

When we deal with the autonomic nervous system, we shall find that it consists *only of efferent neurons.* Whereas the cell bodies of some of these neurons lie in the brain and spinal cord, the cell bodies of others are scattered throughout the body in *autonomic ganglia.* The cell bodies in these ganglia therefore lie outside the confines of the CNS. They develop from neuroectoderm-derived neural crest cells that migrate to these sites early in development.

SPINAL GANGLIA

The bodies of nerve cells here are extremely rounded. Many of them are large—as much as 120 μm in diameter (Fig. 14-30)—but some are small (15 μm). Their central nucleus is large and pale staining, and it commonly contains a single prominent nucleolus (Fig. 14-30). Their cytoplasm contains basophilic Nissl bodies that are characteristically more dispersed than in anterior horn cells. Accumulations of the yellow-brown pigment lipofuscin may be present in the cytoplasm (see Fig. 4-42). Each of the rounded cell bodies of ganglion cells is separated from the connective tissue framework of a ganglion by a single layer of flattened *capsule cells* or *satellite cells* (Fig. 14-30), which are derived from neuroectoderm; as noted, these are the PNS counterparts of the neuroglia of the CNS.

The proximal process of each ganglion cell approaches the bundle of fibers in the posterior root, where it divides, as noted, into two branches. One branch passes into the spinal nerve, which conducts it to a receptor ending (Fig. 14-31). The other branch passes inward by way of the posterior root to reach the posterior column of gray matter on that side of the cord (Fig. 14-31). Both branches have the appearance of axons and both are commonly myelinated. The connective tissue in which the ganglion cells and their processes lie is the counterpart of the connective tissue sheath of nerves, which will be described in the following section.

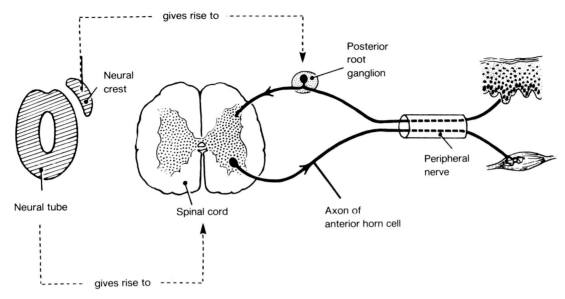

Fig. 14-29. Diagram illustrating the development of the PNS. The neural crest gives rise to posterior root ganglion cells. Processes from each of these grow peripherally and centrally; hence the neural crests give rise to the afferent components of the PNS. The efferent components of the PNS develop from the neural tube by means of axons from anterior horn cells growing out from the developing spinal cord.

PERIPHERAL NERVES

Unlike the CNS, peripheral nerves are fairly strong and resilient. This is because they contain a series of *connective tissue sheaths* of decreasing order of magnitude that consecutively enclose their nerve fibers. Thus an outer fibrous sheath called the *epineurium* (Gr. *epi*, upon) invests a moderate- to large-sized nerve, surrounding the nerve as a whole (Fig. 14-31). Internal to this, a fairly prominent sheath termed the *perineurium* (Gr. *peri*, around) surrounds each *fascicle* (L. *fasciculus*, bundle) of nerve fibers (Fig. 14-31). Then, within a fascicle, a delicate sheath of vascular

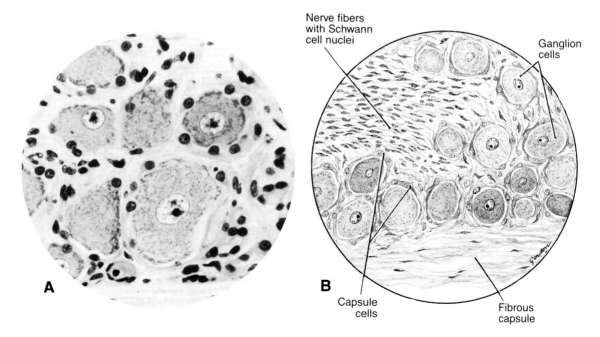

Fig. 14-30. Photomicrograph of part of a spinal ganglion (*A*), with interpretive drawing (*B*).

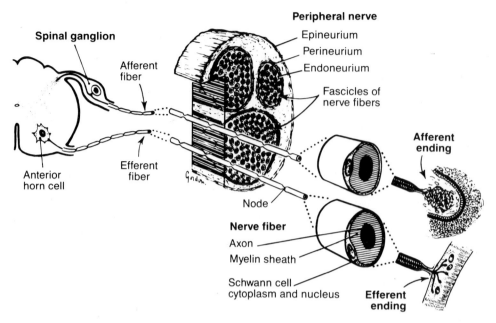

Fig. 14-31. Schematic representation of the organization of the peripheral nervous system.

loose connective tissue known as the *endoneurium* (Gr. *endon*, within) invests each individual nerve fiber (Fig. 14-31). Small peripheral nerves lack an epineurium, possessing only perineurium and endoneurium (see Fig. 14-36). In large peripheral nerves made up of a number of fascicles (as in Fig. 14-31), the fascicles are bound together by inward extensions of the epineurium.

The same three orders of connective tissue wrappings (epi-, peri-, and endoneurial) are found in the cranial and spinal ganglia.

Within its endoneurial sheath, each nerve fiber is intimately invested by a segmented cellular sheath called the *sheath of Schwann* or *neurolemma* (*neurilemma*). This sheath is made up of individual *Schwann cells,* which are neuroglial counterparts derived from neural crest neuroectoderm. In each segment of a *myelinated fiber,* it is possible to distinguish two parts of the Schwann cell sheath even at the LM level: (1) a thin outer layer of *Schwann cell cytoplasm* that contains the cell nucleus, and (2) a thicker inner region that is part of the *myelin sheath* and that represents the myelin made by that particular Schwann cell (Fig. 14-31). All the myelin in the PNS is produced by Schwann cells. However, no Schwann cell can myelinate more than one segment of a single axon, so the myelination of an entire axon requires the participation of a long string of these cells.

As in the CNS, the myelin sheath is interrupted at *nodes of Ranvier* (Fig. 14-31). These nodes are situated between consecutive Schwann cells, and they represent the only branch points in myelinated axons. At each node, the axolemma is exposed to tissue fluid instead of being covered by myelin. However, as may be seen in Figure 14-37, cy-toplasmic processes of neighboring Schwann cells interdigitate at the nodes and some lie fairly closely apposed to the axolemma. A basement membrane surrounds the sheath of Schwann and extends in a continuous manner across each node from one Schwann cell to the next. There is one Schwann cell between consecutive nodes; the distance between consecutive nodes varies from 0.3 mm to 1.5 mm. As noted, nodes are also present in the CNS, but in the CNS, the myelin is produced by oligodendrocytes and no basement membrane is present external to the myelin-forming cells. The role of the nodes in saltatory conduction was described earlier in this chapter, in the section on Nerve Impulses.

Myelin of the PNS Is Derived from Compacted Schwann Cell Membrane. In myelinating an axon, a Schwann cell first enfolds the axon in a groove in its cytoplasm (Fig. 14-32A). It is generally believed that the Schwann cell, or some part of it, then begins to rotate around the axon (Fig. 14-32B). The cell winds around the axon (Fig. 14-32B) until many layers of Schwann cell membrane become built up into a tight spiral (Fig. 14-32C). The cytoplasm initially present between the closely apposed areas of cell membrane is squeezed back mainly into the outer region of the Schwann cell (Fig. 14-32C), with the result that the apposed regions of cell membrane come into contact with each other and fuse. As a consequence, a cross section of the myelin sheath exhibits a highly characteristic pattern of parallel, intensely electron-dense lines (Fig. 14-33). In the PNS, this pattern represents a succession of double thicknesses of compacted Schwann cell membrane.

At high magnification, the myelin sheath shows an al-

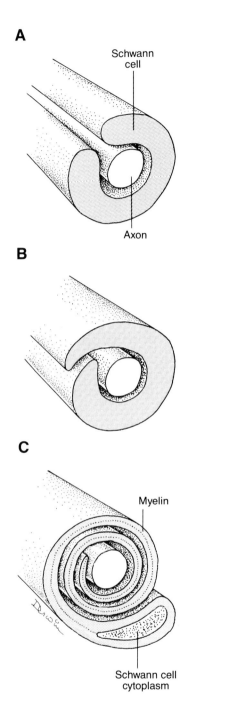

A

Schwann
cell

Axon

B

C

Myelin

Schwann cell
cytoplasm

Fig. 14-32. Diagrammatic representation of three consecutive stages in the myelination of a segment of an axon by a Schwann cell in the peripheral nervous system. See text for details.

ternating pattern of (1) electron-dense *major dense lines* (Fig. 14-33*B*) and (2) lighter stained *intraperiod lines*. The major dense lines indicate where the cytoplasmic surface of the cell membrane has come together, fused, and compacted, whereas the intraperiod lines indicate where the

outer (external) surface of the cell membrane has come into close apposition or fused (Fig. 14-33*B*). The few proteins that are present in myelin are associated with both kinds of electron-dense lines. For further information, see Morell and Norton.

It is still unclear whether the entire cell body of the Schwann cell needs to rotate around the axon for myelination to occur in the PNS. In the CNS, this is clearly not the case because it would be impossible for the cell body of an oligodendrocyte to wind around a number of different axons at the same time (Fig. 14-18). This implies that in the CNS, it is possible for the leading edge of the double thickness of compacting oligodendrocyte cell membrane to grow *under* the myelin that has already formed. It is not known whether the same mechanism applies in the PNS or whether the Schwann cell rotates around the axon, leaving a double thickness of compacting cell membrane behind. A third possibility is that both of these mechanisms could apply in the PNS.

Small channels of cytoplasm that remain in direct communication with the cell body of the Schwann cell are found in the myelin of peripheral nerves. Such discontinuities in the myelin are known as *clefts of Schmidt–Lanterman* (see Fig. 14-37). One idea is that they are not fixed in position and that they provide the Schwann cell with access to the cytoplasmic face of its myelin, facilitating the replacement of macromolecular constituents as necessary to maintain the myelin sheath in good repair. Finally, as in the CNS, myelination in the PNS continues after birth and is rendered necessary by growth of the body.

Microscopic Appearance of Peripheral Nerves. In the preparation of routine H & E sections, the lipid in the myelin surrounding individual nerve fibers, unless specially treated, dissolves away in the dehydrating and clearing agents. Hence cross sections of nerves show the site previously occupied by myelin as little rounded spaces, empty except for the nerve fiber, which may be situated toward one side of the space (see Fig. 14-35*A*). Pale-staining Schwann cell cytoplasm is seen on the outer surface of the myelin space. The nuclei within a nerve bundle belong to Schwann cells, fibroblasts of the endoneurium, or endothelial cells of capillaries (also of the endoneurium). In an osmic acid–stained preparation, the myelin surrounding the nerve fiber is preserved and stains black so that the myelin sheaths appear as blackened rings (Figs. 14-34 and 14-35*B*).

Small peripheral nerves that have been cut in longitudinal or oblique section exhibit a characteristic wavy appearance that is accentuated by waviness of the nuclei of their Schwann cells (Fig. 14-36). This is a feature that enables fascicles of small peripheral nerves to be distinguished from bundles of smooth muscle fibers (compare Fig. 14-36 with Fig. 15-32).

In the EM, a narrow *periaxonal space* (15 nm to 20 nm wide) can be discerned between the axolemma of a myelinated axon and the apposed cell membrane of an investing Schwann cell (Fig. 14-37). Bordering on this part

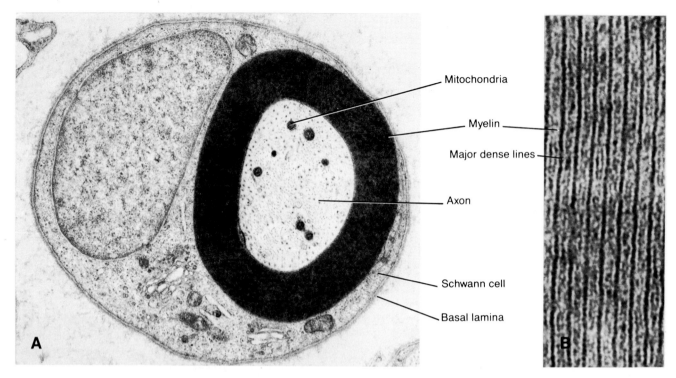

Mitochondria

Myelin

Major dense lines

Axon

Schwann cell

Basal lamina

Fig. 14-33. (*A*) Electron micrograph of a myelinated axon and Schwann cell of peripheral nerve. (*B*) Transverse section of myelin sheath, showing its regular pattern of parallel electron-dense lines under higher magnification. Between the major dense lines, intraperiod lines (double at some sites) can be discerned. (*A*, courtesy of J. Bilbao and S. Briggs; *B*, courtesy of M. Nagai and A. Howatson)

Endoneurium

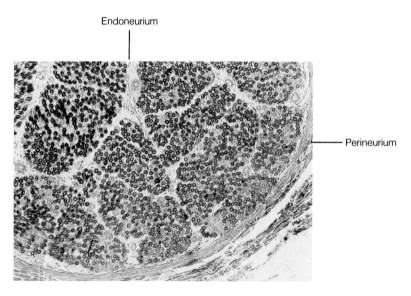

Perineurium

Fig. 14-34. Photomicrograph of a peripheral nerve (stained with osmic acid). Note the substantial perineurium surrounding the fascicle of myelinated nerve fibers, the myelin sheaths of which are stained black. The delicate loose connective tissue constituting the endoneurium can also be seen. (Courtesy of C. P. Leblond)

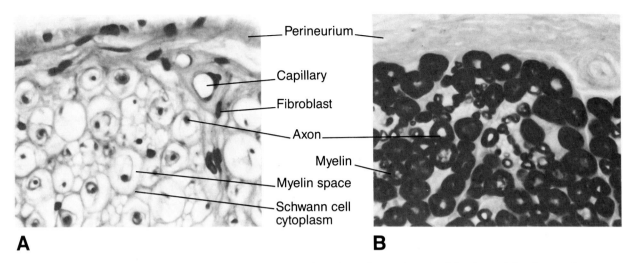

Fig. 14-35. Photomicrograph of myelinated axons in a fascicle of a peripheral nerve (transverse section) (*A*) stained with H & E and (*B*) stained with osmic acid.

of the Schwann cell membrane is a thin *inner layer of Schwann cell cytoplasm*. External to this, layers of compacted Schwann cell membrane constitute the *myelin sheath* (Fig. 14-37). External to the myelin sheath is the bulk of the *Schwann cell cytoplasm* (Fig. 14-37), which is bounded on its outer surface by the cell membrane and the *basement membrane* of the Schwann cell. The periaxonal space is partially sealed from the perinodal extracellular space, facilitating the saltatory conduction of nerve impulses (described earlier in this chapter). The morphological basis of the partial seal is described in the following section.

In the so-called *paranodal region* on each side of a node, there is a series of lateral marginal distensions of the Schwann cell that are commonly described as *paranodal loops* (Fig. 14-37). These loops constitute a longitudinal series because each layer of myelin

that forms in the sheath is slightly longer than the previous one, with the result that its lateral margins overhang those of the previous layer. Within these loops, there is a small amount of cytoplasm. Moreover, their cell membrane is connected to the axolemma by a number of evenly spaced septa that spiral around the axon. The same arrangement of paranodal loops and spiral septa is found between axons and oligodendrocyte processes of the CNS. The periaxonal space under the paranodal loops is reduced to 2 nm to 4 nm, and it is bridged by the three to six spiral septa on each paranodal loop. However, the use of EM tracers has shown that macromolecules (and therefore small molecules as well) are able to penetrate the periaxonal space under the loops, provided that sufficient time is allowed for penetration. Hence the septa do not constitute a typical "all or nothing" occluding junction.

Recent freeze-fracture studies indicate that the spiral septa constitute a fairly uniform annulus at the site of the paranodal loop. It has been suggested that they could be composite structures

Fig. 14-36. Photomicrograph of fascicle of a small peripheral nerve (longitudinal section). Most of the wavy nuclei belong to Schwann cells.

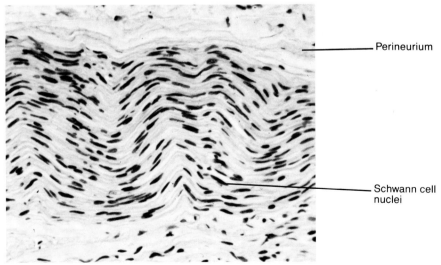

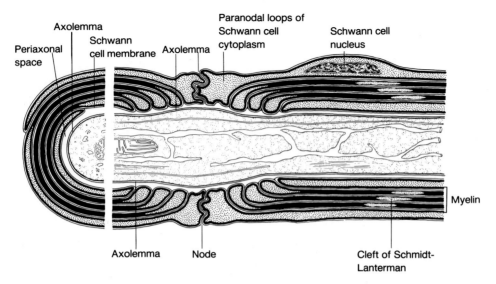

Fig. 14-37. Diagram illustrating the fine structure of a myelinated nerve fiber of a peripheral nerve in cross section (*left*) and longitudinal section (*right*). Surrounding the fiber is a sheath of Schwann, with a node of Ranvier. Between the axolemma and the Schwann cell membrane there is a periaxonal space. At the nodes, the processes of the neighboring Schwann cells interdigitate but do not seal the axolemma from intercellular space. Most of the Schwann cell cytoplasm lies external to the myelin. Clefts of Schmidt–Lanterman consist of pockets of Schwann cell cytoplasm trapped within the myelin. (Courtesy of C. P. Leblond)

consisting of integral membrane proteins of both the investing myelinating cell (oligodendrocyte or Schwann cell) and the axolemma (Ellisman et al). The paranodal junction may represent a unique type of arrangement that is capable of serving two purposes. First, it seems to constitute a partial seal between the internodal periaxonal space and the perinodal extracellular space; in other words, it creates sufficient impedance to make it easier for the high-speed currents associated with action potentials to jump from node to node than to flow from node to internode (Rosenbluth). Second, its unique construction would allow other slower but necessary exchanges to occur between the tissue fluid in the periaxonal space and the surrounding tissue fluid.

Unmyelinated Nerve Fibers. Certain afferent and autonomic nerve fibers possess no myelin sheath. They are nevertheless supported and protected by Schwann cells because a Schwann cell can accommodate one (Fig. 14-13) or a number (Fig. 14-38) of such axons individually invaginated into grooves in its cytoplasm. The protective cellular sheath that enfolds a group of unmyelinated axons is made up of a series of Schwann cells arranged end to end, each interdigitating with the next so as to constitute a continuous column. A basement membrane surrounds the external surface of the Schwann cells in such a way as to cover over their grooves where these open to the exterior (Fig. 14-39). Between the axolemma of each unmyelinated axon and the Schwann cell membrane lining the groove that houses it, there is an intercellular space, 10 nm to 15 nm wide, containing tissue fluid that is involved in impulse conduction.

Variability in Nerve Fascicles. Most peripheral nerves are *mixed,* containing afferent and efferent fibers (Fig. 14-31). However, it is not possible to distinguish between these two types of fibers on the basis of their microscopic appearance. Toward the distal end of nerves, the afferent and efferent fibers tend to segregate, with the result that individual fascicles become predominantly motor or sen-

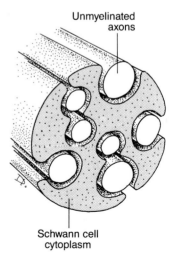

Fig. 14-38. Diagram illustrating the arrangement between unmyelinated axons and a Schwann cell of a peripheral nerve. See text for details.

Myelinated
axon

Unmyelinated
axon

Endoneurial
collagen
fibrils

Schwann
cell
nucleus

Basement membrane

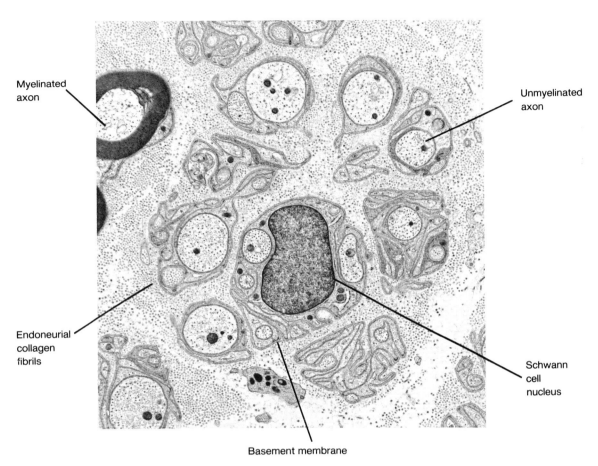

Fig. 14-39. Electron micrograph of unmyelinated axons and Schwann cells of a peripheral nerve. Compare this figure with Figure 14-38.

sory. A large peripheral nerve contains several fascicles, each with a surrounding sheath of perineurium (Fig. 14-31). There is nevertheless much communication between fascicles in that nerve fibers pass from one fascicle to another (Sunderland). Consequently, the relative size and content of the fascicles changes along the course of the nerve. Hence if a small segment of a nerve is destroyed and an attempt is made to rejoin the two stumps, the fascicles in the stumps may fail to match each other.

A peripheral nerve can resist a certain amount of gentle stretch without becoming damaged. This is because the nerve fibers in its fascicles pursue a wavy course along its length (Fig. 14-36). A certain amount of stretch straightens them, and any additional stretch is resisted by the strong perineural sheaths around the fascicles.

Small nerves are composed of only a single fascicle surrounded by a perineurial sheath (Figs. 14-34 and 14-36).

The number of nerve fibers within a fascicle varies greatly, as does the diameter of the nerve fibers in the fascicle, and there are more fibers in the distal parts of some

nerves than at more proximal levels. The increased number of fibers is attributable to the branching of fibers within nerves.

Blood Supply of Nerves. In certain surgical procedures, nerves must be freed of their attachments for some distance, and it is important to know whether this will cause serious damage within them. Fortunately, nerves are supplied by a profusion of vessels that anastomose freely. The vessels are of several orders. There are longitudinally disposed epineurial, interfascicular, perineurial, and intrafascicular arteries and arterioles. The endoneurium contains a capillary network. Nutrient arteries from vessels outside the nerve, and from longitudinally disposed vessels accompanying the nerve, penetrate the nerve at frequent intervals along its course to communicate with the neural vessels. The number of anastomoses between all these vessels is so great that nerves can be freed from their surrounding attachments for considerable distances. Sunderland stresses the importance of preserving superficial vessels when nerves are being freed from adjacent structures because they are important links in the system of anastomoses.

REGENERATION OF PERIPHERAL NERVES

Nerve injuries are of varying degrees of severity, as outlined in the following sections.

First-Degree Injuries. Pressure applied to a nerve for some time can compress its blood vessels sufficiently to cause local hypoxia of axons and *interfere with their function.* Sensory fibers are more affected than motor fibers, and different kinds of sensory fibers vary in susceptibility. After pressure is released, recovery of sensation or motor function may occur in a matter of minutes, hours, or weeks, depending on the severity of the injury. If recovery does not occur in a few weeks, the injury must be regarded as more severe than a first-degree type, as will now be described.

Second-Degree Injuries. Prolonged or severe pressure on some part of a nerve is enough to destroy the axon where it is subjected to pressure. Nerves are sometimes injured purposefully in this manner to bring about temporary paralysis of muscles whose actions are interfering with recovery of some part of the body. For example, the nerves to one side of the diaphragm can be squeezed hard enough to put the lung on that side to rest.

Such severe pressure causes *death of axons* at the site where pressure is applied. In this respect, a second-degree injury has consequences that are fundamentally different from a first-degree injury. When even a small segment of an axon dies, the part of the axon distal to the injury also dies because it is separated from the cell body that maintains it. Accordingly, nerve function in a second-degree injury can only be restored if all parts of the axon distal to the injury are regenerated.

As soon as the cell body recovers from the axon reaction, it regains the capacity to synthesize cytoplasmic proteins. These move along the axon to the site where the axon was crushed, and the axon is now able to grow again. The rate of growth of the regenerating axon, 3.5 mm to 4.5 mm per day, is virtually identical to the rate of axoplasmic flow (slow axonal transport), which was discussed earlier in this chapter. Before discussing the details of what happens to the axon, we shall mention some other consequences of the injury.

When the part of a myelinated axon distal to the site of injury dies, its myelin sheath also degenerates. Such degeneration of the axon and its sheath is known as *Wallerian degeneration.* Macrophages from the endoneurium phagocytose the degenerating material. Schwann cells also seem to become phagocytic and to play a role in clearing away the debris.

It is widely believed that second-degree injuries do not interrupt the continuity of the endoneurial tubes at the site of the injury. Accordingly, when the cell body supplies cytoplasmic proteins to the damaged axon, it *grows along the same endoneurial tube.*

Regeneration Can Occur in Severed Nerves if They Are Surgically Rejoined. Provided the proximal and distal stumps of a severed peripheral nerve are reattached with sutures, some degree of function may be restored to the affected parts of the body after an adequate period has elapsed.

The part of the axon that is distal to the transection (the part shown on the *right* in Fig. 14-40), together with its myelin sheath, degenerates because it is severed from the cell body that maintains it. Similar fragmentation of the axon and its myelin is also seen for a short distance just proximal to the cut (Fig. 14-40A). The surviving Schwann cells (*blue* in Fig. 14-40) then begin to proliferate and become motile. In the form of cords, they grow out along the endoneurial tubes into the site of injury, primarily from the distal stump (Fig. 14-40B). In the meantime, macrophages phagocytose the residual myelin droplets and the remains of dead axons and then move away. Axon sprouts from the viable proximal parts of the severed axons grow into the long slitlike spaces between the cords of Schwann cells, which serve to guide them across the gap from the proximal stump to the distal stump (Fig. 14-40C). The same cells protect and support the regenerating axon sprouts and remyelinate them when necessary to restore their former function. Fibroblasts repair the defects in the connective tissue sheaths, and the damaged nerve becomes as strong as before.

Many of the axon sprouts that grow into the maze of slitlike spaces between the cords of Schwann cells fail to reestablish appropriate connections, but, given enough time, a sufficient number of them grow down the right endoneurial tubes to restore a substantial measure of lost function.

If a long stretch of peripheral nerve has become damaged, it may be necessary to interpose an autologous *nerve transplant* between its two undamaged ends. A segment of some nonessential superficial nerve that can be spared is employed to fill the gap. Many of the Schwann cells in the transplant survive and proliferate. In this respect, the transplant acts very much like the distal stump described above. However, because the axon sprouts are obliged to find their way through two mazes instead of one, the results obtained with a nerve transplant are rarely as satisfactory as those obtained when the cut ends are reattached directly.

To complete our discussion of the three structural components of the PNS, we shall now briefly consider nerve endings.

AFFERENT AND EFFERENT NERVE ENDINGS

The modalities of sensation include touch, pressure, heat, cold, pain, smell, sight, hearing, and an appreciation of the position and movement of the parts of the body. Impulses elicited by stimuli at nerve endings of afferent neurons are conducted by way of ascending tracts in white columns of the spinal cord to sensory areas of the cerebral cortex. Sensation is experienced in the brain; the kind of sensation perceived depends on which general area of the sensory cortex is stimulated. Moreover, the particular region of cortical sensory area receiving the impulses provides an awareness of the location of the receptors that are being stimulated.

Afferent nerve terminals transduce stimulus energy into nerve impulses. In most cases, the stimulus elicits a depolarization of the afferent terminal. Broadly speaking, the

Proximal   **Distal**

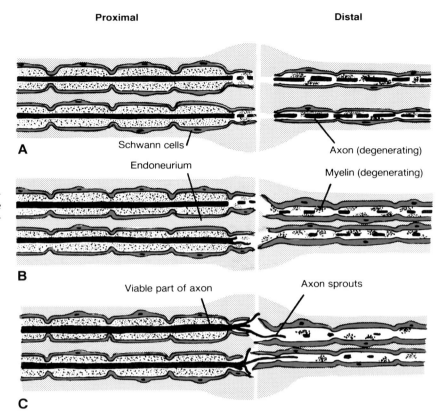

Fig. 14-40. Schematic diagram showing the regeneration of a severed nerve that has been surgically rejoined. For details, see text.

different types of sensory receptors are designed to respond to (1) different kinds of stimulus energy or (2) different intensities of the same type of energy. The receptors that are responsible for the senses of smell, taste, sight, hearing, and the perception of movement and position of the head are brought together in the *organs of special sense*.

As noted, the various types of *afferent nerve endings* will be described in the chapters that deal with the parts of the body in which they are situated.

Efferent nerve endings on muscle cells are described in Chapter 15, and those in glands are dealt with in this chapter at the end of the section on the autonomic nervous system.

THE AUTONOMIC NERVOUS SYSTEM

Although there are many different physiological responses that can be influenced by efferent nerve impulses, only skeletal muscle contraction can be brought about at will. The other responses are not normally under voluntary control. Accordingly, the efferent innervation of exocrine glands, heart muscle, smooth muscle, the viscera, and the circulatory system is collectively referred to as the *autonomic*

nervous system (Gr. *autos*, self; *nomos*, law). The remainder of the PNS is referred to as the *somatic nervous system*.

Cardiac muscle and most smooth muscle and exocrine glands are innervated by both divisions of the autonomic nervous system, which are known as its sympathetic and parasympathetic divisions, respectively. In many cases, the responses elicited by the activity of the one division are functionally antagonistic to those elicited by that of the other. These activities are integrated in the hypothalamus.

Both the *sympathetic* (Gr. *syn*, with; *pathos*, suffering) and the *parasympathetic* (Gr. *para*, beside) divisions of the autonomic nervous system arise in the CNS, but from different parts of it (Figs. 14-41 and 14-42). The fibers of neurons innervating muscle and glands from the two divisions therefore travel along different routes. Moreover, in both divisions, *two efferent neurons* are always required to join the CNS with each gland or muscle innervated. Also, in both divisions, the cell body of the first neuron in each efferent chain is situated in the CNS but that of the second neuron lies outside the CNS in a ganglion of the autonomic nervous system. The two neurons involved in each instance are called *preganglionic* and *postganglionic*, respectively.

We shall now briefly consider the microscopic structure of ganglia of the autonomic nervous system and then consider its two divisions in more detail and describe where the ganglia are located.

(*Text continues on p. 384.*)

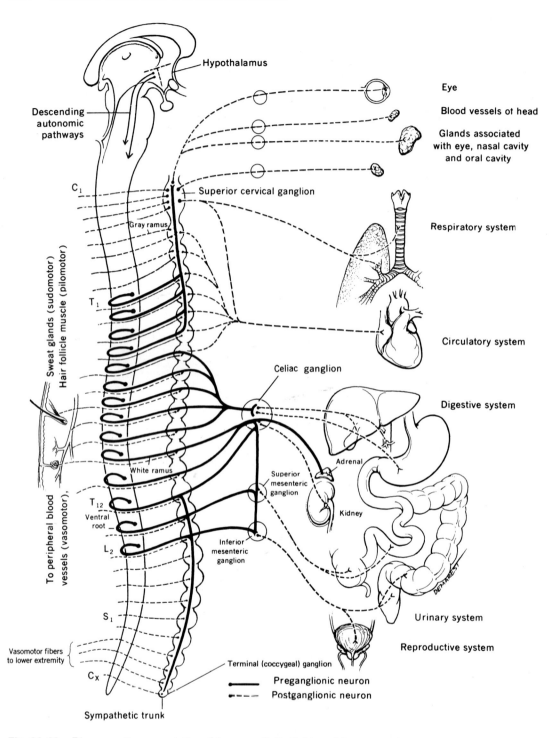

Fig. 14-41. Diagrammatic representation of the sympathetic division of the autonomic nervous system (Noback CR, Demarest RJ: The Nervous System—Introduction and Review, 2nd ed. New York, McGraw-Hill, 1977)

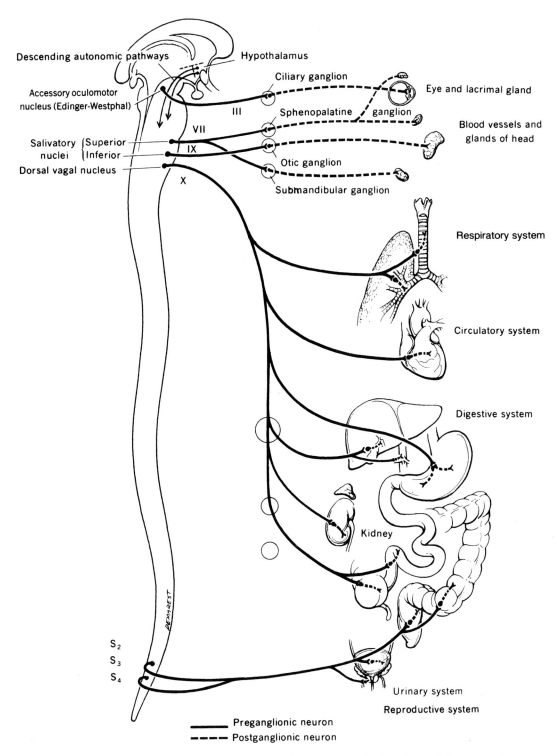

Fig. 14-42. Diagrammatic representation of the parasympathetic division of the autonomic nervous system (Noback CR, Demarest RJ: The Nervous System—Introduction and Review, 2nd ed. New York, McGraw-Hill, 1977)

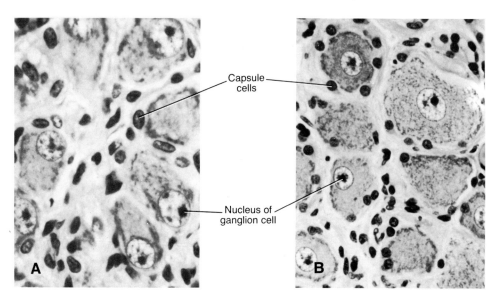

Fig. 14-43. Photomicrograph of ganglion cells in (A) an autonomic (parasympathetic) ganglion and (B) a spinal ganglion. Note the relatively discontinuous layer of capsule cells and the eccentric position of the nuclei of ganglion cells in A.

AUTONOMIC GANGLIA

The ganglia of the autonomic nervous system are generally similar to spinal ganglia in that they have a connective tissue framework and contain ganglion and capsule cells. However, there are certain differences. The nerve cells of autonomic ganglia are *multipolar* and, because they possess many dendrites, have somewhat more irregular and less distinct contours than spinal ganglion cells (Fig. 14-43). Furthermore, their capsule cells constitute a less uniform layer because of the multipolar shape of the ganglion cells. In general, the nerve cells of autonomic ganglia are smaller than those of spinal ganglia and not all of them are surrounded by capsules. Moreover, their nucleus, which resembles that of spinal ganglion cells in that it contains a prominent central nucleolus, is situated more eccentrically than in spinal ganglion cells (Fig. 14-43). The terminal ganglia of the parasympathetic system may be very small and sometimes may contain only a single ganglion cell.

Next we shall give a short account of the anatomy of the sympathetic division of the autonomic nervous system. It is more complex than that of the parasympathetic division, a description of which follows.

SYMPATHETIC DIVISION

In the thoracic and upper lumbar portions of the spinal cord, intermediolateral as well as anterior and posterior columns of gray matter are present. The nerve cell bodies in these intermediolateral columns differ somewhat from those in the anterior columns; they are smaller and their lightly myelinated axons leave the cord by way of the anterior nerve roots. These axons extend into the anterior roots for only a short distance, whereupon they leave by way of little nerve trunks called white *rami communicantes* (L. *ramus*, branch; *communicans*, communicating; white because the axons are myelinated).

The ganglia of the sympathetic division are described as *paravertebral, prevertebral,* or *terminal ganglia* according to their position in the body. The *paravertebral ganglia* (*e.g.,* the superior cervical ganglion) are interconnected to form bilateral *sympathetic chains* (*trunks*) that are situated anterolaterally with respect to the vertebral column and that extend from the upper cervical to the sacral level (Fig. 14-41). In the lumbar and sacral regions, there are also fibers that connect the ganglia on the left with those on the right. The *prevertebral ganglia* comprise an abdominal plexus that lies anterior to the vertebral column, in closer association with the viscera than the paravertebral ganglia. The main prevertebral ganglia are the celiac, superior mesenteric, and inferior mesenteric ganglia (Fig. 14-41). The *terminal ganglia* are peripherally situated close to the organs they innervate.

Axons of cell bodies that are situated in the intermediolateral columns of the spinal cord extend through the white rami and then proceed to synapse with neurons of the paravertebral, prevertebral, or terminal ganglia. These axons are therefore called *preganglionic fibers*. The *postganglionic fibers* that emerge from the ganglia in the sympathetic chains reenter the spinal nerves by way of the gray rami. The postganglionic fibers are unmyelinated.

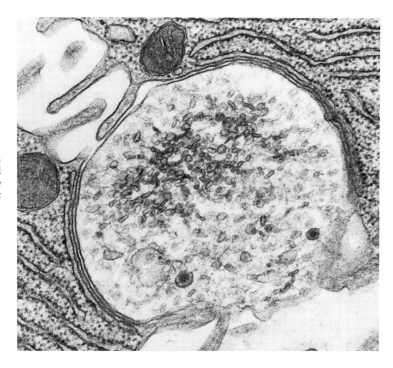

Fig. 14-44. Electron micrograph ($\times$65,750) of an axon bulb lying between two secretory cells of parotid (rat). Within the bulb there are synaptic vesicles. The bulb is not separated from the cells by basement membrane. (Hand AR: J Cell Biol 47:540, 1970)

PARASYMPATHETIC DIVISION

The parasympathetic division supplies most glands and muscles innervated by the sympathetic division. Here again, a chain of two efferent neurons transmits impulses from the CNS to the cells that are innervated (Fig. 14-42), and the preganglionic fibers are lightly myelinated whereas the postganglionic fibers are unmyelinated.

The parasympathetic division originates from two widely separated parts of the CNS. The cell bodies that give rise to some of its preganglionic fibers are situated in nuclei of gray matter in the medulla and the midbrain, and the preganglionic fibers arising from these cell bodies leave the CNS by way of the 3rd, 7th, 9th, and 10th cranial nerves (Fig. 14-42). The cell bodies from which the remainder of the preganglionic fibers arise are found in the lateral columns of the sacral portion of the spinal cord. These fibers exit from the CNS by way of the 2nd, 3rd, and 4th sacral spinal nerves, from which they leave by way of visceral rami of these nerves (Fig. 14-42).

Because the preganglionic fibers of the parasympathetic division emerge by way of cranial and sacral nerves, the parasympathetic division is sometimes referred to as the *craniosacral division* of the autonomic system, in contrast to the *thoracolumbar division* (the other name for the sympathetic division).

The preganglionic fibers of the parasympathetic division are, in general, longer than those in the sympathetic division, and with certain exceptions, they proceed all the way to the muscle or gland with whose innervation they are concerned (Fig. 14-42). Here they generally end in small *terminal ganglia* that are closely associated with the gland or muscle innervated. The postganglionic axons are generally short. However, in the head, the ganglia of the parasympathetic division are not closely associated with the glands or muscles innervated and the postganglionic fibers are correspondingly longer (Fig. 14-42).

AUTONOMIC NERVE ENDINGS

Postganglionic autonomic nerve fibers terminate in certain regions of the heart, in smooth muscle, and in exocrine glands and adipose tissue. The postganglionic autonomic nerve endings on secretory cells of exocrine glands resemble those on smooth muscle cells (described in Chap. 15). At such an ending, the postganglionic fiber becomes distended into a series of varicosities that are closely associated with the cell membrane of the secretory cell but that nevertheless remain separated from it by a synaptic cleft (Fig. 14-44). These varicosities contain mitochondria and numerous synaptic vesicles (Fig. 14-44); their neurotransmitter is norepinephrine or acetylcholine (generally norepinephrine at sympathetic endings and acetylcholine at parasympathetic endings, but the postganglionic sympathetic endings on sweat glands are a notable exception because they are cholinergic). In both divisions of the autonomic nervous system, the preganglionic fibers are cholinergic.

SELECTED REFERENCES

General

ALBERTS B, BRAY D, LEWIS J ET AL: The nervous system. In Molecular Biology of the Cell, p 1013. New York, Garland Publishing, 1983

KOELLE GB: Neurohumoral transmission and the autonomic nervous system. In Goodman LS, Gilman A (eds): The Pharmacological Basis of Therapeutics, 5th ed, p 404. New York, Macmillan, 1975

NOBACK CR, DEMAREST RJ: The Nervous System—Introduction and Review, 2nd ed. New York, McGraw-Hill, 1977

PETERS A, PALAY S, WEBSTER H: The Fine Structure of the Nervous System: The Neurons and Supporting Cells, Philadelphia, WB Saunders, 1976

Central Nervous System, Neurons, Axonal Transport, and Synapses

ADAMS I, JONES DG: Quantitative ultrastructural changes in rat cortical synapses during early-, mid-, and late-adulthood. Brain Res 239:349, 1982

AXELROD J: Neurotransmitters. Sci Am 230 No 6:56, 1974

BUNGE RP: Glial cells and the central myelin sheath. Physiol Rev 48:197, 1968

CHANG DC, TASAKI I, ADELMAN WJ, LEUCHTAG HR (eds): Structure and Function in Excitable Cells. New York, Plenum, 1983

ELAM JS, CANCALON P (eds): Axonal Transport in Neuronal Growth and Regeneration. Advances in Neurochemistry, Vol 6. New York, Plenum, 1984

GRAY EG, GUILLERY RW: Synaptic morphology in the normal and degenerating nervous system. Int Rev Cytol 19:111, 1966

HEUSER JE, REESE TS: Evidence for recycling of synaptic vesicle membrane during transmitter release of the frog neuro-muscular junction. J Cell Biol 57:315, 1973

HEUSER JE, REESE T: Structure of the synapse. In Kandel ER (ed): Handbook of Physiology. The Nervous System, Vol 1, Cellular Biology of Neurons, p 261. Baltimore, Williams & Wilkins, 1977

HIROKAWA N: Cross-linker system between neurofilaments, microtubules, and membranous organelles in frog axons revealed by the quick-freeze, deep-etching method. J Cell Biol 94:129, 1982

HÖKFELT T, FUXE K, GOLDSTEIN M ET AL: Transmitter histochemistry of the central nervous system. In Santini M (ed): Golgi Centennial Symposium. Proceedings, p 401. New York, Raven Press, 1975

HOPKINS WG, BROWN MC: Development of Nerve Cells and Their Connections. London, Cambridge University Press, 1984

HUTTENLOCHER PR: Synaptic density in human frontal cortex—developmental changes and effects of aging. Brain Res 163:195, 1979

JONES DG: Some current concepts of synaptic organization. Advances in Anatomy, Embryology and Cell Biology. Vol 55, Part 4. Berlin, Springer-Verlag, 1978

LASEK RJ, GARNER JA, BRADY ST: Axonal transport of the cytoplasmic matrix. J Cell Biol 99:212s, 1984

LLINÁS RR: The cortex of the cerebellum. Sci Am 232 No 1:56, 1975

LUND RD: Development and Plasticity of the Brain. An Introduction. New York, Oxford University Press, 1978

MILLER RH, LASEK RJ: Cross-bridges mediate anterograde and retrograde vesicle transport along microtubules in squid axoplasm. J Cell Biol 101:2181, 1985

SCHWARTZ JH: The transport of substances in nerve cells. Sci Am 242 No 4:152, 1980

SHEPHERD GM: Microcircuits in the nervous system. Sci Am 238: 93, February, 1978

SOTELO C: Morphological correlates of electronic coupling between neurons in mammalian nervous system. In Santini M (ed): Golgi Centennial Symposium. Proceedings, p 355. New York, Raven Press, 1975

STEVENS CF: The neuron. Sci Am 241 No 3:55, 1979

Neuroglia

ADRIAN EK, SCHELPER RL: Microglia, monocytes, and macrophages. In Fedoroff S (ed): Eleventh International Congress of Anatomy, Part A: Glial and Neuronal Cell Biology, p 113. New York, Alan R Liss, 1981

FEDOROFF S (ed): Glial and Neuronal Cell Biology. Eleventh International Congress of Anatomy, Part A. Progess in Clinical and Biological Research, Vol 59A. New York, Alan R Liss, 1981

FEDOROFF S, NEAL J, OPAS M, KALNINS VI: Astrocyte cell lineage. III. The morphology of differentiating mouse astrocytes in colony culture. J Neurocytol 13:1, 1984

FUJITA S, KITAMURA T: Origin of brain macrophages and the nature of the microglia. In Zimmerman HM (ed): Progress in Neuropathology, Vol 3, p 1. New York, Grune & Stratton, 1976

FUJITA S, TSUCHIHASHI Y, KITAMURA T: Origin, morphology and function of the microglia. In Fedoroff S (ed): Eleventh International Congress of Anatomy, Part A: Glial and Neuronal Cell Biology. Progress in Clinical and Biological Research, Vol 59A, p 141. New York, Alan R Liss, 1981

IMAMOTO K: Origin of microglia: Cell transformation from blood monocytes into macrophagic ameboid cells and microglia. In Fedoroff S (ed): Eleventh International Congress of Anatomy, Part A: Glial and Neuronal Cell Biology, p 125. New York, Alan R Liss, 1981

LING EA, PATTERSON JA, PRIVAT A ET AL: Identification of glial cells in the brain of young rats. J Comp Neurol 149:43, 1973

MATO M, OOKAWARA S, MATO TK, NAMIKI T: An attempt to differentiate further between microglia and fluorescent granular perithelial (FGP) cells by their capacity to incorporate exogenous protein. Am J Anat 172:125, 1985

MORI S, LEBLOND CP: Electron microscopic features and proliferation of astrocytes in the corpus callosum of the rat. J Comp Neurol 157:197, 1969

MORI S, LEBLOND CP: Electron microscopic identification of three classes of oligodendrocytes and a study of their proliferative activity in the corpus callosum of young rats. J Comp Neurol 139:1, 1970

MORI S, LEBLOND CP: Identification of microglia in light and electron microscopy. J Comp Neurol 155:57, 1969

NORTON WT (ed): Oligodendroglia. Advances in Neurochemistry, Vol 5. New York, Plenum, 1984

Blood–Brain Barrier, Choroid Plexuses, Cerebrospinal Fluid, and Meninges

BRADBURY MWB: The structure and function of the blood–brain barrier. Fed Proc 43:186, 1984

BRADBURY MWB: The blood–brain barrier. Transport across the cerebral endothelium. Circ Res 57:213, 1985

BRADBURY MWB, CSERR HF: Drainage of cerebral interstitial fluid and of cerebrospinal fluid into lymphatics. In Johnston MG (ed): Experimental Biology of the Lymphatic Circulation, p 355. Amsterdam, Elsevier Biomedical Press, 1985

BRIGHTMAN MW: The distribution within the brain of ferritin injected into cerebrospinal fluid compartments. II. Parenchymal distribution. Am J Anat 117:193, 1965

BRIGHTMAN MW, REESE TS: Junctions between intimated apposed cell membranes in the vertebrate brain. J Cell Biol 40:648, 1969

GOLDSTEIN GW, BETZ AL: The blood–brain barrier. Sci Am 255 No 3:74, 1986

HUDSON AJ, SMITH CG: The vascular pattern of the choroid plexus of the lateral ventricle. Anat Rec 112:43, 1952

REESE TS, KARNOVSKY MJ: The structural localization of a blood–brain barrier to exogenous peroxidase. J Cell Biol 34:207, 1967

STEER JC, HORNEY FD: Evidence for passage of cerebrospinal fluid along spinal nerves. Can Med Assoc J 98:71, 1968

STEWART PA, COOMBER BL: Astrocytes and the blood–brain barrier. In Fedoroff S, Vernadakis A (eds): Astrocytes. New York, Academic Press, 1986

STEWART PA, WILEY MJ: Developing nervous tissue induces formation of blood–brain barrier characteristics in invading endothelial cells: A study using quail-chick transplantation chimeras. Dev Biol 84:183, 1981

TAUC M, VIGNON X, BOUCHAUD C: Evidence for the effectiveness of the blood–CSF barrier in the fetal rat choroid plexus. A freeze-fracture and peroxidase diffusion study. Tissue Cell 16:65, 1984

WEED LH: Certain anatomical and physiological aspects of the meninges and cerebrospinal fluid. Brain 58:383, 1935

WEED LH: Meninges and cerebrospinal fluid. J Anat 72:181, 1938

WOOLLAM DHM, MILLEN JW: The perivascular spaces of the mammalian central nervous system and their relation to the perineuronal and subarachnoid spaces. J Anat 89:193, 1955

Regeneration in CNS and PNS, and Blood Supply of Nerves

AGUAYO AJ, DAVID S, BRAY G: Influences of the glial environment on the elongation of axons after injury: Transplantation studies in adult rodents. J Exp Biol 95:231, 1981

FINE A: Transplantation in the central nervous system. Sci Am 255 No 2:52, 1986

NESMEYANOVA TA: Experimental Studies on Regeneration of Spinal Neurons. New York, Halsted Press, 1977

POLEZHAEV LV: Loss and Restoration of Regenerative Capacity in Tissues and Organs of Animals, Cambridge, MA, Harvard University Press, 1972

RICHARDSON PM, MCGUINNESS UM, AGUAYO AJ: Peripheral nerve autografts to the rat spinal cord: Studies with axonal tracing methods. Brain Res 237:147, 1982

SUNDERLAND S: Blood supply of peripheral nerves. Arch Neurol Psychiat 54:280, 1945

SUNDERLAND S: A classification of peripheral nerve injuries producing loss of function. Brain 74:491, 1951

SUNDERLAND S: Factors influencing the course of regeneration and the quality of the recovery after nerve suture. Brain 75:19, 1952

SUNDERLAND S: The capacity of regenerating axons to bridge long gaps in nerves. J Comp Neurol 99:481, 1953

Peripheral Nervous System, Peripheral and Central Myelin, and Nerve Endings*

BOEHME DH, MARKS N: Myelin. In Schwartz LM, Azar MM: Advanced Cell Biology, p 163, New York, Van Nostrand Reinhold, 1981

CHOUCHKOV CV: Cutaneous receptors. Advances in Anatomy, Embryology, and Cell Biology, Vol 54, Fasc 5. Berlin, Springer-Verlag, 1978

ELLISMAN MH, LINDSEY JD, WILEY–LIVINGSTON C, LEVINSON SR: Differentiation of axonal membrane systems, the axolemma, and the axoplasmic matrix. In Chang DC, Tasaki I, Adelman WJ, Leuchtag HR (eds): Structure and Function in Excitable Cells, p 3. New York, Plenum, 1983

HALATA Z: The mechanoreceptors of the mammalian skin. Ultrastructure and morphological classification. Advances in Anatomy, Embryology and Cell Biology. Vol 50, Fasc 5. Berlin, Springer-Verlag, 1975

HAND AR: Adrenergic and cholinergic nerve terminals in the rat parotid gland. Electron microscopic observations on permanganate-fixed glands. Anat Rec 173:131, 1972

HAND AR: Nerve-acinar relationships in the rat parotid gland. J Cell Biol 47:540, 1970

IGGO A: Cutaneous and subcutaneous sense organs. Br Med Bull 33:97, 1977

LANDON DN (ed): The Peripheral Nerve. London, Chapman & Hall, 1976

LYNN B: Somatosensory receptors and their CNS connections. Ann Rev Cytol 37:105, 1975

MORELL P, NORTON WT: Myelin. Sci Am 242 No 5:88, 1980

ROSENBLUTH J: Membrane specializations at the nodes of Ranvier and paranodal and juxtaparanodal regions of myelinated central and peripheral nerve fibers. In Zagoren JC, Fedoroff S (eds): The Node of Ranvier, p 31. Orlando, Academic Press, 1984

ROSENBLUTH J: Structure of the node of Ranvier. In Chang DC, Tasaki I, Adelman WJ, Leuchtag HR (eds): Structure and Function in Excitable Cells, p 25. New York, Plenum, 1983

SCHNAPP B, MUGNAINI E: The myelin sheath: Electron microscopic studies with thin sections and freeze-fracture. In Sanitini M (ed): Golgi Centennial Symposium. Proceedings, p 209. New York, Raven Press, 1975

SHANTHAVEERAPPA TR, BOURNE GH: The "perineural epithelium," a metabolically active, continuous, protoplasmic cell barrier surrounding peripheral nerve fasciculi. J Anat 96:527, 1962

SINCLAIR D: Normal anatomy of sensory nerves and receptors. In Jarrett A (ed): The Physiology and Pathophysiology of the Skin. The Nerves and Blood Vessels, Vol 2, p 371. London, Academic Press, 1973

WERNER JK: Trophic influence of nerves on the development and maintenance of sensory receptors. Am J Physical Medicine 53:127, 1974

ZAGOREN JC, FEDOROFF S (eds): The Node of Ranvier. Orlando, FL, Academic Press, 1984

* For references on afferent and efferent endings in muscle, see Selected References, Chapter 15.

15

Muscle Tissue

Epithelial glands, nervous tissue, and muscle tissue are composite tissues, which means that although they consist primarily of the cells that give them their names, they also incorporate at least a minimal amount of connective tissue. Muscle tissue needs its connective tissue component for at least two reasons. First, muscle cells have a very active metabolism and therefore require an abundance of nutrients and oxygen. The capillaries that provide these essentials are situated in the delicate loose connective tissue that lies between individual muscle cells or between bundles of these cells. Second, for the body to gain any advantage from a muscular contraction, the muscle cells need to pull on something. The harness on which they pull is the strong fibrous connective tissue component of the muscle.

Relaxed muscle cells are characteristically long and narrow and are therefore known as *muscle fibers*. This term is also used with reference to heart muscle, but here the term *fiber* is used much more loosely to refer to a series of cardiac muscle cells that are joined end to end (comprising a fiber of indeterminate length) rather than to refer to an individual cell.

For the various kinds of contraction needed in different parts of the body, there are three different types of muscle. The most familiar type is variously known as *skeletal*, *voluntary*, or *striated muscle*. Muscle is described as *skeletal* because its contraction generally moves some part of the skeleton, *voluntary* because its contraction can generally be elicited at will, and *striated* because its fibers exhibit alternating dark and light transverse bands called *striations* when seen under the microscope. It should nevertheless be appreciated that skeletal muscle is capable of functioning without conscious effort (*e.g.*, in maintaining the position of the head). At one time it was more common for *skeletal* muscle to be referred to as *striated* muscle. However, the next type of muscle to be described (cardiac muscle) is also striated, and this can cause confusion, so the current tendency is to avoid using this name. It is nevertheless common to find that, in other disciplines, the term *striated* muscle is used to mean *striated voluntary*, that is, *skeletal* muscle.

Because the second type of muscle constitutes most of the heart, it is called *cardiac muscle*. However, it is not entirely confined to the heart because some cardiac muscle can also be found in the walls of the pulmonary vein and superior vena cava. Its cells also exhibit striations, but in contrast to skeletal muscle, its contraction cannot be brought about at will; in other words, it is *involuntary*. Cardiac muscle also exhibits certain unique ultrastructural features that warrant its classification as a distinctive type of muscle. One of these features is that it is the only kind of muscle with constituent cells that are joined together end to end by complexes containing three different kinds of cell junctions.

Because the third type of muscle does not exhibit striations, it is known as *smooth muscle*. Its contraction cannot be elicited at will, so it represents a second type of *involuntary* muscle. Thus it is possible to initiate the swallowing of food voluntarily, but after the food has reached a certain level, it becomes impossible to control its further passage along the digestive tract by initiating voluntary contractions. In smooth muscle as well as cardiac muscle, contraction is subject to regulation by the autonomic nervous system. Coats made of smooth muscle represent an important component of the walls of (1) most blood vessels and (2) the various tubular or hollow organs (*e.g.*, the intestine and urinary bladder). It is the degree of contraction in this muscle that regulates the luminal diameter of such structures.

It is important to realize that muscles do not necessarily have to contract to their maximal extent. Thus prolonged partial contractions of skeletal muscles are necessary for holding one's head up, and sustained partial contraction of the smooth muscle cells in the walls of arterioles is necessary to achieve an appropriate hydrostatic pressure in the blood capillaries. Such prolonged partial contractions, which are achieved by different means in skeletal and smooth muscles, are referred to as their *tonus*.

SKELETAL MUSCLE

Connective Tissue Component. The connective tissue in a skeletal muscle is arranged as follows (Fig. 15-1). The entire muscle is enclosed by a sheath of dense ordinary connective tissue called the *epimysium* (Gr. *epi*, upon). Blood vessels, lymphatics, and nerves enter or leave the interior

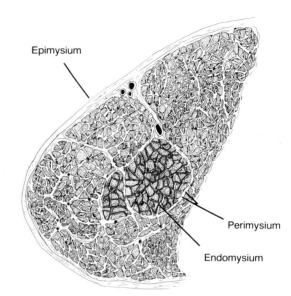

Fig. 15-1. Diagram of part of a small skeletal muscle in cross section under very low magnification, showing its connective tissue components and organization into bundles of muscle fibers. *Epimysium* encloses the entire muscle, *perimysium* surrounds each bundle of fibers, and *endomysium* (indicated in *blue*) lies between the individual muscle fibers.

of the muscle from the epimysium by way of fibrous partitions that extend into the muscle and surround its fascicles (bundles) of muscle fibers. These partitions constitute the *perimysium* (Gr. *peri*, around). Continuous with the perimysium, sheets of delicate connective tissue extend between each muscle fiber and constitute the *endomysium* (Gr. *endon*, within). The endomysium (indicated in *blue* in Fig. 15-1) contains the many capillaries and nerve fibers that supply the muscle fibers.

At each end of the muscle, the connective tissue elements merge into the strong connective tissue structure that anchors the muscle to the structures on which it pulls. Many muscles terminate in tendons that are anchored to bone or cartilage. However, muscles can also have other kinds of attachments, for example, aponeuroses, raphes, direct attachments to periosteum, and even attachments to the dense ordinary connective tissue layer of the skin (reticular layer of dermis).

Skeletal Muscle Fibers. The fibers of skeletal muscles are much larger than most other kinds of cells, and each contains many nuclei. Cylindrical in shape with tapered ends, they are up to several centimeters in length and up to 0.1 mm in diameter. In any given muscle they tend to be of uniform length, but in some muscles they are long and in other muscles they are shorter. In some instances skeletal muscle fibers span the entire length of the muscle, but in other cases they are not as long as the muscle and their

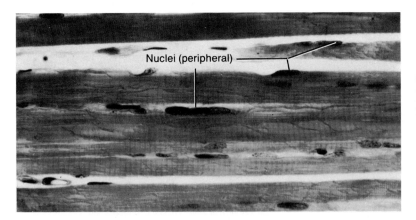

Nuclei (peripheral)

Fig. 15-2. Photomicrograph of skeletal muscle fibers in longitudinal section. Striations can be seen. Muscle nuclei are located at the periphery of the fibers but sometimes appear to lie within them because of the plane of section. Some fibroblast nuclei can also be seen in the endomysium, between the muscle fibers. (Courtesy of E. Schultz and C. P. Leblond)

pull has to be transmitted by the endomysial connective tissue.

The cell membrane of a muscle fiber is called its *sarcolemma* (Gr. *sarkos*, flesh; *lemma*, husk). Between the sarcolemma and the surrounding endomysium, there is a basement membrane (see Fig. 15-22). The elongated ovoid nuclei (*myonuclei*) of the muscle fiber are situated just under its sarcolemma (Figs. 15-2 and 15-3), that is, in the *peripheral* region of its cytoplasm (more commonly called its *sarcoplasm*). Nuclei of endomysial fibrocytes also lie near the surface of muscle fibers (Fig. 15-2), but they can easily be distinguished from myonuclei in cross sections (Fig. 15-3).

Striations Are a Result of Transverse Alignment of the Sarcomeres in Myofibrils. Longitudinal sections of skeletal muscle fibers disclose a distinctive pattern of alternating dark- and light-staining transverse *bands* (Fig. 15-4). When observed under polarized light, the dark-staining bands are birefringent (anisotropic) whereas the light-staining bands are isotropic. Accordingly, the dark bands are called *A bands* (*A* for *a*nisotropic) and the light ones, *I bands* (*I* for *i*sotropic). In addition, dark lines termed *Z lines* (*disks*) traverse the fiber, bisecting the I bands (Fig. 15-4). Sometimes a paler region called the *H zone* can be discerned in the middle of the A band (Fig. 15-4). The functional significance of these striations will soon become apparent.

Skeletal muscle fibers contain component fibrils called *myofibrils* that are longitudinally oriented and that exhibit the same pattern of striations as the fiber does. Moreover, the striations across the fiber are *not continuous* even though they appear to be so because of close packing of the myofibrils and precise lateral registration of their individual striations. The lateral borders of myofibrils can occasionally be distinguished in longitudinal sections (Fig. 15-4), but myofibrils are easier to discern in transverse sections (Fig. 15-3), in which they appear as darker staining entities separated by paler staining regions of sarcoplasm. *Sarcomeres* (Gr. *meros*, part) are the short segments of myofibrils, 2 μm to 3 μm in length, that lie between consecutive Z lines (see Fig. 15-10, in which they are labeled *S*). Sarcomeres represent the *contractile units of striated muscles*. When striated

muscles contract, the component sarcomeres shorten to approximately half their resting length. The mechanism by which this is achieved will now be described.

The Sliding Filament Theory of Muscular Contraction. When it became possible to study skeletal muscle in the electron microscope (EM), the internal structure of the sarcomere was found to be totally different from what had been surmised from light microscopy. Instead of consisting of two different kinds or concentrations of homo-

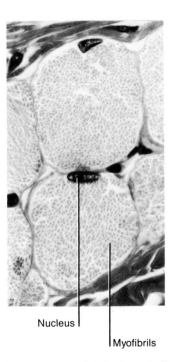

Nucleus

Myofibrils

Fig. 15-3. Photomicrograph of skeletal muscle fibers cut in cross section (high power). Their nuclei lie peripherally in the fibers and are distinguishable, by their position and appearance, from nuclei of fibroblasts in the endomysium lying between the fibers. The myofibrils within the fibers are visible as gray dots in the pale-staining cytoplasm.

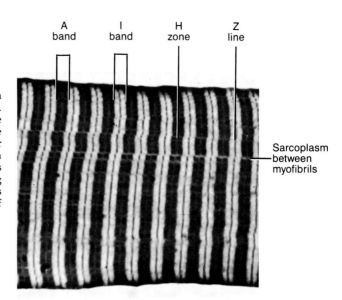

Fig. 15-4. Photomicrograph of a skeletal muscle fiber cut in longitudinal section (oil immersion, stained with toluidine blue). The thick dark vertical stripes are A bands of myofibrils; the light stripes contain the I bands, centered by Z lines. On close inspection, a paler region, the H zone, can be seen in the center of each A band. Note how all the bands of the myofibrils lie in register with one another, giving an impression of continuous striations across the fiber. Note also the pale fine lines running horizontally through the dark A bands; these are narrow regions of sarcoplasm lying between individual myofibrils. (Courtesy of E. Schultz)

geneous proteins, the A and the I bands were found to consist of characteristic arrays of longitudinal rod-shaped structures that became known as *filaments.* Two different kinds of filaments were identified, thick ones and thin ones; their distribution is represented in Figure 15-5.

In the relaxed sarcomere, the thick filaments span the midregion of the sarcomere, that is, the region recognized in the light microscope (LM) as the A band (compare the upper parts of Figs. 15-5 and 15-7). Both ends of the thick filaments are free. In contrast, the thin filaments have only one free end; their other end is attached to a Z line. Thus the thin filaments extend from the Z lines toward the middle of the sarcomere, where they interdigitate with the thick filaments. However, they do not reach the middle of the relaxed sarcomere (Fig. 15-5, *top*). It is now firmly established that the thick filaments contain myosin and the thin filaments contain actin. Thus the thin filaments correspond to the microfilaments that are present in other cell types.

In the contracted sarcomere, the thin filaments extend farther in between the thick filaments, with the result that their free ends almost meet at the middle of the sarcomere (Fig. 15-5, *bottom*). The only way in which the thin filaments can move farther in between the thick ones is by pulling on the Z lines to which they are attached, and this pulls the Z lines of all the sarcomeres closer together, resulting in a contraction.

After it was appreciated that the thick filaments contain myosin and the thin filaments contain actin, it became apparent that some sort of interaction between actin and myosin was responsible for pulling the thin filaments farther in between the thick filaments. The concept of the two arrays of filaments sliding past each other was embodied in the *sliding filament theory* of muscular contraction, which was propounded by H. E. Huxley and his coworkers as an outcome of their EM and x-ray diffraction studies on striated muscle. This theory revolutionized thinking about contraction, and it is now widely accepted as the underlying basis of muscular contraction.

In the next section, we shall consider how the two interdigitating arrays of filaments are related to the striations observed with the LM.

Ultrastructural Basis of Striations in Myofibrils

The various names ascribed to the striations in striated muscle fibers were derived from LM studies. With the LM, it was possible to discern A and I bands and Z lines, and sometimes H zones as well (Fig. 15-4). It was also observed that during contraction, the A bands remain of constant length but the I bands shorten. The EM has now disclosed why this is so.

As may be seen in Figure 15-6A, the darker staining of the A band in relaxed fibers is due to the presence of *thick filaments* that are approximately 1.5 μm long and 12 nm

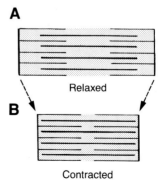

Fig. 15-5. Schematic diagrams of a sarcomere. (*A*) The two sets of thin filaments are attached to the two Z lines, one at each end of the sarcomere. (*B*) During contraction, the two Z lines are pulled closer together.

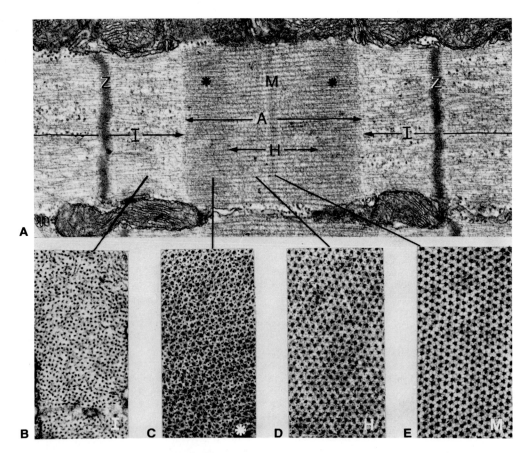

Fig. 15-6. Electron micrographs illustrating a sarcomere of skeletal muscle. *A* shows a *longitudinal section* of a relaxed sarcomere. On either side of the Z lines are halves of lightly stained I bands containing only thin filaments; these filaments extend from the Z lines and interdigitate with thick filaments lying within the darker staining A band. The regions of the A band that are marked (∗) contain both thick and thin filaments and hence appear darker than the region where only thick filaments are present—the H zone (*H*). A darker M line (*M*) lies at the center of the A band.

Cross sections taken at the levels indicated are shown in the lower four micrographs (×33,000). *B* shows thin filaments in the I bands. *C* shows thin filaments interdigitating with thick filaments in the A band, forming hexagonal patterns around them; this section is cut through the region marked (∗) in *A. D* shows thick filaments in the H zone. *E* shows thick filaments at the level of the M line, where fine interconnections link them together. (Courtesy of E. Schultz and C. P. Leblond)

to 15 nm in diameter. The I band is lighter staining because it contains only *thin filaments* that are approximately 1 μm long and 6 nm to 7 nm in diameter. The thin filaments at each end of the relaxed sarcomere project into the A band for about one quarter of its length, leaving a lighter zone in the middle of the A band. This lighter middle region corresponds to the H zone seen in the LM (Fig. 15-4). As may be seen in the lower part of Figure 15-7, the H zone virtually disappears during a contraction because thick and thin filaments both are then present throughout most of the A band. At the M line seen in the middle of the H zone, there are fine filamentous structures that interconnect the thick filaments (Figs. 15-6E and 15-7). These interconnecting filaments contain the enzyme creatine kinase and a protein called myomesin.

EM studies have also shown that the thin filament attachments on one side of the Z line lie opposite spaces between thin filament attachments on the other side; this is why the Z line has a characteristic zigzag appearance in electron micrographs (Fig. 15-8). The Z lines thus interconnect the thin filaments of adjacent sarcomeres. One interpretation of the arrangement is that the thin filaments are attached to a lattice of filaments of another type, which are referred to as Z *filaments*. As can be seen in the electron micrograph in Figure 15-8, these Z filaments pursue a zigzag course across the myofibril. The inset in Figure 15-8 represents a surface view of the Z line and shows diagrammatically how each thin filament (*stippled* circles) in one sarcomere appears to be linked by Z filaments to the four nearest thin filaments (*black* circles) belonging to the ad-

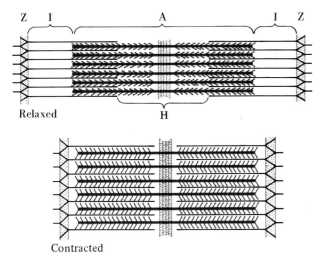

Relaxed

Contracted

Fig. 15-7. Diagrams of a sarcomere of skeletal muscle, showing the detailed arrangement of its components. Its thick filaments are indicated in *blue*. In the relaxed sarcomere, halves of I bands, containing only thin filaments, are evident on either side of the darker A band. In the middle of the A band, there is a lighter region, the H zone, centered by the M line. Interdigitation is at a minimum in the relaxed state, so that both the I bands and H zone are relatively long, but these parts of the sarcomere shorten during contraction caused by the movement of the Z lines toward the free ends of the thick filaments. The change in position of the myosin heads (cross bridges) during contraction is also indicated. (Courtesy of E. Schultz and C. P. Leblond)

jacent sarcomere, at least in the simpler kinds of Z lines that have been studied. Finally, Z lines contain the protein α-actinin, which is believed to be the distinctive amorphous electron-dense material associated with these sites (see Figs. 15-6A and 15-10, *inset*).

Information about the various parts of the sarcomere and their respective filament arrangements can also be ob-

tained from transverse sections of muscle fibers. Thus in a cross section through an I band of a relaxed sarcomere, only thin filaments are present (Fig. 15-6B), whereas in a cross section through one end of the A band, both thick and thin filaments are present (Fig. 15-6C). Cross sections also disclose that the thin filaments conform to a hexagonal pattern with a thick filament in the center of each hexagon. Furthermore, the thick filaments conform to a triangular pattern with a thin filament in the center of each triangle. Cross sections through the H zone contain only thick filaments (Fig. 15-6D). Finally, cross sections through the M line disclose the fine filamentous interconnections between the thick filaments (Fig. 15-6E).

The Various Parts of Sarcomeres Appear to Be Supported by Filament Lattices.

Evidence is accumulating that the Z lines (disks) and the interdigitating arrays of thick and thin filaments within each myofibril are held in place by an elaborate framework of cytoskeletal filaments. In the regions of the sarcoplasm that border on the periphery of the Z lines (disks), ringlike arrangements of intermediate filaments that contain the proteins desmin (skeletin), vimentin, and synemin have been described (Lazarides). An actin-binding protein called filamin exhibits the same distribution, suggesting that it may be bound to the thin filaments at the periphery of the Z disk. A system of extremely fine filaments that is believed to contain the protein titin appears to extend from each Z line to the next or at least to be involved in linking the thick filaments to the Z lines.

These ancillary filament systems are believed to provide the structural support necessary to ensure accurate longitudinal and transverse alignment of the contractile filaments and precise registration of the Z lines. According to a recent proposal, each sarcomere is supported by an *external scaffolding* made of desmin-containing intermediate filaments that interconnects the force-bearing Z lines and M lines of the myofibril. In addition, the sarcomere seems to be supported by a delicate flexible *internal lattice* consisting of extremely fine filaments. This lattice is believed to be made up partly of titin filaments and partly of filaments of yet an-

Fig. 15-8. Electron micrograph (×150,000) of a Z line in a skeletal muscle fiber of a fish (in which a Z line is a comparatively simple structure). Its zigzag appearance is due to Z filaments, to which the thin filaments are attached. (*Inset*) Diagram of a Z line in surface view, showing how the thin filaments are connected to the Z filaments. For details, see text. (Franzini–Armstrong C: J Cell Biol 58:630, 1973)

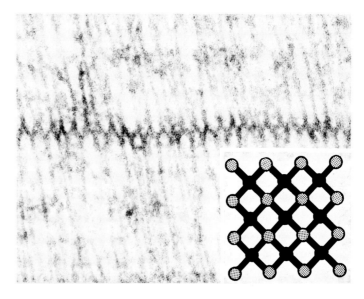

other protein called nebulin, and it is postulated that it, too, spans the whole length of the sarcomere from one Z line to the next. For further details, see Wang.

Red, White, and Intermediate Fibers

The sarcoplasm of skeletal muscle fibers contains a variable number of mitochondria (see Fig. 15-11) and also copious glycogen deposits (see Fig. 15-10, *inset;* glycogen indicated by *arrowheads*). In addition, it contains the protein myoglobin, which is similar to hemoglobin and takes up, stores, or gives up oxygen as needed. Muscle fibers with a high content of myoglobin, the color of which is reddish-brown, are described as *red fibers.* The brown color of muscles that contain large amounts of myoglobin (for example, those of whales, seals, and the dark meat of fowl) is attributed to their high content of myoglobin.

Skeletal muscle fibers show significant variation in diameter and myoglobin content and are accordingly classified as *red, white,* or *intermediate.* Most human muscles incorporate all three types of fibers; their respective proportions depend on the functional role of the muscle.

Red fibers (labeled *R* in Figs. 15-9 and 15-11, *inset*) are characterized by their small diameter and the relative abundance of (1) myoglobin in their cytosol and (2) cytochromes in their numerous mitochondria. *White fibers* (labeled *W* in Figs. 15-9 and 15-11; also shown in Fig. 15-10) are wider and contain less myoglobin and fewer mitochondria. Relative to red and white fibers, *intermediate fibers* (labeled *I* in Fig. 15-11, *inset*) exhibit intermediate characteristics.

Muscles that consist primarily of red fibers can sustain their contractile activity for a longer period than can muscles that are composed primarily of white fibers; this is because they have the equipment necessary to provide a continuing supply of metabolic energy. Even though white fibers are able to contract more rapidly, they also fatigue more rapidly; hence they are better adapted for intermittent bursts of contractile activity.

The difference between red fibers and white fibers becomes obvious if one compares the muscles of domestic fowl with those of their wild counterparts. Thus the red fibers that give the dark meat of chickens its characteristic color predominate in their much-used thigh and leg musculature. In contrast, their pectoral muscles are not used for flying and are composed mainly of white fibers. In wild fowl that are capable of sustained flight, on the other hand, red fibers are the major type of fiber that is present in the pectoral muscles.

Sarcolemmal Depolarization

In tracing the path of impulse conduction to the myofibrils, it should be pointed out that the permeability characteristics of the sarcolemma are essentially similar to those of the axolemma. Hence during relaxation, it is *electrically polarized.* The factors that contribute to the resting potential of

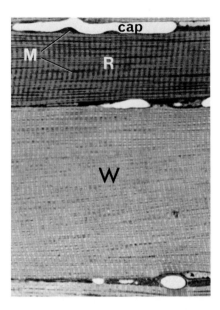

Fig. 15-9. Photomicrograph of skeletal muscle (stained with toluidine blue), showing two of its fiber types. The narrower red fibers (*R*) contain numerous mitochondria (groups of which are indicated by *M*) packed between their myofibrils, and also at their periphery, especially in association with capillaries (*cap*). The wider white fibers (*W*) contain fewer mitochondria. (Courtesy of E. Schultz)

an electrically excitable membrane were discussed in connection with nerve impulses in Chapter 14. Thus during relaxation, the sarcoplasmic side of the sarcolemma is maintained at a negative resting potential with respect to its extracellular side.

Impulses for contraction are propagated as waves of depolarization along a motor axon, the terminals of which are apposed to the sarcolemma of muscle fibers. Where the axolemma lies in intimate apposition with muscle fibers, their sarcolemma is provided with *acetylcholine receptors.* The effect of the motor impulses that arrive at axon terminals is to elicit a *local depolarization* of the sarcolemma. The resulting wave of depolarization spreads from the region under the terminal and sweeps along the sarcolemma, whereupon it passes down tubular invaginations of the sarcolemma that are known as *transverse (T) tubules.* In this manner, impulses are conducted from the surface of the muscle fiber deep into its sarcoplasm. However, before discussing what happens within the muscle fiber, it should be explained how the motor impulses are transmitted across the synapse between the axolemma and the sarcolemma, and this entails explaining how skeletal muscle fibers are arranged with respect to the motor nerve fibers that supply them.

Efferent Innervation of Skeletal Muscles

The peripheral nerve that supplies a given skeletal muscle contains the axons of many motor neurons. Every muscle fiber is supplied by a branch of a motor axon. In some skeletal muscles (*e.g.*, certain extrinsic muscles of the eye that are responsible for very delicate eye movements), every three to five muscle fibers are innervated by the axonal branches of one motor neuron. In most muscles, however, each motor axon branches in such a way that it innervates many muscle fibers. This broader pattern of innervation is seen, for example, in the trunk muscles that are responsible for maintaining posture, in which each motor axon has abundant branches that supply several hundred muscle fibers. In this type of arrangement, the muscle fibers supplied by any given motor neuron are *widely distributed throughout the muscle.*

One motor neuron and its axonal branches, together with the skeletal muscle fibers that it innervates, comprises what is termed a *motor unit.* The extent to which the individual muscle fibers that belong to any given motor unit contract is not subject to voluntary control: they either contract fully (although the force of their contraction can vary under differing circumstances), or they do not contract at all. The strength of any given skeletal muscle contraction therefore depends on *how many* of its motor units participate in the contraction. Because of the wide separation of the individual muscle fibers in any given motor unit, weak contractions that require the participation of relatively few motor units involve the muscle as a whole. In any given motor unit, all the muscle fibers can be either red or white, but not both.

Motor End Plate. Every skeletal muscle fiber is innervated by a terminal branch of a motor axon and hence belongs to a motor unit. A general term for a site where an axon ends on a muscle fiber is a *neuromuscular (myoneural) junction.* The axon, with its covering, approaches the surface of a skeletal muscle fiber from the endomysium at an angle and generally makes contact with the muscle fiber midway between its ends. At the site of contact, the axon and its covering form a small flattened mound on the surface of the muscle fiber, called a *motor end plate.* This may be stained for the LM by impregnation with gold or silver salts (Fig. 15-12) or methylene blue in fresh tissue.

Where the axon branch reaches the mound, its myelin sheath disappears but the Schwann cells investing it remain in the form of a continuous roof over the axon terminals (Figs. 15-13B and 15-14B and C). Near its termination, the axon again branches repeatedly to form a number of short *axon terminals* that are clustered together over the deep central part of the mound. Such terminals can easily be recognized in surface view (Fig. 15-12), but more often they are encountered after being sectioned in a plane that is perpendicular to the sarcolemma (Figs. 15-13C and 15-14A). The axon terminals are accommodated in surface troughs that are lined by sarcolemma (Figs. 15-13B and 15-14C). In these troughs, the axolemma is separated from the sarcolemma by a synaptic cleft that is approximately 50 nm across (Fig. 15-14C). Here the surface area of the

sarcolemma is increased by the presence of sarcolemmal folds that are invaginated into the sarcoplasm. These invaginations are commonly known as *junctional folds* (Figs. 15-13 and 15-14), and they contain extensions of the synaptic cleft that are sometimes referred to as *subneural clefts.* The synaptic cleft and its subneural extensions contain a basement membrane with associated *acetylcholinesterase,* the enzyme that is responsible for inactivating the neurotransmitter acetylcholine when this is liberated at the motor end plate (see below). Histochemical staining for this enzyme unequivocally demonstrates its presence in the synaptic and subneural clefts (Fig. 15-14A). The sarcoplasm associated with the motor end plate is comparatively rich in mitochondria and nuclei (Figs. 15-13C and 15-14C).

Transmission at the Motor End Plate. The axon terminals situated in the sarcolemmal troughs exhibit many mitochondria and numerous *synaptic vesicles* containing *acetylcholine* (Figs. 15-13 and 15-14C). When a wave of depolarization reaches these terminals, the permeability increase associated with the action potential also allows calcium ions to enter the terminals from the intercellular fluid. This causes several hundred synaptic vesicles to establish contact with the axolemma, whereupon they fuse with it and discharge their contents of acetylcholine into the synaptic cleft by exocytosis. The acetylcholine then interacts with its receptors on the sarcolemma, which for the most part are situated along the origins of the junctional folds but also extend down their sides for a short distance. When acetylcholine combines with these receptors, it immediately increases the permeability of the sarcolemma in the end plate region. This permits sodium ions to pass into the sarcoplasm and potassium ions to move out in the reverse direction. As a result, there is a decrease in the resting potential of the sarcolemma in this region, and once this decrease attains a threshold level, a new wave of depolarization is instigated that proceeds to sweep over the sarcolemma, away from the end plate region.

The synaptic vesicles are most numerous at sites that are situated opposite the openings of the sarcolemmal junctional folds. The excess membranous constituents contributed by their fusion with the axolemma are retrieved through the local recycling mechanism that was described in Chapter 14 in the section on Synapses (illustrated in Fig. 14-16). The membrane constituents taken up through endocytosis become added to the smooth-surfaced membranous cisterna from which new synaptic vesicles are produced. The size of this cisterna depends on the activity of the end plate. Because acetylcholine is synthesized in the cisterna utilizing enzymes that are brought to the terminal by axonal transport, it is already present in the synaptic vesicles when these bud from the cisterna.

After acetylcholine has been released into the synaptic cleft, it is promptly degraded to choline and acetate by the enzyme *acetylcholinesterase.* This enzyme is produced by the muscle fiber, and it seems to be anchored to the part

(Text continues on p. 398.)

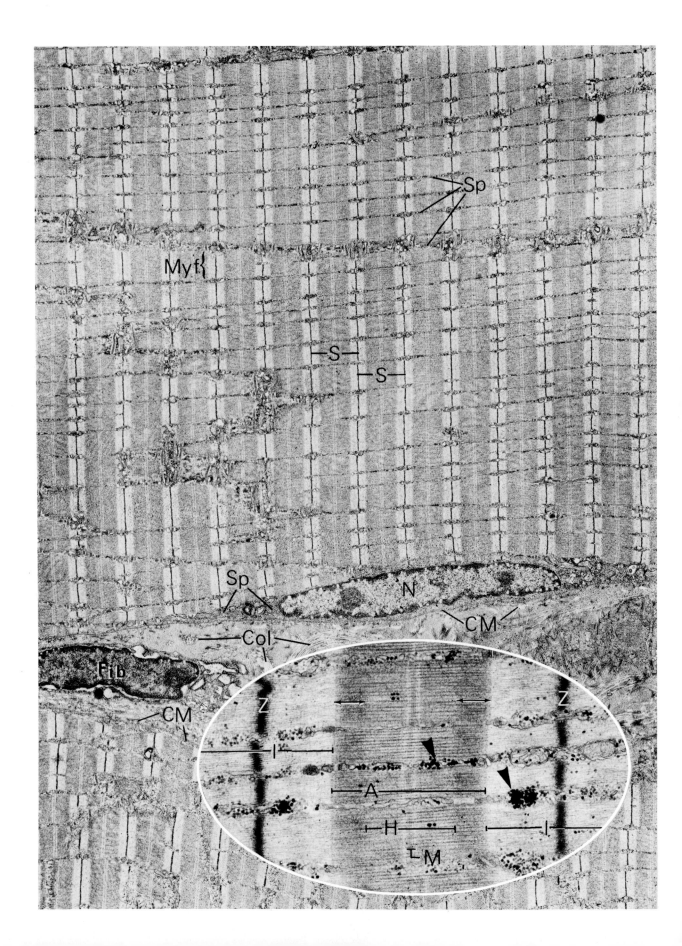

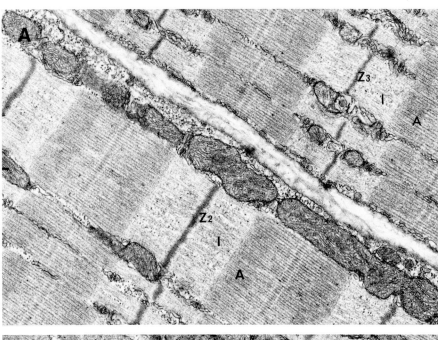

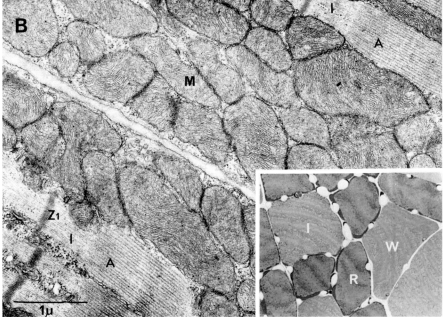

Fig. 15-11. Electron micrographs (×33,000) of skeletal muscle (longitudinal section) showing the three fiber types. (*A*) At upper right, there is a white fiber (Z_3), characterized by relatively few mitochondria lying chiefly between myofibrils at the level of Z lines. At lower left, there is a fiber of the intermediate type (Z_2). (*B*) Red fibers (Z_1) shown here contain an abundance of mitochondria (*M*) at their periphery as well as between myofibrils. (*Inset*) Photomicrograph showing white (*W*), intermediate (*I*), and red (*R*) fibers in cross section. Note their relative diameters. The rounded pale areas between the muscle fibers are blood capillaries. (Courtesy of J. Dadoune)

Fig. 15-10. Electron micrograph of a skeletal muscle fiber (white fiber) taken at a relatively low magnification (×6500) to show its general features. The sarcomeres (*S*) of myofibrils (*Myf*) are precisely aligned across the fiber. The borders of each myofibril are delineated by thin sheaths of sarcoplasm (*Sp*). Transversely oriented T tubules can just be discerned in the patches of sarcoplasm visible at middle left, where myofibrils have been sectioned obliquely. At the periphery of the fiber, there is a muscle cell nucleus (*N*), together with the cell membrane (*CM*) or sarcolemma, a fibroblast (*Fib*), and collagen of the endomysium (*Col*). (*Inset*) Electron micrograph showing the alignment of myofibrils at higher magnification (×30,000). The parts of the sarcomere are labeled, and the arrowheads indicate glycogen deposits in the sarcoplasm between the myofibrils. (Ross MH, Reith EJ: Histology: A Text and Atlas. New York, Harper & Row/JB Lippincott, 1985)

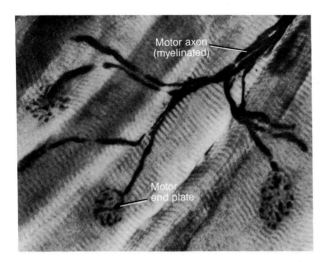

Motor axon
(myelinated)

Motor
end plate

Fig. 15-12. Photomicrograph showing the motor end plates on skeletal muscle fibers (stained with gold chloride).

of the basement membrane that lies in the synaptic and subneural clefts. Because it is interposed between the axolemma and sarcolemma, acetylcholinesterase degrades a substantial proportion of acetylcholine before it ever reaches its receptors in the sarcolemma. This arrangement reduces the risk of spurious contraction as a result of background release of the neurotransmitter. Also, during rapid transmission of impulses to the muscle fiber, fast degradation of receptor-bound neurotransmitter is necessary for the same receptors to respond repeatedly. For further information, see Lester.

It is now established that in *myasthenia gravis* (Gr. *mys,* muscle; *astheneia,* weakness), a condition in which there is profound muscular weakness, the end plate region of the sarcolemma has fewer acetylcholine receptors than normal. As a result, motor nerve impulses fail to elicit contraction of the requisite number of muscle fibers and the muscle executes only feeble contractions. There is clear evidence that this debilitating condition is due to the development of autoimmunity against the patient's acetylcholine receptors. Antibody molecules directed against these receptors are produced that not only block the receptors but also crosslink them and accelerate their rate of degradation, probably by inducing their endocytotic removal from the sarcolemma (Drachman).

Transverse Tubules (T Tubules)

The wave of sarcolemmal depolarization initiated when efferent impulses arrive at the motor end plate now begins to sweep along the sarcolemma. The EM has disclosed a system of narrow tubules known as *T tubules* that extend from the sarcolemma into the fiber at regularly repeated intervals. Studies using ferritin as an extracellular marker clearly show that the lumen of the T tubules is in direct communication with the intercellular space (Fig. 15-15, *inset*). T tubules accordingly represent *tubular invaginations of the sarcolemma* that readily conduct waves of depolarization into the substance of the fiber.

In mammalian skeletal muscle, the T tubules enter the fiber at each site where an A band and an I band meet. They then branch extensively in a transverse plane. As a result, branches of two T tubules encircle each component sarcomere of every myofibril, and these branches lie at the level of its A band–I band junctions. Reference to Figure 15-16 will clarify where the T tubules lie in relation to the striations in the myofibrils. However, in amphibian skeletal muscle (the first kind of skeletal muscle to be described in the literature), the T tubules enter the fiber and branch within it only at the Z lines, with the result that there is only a single T tubule per sarcomere instead of two (Fig. 15-15). This is the arrangement that is found in mammalian *cardiac* muscle, which will be described later in this chapter.

The wave of sarcolemmal depolarization does not affect the myofibrils directly. Instead, it elicits another event in a different compartment of the muscle fiber that is known as its *sarcoplasmic reticulum.* The membrane of the sarcoplasmic reticulum is closely associated with the T tubules in an arrangement that enables the wave of depolarization conveyed by the T tubules to bring about an important permeability change in this membrane.

Sarcoplasmic Reticulum

This organelle of the muscle fiber corresponds to the smooth endoplasmic reticulum of other cell types. It constitutes a separate sarcoplasmic compartment that is made up of (1) flattened cisternae and (2) a system of anastomosing tubules that interconnect them. Together, these two components comprise a collarlike complex that surrounds each myofibril (Fig. 15-16).

Near each end of a sarcomere, there is a *terminal cisterna* of the sarcoplasmic reticulum that is described as terminal because of its position in a sarcomere of amphibian skeletal muscle (Fig. 15-15). These cisternae encircle the sarcomere in the form of paired collars (Fig. 15-16). One pair of terminal cisternae is associated with each of the A band–I band junctions (Fig. 15-16). Furthermore, the neighboring terminal cisternae of each pair lie in close apposition to the T tubule that encircles the myofibril at this level (Fig. 15-16). Each sarcomere is therefore encircled by two T tubules (one at each A band–I band junction), and each T tubule is flanked by two terminal cisternae. Hence mammalian skeletal muscle fibers have a total of four terminal cisternae per sarcomere (Fig. 15-16). At sites where a T tubule with a terminal cisterna on either side has been cut in cross section (as in Fig. 15-16), the three associated structures are described as a *triad.* As might be expected, no direct structural continuity has ever been demonstrated between the lumen of the T tubule, which is continuous with the

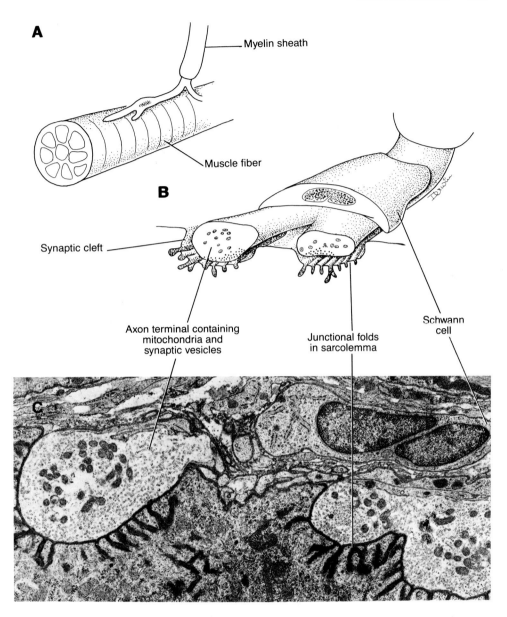

A

Myelin sheath

Muscle fiber

B

Synaptic cleft

Axon terminal containing
mitochondria and
synaptic vesicles

Junctional folds
in sarcolemma

Schwann
cell

C

Fig. 15-13. Electron micrograph and interpretive drawings illustrating the general structure of a motor end plate. (C, courtesy of A. Sima)

extracellular space, and the lumen of the sarcoplasmic reticulum, which represents a separate intracellular compartment.

The remainder of the sarcoplasmic reticulum is made up of anastomosing tubules that are often referred to as *sarcotubules.* This network of tubules interconnects terminal cisternae of consecutive pairs of such cisternae, but it does not interconnect the two associated cisternae of each pair (Fig. 15-16). Over the midregion of the sarcomere, the sarcotubules form an intricate network (Figs. 15-16 and

15-17), but elsewhere they have a primarily longitudinal orientation. The sarcoplasmic reticulum has accordingly been described as having the general appearance of a lacy sleeve (Figs. 15-16 and 15-17).

The stimulus for contraction passes from the T tubules to the terminal cisternae of the sarcoplasmic reticulum at the triads. Here there is a distinctive specialization of the apposed membranes. Rows of electron-dense junctional structures that are commonly described as *junctional feet* appear to bridge the intermembranous (junctional) gap of

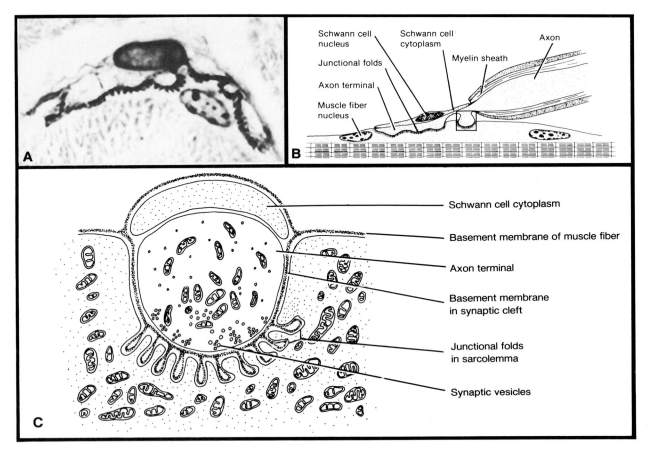

Fig. 15-14. Photomicrograph and interpretive diagrams illustrating the structure of a motor end plate. (*A*) Photomicrograph of a motor end plate (hedgehog), stained by the acetylthiocholine method for cholinesterase; nuclei are counterstained with hematoxylin. The darkly stained nucleus just above center belongs to a Schwann cell; the paler one right of center belongs to the muscle fiber. Dark staining of the cholinesterase in the synaptic cleft outlines the junctional folds. (*B*) EM diagram of a motor end plate in longitudinal section. The terminal axon branches are covered on their exposed side with Schwann cells. (*C*) EM diagram of boxed-in area in *B*, showing an axon terminal in transverse section. For further details, see text. (Photomicrograph courtesy of, and diagrams after, R. Couteaux)

approximately 10 nm to 12 nm between the membrane of the terminal cisterna and that of the T tubule. These rows of electron-dense particles can be seen quite clearly on the left and right sides of Figure 15-15. The particles seem to represent integral protein complexes of the two apposed membranes, with associated electron-dense material, that link the two membranes together. However, their functional significance is not yet clear. For example, the design of this unique intermembranous arrangement differs considerably from that of a typical low-resistance pathway (gap junction), and this raises the question of whether impulses are transmitted electrically from T tubules to the sarcoplasmic reticulum or by some other means.

Muscular Contraction Is Regulated by the Calcium Ion Concentration in the Myofibrils. The primary role of the sarcoplasmic reticulum is to regulate the concentration of calcium ions within the myofibrils. It is this level of calcium ions that determines whether actin will interact with myosin. The principal integral membrane protein of the sarcoplasmic reticulum is the enzyme $Ca^{2+} + Mg^{2+}$–*dependent adenosine triphosphatase (ATPase)*. Using energy provided by adenosine triphosphate (ATP), this enzyme pumps calcium ions from the myofibrils into the lumen of the sarcoplasmic reticulum, where they are stored whenever the muscle fiber is not undergoing contraction. After these ions have entered the sarcoplasmic reticulum, they become bound to calcium-binding proteins, primarily a peripheral (extrinsic) membrane protein called *calsequestrin*.

The intracellular localization of these two major proteins of the sarcoplasmic reticulum has now been established by immunoelectron microscopy. Whereas $Ca^{2+} + Mg^{2+}$–dependent ATPase can be detected throughout the part of the sarcoplasmic reticulum that

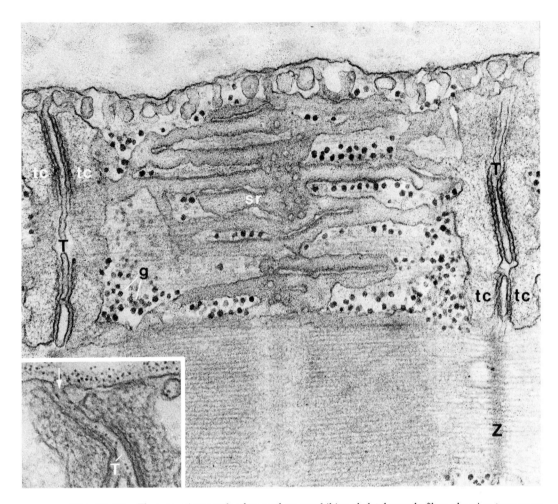

Fig. 15-15. Electron micrograph of part of an amphibian skeletal muscle fiber, showing transverse (*T*) tubules and sarcoplasmic reticulum (*sr*). The top myofibril has been cut tangentially, revealing the sarcoplasmic reticulum in surface view. T tubules enter the fiber at the level of Z lines. These tubules are closely associated with terminal cisternae (*tc*) of the sarcoplasmic reticulum. A unique kind of intracellular junction can be seen between the T tubules and terminal cisternae (see text). Abundant glycogen (*g*) particles lie between the tubules of sarcoplasmic reticulum.

(*Inset*) Part of a similar muscle fiber treated with ferritin before fixation. Ferritin particles are present in the lumen of the T (*T*) tubule, indicating that this is continuous with intercellular space. (Courtesy of R. Birks)

is associated with the I-band region and the middle of the A band, calsequestrin is confined to the interior of the terminal cisternae, which is where the majority of calcium ions are stored during relaxation (Jorgensen et al).

Whenever there is a low concentration of calcium ions in the myofibrils, the active sites on actin molecules are unable to interact with myosin because they are blocked by molecules of the regulatory protein tropomyosin (which is active in the absence of calcium ions). Because the majority of calcium ions are being stored in the sarcoplasmic reticulum during relaxation, actin and myosin are prevented from interacting with each other.

If, on the other hand, a muscle fiber is stimulated to contract, calcium ions are liberated from the sarcoplasmic reticulum and enter the myofibrils, whereupon they release the actin from this constraint. Thus it is the release of calcium ions from the sarcoplasmic reticulum that allows the actin to interact with the myosin. The link between conduction of a wave of depolarization into a muscle fiber and resulting contraction of the fiber is known as *excitation–contraction coupling*.

The following additional information is included for those students who may not yet be familiar with the biochemistry of muscular contraction.

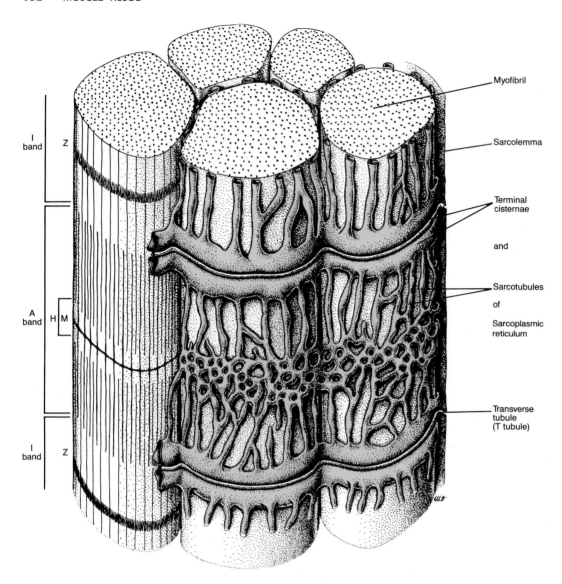

Fig. 15-16. Diagram of part of a mammalian skeletal muscle fiber, illustrating the sarcoplasmic reticulum surrounding its myofibrils. In mammalian skeletal muscle, two transverse (*T*) tubules supply a sarcomere. Each T tubule is situated at the junction between an A and an I band, where it is associated with two terminal cisternae of sarcoplasmic reticulum. Terminal cisternae connect with sarcotubules located around the A band, and these anastomose to form a network in the central region of the A band. The triple structure seen in cross section where terminal cisternae from adjacent sarcomeres flank a transverse tubule is called a triad. (Courtesy of C. P. Leblond)

MOLECULAR BASIS OF MUSCULAR CONTRACTION

Thin Filaments. In addition to actin, the thin filaments of striated muscle fibers contain two other proteins, *tropomyosin* and *troponin*. The manner in which molecules of these proteins fit together to form a thin filament is illustrated in Figure 15-18. Two rows of globular actin molecules are intertwined to form a double-stranded helix that constitutes the backbone of the thin filament (Fig. 15-18). There is thus a spiral groove along each side of the helix. Long, narrow tropomyosin molecules lie end to end in these grooves (Fig. 15-18), so that there are tropomyosin molecules lying along both sides of the helix. Troponin molecules are bound to the tropomyosin molecules in the grooves at regular intervals. In conjunction with troponin, tropomyosin plays a key role in *regulating interaction of actin with myosin*. Troponin is a complex of three subunits, each with its own role in regulating contraction.

Thick Filaments. These are composed primarily of myosin molecules together with a protein known as C-protein. A myosin

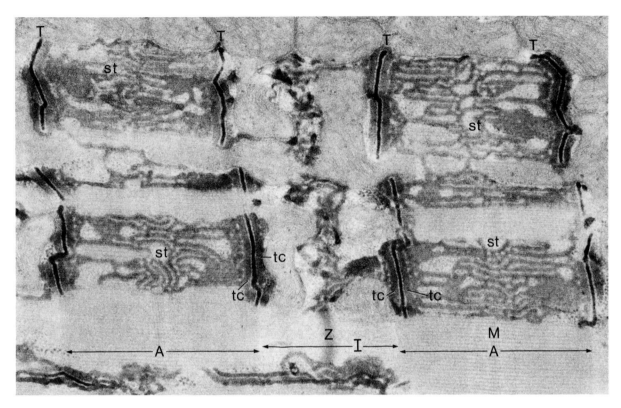

Fig. 15-17. Electron micrograph (×38,000) of part of a mammalian skeletal muscle fiber (mouse) postfixed in osmium ferrocyanide, showing the sarcoplasmic reticulum around adjoining sarcomeres. The T tubules lie at the junctions of A and I bands. Terminal cisternae (*tc*) of the sarcoplasmic reticulum lie alongside the T tubules. The "torn sleeve" appearance of the sarcoplasmic reticulum is due to anastomosis of sarcotubules (*st*). (Forbes MS, Plantholt BA, Sperelakis N: J Ultrastruct Res 60:306, 1977)

Fig. 15-18. Diagram illustrating how the double head of a myosin molecule of a thick filament interacts with actin molecules in a thin filament. A thin filament is made up of a double-stranded helix of G-actin molecules with tropomyosin molecules (shown as rods) and units of troponin complex (shown in *black*) lying along the grooves between the strands. (*Top*) During relaxation, tropomyosin molecules block the active sites (indicated in *blue*) on actin molecules and prevent myosin heads from interacting with them. (*Bottom*) During contraction, the configuration of the troponin complex is altered by calcium ions. This causes the tropomyosin molecules to move away from the active sites on actin molecules so that the sites interact with myosin heads of thick filaments.

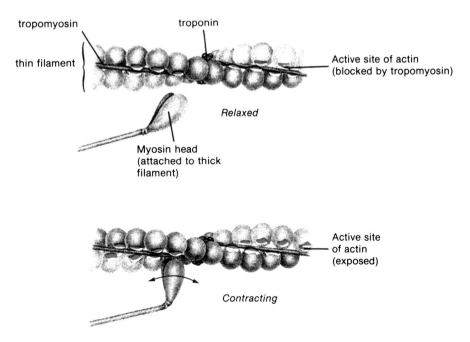

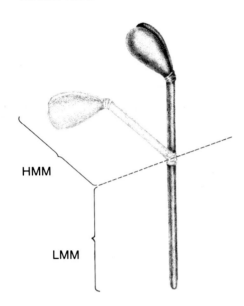

Fig. 15-19. Diagram illustrating the change in shape of a myosin molecule as it interacts with actin. Its two subunits, heavy meromyosin (*HMM*) and light meromyosin (*LMM*), are also indicated. Bending at two hinge regions permits movement of the double head from its position during relaxation (indicated by *solid lines*) to another position (*dotted*) that allows it to interact with an actin molecule in an adjacent thin filament. The two parts of the myosin head oscillate between these two positions very rapidly, interacting with actin molecules and thereby helping to move the actin-containing filament along. Most of the tail region is embedded in a thick filament.

molecule possesses a head and a long tail region and thus resembles a golf club (Fig. 15-19). Its head region, which is a double structure, and the adjacent (proximal) portion of its tail, approximately 60 nm in length, constitute what is termed *heavy meromyosin* (Gr. *meros*, part). The remainder of the tail region (the handle and most of the shaft of the golf club), which totals about 90 nm in length, constitutes its other part, called *light meromyosin*. As shown in Figure 15-19, a myosin molecule is flexible both at the junction of its heavy and light meromyosin portions and also at its neck region, allowing the two parts of the double head and also the proximal tail portion to hinge on the rest of the molecule; the significance of this flexibility will soon become apparent.

The myosin molecules of a thick filament are bundled together as depicted in Figure 15-20. Half have their heads pointing toward one end of the filament and half point in the opposite direction. The significance of this arrangement is that it explains why the two sets of thin filaments in the sarcomere are pulled in *opposite directions*. Moreover, because the myosin molecules have a staggered arrangement, their heads lie at regular intervals along the thick filaments (Fig. 15-20). The midsection of the thick filament is nevertheless devoid of myosin heads, containing only the tail regions of these molecules (Fig. 15-20).

Also termed *cross bridges,* the heads of myosin molecules are distinguishable in the EM (Fig. 15-21). Due to their helical arrangement along the filament (Fig. 15-20), these myosin heads constitute six longitudinal rows of lateral projections. Each row of projections is arranged so that it is directly aligned with one of the six thin filaments associated with the thick filament. Under the conditions outlined below, the myosin heads interact with the actin molecules in the adjacent thin filaments and bring about a contraction.

For further details about these contractile proteins, including their respective arrangements and interactions (which we shall describe in the following section) and a great deal of other useful information as well, see Gröschel–Stewart and Drenckhahn.

The Regulatory Proteins in the Thin Filaments Undergo Conformational Changes in the Presence of Calcium Ions. The troponin complex and tropomyosin molecules cooperate to form a molecular locking device that, during relaxation, *prevents* actin molecules from interacting with myosin heads on adjacent thick filaments. The actin in thin filaments can only be "unlocked" by *calcium ions,* which are liberated from the sarcoplasmic reticulum in response to sarcolemmal depolarization. When the muscle fiber is not being stimulated to contract, calcium ions are quickly withdrawn from myofibrils into the sarcoplasmic reticulum so that their concentration falls below the minimum required to "unlock" actin; the contraction process therefore abruptly ceases. The mechanism by which calcium ions "unlock" actin involves their binding to one kind of troponin. Such binding brings about a change in the configuration of the troponin complex. This, in turn, causes a slight shift in position of the tropomyosin molecules that is sufficient to expose the myosin-interacting sites on the actin molecules (Fig. 15-18). For further details about these regulatory proteins, see Cohen.

It is generally conceded that for contraction to occur, both parts of each double myosin head on the thick filaments swivel independently, serially connecting and then disconnecting with the actin molecules in the thin filaments in such a way as to pull on them. Although there is evidence that the myosin heads alter their position slightly when bringing about a contraction, the precise way in which contractile force is generated from this conformational change in the myosin molecules is still unclear.

ATP Provides the Energy for Muscular Contraction. The energy required for muscular contraction is derived from ATP, which is the essential energy "currency" of the cell. The ATP becomes hydrolyzed due to *actin-activated Mg^{2+}–dependent ATPase* activity of the myosin heads. The liberated energy then causes the myosin heads to alter their position, with the result that they also move the thin filaments to which they have temporarily become attached. Details of the cycle of operation are described in the following section.

The first effect of binding of ATP to myosin heads is extremely rapid. It causes them to *dissociate* from the actin in the thin filaments. The bound ATP is then quickly hydrolyzed, and the myosin heads enter an activated state in which they respond to the regulatory signal. This signal, as already noted, is a critical calcium level in the myofibrils. Provided that this level is high enough for contraction to proceed, the myosin heads interact with the actin in the thin filaments, after which they tilt to a different angle (Fig. 15-18, *bottom*). This is sometimes referred to as the *power stroke.* Once again, ATP binds to the myosin heads, whereupon they dissociate from the thin filaments and, on hydrolysis of the ATP, reassume their untilted position, ready for the next cycle of operation. However, on the next occasion, they will attach themselves to actin molecules that lie approximately 20 nm farther along the thin filaments. Calculations indicate that this cycle is repeated between 5 and 50 times per second.

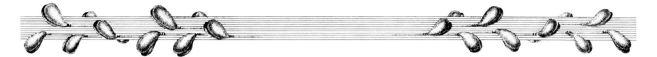

Fig. 15-20. Diagram of the midregion of a thick filament, illustrating the arrangement of its myosin molecules. Their double heads are arranged in pairs, with each one of the pair located on opposite sides of the filament. These heads are helically arranged, and they lie in six longitudinal rows at intervals of 43 nm along the filament. Due to the orientation of the myosin molecules, the middle of the filament is devoid of myosin heads; it consists solely of tail regions.

No more ATP is generated after death, and when none is left to dissociate the myosin heads from the actin in the muscles, these proteins remain permanently locked together. For several hours after death, the muscles therefore remain seized in a fixed position, and it is not until autolysis sets in that they will yield to passive stretch. This rigid state is known as *rigor mortis,* meaning rigidity of death.

When a muscle fiber is being stimulated, it remains contracted as long as impulses keep arriving at the motor end plate. When the impulses cease or the energy reserves of the muscle fiber have become exhausted, the fiber relaxes. In the former case, relaxation is brought about by removal of calcium ions by the sarcoplasmic reticulum until they reach a low concentration in the myofibrils. The energy for pumping calcium ions out of the myofibrils into the sarcoplasmic reticulum is again provided by ATP. Hence ATP plays a role not only in contraction but also in relaxation.

The energy for *resynthesis* of ATP can be derived from the breakdown of glucose, glycogen, or free fatty acids. ATP can also be rapidly resynthesized during exercise by combination of adenosine diphosphate (ADP) with phosphate groups from another high-energy compound called *creatine phosphate* (phosphorylcreatine), which is reconstituted during relaxation. Such use of creatine phosphate as an intermediary may be likened to having additional currency of another denomination in the bank ready for a time of need. Whereas the efficient way of producing ATP from glucose or glycogen is through oxidative phosphorylation, some energy can also be liberated in the absence of oxygen, with the production of lactate and pyruvate as metabolites. This latter pathway is an important alternative in skeletal muscle during sustained exercise, when the oxygen supply may become inadequate to permit continued oxidative phosphorylation. Moreover, the various types of skeletal muscle fibers differ with regard to which pathway predominates. Thus oxidative phosphorylation is more prevalent in red fibers, which have abundant mitochondria, and anaerobic glycolysis is more important in white fibers.

DEVELOPMENT, GROWTH, AND REGENERATION OF SKELETAL MUSCLE FIBERS

The cells that form skeletal muscle fibers in the embryo are called *myoblasts.* These cells have a single nucleus and lack myofibrils. However, after repeated proliferation, they begin to fuse together, forming long multinucleated *myotubes* that, in due course, develop myofibrils and the other organelles characteristic of skeletal muscle fibers. In man, most skeletal muscle fibers develop before birth, and vir-

tually all have formed by the end of the first year of postnatal life. However, these fibers continue to acquire more nuclei as a result of their fusion with small uninucleated cells that seem to represent residual myoblast-derived stem cells. These relatively undifferentiated cells are known as *satellite* (or *myosatellite*) *cells,* and they lie alongside skeletal muscle fibers, enclosed within the same basement membrane (Fig. 15-22).

Postnatal Growth of Skeletal Muscle Fibers. During the postnatal growth period, muscles need to be able to increase in length and width to match the growth of the skeleton. The size they reach depends on the amount of exercise obtained, and much effort is often expended in achieving the desired results. After the first year of life, all growth of skeletal muscles is due to enlargement of the existing muscle fibers (*i.e.,* hypertrophy); it is not due to an increase in the number of muscle fibers (*i.e.,* hyperplasia). Nevertheless, muscle samples obtained at different times during the growth period show an increase in the number of *myofibrils* in each fiber. As skeletal muscle fibers grow, new filaments are added to the periphery of their myofibrils. After their myofibrils attain an optimal diameter (1 μm to 1.2 μm), they appear to split longitudinally to create more myofibrils. Hence most growth in the width of skeletal muscle fibers is due to an increase in the number of myofibrils that they contain.

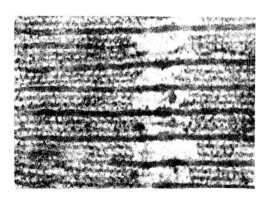

Fig. 15-21. Electron micrograph ($\times$150,000) of part of a sarcomere of a skeletal muscle fiber (rabbit psoas), showing cross bridges on the thick filaments. (Courtesy of H. E. Huxley)

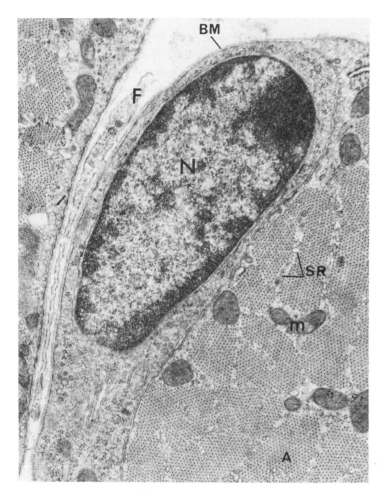

Fig. 15-22. Electron micrograph (×22,000) of a satellite cell, the nucleus of which is labeled N. This cell lies adjacent to a skeletal muscle fiber (*lower right*), enclosed by the same basement membrane (*BM*). The muscle fiber at lower right is cut through an A band; some sarcoplasmic reticulum (*SR*) is also visible. A portion of fibroblast cytoplasm (*F*) lies between the satellite cell and the muscle fiber at upper left. (Courtesy of E. Schultz)

Increase in the length of skeletal muscle fibers can be due to their fusion with satellite cells (or progeny of these cells). Furthermore, myofibrils can lengthen due to the addition of new sarcomeres to their ends, in the regions adjoining the muscle attachments.

Satellite Cells Provide a Basis for Regeneration in Skeletal Muscles.   In addition to providing a mechanism for growth of skeletal muscle fibers, satellite cells are believed to persist throughout adult life as a stem cell population that serves as a potential source of new myoblasts that are capable of fusing to form new muscle fibers. Hence following muscle trauma and in certain dystrophic conditions, an attempt is made to regenerate new muscle fibers to replace damaged or necrotic fibers. This seems to be the only recourse in skeletal muscles because nuclei that have become incorporated into skeletal muscle fibers do not divide. Any large muscle defects resulting from severe trauma, however, become filled in with a disorganized mixture of fibrous scar tissue laid down by fibroblasts and new muscle fibers derived from satellite cells. Furthermore, loss of muscle function due to injury is compensated for primarily by *hypertrophy of the undamaged muscle fibers*,

and only to a lesser degree is it due to the regeneration of new fibers. Successful regeneration depends on preservation of the endomysial connective tissue framework because this serves as an essential scaffolding during the repair process.

Motor Neurons Exert a Trophic Influence on the Muscle Fibers That They Innervate.   Skeletal muscle fibers require their motor nerve supply not only to elicit their contraction but also for their general maintenance. Loss of efferent innervation greatly increases their sensitivity to acetylcholine and can lead to their degeneration or atrophy.

Cross-reinnervation experiments show that when white muscle fibers (faster contracting) are artificially supplied with motor nerves that formerly supplied red fibers (slower to contract), they contract more slowly, like red fibers. Conversely, red fibers contract like white ones when supplied with motor fibers that formerly supplied white fibers. This shows that the physiological characteristics of muscle fibers also are dependent on their efferent innervation.

Motor neurons are therefore said to exert a continuous *trophic influence* on the muscle fibers they innervate. Without this influence, which could prove to be no more than liberation of a neurotrophic factor from the terminals of motor axons, skeletal muscle fibers undergo degenerative changes. Some hold the view that at least some forms of *muscular dystrophy* (Gr. *dys*, bad or difficult), conditions characterized by atrophic changes in individual muscle fibers, may be a result of inadequate production of neurotrophic factors or diminished responsiveness to them. However, a number of other hypotheses have also been proposed to explain this condition.

AFFERENT INNERVATION OF SKELETAL MUSCLES, TENDONS, AND SYNOVIAL JOINTS

In addition to their efferent nerve supply, skeletal muscles are provided with afferent nerve endings that enable them to signal their degree of contraction to the CNS. Within the CNS, this information is integrated with information arriving from tendons, ligaments, and joint capsules to provide an awareness of the positions and rates of movement of the various parts of the body. The sensory receptors that initiate these afferent impulses are the *muscle spindles, tendon organs,* and *joint receptors.*

Muscle Spindles.   Also known as *neuromuscular spindles,* these structures are the length-registering receptors of skeletal muscles. The simplest reflexes in which they participate are described as *stretch reflexes* because they bring about responses to stretch in muscles. A familiar example is the *knee jerk* elicited by striking the patellar tendon so that the quadriceps femoris muscle is stretched. Reflex contraction of this muscle makes the foot kick forward (see Fig. 14-2). To explain how muscle spindles participate in such reflexes, we need to discuss their structure and innervation.

A muscle spindle is fusiform (3 mm to 5 mm long and approximately 0.2 mm in diameter at its middle) and is enclosed by an extensible connective tissue capsule (Figs. 15-23 and 15-24). Muscle spindles are longitudinally oriented and become stretched when the muscle is stretched. They are most numerous in muscles that require fine control. Each muscle spindle contains from 2 to 12 muscle fibers that are narrower than ordinary skeletal muscle fibers and are also different in other ways. These special fibers are termed *intrafusal fibers* (L. *fusus,* spindle) to distinguish them from the *extrafusal fibers* outside the spindle.

Two microscopically distinguishable types of intrafusal fibers are recognized. The larger ones are termed *nuclear bag fibers,* and there are generally one to four of these fibers in the spindle. The others are termed *nuclear chain fibers,* and there are up to ten of them in the spindle. The nuclear bag fibers are both wider and longer than the nuclear chain fibers (Figs. 15-23 and 15-24*B*). They are described as *nuclear bag fibers* because their noncontractile midportions contain so many nuclei that they literally look like bags of nuclei. Nuclear chain fibers do not have an expanded midregion, and they contain nuclei that are lined up in a single row, resembling a chain (Fig. 15-23). For those re-

quiring more information, details of the afferent and efferent innervation of these two types of intrafusal fibers will now be given.

The Afferent Innervation of Nuclear Bag Fibers.   Each nuclear bag fiber receives a terminal branch of a large myelinated sensory fiber (*primary afferent* in Fig. 15-23). As can be seen in Fig. 15-24*A*, the afferent ending of this group IA fiber winds around the nuclear bag more or less spirally and hence is sometimes called an *annulospiral ending*; however, in man it is not as spiral as it is in other vertebrates, and it is now more common to call it a *primary ending*.

The Afferent Innervation of Nuclear Chain Fibers.   Unlike nuclear bag fibers, nuclear chain fibers receive afferent innervation from *two* sources. First, branches of the same large sensory fiber (*primary afferent* in Fig. 15-23) that terminates in primary endings in nuclear bag fibers form similar primary endings in the central regions of nuclear chain fibers. Second, branches of smaller and separate afferent fibers (*secondary afferent* in Fig. 15-23; *II* in Fig. 15-24*A*) terminate in *secondary* (*flower-spray*) endings, one on each side of the primary ending. Thus nuclear chain fibers are supplied with both primary and secondary afferent endings.

The primary ending responds to both the degree and rate of stretch of a muscle, whereas the secondary endings respond only to the degree of stretch. The ways in which impulses from the two kinds of afferent endings participate in different reflexes are complex. Stretching afferent endings, for example by tapping a patellar tendon, initiates impulses that travel up afferent fibers to the spinal cord (see Fig. 14-2), where afferent neurons synapse with large α motor neurons that supply numbers of ordinary (extrafusal) fibers in the muscle involved. The motor neurons thereupon elicit contraction of the extrafusal fibers that they innervate so that the stretch reflex is completed. Stimulation of afferent endings ceases when tension in intrafusal fibers is unloaded by contraction of the extrafusal fibers with which they are in parallel. The afferent neurons synapse in the spinal cord not only with efferent neurons of the same segment but also with intersegmental interneurons that conduct impulses to the parts of the brain concerned with muscular coordination.

The Efferent Innervation of Intrafusal Fibers.   Intrafusal fibers, like extrafusal fibers, also have an *efferent* nerve supply. Efferent stimulation causes the intrafusal fibers to contract and thereby increases their response at any given muscle length. Small motor fibers (*dynamic and static γ efferents* in Fig. 15-23) from γ motor neurons supply the contractile ends of intrafusal fibers. Studies by Boyd's group have shown that nuclear bag fibers may receive either dynamic γ fibers or static γ fibers. Thus there are two functionally different types of nuclear bag fibers. Nuclear chain fibers, however, all receive static γ fibers. As shown in Figure 15-23, γ fibers terminate in either multiple *en grappe* (Fr. *grappe,* cluster) *endings* or in more extensive *trail endings* on contractile portions of intrafusal fibers. Efferent impulses from the γ motor neurons elicit contraction in these regions so as to stretch the afferent endings still further, and this increases their response at any given muscle length. Some of the nuclear bag fibers also receive β efferent fibers (not shown in Fig. 15-23).

It will be appreciated from the foregoing discussion that both the degree and velocity of stretch of skeletal muscles are automatically monitored by their muscle spindles, which operate by signalling to the CNS any temporary

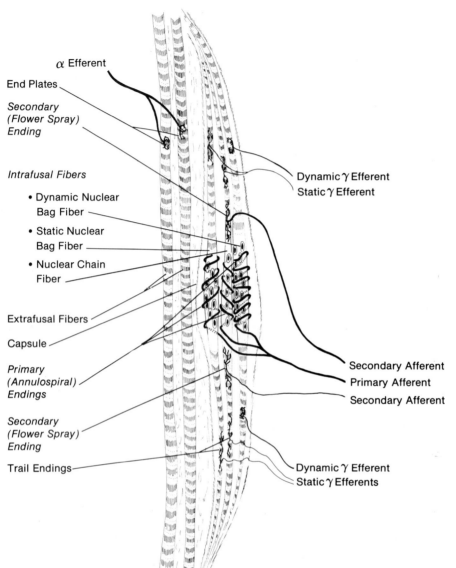

α Efferent

End Plates

Secondary
(Flower Spray)
Ending

Intrafusal Fibers

• Dynamic Nuclear
  Bag Fiber

• Static Nuclear
  Bag Fiber

• Nuclear Chain
  Fiber

Extrafusal Fibers

Capsule

Primary
(Annulospiral)
Endings

Secondary
(Flower Spray)
Ending

Trail Endings

Dynamic γ Efferent
Static γ Efferent

Secondary Afferent
Primary Afferent
Secondary Afferent

Dynamic γ Efferent
Static γ Efferents

Fig. 15-23. Schematic diagram of a muscle spindle showing the innervation of nuclear bag fibers and nuclear chain fibers as determined from cat muscles. Only two nuclear bag fibers and one nuclear chain fiber are shown here for clarity. (See text for details.) The β-innervation is omitted and the diameter of the spindle is expanded to show details.

discrepancies that may exist between the length of the intrafusal fibers and the length of the muscle as a whole. These signals are used to moderate contraction in the extrafusal fibers of the muscles concerned. This constitutes a servomechanism that has been likened to power-assisted steering of motor vehicles, in which misalignment between steering wheel and road wheel positions is measured and applied toward turning the road wheels in the desired direction. Muscle spindles, together with other afferent endings sensitive to tendon tension and joint position and motion, comprise a group of receptors called *proprioceptors* (L. *proprius*, own; *capio*, to take) that are involved in controlling motion and posture. The other types of proprioceptors will now be considered briefly.

Tendon Organs. Also referred to as *Golgi tendon organs* or *neurotendinous organs*, these receptors are found at the junctions between muscles and their tendons and also in aponeuroses (on which muscles pull). They are encapsulated structures that are approximately half the size of muscle spindles. As shown in Figure 15-25, the large myelinated afferent fiber supplying a tendon organ has small nonmyelinated branches that ramify within the tendon organ between the collagen bundles of the tendon. Unlike muscle spindles, tendon organs lack efferent innervation. The afferent endings are probably stimulated by being compressed and twisted between the collagen bundles when the tendon is under tension, because they respond to tension in the muscles with which they are in series.

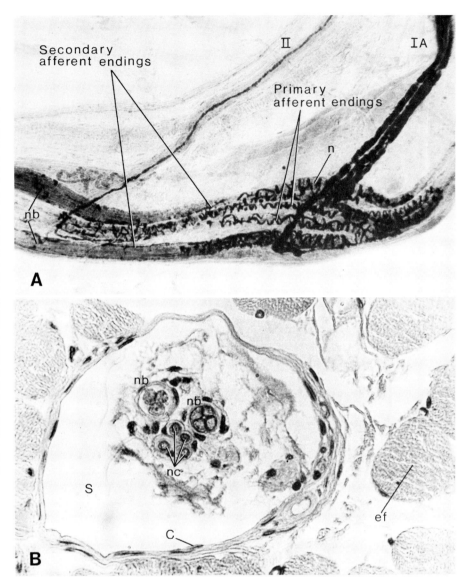

Fig. 15-24. Photomicrographs illustrating the structure and innervation of a muscle spindle (cat). (*A*) Part of a spindle teased from a soleus muscle (stained with gold chloride), showing primary (annulospiral) afferent endings at right and secondary (flower spray) afferent endings at left. The primary endings are supplied by branches of a group IA afferent fiber (*top right*), and the secondary endings are supplied by a group II afferent fiber (*top center*). The top and bottom intrafusal fibers (*nb*) are of the nuclear bag type; closely packed nuclei (*n*) can be discerned beneath the primary ending in the top nuclear bag fiber. Between the two nuclear bag fibers lie four smaller nuclear chain fibers. (*B*) Transverse section of adductor digiti longus muscle showing a muscle spindle sectioned through its midregion. As in *A*, this spindle contains two large nuclear bag fibers (*nb*) and four smaller nuclear chain fibers (*nc*). Note the smaller diameter of intrafusal fibers compared with extrafusal fibers (*ef*). The connective tissue capsule (*C*) of the muscle spindle with its fluid-filled space (*S*) is also evident. (Boyd IA: Philos Trans R Soc Lond [Biol] 245:81, 1962)

Stimulation of a Golgi tendon organ leads to reflex inhibition of firing of the lower motor neurons that supply the muscle; hence it terminates a reflex contraction elicited by stretch.

Joint Receptors. Several types of sensory receptors are associated with synovial joints. The internal and external joint ligaments, for example, are provided with receptors that closely resemble Golgi tendon organs. The fibrous connective tissue capsule of such joints contains numerous free nerve endings and Ruffini-type and paciniform corpuscles (which will be described in Chap. 17). The paciniform corpuscles (which are mechanoreceptors) are positioned at sites that are compressed by joint movements. Together with muscle spindles and tendon organs, they

play a role in *kinesthesia* (Gr. *kinesis*, motion; *aisthesis*, perception), which means conscious perception of the position and movement of the various parts of the body. Kinesthetic sensation in joints such as the hip is not lost after surgical replacement of the joint (and its receptors) by a prosthesis. The importance of the contribution made by the muscle spindles and tendon organs toward the perception of limb position becomes obvious under such circumstances.

CARDIAC MUSCLE

Before cardiac muscle was studied in the EM, it was believed to represent a multinucleated syncytial network made up of branched fibers that had no ends. The LM appearance

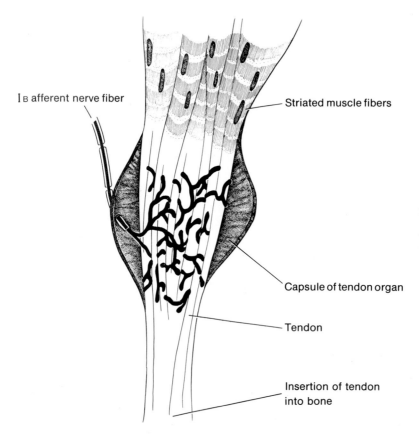

I B afferent nerve fiber

Striated muscle fibers

Capsule of tendon organ

Tendon

Insertion of tendon into bone

Fig. 15-25. Diagram of a Golgi tendon organ with its connective tissue capsule cut open and reflexed to reveal its innervation. A large myelinated afferent fiber (group IB) terminates in unmyelinated branches that ramify between the collagen bundles of the tendon.

that gave this erroneous impression can be seen in Figure 15-26, which shows that cardiac muscle fibers branch and anastomose extensively so as to leave slitlike spaces between them. However, when cardiac muscle was observed in the EM, it became apparent that its fibers are composed of individual muscle cells that are joined together end to end by cell junctions. The slitlike spaces between the fibers contain endomysium that brings capillaries and lymphatic vessels close to the muscle fibers.

Cardiac muscle fibers exhibit the same general pattern of striations as skeletal muscle fibers do. In addition, cardiac muscle fibers are traversed at intervals by dark-staining structures that are unique to cardiac muscle and are called *intercalated disks* (L. *intercalatus,* inserted). In many cases, these structures extend across the fiber in a stepwise manner (Fig. 15-27, *inset*). In the EM, it can be seen that they represent the boundaries between the individual muscle cells that make up a cardiac muscle fiber (see Fig. 15-30). Most of these cells possess one nucleus, but some of them have two. Their nuclei are somewhat larger than those of skeletal muscle fibers, and they occupy a *central* position in the fibers (Fig. 15-26, see also Figs. 15-28 and 15-30).

Even though cardiac muscle is striated, it is *involuntary.* Cardiac muscle will contract spontaneously without any nerve supply whatsoever. However, in life, its contraction is initiated by the spontaneous depolarization of special

pacemaker cells, which are situated in a part of the heart known as its *pacemaker;* the pacemaker is innervated by the autonomic nervous system. It is important to realize that the heartbeat originates in cardiac muscle cells themselves (the pacemaker cells) and that it is only the *rate* of contraction (the *heart rate*) that is regulated by the autonomic nervous system. From the pacemaker, ordinary cardiac muscle fibers and a system of cardiac muscle fibers that are specialized for impulse conduction distribute the impulse for contraction throughout the heart, with the result that first the atria and then the ventricles beat in a synchronized sequence at a resting rate of 70 beats per minute. More details about impulse conduction in the heart will be given in Chapter 16 when we deal with the heart as an organ.

General Structure of Cardiac Muscle Cells. Certain aspects of the fine structure of cardiac muscle fibers are similar to those seen in skeletal muscle. For example, each fiber is surrounded by a basement membrane (see Fig. 15-29), and myofibrils again constitute a major component of the muscle fiber (Fig. 15-28). However, the myofibrils in cardiac muscle fibers anastomose and are of variable diameter instead of being discrete and cylindrical as in skeletal muscle (Figs. 15-28 and 15-29). In the clefts between the myofibrils and at the poles of the nucleus, there are numerous large

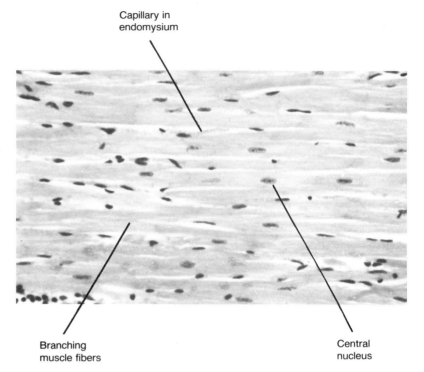

Capillary in
endomysium

Fig. 15-26. Low-power photomicrograph of cardiac muscle (sheep). Note that cardiac muscle fibers branch and anastomose. The light-staining slitlike spaces between them are filled with endomysium conveying blood (and lymph) capillaries.

Branching
muscle fibers

Central
nucleus

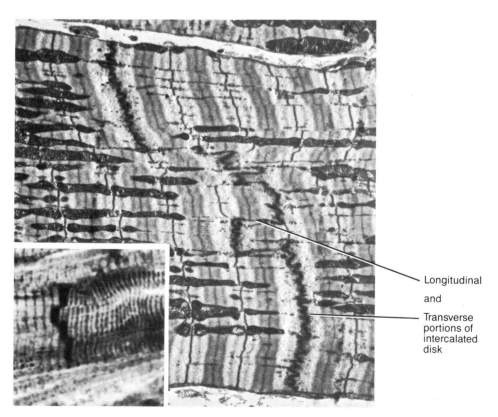

Longitudinal

and

Transverse
portions of
intercalated
disk

Fig. 15-27.   Electron micrograph (×5100) of an intercalated disk in ventricular heart muscle (dog). This disk crosses the fiber in a stepwise fashion. (*Inset*) Photomicrograph of a comparable intercalated disk from the same source. (Courtesy of A. Spiro)

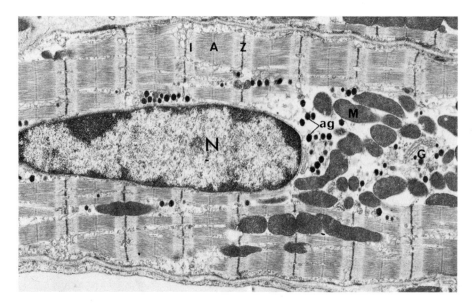

Fig. 15-28. Electron micrograph (×10,300) of an atrial heart muscle cell (hamster). The central nucleus (*N*) is bounded laterally by myofibrils. To the right of the nucleus, there is a region of sarcoplasm containing mitochondria (*M*), a Golgi (*G*), and darkly stained atrial granules (*ag*) that contain atrial natriuretic factor. (Courtesy of M. Cantin)

mitochondria. Their abundance is an indication of the sustained energy requirements of this type of muscle (Figs. 15-28 and 15-29). Granules of glycogen, together with stacks of Golgi saccules and lipid droplets, are also present at the poles of the nucleus (Fig. 15-28). In addition, deposits of the pigment lipofuscin may be present at this site, particularly in older individuals. Atrial granules are an additional feature of the sarcoplasm that is unique to the cells in the walls of the atria. The content of these granules deserves the following special mention because of its physiological importance.

Atrial Muscle Cells Produce a Hormone That Is Involved in the Regulation of Blood Pressure. It was pointed out over 20 years ago that in atrial muscle cells, the sarcoplasm at the poles of the nucleus also contains a number of electron-dense secretory granules with a diameter of 100 nm to 450 nm that have since become known as *atrial granules* (Fig. 15-28). In mammals, these secretory granules are limited to the walls of the atria, and they are more numerous in the walls of the right atrium than the left. It is now established that the atrial granules are the source of an important peptide hormone called *atrial natriuretic factor* (ANF).

It had been known for some time that stretch of the atrial musculature as a result of atrial distension caused increased renal sodium excretion (*natriuresis*), increased renal potassium excretion (*kaliuresis*), and increased renal water excretion (*diuresis*), yet the basis for this regulation was unclear. It has recently been established that the ANF content of the atrial granules is liberated in response to atrial distension and mediates this response. Furthermore, it is evident that this hormone participates in the *regulation of blood pressure and blood volume* through direct and indirect effects on (1) the rate of renal excretion of sodium, potassium, and water; (2) the tonus in the smooth muscle coat of the walls of blood vessels; (3) the rate of secretion of the hormone aldosterone by the adrenal glands; and (4) the control centers in the brain that regulate blood pressure and water excretion.

The multiple actions of ANF are very complex, involving a number of different interactions with other types of regulatory cells and with the various effects that these cells exert on their target cells. For example, the renin–angiotensin system (which will be described in Chaps. 21 and 22) is very much involved. Three of the most important effects of ANF are that it (1) *decreases blood pressure*, (2) *inhibits renin secretion* by the kidneys (see Chap. 21), and (3) *inhibits aldosterone secretion* by the adrenals (see Chap. 22). Currently, there is a great deal of interest in ANF because of the distinct possibility that it will prove to be a useful pharmacological agent in the clinical management of blood pressure disorders such as hypertension (increased blood pressure). For further information about ANF, see Cantin and Genest. More detailed information about this hormone is given in Maack et al.

Intercalated Disks Contain Three Different Types of Cell Junctions. In the EM, it can be seen that at the intercalated disks, the cell membranes that cover the ends of contiguous cardiac muscle cells interdigitate extensively and are interconnected by a distinctive type of junctional complex (Fig. 15-27). Each intercalated disk crosses a cardiac muscle fiber at the Z-line level, even where it traverses the fiber in a stepwise manner (Fig. 15-27). In the latter type of arrangement, the *transverse portions* of the disk that lie at Z-line levels are interconnected by *longitudinal portions* of the disk (Figs. 15-27 and 15-30).

Three different types of cell junctions are present in the transverse portions of such intercalated disks. First, there are abundant myofibrillar interconnections of a design similar to the *zonula adherens* (*intermediate*) type of junction between epithelial cells (see Chap. 6). Here the thin filaments are attached to electron-dense material on the sar-

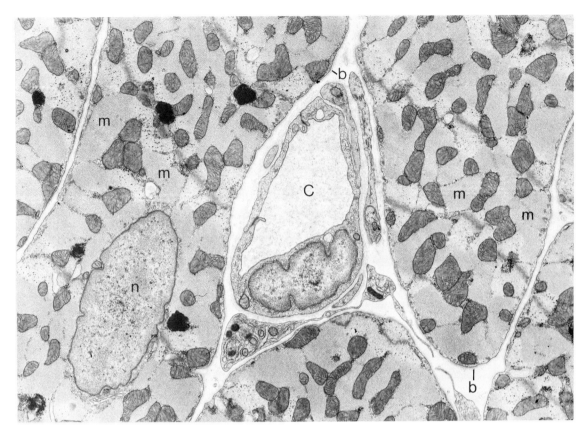

Fig. 15-29. Electron micrograph (low power) of a transverse section of ventricular papillary muscle (cat) showing cardiac muscle cells in cross section. The myofibrils (*m*) have irregular contours in cross section because of anastomosis of the myofibrils. Their filaments are just visible as closely packed dots. Note the abundant mitochondria between myofibrils, the central nucleus (*n*) in the fiber at left, and the basement membrane (*b*) surrounding the fibers. A blood capillary (*C*) lies in the endomysium at center. (Fawcett DW: Bloom and Fawcett: A Textbook of Histology, 11th ed. Philadelphia, WB Saunders, 1986)

coplasmic aspect of the sarcolemma (Fig. 15-30). However, instead of forming continuous beltlike junctions, these intermyofibrillar junctions have the shape of a patch and are therefore sometimes described as *fascia adherens* junctions. Second, there are junctions that represent expanded *desmosomes*. This type of junction is characterized by the presence of a plaque of electron-dense material on the sarcoplasmic aspect of the sarcolemma. The plaque provides anchorage for the desmin- and vimentin-containing intermediate filaments that constitute the scaffolding around each myofibril. These junctions provide sites of particularly strong intercellular adhesion that help to prevent separation of the adjoining muscle cells when they contract. Third, scattered along these transverse portions of the disks, there are small *gap junctions* that provide direct electrical communication between the adjoining muscle cells because junctions of this type are freely permeable to ions. Direct electrical communication is facilitated by even larger gap junctions that are present in the longitudinal portions of the disks (Fig. 15-30B). Intercalated disks therefore (1) pro-

vide the necessary strong attachment between the cells that make up the fiber, (2) transmit their pull, and (3) permit them to communicate electrically so that an impulse for contraction can spread over the heart from one cell to the next.

Sarcoplasmic Reticulum, T Tubules, and the Importance of Extracellular Calcium in Cardiac Contraction

Cardiac muscle cells have a less well-developed sarcoplasmic reticulum that lacks the large terminal cisternae that are seen in skeletal muscle fibers. It consists primarily of an irregular system of narrow anastomosing sarcotubules that is closely associated with the exterior of each myofibril, as in skeletal muscle (Fig. 15-31). However, two other regions of the sarcoplasmic reticulum have also been described. The part that is most closely associated with the sarcolemma and its T tubules and that is connected to them by junctional feet is described as the *junctional sarcoplasmic*

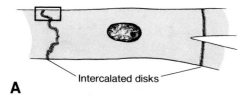

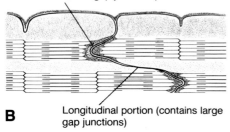

A

Transverse portion (myofibrillar junctions, desmosomes, and gap junctions)

B

Longitudinal portion (contains large gap junctions)

Fig. 15-30. (*A*) Diagram of a cardiac muscle cell with intercalated disks at either end. (*B*) Boxed-in area in *A* as seen in the EM, showing the cell junctions in the two different portions of an intercalated disk. The longitudinal portions possess large gap junctions, and the transverse portions possess small gap junctions.

reticulum. In addition, there are small bulbous and cisternal expansions of the reticulum that are also connected to the sarcolemma by junctional feet; these are called the *corbular sarcoplasmic reticulum* (Sommer and Johnson; Forbes and Sperelakis). The network of sarcotubules that constitutes the main part of the reticulum is sometimes described as the *network sarcoplasmic reticulum*. Calsequestrin is confined

to the lumen of the junctional and corbular sarcoplasmic reticulum (Jorgensen et al).

In mammalian cardiac muscle, the T tubules enter at the level of Z lines, so that, as in amphibian skeletal muscle, there is only one T tubule per sarcomere. The T tubules are considerably wider than those of skeletal muscle. Triads are not evident in cardiac muscle because the terminal elements of junctional sarcoplasmic reticulum associated with the T tubules are relatively small and do not constitute continuous collarlike terminal cisternae around the myofibrils.

In contrast to skeletal muscle fibers, in which the concentration of calcium ions within the myofibrils is regulated solely through the transfer of these ions into and out of their highly developed sarcoplasmic reticulum, cardiac muscle cells contain more limited intracellular reserves of calcium ions because their smaller sarcoplasmic reticulum lacks large terminal cisternae. However, depolarization of the sarcolemma of a cardiac muscle cell allows a certain amount of calcium from the extracellular fluid to enter the cell by way of the sarcolemma and its T tubules. Furthermore, access to the interior of the cell is facilitated by the greater width of the T tubules in this type of muscle. This influx of external calcium then acts as a trigger for the release of the calcium stored in the lumen of the sarcoplasmic reticulum, which on reaching the myofibrils elicits an "all-or-nothing" contraction. Calcium ions are subsequently pumped back into the sarcoplasmic reticulum, leading to relaxation. The importance of the extracellular calcium is such that without it, the heart ceases to beat. Hence extracellular as well as intracellular calcium is involved in cardiac contraction.

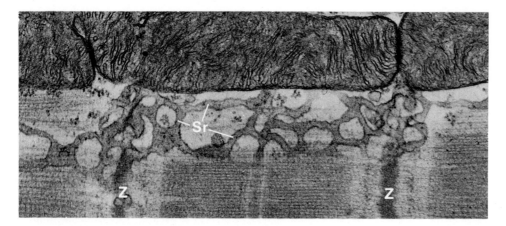

Fig. 15-31. Electron micrograph (×47,000) of part of a cardiac muscle cell (ventricular papillary muscle of cat), showing sarcoplasmic reticulum surrounding a myofibril. Part of the reticulum has been cut tangentially. Narrow tubules of the reticulum (*Sr*) lie between the myofibril extending across the bottom of the micrograph and the row of mitochondria (between myofibrils) extending across the top. In cardiac muscle the sarcoplasmic reticulum consists of an irregular arrangement of narrow tubules. It has no special distribution over A bands or Z lines and lacks the large terminal cisternae seen in skeletal muscle fibers. (Fawcett DW, McNutt NS: J Cell Biol 42:1, 1969)

Growth and Regeneration of Cardiac Muscle

Heart muscle responds to increased functional demands by increasing the size of its existing fibers, that is, by compensatory *hypertrophy*. It is generally believed that cardiac muscle cells have no capacity for mitosis in postnatal life. Moreover, they lack the satellite cells that are responsible for regeneration in skeletal muscle. Nevertheless, there are reports that a few poorly differentiated cardiac muscle cells may form in experimentally traumatized hearts of animals (Polezhaev). This new potential muscle tissue, however, quickly becomes replaced by connective tissue scars. Due to the obvious difficulty in studying regeneration of human heart muscle, it is not known whether a similar (though ineffective) attempt at regeneration might occur in humans. All that can be found at autopsies in regions where heart muscle was damaged is fibrous scar tissue.

SMOOTH MUSCLE

In describing smooth muscle, the term *fiber* is used in the same way that it is used in describing skeletal muscle, that is, to denote a single cell. Each smooth muscle fiber, however, has only one nucleus, and, as in cardiac muscle, it occupies a *central* position in the cell. This type of muscle is characteristically found in the walls of the hollow viscera and in all but the smallest blood vessels. In the walls of the viscera, it is commonly arranged in two layers and, in most cases, the inner layer is circular whereas the outer layer is longitudinal. There are nevertheless some exceptions to this general rule. Smooth muscle fibers are arranged spirally in parts of the digestive and respiratory tracts and also in arteries, but their arrangement is still usually described as circular. Such muscle layers commonly consist of anastomosing bundles of muscle fibers. Each muscle bundle is invested by a sheath of delicate connective tissue that supplies it with capillaries and nerve fibers (Fig. 15-32).

Like cardiac muscle, smooth muscle is innervated by the autonomic nervous system and is *involuntary*. It is able to maintain tonus indefinitely and is of great importance in regulating the luminal diameter of tubular structures. An increase in tonus of circularly arranged smooth muscle decreases the luminal diameter and vice versa. Undue tonic contraction of such muscle can have clinical repercussions. For example, any excessive tonus in the circular layer of smooth muscle in the walls of arterioles can restrict the outflow of blood from arteries to such an extent that blood backs up, raising the blood pressure.

As well as maintaining tonus, the smooth muscle fibers in the walls of blood vessels have the important role of producing elastin and other intercellular constituents of the vessel wall. The significance of this will be discussed in Chapter 16. In the walls of the gastrointestinal tract, and

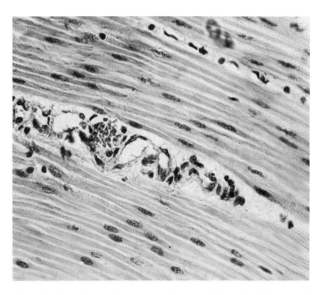

Fig. 15-32. Photomicrograph of part of the wall of the small intestine (dog), showing bundles of smooth muscle fibers cut longitudinally. Loose connective tissue (*center*) invests each bundle, supplying it with capillaries and nerve fibers.

to a lesser extent the oviducts and ureters, smooth muscle fibers undergo rhythmic contractions and give rise to *peristaltic waves* that sweep down these tubes and propel their contents along. The contraction of smooth muscle is usually sluggish compared with that of skeletal muscle, but the smooth muscle fibers of the *sphincter pupillae* (the circular fibers of the iris that constrict a pupil) contract relatively quickly.

As may be seen in Figure 15-32, smooth muscle fibers have an elongated, tapered form. Their size varies considerably with their location. The smallest are approximately 30 μm long and lie in the walls of small blood vessels. The largest are approximately 0.5 mm long and are found in the walls of the uterus during pregnancy. However, most are approximately 0.2 mm long and up to 8 μm wide. The nucleus, which lies in the widest part of the fiber (usually toward its middle), can become passively pleated when the fiber contracts (Fig. 15-33).

In the EM, mitochondria, Golgi saccules, and glycogen, together with a small amount of rough-surfaced endoplasmic reticulum, can be distinguished in the cytoplasm of smooth muscle fibers. However, these organelles and inclusions are largely confined to the perinuclear cytoplasm located at the poles of the nucleus (Fig. 15-34). The sarcoplasmic reticulum of smooth muscle fibers is only poorly developed, consisting of narrow sarcotubules with no terminal cisternae (Fig. 15-35). There are no T tubules, but longitudinal rows of closely associated vesicles opening onto the surface of the fiber are present just under the cell membrane (Fig. 15-35). These vesicles are termed *caveolae*, and they are regarded as the probable counterparts of the T tubules.

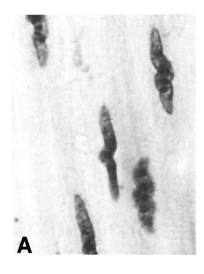
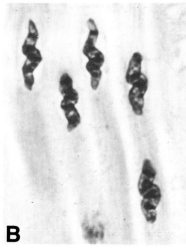

Fig. 15-33. High-power photomicrographs of partly contracted smooth muscle fibers. Note the way their nuclei become progressively pleated as the fibers contract.

Each smooth muscle cell is externally bounded by a basement membrane. Also, contiguous smooth muscle cells are linked by gap junctions, as are cardiac muscle cells. In contrast, skeletal muscle fibers are *not* electrically linked by gap junctions, because this would interfere with voluntary control of their contraction.

Contraction of Smooth Muscle

In good electron micrographs, it is possible to distinguish thick, thin, and intermediate filaments in the cytoplasm of smooth muscle fibers (Fig. 15-36). However, the filaments do not have the arrangement seen in the sarcomeres of skeletal or cardiac muscle, nor are Z lines present. The proportion of actin relative to myosin is greater in smooth than in striated muscle fibers, and the thin filaments of

smooth muscle contain the regulatory protein tropomyosin in addition to actin. The troponin complex, however, is lacking from these filaments.

Hence although the contraction of smooth muscle is again regulated by the intracellular concentration of calcium ions, the mechanism by which the cell responds to the calcium ion concentration is different from that in skeletal and cardiac muscle. It involves a calcium-binding protein called *calmodulin* that, in the presence of calcium, combines with an inactive precursor to produce an active enzyme (*myosin light-chain kinase*) that phosphorylates myosin. This phosphorylation reaction seems to be necessary for interaction between the actin and myosin. In the absence of calcium, the light chain becomes dephosphorylated and relaxation ensues. Tropomyosin and other calcium-dependent enzymatic and nonenzymatic proteins are also involved in the regulatory mechanism.

The intermediate filaments of smooth muscle, which contain primarily desmin (in nonvascular smooth muscle)

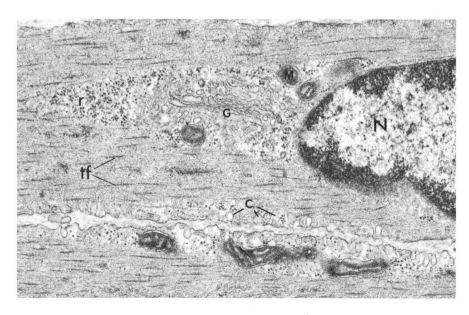

Fig. 15-34. Electron micrograph (×38,000) of part of a smooth muscle fiber in longitudinal section. Numerous thick filaments (*tf*) are visible in the cytoplasm, with thin filaments between them. The sarcoplasm at one end of the central nucleus (*N*) contains ribosomes (*r*), mitochondria (*M*), and Golgi saccules (*G*). Note the caveolae (*c*) in the cytoplasm beneath the cell membrane. (Somlyo AP, Devine CE, Somlyo AV, Rice RV: Philos Trans R Soc Lond [Biol] 265:223, 1973)

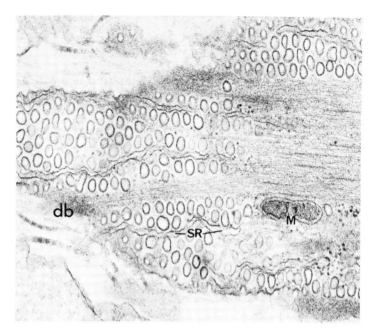

Fig. 15-35. Electron micrograph (×53,000) of a smooth muscle fiber, cut tangentially along its longitudinal axis and disclosing numerous caveolae in the cytoplasm immediately under its cell membrane. These caveolae are intimately associated with tubules of sarcoplasmic reticulum (*SR*). Note also the cell membrane–associated dense body (*db*) at lower left and the bundle of filaments extending from it toward the interior of the cell. (Devine CE, Somlyo AV, Somlyo AP: J Cell Biol 52:690, 1972)

or primarily vimentin (in vascular smooth muscle) together with synemin, appear to comprise a continuous interconnecting system. They are attached to electron-dense structures known as *dense bodies* that contain α-actinin and that are accordingly believed to represent the counterparts of Z lines (Fig. 15-37). These dense bodies are distributed throughout the cytoplasm, and other similar structures variously known as *dense bodies* or *dense areas* adhere to the inner surface of the cell membrane (Fig. 15-37). Bundles of intermediate filaments extend from one dense body to another (Fig. 15-37), comprising a strong cablelike system

that is believed to harness the pull that is generated by the sliding of the thin filaments past the thick ones.

One hypothesis is that this force is transmitted by the intermediate filaments to the dense areas on the cell membrane so that the longitudinal axis of the fiber is shortened in the manner depicted in Figure 15-37. This would explain why the parts of the cell lying between the dense areas bulge during contraction (Figs. 15-37 and 15-38C). However, there are indications that contraction is still possible after the intermediate filaments have been removed, suggesting that the intermediate filaments serve (1) to guide, orient, and align the contractile filaments, and (2) to assist in transmitting

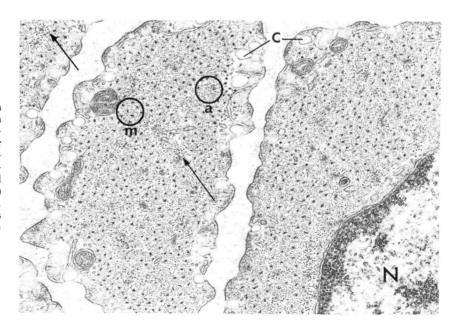

Fig. 15-36. Electron micrograph (×34,000) of smooth muscle fibers in transverse section, showing thick filaments (*m*) and a relatively large number of thin filaments (*a*). Bundles of intermediate filaments are also present (*arrows*). The fiber at right shows a central nucleus (*N*). Note also the caveolae (*c*) beneath the cell membrane. (Somlyo AP, Devine CE, Somlyo AV, Rice RV: Philos Trans R Soc Lond [Biol] 265:223, 1973)

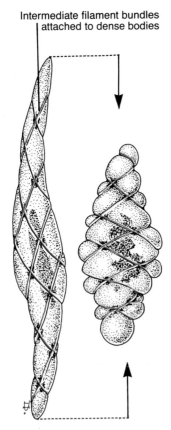

Intermediate filament bundles
attached to dense bodies

Fig. 15-37. Diagram illustrating how contraction seems to be effected in a smooth muscle fiber. Bundles of intermediate filaments are attached to dense bodies that are distributed in the cytoplasm and attached to the cell membrane. Contractile forces are believed to be transmitted through this system of bundles of intermediate filaments to the cell membrane, which, in full contraction, changes shape as shown.

the tensile force that they generate to the dense areas on the cell membrane. Although it is still unclear how the thin filaments might be connected to the dense bodies and their associated intermediate filaments, there is recent evidence that the protein vinculin is involved in securing the thin filaments to the dense areas on the inner aspect of the cell membrane.

Efferent Innervation of Smooth Muscle

Smooth muscles are essentially of two different functional types. First, there are layers of smooth muscle fibers in walls of tubes and hollow viscera that undergo sustained partial contraction or participate in peristaltic waves of contraction. Then there are others like the sphincter pupillae that undergo relatively fast, precisely graded contractions. Those of the former type are called *visceral smooth muscles*, and they have a pattern of innervation different from those of the latter type, which, for reasons given below, are called *multiunit smooth muscles*.

In *visceral smooth muscle* (found, for instance, in the walls of the intestine and uterus), few of the muscle fibers of a bundle are supplied with neuromuscular junctions. Instead, impulses for contraction pass from one muscle cell to the next by way of *gap junctions*, as in cardiac muscle. Here, again, efferent nerve impulses *regulate* contraction instead of initiating it. Furthermore, smooth muscle fibers of this type also contract in response to a variety of non-neural stimuli, including histamine, the hormone oxytocin, and even physical stretch.

In *multiunit smooth muscle* (such as that of the iris and the wall of the vas deferens), every muscle fiber is *individually innervated*. Gap junctions may be present between the fibers, but the extent to which they participate in conducting impulses from one muscle fiber to another has not been established. The pattern of innervation of multiunit smooth muscles is similar to that found in motor units of skeletal muscles, except that the muscle fibers in the unit are *localized* instead of being distributed throughout the muscle. This arrangement allows impulses for contraction to be delivered simultaneously to all the smooth muscle fibers in a given local region so that they participate in a relatively fast local contraction.

In some parts of the body, the smooth muscle is of an *intermediate* type in which approximately 20% to 50% of the muscle fibers are individually innervated.

Neuromuscular Junctions on Smooth Muscle Fibers. The structure of neuromuscular junctions between autonomic nerve fibers and smooth muscle fibers is less complex than that between motor nerves and skeletal muscle fibers. Postganglionic autonomic nerve fibers branch repeatedly, and each branch supplies a number of smooth muscle fibers, making synapses *en passant*. These branches form a series of *axon varicosities* that lie in a groove on the surface of the muscle fiber. There is a synaptic cleft of 20 nm to 100 nm between the axolemma and the sarcolemma. Within the axon varicosities, there are numerous mitochondria and synaptic vesicles containing either *acetylcholine* (parasympathetic fibers) or *norepinephrine* (sympathetic fibers). On stimulation, the neurotransmitter is released by exocytosis into the synaptic cleft and combines with receptors in the sarcolemma. In addition to having receptors for acetylcholine, smooth muscle fibers have two different receptors for norepinephrine and other adrenergic neurotransmitters, referred to as α- and β-adrenergic receptors.

Growth and Regeneration of Smooth Muscle

Like the other two types of muscle, smooth muscle responds to increased demands by undergoing compensatory hypertrophy, but this is not its only response. During pregnancy, for example, the smooth muscle cells in the wall of the uterus increase not only in size (hypertrophy) but also in number (hyperplasia). Smooth muscle cells also increase

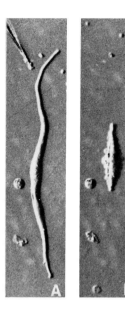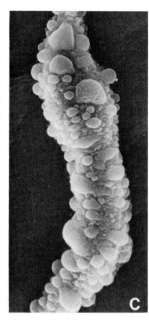

Fig. 15-38. Photomicrographs (*A* and *B*) and scanning electron micrograph (*C*) illustrating how the contours of a smooth muscle fiber change during contraction. The two photomicrographs (×310) are frames from a film, showing a living smooth muscle fiber (*A*) before stimulation and (*B*) undergoing maximal contraction. The scanning electron micrograph (×1800) shows an isolated smooth muscle cell (*C*) contracted to approximately one third of its resting length. Note that in (*B*) and (*C*) the cell membrane of the fiber balloons during contraction. (Fay FS, Delise CM: Proc Natl Acad Sci USA 70:641, 1973)

in number in certain pathological conditions. Thus focal proliferation of smooth muscle cells can be demonstrated in atherosclerosis, a major cause of death that will be described in Chapter 16.

In hormone-treated or pregnant animals, mitotic figures are frequently observed among smooth muscle cells of the uterus, so it is generally accepted that smooth muscle cells retain the capacity for mitosis. Furthermore, new smooth muscle cells can arise at any time of life from pericytes that are distributed along the course of the smallest blood vessels. Hence, compared with cardiac and skeletal muscle, smooth muscle has a great capacity for regeneration.

SELECTED REFERENCES

Skeletal Muscle and Molecular Basis of Muscular Contraction

ALBERTS B, BRAY D, LEWIS J ET AL: Muscle contraction. In Molecular Biology of the Cell, p 550. New York, Garland Publishing, 1983

CARAFOLI E, PENNISTON JT: The calcium signal. Sci Am 253 No 5: 70, 1985

CARLSON BM: The regeneration of skeletal muscle. A review. Am J Anat 137:119, 1973

COHEN C: The protein switch of muscle contraction. Sci Am 233 No 5:36, May, 1975

FORBES MS, PLANTHOLT BA, SPERELAKIS N: Cytochemical staining procedures selective for sarcotubular systems of muscle: Modifications and applications. J Ultrastruct Res 60:306, 1977

FRANZINI-ARMSTRONG C: The structure of a simple Z line. J Cell Biol 58:630, 1973

FRANZINI-ARMSTRONG C: Studies of the triad. I. Structure of the junction in frog twitch fibers. J Cell Biol 47:488, 1970

FRANZINI-ARMSTRONG C, PEACHEY LD: Striated muscle—Contractile and control mechanisms. J Cell Biol 91:166s, 1981

GOLDMAN R, POLLARD T, ROSENBAUM J (eds): Cell Motility. Book A, Motility, Muscle and Non-Muscle Cells; and Book B, Actin, Myosin and Associated Proteins. Cold Spring Harbor Conferences on Cell Proliferation, Vol 3. Cold Spring Harbor, NY, Cold Spring Harbor Laboratory, 1976

GRANGER BL, LAZARIDES E: The existence of an insoluble Z disc scaffold in chicken skeletal muscle. Cell 15:1253, 1978

GRÖSCHEL-STEWART U, DRENCKHAHN D: Muscular and cytoplasmic contractile proteins. Coll Relat Res 2:381, 1982

HANSON J, HUXLEY HE: The structural basis of contraction in striated muscle. Symp Soc Exp Biol 9:228, 1955

HUDDART H: The Comparative Structure and Function of Muscle. Oxford, Pergamon Press, 1975

HUXLEY HE: Introductory remarks: The relevance of studies on muscle to problems of cell motility. In Goldman R, Pollard T, Rosenbaum J (eds): Cell Motility. Book A, Motility, Muscle and Non-Muscle Cells, p 115. Cold Spring Harbor Conference on Cell Proliferation. Cold Spring Harbor, NY, Cold Spring Harbor Laboratory, 1976

HUXLEY HE: The mechanism of muscular contraction. Science 164: 1356, 1969

HUXLEY HE: The structural basis of muscular contraction. Proc R Soc Lond [Biol] 178:131, 1971

ISHIKAWA H: Fine structure of skeletal muscle. In Dowben RM, Shay JW (eds): Cell and Muscle Motility, Vol 4, p 1. New York, Plenum, 1983

JORGENSEN AO, KALNINS V, MACLENNAN DH: Localization of sarcoplasmic reticulum proteins in rat skeletal muscle by immunofluorescence. J Cell Biol 80:372, 1979

JORGENSEN AO, SHEN ACY, CAMPBELL KP, MACLENNAN DH: Ultrastructural localization of calsequestrin in rat skeletal muscle by immunoferritin labeling of ultrathin frozen sections. J Cell Biol 97: 1573, 1983

LANDON DN: Skeletal muscle—normal morphology, development and innervation. In Mastaglia FL, Walton J (eds): Skeletal Muscle Pathology, p 1. Edinburgh, Churchill Livingstone, 1982

LAZARIDES E: Molecular morphogenesis of the Z-disc in muscle cells. In Schweiger HG (ed): International Cell Biology 1980–1981, p 392. Berlin, Springer-Verlag, 1981

MOSS FP, LEBLOND CP: Satellite cells as the source of nuclei in muscles of growing rats. Anat Rec 170:471, 1971

MURRAY JM, WEBER A: The cooperative action of muscle proteins. Sci Am 230 No 2:59, February, 1974

SQUIRE J: The Structural Basis of Muscle Contraction. New York, Plenum, 1981

STRACHER A (ed): Muscle and Nonmuscle Motility, Vol 2. New York, Academic Press, 1983

WANG K: Sarcomere-associated cytoskeletal lattices in striated muscle—Review and hypothesis. In Shay JW (ed): Cell and Muscle Motility, Vol 6, p 315. New York, Plenum, 1985

Efferent and Afferent Innervation of Skeletal Muscle and Tendons*

BOYD IA: The response of fast and slow nuclear bag fibers and nuclear chain fibers in isolated cat muscle spindles to fusimotor stimulation, and the effect of intrafusal contraction on the sensory endings. Q J Exp Physiol 61:203, 1976

BOYD IA, WARD J: Motor control of nuclear bag and nuclear chain intrafusal fibers in isolated living muscle spindles from the cat. J Physiol 244:83, 1975

BRIDGMAN CF: Comparisons in structure of tendon organs in the rat, cat and man. J Comp Neurol 138:369, 1970

COUTEAUX R: Motor end plate structure. In Bourne GH (ed): The Structure and Function of Muscle. Vol 1, p 337. New York, Academic Press, 1960

DRACHMAN DB: Myasthenia gravis. N Engl J Med 298:136, 186; 1978

DRACHMAN DB: Myasthenia gravis and acetylcholine receptors. In Bearn AG, Choppin PW (eds): Receptors and Human Disease, p 197. New York, Josiah Macy, Jr Foundation, 1979

KENNEDY WR: Innervation of normal human muscle spindles. Neurology 20:463, 1970

LESTER HA: The response to acetylcholine. Sci Am 236 No 2:106, 1977

MATTHEWS PBC: Mammalian Muscle Receptors and Their Central Actions. London, Edward Arnold, 1972

MERTON PA: How we control the contraction of our muscles. Sci Am 226 No 5:30, 1972

MOORE JC: The Golgi tendon organ and the muscle spindle. Am J Occup Ther 28:415, 1974

Cardiac Muscle and Atrial Natriuretic Factor

CANTIN M, GENEST J: The heart as an endocrine gland. Sci Am 254 No 2:76, 1986

CHALLICE CE, VIRÁGH S (eds): Ultrastructure of the Mammalian Heart. Ultrastructure in Biological Systems. Vol 6. New York, Academic Press, 1973

FAWCETT DW, MCNUTT NS: The ultrastructure of the cat myocardium. I. Ventricular papillary muscle. J Cell Biol 42:1, 1969

FORBES MS, SPERELAKIS N: The membrane systems and cytoskeletal elements of mammalian myocardial cells. Cell and Muscle Motility 3:89, 1983

FORSSMANN WG, GIRARDIER L: A study of the T-system in rat heart. J Cell Biol 44:1, 1970

JAMIESON JD, PALADE GE: Specific granules in atrial muscle. J Cell Biol 23:151, 1964

JORGENSEN AO, SHEN ACY, CAMPBELL KP: Ultrastructural localization of calsequestrin in adult rat atrial and ventricular muscle cells. J Cell Biol 101:257, 1985

MAACK T, CAMARGO MJF, KLEINERT HD ET AL: Atrial natriuretic factor: Structure and functional properties. Kidney Int 27:607, 1985

MCNUTT NS, FAWCETT DW: The ultrastructure of the cat myocardium. II. Atrial Muscle. J Cell Biol 42:46, 1969

POLEZHAEV LV: Organ Regeneration in Animals, chap. 6, p 100. Springfield, IL, Charles C Thomas, 1972

RUMYANTSEV PP: Interrelations of the proliferation and differentiation processes during cardiac myogenesis and regeneration. Int Rev Cytol 51:188, 1977

SOMMER JR, JOHNSON EA: Ultrastructure of cardiac muscle. In Berne RM, Sperelakis N, Geiger SR (eds): Handbook of Physiology, Section 2: The Cardiovascular System. Vol I—The Heart, p 113. Bethesda, American Physiological Society, 1979

Smooth Muscle and Its Efferent Innervation*

COOKE P: A filamentous cytoskeleton in vertebrate smooth muscle fibers. J Cell Biol 68:539, 1976

COOKE PH, FAY FS: Correlation between fiber length, ultrastructure and the length-tension relationships of mammalian smooth muscle. J Cell Biol 52:105, 1972

DEVINE CE: Vascular smooth muscle, morphology and ultrastructure. In Kaley G, Altura BM (eds): Microcirculation. Vol 2. Baltimore, University Park Press, 1978

DEVINE CE, SOMLYO AP: Thick filaments in vascular smooth muscle. J Cell Biol 49:636, 1971

DEVINE CE, SOMLYO AV, SOMLYO AP: Sarcoplasmic reticulum and mitochondria as cation accumulation sites in smooth muscle. Philos Trans R Soc Lond [Biol] 265:17, 1973

FAY FS: Structural and functional features of isolated smooth muscle cells. In Goldman R, Pollard T, Rosenbaum J (eds): Cell Motility. Book A, Motility, Muscle and Non-Muscle Cells, p 185. Cold Spring Harbor Conference on Cell Proliferation. Cold Spring Harbor, NY, Cold Spring Harbor Laboratory, 1976

FAY FS, DELISE CM: Contraction of isolated smooth muscle cells—structural changes. Proc Natl Acad Sci USA 70:641, 1973

GABELLA G: Fine structure of smooth muscle. Proc Trans R Soc Lond [Biol], 265:7, 1973

GABELLA G: Smooth muscle cell junctions and structural aspects of contraction. Brit Med Bull 35, No 3:213, 1979

MCGEACHIE JK: Smooth muscle regeneration. Monographs in Developmental Biology, 9. Basel, S Karger, 1975

RHODIN JAG: Architecture of the vessel wall. In Bohr DF, Somlyo AP, Sparks HV (eds): Handbook of Physiology, Section 2: The Cardiovascular System, Vol II—Vascular Smooth Muscle, p 1. Bethesda, American Physiological Society, 1980

RICE RV, MOSES JA, MCMANUS GM ET AL: The organization of contractile filaments in a mammalian smooth muscle. J Cell Biol 47:183, 1970

RICHARDSON KC: The fine structure of autonomic nerve endings in smooth muscle of the rat vas deferens. J Anat 96:427, 1962

SOMLYO AP, DEVINE CE, SOMLYO AV, RICE RV: Filament organization in vertebrate smooth muscle. Philos Trans R Soc Lond [Biol] 265:223, 1973

SOMLYO AP, SOMLYO AV, ASHTON FT, VALLIÈRES J: Vertebrate smooth muscle: Ultrastructure and function. In Goldman R, Pollard T, Rosenbaum J (eds): Cell Motility. Book A, Motility, Muscle and Non-Muscle Cells, p 165. Cold Spring Harbor Conference on Cell Proliferation. Cold Spring Harbor, NY, Cold Spring Harbor Laboratory, 1976

---

* References on sensory receptors in joints are listed under Selected References, Nerve Endings, in Chapter 14.

* Further references on smooth muscle are listed in connection with arteries and atherosclerosis under Selected References in Chapter 16.

PART FOUR

THE SYSTEMS OF THE BODY

The fourth portion of this book deals with the remainder of the body systems. The term *system* is used in medical subjects to denote a group of organs or structures that collectively carry out some useful function for the body as a whole. The circulatory system, for example, consists of the heart and the various types of vessels involved in blood circulation and lymph drainage. Since the immune system was considered in Chapter 10 and the nervous system was described in Chapter 14, no further chapters on these two systems are included.

16

The Circulatory System

The circulatory system is actually made up of two distinct systems that complement each other and operate in parallel. However, through convention they are regarded as components of a single system. First, there is the *blood circulatory (cardiovascular) system,* which is made up of the heart and the various types of blood vessels, that distributes blood to virtually every part of the body and then returns it to the heart for redistribution. Second, there is the *lymphatic system,* which is made up of an independent set of vessels, that collects the excess tissue fluid from the body tissues and returns it to the blood circulatory system. The blood circulatory system serves as a medium for the rapid and efficient dissemination of oxygen, nutrients, and various cell products throughout the body, and it also facilitates the removal of metabolic waste substances from their sites of production. All the cells of the body have at least indirect access to the contents of the bloodstream through tissue fluid, and in virtually every case, their survival is ultimately dependent on an adequate blood circulation. The lymphatic system, on the other hand, serves as an adjunct drainage system that is needed to prevent undue accumulation of tissue fluid in the interstitial spaces. Furthermore, as noted in Chapter 10, the lymphatic tissue associated with this part of the circulatory system is substantially involved in the immune defenses of the body.

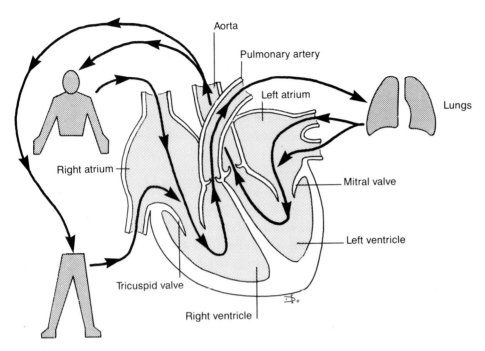

Fig. 16-1. Schematic representation of the heart in relation to the blood circulatory system. The pulmonary circulation is shown on the right and the systemic circulation is shown on the left.

THE BLOOD CIRCULATORY (CARDIOVASCULAR) SYSTEM

The heart consists of two pumps arranged side by side that move blood through the two circuits depicted in Figure 16-1. Because these pumps correspond to the right and left sides of the heart, they are commonly referred to as the right and left hearts. The *right heart* pumps blood through the *pulmonary* circuit (L. *pulmo,* lung) and maintains the *pulmonary circulation.* The *left heart* pumps blood through the remainder of the body and maintains the *systemic circulation.*

In each circuit, the pump delivers blood under pressure into thick-walled vessels called *arteries.* The arteries then branch repeatedly and terminate in thick-walled vessels with a narrow lumen that are termed *arterioles.* An important role of arterioles is to reduce the hydrostatic pressure of the blood before they deliver it to the thin-walled *capillaries.* From the capillary beds, blood is delivered first into *venules* and then into *veins.* The veins are arranged so that the blood received from the *lungs* is delivered to the *left heart,* which can then pump it through the systemic circulation, whereas the blood returned from the *systemic* circuit is delivered to the *right heart,* which pumps it through the lungs, where it is oxygenated and cleared of carbon dioxide.

The right and left hearts each have two main parts: an *atrium* (Gr. *atrion,* hall) in which the blood being returned to that side of the heart collects and a *ventricle* (L. for cavity). Both the atria and the ventricles are saclike structures, the walls of which consist primarily of cardiac muscle. The walls of the ventricles are much thicker and stronger than those of the *atria* are (Fig. 16-1). The chief function of the atria is to act as reservoirs between contractions of the heart. However, most of the blood that, between heartbeats, enters an atrium passes through the valve that guards the passageway into the ventricle below it. The valve between the right atrium and the right ventricle is termed the *tricuspid valve* and the one between the left atrium and ventricle is called the *mitral valve* (Fig. 16-1). Both these valves are open when the heart fills between beats, and they remain open as the atria contract. But when the ventricles contract, both valves are forced closed by pressure being built up in the contracting ventricles. This pressure, however, forces the pulmonary valve (shown at the base of the pulmonary artery in Fig. 16-1) to open so that the right ventricle can pump its contents through the pulmonary circulation, and it forces open the aortic valve (shown at the base of the aorta in Fig. 16-1) so the blood in the left ventricle can be pumped throughout the body.

When the ventricles finish their contraction and begin to relax, the pressure within them drops below that in the arteries into which they have pumped most of their con-

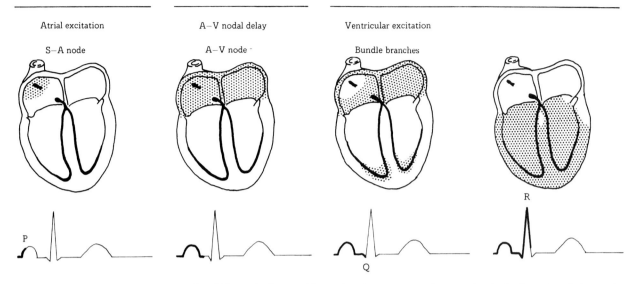

Atrial excitation   A–V nodal delay   Ventricular excitation

S–A node   A–V node   Bundle branches

Fig. 16-2. Schematic diagram illustrating the sequence of contraction in the heart in relation to the cardiac cycle. Below each stage, in which the contracting region is shown stippled, the corresponding wave that appears on an electrocardiogram at this time is indicated by a heavy line. (Shepard RS: Human Physiology. Philadelphia, JB Lippincott, 1971)

tents. So the pulmonary and aortic valves are both forced, by the pressure in the arteries above them, into the closed position, in which they remain until the ventricles are refilled and contract again. While the relaxing ventricles are being refilled, the tricuspid and mitral valves open because the pressure of the venous blood emptying into them is then greater than that existing in the relaxing ventricles.

In arteries, blood is under considerable hydrostatic pressure; the pressure is higher in the systemic circulation than in the pulmonary circulation. Because artery walls have elastin and smooth muscle as their chief components, they accommodate the pressure inside them. The elastin, moreover, is stretched by ventricular contractions, and in returning to a less stretched state, it maintains pressure in the arteries between heartbeats as will be described later in this chapter.

Each of the different parts of the blood circulatory system will now be described.

HEART

The muscular walls of the atria and ventricles comprise the *myocardium*. The myocardium consists of a network of anastomosing cardiac muscle fibers with endomysium in its interstices (see Fig. 15-26). It will be recalled from Chapter 15 that cardiac muscle fibers are made up of individual muscle cells and that these are interconnected end to end by intercalated disks that include gap junctions. This arrangement ensures the spread of each wave of depolarization throughout the myocardium as described in the following section.

Cardiac Cycle.   A repeated succession of events occurs in the heart from the beginning of one beat to the beginning of the next. In one phase of the cycle, the heart is relaxing. In this phase, blood is flowing from the venae cavae into the relaxing right atrium and from there through the open tricuspid valve into the relaxing right ventricle. Simultaneously, blood from the pulmonary vein is flowing into the relaxing left atrium and through the open mitral valve into the relaxing left ventricle. In the next phase of the cycle, the two atria contract; the process of contraction begins in the right atrium near the opening of the superior vena cava (*stippled* area in the *left* diagram in Fig. 16-2). The contraction spreads over both atria so that most of the blood they contain is forced into the ventricles. The wave of contraction that sweeps over the atria *is not, however, immediately transmitted to the ventricles*. There is a brief enough delay to allow the atria to finish their contraction. Furthermore, when contraction occurs in the ventricles, it does not begin, as might be thought, next to the atria but near the apex of the heart (*stippled* area in third diagram from *left* in Fig. 16-2). From here it spreads rapidly throughout the myocardium of both ventricles, causing them to deliver their contents into the pulmonary artery and aorta, respectively. We shall now describe how the impulse for contraction originates and spreads through the heart.

Impulse-Conducting System of the Heart

Efficiency of the heart as a dual pump is dependent on synchronous contraction of the left and right hearts and on the consecutive stages of the cardiac cycle following

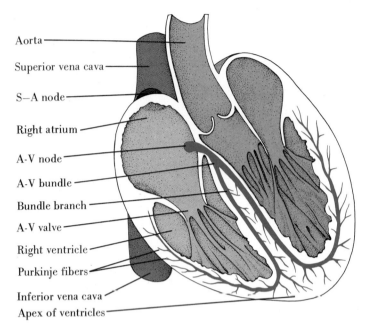

Aorta

Superior vena cava

S—A node

Right atrium

A-V node

A-V bundle

Bundle branch

A-V valve

Right ventricle

Purkinje fibers

Inferior vena cava

Apex of ventricles

Fig. 16-3.   Diagram of the impulse-conducting system of the heart. The heart has been cut open in the coronal plane to expose its interior and the main parts of its impulse-conducting system (indicated in *blue*). For details, see text. (Shepard RS: Human Physiology. Philadelphia, JB Lippincott, 1971)

one another in the proper sequence. Coordination depends on the wave of excitation sweeping through the heart by way of its *impulse-conducting system* (Fig. 16-3). This system is composed of cardiac muscle cells that are specialized for initiating impulses for contraction and conducting them through the heart.

The Impulse for Contraction Arises in the Sinoatrial Node.   The *sinoatrial* (S-A) *node* is a small mass of specialized cardiac muscle fibers contained in substantial amounts of fibroelastic connective tissue that is richly supplied with capillaries. Located in the right-hand wall of the superior vena cava at its junction with the right atrium (Figs. 16-3 and 16-4*A*), the S-A node is supplied by a *nodal artery* (Fig. 16-4) and numerous nerve fibers belonging to both divisions of the autonomic nervous system. The fibers that are responsible for its specialized function are like ordinary cardiac muscle fibers, but they are narrower (Fig. 16-4*B*), and like the fibers of other parts of the system (to be illustrated shortly), they contain fewer myofibrils than ordinary cardiac muscle fibers.

The S-A node is termed the *pacemaker* of the heart. It generates cardiac impulses at an intrinsic rate of about 70 depolarizations per minute. These impulses are then conducted throughout the heart in such a way that they bring about contraction of its constituent parts in the necessary sequence.

Pacemaker Cells.   In certain cardiac muscle cells known as *pacemaker cells*, the resting potential (the ionic basis for which was considered under Nerve Impulses in Chap. 14) is unstable. The primary reason for this instability is that during the resting phase (*i.e.*, between heartbeats), the cell membrane of these cells shows a progressive decline in its permeability to potassium ions. The resulting progressive decrease in potassium loss from the

cytoplasm becomes manifested as a steady decline in the negative resting potential. After only a fraction of a second has elapsed, the resting potential becomes so diminished that it reaches the threshold level at which an action potential is triggered.

As noted, spontaneous depolarization of the pacemaker cells in the S-A node results in the generation of repeated waves of excitation that spread through the heart at a resting rate of about 70 impulses per minute. However, the frequency with which this depolarization occurs is influenced by nerve impulses arriving by way of the autonomic nervous system. *Sympathetic* stimulation *accelerates* the heart rate (and also increases the force of cardiac contraction), and *parasympathetic* stimulation causes it to *slow down*. Thus during sleep, the heart rate may be as low as 35 beats per minute whereas during strenuous exercise it may rise to 200 beats per minute.

The Wave of Excitation Spreads Through the Heart by Way of a Specialized Cardiac Conduction System.   From the S-A node, the wave of depolarization is conducted by way of gap junctions along *internodal atrial pathways* to a second node of specialized cells called the *atrioventricular* (A-V) *node* (Fig. 16-3). Three such preferred pathways of internodal impulse conduction have now been identified within the atrial musculature.

The A-V node lies in the lower part of the interatrial septum, immediately above the attachment of the septal cusp of the tricuspid valve (labeled *A-V valve* in Fig. 16-3). It constitutes the only bridge of cardiac muscle between the atrial and the ventricular musculature. On reaching this node, the wave of depolarization—which by now has spread over most of the atrial musculature—is momentarily delayed by the nodal cells before being conducted to the ventricles (second diagram from the *left* in

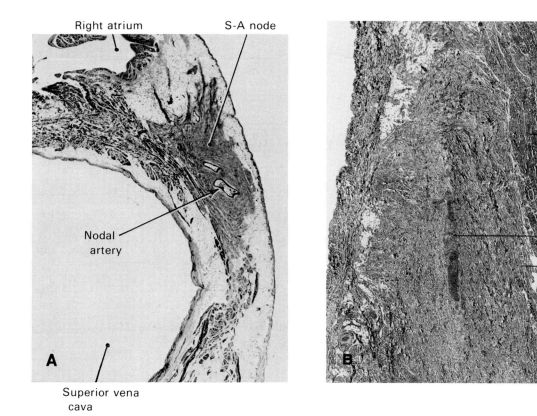

Right atrium   S-A node

Nodal
artery

Superior vena
cava

— af

— na

— nf

Fig. 16-4. (*A*) Very low-power photomicrograph of a cross section of the right-hand wall of the superior vena cava at its junction with the right atrium. This shows the sinoatrial (*S-A*) node, the pacemaker of the heart. (*B*) Low-power photomicrograph showing the S-A node in longitudinal section. A small area of the lumen of the superior vena cava is seen as a white space at upper left, and atrial muscle is the darker tissue at right. Note that the nodal fibers (*nf*) of the node, which occupies the middle part of the illustration are narrower than the darker staining atrial fibers (*af*) at right. The nodal fibers are embedded in abundant collagen fibers. Part of the wall of the nodal artery (*na*) is seen near center. (Courtesy of J. Duckworth)

Fig. 16-2). As in the S-A node, the A-V node is provided with its own artery and is richly supplied with autonomic nerve fibers. In addition, its microscopic structure resembles that of the S-A node (Fig. 16-5). Thus it is made up of narrow cardiac muscle fibers that anastomose extensively. On their atrial side, these nodal fibers connect with atrial muscle fibers, and near the A-V septum, they connect with specialized cardiac muscle cells of the A-V bundle (Fig. 16-5; *bottom left*).

As in other cells of the cardiac conduction system, the cells of the A-V node contain only a small number of poorly organized myofibrils (Fig. 16-6). Normally, the cells of the A-V node do not function as pacemaker cells, but under certain circumstances, they can take over pacemaker function, so it would seem that the fine structure of the cells illustrated in Figure 16-6 would be fairly representative of pacemaker cells in general.

The Atrioventricular (A-V) Bundle. From the A-V node, the wave of depolarization passes along a bundle of spe-

cialized conducting cardiac muscle fibers called the *atrioventricular (A-V) bundle* or *bundle of His* (Figs. 16-3 and 16-5). This single conduction path extends anteriorly from the A-V node. It penetrates the fibrous partition that separates the atrial from the ventricular musculature and enters the interventricular septum, where it becomes subdivided into right and left branches (Fig. 16-3). Roughly halfway down this septum, the two bundle branches become bundles of wide, rapidly conducting *Purkinje fibers* (Fig. 16-3).

Purkinje Fibers. These specialized conducting muscle fibers are wider than ordinary cardiac muscle fibers, and for the most part, they lie in the deepest layer of the endocardium, which is the lining layer of the heart. They are particularly large and prominent in the sheep's heart (Fig. 16-7A). Purkinje fibers have centrally located nuclei, and they possess relatively few myofibrils that are peripherally arranged around a central clear core of sarcoplasm containing considerable quantities of stored glycogen (Fig. 16-7).

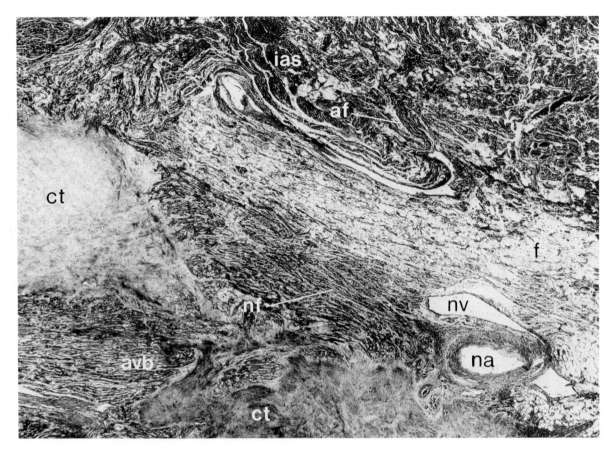

Fig. 16-5. Low-power photomicrograph of a sagittal section of the atrioventricular (*A-V*) node of the heart. The left-hand side of the illustration is anterior, the right posterior. Atrial muscle of the interatrial septum (*ias*) extends along the top. The grayish areas at left and bottom are fibrous connective tissue (*ct*) of the skeleton of the heart. Pale areas containing fat cells (*f*) are present at middle and lower right. Both the nodal artery (*na*) and the nodal vein (*nv*) are included in the section at lower right, posterior to the node. The darkly staining A-V node lies anterior to these vessels, between them and the fibrous tissue at bottom and left and the fatty connective tissue above. The nodal fibers (*nf*) are narrower than the atrial fibers (*af*) of the interatrial septum above the node. Nodal fibers extend anteriorly at lower left to join the A-V bundle (*avb*), which runs anteriorly from the node. The fibers of the A-V bundle are also narrower than ordinary cardiac muscle fibers. (Courtesy of J. Duckworth)

It is important to realize that Purkinje fibers supply the papillary muscles before they supply the lateral walls of the ventricles; they spread up the ventricles as a subendocardial network. Because these fibers conduct the impulse for contraction much more rapidly than the ordinary heart muscle does, this arrangement ensures that the *papillary muscles* will *take up the strain* on the leaflets of the mitral and the tricuspid valves before the full force of ventricular contraction is thrown against them. It should also be noted by referring to Figures 16-2 and 16-3 that the distribution of the branches of the rapidly conducting Purkinje system is such that the relatively thick exterior walls of the ventricles near the apex of the heart are depolarized before the impulse reaches the ventricular walls at the base of the heart. Hence, in general, the apical parts of the ventricles

contract before their basal parts (see third diagram from *left* in Fig. 16-2 and compare it with the diagram on its *right*).

The fine structure of Purkinje fibers corresponds to what would be anticipated from their light microscope (LM) appearance. Thus they contain relatively few myofibrils (which demonstrate striations similar to those seen in ordinary cardiac muscle and are peripherally disposed), many mitochondria, and much glycogen. The sarcoplasmic reticulum is not as well developed as in ordinary cardiac fibers, and Purkinje fibers are relatively, if not completely, deficient in transverse tubules.

Electrocardiograms. Electrical activity of the heart is monitored by means of *electrocardiograms* (Fig. 16-8). These are records, made on moving paper, of the fields of electrical potential

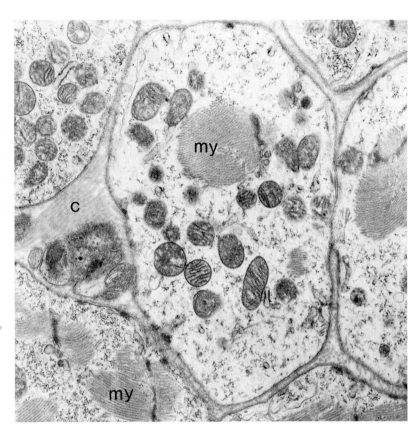

Fig. 16-6. Electron micrograph (×9000) of a cross section of nodal cells in the lower part of the A-V node (ferret heart) at a level at which conducting cardiac muscle fibers leave the node anteriorly to enter the A-V bundle. These are all cells of nodal fibers. Very few myofibrils (*my*) are present in the pale type of cell seen at middle and right. The cells at top left, bottom left, and bottom right more closely resemble ordinary cardiac muscle cells but have fewer myofibrils (although slightly more than pale fibers). The irregular orientation of the myofibrils in both kinds of nodal cells accounts for the myofibrils being cut in oblique section. Some collagen fibrils (*c*) are visible between the muscle fibers, situated in the endomysium (together with small nerve fibers) at middle left. (Courtesy of I. Taylor)

that extend from the heart into the surrounding tissues during the cardiac cycle. Such electrical fields can be detected by electrodes placed at convenient sites on the body surface that represent projections of the different parts of the heart. Electrocardiograms are of sufficient importance in clinical medicine to warrant the following brief introduction.

First, the *P* wave (Figs. 16-2 and 16-8) is due to depolarization of the atria. The next obvious wave is the *R* wave (Fig. 16-8), which results from depolarization of the bulk of the ventricular myocardium. The minor *Q* and *S* waves (Fig. 16-8) represent the respective depolarizations of the first and the last parts of the ventricular musculature to become depolarized. The *T* wave indicates repolarization of the ventricular myocardium. Figure 16-2 shows how these waves are related to the cardiac cycle.

Electrocardiograms greatly facilitate the detection and diagnosis of heart muscle damage and malfunctions of the cardiac conduction system. A substantial proportion of the heart conditions with which the physician is confronted concern the impulse-conducting system of the heart.

Latent Pacemaker Cells Can Assume Pacemaker Function. There is also evidence that a hierarchy of *subsidiary pacemaker cells* exists outside the S-A node, but their rate of spontaneous depolarization is less rapid than that of the pacemaker cells in the S-A node. However, such latent pacemaker cells can make their presence felt if conduction is either permanently or intermittently blocked in the A-V bundle. Under such conditions, waves of depolarization arise in the S-A node but fail to reach the ventricles. Such an occurrence would lead to death if it were not for the presence of

latent pacemaker cells among the ordinary ventricular muscle cells. However, the rate of spontaneous depolarization of these subsidiary cells is slow compared with their counterparts in the S-A node.

Patients Can Be Maintained with an Artificial Pacemaker. It is now possible to equip patients who have heart conduction problems with an *artificial pacemaker.* Connected to the ventricular myocardium, this device takes over pacemaker function from the slowly depolarizing latent pacemaker cells of the ventricles and elicits ventricular contraction at a normal rate (*e.g.*, 70 beats per minute). In patients with intermittent bundle block, impulses occasionally reach the ventricles from the S-A node. Such patients can be given a *standby pacemaker* that is designed to detect whether ventricular contraction (sensed as an R wave) has occurred during the cardiac cycle. If none is forthcoming, the pacemaker triggers it artificially.

Lining and Covering Membranes of the Heart

Endocardium. This connective tissue membrane forms a complete lining for the atria and ventricles and covers all the structures projecting into them, such as valves, chordae tendineae, and papillary muscles, which will be described later in this chapter. In general, the thickness of the endocardium varies inversely with the thickness of the myocardium it lines. The endocardium consists of three layers.

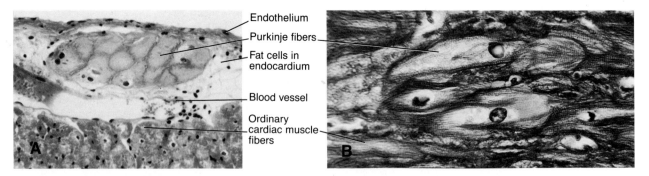

Endothelium

Purkinje fibers

Fat cells in endocardium

Blood vessel

Ordinary cardiac muscle fibers

Fig. 16-7. Photomicrographs of Purkinje fibers of the heart. (*A*) Transverse section (sheep's heart). (*B*) Longitudinal section (human heart). (*B*, courtesy of J. Duckworth)

The innermost comprises an endothelium that is supported by delicate connective tissue; this layer is continuous with the lining of the blood vessels opening into the heart. The next (middle) layer is the thickest. It consists of dense connective tissue in which many elastic fibers are present, particularly in its inner part. These fibers are commonly arranged parallel with the surface, and in some sites where they are abundant, they alternate with layers of collagen fibers. In the outer part of this layer, some smooth muscle fibers may also be present. The third (deepest) layer of the endocardium consists of more irregularly arranged connective tissue. Fat cells may be present here (Fig. 16-7*A*). This layer contains blood vessels, and in certain sites, it also contains branches of the impulse-conducting system (Purkinje fibers, Fig. 16-7), described above. The connective tissue of this layer is continuous with the endomysium of the myocardium.

Epicardium. This connective tissue membrane forms the intimate covering of the heart. It is made up of two layers. First, there is a deeper layer that is made of fibroelastic connective tissue and that merges with the endomysium of the underlying cardiac muscle. This layer contains blood

vessels, lymphatics, nerve fibers, and a variable amount of fat tissue. The second layer is a superficial mesothelial membrane that is made up of squamous mesothelial cells.

Anatomical Relation Between the Epicardium and the Pericardium. External to the heart, there is an additional protective connective tissue sac termed the *pericardium,* the walls of which are made up of (1) a strong outer layer of fibroelastic connective tissue called the *fibrous pericardium* and (2) a delicate inner mesothelial membrane called the *serous pericardium* (Fig. 16-9). As the heart develops, it invaginates into the serous pericardium, with the result that it becomes covered by a visceral layer of serous pericardium (Fig. 16-9). At the roots of the great vessels that enter or leave the heart, the investing *visceral layer of serous pericardium* is therefore continuous with a *parietal layer of serous pericardium* that lines the inner aspect of the fibrous pericardium (Fig. 16-9). The narrow potential space enclosed by the serous pericardium is termed the *pericardial cavity* (Fig. 16-9). It contains a thin film of fluid (normally no more than 50 ml) that facilitates the free movement of the heart during its contraction. Hence the superficial mesothelial membrane of the epicardium represents a part of the serous lining of the pericardial cavity (*i.e.,* the visceral layer of serous pericardium) as well (Fig. 16-9).

Skeleton of the Heart

The origin of the aorta and the origin of the pulmonary artery (from the left and the right ventricles, respectively) are each supported by a ring of fibrous connective tissue. The dense connective tissue of these rings is continuous with a roughly triangular mass of fibrous connective tissue known as a *trigonum fibrosum*. Similarly, rings of fibrous connective tissue surround the atrioventricular orifices. The role of these four fibrous rings that surround the valve-containing outlets is to prevent their dilatation when the ventricles contract and force their contents through the orifices. These fibrous rings and trigona, together with the membranous part of the interventricular septum, also pro-

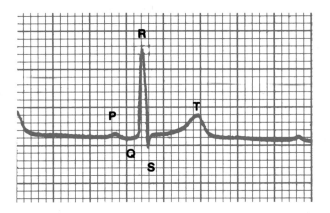

Fig. 16-8. An electrocardiogram obtained from a normal human heart. For details, see text.

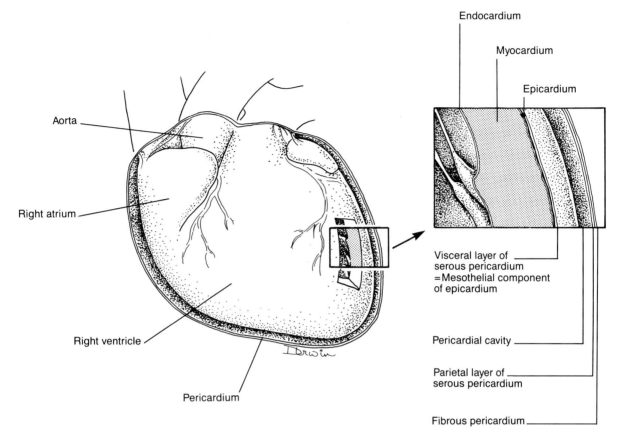

Fig. 16-9. Schematic diagram showing the anatomical relation between the epicardium and the pericardium and indicating the terms used in describing the heart wall and pericardium. This diagram shows the anterior aspect of the heart, with the pericardium and a block of the heart wall dissected away.

vide the means for insertion of the free ends of cardiac muscle fibers and, for this reason, are often referred to as the fibrous *skeleton* of the heart (Fig. 16-10).

Valves of the Heart

Each ventricle is provided with an intake valve and an exhaust valve, both of which are of the leaflet (flap) type (Figs. 16-10 and 16-11). The intake valve of the right ventricle consists of three leaflets and is called the *tricuspid valve.* The intake valve of the left ventricle consists of only two leaflets and is therefore sometimes referred to as the *bicuspid valve,* but its more common name is the *mitral valve,* which denotes its resemblance to a bishop's miter (tall cap). The leaflets of both atrioventricular valves have a similar histological structure. They are covered on both sides with endocardium and have a middle supporting layer of dense connective tissue containing numerous elastic fibers (Fig. 16-10).

At the base of the leaflet, the middle supporting layer becomes continuous with the dense connective tissue of the fibrous rings surrounding the orifices. Capillaries and

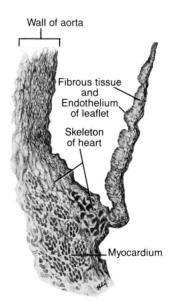

Fig. 16-10. Drawing of one leaflet of the aortic valve in longitudinal section, including a portion of the fibrous skeleton of the heart.

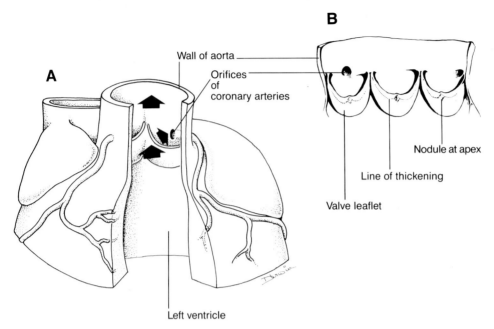

Fig. 16-11. Diagrammatic representation of the aortic valve. Its position at the base of the ascending aorta is indicated in *A*, and the appearance of its three leaflets when the aorta is cut open and spread out flat is depicted in *B*.

smooth muscle cells may be present at the base of the leaflet but do not extend up into the valves in man. The cells in the dense connective tissue of the valves are maintained by tissue fluid derived from the blood that bathes the valves.

Tendinous cords of dense connective tissue called *chordae tendineae,* which are covered with thin endocardium, extend from the papillary muscles and connect with the ventricular surface of the middle supporting layer of each leaflet. It should be realized that the exhaust valves of the ventricles (the aortic and the pulmonary valves) open on ventricular contraction and that only the closed intake (the tricuspid and mitral) valves have to withstand the full pressure of ventricular contraction. There is a danger, then, that unless they were specially protected, they might, during strong ventricular contraction, behave like umbrellas on windy days and be blown inside out. The chordae tendineae and the papillary muscles from which they arise limit the extent to which the portions of the valves near their free margins can be "blown" toward the atria (Fig. 16-3).

The exhaust valve of the right ventricle is termed the *pulmonary semilunar* (L. *semi,* half; *luna,* moon) *valve* because its leaflets are crescent-shaped. The exhaust valve of the left ventricle is termed the *aortic semilunar valve,* and it, too, has three leaflets (Fig. 16-11). The leaflets of these valves are thinner than those of the atrioventricular valves. However, they are of the same general construction, being composed essentially of folds of endocardium reinforced with a middle layer of dense connective tissue; the folds of endocardium at their bases become continuous with the

skeleton of the heart (Fig. 16-10). They have no chordae tendineae. The leaflets contain a considerable amount of elastic tissue on their ventricular side.

In a semilunar valve leaflet, the dense middle layer is thickened along a line close to, and parallel with, its free margin, particularly near the middle of the leaflet (Fig. 16-11*B*). This thickened line, not the free margin, is the line along which the leaflets touch one another when the valves close. Between this line of thickened tissue and their free margins, the leaflets are more flimsy and filmlike. These very pliable free margins ensure an effective seal.

In children suffering from rheumatic fever, the leaflets may become the seat of an inflammatory process that can deform their line of closure. The healing of the leaflets is often associated with considerable increase in their collagen content; as a result, they become stiffer and shorter or deformed in other ways. Leaflets can even adhere to one another. In any event, the end result is likely to be a valve that does not open or close properly. In his clinical training, the student will see many examples of valves affected in this way. It is now possible to replace certain diseased valves with artificial ones.

ARTERIES AND ARTERIOLES

Arterial vessels are classified as (1) elastic arteries, (2) muscular (distributing) arteries, and (3) arterioles. We shall start by considering the respective functions of these three different types of vessels.

During contraction of the ventricles, a relatively high blood pressure is generated. However, blood pressure also needs to be maintained during the period between ventricular contractions. For this reason, the walls of the great arteries leading from the ventricles are constructed chiefly of elastic laminae. Such arteries are known as *elastic arteries.* Blood delivered to them by the contracting ventricles stretches the elastin in their walls. Following ventricular contraction, the elastic recoil of their walls then maintains the blood pressure until the ventricles undergo their next contraction.

The pressure generated within the arterial system during ventricular contraction is called the *systolic blood pressure* (Gr. *systolē,* contraction), and it is half as much again as the pressure maintained between ventricular contractions, which is called the *diastolic blood pressure* (Gr. *diastolē,* dilatation). Normal arterial blood pressure taken at rest is 120/80 mm Hg (systolic/diastolic). A sustained resting blood pressure in excess of 150/90 mm Hg is an indication of *primary (essential) hypertension* (high blood pressure).

In contrast to the largest arteries, the primary function of which is to maintain diastolic blood pressure, the main function of the arteries that arise from them is to distribute blood to the various parts of the body. Because different parts of the body, under varied conditions of activity, require unequal amounts of blood, the luminal diameter of the arteries supplying them requires continuous regulation to ensure that appropriate quantities of blood reach them at any given time. The luminal diameter of these *distributing arteries* is regulated by the sympathetic division of the autonomic nervous system. The walls of such arteries consist chiefly of smooth muscle cells that are arranged in so-called circular layers (in which they actually take a helical path). Because the important component of their walls is smooth muscle, distributing arteries are also known as *muscular arteries.*

Arterioles deliver arterial blood to capillary beds under relatively low hydrostatic pressure. These vessels, as their name implies, are essentially very small arteries, but they have a relatively narrow lumen and thick muscular walls. Because blood is viscous, their narrow lumen offers considerable resistance to blood flow, and this enables a relatively high arterial blood pressure to be maintained. The pressure within the arterial system as a whole is regulated mainly by the *tonus of the smooth muscle cells in the walls of arterioles,* and this, in turn, is subject to autonomic and hormonal regulation. If the tonus of these smooth muscle cells becomes increased above the normal range, *hypertension* results.

Before describing the detailed wall structure of the various types of blood vessels, we should explain that their walls are conventionally regarded as conforming to a generalized plan in which they are made up of three coats called *tunicae.* However, these coats are not always as clearcut as their descriptions make them out to be. They are called (1) the *tunica intima* (the innermost coat), (2) the

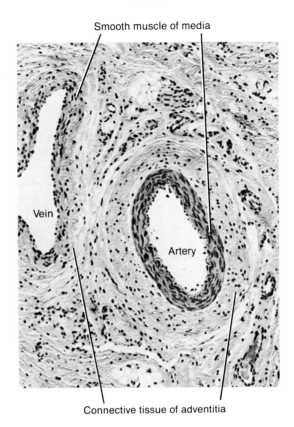

Smooth muscle of media

Vein

Artery

Connective tissue of adventitia

Fig. 16-12. Photomicrograph of a muscular (distributing) artery and its companion vein (from groove between trachea and esophagus of a child).

tunica media (the middle coat), and (3) the *tunica adventitia* (the outermost coat). As we shall see, the relative thickness of each coat and the tissues it contains depend on the type of vessel concerned. The three coats are more readily recognized in muscular arteries than in elastic arteries, so we shall begin with these.

Muscular (Distributing) Arteries

Almost all the fairly large to medium-sized blood vessels seen in routine sections are either muscular arteries or veins. Such vessels can readily be distinguished from one another by observing their relative wall thickness and the shape and size of their lumen. Arterial walls are comparatively thick because they need to be able to withstand arterial blood pressure. Furthermore, the lumen of an artery remains more or less round because the walls of the vessel are thick enough to resist collapse at death (Fig. 16-12). In comparison, the walls of a vein are much thinner in relation to the overall diameter of the vessel because they are only required to withstand venous blood pressure, and the lumen is relatively wide and generally flattens because of collapse of the vessel at death (Fig. 16-12).

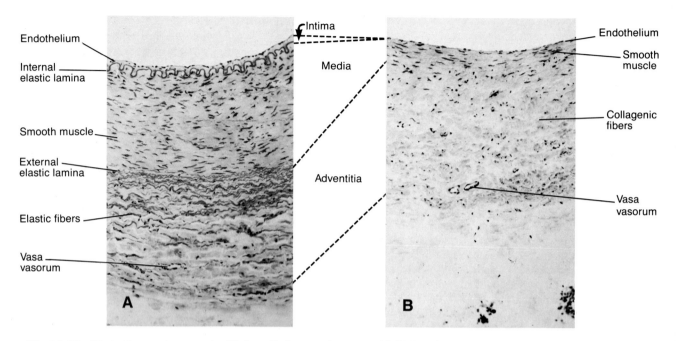

Fig. 16-13. Photomicrographs comparing (*A*) the wall of a muscular artery with (*B*) that of a companion vein (transverse section).

The *intima* of a muscular artery is bounded on its inner surface by the *endothelium* and the underlying basement membrane (both of which are included with the intima) and on its outer surface by a substantial lamina of elastin termed the *internal elastic lamina;* this lamina, too, is regarded as part of the intima. Generally, it is seen as a wavy pink line just beneath the endothelium (Fig. 16-13*A*). In many muscular arteries, the endothelium seems to lie directly on the internal elastic lamina. Sometimes the internal elastic lamina is duplicated, in which case it is described as a *split internal elastic lamina.*

The *media* of a muscular artery is composed of circularly (helically) arranged smooth muscle cells (Fig. 16-13*A*). The intercellular substance holding the smooth muscle cells together is made by the smooth muscle cells themselves and is chiefly *elastin.* There is relatively more elastin in the media of a large muscular artery than in a small one. The outer border of the media of a muscular artery is marked by a substantial lamina of elastin, called the *external elastic lamina.*

The *adventitia* of a muscular artery varies but is commonly comparable in thickness to the media (Fig. 16-13*A*). It consists chiefly of elastic fibers (darkly stained in Fig. 16-13*A*) but also contains collagen fibers. Hence most of the elastin in the wall of a muscular artery lies in the tunica adventitia. Tiny blood vessels called *vasa vasorum* (vessels of vessels) supply the adventitia, particularly in larger arteries, and may reach the periphery of the media. Lymphatics are also present in the adventitia.

The coronary arteries, which supply blood to the mus-

culature of the heart, and certain other arteries found in the reproductive organs (namely, the helicine arteries of the uterus, ovaries, and penis) have an additional feature that sets them apart from the usual type of muscular artery. The endothelium of a small muscular artery generally lies directly on the internal elastic lamina, but this is not true for some parts of these atypical arteries. Thus intimal thickenings occasionally referred to as musculoskeletal cushions can be found even in newborn babies at sites of bifurcation of the coronary arteries. Here smooth muscle cells assume a subendothelial position and produce elastin and other types of intercellular substances. Such intimal thickenings subsequently become more general along the coronary arteries, although they also become somewhat less pronounced. In contrast to the circular (helical) arrangement of the smooth muscle cells that are present in the media, the arrangement of the additional smooth muscle cells in the intima of such atypical muscular arteries is longitudinal.

Elastic Arteries

The *intima* of an elastic artery is much thicker than is its counterpart in a muscular artery. In the aorta, for example, the intima makes up about 20% of the total thickness of the wall (Fig. 16-14). In the hematoxylin and eosin (H & E) section shown in Figure 16-14*A*, the intima appears paler than the media, and in the section stained for elastin (Fig. 16-14*B*), it can be seen that the intima contains much elastin. This component is present in the form of fibers and

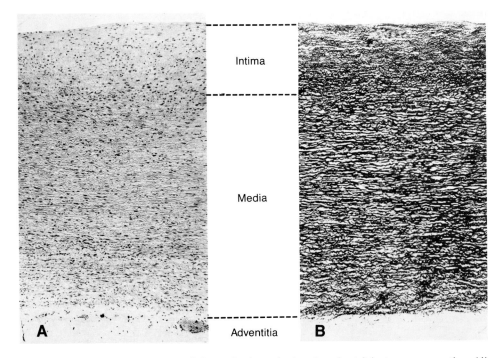

Fig. 16-14. Photomicrographs of the wall of an elastic artery (aorta) in transverse section. (*A*) H & E section; (*B*) stained for elastin.

incomplete fenestrated laminae that are embedded, along with collagen fibers and cells, in amorphous ground substance. The main type of cell in the intima is the smooth muscle cell, and this produces the various types of intercellular substances that are present in the intima. However, other types of cells are also seen in the intima of elastic arteries—for example, fibroblasts and macrophages. The intima increases in thickness with age and can become considerably thickened by the atherosclerotic process, which will be described later in this chapter.

The external border of the intima is delineated by an internal elastic lamina; this is considered to be part of the intima, but it is similar to the other laminae that are such a prominent feature of the media (Fig. 16-14*B*). It is not always easy to distinguish the internal elastic lamina because there is so much elastin in the intima (Fig. 16-14*B*). The process of elastin formation was described in Chapter 7; an electron micrograph of the internal elastic lamina at the stage during which it is being formed by smooth muscle cells is shown in Figure 16-15.

The *media* of an elastic artery constitutes the bulk of its wall and consists chiefly of concentric fenestrated laminae of elastin (Fig. 16-14*B*) together with collagen fibers and smooth muscle cells. The number of elastic laminae in the wall increases until the age of approximately 35 years, reaching almost 60 laminae in the thoracic aorta and almost 30 laminae in the abdominal aorta. The aortic laminae also thicken in adult life. Then beginning at the age of approx-

imately 50 years, they begin to show signs of degeneration (fraying, fragmentation, etc.) and gradually become replaced by collagen. As a result, there is a gradual loss of elasticity but an overall increase in the strength of the aortic wall. The numerous smooth muscle cells situated between neighboring laminae produce the elastin, collagen, and proteoglycans of the media. At the outermost limit of the media, there is an external elastic lamina, but in the aorta this is very indistinct (Fig. 16-14).

The *adventitia* of an elastic artery is thin (Fig. 16-14*A*). It consists of irregularly arranged connective tissue with both collagen and elastic fibers, and it contains fibroblasts, a few smooth musle cells near the media, and other types of connective tissue cells. Lymphatic capillaries can be found in this layer of the wall. The presence of much collagen in the adventitia probably helps to prevent the vessel from becoming overdilated during systole.

A number of small nutritive blood vessels are present in the adventitia, and in the thoracic aorta, they also supply at least the outer half of the media. These vessels constitute the *vasa vasorum* of the aorta. Certain studies suggest that the extent to which these small vessels nourish the media is a function of the total number of elastic laminae in the vessel wall. Such studies indicate that approximately the inner 30 lamellae are devoid of any significant supply of vasa vasorum in adult life. This being the case, because the abdominal aorta possesses a maximum of 30 or so lamellae, its media would probably have to be nourished

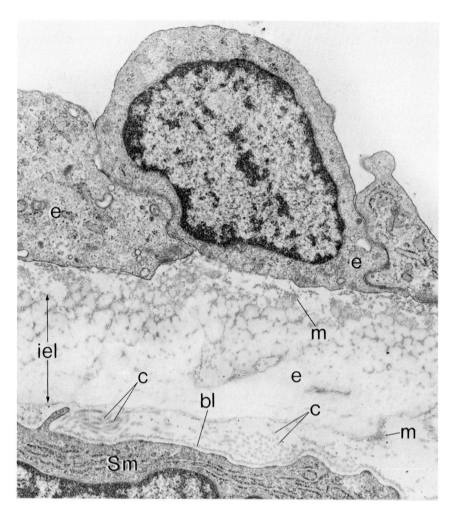

Fig. 16-15. Electron micrograph (×16,000) of intima of developing aorta (human fetus), showing the internal elastic lamina (*iel*) beneath the endothelial cells (*e*). At bottom left, part of a smooth muscle cell (*Sm*) is present; this cell is producing elastin and other intercellular constituents of the wall. It is enclosed in a basement membrane (*bl*) and also has collagen fibrils (*c*) associated with it. Note also that microfibrils (*m*) form a scaffolding for the amorphous elastin (*e*) of the internal elastic lamina. (Courtesy of M. D. Haust)

entirely by diffusion from the lumen. However, other investigators have concluded that the outer two thirds of the media of the abdominal aorta is provided with vasa vasorum (for further discussion, see Lindsay and Hurst). Resolution of this matter could help to explain why the media of the abdominal aorta is particularly prone to degenerative *arteriosclerotic* changes (Gr. *sclerosis*, hardening; *i.e.,* hardening of the arterial wall due to thickening and loss of elasticity); such changes can result in the formation of arteriosclerotic *aortic aneurysms* (saclike dilatations of the vessel wall). In any event, it is generally conceded that the intima and at least the inner third of the media must rely on the diffusion of nutrients and oxygen from the lumen of the vessel because arterial blood pressure transmitted through the vessel wall would not allow any blood to fill the vasa vasorum even if they were present.

Some implications of the absence of vasa vasorum and the lack of a lymphatic drainage from the innermost region of the arterial wall will become evident in the following discussion of a common type of degeneration that affects the inner part of the arterial wall.

What Is It About the Design of the Arterial Wall That Makes Arteries So Susceptible to Atherosclerosis? Of profound clinical importance is a form of *arteriosclerosis* (thickening and hardening of the arterial walls) known as *atherosclerosis*—a disease characterized by the presence of intimal focal lesions (*atheromatous plaques*) that, at one stage in their development, acquire a distinctly gruel-like appearance (Gr. *athere*, gruel; *i.e.,* sloppy oatmeal porridge). The reason for its clinical importance is that atherosclerosis is the main underlying cause of ischemic heart disease, cerebrovascular disease, and arteriosclerotic aortic aneurysms. Epidemiological and health statistics indicate that atherosclerosis is the primary contributing factor to deaths in the United States and is a prevalent cause of death in certain other affluent nations with high standards of living.

Atherosclerotic lesions are patchy in distribution, affecting both muscular (distributing) arteries and elastic arteries. The most serious consequences result from atherosclerotic involvement of coronary or cerebral arteries (which can lead to a heart attack or a stroke) or the aorta (which can develop an aneurysm and rupture). *Atheromatous* (*ath-*

erosclerotic) *plaques,* which are also known as *fibrous* or *fibrofatty plaques,* are elevations of the intima that generally develop a central core of fatty necrotic debris. Present evidence suggests that they may be a consequence of a multi-staged interactive tissue response to focal injury or loss of integrity of the endothelium, which normally constitutes a permeability barrier to leukocytes and plasma-borne macromolecules (Ross). Such damage elicits a number of interrelated changes that include those described in the following paragraphs.

At an early stage in the formation of diet-induced atherosclerotic plaques, monocytes adhere to the endothelium and then migrate to a subendothelial position where they become macrophages and begin to accumulate lipids. In addition, smooth muscle cells begin to migrate from the media to the intima of the affected site. The smooth muscle cells that enter the intima undergo marked proliferation and accumulate low-density lipoprotein (LDL)-derived cholesteryl esters in their cytoplasm. LDL-derived cholesterol and its esters similarly accumulate in the macrophages that appear in the intima. Furthermore, a substantial quantity of cholesterol is deposited extracellularly in the amorphous intercellular component of the intima. It is at this stage that the plaque acquires its characteristic gruel-like appearance because of the presence of cholesterol-laden cells (known collectively as *foam cells*), necrotic cell debris, and extracellular cholesterol deposits. In this connection, it should be noted that there are no lymphatics or vasa vasorum in the inner part of the arterial wall to facilitate removal of such extracellular deposits or products of degradation. Commonly, the accumulated material undergoes subsequent calcification, resulting in hardening of the plaque. The net result is that the atherosclerotic lesion damages and weakens the arterial wall.

While all this is happening, platelets can come into contact with exposed intimal collagen, whereupon they aggregate on the denuded surface of the lesion. They undergo the release reaction (see Chap. 8) and liberate platelet-derived growth factor (PDGF), which can induce smooth muscle cells to proliferate. Moreover, they have the potential to trigger the formation of a thrombus that may be large enough to occlude the entire arterial lumen. If this happens in a coronary artery, it can result in ischemic necrosis of an entire portion of the myocardium (a *myocardial infarct*). Furthermore, there is the added danger that the thrombus, or some part of it, will detach and circulate to an important artery elsewhere in the body, where it may obstruct that artery as well. An obstructed cerebral artery, for example, can result in a *cerebral infarct* that is manifested as a stroke. Such blockage by a circulating blood clot is termed *thromboembolism*.

The pathogenesis of atherosclerosis nevertheless remains poorly understood. A hypothesis that is currently finding wide acceptance is that the atherosclerotic process stems from chronic or repeated structural or functional insults to the integrity of the arterial endothelial cell barrier with the result that, in hypercholesterolemic individuals, it admits monocytes, cell-derived and plasma-borne mitogens, and mitogen promoters to the subendothelial layer of the intima. Furthermore, it has been found that PDGF is chemotactic for arterial smooth muscle cells, suggesting that at least under certain circumstances, PDGF can play a major role in inducing smooth muscle cells to migrate through the fenestrated internal elastic lamina, promoting focal invasion of the intima. There is also some evidence to indicate that a PDGF-like growth factor is secreted by the intimal vascular smooth muscle cells themselves. Apparently in response to a considerable variety of cell-derived mitogenic growth factors that includes PDGF, macrophage-derived growth factor (MDGF), and endothelial cell–derived growth factor (EDGF), these smooth muscle cells proliferate, and they begin to produce substantial quantities of intercellular substances, with the result that these build up and the intima begins to thicken. There are indications that such smooth muscle cells have entered a PDGF-responsive *synthetic state* (in which they produce elastin, collagen, and proteoglycans) that is distinct from the PDGF-insensitive *contractile state* that ordinarily characterizes the smooth muscle cells in the media (Ross). As the intima thickens, it encroaches on the lumen until this becomes reduced to a very narrow opening (Fig. 16-16). The amount of blood that such a vessel is able to deliver is thereby greatly diminished, and the risk that the lumen will become occluded by a thrombus increases.

The ways in which LDL is implicated in this process are still being elucidated. However, there is evidence to suggest that chronically elevated LDL levels can damage arterial endothelium, and LDL from hypercholesterolemic plasma has been found to promote the proliferation of smooth muscle cells, perhaps by enhancing their responsiveness to mitogens. Furthermore, elevated levels of LDL promote the accumulation of cholesteryl esters in foam cells. Hence it seems likely that LDL participates at several different levels in the development of atherosclerotic plaques.

For a recent review of the respective roles of arterial endothelium, macrophages, smooth muscle cells, platelets, and growth factors in the pathogenesis of atherosclerosis, see Ross (1986).

Arterioles

Arterial vessels with an overall diameter of less than 100 μm and an internal diameter of approximately 30 μm are called *arterioles.* As may be seen from Figure 16-17, the wall thickness of an arteriole is generally only slightly less than the diameter of its lumen. In small arterioles, the *intima* consists only of the endothelium and its basement membrane, but in larger arterioles, there is also an internal elastic lamina. The *media* generally consists of *only one or two circular (helical) layers of smooth muscle* (Fig. 16-17); however, in the larger arterioles, an external elastic lamina is present as well. The *adventitia* may be as thick as the media; it contains a mixture of collagen and elastic fibers.

As arterioles branch and become smaller, their walls become thinner and their lumen becomes smaller. The ratio between the wall thickness and the diameter of the lumen, however, remains approximately the same, and this, together with an estimate of the number of layers of smooth muscle cells in the media, are criteria that are used for

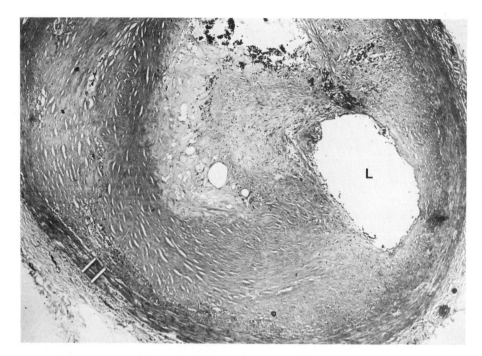

Fig. 16-16. Photomicrograph of a coronary artery with a reduced luminal diameter caused by the development of an atherosclerotic plaque. The width of the media is indicated by the white lines at lower left; external to this layer lies the adventitia. The remainder of the wall represents a greatly thickened intima. (Gotlieb AI: Can Med Assoc J 126:903, 1982)

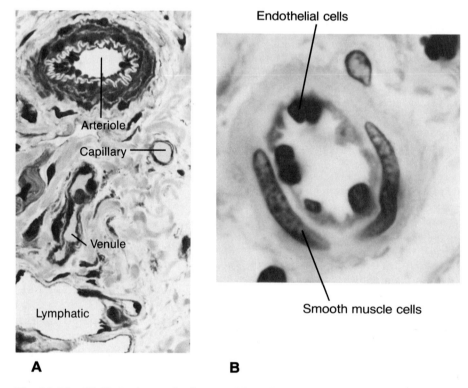

A   **B**

Fig. 16-17. (*A*) Photomicrograph of an arteriole and venule, together with a capillary and lymphatic, in a semithin (2 μm) section of subcutaneous connective tissue (rabbit). The corrugated pale-staining layer deep to the endothelium of the arteriole is its internal elastic lamina. (*B*) Photomicrograph of a small arteriole in a routine H & E section (oil immersion). (*A*, courtesty of H. Z. Movat)

recognizing arterioles. The internal and external elastic laminae become very thin in smaller arterioles; and in the smallest (those less than 35 μm in diameter), these two components are absent. The adventitia of small arterioles is very thin and consists chiefly of collagen fibers.

CAPILLARIES

Thin-walled vessels with a luminal diameter of only 8 μm to 10 μm (*i.e.,* that are only slightly wider than an erythrocyte) are known as *capillaries.* Networks of these vessels known as *capillary beds* supply tissue fluid, nutrients, and oxygen to the component cells of body tissues.

The LM appearance of capillaries can be seen to advantage in a cross section of skeletal muscle (because these blood vessels run parallel to the muscle fibers). Such a section (Fig. 16-18) cuts through most capillaries without passing through nuclei of their endothelial cells (which is the case in Fig. 16-17A). However, in cases in which the nuclei of endothelial cells are included, these appear as dark crescents that partly encircle the lumen and they generally create a bulge in the capillary wall (Fig. 16-18, *lower left*). Cross sections of capillaries sometimes also include a central erythrocyte or leukocyte (Fig. 16-18).

In the electron microscope (EM), it can be seen that the cytoplasm of capillary endothelial cells contains all the usual organelles; in most of these vessels, it is replete with endocytotic pits and vesicles (some coated pits are indicated by *arrowheads* in Fig. 16-19). Such pits and vesicles form on both the inner and the outer surfaces of the capillary endothelial cells, and they are presumed to fuse with each other from time to time so as to establish temporary tortuous tubular channels across the attenuated cytoplasm. These channels are believed to provide the means for bidirectional macromolecular exchanges between the blood plasma and tissue fluid.

In most parts of the body, the edges of contiguous capillary endothelial cells are joined together by tight junctions of the *fascia occludens* type (described in Chap. 6). Because these junctions do not occupy the entire margin of the cells, there are slitlike clefts between them through which tissue fluid can pass. In most regions of the brain, however, the tight junctions between capillary endothelial cells extend all the way around their margins and are of the *zonula occludens* type; hence there is a blood–brain barrier (see Chap. 14). The capillary as a whole is enclosed by a prominent basement membrane (Fig. 16-19). Furthermore, scattered along its course, there are pericytes which, as noted in Chapter 7, are relatively undifferentiated pluripotential cells of mesenchymal origin that represent a potential source of fibroblasts and smooth muscle cells. As with smooth muscle cells, pericytes have a surrounding basement membrane and they lie so close to the endothelium that they are sometimes described as being insinuated into

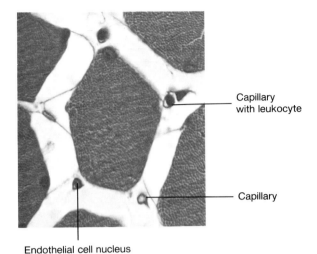

Fig. 16-18. Photomicrograph showing representative sections through capillaries in a cross section of skeletal muscle (oil immersion).

the basement membrane of the capillary (Fig. 16-19, see also Figs. 7-12 and 14-26).

There are two main types of capillaries. These are classified as *continuous* or *fenestrated,* as will be described in the following sections.

Continuous Capillaries. Each individual endothelial cell that lines a capillary is generally large enough to encircle its entire lumen. Due to interdigitation of the cell margins, it is nevertheless quite common to see parts of more than one endothelial cell in a cross section of a capillary. Continuous capillaries represent the common type of capillary encountered in sections of body tissues, and they are continuous in the sense that they possess a continuous and uninterrupted (*i.e.,* unfenestrated) lining.

Fenestrated Capillaries. Capillaries of this type are essentially similar to capillaries of the continuous variety except that some of the attenuated regions of endothelial cell cytoplasm are provided with permanent circular fenestrae (Fig. 16-20). These fenestrae are covered by a thin diaphragm in all capillaries other than those of the kidney glomeruli, which seem to lack diaphragms and hence represent true openings. The endothelial cells that line the liver sinusoids (unusually wide, thin-walled venous vessels) are similarly provided with permanent open fenestrae that are not covered by a diaphragm. It is widely believed that the presence of open or of closed fenestrae facilitates exchanges across the endothelial lining.

The diaphragm that covers a fenestra appears in the EM as a single structure that is described as being somewhat thinner than a single cell membrane and as possessing a central thickening that is approximately 10 nm to 15 nm across. Rather than being a circumscribed region of ordinary

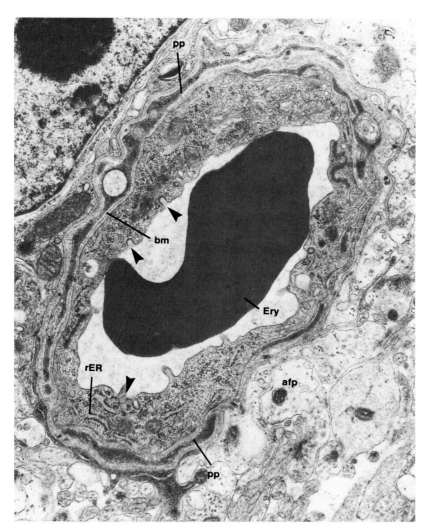

Fig. 16-19. Electron micrograph of a continuous capillary (from brain of immature chick). The diameter of its lumen can readily be estimated from that of the erythrocyte (*Ery*) in its lumen. The lining endothelial cells exhibit coated pits (*arrowheads*), coated vesicles, free ribosomes, and cisternae of rough-surfaced endoplasmic reticulum (*rER*). External to the endothelium, there is a prominent basement membrane (*bm*). Dark-stained pericyte processes (*pp*) can also be distinguished. Most of the external surface of the vessel is covered with astrocyte foot processes (*afp*). (Courtesy of P. A. Stewart and M. J. Wiley)

cell membrane, it is more likely to be a special structure that is inserted, as it were, into the attenuated cytoplasm. Hence all around the periphery of the fenestra, the cell membrane on the luminal side of the endothelial cell would be in direct continuity with the part of the cell membrane on the surface facing the surrounding tissue. If it were otherwise, with the cell membrane extending across the fenestra instead of meeting around it, the diaphragm might be expected to be a double structure made up of two thicknesses of cell membrane.

How Is Blood Flow Through the Terminal Vascular Bed Regulated?   Only vessels with smooth muscle cells in their walls are able to regulate the distribution and rate of flow of blood through capillary beds. This regulation is effected by narrowing (*vasoconstriction*) or widening (*vasodilatation*) of the lumen of these vessels. Continuous adjustment of the caliber of their lumina, which is referred to as *vasomotor activity,* is mediated by autonomic nervous impulses and also by chemical mediators and metabolites.

There are several levels at which blood flow is regulated in the terminal vascular bed. The first is the level of the *terminal arterioles* delivering blood to the capillary networks. These vessels are small in diameter (30 μm to 50 μm) but still have a single continuous layer of smooth muscle cells in the media of their walls, and it is the degree of tonus in these cells that determines the diameter of their lumina at any given moment.

As may be seen in Figure 16-21, a terminal arteriole opens into vessels of two distinct types. At top left and also at top right in this diagram, it opens into *capillaries*. Although there are no smooth muscle cells along the course of a capillary, these cells do encircle each capillary at its site of origin from an arteriole. As shown in Figure 16-21, such smooth muscle cells constitute what are termed *precapillary sphincters*. The degree of tonus in these tiny sphincters regulates the amount of blood that can enter the capillaries. Also arising from terminal arterioles are larger vessels termed *metarterioles* (Fig. 16-21). Such vessels pursue a

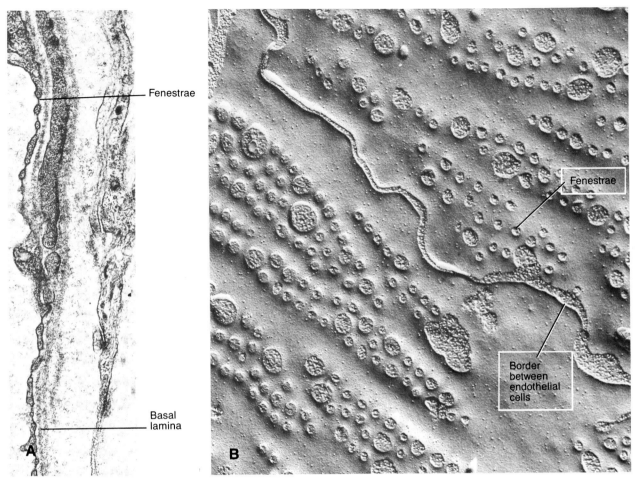

Fig. 16-20. Electron micrographs of fenestrated capillaries (*A*) in longitudinal section, and (*B*) in surface view (freeze-fracture replica). Note the thin diaphragms closing over the fenestrae in *A* and the tracts of fenestrae in *B*. The biggest fenestrae here (in the adrenal cortex) are 166 nm in diameter, which is uncommonly large for fenestrated capillaries in general. (*A*, courtesy of J. Bilbao and S. Briggs; *B*, Ryan US, Ryan JW, Smith DS, Winkler H: Tissue Cell 7:181, 1975)

course that traverses the capillary bed and then drains into a venule, shown at the bottom of Figure 16-21. Many of the capillaries in the capillary bed arise from the proximal portion of the metarteriole, so this part of the vessel is also provided with precapillary sphincters (Fig. 16-21). Furthermore, many of the capillaries drain into its distal part (the portion known, for reasons that will be explained shortly, as a *thoroughfare channel*; labeled in Fig. 16-21). A metarteriole is wider than a capillary, and it is encircled by smooth muscle cells at many scattered sites along the first half of its course (these smooth muscle cells are indicated by *black semicircles* in Fig. 16-21). Hence the volume of blood entering a capillary bed is regulated by precapillary sphincters at sites where capillaries originate from terminal arterioles or metarterioles. Furthermore, the volume of blood flowing along a metarteriole itself is controlled by the tonus in the encircling smooth muscle cells scattered

along its course. In some tissues, however, vasomotor activity in terminal arterioles is the main factor controlling local blood flow in capillary beds. Moreover, vasomotor activity of precapillary sphincters can be independent of that of the terminal arterioles and metarterioles from which the capillaries originate.

The metarterioles in some sites can serve another purpose, namely, that of acting as low-resistance channels for an increased blood flow. This occurs especially in mesenteries and body sites where thermoregulation is important, such as in the skin and ear. As can be seen in Figure 16-21, these low-resistance pathways, which are called *preferential (thoroughfare) channels*, represent continuations of the distal ends of metarterioles and empty into venules. Preferential channels (which are not present to the same extent in all tissues) open when constriction of precapillary sphincters reduces blood flow through the local capillary

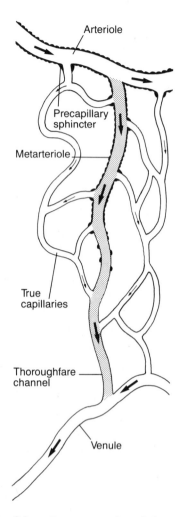

Fig. 16-21. Schematic representation of the arrangement of vessels in the terminal vascular bed. See text for details. (After Zweifach)

network; the channels thus bypass the capillary bed and sustain blood flow through the region when the capillaries are not being utilized. In sections, these channels would be indistinguishable from large capillaries or postcapillary venules (see below).

Most knowledge of the terminal vascular bed has come from studies on flattened tissues such as mesenteries. However, microvascular beds extend in three dimensions at other sites and hence are a good deal more complex. For information about the microcirculation in such terminal vascular beds, see Sobin and Tremer, and also Baez.

ARTERIOVENOUS ANASTOMOSES (AV SHUNTS)

Not all the circulating blood is required to pass through the terminal vascular bed. In certain regions of the body,

there are alternative channels called *arteriovenous anastomoses* (*AV shunts*) that permit blood to pass directly from the arterial to the venous side of the circulation, without its having to go through capillaries, metarterioles, or preferential channels.

In the liver, for example, short unbranched vessels (up to 45 μm in diameter) connect some of the arteries directly to veins. Elsewhere, anastomoses may be longer and narrower (5 μm to 18 μm in diameter) and connect arterioles to venules. The proximal half or two thirds of such vesels has a well-developed smooth muscle layer in its walls, and the distal segment has a somewhat wider lumen.

Arteriovenous anastomoses exhibit vasomotor activity and are extremely responsive to thermal, mechanical, and chemical stimuli. They are fairly numerous in the skin, where they are considered to be of importance in bypassing the capillary beds of the dermis in order to conserve heat as will be explained in Chapter 17.

VENULES

Capillaries and thoroughfare channels open at their venous end into *postcapillary venules* (8 μm to 30 μm in diameter), which have increasing numbers of pericytes associated with them as their diameter increases. These vessels, in turn, open into *collecting venules* (30 μm to 50 μm in diameter) that, as well as having pericytes, also possess an adventitia consisting of fibroblasts and collagen fibers. The *muscular venules* (50 μm to 100 μm in diameter) into which the collecting venules empty have one or two layers of smooth muscle cells in their media, and their adventitia is relatively well developed. In routine sections, however, all venules tend to look alike except for the size of their lumen. The venules empty the venous blood that they collect from the microcirculation into small *collecting veins* (100 μm to 300 μm in diameter) that have several layers of smooth muscle cells in their media.

Venules are very much involved in inflammation because they are the vessels from which leukocytes and fluid exudate enter tissues during the acute inflammatory reaction (see Figs. 8-12 and 8-13). Even under normal conditions, there is believed to be a continuous interchange of water and small molecules between blood plasma and the interstitial fluid by way of the relatively extensive intercellular clefts present between the endothelial cells that line these vessels.

External to the endothelium lies its basement membrane (Fig. 16-22). The cytoplasmic processes of associated pericytes are commonly seen cut in oblique or transverse section, where they extend around or along the vessel (Fig. 16-22A). Pericytes and their processes also have a surrounding basement membrane that, as in capillaries, is continuous with that of the endothelium. Some supporting collagen fibrils are seen external to the basement membrane (Fig. 16-22A).

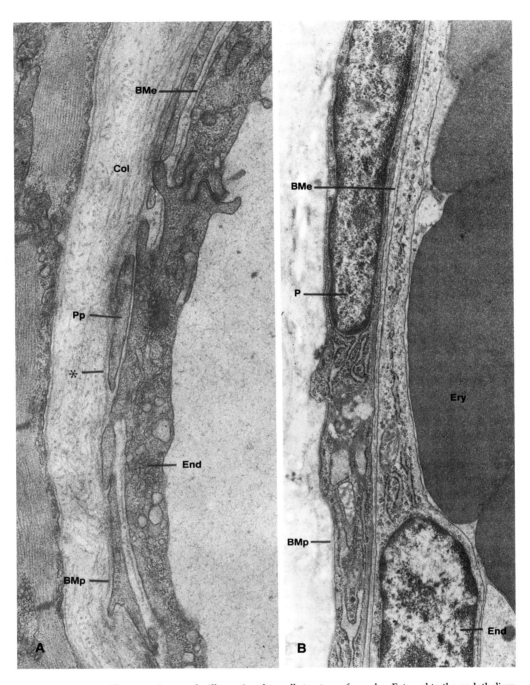

Fig. 16-22. Electron micrographs illustrating the wall structure of venules. External to the endothelium (*End*) lies its basement membrane (*BMe*) and an investment of pericytes (*P*) with their cytoplasmic processes (*Pp*). The pericytes are surrounded by a basement membrane (*BMp*) that, at some sites (*asterisk* in *A*), merges with that of the endothelium. Adventitial collagen fibrils (*Col*) are present external to the pericyte basement membrane in *A*. Erythrocytes (*Ery*) are seen in the lumen in *B*. (Courtesy of H. Z. Movat)

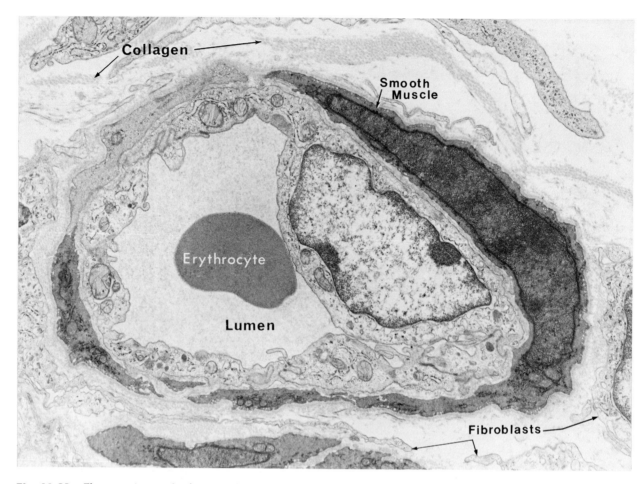

Fig. 16-23. Electron micrograph of a muscular venule. Smooth muscle cells do not surround the lumen completely as they do in arterioles. To the right of the erythrocyte, the nucleus of an endothelial cell is seen. A basement membrane is present between the endothelium and the smooth muscle cell, and also surrounding the smooth muscle cell. (Courtesy of M. Weinstock)

Where venules increase in diameter and merge into small veins, the pericytes become replaced by fully differentiated smooth muscle cells, and the vessels are termed *muscular venules* (Fig. 16-23).

VEINS

Small and Medium-Sized Veins. The *intima* of a vein consists of an endothelium and its basement membrane, which either rests directly on a poorly defined internal elastic lamina or is separated from it by only a small amount of subendothelial connective tissue. The *media* is generally much thinner than that of a companion artery, and it consists chiefly of a circular layer of smooth muscle fibers (Figs. 16-12 and 16-13). More collagen fibers and fewer elastic fibers lie between them than in arteries. In some veins, the innermost smooth muscle cells of the media have a longitudinal orientation. In general, the media is thinner and

less muscular in veins that are protected by muscles or by the pressure of abdominal contents than it is in more superficial veins. The cerebral and meningeal veins have almost no smooth muscle cells in their walls. The *adventitia* of medium-sized veins, which consists chiefly of collagen, is generally their thickest coat (Fig. 16-13B). However, certain veins of the limbs, exemplified by the superficial veins of the legs, possess a highly developed muscular media that counteracts the tendency to distension as a result of venous return against the force of gravity. This modification is particularly noticeable in the great saphenous veins, which because of their superficial position are poorly supported by subcutaneous adipose tissue. These veins possess inner longitudinal as well as outer circular layers of smooth muscle in their media (Fig. 16-24).

Large Veins. In general, the tunica intima of large veins resembles that of medium-sized veins, but the subendothelial connective tissue layer is thicker. In most of the

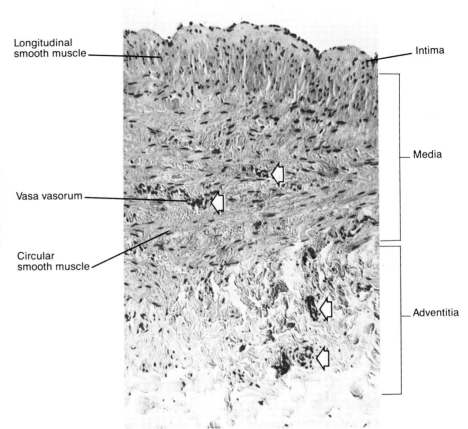

Longitudinal smooth muscle

Intima

Media

Vasa vasorum

Circular smooth muscle

Adventitia

Fig. 16-24. Photomicrograph showing the wall structure of a large vein (saphenous vein). Vasa vasorum (*arrows*) extend a fair distance into the media. The muscular media contains an inner longitudinal layer of smooth muscle in addition to its thick outer circular layer of smooth muscle.

largest veins, there is hardly any smooth muscle in the media; hence the *adventitia is by far the thickest* of the three coats (Fig. 16-25). This layer contains collagen and elastic fibers. In some instances (*e.g.,* the inferior vena cava) the innermost region of the adventitia also contains prominent longitudinal bundles of smooth muscle fibers (Fig. 16-25).

Vasa Vasorum and Lymphatics of Veins. Veins are *supplied much more abundantly* with vasa vasorum than are arteries. Because veins contain poorly oxygenated blood, the cells in the walls of veins need more oxygen than can be obtained by diffusion from the lumen of the vessel. Vasa vasorum carrying arterial blood into the walls supply this need. Furthermore, because the blood in veins is under low pressure, vasa vasorum can approach the intima of the walls of veins without collapsing because of the pressure within the vein. Hence the vasa vasorum of veins penetrate much closer to the intima than do those of arteries. They are seen to advantage in the thick walls of the saphenous vein (Fig. 16-24, indicated by *arrows*).

Because the walls of veins do not have to withstand great pressures, as do the walls of arteries, lymphatics, as well as vasa vasorum, can be present in a patent state within the substance of their walls. The walls of veins are *supplied much more abundantly* with lymphatic capillaries than are

the walls of arteries. Indeed, this probably explains why tumors that spread by way of lymphatics invade the walls of veins but not the walls of arteries.

Valves of Veins. Veins are provided with valves of the leaflet (flap) type that are arranged so as to permit blood to flow toward the heart but not in the opposite direction. The leaflets are folds of intima with central reinforcements of connective tissue. Elastic fibers are present on the side of the leaflet that faces the lumen of the vessel.

Valves are especially abundant in the veins of the extremities, but they are generally absent from the veins of the thorax and the abdomen. Valves are commonly located immediately distal to sites where tributaries join veins. Immediately proximal to the attachment of a valve, a vein is dilated slightly to form a pouch or sinus. Hence in distended superficial veins, localized swellings indicate the sites of valves.

The roles of valves in veins are several. First, they help to overcome the force of gravity by preventing backflow. But they may also act in other ways. For example, valves enable veins that are squeezed when surrounding muscles contract to serve as pumps. Moreover, they prevent the force of muscular contraction from creating back pressure on the capillary beds drained by the veins.

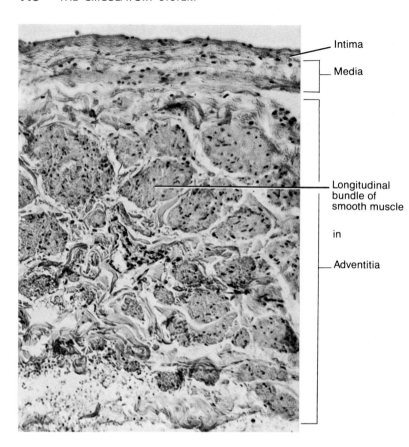

Intima

Media

Longitudinal
bundle of
smooth muscle

in

Adventitia

Fig. 16-25. Photomicrograph showing the wall structure of the inferior vena cava. The large longitudinal bundles of smooth muscle in its walls are situated in its adventitia.

Varicose Veins. Superficial veins, as noted, are relatively unsupported, and the weight of the blood within those veins that are situated below the heart is a factor that tends to cause their dilatation. Under conditions in which there is some resistance or obstruction to the return of blood from a part of the body, or in which the walls of the veins are not as strong as usual (*e.g.,* due to degeneration or disease), superficial veins gradually dilate. As dilatation proceeds, the valves become incompetent and, as a result, gravity exerts a still greater dilating force on their walls. Superficial veins that under these conditions become tortuous, irregular, and wider than usual are called *varicose veins.*

EFFERENT AND AFFERENT INNERVATION OF BLOOD VESSELS

The important efferent innervation of blood vessels is their *sympathetic vasoconstrictor innervation.* Release of norepinephrine from the axon terminals of these sympathetic fibers elicits vasoconstriction through an adrenergic-mediated effect on the circular smooth muscle cells in the vessel walls.

Some of the blood vessels in skeletal muscle have a subsidiary cholinergic *sympathetic vasodilator innervation.* However, there are a few other parts of the body in which the vasodilator innervation is *parasympathetic,* the best known example being the penis.

The carotid sinuses and the carotid bodies are sites where sensory receptors that are involved in reflex regulation of the blood circulation are located. Each *carotid sinus* is a small dilatation of the carotid artery (generally a dilatation of the internal carotid artery at a site immediately above the bifurcation of the common carotid artery). Here the arterial wall has a thin media and a thicker adventitia. Furthermore, the adventitia is provided with numerous endings of afferent nerve fibers that enter the carotid branch of the glossopharyngeal nerve. Because the media is so thin, these endings in the adventitia are able to provide information about the blood pressure in the carotid artery. This information is relayed to the control centers in the brain where the motor activities of the heart and arteries are regulated. The walls of the aortic arch and of the great veins close to the heart are similarly provided with *baroreceptors* (pressure receptors).

Each *carotid body* is a small condensation of tissue that is situated just above the bifurcation of the common carotid artery. It is abundantly supplied with wide, capillarylike vessels. In addition, it contains cords and clumps of ovoid cells that are richly supplied with *chemoreceptive* nerve endings that are capable of responding to changing blood levels of carbon dioxide, oxygen, and *p*H. The aortic arch, the pulmonary artery, and the origin of the right subclavian artery are similarly provided with such chemoreceptive endings.

THE LYMPHATIC SYSTEM

Excess interstitial fluid and protein drain from most parts of the body as *lymph.* There are nevertheless some sites in the body that lack a lymphatic drainage. These include the central nervous system, the cornea and lens of the eye, epithelial tissue, cartilage, and the inner region of the arterial wall. The vessels that convey lymph from its sites of origin are known as *lymphatics* or *lymphatic vessels.* They commonly extend through tissue along with an arteriole and venule (Fig. 16-17*A*) or an artery and its companion vein. Several lymphatics may be associated with an artery and its companion vein.

LYMPHATIC VESSELS (LYMPHATICS)

The walls of lymphatics (*i.e.,* the vessels into which lymphatic capillaries empty) are made up of a thin layer of connective tissue with an endothelial lining. The walls of large lymphatics (0.2 mm to 0.5 mm in diameter) show indications of being made up of an intima, media, and adventitia, but these three coats are not readily distinguishable in medium-sized and small lymphatics (Fig. 16-26). The *intima* commonly contains elastic fibers as well as an endothelium. The *media* of a collecting lymphatic consists of two or three layers of circular or oblique smooth muscle that are supported by connective tissue with elastic fibers. The *adventitia* is relatively well developed, particularly in smaller lymphatics; it contains smooth muscle cells that run longitudinally as well as obliquely. Small blood vessels are present in the outer coats of medium-sized and large lymphatics.

Lymphatics are provided with funnel-shaped valves of the leaflet (flap) type. The valves can be so close to one another that a distended lymphatic can take on a beaded appearance when the segments between its valves become distended. A lymphatic valve consists of a fold of intima reinforced with a central sheet of delicate connective tissue (Fig. 16-27).

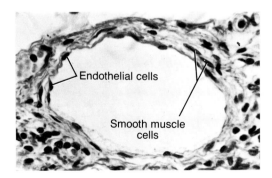

Fig. 16-26. Photomicrograph of a small lymphatic. The nuclei of a few smooth muscle cells can be seen in its wall, but the various layers of the wall are not clearly defined in lymphatics.

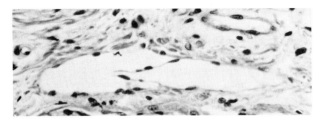

Fig. 16-27. Photomicrograph of an oblique section of a small lymphatic, showing one of its valves. (Courtesy of Y. Clermont)

It is not difficult to visualize how each segment between two one-way valves would act as a pump if (1) the walls of the segment contracted or (2) the segment were subjected to external compression. It is now evident that lymph can be actively propelled along lymphatics by intrinsic peristaltic contractions of the smooth muscle cells in their walls. Compression of lymphatics by pulsating blood vessels in their vicinity, or by active or passive movements of the body parts in which they are situated, also causes the segments of lymphatics to serve as pumps, aiding the one-way propulsion of lymph along them. This is why massage can be employed to improve lymphatic drainage from certain parts of the body. In addition, we shall find that the lymphatics draining the intestine participate in the process of fat absorption. Lymph draining from the intestine after a fatty meal appears milky and is called *chyle.*

Lymph draining from the body is returned to the bloodstream by way of two large lymphatic ducts called the *thoracic duct* and the *right lymphatic duct.* At its origin in the abdomen, the thoracic duct is dilated as the *cisterna chyli.* From there it extends and opens into the junction between the left internal jugular and subclavian veins. In some cases, it is represented by several smaller ducts. The right lymphatic duct (or its several smaller representations) opens into the junction between the right internal jugular and subclavian veins.

Lymphatic Capillaries

Also known as *terminal lymphatics,* these vessels resemble blood capillaries in many respects, but there are a few significant differences. As may be seen in Figure 16-28, lymphatic capillaries lack a well-developed basement membrane; where one is present, it is only poorly developed, and hence it does not impede the entry of macromolecules. Furthermore, lymphatic capillaries begin blindly whereas all blood capillaries have an arterial and a venous end. Also, lymphatic capillaries do not have pericytes associated with them (Fig. 16-28). Lastly, and perhaps most importantly, attached to the outer surface of the endothelial cells of lymphatic capillaries, there are small bundles of intercellular filaments. These filaments are 5 nm to 10 nm in diameter, and at least some of them are believed to represent very fine collagen fibrils. They are anchored to substantial intercellular fibers of the surrounding connective tissue and are accordingly known as *anchoring filaments*

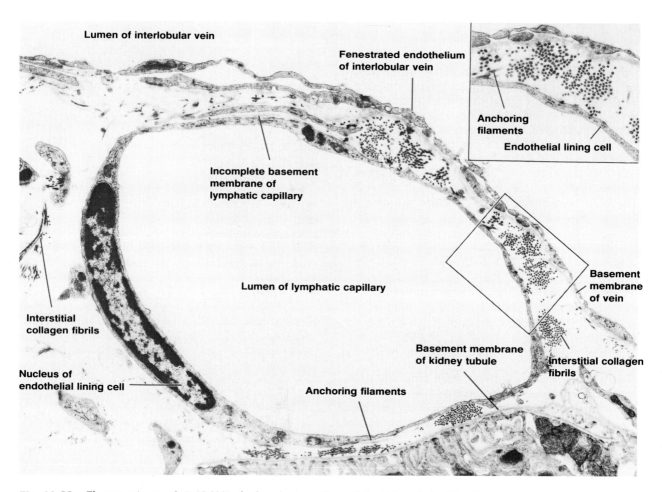

Fig. 16-28. Electron micrograph (×10,000) of a lymphatic capillary of the kidney (rat). Extending along the top and right-hand margins of the micrograph is the lumen of an interlobular vein, the endothelium of which is fenestrated. Unlike the basement membrane of the tubular epithelial cell (*lower right*) and vein (*right*), the basement membrane of the lymphatic capillary (seen above *center*) is only poorly developed. (*Inset*) Higher magnification (×20,000) of boxed-in area, showing anchoring filaments attached to an electron-dense area on the surface of the unfenestrated endothelial cell. These filaments attach the endothelial cell to the collagen fibrils that are seen here in the interstitial space, and they transmit tensile forces to the cell under conditions of edema. (Courtesy of C. C. C. O'Morchoe, P. J. O'Morchoe, and W. R. Jones)

(Fig. 16-28, *inset*). Their role seems to be that of holding these vessels open under conditions of edema, when hydrostatic pressure in the surrounding tissue would otherwise cause them to collapse.

Excess tissue fluid, including interstitial protein and any suspended particulate matter that may also be present, enters lymphatic capillaries through flap-valve–like slits, 15 nm to 20 nm wide, between the endothelial lining cells. It also enters as a result of transcellular channel-mediated or vesicular transport across their cytoplasm. The negative intraluminal hydrostatic pressure that draws tissue fluid into these capillaries is thought to be generated by contractile activity of the lymphatic capillaries themselves. This same activity—which is presumably a function of the endothelial lining cells—would also serve to start the lymph on its journey back to the bloodstream. For further information, see Johnston.

SELECTED REFERENCES

Impulse Conducting System of the Heart*

HERMAN L, STUCKEY JW, HOFFMAN BF: Electron microscopy of Purkinje fibers and ventricular muscle of dog heart. Circulation 24:954, 1961

RHODIN JAG, DELMISSIER P, REID LC: The structure of the specialized conducting system of the steer heart. Circulation 24:349, 1961

VIRÁGH S, CHALLICE CE: The impulse generation and conduction system of the heart. In Challice CE, Virágh S (eds): Ultrastructure of the Human Heart. New York, Academic Press, 1973

WELLENS HJJ, LIE KI, JANSE MJ (eds): The Conduction System of the

* References on Cardiac Muscle and Atrial Natriuretic Factor are listed under Selected References, Chap. 15.

Heart. Structure, Function and Clinical Implications. Leiden, Stenfert Kroese, 1976

Blood Vessels

BOSS J, GREEN JH: The histology of the common carotid baroceptor areas of the cat. Circ Res 4:12, 1956

CERVÓS-NAVARRO J, MATAKAS F (eds): The Cerebral Vessel Wall. New York, Raven Press, 1975

HAUST MD, MORE RH, BENCOSME SA, BALIS JU: Elastogenesis in human aorta: An electron microscope study. Exp Mol Pathol 4:508, 1965

JAFFÉ D, HARTROFT WS, MANNING M, ELETA G: Coronary arteries in newborn children. Acta Paediatr Scand (Suppl) 219:1, 1971

KEECH MK: Electron microscope study of the normal rat aorta. J Biophys Biochem Cytol 7:533, 1960

LINDSAY J, HURST JW (eds): The Aorta. New York, Grune & Stratton, 1979

PAULE WJ: Electron microscopy of the newborn rat aorta. J Ultrastruct Res 8:219, 1965

PEASE DC, MOLINARI S: Electron microsopy of muscular arteries: Pial vessels of the cat and monkey. J Ultrastruct Res 3:447, 1960

PEASE DC, PAULE WJ: Electron microscopy of elastic arteries: The thoracic aorta of the rat. J Ultrastruct Res 3:469, 1960

PRITCHARD MML, DANIEL PM: Arterio-venous anastomoses in the human external ear. J Anat 90:309, 1956

RHODIN JAG: Architecture of the vessel wall. In Bohr DF, Somlyo AP, Sparks HV (eds): Handbook of Physiology, Section 2: The Cardiovascular System, Vol II—Vascular Smooth Muscle, p 1. Bethesda, American Physiological Society, 1980

RHODIN JAG: Fine structure of the vascular wall in mammals. Physiol Rev (Suppl 5)42:48, 1962

RHODIN JAG: Fine structure of vascular walls in mammals with special reference to smooth muscle component. Physiol Rev 42(5):447, 1962

RYAN TJ: Structure and shape of blood vessels of skin. In Jarrett A (ed): The Physiology and Pathophysiology of the Skin. The Nerves and Blood Vessels. Vol 2. London, Academic Press, 1973

SIMIONESCU M, SIMIONESCU N, PALADE GE: Segmental differentiations of cell junctions in the vascular endothelium. Arteries and Veins. J Cell Biol 68:705, 1976

Atherosclerosis

BENDITT EP: The origin of atherosclerosis. Sci Am 236:74, February 1977

BENDITT EP, BENDITT JM: Evidence for a monoclonal origin of human atherosclerotic plaques. Proc Natl Acad Sci USA 70:1753, 1973

BROWN MS, GOLDSTEIN JL: How LDL receptors influence cholesterol and atherosclerosis. Sci Am 251, No 5:58, 1984

CAMPBELL GR, CAMPBELL JH: Smooth muscle phenotypic changes in arterial wall homeostasis: Implications for the pathogenesis of atherosclerosis. Exp Mol Pathol 42:139, 1985

GOTLIEB AI: Smooth muscle and endothelial cell function in the pathogenesis of atherosclerosis. Can Med Assoc J 126:903, 1982

MUSTARD JF, PACKHAM MA, KINLOUGH-RATHBONE RL: Platelets and atherosclerosis. In Miller NE (ed): Atherosclerosis: Mechanisms and Approach to Therapy, p 29. New York, Raven Press, 1983

PAOLETTI R, GOTTO AM JR (eds): Atherosclerosis Reviews. Vol. 1. New York, Raven Press, 1976

ROSS R: Atherosclerosis: A problem of the biology of arterial wall cells and their interactions with blood cell components. Arteriosclerosis 1:293, 1981

ROSS R: The pathogenesis of atherosclerosis—An update. N Engl J Med 314:488, 1986

ROSS R, GLOMSET JA: The pathogenesis of atherosclerosis. N Engl J Med 295:369 (Part I), 420 (Part II), 1976

Capillaries and Microcirculation

BAEZ S: Skeletal muscle and gastrointestinal microvascular morphology. In Kaley G, Altura BM (eds): Microcirculation. Vol 1, p 69. Baltimore, University Park Press, 1977

BEACHAM WS, KONISHI A, HUNT CC: Observations on the microcirculatory bed in rat mesocecum using differential interference contrast microscopy in vivo and electron microscopy. Am J Anat 146:385, 1976

FAWCETT DW: Comparative observations on the fine structure of blood capillaries. In The Peripheral Vessels, Internat Acad Pathol Monograph No 4, p 17. Baltimore, Williams & Wilkins, 1963

FERNANDO NVP, MOVAT HZ: The capillaries. Exp Mol Pathol 3:87, 1964

FERNANDO NVP, MOVAT HZ: The smallest arterial vessels: Terminal arterioles and metarterioles. Exp Mol Pathol 3:1, 1964

FRØKJAER-JENSEN J: The plasmalemmal vesicular system in striated muscle capillaries and in pericytes. Tissue Cell 16:31, 1984

KALEY G, ALTURA BM (eds): Microcirculation. Vols 1, 2, and 3. Baltimore, University Park Press, 1977 to 1978

MAJNO G, PALADE GE, SCHOEFL GI: Studies on inflammation. II. The site of action of histamine and serotonin along the vascular tree: A topographic study. J Biophys Biochem Cytol 11:607, 1961

MOVAT HZ, FERNANDO NVP: Small arteries with an internal elastic lamina. Exp Mol Pathol 2:549, 1963

MOVAT HZ, FERNANDO NVP: The venules and their perivascular cells. Exp Mol Pathol 3:98, 1964

PALADE GE: Blood capillaries of the heart and other organs. Circulation 24:368, 1961

RYAN US, RYAN JW, SMITH DS, WINKLER H: Fenestrated endothelium of the adrenal gland: Freeze-fracture studies. Tissue Cell 7:181, 1975

SIMIONESCU M, SIMIONESCU N, PALADE GE: Segmental differentiations of cell junctions in the vascular endothelium. The microvasculature. J Cell Biol 67:863, 1975

SOBIN SS, TREMER HM: Three-dimensional organizational organization of microvascular beds as related to function. In Kaley G, Altura BM (eds): Microcirculation. Vol 1, p 43. Baltimore, University Park Press, 1977

ZWEIFACH BW: Introduction: Perspectives in microcirculation. In Kaley G, Altura BM (eds): Microcirculation. Vol 1. Baltimore, University Park Press, 1977

Lymphatic System

ABRAMSON DI (ed): Blood Vessels and Lymphatics. New York, Academic Press, 1962

JOHNSTON MG (ed): Experimental Biology of the Lymphatic Circulation. Research Monographs in Cell and Tissue Physiology, Vol 9. Amsterdam, Elsevier, 1985

LEAK LV: Electron microscopic observations on lymphatic capillaries and the structural components of the connective tissue–lymph interface. Microvasc Res 2:391, 1970

17

The Integumentary System

The *skin* has a greater total mass than any other organ in the body. It is made up of two layers that are strongly attached to each other. Its outer layer, the *epidermis* (Gr. *epi,* upon), is composed of *stratified squamous keratinizing epithelium* derived from ectoderm. Because this layer is avascular, it has to be nourished by tissue fluid from the *dermis* (Gr. for skin), the second and deeper layer of the skin. The dermis is composed of vascularized and irregularly arranged fibroelastic *connective tissue* derived from mesenchyme.

The cells in the basal layer of the epidermis are able to proliferate throughout life. As their progeny cells become displaced farther and farther away from their source of nutrients in the dermis, these cells die and become transformed into a superficial layer of dead keratin. Based on the relative thickness of the keratin thereby formed, skin is classified as thick or thin. However, it should be pointed out that these terms refer to the *thickness of the epidermis* and not to the thickness of the skin as a whole.

Thick skin covers the palms of the hands and the soles of the feet; thin skin covers the remainder of the body. Thick skin is characterized by having a relatively *thick epidermis* (0.4 mm to 0.6 mm) that possesses a particularly thick layer of keratin (stratum corneum) on its outer surface (Fig. 17-1A). Even though the dermis of the skin that covers the remainder of the body is comparatively thick, especially at some sites (*e.g.,* 4 mm over the back), it has a relatively *thin epidermis* (75 μm to 150 μm) and the layer of keratin on its outer surface is rather thin (Fig. 17-1B).

The *subcutaneous tissue* (*hypodermis*) beneath the skin, also known as the *superficial fascia,* is composed of loose connective tissue with a variable and usually substantial proportion of adipose tissue (Fig. 17-1). Fibrous bands that are composed primarily of collagen anchor the deep layers of the dermis to underlying fibrous fascial sheets or periosteum, providing an arrangement that, in most parts of the body, permits a limited amount of free movement of the skin over the underlying tissues.

During development, epidermal cells grow down into the dermis to form sweat glands, hair follicles, sebaceous glands, and the epidermal grooves that produce the

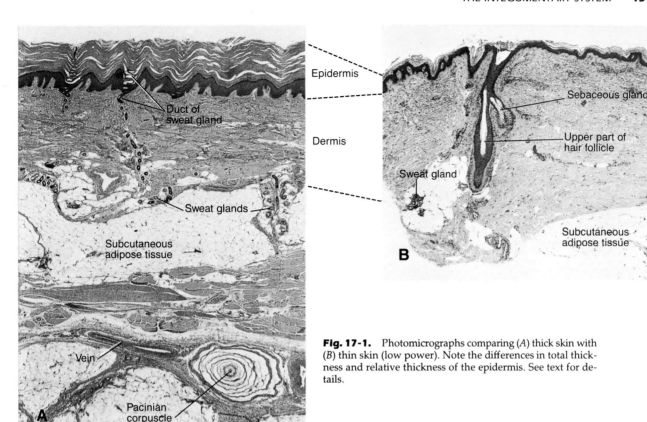

Fig. 17-1. Photomicrographs comparing (*A*) thick skin with (*B*) thin skin (low power). Note the differences in total thickness and relative thickness of the epidermis. See text for details.

fingernails and toenails. Hence our study of the integumentary system will include the *epidermal appendages*, namely, the sweat glands, hairs, sebaceous glands, and nails.

The Skin Has Many Important Functions. Primarily because of the layer of keratin on its outer surface, the epidermis constitutes an effective barrier against pathogenic organisms. Because this layer is almost waterproof, the body does not become dessicated in a dry atmosphere, nor does it imbibe water in the bath. However, the epidermis is not entirely impervious. Chemicals, for example, can be absorbed directly into the capillaries and lymphatics of the underlying dermis. Accordingly, care should be taken to prevent harmful chemicals from coming into direct contact with the epidermis. Furthermore, the epidermis contains cells that produce the pigment melanin, which can protect the body from the harmful effects of too much penetrating ultraviolet light.

The skin also has many other useful functions. It is of the greatest importance in the regulation of body temperature, and by sweating, the skin functions as an ancillary excretory organ. Vitamin D is made in skin that is exposed to ultraviolet light. Hence without vitamin D from other sources, babies kept shielded from sunshine can develop rickets. The skin contains afferent nerve endings that are sensitive to stimuli that evoke various types of sensation (touch, pressure, heat, cold, and pain). Hence, in many ways, the skin enables the body to adapt to its environment.

Medical students will appreciate the value of observing the skin as part of the patient's routine physical examination. Without resorting to exploratory procedures, the skin's appearance can reflect the existence of general disease just as accurately as that of the internal organs. Furthermore, its appearance gives the physician a general indication of the accuracy of the patient's verbal declaration of his or her age. The color and texture of the skin can indicate a variety of conditions: it becomes yellow in jaundice, bronzed in certain glandular deficiencies, dry and hard in others, and warm and moist in still others. Babies who are allowed to consume voluminous quantities of vegetable juices can turn a rather vivid orange-yellow color (carotenemia). Cyanosis can give the skin a blue-gray appearance, which reflects generalized impairment of circulatory or respiratory functions. In vitamin A deficiencies, the skin of extensor surfaces may lose its hair and become rough, like sandpaper. In certain other vitamin deficiencies, the skin around the corners of the mouth may become cracked and scaly. Many infectious diseases that affect the whole body produce characteristic rashes or other kinds of lesions on the skin (*e.g.*, scarlet fever, measles, chickenpox, syphilis,

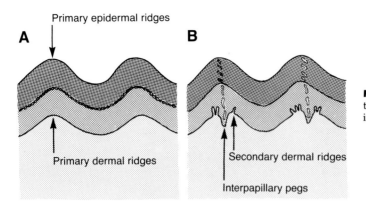

A Primary epidermal ridges

B

Primary dermal ridges

Secondary dermal ridges

Interpapillary pegs

Fig. 17-2. Diagrammatic representations of the ridges on thick skin. The actual arrangement of these ridges, depicted in *B*, is shown in simplified form in *A*.

and others). The skin can also manifest certain kinds of hypersensitivity reactions; for example, some women develop rashes from certain kinds of makeup. In addition to involvement of the skin in conditions and diseases of fairly general character, there is a whole host of skin diseases proper.

Because the skin is the most exposed part of the body, it is very susceptible to various kinds of injuries. The treatment of cuts, abrasions, and burns is part of routine medical and paramedical practice. Skin is often destroyed in accidents, and it is fortunate that it can be readily grafted from one part of the body to another.

THICK SKIN

The palms of the hands (including the fingers) and the soles of the feet (including the toes) are covered with ridges and grooves that develop during the third and fourth months of prenatal development. Distinctive for each individual, this so-called *dermatoglyphic pattern* is determined chiefly by hereditary factors. However, it can be greatly modified by any growth disturbances occurring in the fetus during the prenatal period. This becomes strikingly evident in babies born with Down syndrome (described under Chromosomal Anomalies in Chap. 3). Some 70% of such babies exhibit unusual combinations of ridge patterns and flexion creases; hence observation of the dermatoglyphic patterns of newborn babies can provide useful information regarding the occurrence of this anomaly.

Under each *primary epidermal ridge* that can be seen on the surface of thick skin even with the unaided eye, there is a corresponding *primary dermal ridge* (Fig. 17-2A). However, every primary dermal ridge is subdivided into two *secondary dermal ridges* as a result of downgrowth of the epidermis along its crest (Fig. 17-2B). Furthermore, projecting from the top of each secondary dermal ridge, there are several rows of relatively tall conical projections, up to 0.2 mm high, that are known as *dermal papillae* (Figs. 17-3A and 17-4). The central epidermal downgrowth that separates the two secondary dermal ridges is called an *in-*

terpapillary peg (Figs. 17-2B and 17-3A) even though in three dimensions it is a tapered partition and not a conical structure (Fig. 17-3A).

Much of the following description of the epidermis of thick skin applies to that of thin skin also.

Epidermis

In approaching a study of the epidermis, it is important to appreciate that the keratin that constitutes the outer layer of this component is not a cellular secretion but the end result of *transformation* of ectoderm-derived epithelial cells known as *keratinocytes* into *squames* (scales) of keratin. When these scales are worn away or desquamate from the surface, they can be replaced only by keratinization of the underlying living cells, and this means that there must be as much cellular proliferation in the deepest layers of the epidermis as there is loss of keratinized cells from its surface. It takes approximately 2 weeks for keratinocytes to move from the basal layer (stratum germinativum) to the cornified layer (stratum corneum), after which they remain in the stratum corneum for approximately 2 weeks more, giving a total transit time of approximately 1 month. Because the appearance of keratinocytes changes as they become displaced from the bottom to the top of the epidermis, this epithelial component of the skin has the microscopic appearance of being composed of five different layers, each of which will be described below.

Stratum Germinativum. The deepest epidermal layer, which is attached to the underlying prominent basement membrane by hemidesmosomes (see Fig. 6-14), is made up of low columnar cells and is known as the *stratum germinativum* (Fig. 17-4) because it generates new cells. Hence new keratinocytes are displaced from this layer into the layer above it.

In the electron microscope (EM), it can be seen that the cells in this basal layer (labeled *ger* in Fig. 17-5A) have a considerable content of free ribosomes and polysomes, together with substantial numbers of intermediate filaments of the prekeratin type (*pk* in Fig. 17-5A). Known also as

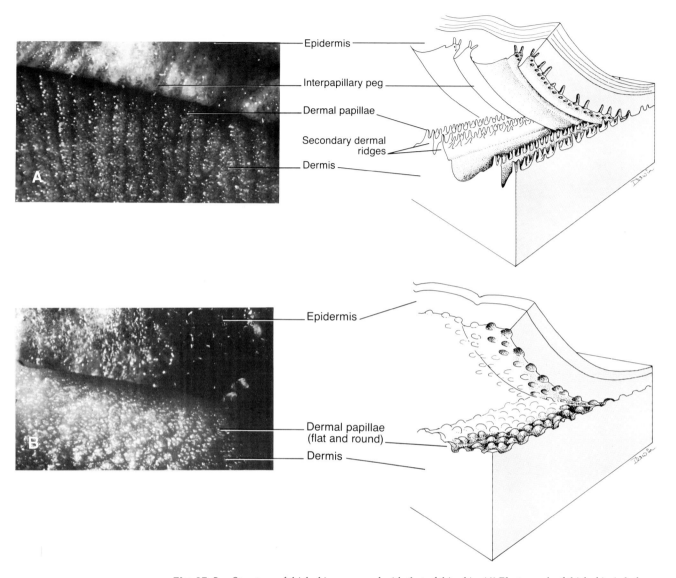

Epidermis

Interpapillary peg

Dermal papillae

Secondary dermal ridges

Dermis

Epidermis

Dermal papillae (flat and round)

Dermis

Fig. 17-3. Structure of thick skin compared with that of thin skin. (*A*) Photograph of thick skin (whole preparation) with its epidermis peeled away to expose its dermal ridges and papillae, together with interpretive drawing. (*B*) Identical preparation of thin skin, with interpretive drawing.

tonofilaments, these filaments are destined to become part of the keratin. By the time the cells reach the next layer, bundles of prekeratin filaments have become wide enough to be seen in the light microscope (LM). These bundles were originally termed *tonofibrils,* and they account for the second epidermal layer being called the *prickle cell layer* or *stratum spinosum.*

Stratum Spinosum.   The cells of this second layer are polyhedral, and, as may be seen in Figure 17-5*B,* in LM sections their borders appear to be separated from one another by small spaces that are traversed by fine spinelike processes; this gives the cells the prickly appearance from

which the name of the layer was derived. With the EM, it can be seen that each of these spinelike processes represents a site where a *desmosome* holds the contiguous cell membranes together, and that the typically scalloped contour of each cell can be attributed to shrinkage artifact (Fig. 17-5*A* and *C*). As described under Adhering Junctions in Chapter 6, bundles of tonofilaments (prekeratin filaments) that are anchored to the plaques of desmosomes (see Fig. 6-10, second from *bottom,* and Fig. 6-13) distribute tensile forces from one cell to the next and thereby enable epidermal cells to withstand fairly rough treatment. As noted, these filament bundles can be discerned as tonofibrils in the LM (Fig. 17-5*B*).

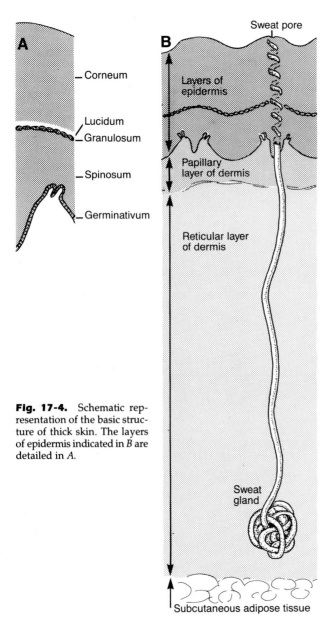

Fig. 17-4. Schematic representation of the basic structure of thick skin. The layers of epidermis indicated in *B* are detailed in *A*.

In the upper levels of the stratum spinosum, lipid-containing granules with a laminated internal structure (*lamellar granules*) are formed. The contents of these granules are extruded into the intercellular space as the cells pass through the next layer.

Stratum Granulosum. In thick skin, this layer (labeled *gr* in Fig. 17-5A) is from two to four cells thick. It lies immediately superficial to the stratum spinosum (Fig. 17-4A). Its flat diamond-shaped cells are characterized by the presence of granules that stain deeply with hematoxylin (see Fig. 17-9); these are called *keratohyalin* granules. In the EM, such granules appear as stellate or angular electron-dense masses (*khg* in Fig. 17-5A).

Stratum Lucidum. This fourth layer is not always seen to advantage. When discernible, it is thin and appears as a clear, bright, homogeneous line (Fig. 17-4A). For this reason, it is called the *stratum lucidum*. Its closely packed flattened cells are dead, and their nuclei are well on the way to disappearing through karyolysis. These cells are now little more than a cell membrane containing prekeratin filaments complexed with amorphous protein.

Stratum Corneum. The fifth and final layer, which is from 15 to 20 cells thick, is known as the *stratum corneum*. It represents the superficial layer of keratin (Figs. 17-4 and 17-5A, labeled *cor*). Here the nuclei and cytoplasmic organelles disappear, but the desmosomes connecting the keratinized squames (formerly living cells) can still be distinguished in the EM. The keratohyalin granules transform into an amorphous matrix in which the prekeratin filaments become embedded. In this manner, each cell is transformed into one of the squames of keratin, 30 μm to 40 μm in diameter, that constitute the stratum corneum. Between the lowermost constituent layers of the stratum corneum, there are layers of extracellular lipid that are thought to be derived from the lamellar granules of keratinocytes. For further information about the keratin complex, see Fraser and MacRae.

It has recently become evident that the hexagonal squames of the stratum corneum of mouse skin are arranged in vertical stacks (Figs. 17-6 and 17-7). Each squame has the shape of a flattened tetrakaidecahedron that interlocks with neighboring squames as shown in Figure 17-7 (Menton). This arrangement helps to render the keratin layer comparatively impervious to exogenous substances. It also represents the most efficient way in which to pack solid shapes together without wasting any space. To some extent, this distinctive organization reflects the way in which new keratinocytes are generated in the basal layer of the epidermis, a matter that is described in the following section.

The Columnar Arrangement of Keratinizing Cells Reflects Functional Grouping of the Cells in the Basal Layer. The pattern of proliferation and differentiation in the epidermis is far from random. From studies in the mouse, it is now known that the epidermal keratinocytes are derived from groups of 10 to 11 basal epidermal cells that constitute the basal compartment of what is termed an *epidermal proliferative unit* or EPU (Potten). Each EPU seems to contain one stem cell that occupies a more or less central position in the basal layer of the unit. As progeny cells in the basal layer begin to differentiate, they are laterally displaced to the periphery of the EPU. Continuing proliferation eventually results in the ejection of such cells into the overlying layer, where they continue to mature and gradually flatten so that they eventually cover the area occupied by the EPU. Studies in mice indicate that the rate at which the maturing postmitotic cells move up the EPU from its basal layer is approximately one cell per day. Most of the cellular proliferation occurs in the basal layer of the epidermis (*i.e.,* the stratum germinativum), but in human skin, mitotic fig-

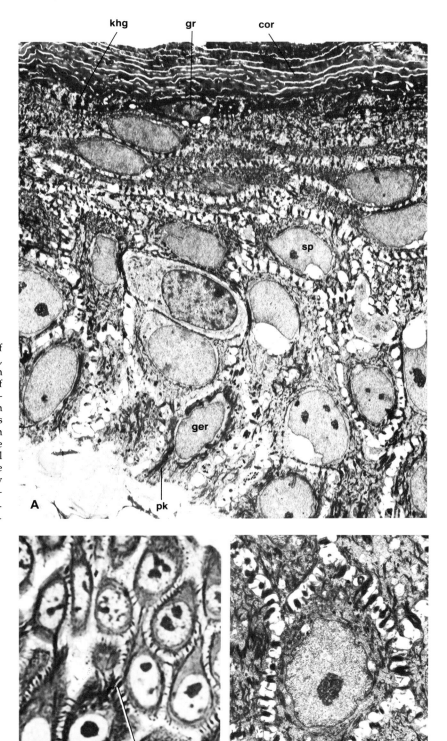

Fig. 17-5. (*A*) Electron micrograph of epidermis of thin skin (human skin biopsy), showing cells of the stratum germinativum (*ger*) with prekeratin filaments (*pk*), cells of the stratum spinosum (*sp*) with interconnecting desmosomes, cells of the stratum granulosum (*gr*) with keratohyalin granules (*khg*), and keratin squames of the stratum corneum (*cor*). (*B* and *C*) Prickle cells of the stratum spinosum, seen (*B*) in the LM (oil immersion) and (*C*) in the EM. The spinelike processes of these cells indicate where they are joined by desmosomes, and the intervening spaces represent shrinkage artifact. (*A*, courtesy of P. Lea; *C*, courtesy of A. Chalvardjian)

Tonofibrils (tonofilament bundles) anchored to desmosome

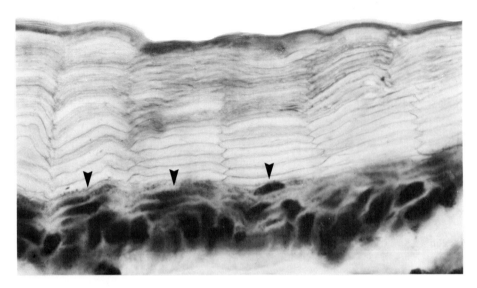

Fig. 17-6. Photomicrograph of thin skin (ear of mouse). This is a frozen section stained with methylene blue after alkali treatment to swell the cells. Note the stacking of the cells, which is particularly evident in the pale-staining stratum corneum. Arrowheads indicate the most superficial nucleated cell in each vertical column. The cells in each column interlock with those in adjacent columns. (Menton DN: Am J Anat 145:1, 1976)

ures are also occasionally observed in the suprabasal layers, indicating that at least some of the cells that enter these layers are still capable of mitosis.

Psoriasis Is a Manifestation of Accelerated Keratinocyte Turnover. The chronic skin condition *psoriasis*, which is characterized by clearly demarcated red-to-brown areas of skin with superficial fine silvery scales, is primarily due to excessive epidermal proliferation. This condition seems to stem from accelerated and presumably misregulated turnover of the epidermal keratinocytes. Whereas in normal epidermis the transit time for cell displacement from the stratum germinativum to the outer surface of the skin is approximately 4 weeks, in cases of psoriasis it is only approximately 1 week. This seems to be because proliferation occurs in the bottom three layers of the epidermis instead of being largely confined to the stratum germinativum. Also, the intercellular spaces in psoriatic epidermis remain unusually wide, presumably because there is insufficient time to allow full maturation of its keratinocytes.

Dermis

The dermis is made up of two layers of connective tissue that merge with each other. The outer layer, which is by far the thinner of the two, is composed of loose connective tissue. It is called the *papillary layer* because it is represented primarily by the connective tissue papillae that project up into the epidermis (Fig. 17-4B). This layer extends for a short distance below the papillae and then merges with the thicker *reticular layer*, which consists of dense, irregularly arranged connective tissue and comprises the remainder of the dermis (Fig. 17-4B). This second layer is called the reticular layer of the dermis because it is composed of thick bundles of collagen fibers that interlace with

one another in a netlike manner. Most of the dermal collagen is type I collagen; approximately 15% of it is type III collagen.

Whereas fine elastic fibers are arranged as a network in the papillary layer, coarser elastic fibers are randomly distributed in the reticular layer. The elastin content of the dermis, however, is relatively low.

The papillary layer also differs from the reticular layer in the number of capillaries it contains. The relatively abundant capillaries in the papillary layer extend up into its papillae and provide nourishment for the epidermis. In the reticular layer, capillaries are not numerous except in association with epidermal appendages that extend down into the reticular layer.

Most of the cells in the dermis of thick skin are fibrocytes, and these are sparingly distributed. A few macrophages are also present. In addition, there are generally some adipocytes.

Eccrine Sweat Glands

Eccrine sweat glands are the type of sweat gland commonly found in man. They are simple tubular glands that are distributed over the body except in a very few sites (lips and certain parts of external genitalia of both males and females). It has been estimated that there are approximately 3 million of them in the skin. They are particularly numerous in thick skin (it has been estimated that there are 3000 per square inch in the palm of the hand). Each consists of a secretory part and an excretory duct. The secretory part of most eccrine sweat glands is situated immediately below the dermis *in the subcutaneous tissue* (Fig. 17-1A). The secretory part of the tubule is coiled on itself; hence in sections, it appears as a little cluster of tubes cut in cross

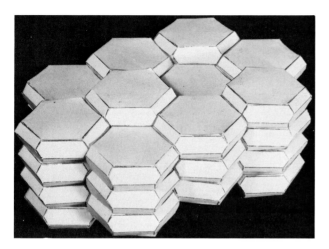

Fig. 17-7. Photograph of model illustrating the cells of stratum corneum packed together in interlocking columns, each cell having the shape of a flattened tetrakaidecahedron. (Menton DN: J Invest Dermatol 57:925, 1971)

epidermis constitute the walls of the duct. After pursuing a markedly helical course through the epidermis, the duct of an eccrine sweat gland opens at a *sweat pore* on the crest of an epidermal ridge.

Sweat contains sodium, potassium, and chloride ions; water; and certain metabolites and nitrogenous waste substances. Some sodium chloride is resorbed as the secretion passes along the duct. Such sodium resorption is increased by the steroid hormone *aldosterone*, which is produced by the outermost zone of the adrenal cortex.

The autonomic regulation of sweat secretion and the role of sweating in the regulation of body temperature will be considered after we have dealt with the blood supply of the skin.

THIN SKIN

Thin skin covers all parts of the body except for the palms of the hands and the soles of the feet. It will be recalled

and oblique section (Fig. 17-8). The secretory cells are of two types. Most are cuboidal or columnar and have pale cytoplasm containing some glycogen. These cells are wider at their base than at their luminal surface. Canaliculi between cells of this type convey sweat to the lumen. Cells of the second type are commonly narrower at their base than at their luminal surface. Their cytoplasm contains granules that stain darkly enough for them to be described as *dark cells,* which distinguishes them from the *clear cells* just described.

The luminal diameter of the *secretory portion* of a sweat gland is roughly equal to the thickness of its walls. Spindle-shaped myoepithelial cells, which resemble smooth muscle cells but are derived from ectoderm, are wrapped around this secretory portion on the inner aspect of its basement membrane. It is widely assumed that, at least under certain circumstances, contraction of these cells assists in expelling sweat. The connective tissue that immediately surrounds the basement membrane of the secretory portion of the gland is condensed so as to form a supporting sheath.

From the secretory portion of the gland, the *duct* ascends to the skin surface. Here it should be pointed out that, *in a sweat gland, the duct cells stain more deeply than the secretory cells.* This is mainly because the duct possesses *two layers* of lining cells that are noticeably smaller than those of the secretory portion. Hence compared with the secretory portion, the duct has more nuclei in its walls to take up stain, and it is more prominent in sections because it stains more darkly (Fig. 17-8). Also, the lumen of the duct is *narrower* than that of the secretory portion. This is unusual because, in most glands, the luminal diameter of ducts exceeds that of secretory units. The duct follows a slightly helical path through the dermis and enters an interpapillary peg (Fig. 17-4*B*). From this point on, keratinocytes of the

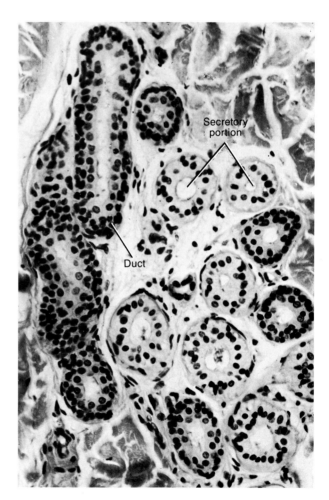

Fig. 17-8. Photomicrograph of an eccrine sweat gland, showing the distinction between its secretory portion and duct.

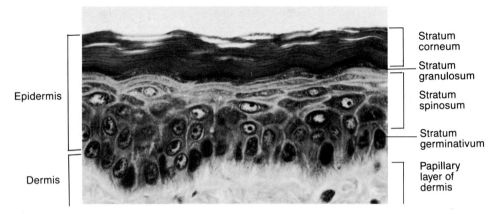

Epidermis

Dermis

Stratum corneum

Stratum granulosum

Stratum spinosum

Stratum germinativum

Papillary layer of dermis

Fig. 17-9.   Photomicrograph showing the layers of the epidermis of thin skin (ear of monkey).

that "thick" and "thin" apply to the epidermis only and not to the skin as a whole. Actually, thin skin varies greatly in thickness in different parts of the body. These variations are due almost entirely to variation in the thickness of the dermis. The skin covering extensor surfaces is usually thicker than that covering flexor surfaces. The skin covering the eyelid is the thinnest in the body and that covering the back is the thickest.

Thin skin contains sweat glands (Fig. 17-1B), but they are less numerous than in thick skin. Thin skin differs from thick skin in that it contains *hair follicles*. These structures are highly developed in the scalp and certain other regions but are also present in thin skin over most of the body surface.

The external surface of thin skin lacks the pattern of ridges and grooves seen on thick skin. Also, the epidermis exhibits fewer layers than thick skin (Fig. 17-9). The stratum germinativum is similar to that of thick skin, but the stratum spinosum is thinner. The stratum granulosum (Fig. 17-9) may be represented only by a discontinuous layer. No stratum lucidum is present, and the stratum corneum is relatively thin (Fig. 17-9).

The superficial surface of the dermis of thin skin (*i.e.*, the aspect presented to the epidermis) is considerably different from that of thick skin. The dermal papillae that nourish the epidermis are lower, broader, and fewer in number than in thick skin (compare Figs. 17-3B and 17-3A), and there are no external signs of where these papillae lie. The pattern of tiny creases that can be seen on the surface of thin skin does not indicate the position of underlying dermal papillae; it is more closely related to the position of hair follicles. In most other respects, the dermis of thin skin is similar to that of thick skin except that it is thicker.

Before we discuss the other skin appendages that are associated with thin skin (namely hairs, sebaceous glands, apocrine sweat glands, and nails), it is necessary to consider two other important cell types that are also constituents of

the epidermis. In addition to the *keratinocytes* mentioned previously, there are *melanocytes*, which are cells of neural crest origin that produce the skin pigment melanin, and *Langerhans cells*, which are cells of myeloid origin that are now known to be involved in cutaneous immune responses. These two cell types are of sufficient medical importance to warrant a more detailed description. Specialized epidermal cells of a fourth type, known as *Merkel cells*, are individually supplied with afferent nerve endings and will be described in connection with cutaneous sensory receptors at the end of this chapter.

PIGMENTATION OF SKIN

The important endogenous pigment of the skin is *melanin* (Gr. *melas*, black). In white races, melanin occurs chiefly in the basal layers of the epidermis (Fig. 17-10). The relative content of melanin in the epidermis accounts for different skin colors in the various races of man (black, brown, yellow, or white). People of all races, however, normally have *some* melanin in their skin. An inherent incapacity of any individual (regardless of race) to produce melanin is manifested as the *albino* condition (L. *albus*, white). Increased amounts of melanin are produced in the epidermis as a response to exposure to ultraviolet light. It is this component of sunlight that causes a suntan to develop. Brunettes generally tan more readily than blondes. In some people, however, the epidermal melanin tends to be distributed in little patches (freckles).

The cells that produce melanin are dendritic cells called *melanocytes*. Precursor cells that are destined to become melanocytes arise from neural crest and migrate during prenatal life to the epidermal–dermal border. Here they assume a position at or in the basal layer of the epidermis and differentiate into melanocytes. The cell bodies of melanocytes lie either just below or between the cells of the stratum germinativum (see Fig. 17-12). In either position,

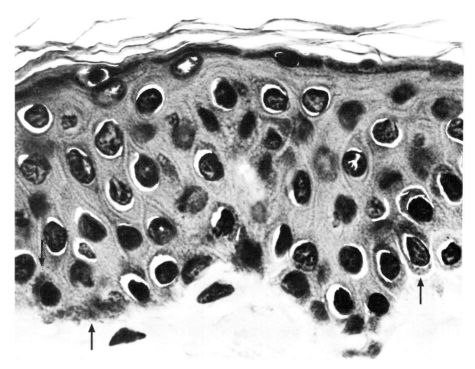

Fig. 17-10. Photomicrograph of thin skin showing melanin (*arrows*) in the stratum germinativum.

they extend long dendritic processes between or under the epidermal keratinocytes, primarily those of the basal layer (Fig. 17-11). Melanin synthesized by melanocytes can apparently be transferred directly to keratinocytes as a result of phagocytosis of the tips of melanocyte processes. By this means, the keratinocytes in the basal layer also come to acquire melanin pigment. The ability of melanocytes to produce melanin depends on their ability to synthesize the enzyme *tyrosinase*.

If dihydroxyphenylalanine, which is more commonly known as *dopa*, is added to a suitable epidermal preparation, the tyrosinase within melanocytes converts the dopa into melanin that thereupon becomes visible in the cytoplasm as dark pigment. Known as the *dopa reaction*, this test is useful for distinguishing between cells that have the ability to *make* melanin and cells that merely *take up* this pigment. In life, the tyrosinase in melanocytes is also thought to be utilized for producing dopa from tyrosine.

The tyrosinase is synthesized in the rather minimal rough-surfaced endoplasmic reticulum (rER) of the cell and then is transferred to Golgi saccules where it is packaged in membranous vesicles known as *premelanosomes*. Active tyrosinase now appears in the content of the vesicles and melanin is synthesized, at which stage the vesicles become known as *melanosomes*. These are ovoid membrane-bounded granules with a length of up to 0.7 μm (Fig. 17-12). Before melanin deposition obscures everything in these granules, they exhibit a lamellar or gridlike filamentous internal structure that is characterized by a distinctive periodicity. Any type of melanin-containing particle that can be recognized in the LM is described as a *melanin granule*.

A melanocyte and the group of keratinocytes that it pro-

vides with melanin are sometimes collectively described as an *epidermal melanin unit*. The melanosomes in these keratinocytes either remain widely dispersed as discrete structures or become aggregated into membrane-bounded *me-*

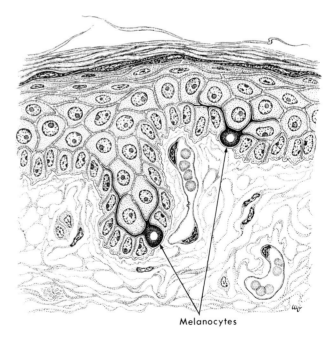

Melanocytes

Fig. 17-11. Diagrammatic representation of melanocytes in the stratum germinativum of thin skin, showing how their branched processes ramify between keratinocytes to supply them with melanin.

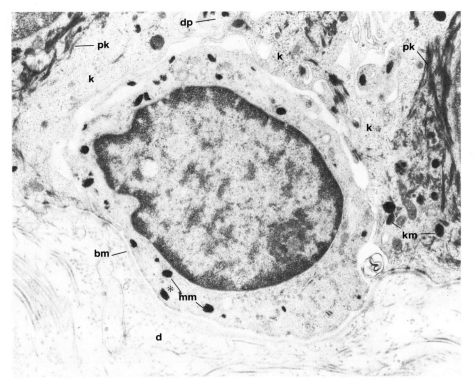

Fig. 17-12. Electron micrograph of a melanocyte (human skin biopsy). This cell is bordered laterally and superficially by keratinocytes (*k*), and beneath it there is part of the superficial region of the underlying dermis (*d*). Extending along the epidermal–dermal border is a prominent basement membrane (*bm*). Melanosomes (*mm*) are synthesized by melanocytes and then are taken up by keratinocytes (*km*). Their characteristic ovoid shape and limiting membrane can be seen at the asterisk. The long electron-dense structures at right and top left are bundles of prekeratin filaments (*pk*). A dendritic process of the melanocyte (*dp*) is seen at top center. (Courtesy of P. Lea)

lanosome complexes, particularly if the melanosomes are rather small. Acid phosphatase activity is sometimes detectable in association with the two or three melanosomes that are present in each complex, and these melanosomes may also show signs of degeneration, indicating that melanosome complexes may represent residual bodies that result from lysosomal degradation. Whereas in the white (Caucasian) and the Mongol races, melanosome complexes predominate in epidermal keratinocytes, in black (Negroid) races, and also in all kinds of black hair, the melanosomes are generally somewhat larger, more numerous, and more heavily melanized, and they show a greater tendency to remain dispersed as discrete structures in the cytoplasm. Furthermore, in Negroids melanosomes are distributed throughout the epidermis (even the stratum corneum) whereas in nonexposed skin of Caucasians they are confined to the stratum germinativum and, to a minor extent, to the first layer of keratinocytes above this. Finally, although the number of melanocytes per unit area of the skin may show an almost threefold variation from one part of the body to another, there is no significant variation between corresponding regions in individuals of light- and dark-skinned races.

Epidermal Melanin Protects the Body from Ultraviolet Light. In man the most important role of epidermal melanin is to protect the cells in the deepest layers of the epidermis and underlying dermis from the harmful effects of

excessive ultraviolet light by scattering it. When a person becomes suntanned, an increased amount of melanin is produced by melanocytes for this purpose. The effect of ultraviolet light on the skin is beneficial to some extent, because it irradiates ergosterol (a cholesterol derivative) and thereby produces a form of vitamin D. However, now there is a great deal of clinical and epidemiological evidence that overexposure to ultraviolet light, particularly between wavelengths of 280 nm and 320 nm, is closely associated with the development of epithelial skin cancers. Experimental studies have shown that ultraviolet light can damage DNA in many different ways and can act both as a carcinogen and as a mutagen. In addition to acting as an initiator of skin cancer, this form of radiation can act as a tumor promoter, causing the effects of a carcinogen to be manifested as a malignancy.

Melanin-Containing Cells Can Also Be Present in the Dermis. Only a few melanin-containing cells are normally present in the dermis. With one exception, they represent cells that have phagocytosed melanin instead of producing it. The one exception is infants of the Mongol race, in whom melanocytes can be present in the deep dermis of the sacral region. Seen through the overlying tissues, the melanin in these cells can appear bluish-gray. Such a bluish-gray to brown area over the sacral region is called a *mongolian spot.* Melanocytes are rarely evident in this position in children of other races.

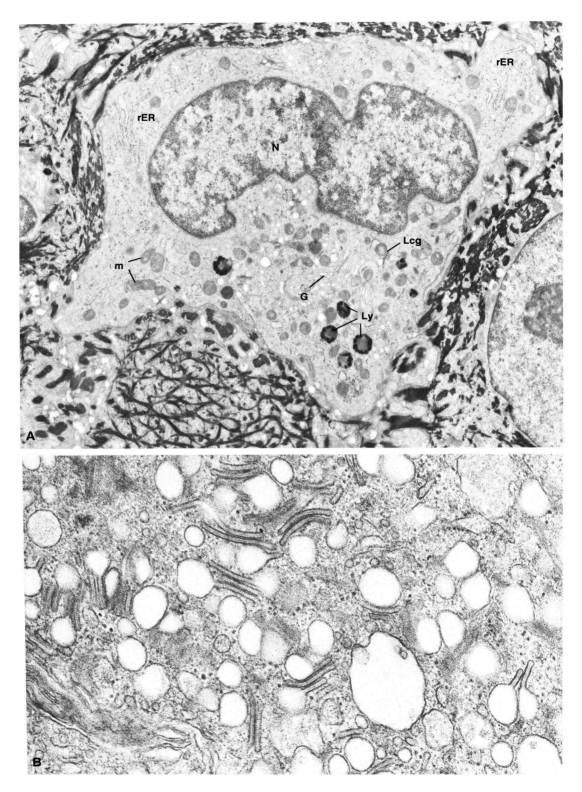

Fig. 17-13. (*A*) Electron micrograph (×9000) of a Langerhans cell of adult epidermis. The cell has an irregularly shaped nucleus (*N*). Its cytoplasm contains characteristic Langerhans cell granules (*Lcg*) that are particularly abundant in the region of the Golgi complex (*G*). Secondary lysosomes (*Ly*), a moderate number of mitochondria (*m*), and small patches of rough-surfaced endoplasmic reticulum (*rER*) are also discernible in the cytoplasm. Dark-staining bundles of prekeratin filaments are seen in the surrounding keratinocytes. (*B*) Electron micrograph (×50,000) of some representative Langerhans cell granules. For a description, see text. (*A,* Holbrook KA: Structure and development of the skin. In Soter NA, Baden HP: Pathophysiology of Dermatologic Diseases. New York, McGraw-Hill, 1984; *B,* courtesy of K. A. Holbrook)

IMMUNE RESPONSES IN SKIN

Langerhans cells are another type of dendritic cell that have a somewhat irregular shape (Fig. 17-13A). They are insinuated between keratinocytes but are not joined to them by cell junctions. In the EM, Langerhans cells can readily be distinguished from keratinocytes by their obvious lack of prekeratin filament bundles (Fig. 17-13A). Also, their nucleus generally exhibits irregular indentations (Fig. 17-13A). Their cytoplasm contains a prominent Golgi complex without very much rER; secondary lysosomes and a moderate number of mitochondria are also present (Fig. 17-13A). The most distinctive feature of their cytoplasm, however, is the presence of unique granules variously known as *Langerhans cell granules* or *Birbeck granules*, which are particularly abundant in the vicinity of the Golgi complex in Figure 17-13A. Most of these are cupped disk-shaped structures that exhibit a central linear density when cut in certain planes of section (Fig. 17-13B). Furthermore, the central linear density (visible in the granules *above* and *below center* in Fig. 17-13B) can exhibit a zipper-like pattern of periodic striations that is suggestive of a latticework of intragranular particles. Also, many of these granules have the two-dimensional appearance of a tennis racket because of the presence of a vesicular expansion of their limiting membrane at one end of the linear density (Fig. 17-13B). Despite the extraordinary appearance of these curious structures, neither their origin nor their functional significance is clear. Nevertheless, the functional role of Langerhans cells has recently been established, as described in the following section.

Langerhans Cells Are the Antigen-Presenting Cells That Promote Cutaneous Delayed Hypersensitivity Reactions. Present evidence indicates that immature Langerhans cells or their marrow-derived precursors arrive by way of dermal blood vessels and then invade the epidermis. Most Langerhans cells become situated in the stratum germinativum, where some have been found to come into close apposition with small lymphocytes. They possess surface Fc receptors (for IgG) and C3 receptors, which also characterize the monocyte–macrophage lineage (together with many—but not all—lymphocyte lineages). In addition, they are positive for T6 (OKT6), which is a surface antigen expressed by immature T-lymphocytes during their intrathymic differentiation but that is not expressed by postthymic T-lymphocytes (Edelson and Fink). At present it is not known whether this implies that Langerhans cells produce or strongly absorb this antigen. Like other types of antigen-presenting cells, Langerhans cells also express HLA class II histocompatibility antigens on their surface. Their role seems to be to serve as antigen-presenting cells in the initiation of *cutaneous contact hypersensitivity reactions* (i.e., contact allergic dermatitis).

Langerhans cells (or immature forms of these cells) are believed to be motile because in addition to being present in the epidermis, they are found in wet stratified squamous epithelia such as those lining the oral cavity, esophagus, vagina, and rectum. Furthermore, they are found in the local lymph nodes that drain areas of cutaneous application of allergens or sites of intradermal injection of such antigens.

Some exciting new findings indicate that cutaneous responses to antigens may also involve a second type of antigen-presenting cell and keratinocytes as well. This second type of antigen-presenting cell is believed to present antigen to T-suppressor cells whereas Langerhans cells present it to T-helper cells (these two subsets of T-lymphocytes are described in Chap. 10). The chief role of the keratinocytes in promoting cutaneous immune responses seems to be that, like macrophages, they produce IL-1, which in turn stimulates T-lymphocytes to release IL-2, the interleukin that causes T-lymphocytes to proliferate (see Chap. 10 under B-Lymphocytes and Their Involvement in the Humoral Antibody Response and also under Lymphokines). Keratinocytes are also suspected of bringing about postthymic functional maturation of skin-localizing T-lymphocytes. Evidence for this hypothesis comes from a recent finding that the cells of the stratum germinativum contain a cytoplasmic constituent that is antigenically similar to thymopoietin, a thymic hormone that promotes T-cell differentiation (see Chap. 10 under Thymic Hormones). For a fascinating account of this recently elucidated role of the skin, see Edelson and Fink.

HAIR

Hair follicles develop during the third month of gestation as downgrowths of the epidermis into the dermis and subcutaneous tissue. By the fifth or sixth month, the fetus becomes covered with very delicate hairs that are described as *lanugo* (L. *lana*, wool). This hair is shed before birth except in the region of the eyebrows, eyelids, and scalp, where the hairs persist and become somewhat stronger. A few months after birth, these hairs are shed and replaced by slightly thicker ones, whereas over the remainder of the body a new growth of hair occurs, and the body of the infant becomes covered with a downy coat called *vellus* (L. for fleece). No hair follicles are formed after birth. Because of the influence of male sex hormone at puberty, coarse hairs develop in the axillary and pubic regions and, in males, also on the face and (to a variable extent) other parts of the body. The coarse hairs of the scalp and the eyebrows and those that develop at puberty are termed *terminal hairs* to distinguish them from vellus. Approximately 95% of the body hair on men is terminal hair and about 65% of the body hair on women is vellus.

There are two different forms of keratin that are present in hair follicles. *Soft keratin* can be distinguished from *hard keratin* by its microscopic appearance as well as by its physical and chemical properties. Chemically, hard keratin is relatively unreactive and contains more cystine and disulfide bonds than soft keratin does. Whereas soft keratin covers the skin as a whole, hard keratin exists only in the cortex and cuticle of hairs and in the nail plates of fingers and toes. The formation of hard keratin involves a steady transition from living epidermal cells to keratin without the formation of keratohyalin granules. Hard keratin is solid and does not desquamate; hence it is more permanent than soft keratin.

Hair Follicles.   The deepest part of a developing hair follicle gives rise to an important group of cells called the hair *matrix* (Fig. 17-14). This matrix fits over a tiny connective tissue *papilla* (Fig. 17-14) containing capillaries that serve as a source of tissue fluid.

The part of the epidermal downgrowth that connects the matrix with the surface becomes canalized and thereafter is called the *external root sheath* of the hair follicle (Figs. 17-14 and 17-15). Near the surface of the skin, the external root sheath exhibits all the layers seen in the epidermis of thin skin (Fig. 17-14, *top*). The external root sheath near the surface of the skin is therefore lined with soft keratin that is continuous at the follicle orifice with the soft keratin of the epidermis (Fig. 17-14). Deep down in the follicle, the external root sheath becomes thinner and does not exhibit some of the more superficial layers of the epidermis. At the bottom of the follicle, where the external root sheath surrounds and becomes continuous with the matrix, the external root sheath consists of only the *stratum germinativum* (Fig. 17-14). Investing the external root sheath, there is also a *connective tissue sheath* (Figs. 17-14 and 17-15).

Growth of hair in a follicle is due to proliferation of the cells in the hair matrix. As the uppermost cells in the matrix become displaced farther away from the papilla, they become transformed into keratin. The cells that give rise to the cortex and cuticle of the hair, which are made of hard keratin, do so without forming keratohyalin granules. The cellular region where the transition from cells to hard keratin occurs is called the *keratogenous zone* (Fig. 17-14). Hairs grow because of continuing proliferation of matrix cells and continuing conversion of their progeny into keratin.

The proliferating matrix cells also produce another structure called the *internal root sheath* (Figs. 17-14 and 17-15). This is a cellular sheath that surrounds and grows up along with the hair, separating the hair from the external root sheath. The internal root sheath extends only partway up the follicle (Fig. 17-14), and it is made of *soft keratin* (Fig. 17-14). Granules are therefore seen in the cells that are becoming keratinized (Fig. 17-14), but instead of being basophilic, they stain a bright red color. They are known as *trichohyalin granules* (Gr. *thrix*, hair).

Hair Color.   As in the epidermis, the endogenous pigment in hair is *melanin* that is synthesized by *melanocytes;* these are distributed in the hair matrix close to the papilla. The melanocytes in this region possess dendritic processes that provide melanin for the epithelial cells that will become the cortex of the hair. As a result, melanin becomes incorporated into the hair cortex and gives it color.

As people become older, their hair turns "gray." The

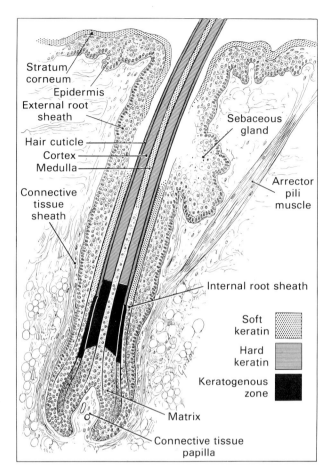

Fig. 17-14.   Diagram of a hair follicle, showing the distribution of soft and hard keratin and the keratogenous zone in which the hard keratin of the hair is produced. (After Leblond CP: Ann NY Acad Sci 53:464, 1951)

lack of pigment in the hair of older people is ascribed to an increasing inability of the melanocytes of the bulbs of their hair follicles to make tyrosinase.

Although hair has many different colors, hair *pigments* of only three different colors can be seen with the microscope; these are black, brown, and yellow. The yellow melanin is known as *pheomelanin,* and the brown and black melanins are known as *eumelanin.* Pheomelanin and eumelanin levels and the type of eumelanin produced are genetically controlled.

Hair Structure.   The cross-sectional shape and other features of terminal hairs vary in relation to race. Three chief types of hair are recognized: straight, wavy, and woolly. Straight hair is found in the Mongol races, Chinese, Eskimos, and the Indians of America; it is characteristically coarse and is round in cross section. Wavy hair is found in a number of ethnic groups, including Europeans, and woolly hair is characteristic of nearly all black races. A

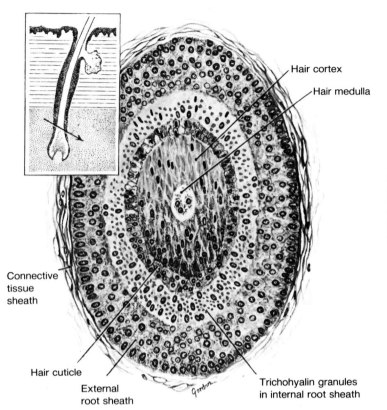

Fig. 17-15. Diagrammatic representation of a slightly oblique section of a hair within its follicle. The plane of section is through the subcutaneous tissue at the level of the keratogenous zone of the hair, as indicated by the arrow in the inset. See text for details.

Hair cortex

Hair medulla

Connective tissue sheath

Hair cuticle

External root sheath

Trichohyalin granules in internal root sheath

cross section of a wavy hair is oval and that of a woolly hair is elliptical or kidney-shaped.

Typically, a terminal hair consists of a central *medulla* of soft keratin and a *cuticle* and *cortex* of hard keratin (Figs. 17-14 and 17-15). However, some hairs contain virtually no medulla; hence they show only a cuticle and a cortex of hard keratin.

The cuticle consists of thin, flat, scalelike cells arranged on the surface of a hair, like shingles on the side of a house, except that their free edges point upward instead of downward (Fig. 17-16). The free edges of these cells interlock with the free edges of similar cells that line the internal root sheath and whose free edges point downward. This arrangement makes it difficult to pull out a hair without removing at least part of the internal root sheath with it. This can be of medicolegal interest.

Where present, the medulla consists of soft keratin. In it, cornified cells are commonly separated from one another. Air or liquid may be present between the cells of the medulla.

Hair Growth Is Cyclic. Hair coming out on a brush or comb is not an omen of imminent baldness. Reassurance for worried patients is gained by informing them that hair growth is cyclic. Each hair follicle alternates between *growing* and *resting phases*. During the former, the cells of the matrix continue to proliferate and the hair elongates. However, in the resting phase, the matrix becomes inactive and atrophies. The root of the hair then becomes detached from its matrix and gradually moves up the follicle, gaining for a time a secondary attachment to the external root sheath as the lower end of the hair approaches the neck of the follicle. Eventually, the hair falls out of the follicle. A new matrix then develops and this leads to a new hair beginning to grow in the same follicle.

The hairs of the scalp last approximately 2 to 3 years before entering their short resting phase of 3 to 4 months. This enables some people to attain a hair length of 50 cm or more. In other parts of the body, however, the growing phase is shorter than this and the resting phase is relatively long. The hairs of the eyebrows, for example, grow for 1 to 2 months and then their follicles rest for 3 to 4 months. However, because neighboring hair follicles are commonly in different phases of their growth cycle at any given time, the renewal of hair usually goes unnoticed.

Factors That Influence Hair Growth. By the time of birth, the number and distribution of hair follicles are already determined. Yet there are noticeable differences in the amount, texture, and distribution of terminal body hair between the two sexes and even between different individuals of the same sex. There are also marked racial differences in the amount and distribution of the terminal body hair that appears at puberty. In both males and females, growth of this extra hair is mainly due to an increase

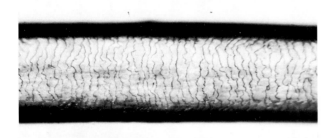

Fig. 17-16. Photomicrograph of a hair showing the cuticle on its surface (oil immersion).

in the blood level of male sex hormone (*androgen*), primarily testosterone, at the time of puberty. The fairly obvious racial differences that exist in the amount and texture of the body hair that develops in individuals who fall within the normal range of androgen levels suggest that there is also an inherited component that may be expressed as androgen responsiveness on the part of the hair follicles. A clear-cut example of the importance of such responsiveness by hair follicles is seen in the *testicular feminization syndrome*, which was described under Chromosomal Anomalies in Chapter 3.

The role of androgen in stimulating growth of terminal hair becomes particularly obvious when males are castrated prior to puberty. Such individuals fail to develop facial, pubic, or axillary hair, and their scalp hair remains silky soft. Postpubertal castration leads to less rapid growth of facial hair and a gradual disappearance of body hair. A more common problem, however, is the progressive replacement of terminal scalp hair by much less evident vellus in males who have not been castrated. Paradoxically, the testosterone level in such bald men is also responsible for their baldness. This is because they have inherited an autosomal-dominant predisposition to developing baldness that is maximally expressed only in the presence of substantial levels of androgen. Hence testosterone is responsible for both hair growth and hair loss, and men are much more likely than women to manifest the trait for common baldness (*male pattern alopecia*).

Finally, there is no sound evidence to substantiate the notion sometimes overheard in the barber's chair that haircuts or too much shaving accelerate the rate of hair growth, which is estimated to be 0.4 mm to 0.5 mm per day in the case of scalp hair.

SEBACEOUS GLANDS AND ARRECTOR PILI MUSCLES

Most hair follicles slant to one side, their hairs pointing in one particular direction (Fig. 17-14). On the side of the hair follicle indicated by the tip of the hair, there are generally

several *sebaceous glands* (Figs. 17-15, *inset*, and 17-17). These simple alveolar glands empty into the upper third of the hair follicle (Fig. 17-14). Sebaceous glands are readily recognizable in sections as pale-staining, flask-shaped areas (Fig. 17-17). They secrete a complex oily product known as *sebum* that helps to keep thin skin and its hairs (notably those of the scalp) soft, supple, and waterproof. As was explained in Chapter 6, these glands produce their secretion by the *holocrine* mechanism; in other words, all parts of the cell contribute to the secretion. Thus progeny cells formed through mitosis in the basal layer of the gland synthesize and accumulate lipids, and at the same time, they become progressively displaced toward the interior of the gland. At this point, far away from their source of nutrients (the capillaries of the investing connective tissue), they die and disintegrate (see Figs. 6-19 and 17-17) and become the oily secretion *sebum*.

Most sebaceous glands develop from hair follicles, and none of these glands is present in the thick skin on the soles of the feet and the palms of the hands. However, sebaceous glands also develop in a few sites that are devoid of hair follicles (the eyelids, nipples, labia minora, and sometimes the corners of the lips near the red margins). Furthermore, in some sites, particularly the skin that covers the nose, the sebaceous glands that develop from hair follicles become much more prominent than the follicles themselves.

Acne Is a Manifestation of Hyperactive Secretion by Sebaceous Glands. Sex hormones become secreted into the bloodstream in increased amounts at puberty. Although the secretion of male sex hormone is predominant in males and female sex hormone is predominant in females, the chemistry of the sex hormones is interrelated and there is some male sex hormone activity in females and some female sex hormone activity in males. There is a substantial increase in sebum secretion at the time of puberty because of increased levels of male sex hormone. This increased output of sebum is the result of increased mitotic activity that brings about a more rapid turnover of the cell population in sebaceous glands. Limitations in the structural arrangements that deliver sebum to the skin surface make it difficult for so much sebum to be expressed through hair follicles. Instead, the sebum-filled glands tend to bulge into the dermis, leading to the development of pimples (*acne*). This condition predisposes the dermis to further problems such as local infection and can require medical attention. Although female sex hormone may depress sebum output by sebaceous glands to some extent, it apparently does not suppress mitosis; hence girls, too, are susceptible to acne at puberty.

Arrector Pili Muscles. In most areas of thin skin, each of the hair follicles has an associated bundle of smooth muscle called an *arrector pili* muscle (Fig. 17-14). The muscle received this name because its contraction can make the hair "stand on end." The arrector pili muscle extends from an

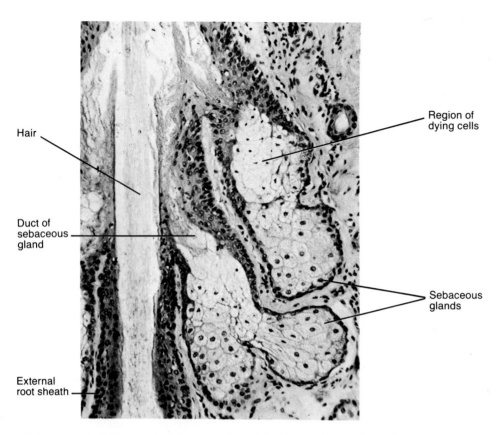

Hair

Duct of
sebaceous
gland

External
root sheath

Region of
dying cells

Sebaceous
glands

Fig. 17-17. Photomicrograph of the top part of a hair follicle cut in longitudinal section, showing sebaceous glands near its upper end. Note the region of dying cells within the gland.

attachment near the base of the connective tissue sheath of the follicle to the papillary layer of the dermis and hence traverses the dermis obliquely (Fig. 17-14). Together with the sebaceous glands, it is situated on the side that is pointed to by the hair in the follicle. Because of this arrangement, when the arrector pili muscle contracts, it not only causes the hair to stand up a little straighter but also gives the sebaceous glands a gentle squeeze, helping to express more of their oily secretory product onto the hair and the skin surface. The arrector pili muscles are innervated by the sympathetic division of the autonomic nervous system, and cold is a well-known stimulus for the reflex that leads to their contraction. Inexperienced rush-hour drivers will also know that sudden panic can literally make one's hair stand on end. This is due to a release of epinephrine into the bloodstream as part of the body-wide sympathetic response to emergency situations.

APOCRINE SWEAT GLANDS

Apocrine sweat glands are microscopically similar to eccrine sweat glands except that, like sebaceous glands, they open into the upper part of hair follicles. However, their distribution is limited to the axillae, the areolae of the breasts, and the pubic and perineal regions, and they only secrete after puberty. When produced, their slightly cloudy-looking secretion does not give off any odor. However, as soon as certain of its constituents have been acted upon by bacteria, they liberate rather noticeable and sometimes distinctly unpleasant odors. Such odors seem to have evolved as species recognition signals and sex attractants, but offensive body odors are no longer socially acceptable and for the most part they are kept under control as a matter of personal hygiene. Apocrine sweat glands have a relatively large secretory portion with a wide lumen, and their duct is fairly narrow. The coiled secretory portion is made up of low-to-high columnar secretory cells, and it is surrounded by myoepithelial cells that are innervated by the autonomic nervous system. Contraction of these cells can bring about expression of the secretory product under conditions of aroused emotion, sexual excitement, or stress. Lastly, we should point out that the names of the two types of sweat glands are quite misleading because it is now known that so-called apocrine and eccrine sweat glands secrete by the usual merocrine mechanism, which was described in Chapter 6.

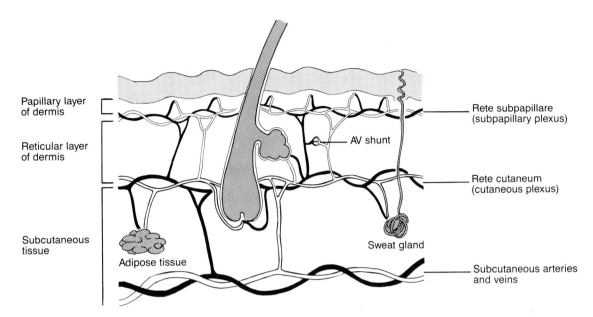

Fig. 17-18. Schematic representation of the blood supply of the skin. See text for details.

BLOOD SUPPLY OF SKIN

The skin is provided with cutaneous branches of subcutaneous musculocutaneous arteries. Branches of these arteries supply a flat network of vessels called the *rete cutaneum* or *cutaneous plexus* that lies at the border between the dermis and the subcutaneous tissue (Fig. 17-18). From the cutaneous plexus, branches descend more deeply or ascend toward the surface. Those branches that pass more deeply supply the more superficial parts of the subcutaneous adipose tissue, the deeper parts of hair follicles, and the secretory portions of sweat glands. Those branches that pass superficially supply the skin, the ducts of sweat glands, the more superficial parts of hair follicles, and the sebaceous glands (Fig. 17-18). On reaching the junction between the reticular and the papillary layers of the dermis, these branches supply a second flat network consisting of arterioles, venules, and capillaries called the *rete subpapillare* or *subpapillary plexus* (Fig. 17-18).

It is also helpful to know where extensive capillary beds are located in the skin because this facilitates an understanding of how body temperature is regulated and also of where fluid loss is likely to occur as a result of burns. The capillary beds of skin are extensive only in the regions of loose connective tissue immediately below the epidermis, surrounding the hair matrix in hair follicles, and around the sweat and sebaceous glands.

From the subpapillary plexus, capillaries extend toward the epidermis as capillary loops within the overlying dermal papillae (Fig. 17-18). Such papillary loops supply tissue fluid to the basal cells of the epidermis, but they contain too little blood to cause the pink color of skin. This color

is chiefly due to the blood in the wide venules of the subpapillary plexus. The venules of the subpapillary plexus eventually drain into small veins that, in most cases, leave the skin along with arteries.

Superficial Dermal Capillaries and Venules Play an Important Role in Regulating Body Temperature. Body heat is lost directly through the skin. If the air temperature is lower than body temperature, heat loss through the skin can be regulated by varying the extent to which its papillary and subpapillary capillaries and venules are open to the circulation. This regulation is due to the smooth muscle tonus in the various vessels that regulate blood flow through the terminal vascular bed, including the relatively numerous arteriovenous anastomoses that enable blood to bypass capillary beds (see Chap. 16), and it conserves as much heat as is necessary.

If the air temperature is similar to or exceeds body temperature, the *effect* of a lower external temperature is achieved by sweat glands, which pour sweat onto the surface of the body, where it evaporates and so cools the skin. Hence blood circulating through the papillary and subpapillary regions of skin from which sweat is evaporating loses heat. To keep down the temperature of an individual who performs violent muscular exercise on a very hot day and so generates a great deal of heat, both profuse sweating and dilation of the superficial blood vessels are needed.

It will be recalled from Chapter 14 that eccrine sweat glands are innervated by postganglionic sympathetic nerve fibers that release acetylcholine instead of the usual neurotransmitter, norepinephrine. The secretory activity of these sweat glands is controlled by heat-regulating centers in the hypothalamus. Anxiety, fear, or emotional stress can also cause a "cold sweat" response in eccrine sweat glands

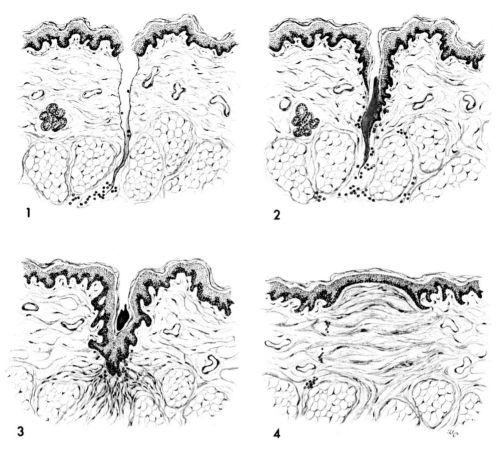

Fig. 17-19. Drawings showing four stages in the healing of a skin incision following approximation of its edges with sutures. (*1*) A few hours after incision; (*2*) after 1 week; (*3*) after 2 weeks; and (*4*) after 1 month. For details, see text. (After Lindsay WK, Birch JR: Can J Surg 7:297, 1964)

of the palms, soles of the feet, and forehead. Sweaty palms and other evidence of epinephrine-mediated nervous sweating can be unrelated to the cutaneous responses involved in regulating body temperature.

How Does the Skin React to Burns?   A light to moderate sunburn results in enough ultraviolet injury to cause capillaries and venules in the papillary and subpapillary regions of the skin to dilate, making the skin turn red (*erythema*). With a slightly more severe burn, such capillaries and venules also allow plasma to leak from them. This causes an edema in the outer part of the dermis and can result in the formation of blisters. In thin skin, the common site of burns, blisters are the result of accumulations of plasma between the dermis and the epidermis. In thick skin, blisters are sometimes due to intraepidermal accumulations of plasma.

When thin skin is burned severely enough for a blister to form, epidermis regenerates over the blister from epidermal cells that survive in the lower parts of hair follicles. Even if the burn destroys the more superficial part of the dermis as well, epithelial cells from the deep parts of hair follicles will grow along the interface between the living dermis and the dead dermis and will form new epidermis at this level. However, if the inflicted damage extends below the bases of the hair follicles, regrowth of the epidermis can occur only at the perimeter of the burn, and it occurs so slowly that a skin graft is necessary.

HEALING OF SKIN INCISIONS AND LACERATIONS

Incisions and lacerations generally heal in a matter of weeks, provided they are managed properly and infection is avoided. The edges of surgical incisions or deep lacerations need to be approximated with sutures to promote healing and to minimize scarring. Under such conditions, the cut edges of the epidermis grow down the edges of the V-shaped cleft extending down into the subcutaneous tissue (Fig. 17-19, stage 2). They grow toward each other fairly rapidly under the scab that has formed as a result of hemorrhage, with the result that epidermal continuity is soon

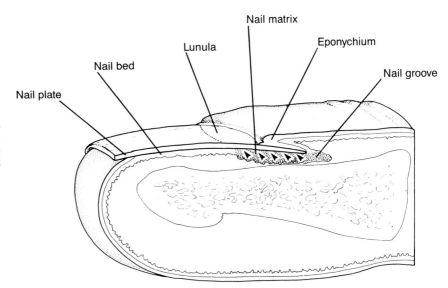

Fig. 17-20. Diagrammatic representation of the parts of a fingernail. Arrowheads indicate displacement of matrix cells as they contribute to the nail plate. See text for details.

restored (Fig. 17-19, stage 3). In the meantime, there is an abundant growth of new fibroblasts that are thought to be derived primarily from the pericytes associated with the capillaries and venules in the subcutaneous tissue (Fig. 17-19, stage 3). The fibroblasts produce new collagen at the site, and this eventually restores the damaged dermis to its former strength (Fig. 17-19, stage 4). The dermis is unlikely to be a major source of such fibroblasts because the reticular layer of dermis consists primarily of collagen bundles and it is not very vascular. For a long time, the new epidermis remains relatively thin; it also lacks the uneven undersurface created by the connective tissue papillae that normally project up into the epidermis (Fig. 17-19, stage 4).

Skin Grafting.   Advantage can be taken of the skin's considerable capacity for regeneration in making autologous skin grafts, that is, in transplanting areas of skin from one body site to another. Where feasible, this can even be done without severing the skin graft from its original blood supply until it has become revascularized from the denuded area. However, under most circumstances, a free skin graft is necessary. In this case, until the graft becomes revascularized, it has to derive its nutrients from the tissue fluid exuding from the raw surface on which it is placed. Commonly, only the epidermis and the superficial part of the dermis are transplanted. In this case, the site from which the grafted skin was taken heals and becomes covered with new skin. The sources from which the new epidermal cells can be derived include the deeper parts of hair follicles and sweat glands, which are left at the site and can be long enough to extend down through the entire thickness of the dermis into the subcutaneous tissue (see Figs. 17-1 and 17-15, *inset*). In addition, slow regrowth of epidermis occurs at the periphery of the site.

NAILS

The nails develop in the fetus toward the end of the first trimester of pregnancy. The epidermis of each terminal phalanx invades the underlying dermis and forms a *nail groove*. The cells that form the floor of this groove become the *nail matrix* Fig. 17-20). Proliferation of the cells in the nail matrix results in formation and growth the *nail plate* (Figs. 17-20 and 17-21), which is made of hard keratin. The epidermis over which the nail plate grows is called the *nail bed* (Figs. 17-20 and 17-21); it consists of only the deeper layers of the epidermis, with the nail plate taking the place of the stratum corneum. *Lateral nail grooves* extend along each side of the nail plate. The crescent-shaped white area at the base of the nail is called the *lunula,* and it indicates the general extent of the underlying nail matrix (Fig. 17-20). Under the nail bed, the dermis is characterized by a pattern of longitudinal ridges and grooves (Fig. 17-21). The soft ''cuticle'' that overlaps the proximal border of the nail plate is known as the *eponychium* (Fig. 17-20).

Nails grow at a rate of approximately 0.5 mm per week. Fingernails grow more rapidly than toenails, and both grow faster in summer than in winter.

Infections of the eponychium or lateral nail grooves are fairly common. Also, severe pinching of a fingernail or toenail as a result of an accident can result in subsequent loss of the nail plate. However, provided the matrix is not destroyed, a new nail plate will still grow from the nail groove. If the nail matrix becomes badly damaged, a new nail will not form. Sometimes, usually from wearing shoes that are too tight, the curvature of a toenail becomes accentuated and the nail plate pierces the epidermis along a lateral groove. This painful condition is known as an *ingrown toenail.* To correct it and to relieve the pain, it may become

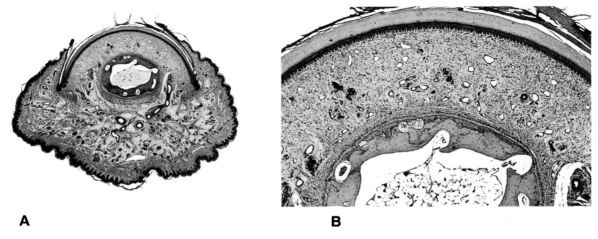

Fig. 17-21. (*A*) Photomicrograph of a child's finger cut in transverse section at the level of the nail plate (very low power). The thin skin on the dorsal surface (which is *uppermost* in this illustration) forms a lateral nail groove on each side of the nail plate. A layer of dermis lies between the nail plate and the central terminal phalanx. The thick skin on the palmar surface of the finger has characteristic ridges and tall dermal papillae. (*B*) Enlarged view showing the hard keratin of the nail plate (*uppermost*), the darker staining nail bed beneath it, and the regular longitudinal pattern of fine dermal ridges projecting into the undersurface of the nail bed. Many thin-walled venules and small veins can be distinguished in the underlying dermis. The thicker walled vessels are small arteries and arteriovenous anastomoses. Part of the cortex of the terminal phalanx, with yellow marrow in its medullary cavity, is seen at bottom.

necessary to cut away some of the nail matrix on the affected side of the nail.

SENSORY RECEPTORS OF SKIN

The skin possesses a remarkable assortment of different *sensory receptors.* Each type of receptor is basically made up of afferent nerve endings in a special kind of association with cells of the surrounding tissue that transduces stimulus energy into afferent nerve impulses. At least six morphologically distinct types of sensory receptors exist in the skin; some are fairly elaborate and contain cells of other types, in addition to afferent nerve endings. The different types of cutaneous sensory receptors are sensitive to a number of different stimuli (*e.g.,* the amount of pressure or tension being exerted on a given region of skin, its local temperature, and so forth), and the sensory areas of the cerebral cortex are able to localize the resulting sensations to the area of body surface involved. The more complex types of cutaneous sensory receptors are constructed in such a way that they respond to specific kinds of stimulus energy that reaches them in particular ways, whereas the simpler receptors can probably respond to stimulus energy of more than one kind. Cutaneous sensory receptors are functionally classified as (1) *mechanoreceptors,* which respond to displacement as a result of touch, pressure, or stretch; (2) *thermoreceptors,* which respond to temperature changes; or (3) *nociceptors* (L. *nocere,* to injure), which respond to injurious agents and irritants that are capable of eliciting pain or

itch. However, in certain cases, it has proved difficult to relate these functional differences to the morphological differences that are seen between cutaneous sensory receptors, and it would appear that morphologically different receptors can register the same kind of stimulus energy and perhaps even perform the same functions. From the structural point of view, cutaneous afferent endings fall into two broad categories: *free nerve endings* and *encapsulated nerve endings.* For students who need detailed information, these categories of nerve endings will now be described.

Free Nerve Endings. Some small unmyelinated and myelinated afferent nerve fibers enter the epidermis and become free of their investing Schwann cells and myelin (Fig. 17-22A). They continue on as so-called *free endings* into the basal layers of the epidermis, where they lie between the cell membranes of contiguous epithelial cells (Fig. 17-22A).

Similar free endings in the papillary layer of the dermis lie parallel with the dermal–epidermal border instead of perpendicular to the skin surface. They are also more bulbous and run a more tortuous course than do free endings in the epidermis. The function of free endings in skin is not entirely clear. However, it is probable that they serve as *thermoreceptors* and *nociceptors.*

Basketlike arrangements of free nerve endings surround hair follicles, and free endings enter the external root sheath, particularly in tactile hairs such as cat whiskers and other long, coarse hairs on the snouts of animals. Because these respond to displacement of the hairs, they are *mechanoreceptors.*

Merkel Endings. These are present in the deep layers of the epidermis of the palmar surface of the hands and the plantar surface of the feet. Here free nerve endings are attached to specialized cells called *Merkel cells* in the stratum germinativum (Fig.

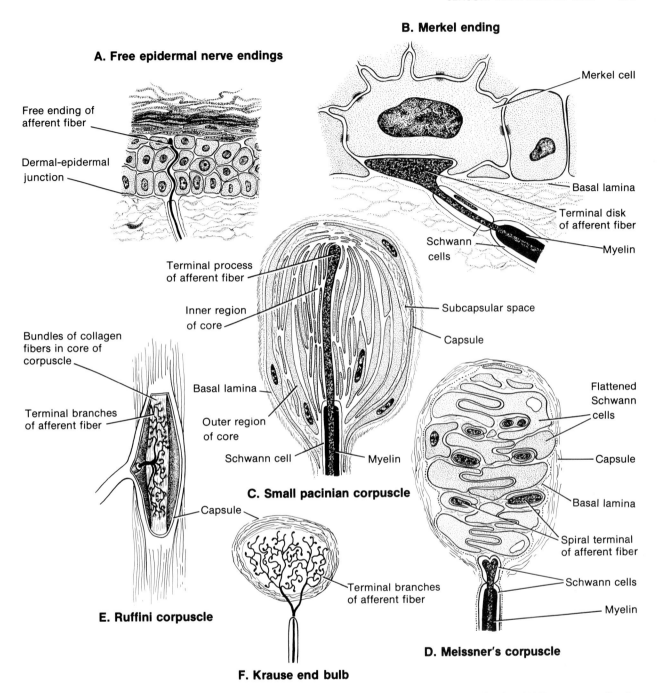

A. Free epidermal nerve endings

Free ending of afferent fiber

Dermal-epidermal junction

B. Merkel ending

Merkel cell

Basal lamina

Terminal disk of afferent fiber

Schwann cells

Myelin

Terminal process of afferent fiber

Inner region of core

Subcapsular space

Capsule

Bundles of collagen fibers in core of corpuscle

Basal lamina

Outer region of core

Terminal branches of afferent fiber

Schwann cell

Myelin

C. Small pacinian corpuscle

Flattened Schwann cells

Capsule

Basal lamina

Spiral terminal of afferent fiber

Schwann cells

Myelin

Capsule

E. Ruffini corpuscle

Terminal branches of afferent fiber

D. Meissner's corpuscle

F. Krause end bulb

Fig. 17-22. Diagram of the sensory receptors that are present in the skin. (*A*) Free nerve ending in epidermis. (*B*) Merkel ending in epidermis. (*C*) Small pacinian corpuscle in dermis. (*D*) Meissner's corpuscle in dermis. (*E*) Ruffini corpuscle in dermis. (*F*) Krause end bulb (mucocutaneous corpuscle) in dermis. For details see text.

17-23). Merkel cells have fingerlike cytoplasmic projections that indent or are insinuated between the keratinocytes to which they are anchored by desmosomes. As shown in Figure 17-22*B,* each of the unmyelinated terminal branches of myelinated afferent nerve fibers penetrates the basal layer of the epidermis, loses its investment of Schwann cells, and becomes expanded into a terminal disk that is apposed to the base of a Merkel cell. Electron-dense granules (80 nm to 100 nm in diameter) are present in the cytoplasm of the Merkel cell (Fig. 17-23), including the part of the cell that is adjacent to the terminal disk. They are widely believed to be synaptic vesicles, but there is no conclusive evidence to support this. The Merkel endings are regarded as mechanoreceptors.

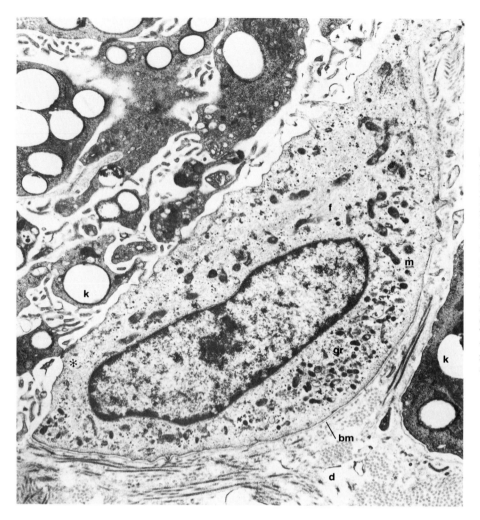

Fig. 17-23. Electron micrograph of a Merkel cell in the stratum germinativum (human skin biopsy). Keratinocytes (*k*) are seen at upper left and lower right. Below the cell is the basement membrane (*bm*) at the epidermal–dermal border. Collagen fibrils are present in the underlying dermis (*d*). Within the cytoplasm of the pale-staining Merkel cell, some intermediate filaments (*f*), a few mitochondria (*m*), free ribosomes, and the characteristic electron-dense granules (*gr*) of these cells can be discerned. The asterisk probably indicates where the cell is attached to a neighboring keratinocyte by way of a desmosome. (Courtesy of P. Lea)

Pacinian Corpuscles. These are encapsulated mechanoreceptors that are distributed throughout the dermis and subcutaneous tissue, particularly in the fingers, external genitalia, and breasts. They are also present in other sites that may be deformed by pressure (*e.g.,* joint capsules, mesenteries, and the wall of the urinary bladder).

A pacinian corpuscle is an ovoid structure, 1 mm to 2 mm long and 0.5 mm to 1 mm in diameter. It is supplied by a myelinated afferent nerve fiber that enters at one pole and loses its myelin sheath at a node of Ranvier just inside the corpuscle (Fig. 17-22C). The fiber then extends axially through the corpuscle and becomes expanded terminally into several clublike processes. Within the corpuscle, the nerve fiber is covered by numerous concentric layers of flattened cells, and hence in longitudinal section, a pacinian corpuscle has the appearance of a longitudinally sliced onion (Fig. 17-22C).

The region immediately surrounding the nerve fiber is described as a *core* with an inner and outer part. The *capsule* surrounds this core. The flattened cells forming the core probably correspond to modified Schwann cells. In the inner part of the core (which contains up to 60 lamellae), the cells alternate with one another on opposite sides of the nerve fiber so as to form a series of concentric sem-

icircles when seen in cross section. The cells in the inner part of the core are extremely flattened and packed together closely so that the intercellular spaces between them are narrow. However, the cells in the outer part of the core entirely surround the nerve fiber, forming approximately 60 complete concentric layers. The peripheral cells in the outer part of the core are somewhat thicker and more widely separated than the deeper ones. Desmosomelike junctions join all the cells that form the core, and there are sparsely distributed collagen fibers and tissue fluid, as well as basement membranes, in the intercellular spaces between them.

External to the core of the corpuscle lies the connective tissue capsule, which is derived from the perineurium. Between the capsule and the core there is a *subcapsular space* that is continuous with the endoneurial sheath of the afferent fiber supplying the corpuscle. The thickness of the capsule is variable; in large corpuscles, it may contain as many as 70 concentric layers of flattened cells, but in small ones, such as that depicted in Figure 17-22C, it consists of only a few layers. These cells also are joined together by desmosomes. The intercellular spaces between them contain bundles of collagen fibers, tissue fluid, and basement membranes. The deeper the position of the pacinian corpuscle in the skin, the greater the number of layers in the corpuscle. The narrow subcapsular space contains amorphous ground substance, collagen fibers, fibroblasts, and some macrophages.

The manner in which the structural arrangements described above facilitate response of pacinian corpuscles to mechanical displacement of the skin due to pressure is not clear. Pacinian corpuscles can also detect vibrations.

Meissner's Corpuscles.   These receptors are most numerous on the palmar surface of the fingers, the plantar surface of the feet, the lips, eyelids, external genitalia, and nipples. They lie just below the epidermal–dermal border in the papillary layer of the dermis. They are almost certainly mechanoreceptors, responding to skin displacement due to touch. It is significant that Meissner's corpuscles are situated in regions of substantial tactile sensitivity.

Each Meissner's corpuscle is an ovoid structure approximately 150 μm long and 30 μm in diameter, lying with its long axis perpendicular to the skin surface. It contains a stack of flattened cells that, for the most part, lie transversely in the corpuscle (Fig. 17-22D) and interleave with one another. These flattened cells are probably modified Schwann cells. The expanded nerve endings are so arranged that they lie parallel with the skin surface. As shown in Figure 17-22D, the myelinated afferent nerve fiber supplying the corpuscle loses its myelin sheath where it branches. From two to six branches enter at the base of the corpuscle and then branch repeatedly. The terminal branches may pursue a tortuous course through the corpuscle but are commonly helically arranged. There are collagen fibers in the intercellular spaces between the nerve endings and flattened Schwann cells.

Surrounding the core of flattened cells and the expanded nerve endings interleaved with them, there is a well-developed connective tissue *capsule* that is anchored to the epidermal–dermal border by bundles of collagen fibers.

Ruffini Corpuscles.   These receptors lie parallel to the epidermal–dermal border deep in the dermis and subcutaneous tissue. They are particularly numerous on the plantar surface of the feet. Each is a small spindle-shaped structure approximately 1 mm long and 0.1 mm in diameter. The large myelinated afferent nerve fiber that supplies the corpuscle branches repeatedly to form a diffuse arborization of unmyelinated terminal branches. These end in flattened terminals ramifying extensively between bundles of collagen fibers in the core of the corpuscle (Fig. 17-22E). The terminals are only incompletely covered by a few modified Schwann cells. The nerve endings in Ruffini corpuscles appear to be stimulated by displacement of the collagen fibers with which they are intertwined. These collagen fibers run axially through the core of the corpuscle and pass through both ends of the corpuscle (Fig. 17-22E) to merge with the collagen in the surrounding regions of the dermis. The *capsule* is relatively thin and surrounds a relatively wide *subcapsular space* that contains fluid, collagen fibrils, fibroblasts, and macrophages.

There is a striking resemblance between Ruffini corpuscles and Golgi tendon organs (see Fig. 15-25), so they are thought to be mechanoreceptors that respond to tension in the collagen fibers in the surrounding connective tissue, much as tendon organs respond to pull in tendons.

Krause End Bulbs (Mucocutaneous Corpuscles).   These receptors are situated in the papillary layer of the dermis of the conjunctiva (the covering of the whites of the eyes and the lining of the eyelids), tongue, mucosa of the mouth and pharynx, and external genitalia. They are lightly encapsulated compared with the other types of encapsulated receptors.

The afferent myelinated fiber branches repeatedly within the capsule, forming a network of coiled unmyelinated endings (Fig. 17-22F).

The function of the end bulb receptors has not been established, but it appears likely that they are mechanoreceptors.

SELECTED REFERENCES

Skin and Sweat Glands

ALLEN TD, POTTER CS: Desmosomal form, fate and function in mammalian epidermis. J Ultrastruct Res 51:94, 1975

CHACKO LW, VAIDYA MC: The dermal papillae and ridge patterns in human volar skin. Acta Anat 70:99, 1968

CHAMPION RH, GILLMAN T, ROOK AJ, SIMS RT (eds): An Introduction to the Biology of the Skin. Oxford and Edinburgh, Blackwell, 1970

GOLDSMITH LA (ed): Biochemistry and Physiology of the Skin. New York, Oxford University Press, 1983

LEVER WF, SCHAUMBURG–LEVER GS: Histopathology of the Skin, 6th ed. Philadelphia, JB Lippincott, 1983

MARKS R, CHRISTOPHERS E (eds): The Epidermis in Disease. Lancaster, England, MTP Press, 1981

MONTAGNA W: The skin. Sci Am 212 No 2:56, 1965

MONTAGNA W, BENTLEY JP, DOBSON RL (eds): The Dermis. Advances in Biology of Skin. New York, Appleton-Century-Crofts, 1970

MONTAGNA W, PARAKKAL PF: The Structure and Function of Skin, 3rd ed. New York, Academic Press, 1974

ODLAND GF: Structure of the skin. In Goldsmith LA (ed): Biochemistry and Physiology of the Skin, Vol 1, p 3. New York, Oxford University Press, 1983

ZELICKSON AS (ed): Ultrastructure of Normal and Abnormal Skin. Philadelphia, Lea & Febiger, 1967

Keratinocytes, Keratin, and Their Formation

FOWLER J, DENEKAMP J: Regulation of epidermal stem cells. In Cairnie AB, Lala PK, Osmond DG (eds): Stem Cells of Renewing Cell Populations. New York, Academic Press, 1976

FRASER RDB, MACRAE TP: Current views on the keratin complex. In Spearman RIC, Riley PA (eds): The Skin of Vertebrates. Linnean Society Symposium Series No 9, p 67. London, Academic Press, 1980

GREEN H: The keratinocyte as differentiated cell type. In The Harvey Lectures, Series 74, p 101. New York, Academic Press, 1980

LAURENCE EB, THORNLEY AL: The influence of epidermal chalone on cell proliferation. In Cairnie AB, Lala PK, Osmond DG (eds): Stem Cells of Renewing Cell Populations. New York, Academic Press, 1976

MENTON DN: A minimum-surface mechanism to account for the organization of cells into columns in the mammalian epidermis. Am J Anat 145:1, 1976

POTTEN CS: Identification of clonogenic cells in the epidermis and the structural arrangement of the epidermal proliferative unit (EPU). In Cairnie AB, Lala PK, Osmond DG (eds): Stem Cells of Renewing Cell Populations. New York, Academic Press, 1976

POTTEN CS: Keratopoiesis in normal epidermis. In Marks R, Christophers E (eds): The Epidermis in Disease, p 171. Lancaster, England, MTP Press, 1981

POTTEN CS, ALLEN TD: The fine structure and cell kinetics of mouse epidermis after wounding. J Cell Sci 17:413, 1975

SEIJI M, BERNSTEIN IA: Biochemistry of Cutaneous Epidermal Differentiation. Baltimore, University Park Press, 1977

Pigmentation of Skin

DELLA PORTA G, MUHLBOCK O (eds): Structure and Control of the Melanocyte. New York, Springer Verlag, 1966

FITZPATRICK TB, KUKITA A, MORIKAWA F ET AL (eds): Biology and Diseases of Dermal Pigmentation. Tokyo, University of Tokyo Press, 1981

FITZPATRICK TB, SZABO G, WICK MM: Biochemistry and physiology of melanin pigmentation. In Goldsmith LA (ed): Biochemistry and Physiology of the Skin, Vol 2, p 687. New York, Oxford University Press, 1983

SEIJI M, SHIMAO K, BIRBECK MSC, FITZPATRICK TB: Subcellular localization of melanin biosynthesis. Ann NY Acad Sci 100:497, 1963

SZABO G, GERALD AB, PATHAK MA, FITZPATRICK TB: Racial differences in the fate of melanosomes in human epidermis. Nature 222: 1081, 1969

WOLFF K, KONRAD K: Melanin pigmentation: An in vivo model for studies of melanosome kinetics within keratinocytes. Science 174:1034, 1971

Cutaneous Immune Responses and Langerhans Cells

BRAATHEN LR, BJERCKE S, THORSBY E: The antigen-presenting function of human Langerhans cells. Immunobiology 168:301, 1984

EDELSON RL, FINK JM: The immunologic function of skin. Sci Am 252 No 6:46, 1985

FRIEDMANN PS: The immunobiology of Langerhans cells. Immunology Today 2 No 7:124, 1981

SILBERBERG–SINAKIN I, GIGLI I, BAER RL, THORBECKE GJ: Langerhans cells: Role in contact hypersensitivity and relationship to lymphoid dendritic cells and to macrophages. Immunol Rev 53: 203, 1980

STINGL G, TAMAKI K, KATZ SI: Origin and function of epidermal Langerhans cells. Immunol Rev 53:149, 1980

STREILEIN JW, BERGSTRESSER PR: Langerhans cells: Antigen presenting cells of the epidermis. Immunobiology 168:285, 1984

Hair Follicles, Hair, and Nails

ACHTEN G, PARENT D: The normal and pathologic nail. Int J Dermatol 22:556, 1983

CHASE HB: Growth of the hair. Physiol Rev 34:113, 1954

HAMILTON JB: Patterned loss of hair in man: Types and incidence. Ann NY Acad Sci 53:395, 1968

JARRETT A (ed): The Physiology and Pathophysiology of the Skin, Vol 4. The Hair Follicle. London, Academic Press, 1977

MONTAGNA W, ELLIS RA (eds): The Biology of Hair Growth. New York, Academic Press, 1958

PRICE ML, GRIFFITHS WA: Normal body hair—a review. Clin Exp Dermatol 10:87, 1985

ZAIAS N, ALVAREZ J: The formation of the primate nail plate. J Invest Dermatol 51:120, 1968

Blood Supply of Skin

ELLIS RA: Vascular patterns of the skin. In Montagna W, Ellis RA (eds): Advances in Biology of the Skin. Vol 2, p 20. New York, Pergamon Press, 1961

JARRETT A (ed): The Physiology and Pathophysiology of the Skin, Vol 2. The Nerves and Blood Vessels. London, Academic Press, 1973

RYAN TJ: Structure and shape of blood vessels of skin. In Jarrett A (ed): The Physiology and Pathophysiology of the Skin. Vol 2. The Nerves and Blood Vessels. London, Academic Press, 1973

Healing of Skin

CROFT CB, TARIN D: Ultrastructural studies of wound healing in mouse skin. I. Epithelial behaviour. J Anat 106:63, 1970

GILLMAN T ET AL: A re-examination of certain aspects of the histogenesis of the healing of cutaneous wounds: A preliminary report. Br J Surg 43:141, 1955

LINDSAY WK, BIRCH JR: Thin skin healing. Can J Surg 7:297, 1964

TARIN D, CROFT CB: Ultrastructural studies of wound healing in mouse skin. II. Dermo-epidermal interrelationships. J Anat 106: 79, 1970

Sensory Receptors of Skin*

BREATHNACH AS: The mammalian and avian Merkel cell. In Spearman RIC, Riley PA (eds): The Skin of Vertebrates. Linnean Society Symposium Series No 9, p 283. London, Academic Press, 1980

*See also Selected References, Chapter 14, under Peripheral Nervous System, Peripheral and Central Myelin, and Nerve Endings.

18

The Digestive System

The *digestive system* consists primarily of the *digestive tract* (*gut*), a long muscular-walled tube beginning at the mouth and terminating at the anus (Fig. 18-1). At these two sites, the ectoderm-derived epidermal covering of the body becomes continuous with the endoderm-derived epithelial lining of the gut. From the *oral cavity*, the digestive tract extends through the body as the *pharynx, esophagus, stomach*, and *small* and *large intestines*. The other important components of the digestive system that will be described

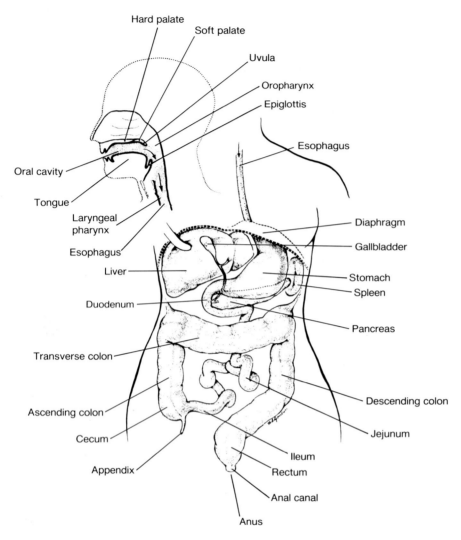

Fig. 18-1. Diagrammatic representation showing the constituent parts of the digestive system. (After Grant)

in this chapter and in Chapter 19 are its various *accessory glands* (namely, the *salivary glands, liver* and *gallbladder,* and *pancreas*). These glands are not situated in the walls of the digestive tract itself, but they deliver their secretory products into its lumen.

Within the lumen of the digestive tract, foodstuffs are still outside the body. To gain access to the interior of the body, substances have to be absorbed through the gut epithelium. However, most of the foodstuffs that are eaten cannot be utilized directly by cells. Thus complex carbohydrates need to be broken down to glucose before they can be absorbed. Proteins need to be degraded to their constituent amino acids, and ingested fats need to be split into monoglycerides, fatty acids, and glycerol. The intraluminal processing to which ingested foods are submitted in order to convert them into products that are suitable for

use by cells is known as food *digestion.* This is brought about by digestive enzymes that are secreted by glands situated either in the walls of the gut or outside its walls but emptying into it. Useful products of digestion are then absorbed by epithelial lining cells of the intestine.

The wet epithelial lining of the digestive tract or of any other internal passageway opening onto the body surface constitutes an important part of the body's barrier between its internal environment and the outside world. Furthermore, a substantial proportion of the lining of the digestive tract needs to be thin enough to facilitate nutrient absorption, so there is a need for effective protective measures along its vast expanse. Protection against the action of stomach acid and digestive enzymes as well as resistance to abrasion is afforded by the secretion of abundant mucus by numerous surface epithelial cells, goblet cells, or underlying mucous glands. Wet epithelial membranes that are able to cover themselves with a protective coating of mucus are described as *mucous membranes.* Included in this term is the underlying layer of loose connective tissue that supports the epithelium. Known as the *lamina propria* (L. *proprius,* one's own), this layer commonly contains mucus-secreting or mixed *mucosal glands.* Beneath the lamina propria of the digestive tract, there is also a delicate layer of smooth muscle called the *muscularis mucosae.* These three components of the mucous membrane are depicted schematically in Figure 18-15.

ORAL CAVITY AND TONGUE

Lips and Cheeks

Each lip is made up mainly of skeletal muscle (the orbicularis oris muscle) together with fibroelastic connective tissue. Its outer surface is covered with thin skin that is provided with hair follicles, sebaceous glands, and sweat glands. The red free margin of the lip is covered with modified skin that represents a transition zone from skin to mucous membrane and that is relatively transparent. The connective tissue papillae of the dermis beneath it are numerous, high, and vascular, and, as a result, the blood in their capillaries readily shows through the transparent epidermis to make the lips appear red. No sweat glands or hair follicles are present in the skin of the red free margin of the lip. Sebaceous glands are not numerous and, where present, are almost entirely confined to the upper lip, with a few at the corners of the lips near the red margin. Because the epithelium is neither heavily keratinized nor adequately provided with sebum, it must occasionally be wetted with saliva by the tongue to avoid ''chapped'' and ''cracked'' lips.

As the skin of the red free margin passes onto the inner surface of the lip, it becomes transformed into mucous membrane. Thicker than the epidermis that covers the outer surface of the lip, the epithelium on this surface is of the stratified squamous nonkeratinizing type. However, some granules of keratohyalin may be found in the cells of the more superficial layers. High papillae of connective tissue of the lamina propria (which, in mucous membranes, replaces the dermis of skin) extend into it. Minor salivary glands called the *labial glands* are embedded in the lamina propria and connect with the surface by means of little ducts.

The mucous membrane lining the cheeks also has a fairly thick stratified squamous nonkeratinizing epithelium. This is the kind of epithelium that is characteristically found on wet epithelial surfaces where there is considerable wear and tear and from which no absorption occurs.

The lamina propria of the cheeks consists of fairly dense fibroelastic tissue and extends into the epithelium in the form of high papillae. The deeper part of it merges into what is termed the *submucosa* of the cheek. This layer contains elastic fibers and many blood vessels. Strands of fibroelastic tissue from the lamina propria penetrate through the submucosa, attaching the mucous membrane to the underlying muscle. This arrangement enables the mucous membrane to pucker into several small folds instead of a single large one.

The submucosal layer beneath the mucous membrane of the cheeks contains many small mucous glands, some with a few serous demilunes. These produce a portion of the saliva and therefore constitute a second group of minor salivary glands.

Tongue

Most of the substance of the tongue is made up of interlacing bundles of skeletal muscle arranged in three different planes. The mucous membrane on the undersurface of the tongue is unkeratinized, smooth, and thin whereas that on the dorsal surface is mostly keratinized and raised into small projections known as papillae (Fig. 18-2). Certain diseases (*e.g.,* scarlet fever and pernicious anemia) can be associated with a changed appearance of the dorsal surface that facilitates their diagnosis.

A V-shaped groove termed the *sulcus terminalis* extends across the dorsal surface of the tongue, subdividing it into (1) the anterior two thirds or *palatine portion* (which corresponds to the *body* of the tongue) and (2) the posterior one third or *pharyngeal portion* (which corresponds to the *base* of the tongue). This groove lies immediately anterior to the row of vallate papillae seen in the drawing at the top left of Figure 18-2. The palatine portion of the tongue is so named because it presses against the hard palate during swallowing. As noted, the dorsal surface of its mucous membrane is covered with small projections. These *papillae* are of four different shapes, as will now be described.

Filiform papillae (L. *filum,* thread) are tapered, threadlike structures that are composed of epithelium and underlying lamina propria (Fig. 18-2, *bottom*). They lie in oblique, transverse rows that become parallel to the sulcus terminalis toward the base of the tongue (Fig. 18-2, *top left*). Each of these papillae has a core of lamina propria that consists of a primary papilla with smaller secondary papillae extending from it toward the surface. Filiform papillae are capped with stratified squamous keratinizing epithelium. On occasion, an unsightly white coating develops on the dorsal surface of the tongue. Sometimes greeted with unnecessary dismay as an omen of imminent poor health, this coating reflects a reduced rate of desquamation of the keratin squames from the filiform papillae.

Fungiform papillae have a narrower base and a rounded top, giving them a shape similar to that of little fungi (Fig. 18-2, *bottom*). Less numerous than the filiform papillae, fungiform papillae lie scattered between them, particularly at the tip of the tongue. Their central core of lamina propria is again made up of a primary papilla, with secondary pa-

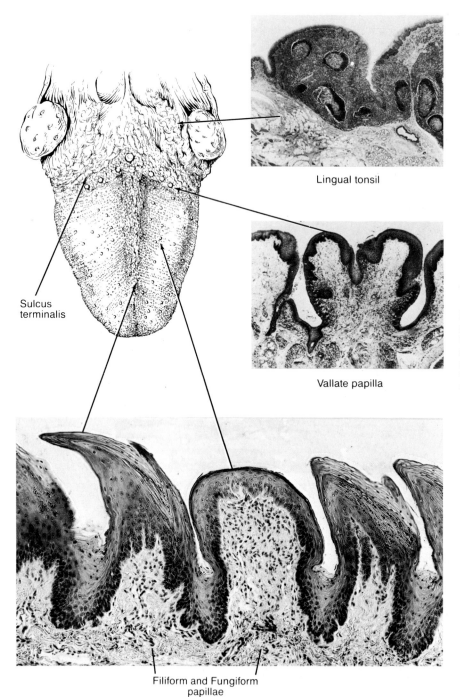

Lingual tonsil

Vallate papilla

Filiform and Fungiform
papillae

Fig. 18-2. Drawing and photomicrographs of the dorsal surface of the tongue, showing the gross anatomical and microscopic appearance of the lingual papillae and lingual tonsil. (Photomicrograph at *bottom,* courtesy of C. P. Leblond)

Sulcus
terminalis

pillae projecting up into the epithelium. In this type of papilla, the covering epithelium is unkeratinized and relatively translucent; this permits capillaries in the underlying tall secondary papillae to show through it, with the result that fungiform papillae appear red.

Vallate papillae, which are also known as *circumvallate papillae,* are distributed along the V-shaped sulcus termin-

alis that lies between the base and body of the tongue (Fig. 18-2, *top left*). There are from 8 to 12 of these papillae. Each is surrounded by a moatlike trough (Figs. 18-2 and 18-3A) that can be flushed out and cleared by the secretory activity of underlying serous glands with ducts that open into the bottom of the trough. Vallate papillae are narrower at their base than at their top; hence their shape is not

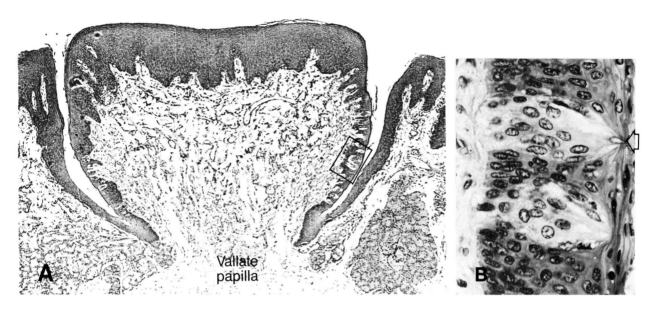

Fig. 18-3. Photomicrographs of (*A*) a vallate papilla with taste buds and (*B*) taste buds under higher magnification (monkey). Arrow indicates the taste pore. (*B*, courtesy of C. P. Leblond)

unlike that of fungiform papillae. Whereas their dorsal surface is keratinized, their lateral walls are not keratinized.

Foliate papillae are ridge-shaped lateral folds of the mucosa that can be present near the base of the tongue along its lateral margins. However, they are not prominent in man.

Human filiform papillae are less well developed than those of some other mammals. They are nevertheless sufficiently well represented to enable children to lick ice cream satisfactorily. This type of papilla contains sensory endings that can respond to touch. Most fungiform papillae and all vallate papillae, on the other hand, are provided with taste buds that have receptor cells that respond to taste stimuli. These receptors will be described in the following section.

Taste Buds and Taste Receptors. The taste receptor cells are protected within small bud- or barrel-shaped structures known as *taste buds* that are arranged perpendicular to the free surface of the epithelial covering of the tongue and the linings of the oral cavity and pharynx. Taste buds are most numerous on the dorsal surface of the tongue, particularly along the sides of the vallate papillae (Fig. 18-3). They are also present in foliate papillae and most fungiform papillae.

From light microscope (LM) studies, it became evident that taste buds contain a number of slightly curved columnar cells arranged beneath a small *taste chamber* that communicates with the surface by way of a *taste pore* (indicated by *arrow* in Fig. 18-3*B*). These cells include both the chemoreceptors (*taste receptor cells*) and their supporting cells (*sustentacular cells*). In the electron microscope (EM), it can be seen that there are long microvilli on the apical surfaces

of both types of cells. The cytoplasm of the putative supporting cells is slightly more electron dense, and they secrete glycosaminoglycan into the taste chamber.

Experimental evidence indicates that both of these cell types can arise from relatively undifferentiated cells that are basally situated in the taste bud (Beidler and Smallman). There is a steady turnover of the cell population in the taste bud because the average lifespan of the columnar cells is only approximately 10 days. Replacements arrive from the periphery of the taste bud, which is where they are formed. Taste receptor cells are as vulnerable to hazards as is the epithelium with which they are associated, so it is understandable that there should be such a mechanism for their replacement. Their renewal seems to occur on a continuous basis from basally situated stem cells.

A fourth cell type has been described in rabbit taste buds (Murray). In this type of cell, the basal cell membrane synapses with nerve terminals and exhibits presynaptic densities with associated synaptic vesicles. It therefore seems likely that this type of cell represents the taste receptor cell.

For a substance to be tasted, it needs to be present in solution and it has to pass through the taste pore into the taste chamber. Its effect is to reduce the negative resting potential of the chemoreceptors, initiating afferent impulses in the taste fibers. There are only four basic tastes (sweet, sour, salty, and bitter), so the great variety of subtle flavors that we can appreciate is due to various combinations of these four basic tastes. Certain parts of the tongue can discern some tastes more readily than other tastes, and some substances are smelled at the same time that they are being tasted. The functional basis of flavor discrimination is poorly understood. However, individual taste receptor cells

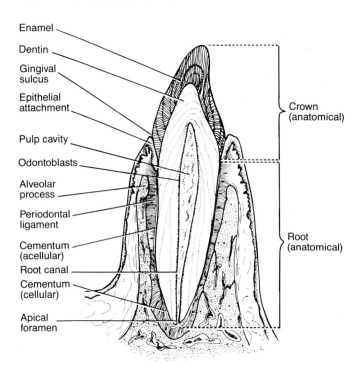

Enamel
Dentin
Gingival sulcus
Epithelial attachment
Pulp cavity
Odontoblasts
Alveolar process
Periodontal ligament
Cementum (acellular)
Root canal
Cementum (cellular)
Apical foramen

Crown (anatomical)

Root (anatomical)

Fig. 18-4. Diagrammatic representation of longitudinal section of a tooth (lower central incisor).

have been found to respond to several different primary taste stimuli. Hence flavor discrimination is thought to involve the recognition of distinctive patterns of nerve impulses coming from numerous receptor cells.

Afferent taste impulses arising from the anterior two thirds of the tongue are carried by the chorda tympani division of the facial nerve, whereas those arising from the posterior third are carried by the glossopharyngeal nerve. Unmyelinated afferent fibers of these nerves enter the proximal end of taste buds and synapse with at least one type of taste receptor cell, as mentioned above.

Lingual Tonsil. The mucous membrane covering the pharyngeal portion (base) of the tongue lacks papillae. The small bumps that can be observed on this part of the tongue are due to the presence of discrete aggregates of lymphatic nodules in the underlying lamina propria (Fig. 18-2, *top right*). This arrangement is termed the *lingual tonsil*. The lymphatic nodules in the lingual tonsil commonly exhibit germinal centers, and in the connective tissue between these nodules, there are abundant small lymphocytes and plasma cells. The stratified squamous nonkeratinizing epithelium that overlies the lymphatic tissue extends down into it as crypts (Fig. 18-2, *top right*). Lymphocytes migrate through the covering epithelium and the walls of the crypts. When the superficial lining cells of the crypts desquamate, lymphocytes and the desquamated epithelial cells enter the crypts. However, the ducts of underlying mucous glands open into the bottoms of many of these crypts, and this arrangement keeps such crypts flushed out and free of debris. Infected crypts are accordingly less common in the

lingual tonsil than in the palatine tonsils, which do not have any glands under their crypts.

TEETH AND GINGIVA

The hard tissue in a *tooth* is mainly a special type of calcified but slightly resilient connective tissue called *dentin*. Two other calcified tissues cover different areas of the dentin. Over the visible portion of the tooth that projects from the gums, the dentin is covered by a highly calcified and extremely hard tissue known as *enamel* (Fig. 18-4). The enamel-covered part of the tooth is called the *anatomical crown*. The remainder of it, known as the *anatomical root* (Fig. 18-4), is covered by a third calcified connective tissue called *cementum*. All three of these dental hard tissues are avascular. The junction between the crown and the root is termed the *cervix* of the tooth, and the term *cervical line* is used to describe the line of demarcation between the enamel and the cementum.

Within each tooth, there is a central soft tissue space that has the same general shape as the tooth itself; this is known as the *pulp cavity* (Fig. 18-4). Its more expanded coronal portion is called the *pulp chamber,* and the narrower part that extends through its root is called the *root canal.* The pulp cavity contains loose connective tissue and is richly provided with small nerve fibers and blood vessels entering by way of the *apical foramen* of the root canal (Fig. 18-4). The dentin that surrounds the pulp cavity is lined by a layer of *odontoblasts* (Fig. 18-4), which are the cells that produce the dentin. Odontoblasts bear the same relation to dentin as osteoblasts do to bone, and they resemble osteoblasts in certain respects.

Bony ridges called *alveolar processes* project from the maxilla and mandible and support the teeth. In these processes, there are sockets termed *alveoli*, one for each root of a tooth (certain teeth posssess more than one root, as will be described later in this chapter). The tooth is suspended in its alveolus by the *periodontal ligament* (Fig. 18-4), which is made up of bundles of collagen fibers that extend from the alveolar bone to the cementum covering the root. The mucous membrane that lines the oral cavity covers the alveolar processes as the *gums*. The portion of the gum mucosa that is strongly bound to the crest of the alveolar process (Fig. 18-4) and that is also tightly attached to the base of the teeth is known as the *gingiva*. It consists of stratified squamous keratinizing epithelium that is firmly attached by lamina propria to the periosteal covering of the underlying alveolar process. Bordering on the gingiva proper, there is a more flexible lining mucosa consisting of nonkeratinizing epithelium with underlying loose connective tissue; this part of the oral mucosa is sometimes referred to as the *loosely attached gingiva*. The part of the tooth that extends into the oral cavity beyond the gingiva is termed the *clinical crown* (which is distinct from the *anatomical crown* mentioned earlier). The clinical crown does not necessarily correspond to the anatomical crown. For a while after eruption, the gingiva remains attached to the anatomical crown. The gingival attachment then recedes to the cervical line and eventually reaches the cementum, with the result that the clinical crown becomes longer than the anatomical crown.

Two separate sets of teeth, described as *dentitions*, are acquired during one's lifetime. These two dentitions and the process by which they develop will be described in the following section.

Primary and Secondary Dentitions

The *primary dentition* that serves during childhood consists of *20 deciduous* (*baby* or *milk*) *teeth*—10 in each jaw. On both sides of the midline of each jaw, there are *central* and *lateral incisors* that generally appear at the age of approximately 6 months. Lateral to the two incisors in each dental quadrant lies the *canine*, which has a single *cusp* (conical projection). Posteriorly, there are only *two molars* with wide occlusal (biting) surfaces made up of three or more cusps, an adaptation for grinding food. Replacement of the primary teeth begins at the age of approximately 6 years, and it culminates in eruption of the third molars by the age of approximately 18 years.

The *permanent dentition* consists of *32 secondary teeth*—16 in each jaw. As was the case in the primary dentition, the anterior group of teeth in each quadrant is made up of the *central* and *lateral incisors* and the *canine*. Immediately lateral to the canine are the *first* and *second premolars,* which are lacking from the primary dentition because they are the teeth that replace the primary molars. Each premolar possesses two cusps and has a single root that bifurcates. Posterior to the premolars there are *three molars.* The molars of the lower jaw are provided with two roots whereas those of the upper jaw have three roots. The first, second, and third molars have no counterparts in the primary dentition. They erupt behind the most posterior primary teeth in order at approximately 6-year intervals, beginning with the first molars at the age of approximately 6 years. The third molars (wisdom teeth) have to wait so long that, in some cases, they become impacted within the jaw because of crowding of the teeth.

Development of the Teeth

Whereas tooth enamel is derived from ectoderm, the dentin, cementum, and pulp of the tooth are derived from mesenchyme. Tooth development begins at week 6 of gestation with oral ectoderm growing into the underlying mesenchyme and then forming a bell-shaped structure that becomes lined with *ameloblasts,* the cells that produce enamel. The mesenchymal cells adjacent to the ameloblasts become *odontoblasts* that form dentin. Hence the crown of the tooth develops from two different germ layers. The details are described below.

From a line of thickening of the oral ectoderm, an epithelial shelf called a *dental lamina* (Fig. 18-5A) grows into the mesenchyme. This lamina gives rise to the epithelial *tooth buds* from which the deciduous teeth will form (Fig. 18-5A). As each tooth bud grows, it assumes the shape of a bell (Fig. 18-5B), becoming the *enamel (dental) organ.* The mesenchyme that fills the bell becomes the *dental papilla* (Fig. 18-5B). The alveolar process begins to enfold the developing tooth (Fig. 18-5C), and the enamel organ loses its connection with the oral epithelium (Fig. 18-5D). In the meantime, a bud of epithelial cells from which the permanent tooth will develop arises from the dental lamina (Fig. 18-5C and D). Also, the dental papilla that gives rise to the pulp of the tooth becomes increasingly vascular.

Ameloblasts (Fig. 18-6) first differentiate adjacent to the tip of the dental papilla and then also down the sides of the developing crown, whereupon they begin producing enamel (Fig. 18-5C and D). Meanwhile, the mesenchymal cells immediately adjacent to them differentiate into *odontoblasts* that begin laying down dentin. The deposition of dentin commences before the ameloblasts have produced any enamel (Fig. 18-6). Dentin, too, is first produced at the tip of the dental papilla (Fig. 18-5C). During dentin and enamel formation, the formative cells are not trapped within the matrix that they produce; instead, they are displaced by it, with the ameloblasts moving outward and the odontoblasts moving inward.

Ameloblasts and the enamel that they produce extend down as far as the base of the developing anatomical crown (Fig. 18-5C and D). From the lower border of the developing crown, epithelial cells grow into the underlying mesenchyme in the form of a sheath called *Hertwig's epithelial root sheath* that induces the mesenchymal cells inside it to differentiate into odontoblasts. This root sheath determines the shape of the root. However, enough space for the root to develop can only be created by emergence of the crown through the gingiva (Fig. 18-5E). Hence root formation is an important factor leading to tooth eruption. The epithelial root sheath then fragments, and mesenchyme-derived cementoblasts begin to deposit cementum on the outer surface of the dentin. As the ce-

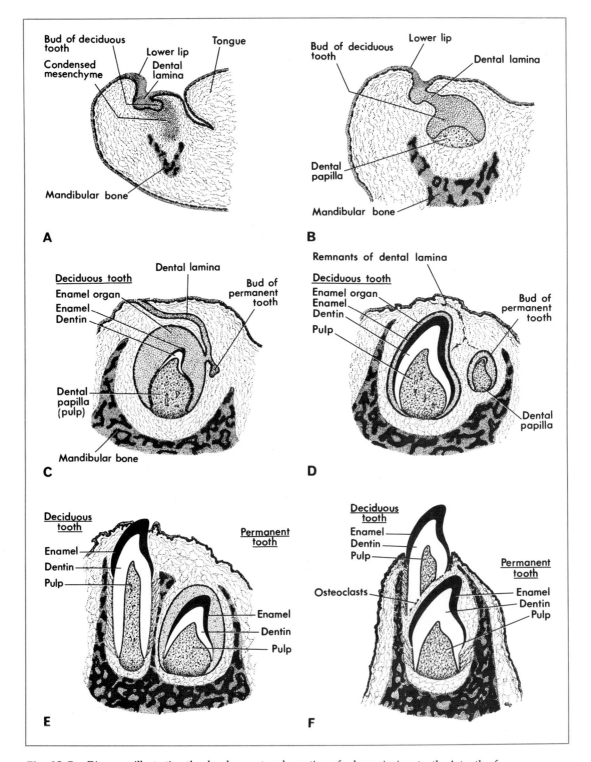

Fig. 18-5. Diagrams illustrating the development and eruption of a lower incisor tooth. A tooth of the permanent dentition develops and erupts, replacing the deciduous tooth.

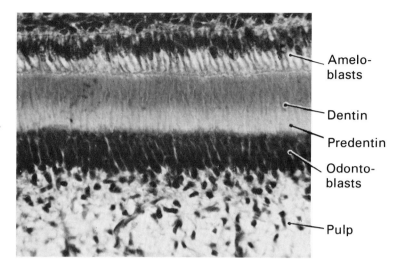

Amelo-
blasts

Dentin

Predentin

Odonto-
blasts

Pulp

Fig. 18-6. Photomicrograph of the dentino-enamel junction of a developing tooth, shortly after dentin formation has begun. Light-staining predentin is present between the odontoblasts and the dentin.

mentum is laid down, it traps the ends of collagen fibers of the periodontal ligament, resulting in a strong ligament attachment. The remnants of the fragmented epithelial root sheath remain scattered within the periodontal ligament as epithelial *cell rests of Malassez*. A clinical consequence of this pattern of development is that such cell rests can subsequently give rise to *dental cysts*.

Eruption of the Permanent Teeth.   When a deciduous tooth erupts, the crown of the permanent tooth that will subsequently occupy the same position has already been formed (Fig. 18-5*E*). In due course, the growing unerupted permanent tooth exerts enough pressure on the root of its associated deciduous tooth to elicit resorption of the root dentin by osteoclasts (Fig. 18-5*F*; see also Fig. 12-17). As a result, the root of the deciduous tooth is already resorbed by the time the permanent tooth is ready to erupt. The deciduous tooth is then shed and is replaced by the permanent tooth.

We shall now describe in more detail the three mineralized tissues of the teeth and the cells that form them.

Dentin and Odontoblasts

Bone, it will be recalled, grows by apposition. The same is true for dentin, but its growth is limited by the fact that odontoblasts are confined to the inner (pulpal) side of the dentin. Hence new layers of dentin can only be added to its pulpal surface, encroaching on the pulp. Also, whereas an osteoblast possesses a number of long cytoplasmic processes that become enclosed within bone canaliculi, an odontoblast possesses only one comparable process termed the *odontoblast process* (Fig. 18-7). This process, which extends from the cell apex to (1) the dentino-enamel junction of the crown or (2) the dentino-cemental junction of the root, becomes enclosed within a narrow canal known as a *dentinal tubule*. With the addition of more layers of dentin, the odontoblasts become displaced progressively farther away from the dentino-enamel or dentino-cemental junction, and the odontoblast processes lengthen along with the dentinal tubules in which they are enclosed. As a result,

dentin is permeated by countless tissue fluid–filled channels that provide a potential access route whereby bacteria can reach the pulp cavity.

Along the pulpal surface of the dentin, there is a continuous layer of odontoblasts that is irregularly penetrated by connective tissue components such as collagen fibrils and capillaries (Fig. 18-7*A*). These cells are nevertheless held together by junctional complexes at the level of the terminal web (Fig. 18-7*B*). When seen in the EM (Fig. 18-7*B*), odontoblasts are made up of an elongated cell body and a long odontoblast process that is situated within the dentin. The cell body contains abundant rough-surfaced endoplasmic reticulum (rER), and its prominent Golgi complex is located near the middle of the cell (Fig. 18-7*B*). The odontoblast process, which branches proximally (Fig. 18-7*B*), lacks rER but contains secretory granules, a few vesicles, microtubules, and microfilaments.

What Makes Exposed Dentin So Sensitive? It is well known that the teeth are highly sensitive to certain kinds of stimuli when these affect an exposed dentinal surface. Several hypotheses have been advanced to account for this sensitivity. According to one theory, the long threadlike odontoblast processes in the dentinal tubules respond to such stimuli, whereupon afferent impulses arise either in the odontoblasts or in the afferent nerve fibers that are associated with these cells at the pulp border. Another acceptable hypothesis is that afferent nerve fibers or nerve endings, which in the pulp cavity are particularly plentiful near the pulp border, respond to thermal and mechanical stimuli that include fluid displacement as a result of the movement of tissue fluid along the dentinal tubules. Dentinal sensitivity fortunately tends to lessen with age, apparently as a consequence of progressive occlusion of the dentinal tubules caused by continuing calcification of their walls.

Although odontoblasts do not divide in postnatal life, they persist and remain capable of laying down more dentin if this becomes necessary to compensate for attrition at occlusal surfaces, accidental loss of part of a tooth, or loss of hard tissue because of dental caries. Over the years, odontoblasts also slowly produce enough additional dentin

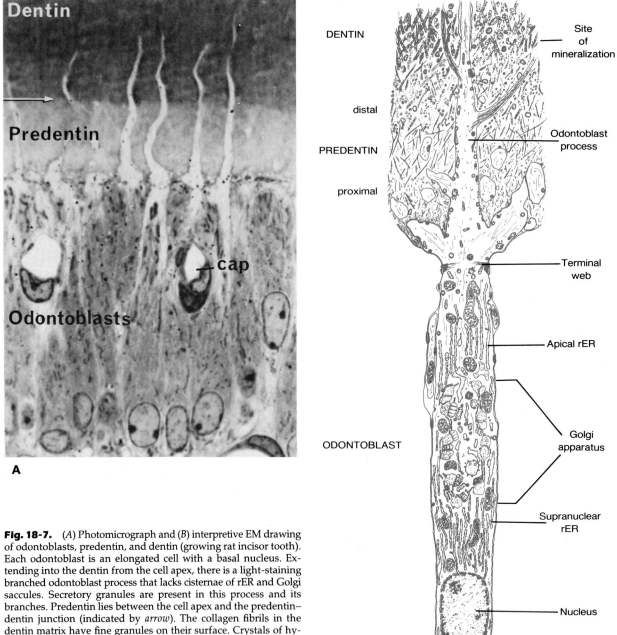

Fig. 18-7. (*A*) Photomicrograph and (*B*) interpretive EM drawing of odontoblasts, predentin, and dentin (growing rat incisor tooth). Each odontoblast is an elongated cell with a basal nucleus. Extending into the dentin from the cell apex, there is a light-staining branched odontoblast process that lacks cisternae of rER and Golgi saccules. Secretory granules are present in this process and its branches. Predentin lies between the cell apex and the predentin–dentin junction (indicated by *arrow*). The collagen fibrils in the dentin matrix have fine granules on their surface. Crystals of hydroxyapatite are also present in dentin matrix (not shown). (*A*, courtesy of M. Weinstock; *B*, Weinstock M, Leblond CP: J Cell Biol 60:92, 1974)

to reduce the overall dimensions of the pulp cavity. Further details will be given when we consider dental pulp.

Dentin Is Formed as Predentin. Several hours after dentin matrix is formed, it calcifies. A layer of uncalcified dentin matrix, which is known as *predentin,* is therefore found between the apex of odontoblasts and calcified dentin (Fig. 18-7). Hence the base of the odontoblast process is surrounded by predentin matrix. Initially, this consists largely of amorphous ground substance with a few collagen fibrils forming within it (Fig. 18-7B). The collagen fibrils become more tightly packed at the predentin–dentin border (Fig. 18-7B). Once dentin calcifies, its fine structure becomes obscured by hydroxyapatite crystals, but decalcified sections show some granular material on the collagen fibrils.

The process of procollagen synthesis and secretion was described in detail in Chapter 7. Type I collagen accounts for almost 90% of the organic content of dentin matrix. The remainder consists of phosphoprotein with small amounts of glycoprotein and glycosaminoglycan. Phosphoprotein synthesized by odontoblasts is released into predentin but then becomes localized on the dentinal side of the predentin–dentin border where it constitutes the granular material seen on the surface of the collagen fibrils (Weinstock and Leblond). This border represents the calcification front in dentin. Once dentin is calcified, it becomes even harder than bone; hydroxyapatite then accounts for approximately 70% of its wet weight. Dentin is nevertheless not as hard as enamel, which has a mineral content of 96%.

Enamel and Ameloblasts

Enamel is an acellular material that is produced by ameloblasts prior to tooth eruption. It is an extremely hard and brittle substance that, because of its high mineral content, is almost always lost during the decalcification step necessary for the preparation of hematoxylin and eosin (H & E) sections. Nevertheless enamel can be seen to advantage in ground sections of teeth. Such sections disclose that it is made up of distinctive structural units known as *enamel rods* that are also sometimes referred to as *enamel prisms.* However, before describing enamel matrix in further detail, it is necessary to consider briefly the cells that produce it.

For histological study, *ameloblasts* can conveniently be found at the periphery of the crown of the developing unerupted permanent tooth associated with each deciduous tooth. These are tall columnar cells with a basal nucleus and an apical conical projection known as a *Tomes' process* that borders on the enamel matrix (Fig. 18-8). The Tomes' process is the part of the cell that secretes the organic matrix of an enamel rod. Thus each ameloblast produces one enamel rod. At the base of the Tomes' process, there are also a few smaller apical processes (Fig. 18-8) that secrete the organic matrix of the so-called *inter-rod component* of the enamel. These rod and inter-rod constituents of the enamel

nevertheless have the same chemical composition and differ only with respect to the pattern in which their mineral is deposited.

In rat ameloblasts (but not human ameloblasts), most of the mitochondria are basally situated in the cell (Fig. 18-8). The rER extends to just below the apical (distal) terminal web (Fig. 18-8). The prominent Golgi complex and a few associated peripheral cisternae of rER are present above the nucleus (Fig. 18-8). Secretory granules formed from the innermost Golgi saccules collect mainly in the Tomes' process (Fig. 18-8). However, a few secretory granules can also be found in the smaller apical ameloblast processes seen at the base of each Tomes' process (Fig. 18-8). Junctional complexes are situated between ameloblasts at the levels of their two terminal webs, one of which is apical (distal) and the other basal (Fig. 18-8).

Enamel matrix consists of calcium phosphate in the form of *hydroxyapatite* (described in connection with Bone Matrix and Calcification in Chap. 12) in an organic matrix that contains protein and polysaccharide. The secretory proteins of ameloblasts are packaged into secretory granules by the Golgi complex. The content of these granules, primarily a water-binding protein called *amelogenin* together with an acidic glycosylated protein called *enamelin*, is released by exocytosis and becomes part of the gel-like organic matrix of enamel. Calcification occurs relatively rapidly; the first-formed hydroxyapatite crystals appear long, thin, and platelike. Their deposition is accompanied by loss of water and decreased organic content of the matrix. The mineral content of the matrix ultimately reaches 96%, making enamel the hardest material in the body.

Each Tomes' process gives rise to organic rod matrix, and the smaller apical extensions around its base (Fig. 18-8) produce organic inter-rod matrix. Although identical in composition, these two forms of the matrix acquire slightly different arrangements of hydroxyapatite crystals. The orientation of their crystals is illustrated in Figures 18-9 and 18-10; the captions to these figures should be consulted for details.

Fully formed enamel is relatively inert; no cells are associated with it because ameloblasts degenerate after they have formed enamel and the tooth erupts. Thus enamel is incapable of undergoing repair if it is damaged by decay, fracture, or other means. However, there is some exchange of mineral ions between enamel and saliva, and this can effect minimal recalcification at the surface, although this effect is negligible deeper in the enamel.

Relation to Dental Caries (Tooth Decay). Tooth minerals are readily dissolved by acids, so that the acids in food and certain drinks in particular may produce tiny pits and crevices on the surface of enamel. Food debris commonly becomes trapped in such areas and acts as a substrate for acid-producing bacteria. Furthermore, sugar in sweet foods, candy, and beverages also acts as a substrate for these bacteria. Progressive loss of enamel as a result of decalcification by the acids that are produced leads to the formation of dental *cavities.* Unless such cavities are properly filled

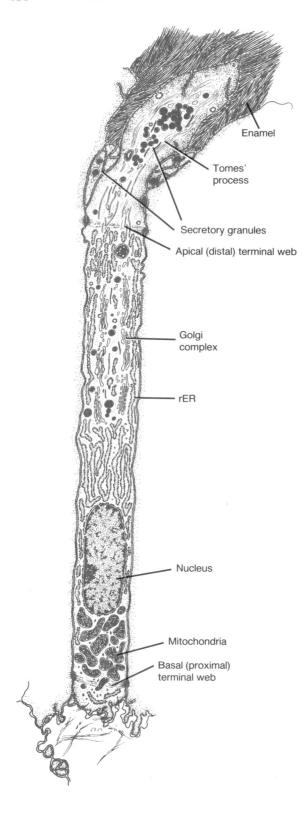

Enamel

Tomes' process

Secretory granules

Apical (distal) terminal web

Golgi complex

rER

Nucleus

Mitochondria

Basal (proximal) terminal web

with a restorative material (a dentist's filling), the carious process reaches the porous dentin and extends along its dentinal tubules to the pulp of the tooth. Pulpal involvement becomes manifested as inflammation that can lead to death of the pulp, as will be explained later in this chapter. Provided a developing cavity remains confined to the enamel, it is painless. When it reaches the dentin, however, it is more likely to be noticed because of increased sensitivity of the tooth. Dental fillings must be used for restoration because there are no cells to produce any new enamel or surface dentin. The topical application of *fluoride* helps to decrease the incidence of dental caries by combining with the hydroxyapatite in enamel, rendering it less susceptible to attack by acids.

Cementum

The cementum covering the root is a calcified, collagen-containing hard tissue that lacks blood vessels but in other respects resembles bone tissue. It is laid down as an organic matrix called *cementoid* that subsequently becomes mineralized. *Cementoblasts,* the cells that form it, closely resemble osteoblasts. The role of cementum, as noted, is to anchor the collagen fibers of the periodontal ligament, securing them to the tooth (Fig. 18-11, *left*). On the upper part of the root, the cementum is *acellular,* but on the lower part, there are cells in its matrix (Fig. 18-4). Like osteocytes, these *cementocytes* occupy lacunae within the calcified matrix and receive their nourishment by way of canaliculi. Cementum is another dental tissue that continues to be formed in adult life, but its deposition tends to be intermittent. As in the case of bone, it grows only by apposition.

Periodontal Ligament

The periodontal ligament consists of wide bundles of collagen fibers that are embedded in amorphous ground substance. These bundles are arranged in the form of a suspensory ligament between the cementum covering the root of the tooth and the bony wall of its alveolus. They are embedded in cementum at one end and in alveolar bone at the other (Fig. 18-11). The turnover rate of the collagen in the periodontal ligament is unusually high and can indicate periodontal deterioration or frequent active remodeling of the ligament. When forces are exerted on the teeth during biting and chewing (*mastication*) or clenching of the

Fig. 18-8. EM drawing of an ameloblast (rat). Mitochondria are located below the basal nucleus in rat ameloblasts but not in human ameloblasts. Cisternae of rER and a tubular Golgi complex are present in the supranuclear region. A large apical projection, the Tomes' process, extends into the newly formed enamel matrix. It contains numerous secretory granules. A few secretory granules are also present in the smaller processes around the base of the Tomes' process. The ameloblast has a basal terminal web as well as an apical terminal web. The latter lies at the base of the Tomes' process. (Courtesy of H. Warshawsky)

Fig. 18-9. Electron micrographs of enamel rods, illustrating the appearance of their electron-dense hydroxyapatite crystals in undecalcified enamel cut in cross section (*large micrograph*) and longitudinal section (*inset*). The upper, rounded part of each fan-shaped area is rod matrix; here the crystals have a predominantly longitudinal orientation (see *inset*). Along the lower (cervical) aspect of each rod, there is a V-shaped ridge of inter-rod matrix; this appears as the handle of the fan-shaped area. In the inter-rod matrix, the crystals become increasingly oblique with increasing distance from the rod matrix (see *inset*). The white line that delineates each fan-shaped area is called the rod sheath; its organic content is higher than that of the rod and inter-rod matrix. (*Inset*) One rod sectioned longitudinally along its midline. Inter-rod matrix extends along its cervical aspect but is not delimited from the rod matrix. It is recognizable only by the gradual change in orientation of its hydroxyapatite crystals. (Courtesy of A. R. Ten Cate)

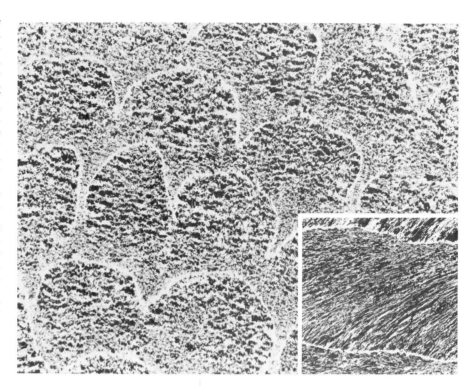

teeth, the collagen fibers in the ligament permit limited tooth movement and bear most of the strain. However, they do so in conjunction with the incompressible fluid-containing ground substance that is present between the fibers, with the whole arrangement working on the same principle as a hydraulic shock absorber. Because the periodontal ligament is also richly supplied with afferent nerve endings that respond to pressure, hard particles in soft foods, for example, can be detected very readily.

Epithelial Attachment

The gingiva forms a collar around each tooth, and when the gums are healthy, the inner surface of this collar is tightly attached to the tooth. Where it borders on the tooth, the gingiva dips down in the form of a shallow crevice called the *gingival sulcus* (Fig. 18-4). This sulcus is normally only 1 mm to 3 mm deep. Along its *epithelial attachment* below the sulcus (Fig. 18-4), the gingival epithelium is

Fig. 18-10. Interpretive drawing of the enamel rods illustrated in Figure 18-9, indicating the orientation of their hydroxyapatite crystals. Alignment of these crystals is more oblique with respect to the rod axis in the inter-rod matrix (*Irm*) than in the rod matrix (*Rm*). In the upper part of a rod (*top right*), it can be seen that the crystals have a predominantly longitudinal orientation. The plane depicted at lower right corresponds to that of the inset in Figure 18-9.

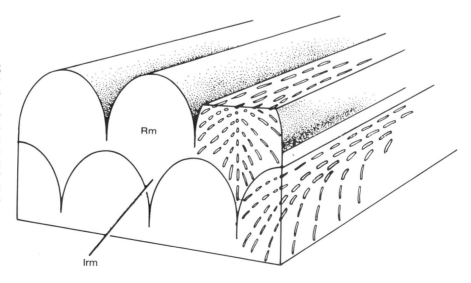

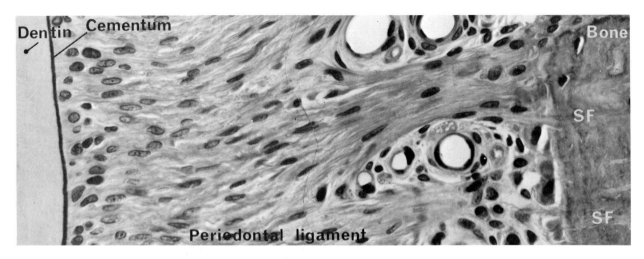

Fig. 18-11.   Photomicrograph of periodontal ligament (rat). From left to right, note the dentin, cementum (acellular), periodontal ligament, and alveolar bone. The collagen fibers of the ligament abut on the cementum at left and extend between blood vessels and reach the alveolar bone. Collagen fibers seen within bone are known as Sharpey's fibers (*SF*). (Courtesy of H. Warshawsky)

tightly adherent to the tooth enamel (or to the cementum if the gums have receded). This attachment is effected by the substantial basement membrane of this type of epithelium together with its associated hemidesmosomes. Nevertheless, this arrangement is vulnerable to disruption, as will be explained in the following section.

Subgingival Accumulation of Calculus Can Result in Periodontal Disease. Each day, the teeth become covered with a coating of *dental plaque.* This is a bacteria-containing film that requires daily removal through brushing because with the ions normally present in the saliva, plaque becomes converted into a strongly adherent calcified material known as *calculus* (L. for pebble). If calculus is allowed to accumulate in the gingival sulcus, it gradually separates the epithelial attachments from the teeth. Once the epithelial seal around the base of the teeth has been disrupted, bacteria gain access to the gingival connective tissue; hence the gingival sulcus is potentially a danger zone. Before long, *periodontal pockets* that are more than 3 mm deep begin to develop down the sides of the teeth, and as these become larger, they harbor anaerobic bacteria that are capable of eliciting inflammation of the gums (*gingivitis*) or inflammation of all the periodontal tissues (*periodontitis*). This latter condition is accompanied by immune responses to bacterial and other antigens, the combined effect of which is that the teeth become loosened because of the resorption of alveolar bone. More teeth are lost as a result of such *periodontal disease* than through any other cause. In recent years, however, it has become feasible to postpone or avoid such loss of teeth from periodontitis through a combined approach of oral surgery to remove the pockets, strict plaque control, and regular removal of recurring subgingival calculus. In discussing periodontitis, it should also be mentioned that a lymphokine called *osteoclast-activating factor* (OAF) made by T- and B-lymphocytes induces osteoclastic bone resorption (see Chap. 10 under Lymphokines); it seems likely that this factor is involved in mediating alveolar bone resorption.

Pulp

The dental pulp that occupies the pulp chamber and the root canal is a soft loose connective tissue that contains some collagen fibers, amorphous ground substance, and fibroblasts. However, it tends to have a mesenchymal appearance because many of its cells are stellate and are interconnected by long cytoplasmic extensions (Fig. 18-12, *left*). Pulp is highly vascular; its vessels enter by way of the apical foramen. However, the vessels in the pulp have very thin walls (Fig. 18-12, *left*). This, of course, renders the tissue very susceptible to changes in hydrostatic pressure because the walls of the pulp chamber are totally rigid. Even a fairly mild inflammatory edema can cause compression of these vessels and resulting necrosis of the pulp. In some cases of pulp death, the pulp can be surgically removed and the space it occupied can be filled with an inert material. Such a tooth is commonly known as a "dead" tooth.

The pulp is also richly supplied with nerves, and nerve endings are present in association with the odontoblast layer between the pulp and the dentin. There are reports of nerve fibers entering some of the dentinal tubules, but they do not extend the full length of these tubules.

Dentin Progressively Encroaches on the Pulp Cavity. The dentin that forms during tooth development is known as *primary dentin.* In addition, *secondary dentin* is gradually deposited during adult life on the dentinal surface bordering on the pulp, which is the only site where odontoblasts are present. Furthermore, *tertiary (reparative) dentin* can be produced at any time during life to compensate for the loss of enamel and dentin that occurs in dental caries or that results from restorative procedures such as filling a cavity.

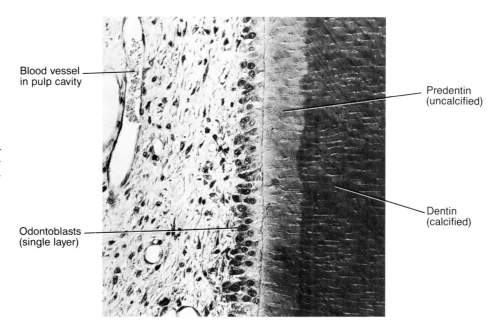

Blood vessel in pulp cavity

Predentin (uncalcified)

Dentin (calcified)

Odontoblasts (single layer)

Fig. 18-12. Photomicrograph of dental pulp and forming dentin (child's tooth). (Courtesy of E. Freeman)

Under certain conditions, it can form quite rapidly (under a cavity, for example), in which case it appears more irregular. The deposition of secondary dentin slowly reduces the size of the pulp chamber and root canal; hence these are much smaller in older people. The microscopic appearance of the pulp also changes in that it becomes less cellular and more fibrous.

SALIVARY GLANDS

The major salivary glands are the paired *parotid, submandibular* (occasionally referred to as the *submaxillary*), and *sublingual glands.*

Parotid Glands

The parotid glands are the largest of the salivary glands. On each side of the mandible, they lie packed into the space between the mastoid process and the ramus of the mandible, and they extend below the zygomatic arch. The orifices of their ducts lie on the mucosal surface of the cheeks opposite the second molars of the upper jaw. Each parotid is enclosed within a strong fibrous capsule and is a compound tubuloalveolar gland of the *serous* type (Fig. 18-13). The secretory units and general features of such glands were described under Exocrine Glands in Chapter 6 and are illustrated in Figures 6-16 and 6-20. In addition to the usual features seen in a gland of this type, the parotid is characterized by having *many prominent intralobular ducts*

(Fig. 18-13). Also, accumulations of fat cells are commonly present in the connective tissue septa of this gland. The secretory granules are believed to contain mucus in addition to enzymes.

Submandibular Glands

The submandibular glands lie against the inner aspect of the body of the mandible, with their ducts opening into the floor of the oral cavity posterior to the incisor teeth of the lower jaw, adjacent to the lingual frenulum. They are compound alveolar or tubuloalveolar glands of the *mixed* type, and the majority of their secretory units are *serous*. Generally, mucous units are also present, but most of these units are capped with serous demilunes (see Fig. 6-17). As in the parotid glands, the submandibular glands have a well-developed capsule and a fairly prominent duct system.

Sublingual Glands

Unlike the other salivary glands, the sublingual glands are not very strongly encapsulated. They lie near the midline, below the mucous membrane of the floor of the mouth, and their several ducts open along a line posterior to the orifices of the submandibular ducts. They are compound tubuloalveolar glands of the *mixed* type, but they differ from the submandibular glands in that most of their secretory units are generally *mucous* secretory units, some with *serous demilunes*. Also, the septa tend to be more prominent than in the parotid or submandibular glands.

Serous secretory units   Fat cells   Intralobular ducts

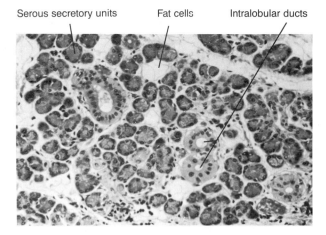

Fig. 18-13.   Photomicrograph of parotid gland, showing its serous secretory units and prominent intralobular ducts.

Salivary Secretion

The mixed secretion of the major and also the numerous minor salivary glands is known as *saliva*. It contains the enzyme *salivary amylase (ptyalin)*, mucus, and also some cellular and bacterial debris and leukocytes. Some of its functions are as follows:

1. It lubricates and moistens the oral mucosa and lips. Such moistening needs to be continuous because of evaporation and the swallowing of saliva.
2. It rinses the oral cavity of food particles and cellular debris.
3. It moistens ingested food so that this acquires a semisolid consistency and can be swallowed easily. This also allows food to be tasted.
4. It buffers the natural acidity of the oral cavity.
5. It contains secretory IgA, which helps to protect against microbial attachment and invasion of the mucosa.
6. It contains at least one digestive enzyme, but the extent to which such enzymes participate in the digestive process is extremely limited. Thus salivary amylase can convert starch to maltose, but food is not retained in the mouth and esophagus long enough for any significant digestion to occur there.

Salivary secretion is generally a reflex response to some stimulus such as the smell or taste of food. It is stimulated by efferent impulses from the autonomic nervous system. Parasympathetic stimulation causes a copious watery secretion to be produced, whereas sympathetic stimulation (which is often due to stress) causes smaller amounts of a thick viscid secretion to be formed, which, as nervous lecturers and dental patients know, can result in the mouth feeling as if it were drying up. (An autonomic nerve ending in a parotid gland is illustrated in Figure 14-44). The activities of both the secretory cells and their surrounding myoepithelial cells are under autonomic control.

PALATE AND PHARYNX

Palate

The roof of the oral cavity has to be strong enough to withstand the pressure of the tongue during mastication and the swallowing of food. It is therefore lined with a mucous membrane that is strongly bound by its lamina propria to the periosteum of the overlying palatine bones and maxillae. Its tough epithelial lining is stratified squamous keratinizing epithelium. Together, these various components constitute the *hard palate* (Fig. 18-1). Along the midline, there is a ridge of bone to which the epithelium is attached by a very thin lamina propria. This ridge is called the *raphe*. Low transverse rugae with connective tissue cores extend across the hard palate from the raphe. Laterally, the mucous membrane is not as evenly adherent to the bony roof; here it is attached by strong bundles of connective tissue that are separated anteriorly by adipose tissue and posteriorly by glands.

Extending posteriorly from the hard palate is the *soft palate* (Fig. 18-1). Not pressed on by the tongue, this part of the palate has to be strong and movable so that it can be drawn upward during swallowing. This action closes off the nasopharynx and prevents food from being pushed up into the nasal cavities. The soft palate therefore contains skeletal muscle, and its strong connective tissue is arranged as in an aponeurosis. Posteriorly, the mucous membrane of the soft palate becomes continuous with that of the nasopharynx and oropharynx. Superiorly, the soft palate is covered with stratified squamous or pseudostratified ciliated columnar epithelium. The lamina propria below this contains a few glands and has the form of an aponeurosis near the hard palate. In the more posterior part of the soft palate, there is a central muscular layer. The inferior surface of the soft palate is covered with stratified squamous nonkeratinizing epithelium that is supported by a thick lamina propria containing many glands.

Pharynx

The pharynx serves as a shared passageway for both the respiratory and digestive tracts. During nose breathing, it conducts air from the nasal cavities to the larynx and also to the auditory (eustachian) tubes (see Fig. 20-1). It also conveys food from the oral cavity to the esophagus, into which it opens (Fig. 18-1). Furthermore, because the pharynx is common to both the respiratory and the digestive tracts, it is possible to breathe through the mouth and, when necessary, to be fed by way of a tube through the nose.

The pharynx is made up of three parts. The *nasopharynx*, which lies above the level of the soft palate, is lined with pseudostratified ciliated columnar epithelium, as are the nasal cavities. The posterior limit of the oral cavity is indicated by the glossopalatine arches, and the part of the

Lymphatic nodule with
germinal center

Primary
crypt

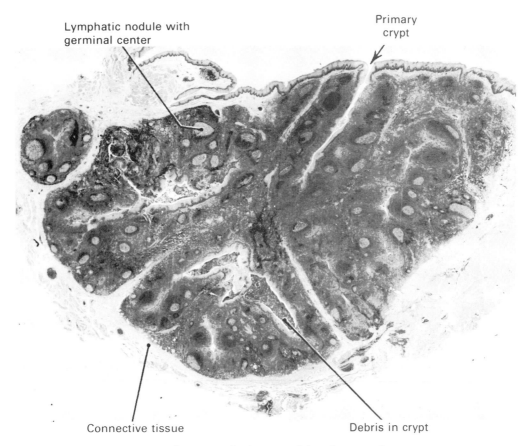

Connective tissue

Debris in crypt

Fig. 18-14. Photomicrograph of a section of palatine tonsil (very low power).

pharynx posterior to these arches is called the *oropharynx* (Fig. 18-1). The *laryngeal pharynx* continues on from the oropharynx, from below the level of the hyoid bone to the esophagus (Fig. 18-1). Like the oral cavity, both the oropharynx and the laryngeal pharynx are lined with stratified squamous nonkeratinizing epithelium.

The lamina propria supporting the epithelial lining is a fairly dense fibroelastic connective tissue with many elastic fibers as well as collagen fibers. External to this connective tissue layer lie the longitudinal and constrictor muscles of the pharynx. Also present under the epithelium of some parts of the pharynx are glands that may extend into the muscle layer.

Pharyngeal and Palatine Tonsils

Along the midline of the posterior wall of the nasopharynx, there is a single *pharyngeal tonsil* that is made up of a group of lymphatic nodules and loose lymphatic tissue in intimate association with the pseudostratified columnar epithelial lining of the nasopharynx. Far more prominent than the pharyngeal and lingual tonsils, however, are the two *palatine* tonsils. These ovoid masses of lymphatic tissue thicken the lamina propria of the mucous membrane that extends

between the glossopalatine and the pharyngopalatine arches. The epithelium here is of the stratified squamous nonkeratinizing type and dips into the underlying lymphatic tissue to form 10 to 20 *primary crypts* in each palatine tonsil (Fig. 18-14). The epithelial lining of the primary crypts may extend into the adjacent lymphatic tissue to form secondary crypts. Either primary or secondary crypts may extend deeply enough to reach the outer limits of the tonsil.

The lymphatic tissue in the tonsil mostly lies directly below the epithelium and extends down along the sides of the crypts. It consists of lymphatic nodules, with or without germinal centers, that may be so close together that they fuse, or they may be separated by looser lymphatic tissue. In addition to small lymphocytes, there are generally many plasma cells in this tissue. The small lymphocytes are able to migrate directly through the crypt epithelium.

Strategic positioning of the pharyngeal, palatine, and lingual tonsils at the crossover point between the respiratory tract and the digestive tract increases the likelihood that their lymphocytes will encounter antigens of potentially infective agents against which antibodies should be produced as rapidly as possible. However, such positioning of the tonsils also renders them vulnerable to infections that, in the case of the palatine tonsils, sometimes become

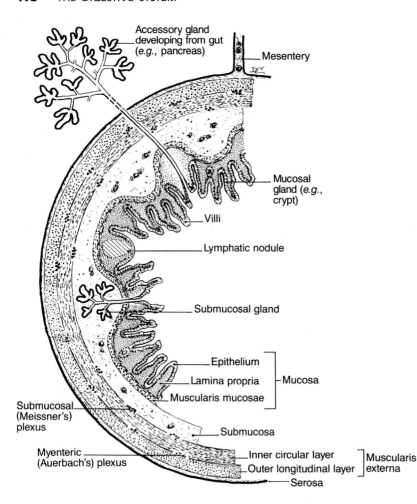

Accessory gland developing from gut (*e.g.,* pancreas)

Mesentery

Mucosal gland (*e.g.,* crypt)

Villi

Lymphatic nodule

Submucosal gland

Epithelium
Lamina propria — Mucosa
Muscularis mucosae

Submucosal (Meissner's) plexus

Submucosa

Myenteric (Auerbach's) plexus

Inner circular layer — Muscularis externa
Outer longitudinal layer

Serosa

Fig. 18-15. Schematic representation of the wall structure of the digestive tract.

sufficiently entrenched to warrant *tonsillectomy* (*i.e.,* their surgical removal). This susceptibility of the palatine tonsils to infections is, in large part, due to the fact that the ducts of their associated mucus-secreting glands do not open into their crypts. Because their crypts are not flushed out as in the lingual tonsil, debris accumulates in them and predisposes them to infection. The nature of tonsillar tissue and the contribution it makes to the immune defenses of the body were considered in Chapter 10 under Lymphatic Nodules.

GENERAL PLAN OF THE DIGESTIVE TRACT

The walls of the remainder of the digestive tract consist of four major layers termed the *mucosa (mucous membrane), submucosa, muscularis externa,* and *serosa* (Fig. 18-15). The main features of these four layers are described in the following sections.

Mucosa (Mucous Membrane)

The mucosa is, in turn, made up of three layers: an *epithelial lining,* a supporting *lamina propria,* and a thin layer of smooth muscle, the *muscularis mucosae* (Fig. 18-15).

Epithelium. The type of epithelium that is present depends on the functions of the part of the tract that it lines. At some sites it is essentially protective (*e.g.,* the stratified squamous epithelium of the esophagus and anus). At other sites it is secretory (*e.g.,* the mucus-secreting epithelium of the stomach) or absorptive (*e.g.,* the columnar epithelium of the small and large intestines). Individual secretory cells may also be scattered throughout the epithelial lining (*e.g.,* the mucus-secreting goblet cells in the intestinal lining). In addition, secretory epithelial cells may be invaginated into the lamina propria in the form of mucosal glands (*e.g.,* in the stomach and the small and large intestines). Submucosal glands (Fig. 18-15, *left*) are also present in the esophagus and duodenum. Finally, glands arising from the lining of the digestive tract may be located outside the walls of the tract itself. The salivary glands, liver, and pancreas are all accessory digestive glands of this type (Fig. 18-15, *upper left*).

Lamina Propria and Its Associated Lymphatic Tissue. The lamina propria supports the epithelium and attaches it to the muscularis mucosae. It also contains many lymphocytes and unencapsulated lymphatic nodules (Fig. 18-15, *left*) that are collectively referred to as the *gut-associated lymphoid tissue* (GALT), the nature and role of which were described in Chapter 10 under Lymphatic Nodules. Such lymphoid tissue is a major source of IgA, a class of immunoglobulins that can be transported into the gut lumen by the mucosal epithelium. (A description of these immunoglobulins may be found in the section on Lymph Nodes in Chap. 10, and their functional role is discussed in the section on Lymphatic Nodules in the same chapter.) In addition, the lamina propria brings fenestrated blood capillaries as well as lymphatic capillaries close to the surface epithelium, particularly within projecting villi of the small intestine (Fig. 18-15). Hence products of digestion do not have to diffuse very far before gaining access to either type of capillary.

Muscularis Mucosae.   This outermost layer of the mucosa typically consists of two thin layers of smooth muscle fibers that are arranged circularly or helically in the inner layer and longitudinally in the outer layer (Fig. 18-15). Its contractile activity permits independent movement and folding of the mucosa, aiding digestion and absorption. Smooth muscle fibers extend from the muscularis mucosae of the small intestine to the tip of each villus; their tonus determines the height of the villi.

Submucosa

The submucosa attaches the mucosa to the muscularis externa. Consisting of loose connective tissue, it conveys larger blood vessels (Fig. 18-15). This layer has a substantial content of elastic fibers and forms the cores of mucosal folds. In the duodenum and esophagus, the submucosa also contains *mucus-secreting glands* (Fig. 18-15, *left*). Deep in the submucosa lies a plexus of autonomic nerve fibers and ganglion cells known as the *submucosal (Meissner's) plexus* (Fig. 18-15, *bottom left*). Many of its mostly unmyelinated fibers are derived from the superior mesenteric plexus (a prevertebral plexus) and represent sympathetic postganglionic fibers. The relatively few ganglion cells in this plexus include interneurons and parasympathetic terminal ganglion cells that synapse with parasympathetic preganglionic fibers derived from the vagus nerve (cranial outflow). The postganglionic fibers that emerge from this plexus supply the smooth muscle cells of the muscularis mucosae and blood vessels and also the secretory cells of the mucosal glands.

Muscularis Externa

The muscularis externa consists of two substantial layers of smooth muscle; the inner one is circular and the outer one longitudinal (Fig. 18-15). However, in both layers, the muscle fibers pursue a somewhat helical path. The tonus of the inner circular layer determines the overall luminal diameter of the bowel. In addition, the muscularis externa undergoes peristaltic contractions that propel the gut contents toward the anus. These peristaltic waves are coordinated by efferent impulses from a second autonomic plexus known as the *myenteric (Auerbach's) plexus* that is situated between the circular and the longitudinal layer of the muscularis externa (Fig. 18-15, *bottom left*). The myenteric plexus contains parasympathetic preganglionic fibers that are derived, for the most part, from the vagus nerve. These fibers synapse with parasympathetic terminal ganglion cells, the postganglionic fibers of which supply the smooth muscle cells. As in the submucosal plexus, sympathetic postganglionic fibers, most of which arise from prevertebral ganglion cells, also contribute to this plexus en route to the muscle cells that they supply. More will be said about the submucosal and myenteric plexuses later in this chapter when we consider gastrointestinal hormones. Parasympathetic stimulation augments tone and peristaltic activity, and sympathetic stimulation has the opposite effect.

Serosa

The outermost layer of the gut wall is a serous membrane known as the *serosa* that consists of loose connective tissue covered by a layer of squamous mesothelium. In regions of the gut that are attached to the adjacent tissues, the connective tissue is not covered by mesothelial cells but merges with the connective tissue associated with the surrounding structures. In this case, it is known as an *adventitia* instead.

Gut *mesenteries* (Fig. 18-15, *top*) are mesothelium-covered serous membranes with a core of loose connective tissue that contains a variable number of fat cells, together with blood vessels, nerves, and lymphatics.

We shall now proceed with the remainder of the digestive tract, the walls of which conform to this general plan.

ESOPHAGUS

The esophagus, which extends from the pharynx to the stomach (Fig. 18-1), is a fairly straight, muscular-walled tube with walls that contain the various layers described above. For protection against coarse-textured foods, it is lined with stratified squamous epithelium. In man and other primates, this epithelium is of the nonkeratinizing type (Fig. 18-16), but in animals that swallow rougher foods, the

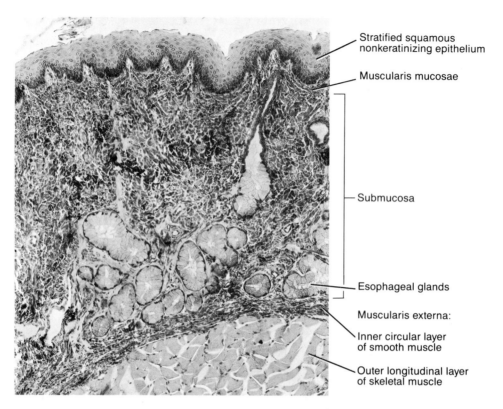

Stratified squamous
nonkeratinizing epithelium

Muscularis mucosae

Submucosa

Esophageal glands

Muscularis externa:

Inner circular layer
of smooth muscle

Outer longitudinal layer
of skeletal muscle

Fig. 18-16. Photomicrograph illustrating the wall structure of the middle third of the esophagus (monkey). (Courtesy of C. P. Leblond)

keratinized type is present. The epithelium undergoes continuous renewal. Mitosis occurs in the lowermost two or three layers, and as the progeny cells become displaced toward the lumen, they lose their proliferative capacity. At the same time, tonofilaments are formed and the cells enlarge. Differentiation is eventually followed by desquamation of the cells from the epithelial surface.

A few mucous glands called *esophageal glands* are scattered through the submucosa (Fig. 18-16). Some glands are also present in the lamina propria in the upper part of the esophagus and near the stomach. Because glands of the latter type resemble the glands in the cardiac portion of the stomach, they are known as *cardiac glands.* However, the amount of mucus secreted at the lower end of the esophagus is not enough to prevent mucosal damage if the gastric contents become regurgitated, so this results in heartburn (*pyrosis*).

Skeletal muscle continues on from the pharynx as the muscularis externa of the upper third of the esophagus. Smooth muscle then begins to take the place of skeletal muscle in the middle third of the esophagus, and the muscularis externa of the lower third contains only smooth muscle. The section in Figure 18-16, taken from the middle third of the esophagus, shows both kinds of muscle in the muscularis externa. The muscularis externa is innervated mainly by parasympathetic fibers from the vagi. Hence swallowing is partly an involuntary reflex action that is set in motion by stimulation of afferent endings distributed chiefly in the posterior wall of the pharynx. Swallowing can be initiated voluntarily, but its continuation from the pharynx onward is involuntary and automatically regulated by the deglutition (swallowing) center in the medulla and lower pons. Where the esophagus joins the stomach, its muscularis externa remains unthickened even though it constitutes the lower esophageal (gastroesophageal) sphincter. Finally, the esophagus possesses an adventitia instead of a serosa. This consists of loose connective tissue that binds it to the surrounding structures.

STOMACH

Between the esophagus and the duodenum lies the stomach, the most extensible part of the digestive tract (Fig. 18-1). Its function as a food reservoir is facilitated by distensibility of its walls and retention of its contents by the prominent pyloric sphincter at its outlet. Its mucosal glands secrete a *gastric juice* that contains hydrochloric acid, three enzymes, and mucus. Of the three enzymes, *pepsin* is the most important. This is a proteolytic enzyme that is secreted

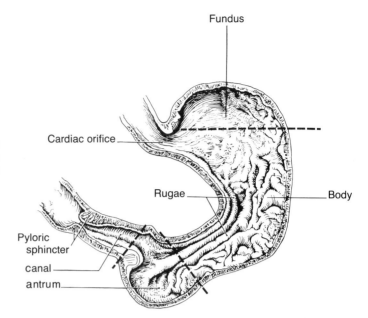

Fig. 18-17. Diagrammatic drawing of the main features of the stomach (internal aspect of posterior wall). (Moore KL: Clinically Oriented Anatomy. Baltimore, Williams & Wilkins, 1980; adapted with permission)

in the form of a precursor called *pepsinogen.* In the acidic environment of the stomach, pepsinogen is converted to pepsin, which thereupon begins the digestion of proteins. The other two enzymes are *rennin,* which curdles milk, and *lipase,* which splits fats, However, this last action is not extensive in the stomach.

The combination of hydrochloric acid and pepsin in the gastric secretion is sufficient to kill living cells in uncooked food (fruit, oysters, etc.), yet the stomach ulcerates only under pathological conditions. Obviously, there are protective mechanisms operating in the gastric mucosa that normally can prevent this from happening. To some extent, the exceptionally thick coating of viscid mucus that is secreted by the stomach's surface epithelial cells has a protective function, but this cannot prevent toxic damage. Another form of protection is that the epithelial lining is renewed every 2 to 6 days, but again this is not fast enough to compensate for acute toxic damage. More will be said about this later in this chapter when we discuss cell renewal in the acid-producing part of the stomach.

The stomach acts as an efficient mixer by virtue of its muscular contractions. Its contents, diluted with gastric juice, become semifluid and are called *chyme.* The stomach also produces an intrinsic factor that is necessary for the absorption of vitamin B_{12}, and it serves to some extent as an absorptive organ, but its function in this respect is more or less limited to the absorption of water, salts, alcohol, and certain drugs.

The parts of the stomach are illustrated in Figure 18-17. Anatomically, the fundus is that part lying above a horizontal line drawn through the lower end of the esophagus. Approximately two thirds of the remainder is called the *body of the stomach.* The distal part of the organ comprises

the *pyloric antrum, pyloric canal,* and *pylorus.* Together, these last three portions are often collectively referred to as the *pylorus* or *pyloric region.* Histologically, three regions are described: (1) the *cardiac* region, which surrounds the cardiac orifice; (2) the acid-secreting *body* or *fundic* region, which includes the anatomical body and fundus; and (3) the *pyloric* region, which is comprised of antrum, canal, and pyloric sphincter.

If an empty (contracted) stomach is opened, its mucous membrane shows branching folds, most of which are longitudinal; these folds are termed *rugae.* Their cores consist of submucosa (Fig. 18-18A). When the stomach is full, however, the rugae are almost completely "ironed out."

The relatively thick gastric mucosa contains numerous simple tubular glands, which will be described in the following section. In some sites, the muscularis mucosae is made up of three layers instead of the usual two. There are no glands in the submucosa except in the pyloric part that is adjacent to the duodenum. The muscularis externa also consists of three layers instead of two; the innermost layer is oblique, the middle layer is circular, and the outermost layer is longitudinal. A serosa is present on the outer surface of the stomach.

Mucosal Epithelium, Pits, and Glands

Whereas in the small and large intestines, goblet cells alternate with absorptive columnar cells that do not produce mucus, the epithelium that lines the stomach is made up of *mucous columnar cells* that are alike. The apical part of these surface epithelial cells is filled with secretory vesicles that contain mucus. Opening onto the surface epithelium are *gastric pits* or *foveolae* that descend into the lamina

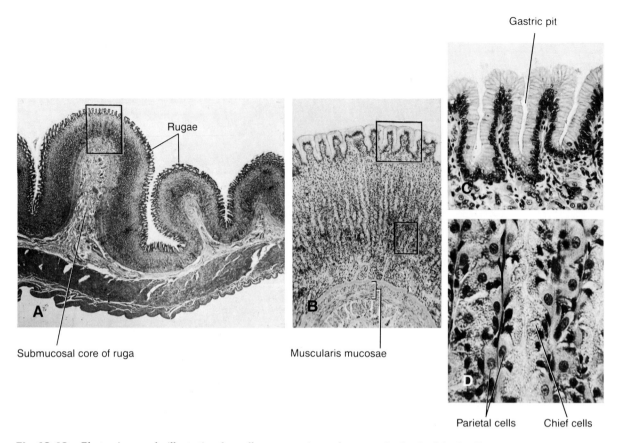

Fig. 18-18.   Photomicrographs illustrating the wall structure, pits, and zymogenic glands of the fundic region of the stomach at increasing magnifications. *B* shows the boxed-in area in *A,* and *C* and *D* show the upper and lower boxed-in areas in *B.*

propria and become continuous with the upper ends of the gastric glands. Two or three glands deliver gastric juice into each gastric pit, which is lined with the same kind of mucus-secreting epithelium as the remainder of the stomach surface. The *gastric glands,* however, differ in different regions of the stomach and are accordingly subdivided into *cardiac, fundic,* and *pyloric glands.* The lamina propria contains smooth muscle fibers, blood vessels, lymphatics, and the usual connective tissue components.

Mucous and Mucoparietal Glands Are Present in the Cardiac Region.   The region that borders on the gastroesophageal junction is characterized by having small *mucous glands* composed of mucus-secreting cells with pale-staining cytoplasm. However, some of these glands, described as *mucoparietal glands,* also contain a variable number of acid-producing parietal cells (which will be described in the following section).

Zymogenic Glands Are Present in the Fundic Region. *Zymogenic glands* produce most of the hydrochloric acid and enzymes that are secreted in the stomach; they also produce some of the mucus. In the body of the stomach,

the glands extending from the pits to the muscularis mucosae appear fairly long in proportion to the pits. Some of these glands branch as they approach the muscularis mucosae (see Fig. 18-20). Each gland is made up of a deep part called its *base,* a middle part known as its *neck,* and an upper part termed its *isthmus* (Fig. 18-19). The isthmus is continuous with a pit. It should be noted that *pits* are not part of glands; they are small depressions of the surface that are lined with surface epithelial cells.

The *isthmus* of a zymogenic gland contains *surface epithelial cells* and *parietal (oxyntic) cells.* Along the sides of the pits, the surface epithelial cells have a substantial content of apical mucus. Deep down in the pits, their mucus content is not as great, and in the isthmus, they contain relatively few vesicles of mucus. Scattered between these cells are large and typically rounded *parietal cells* (Figs. 18-19 and 18-20). These have a spherical and generally central nucleus; their fine structure and functions are considered in the next section.

The *neck* of a zymogenic gland is made up of *mucous neck cells* interspersed with *parietal cells* (Fig. 18-19). The

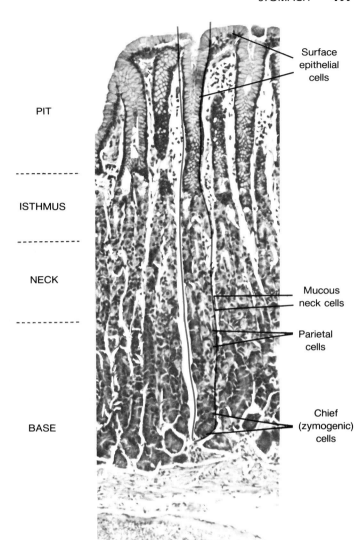

PIT

ISTHMUS

NECK

BASE

Surface
epithelial
cells

Mucous
neck cells

Parietal
cells

Chief
(zymogenic)
cells

Fig. 18-19. Photomicrograph of gastric pits and zymogenic glands in the fundic region of the stomach.

nucleus of a mucous neck cell often appears pressed against the base of the cell by an abundant cytoplasmic content of mucus.

The *base* of a zymogenic gland contains mostly *chief (zymogenic) cells.* The basal cytoplasm of these cells is basophilic, and their apical cytoplasm may appear granular when they are well fixed. They produce the enzymes of the gastric secretion. Scattered among the chief cells are *parietal cells* (Fig. 18-19). These produce the hydrochloric acid. The other types of cells produce only mucus.

Parietal (Oxyntic) Cells.   With the EM, it can be seen that each parietal cell has a branching *canaliculus* extending into it from its apex (Fig. 18-21). This canaliculus delivers the cell's secretion to the lumen of a gastric gland. In addition to intracellular canaliculi, intercellular canaliculi can exist between adjacent parietal cells. A prominent feature

of the intracellular canaliculus is the numerous microvilli that project into it (Fig. 18-21). There are also tubular invaginations between the bases of the microvilli. It has been suggested that such invaginations might evert to become microvilli and vice versa, depending on the level of secretory activity. The relatively small amount of cytoplasm is tightly packed with mitochondria (Fig. 18-21). There are also a few ribosomes, a small amount of rER, and a small Golgi apparatus.

The use of indicators has shown that the cytoplasm of a parietal cell has a normal pH. However, the canaliculi have a pH of 0.8, which, of course, is extremely acidic. The enzyme carbonic anhydrase, which catalyzes the formation of carbonic acid, is abundant in parietal cells.

A currently favored hypothesis of how the parietal cell produces acid is that hydrogen ions from carbonic acid are transported, by an active transport mechanism, through the membrane that lines

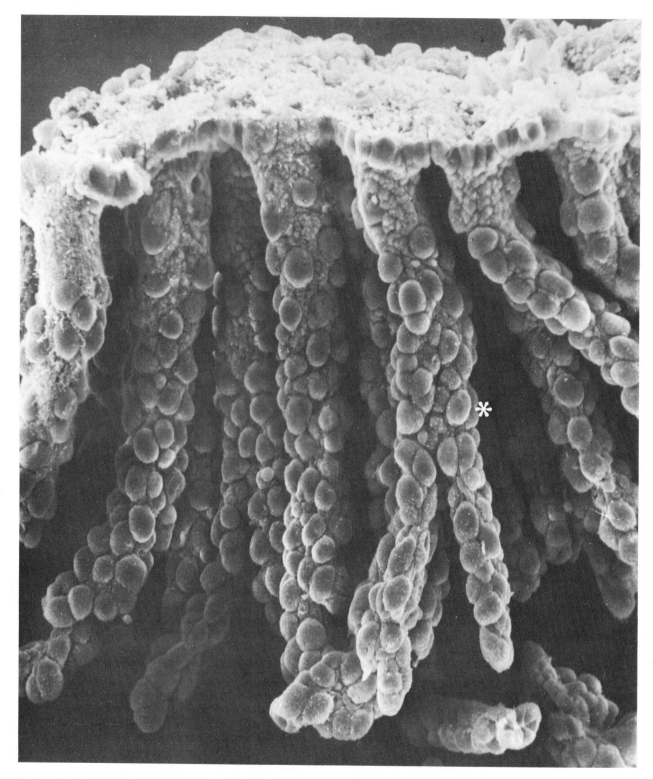

Fig. 18-20.   Scanning electron micrograph (×400) of gastric pits and glands isolated from the fundic region of the stomach (mouse). The large bulging cells on these glands (indicated by *asterisk*) are parietal cells. Note that this particular gland branches at its base. (Courtesy of J. Magney and S. Erlandsen)

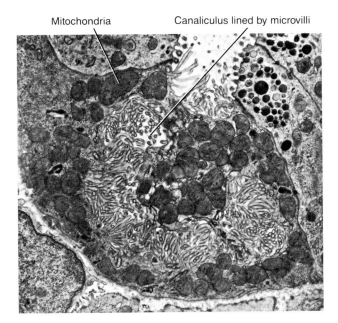

Mitochondria   Canaliculus lined by microvilli

Fig. 18-21. Electron micrograph (×9500) of a parietal cell (bat). The intracellular canaliculus is filled with numerous long microvilli, and these also project from the surface of the cell. The other cells seen at upper right are mucous neck cells, which are characterized by having mucus globules in their apical cytoplasm and short microvilli on their apical surface. (Courtesy of S. Ito, R. Winchester, and D. Fawcett)

the tubular invaginations and covers the microvilli. The bicarbonate ions that are also produced as a result of dissociation of carbonic acid diffuse from the remainder of the cell membrane into the interstitial space and eventually into the bloodstream. Their presence in the interstitial space of the mucosa is thought to provide protection against any leakage of hydrogen ions that may occur through the mucosal epithelium. Also, the mucus coating the inner surface of the stomach provides an unstirred layer that retards the mixing of intraluminal hydrogen ions with mucosal bicarbonate (for further information, see Carter). At the same time that the hydrogen ions are being secreted, chloride ions are transported through the canalicular membrane, accompanied initially by potassium ions that are later retrieved in exhange for hydrogen ions through the activity of a cell membrane-associated H^+-K^+ ATPase.

Besides producing hydrochloric acid, parietal cells secrete *intrinsic factor*, a glycoprotein that is necessary for the absorption of vitamin B_{12} from the small intestine. Adequate amounts of this vitamin are required for normal levels of erythropoiesis in myeloid tissue, and a deficiency of it causes *pernicious anemia* (see Chap. 8 under Anemias). Parietal cells have also been reported to contain appreciable quantities of histamine, which is itself a potent stimulus for acid secretion in the stomach.

The other common cell type found in the base of zymogenic glands of the fundic region is the enzyme-secreting chief (zymogenic) cell. At the EM level, chief cells can readily be distinguished from parietal cells by the fact that

they possess abundant rER and secretory vesicles and lack intracellular canaliculi (Fig. 18-22).

Enteroendocrine Cells Play a Key Role in the Regulation of Gastrointestinal Motility. In addition to the cell types described above, gastric glands contain small numbers of gut endocrine cells that secrete gastrointestinal peptide hormones or other hormonelike substances. For example, the *EC (enterochromaffin) cell* produces *serotonin* and also, according to recent work, *endorphin*, a morphinelike substance that was first identified in the brain. This cell, like most other so-called *enteroendocrine* cells, is characterized by the presence of basal secretory granules that discharge their contents into the circulation by way of the lamina propria.

Many types of enteroendocrine cells are now recognized, and further examples will be cited later in this chapter. An unexpected finding that has emerged from the study of their secretory products is that, in many cases, these products serve a dual purpose in the body, acting not only as gastrointestinal hormones but also as neurotransmitters. Hence their information potential is just as valuable for short-range *synaptic* transmission between neurons as it is for long-range (*hormonal*) or shorter range lateral (*paracrine*) communication between cells that are farther apart.

Thus endorphin has opiatelike activity in the central nervous system (CNS) as well as contraction-regulating activity in the digestive tract, and serotonin serves both as a neurotransmitter in the CNS and as a gastrointestinal hormone. In addition, there is evidence that serotonin and many of the gut peptides (including endorphin) act as neurotransmitters in the two nerve plexuses of

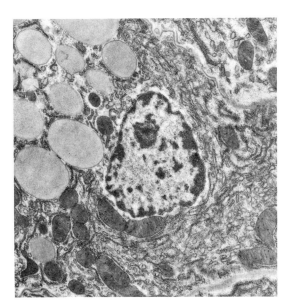

Fig. 18-22. Electron micrograph (×14,000) of part of a chief (zymogenic) cell of a zymogenic gland (stomach of bat). The central nucleus exhibits a prominent nucleolus. Mitochondria are seen at lower left, rER at lower right, and pale-staining zymogen granules at upper left. (Courtesy of S. Ito, R. Winchester, and D. Fawcett)

the gastrointestinal wall. Hence the neurons of these two interconnected plexuses are more than just relay stations for the autonomic nervous system. They are probably responsible for the generation of intrinsic rhythmic activity that takes into account local receptor information about the position, consistency, and composition of the luminal contents of the gut. As well as innervating the smooth muscle layers of the gastrointestinal wall, the neurons of these two plexuses innervate exocrine glands and enteroendocrine cells that produce gastrointestinal hormones, implying that there are complex local interactions that provide the gut with a substantial measure of autonomous intrinsic regulation. A somewhat belated appreciation of the local coordinated activity in the gut wall now makes it easier to understand why the same peptides can behave as gastrointestinal hormones and neurotransmitters of the nervous system.

Epithelial Cell Renewal in the Fundic Region. The surface epithelium of the stomach is believed to undergo renewal every 2 to 6 days as a result of cellular proliferation in the isthmus region of the gastric glands followed by migration of progeny cells up the sides of the pits to replace those lost from the surface. Present evidence suggests that in the region of the isthmus, stem cells and their differentiating progeny give rise to surface epithelial and mucous neck cells and also to the parietal, chief, and enteroendocrine cells that are found lower in the glands. However, the situation is not as clear here as in the pyloric region and in the small intestine, where cell renewal has been studied in more detail.

The Gastric Mucosal Barrier Begins to Restore Itself Within Minutes of Becoming Damaged. Certain substances are notorious for injuring the lining epithelium of the stomach. These damaging agents include aspirin (acetylsalicylic acid), bile salts (which possess detergentlike activity and can become regurgitated into the stomach from the duodenum), and a relatively high concentration of alcohol (the very reason why some people are obliged to take aspirin). Alcohol is not too damaging at the concentrations generally consumed (approximately 10% or less), but at higher concentrations (*e.g.*, straight liquor) it is. Furthermore, the presence of alcohol increases the amount of damage done to the gastric mucosal barrier by salicylates. This damage is sufficient to kill epithelial cells, which are rapidly sloughed off but generally leave the underlying basement membrane fairly intact. Fortunately, the stomach lining possesses a substantial capacity for self-repair because the cells responsible for the high intrinsic rate of renewal of the surface epithelial cells are well protected in the gastric glands. What has recently come to light, however, is the remarkable rapidity with which epithelial continuity is restored, even in the presence of alcohol, following inflicted injury of the gastric epithelium. Signs of re-epithelialization are seen within 5 minutes, and epithelial continuity is essentially regained in 1 hour.

This, of course, rules out cellular proliferation as the underlying mechanism of repair. EM studies indicate that epithelial cells adjacent to the denuded areas extend flat cytoplasmic processes

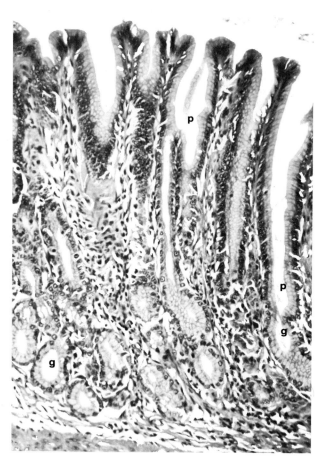

Fig. 18-23. Photomicrograph of the pyloric region of the stomach, showing its gastric pits (*p*) and mucous glands (*g*).

(lamellipodia) and begin to migrate relatively rapidly over the exposed basement membrane until the defect is covered. Microfilaments clearly play an important role in this migration because cytochalasin B inhibits re-epithelialization. The source of these actively migrating cells seems to be viable cells in the bottoms of the gastric pits. The cells deep in the gastric pits and below the orifices of the gastric glands are evidently spared from destruction, probably as a result of focal dilution by fluid exudate that escapes from damaged capillaries in the lamina propria. Because the epithelium has such a high intrinsic rate of renewal, it is not long before there are enough new cells to compensate for the deficit and some to spare in case the same conditions recur. For further details, see Silen and Ito, also Ito and Lacy.

Mucous and Mucoparietal Glands Are Present in the Pyloric Region. The pits in the pyloric region are deeper than those in the fundic region, and their associated glands are correspondingly shorter (compare Figs. 18-18B and 18-23). Furthermore, most of the cells in the pyloric glands are *mucus-secreting cells* that are essentially similar to the mucous neck cells in the fundic region. In this case, however, the mucous secretory granules contain a relatively electron-dense protein core (Fig. 18-24) that contains pep-

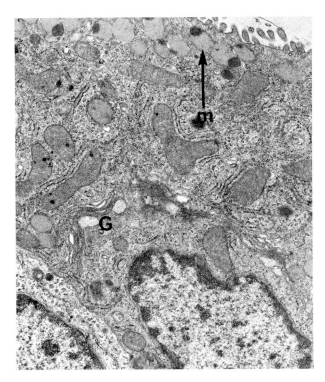

Fig. 18-24. Electron micrograph of a mucus-secreting cell in a pyloric gland of the stomach. Secretory vesicles containing mucus (*m*) are present in the apical cytoplasm of the cell. Their contents are light staining except for a dark-staining core that contains pepsinogen. Note also the abundant mitochondria and prominent Golgi apparatus (*G*) between the nucleus and the apical surface, and the well-developed rER. A portion of the lumen of the gland is seen at top right, with microvilli projecting into it. (Courtesy of C. P. Leblond and E. Lee)

sinogen (Zeitoun et al). Hence their secretory activity results in the release of the precursor of pepsin along with mucus. As in the cardiac region, the pyloric glands also include some mucoparietal glands; these are distributed along the proximal border of the pyloric region, along with the pure mucous glands (Lee et al).

Small numbers of enteroendocrine cells are also present in the pyloric glands and, less commonly, in the lining of the pits into which they open. These cells generally include *EC cells* (as in the fundus) and two other cell types. *D cells* secrete *somatostatin,* a peptide hormone that strongly inhibits the release of many hormones, including growth hormone (somatotrophin), insulin, glucagon, and gastrin, and that therefore participates in the regulation of pancreatic and gastric endocrine secretion. In the stomach, these cells have long cytoplasmic processes that reach other enteroendocrine cells such as G cells. *G (gastrin) cells* produce *gastrin,* a peptide that stimulates secretion of hydrochloric acid by parietal cells. Gastrin is also thought to induce the release of histamine, which is a stimulus for gastric secretion. The secretory granules of G cells are characteristically

pale-staining and have a fairly uniform distribution throughout their cytoplasm (Fig. 18-25).

A few parietal cells are also present in some pyloric glands, but chief (zymogenic) cells are fairly rare.

Epithelial Cell Renewal in the Pyloric Region. As in the fundic region, new pit and gland cells arise from the isthmus region of the pyloric glands, where there are believed to be stem cells. As the pit cells mature, they stop dividing and migrate up the walls of the pit, reaching the surface from which they are subsequently lost. Maturation of the gland cells is accompanied by a decrease in the rates of proliferation and migration. Many of the cells that are generated are extruded, particularly from the neck region, and are lost to the lumen before reaching the base of the gland. Other cells become pyknotic and are phagocytosed somewhere along their migration path. So many cells are lost in this manner that their lifespan can be shorter than a day or longer than 2 months. For further details, see Lee, also Lee and Leblond.

Pyloric Muscularis Externa

The Pyloric Sphincter Regulates Access to the Small Intestine. At the pylorus, the circular middle layer of smooth muscle of the muscularis externa forms a thickened band called the *pyloric sphincter* that encircles the stomach outlet. This raises the mucosa and submucosa so as to constitute a prominent transverse (circular) thickening of the stomach wall (Fig. 18-17). Peristaltic contractions arise near the middle of the stomach and spread toward the pylorus. The pyloric sphincter opens automatically and admits partly digested food when it is sufficiently fluid to enter the small intestine, and at the same time, it retains any food that is still solid and undigested.

SMALL INTESTINE

The small intestine is approximately 20 feet long. Its first foot or so is called the *duodenum,* which pursues a horseshoelike course around the head of the pancreas and then becomes continuous with the *jejunum,* the next part of the small intestine. The last portion is termed the *ileum* (Fig. 18-1).

The main functions of the small intestine are to complete the digestion of food from the stomach, to absorb useful products of digestion into blood capillaries or lymphatic capillaries, and to produce gastrointestinal hormones. Some features that augment its capacity for absorption are described in the following section.

Folds, Villi, and Microvilli Increase the Absorptive Area in the Small Intestine. Absorption from the small intestine is greatly enhanced by the presence of various kinds of folds and mucosal projections that extend into its lumen. Thus beginning a few centimeters from the pylorus, there

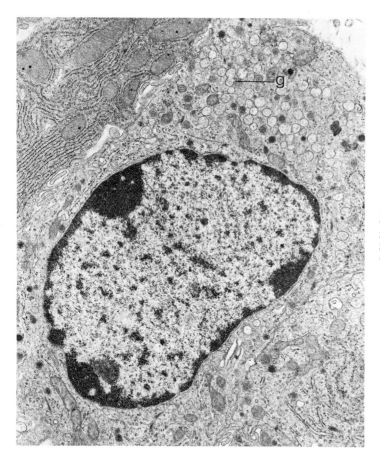

Fig. 18-25. Electron micrograph of a G cell (gastrin cell) in a pyloric gland of the stomach. The secretory granules (*g*) of this type of enteroendocrine cell contain gastrin and appear pale. Some cisternae of rER are seen at bottom right. (Courtesy of C. P. Leblond and E. Lee)

are circular or spiral mucosal folds with submucosal cores (Fig. 18-26). These folds are known as *plicae circulares* (valves of Kerckring), and they are most numerous in the proximal region of the small intestine.

Another adaptation is that the mucosa is raised into *intestinal villi* (Fig. 18-27). These are small leaf-shaped, tongue-shaped, or fingerlike projections with a normal height of 300 μm to 500 μm. Because they are projections of the mucosa, they have cores of lamina propria; muscularis mucosae and submucosa do not extend into villi as they do into the plicae circulares. The villi of the duodenum are broader than elsewhere, and many examples of leaf-shaped ones can be found, particularly in the proximal duodenum (Figs. 18-28*A* and 18-29). The villi in the upper part of the jejunum are more tongue-shaped (Figs. 18-28*B* and 18-30). Farther along the small intestine, most villi are slender and finger shaped (Fig. 18-28*C*). However, these shapes vary in different individuals and in different climates; those described here are typical for temperate climates (Lee and Toner). More consistent are the length and the surface area of the villi, which are both maximal next to the pylorus and minimal at the ileocecal junction.

The height of villi does not depend solely on the amount of absorption they perform. The large size of duodenal villi, for example,

seems to be partly due to factors that arise locally and partly due to factors that come from the stomach and pancreas, because if the duodenum is surgically attached to the terminal ileum, the ileal villi lengthen and the duodenal villi shorten (Altmann and Leblond). In this connection, it should be mentioned that intestinal villi also tend to lengthen following resection of a segment of the bowel, and they shorten when exposure to cytotoxic drugs or ionizing radiation interferes with cell proliferation in the crypts. Growth and recovery following injury is often associated with the replication of existing crypts as a result of their bifurcation, and the increased number of crypts can produce enough cells for new villi to be formed.

Finally, the absorptive surface is further increased by the presence of microvilli on the free surface of the absorptive epithelial cells (see Fig. 18-33).

Digestive Enzymes Come from Three Sets of Glands. To complete the digestion of food, the small intestine requires digestive enzymes and mucus. The digestive enzymes are provided by glands; mucus is provided by glands and innumerable goblet cells. The glands are distributed (1) outside the intestine, but connected to it by ducts, (2) in the submucosa, and (3) in the lamina propria.

The *pancreas* and *liver*, two glands situated outside the small intestine that deliver their secretions into it, will be considered in Chapter 19. Here we are concerned only with

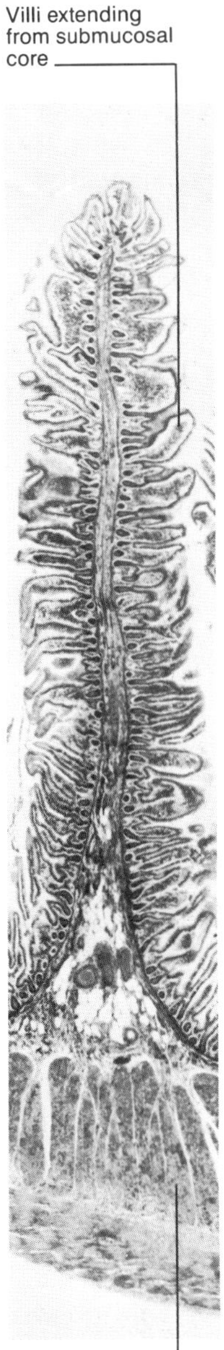

Villi extending
from submucosal
core

Muscularis
externa

Fig. 18-26. Photomicrograph (very low power) of a circular intestinal fold (plica) cut in cross section, from a longitudinal section of jejunum. Such folds have a submucosal core.

their involvement in the digestive process. Their conjoined ducts open into the duodenum approximately 3 inches from the pylorus (Fig. 18-1). The pancreatic exocrine secretion that is delivered into the duodenum at this site is alkaline and therefore helps to neutralize the acidity of the stomach contents. It also contains enzymes that are responsible for the digestion of proteins, carbohydrates, fats, and nucleic acids. These enzymes are active as soon as they reach the

intestinal lumen, degrading proteins to amino acids and starch to sugars. Some sugars (*e.g.*, maltose) must be acted upon by enzymes that are integral membrane glycoproteins of villous epithelial cells and thereby be converted into monosaccharides before they are absorbed. Pancreatic juice also contains a lipase that can break down fats as far as monoglycerides or free fatty acids. The effectiveness of the lipase is increased by the presence of bile, which is the exocrine secretion of the liver.

The second group of glands are those situated in the submucosa. Glands are found in this position in the *duodenum*. Mucus-secreting compound tubular glands, the *glands of Brunner* (Fig. 18-31), are most numerous in its proximal part. Their ducts extend through the muscularis mucosae and open into the intestinal crypts (Fig. 18-31).

The third set of glands are the *intestinal crypts (crypts of Lieberkühn)*. Ranging from 100 μm to 250 μm in length, these simple tubular glands extend from the surface almost to the muscularis mucosae (Figs. 18-15, 18-27, and 18-32). Of the various enzymes secreted by the small intestine, one is exclusively produced within the crypts; this is *lysozyme*, a bactericidal enzyme elaborated by Paneth cells (which are described below). Most of the enzymes produced by the small intestine, however, are associated with the microvilli of the absorptive villous columnar cells, as explained in the following section.

Villous Epithelium. Whereas the surface epithelial cells lining the stomach secrete mucus and are all of one type, the surface epithelial cells covering the villi are of two main types. Most of them are tall cylindrical cells known as *absorptive columnar cells* or *villous columnar cells* that possess a prominent striated (brush) border (labeled in Fig. 18-32*B*,

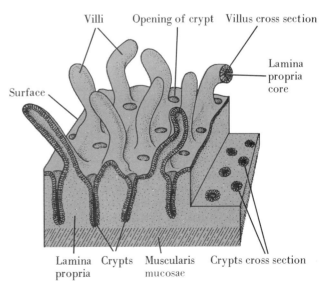

Fig. 18-27. Schematic diagram of the general arrangement of crypts and villi of the small intestine.

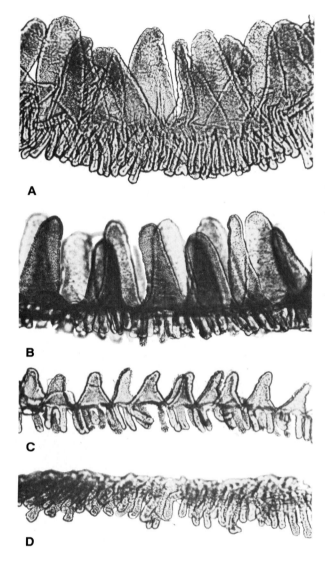

Fig. 18-28. Photomicrographs of intestinal villi and crypts (isolated from a mouse; all taken at the same magnification). (*A*) Duodenum, (*B*) jejunum, (*C*) ileum, and (*D*) colon. The villi (*uppermost*) decrease in height along the length of the small intestine and are completely lacking from the colon. (Bjerknes M, Cheng H: Anat Rec 199:565, 1981)

also described in Chap. 4 and illustrated in Fig. 4-37). This border is composed of a remarkably regular and compact array of microvilli (Fig. 18-33). The other epithelial cells covering the villi are mostly mucus-secreting *goblet cells,* but occasional *enteroendocrine cells* are also present.

The *villous columnar cells* have interdigitating lateral borders and abundant mitochondria but few free ribosomes (Fig. 18-33). Cisternae of rER and Golgi saccules are also prominent in the columnar cells that are situated on the bases of villi. Some of the glycoproteins in the thick cell

coat of the villous columnar cells are hydrolytic enzymes. In addition to alkaline phosphatase, there are enzymes that convert disaccharides into monosaccharides. Thus suckling infants require lactase in order to digest milk lactose, and once they have been weaned onto solid foods, they require the complex of sucrase and isomaltase as well. Continuous renewal of these enzymes compensates for their loss into the intestinal lumen.

The *goblet cells* are of two types. In the common type, the Golgi apparatus is prominent and the apical cytoplasm is distended with mucus-filled secretory vesicles known also as mucus globules (Fig. 18-34*A*). In the less common type, there are small electron-dense granules within these mucus globules (Fig. 18-34*B*).

Crypt Epithelium. In the crypt base there are *Paneth cells,* which are cells that contain relatively large acidophilic secretory granules (Fig. 18-32). Insinuated between the Paneth cells, there are narrow *crypt base columnar cells* (Figs. 18-32 and 18-35). Unlike the villous columnar cells, these crypt base columnar cells have smooth lateral borders. Their cytoplasm contains cisternae of rER, a small Golgi apparatus, and abundant free ribosomes, but few mitochondria (Fig. 18-35). These relatively undifferentiated columnar cells are thought to represent the stem cells from which the other constituent cell types of the intestinal epithelium arise (for the evidence, see Cheng and Leblond). The *Paneth cells,* on the other hand, are differentiated secretory cells with abundant rER, a prominent Golgi complex, and large zymogen granules (Fig. 18-35), the contents of which are discharged into the lumen of the crypt by exocytosis. Paneth cells also contain zinc, but the reason for this is obscure. Nor is the identity of the enzymes they secrete known with certainty, except for the fact that they elaborate lysozyme.

The cells that are present above the crypt base are mostly columnar in shape and show a gradual transition from crypt base columnar cells to villous columnar cells. Next to the Paneth cell region, *oligomucous cells* containing only a few mucus globules are also seen. As these cells produce more mucus globules, they lose their capacity to divide. In the upper half of the crypt, there are typical goblet cells (Fig. 18-34*A*) and some goblet cells with electron-dense granules in their mucus globules (Fig. 18-34*B*). In addition, a few granulated *enteroendocrine cells* are present. These cells produce a variety of gastrointestinal peptide hormones that include *somatostatin, secretin, cholecystokinin-pancreozymin* (CCK-PZ), and the enteric equivalent of pancreatic *glucagon.* EC cells, which were mentioned previously, produce *serotonin* and *endorphin.*

There is also an uncommon type of cell called the *caveolated (tuft) cell* that has irregular tubules termed *caveolae* extending into its cytoplasm. Polyplike projections on the walls of the caveolae detach as small spheres and eventually emerge to join the chyme. This type of cell also has a distinctive tuft of long thick microvilli with long bundles of filaments extending from their cores deep

(*Text continues on p. 508.*)

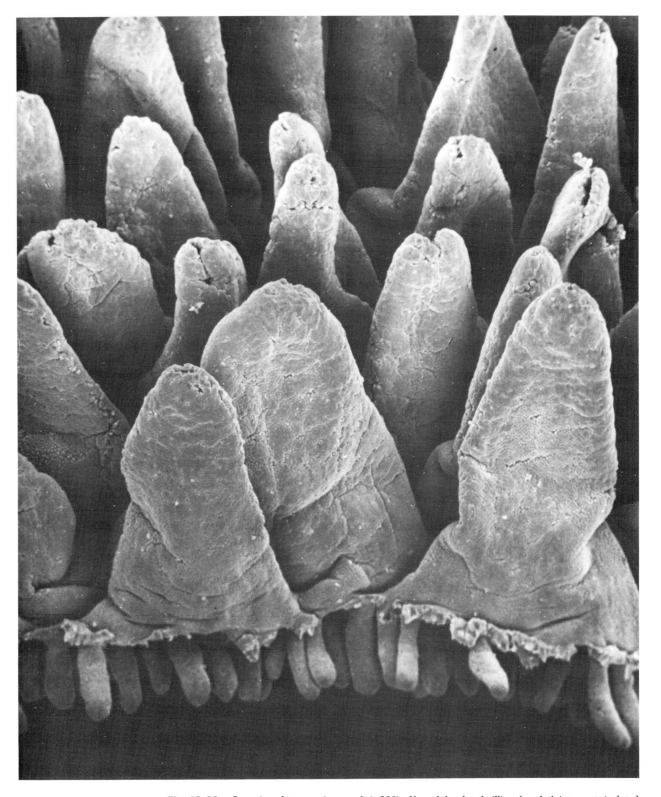

Fig. 18-29.   Scanning electron micrograph (×200) of broad duodenal villi and underlying crypts isolated from the duodenum (mouse). (Courtesy of J. Magney and S. Erlandsen)

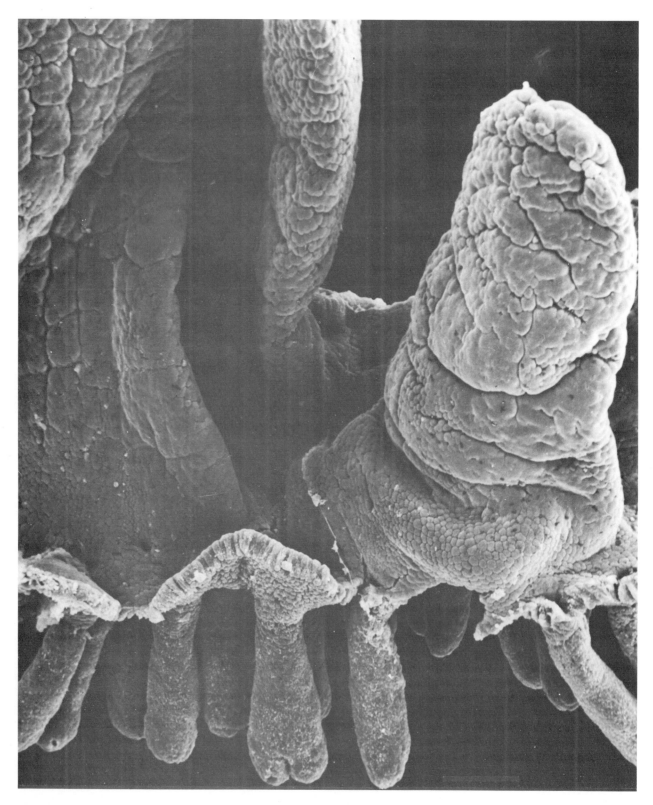

Fig. 18-30. Scanning electron micrograph (×300) of a jejunal villus and crypts isolated from the jejunum (mouse). A villus is seen projecting up at right; crypts, one of which is showing a bifurcation at its base, are seen at lower left. (Courtesy of J. Magney and S. Erlandsen)

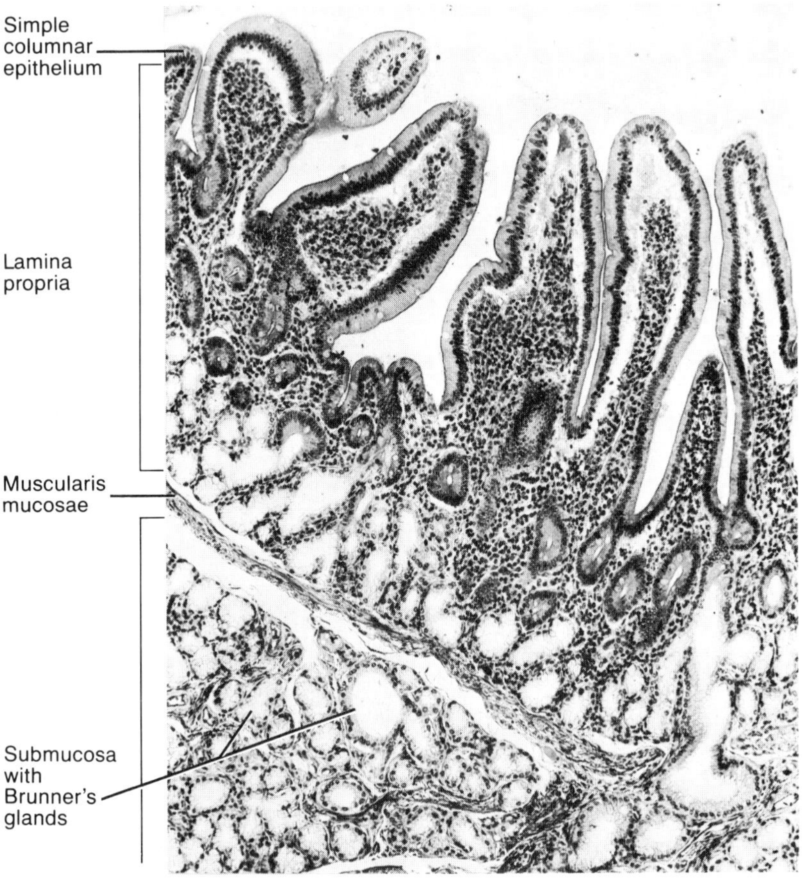

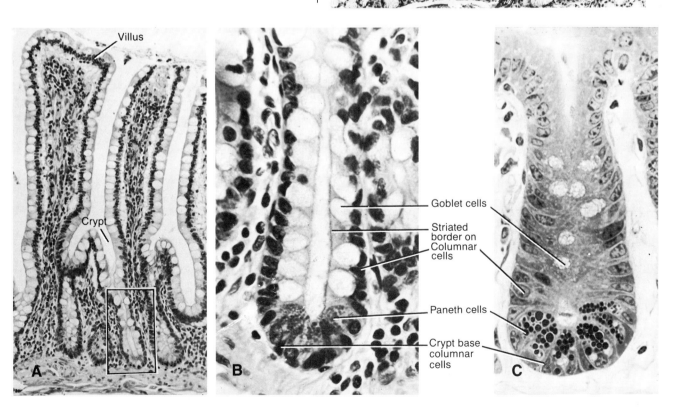

Simple
columnar
epithelium

Lamina
propria

Fig. 18-31. Photomicrograph illustrating part of the wall structure of the duodenum. Mucus-secreting glands are present in the submucosa. They extend through the muscularis mucosae (*bottom right*) and open into the crypts. The simple columnar epithelium also contains goblet cells (discernible on the second villus from the *left*). (Courtesy of C. P. Leblond)

Muscularis
mucosae

Submucosa
with
Brunner's
glands

Villus

Crypt

A

Goblet cells

Striated
border on
Columnar
cells

B

Paneth cells

Crypt base
columnar
cells

C

Fig. 18-32. (*A*) Photomicrograph showing intestinal crypts and villi cut in longitudinal section (small intestine of child). (*B*) High-power view of crypt. (*C*) Component cell types in crypt base (mouse small intestine). *A* and *B* are H & E sections; *C* is a semithin section stained with iron hematoxylin and safranin O. (*C*, courtesy of H. Cheng, J. Merzel, and C. P. Leblond)

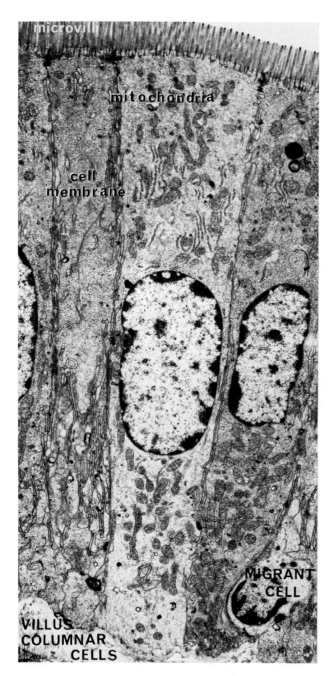

Fig. 18-33. Electron micrograph showing at middle a villus columnar cell of the small intestine (mouse). This tall cylindrical cell has numerous microvilli along its luminal border and complex lateral interdigitations (well seen at *left*, particularly in the columnar cell showing no nucleus). A few cisternae of rER are seen between mitochondria in the supranuclear region of the cell. (Courtesy of H. Cheng and C. P. Leblond)

into their cytoplasm. Although caveolated cells are rare, they can be found in both the crypts and the villi of the small intestine and they are also present in the stomach and the large intestine (Nabeyama and Leblond). Their role remains undetermined.

Mention should also be made of migrating cells found within the epithelium. These include large numbers of intraepithelial *lymphocytes* (which can represent as much as 30% of the cell population of the epithelial layer) as well as some other kinds of leukocytes. In addition, there is a type of cell known as the *globule leukocyte* that is present in the epithelia of normal and, more commonly, of parasite-infested individuals. The globule leukocyte is characterized by having large metachromatic inclusions, but its origin and significance are unclear.

Epithelial Cell Renewal in the Small Intestine.   Columnar cells dividing in the crypts reach the villous surface within 1 day. In 2 to 3 days, they reach the villous tips and are lost into the intestinal lumen. In the mouse, the intestinal epithelium is renewed every third day; in man, this turnover is believed to occur every 3 to 5 days.

The movement of cells out of the crypts is largely a matter of displacement due to proliferation deep in the crypts. However, the migration of villous columnar cells up the villi is at least partly a result of active cell motility because if cell proliferation is blocked, cells continue to leave the crypts and ascend the villi.

Goblet cells also arise in the crypts. Mitosis occurs in the oligomucous cells mentioned above, and these later become goblet cells that migrate from crypts to villi at the same rate as the columnar cells to which they are attached by junctional complexes. Enteroendocrine cells are renewed at approximately the same rate as the other cells (Ferreira and Leblond), and they are similarly attached to them by junctional complexes. Finally, we might also mention that enteroendocrine cells can give rise to small tumors called *carcinoids* that are not uncommon in the appendix.

Other Layers in the Intestinal Wall.   The cores of villi are composed of lamina propria that consists of loose connective tissue with many reticular fibers. Commonly, small lymphocytes, plasma cells, and eosinophils are also present. Smooth muscle fibers extend along the axis of each villus from the muscularis mucosae, usually around a prominent central lymphatic capillary known as a *lacteal* that ends blindly near the tip of the villus. Rhythmic or intermittent contractions of the smooth muscle fibers in the villus are thought to promote the drainage of lymph from the lacteal. A single branch of a submucosal artery and nerve fibers from the submucosal plexus penetrate the muscularis mucosae to supply each villus.

Solitary lymphatic nodules are very common in the walls of the small intestine, especially that of the ileum (Fig. 18-36). They are either confined to the lamina propria or extend through the muscularis mucosae into the submucosa (Fig. 18-36). There are also distinctive large aggregates of confluent lymphatic nodules known as *Peyer's patches* that have an elongated oval outline and that are confined to the side of the intestine that lies opposite its mesenteric attachment. Peyer's patches are present mainly in the lower part of the *ileum*, where they are largest (Fig. 18-36), but they are also

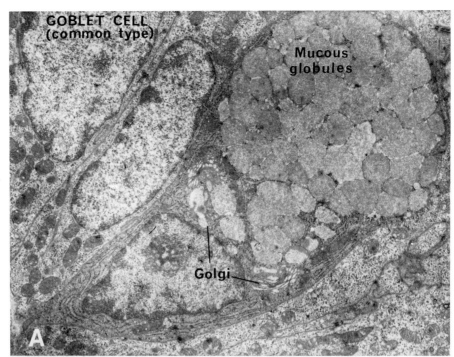

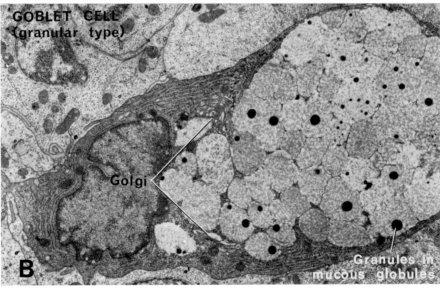

Fig. 18-34. Electron micrographs of the two types of goblet cells in the upper part of intestinal crypts (mouse small intestine). Their apex is distended by mucus globules to form a goblet shape. The Golgi complex is prominent. In approximately 25% of the mucous cells of the crypts, dense granules are present within the globules, as shown in *B*. As these granular mucous cells migrate from the crypts and along the villus walls, they secrete the granule-containing globules and elaborate new mucus globules that are free of granules. (Courtesy of H. Cheng)

found in the upper part of the ileum, the lower part of the jejunum, and even the lower part of the duodenum. Overlying villi are generally absent (as can be seen at *left* in Fig. 18-36), and a distinctive cell type called the *M cell* (described under Lymphatic Nodules in Chap. 10 and illustrated in Fig. 10-6) is found there instead. Peyer's patches become less prominent with increasing age. Their antigen-sampling role in the maintenance of mucosal immunity was described in Chapter 10 under Lymphatic Nodules.

The *muscularis mucosae* and *submucosa* of the small intestine are typical of the digestive tract as a whole. Although

the *muscularis externa* does not exhibit any special features, sections of the small intestine are a good place to look for ganglion cells and nerve fibers of the *myenteric plexus,* which is situated between the internal and external layers of the muscularis externa (Fig. 18-37).

Absorption from the Small Intestine

Sugars. Pancreatic amylase hydrolyzes polysaccharides, but the hydrolysis reaction proceeds only as far as disaccharides.

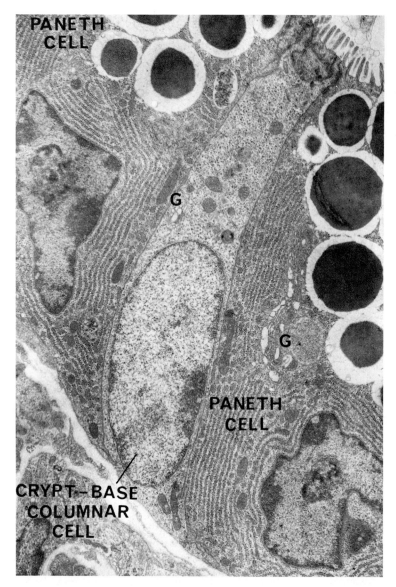

Fig. 18-35. Electron micrograph of a crypt base (mouse small intestine), showing a crypt base columnar cell between Paneth cells. The crypt base columnar cell (*middle*) has smooth lateral borders. Its cytoplasm is packed with free ribosomes and also contains a poorly developed Golgi (*G*) and a few other organelles.

The Paneth cells on either side contain large zymogen granules that have clear halos in the mouse. The Golgi apparatus (*G*) is extensive. To its right, a pale ovoid prosecretory granule lies between the Golgi region and the dark secretory granules. (Courtesy of H. Cheng and C. P. Leblond)

Degradation to monosaccharides requires the additional participation of disaccharidases that are situated on the external surface of microvilli of the villous columnar cells. Such enzymes are therefore known as *brush border enzymes.* Monosaccharides are readily absorbed by these cells and pass into blood capillaries in the underlying lamina propria.

Proteins. Several proteolytic enzymes degrade proteins to amino acids; in this form they can be readily absorbed by the columnar absorptive cells.

Fats. The essentials of fat digestion and fat absorption and the formation of chylomicrons were discussed in connection with Adipose Tissue in Chapter 7. Triglycerides are not absorbed, but with the help of small particles called *micelles* that form from *bile salts,* their breakdown products (monoglycerides and free fatty

acids) enter absorptive columnar cells by diffusing through the cell membrane that covers the luminal striated border.

Monoglycerides and free fatty acids become reincorporated into lipids in the smooth-surfaced endoplasmic reticulum of the absorptive columnar cells. The lipid-containing secretory vesicles that are produced discharge their contents along the *lateral* borders of these cells, releasing their contents into the intercellular spaces. The fat globules that leave these cells possess a delicate protein-containing limiting layer. Known as *chylomicrons,* they are made up of triglycerides, phospholipids, cholesteryl ester, and protein in the form of lipoprotein. Chylomicrons enter the *lacteals* and other *lymphatic capillaries* of the lamina propria and

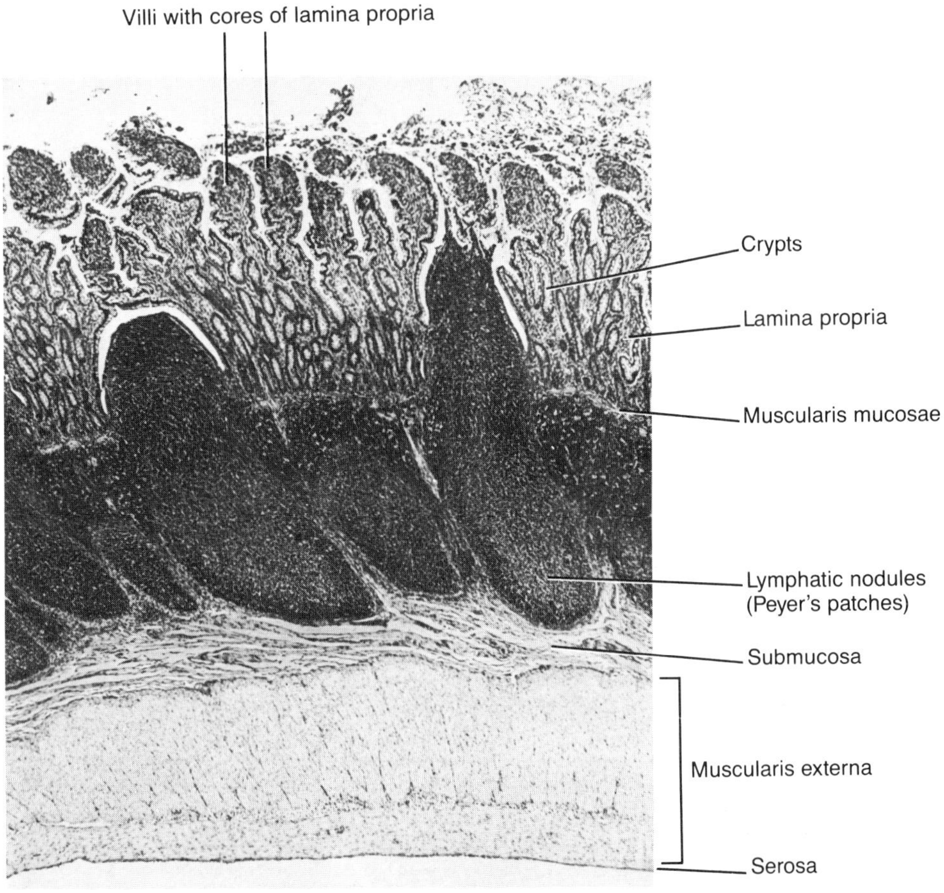

Villi with cores of lamina propria

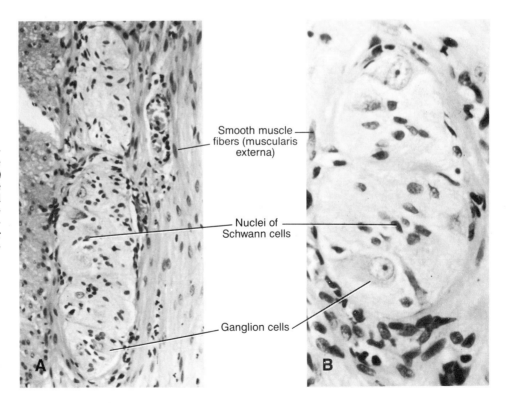

Crypts

Lamina propria

Muscularis mucosae

Lymphatic nodules (Peyer's patches)

Submucosa

Muscularis externa

Serosa

Fig. 18-36. Photomicrograph illustrating the wall structure of the ileum. Peyer's patches that are not covered by villi are seen extending down from the lamina propria through the muscularis mucosae into the submucosa.

Fig. 18-37. Photomicrographs of ganglion cells of the myenteric (Auerbach's) plexus of the small intestine under (A) medium power and (B) high power. This autonomic plexus is situated between the inner and outer layers of the muscularis externa.

Smooth muscle fibers (muscularis externa)

Nuclei of Schwann cells

Ganglion cells

A

B

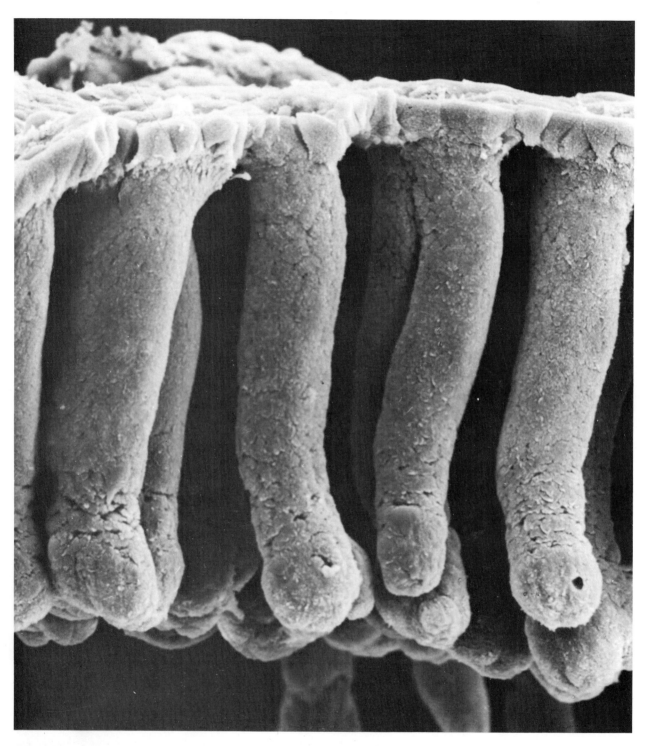

Fig. 18-38.   Scanning electron micrograph (×450) of lining epithelium and underlying crypts isolated from the colon (mouse). Villi are absent from the flat epithelium extending across the top of the micrograph. (Courtesy of J. Magney and S. Erlandsen)

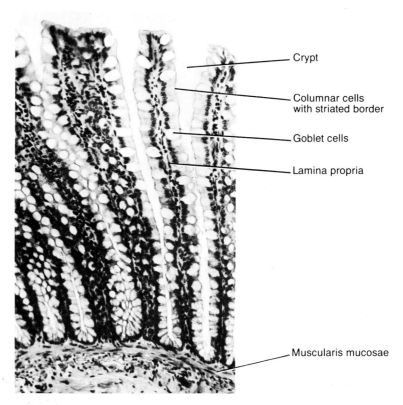

Crypt

Columnar cells
with striated border

Goblet cells

Lamina propria

Muscularis mucosae

Fig. 18-39. Photomicrograph illustrating part of the wall structure of the large intestine. Crypts are present, but there are no villi. Goblet cells are numerous in the large intestine.

reach the bloodstream *indirectly* mainly by way of the thoracic duct lymph. Their fate was discussed in Chapter 7 under White Fat. The lymph draining from the intestine after a fatty meal can contain substantial amounts of emulsified fat and is sometimes referred to as *chyle*.

LARGE INTESTINE

The large intestine consists of the *cecum;* the *appendix;* the *ascending, transverse, descending,* and *pelvic colons;* and the *rectum* (including the *anal canal*). It terminates at the *anus* (Fig. 18-1).

The unabsorbed residue from the small intestine is emptied into the cecum in a fluid state. By the time the contents reach the descending colon, however, they have acquired the consistency of feces. Hence a major function of the large intestine is fluid retrieval.

Although a great deal of mucus is present in the alkaline secretion of the large intestine, no enzymes of importance are secreted along with it. Nevertheless, some digestion occurs in the lumen. Part of this digestion is due to the residual activity of enzymes derived from the small intestine. However, some of it is due to the putrefactive action of bacteria that thrive in the lumen. These bacteria can break down cellulose, which reaches the large intestine because the human intestine secretes no enzymes that are

capable of degrading cellulose. Feces consist of bacteria, products of bacterial putrefaction, undigested material that endures passage through the large intestine, cellular debris from the lining of the intestine, mucus, and a few other substances.

Mucosa. This differs from the mucosa of the small intestine in several respects. It has *no villi* in postnatal life (Fig. 18-38). Also it is thicker; hence the crypts are deeper (Fig. 18-39). In adult life, the crypts *lack Paneth cells,* but they generally have *more goblet cells* than are present in the small intestine (Fig. 18-39) and the proportion of goblet cells increases from the beginning of the colon to the rectum. The ordinary surface epithelial cells have striated borders as do those of the small intestine. Enteroendocrine cells are also present.

New epithelial cells arise in the lower half of the crypts and migrate to the surface, where they are eventually lost to the lumen.

At the base of the crypts, there are immature cells that are believed to represent the stem cells of the epithelium. However, whereas the putative stem cells of the ascending colon appear to be small columnar cells, those of the descending colon and rectum contain secretory vesicles in their apex and are, in fact, often called *vacuolated cells* (*V* in Fig. 18-40). As these cells migrate toward the crypt orifice, they at first become filled with secretory vesicles. However,

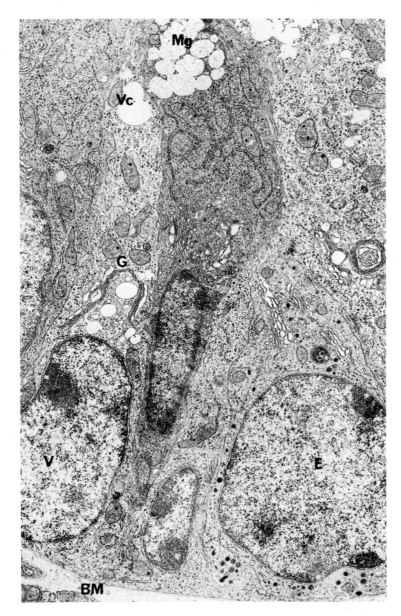

Fig. 18-40. Electron micrograph of a crypt base of descending colon. The columnar cells contain pale secretory vesicles (*Vc*) and are often referred to as vacuolated cells (*V*). The Golgi apparatus (*G*) shows developing secretory vesicles. The cytoplasm of these cells is lighter than that of the oligomucous cell seen at middle, in which a group of mucus globules (*Mg*) may be distinguished. At lower right, a young enteroendocrine cell (*E*) contains only a few dense granules. The crypt epithelium has an underlying basement membrane (*BM*).

As vacuolated cells migrate toward the crypt mouth, they become typical columnar cells with microvilli packed into a striated border. (Courtesy of A. Nabeyama)

before reaching the surface, they lose these vesicles and become typical columnar cells with a striated border (Chang and Leblond).

Crypts are lacking at the junction of the rectal and anal epithelium in the anorectal canal. The stratified squamous anal epithelium extends over approximately 2 cm and is not keratinized. Its distal border is continuous with the stratified keratinized epidermis of the skin, and its proximal border is continuous with the simple columnar epithelium that lines the remainder of the rectum. At the junction between the anal and the columnar epithelium, there are branched tubular glands known as *circumanal glands.* These seem to be inactive in man and are thought to represent nonfunctional counterparts of the functional glands that are present in other mammals. The mucosa of the anorectal canal forms longitudinal folds called *rectal columns* (columns of Morgagni). Adjacent columns are interconnected by membranous folds, forming an arrangement of so-called anal valves.

The muscularis mucosae continues as far as the rectal columns, where it subdivides into bundles and then disappears. The merging lamina propria and submucosa contain many small convoluted veins. A common condition called *internal hemorrhoids* results from dilatation of these veins, which causes the mucous membrane to bulge inward, encroaching on the anal canal. *External hemorrhoids* result from dilatation of similar veins that are situated closer to the anus.

Muscularis Externa and Serosa. Beginning at the cecum, the longitudinal outer layer of the muscularis externa thickens to form three flat bands called the *teniae coli.* The tonus in these three bundles of smooth muscle causes this

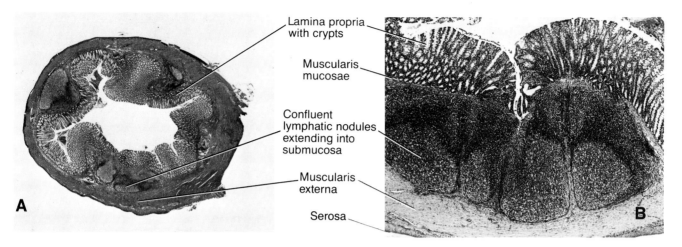

Lamina propria with crypts

Muscularis mucosae

Confluent lymphatic nodules extending into submucosa

Muscularis externa

Serosa

Fig. 18-41. Photomicrograph illustrating the wall structure of the appendix. (*A*) Very low power. (*B*) High power.

part of the bowel to sacculate. Similarly, the walls of the rectum are provided with anterior and posterior thickenings of the same smooth muscle layer that cause the rectal walls to sacculate. In addition, the rectal walls project inward as two transverse shelves called *plicae transversales* that support some of the weight of the rectal contents. The circular inner layer of smooth muscle of the muscularis externa forms the *internal sphincter* of the anus.

Along the colon and the upper part of the rectum, the serosa forms little sacs that enclose small external masses of adipose tissue or loose connective tissue. These peritoneal redundancies hang from the external surface of the bowel and are termed *appendices epiploicae*.

Appendix

The appendix is a small worm-shaped (vermiform) diverticulum of the cecum originating a few centimeters distal to the ileocecal junction (Fig. 18-1). Whereas in some mammals it is a comparatively large structure in which cellulose is subjected to prolonged digestion, in man it is too small to have this function. Furthermore, twisting of this diverticulum can cause its small lumen to become obstructed, predisposing it to bacterial infections and acute inflammation dangerous enough to warrant its surgical removal (*appendectomy*). An accumulation of neutrophils in any layer of its wall is considered to be an indication of *acute appendicitis.*

The wall structure of the appendix conforms to the general plan described earlier in this chapter (Fig. 18-41*A*). However, the wall has a distinctive microscopic appearance because of the presence of *permanent confluent lymphatic nodules* (Fig. 18-41*A*) situated beneath overlying M cells (see Fig. 10-6). The lymphatic nodules are initially confined to the lamina propria, but they soon become large enough to extend far down into the submucosa (Fig. 18-41*B*). In

the earlier decades of life, they are generally large, multiple, and confluent and lie on all sides of the lumen, but with increasing age, they gradually become smaller again.

Because of its position close to the ileocecal junction, the appendix is strategically situated for sampling microbial or parasite antigens refluxing from the ileocecal valve. The role of the gut-associated lymphatic tissue of the appendix in maintaining mucosal immunity was discussed in Chapter 10 under Lymphatic Nodules.

SELECTED REFERENCES

Teeth and Gingiva

ANDERSON DJ, ESTOE JE, MELCHER AH, PICTON DCA (eds): The Mechanism of Tooth Support—A Symposium. Bristol, John Wright, 1967

EISENMANN DR: Enamel structure. In Ten Cate AR: Oral Histology: Development, Structure, and Function, 2nd ed, p 198. St. Louis, CV Mosby, 1985

GARANT PR, NALBANDIAN J: Observations on the ultrastructure of ameloblasts with special reference to the Golgi complex and related components. J Ultrastruct Res 23:427, 1968

GARANT P, SZABO G, NALBANDIAN J: The fine structure of the mouse odontoblast. Arch Oral Biol 13:857, 1968

KALLENBACH E: The cell web in the ameloblasts of the rat incisor. Anat Rec 153:55, 1963

LEBLOND CP, WEINSTOCK M: A comparative study of dentin and bone formation. In Bourne GH (ed): Biochemistry and Physiology of Bone. Vol 4, p 517. New York, Academic Press, 1976

REITH EJ: The ultrastructure of ameloblasts during early stages of maturation of enamel. J Cell Biol 18:691, 1963

SIGAL MJ, AUBIN JE, TEN CATE AR, PITARU S: The odontoblast process extends to the dentinoenamel junction: An immunocytochemical study of rat dentine. J Histochem Cytochem 32:872, 1984

SLAVEN HC, BAVETTA LA (eds): Developmental Aspects of Oral Biology. New York, Academic Press, 1972

STACK MV, FERNHEAD RW (ed): Tooth Enamel. Its Composition, Properties and Fundamental Structure. Bristol, John Wright, 1965

SYMONS NBB (ed): Dentine and Pulp: Their Structure and Reactions. Edinburgh, Churchill Livingstone, 1967

TEN CATE AR: Oral Histology: Development, Structure, and Function, 2nd ed. St. Louis, CV Mosby, 1985

VEIS A: Bones and teeth. In Piez KA, Reddi AH (eds): Extracellular Matrix Biochemistry, p 329. New York, Elsevier North-Holland, 1984

WARSHAWSKY H: The fine structure of secretory ameloblasts in rat incisors. Anat Rec 161:211, 1968

WARSHAWSKY H: A light and electron microscope study of the nearly mature enamel of rat incisors. Anat Rec 169:559, 1971

WEINSTOCK M, LEBLOND CP: Radioautographic visualization of the deposition of a phosphoprotein at the mineralization front in the dentin of the rat incisor. J Cell Biol 56:838, 1973

WEINSTOCK M, LEBLOND CP: Synthesis, migration and release of precursor collagen by odontoblasts as visualized by radioautography after ^{3}H-proline administration. J Cell Biol 60:92, 1974

Oral Cavity, Tonsils, Pharynx, and Esophagus

BARATZ RS, FARBMAN AI: Morphogenesis of rat lingual filiform papillae. Am J Anat 143:283, 1975

BEIDLER LN, SMALLMAN RLS: Renewal of cells within taste buds. J Cell Biol 27:263, 1965

BRANDTZAEG P: Immune functions of human nasal mucosa and tonsils in health and disease. In Bienenstock J (ed): Immunology of the Lung and Upper Respiratory Tract, p 28. New York, McGraw-Hill, 1984

DALE AC: Salivary glands. In Ten Cate AR: Oral Histology: Development, Structure, and Function, 2nd ed, p 303. St Louis, CV Mosby, 1985

GARRETT JR, HARRISON JD, STOWARD PJ: Histochemistry of Secretory Process. London, Chapman & Hall, 1977

MURRAY RG: The ultrastructure of taste buds. In Friedmann J (ed): The Ultrastructure of Sensory Organs, p 1. Amsterdam, North Holland Publishing, 1973

PARKS HF: Morphological study of the extrusion of secretory materials by the parotid glands of mouse and rat. J Ultrastruct Res 6:449, 1962

Stomach, Small and Large Intestine, and Gastrointestinal Hormones

ALTMANN GG: Factors involved in the differentiation of the epithelial cells in the adult rat small intestine. In Cairnie AB, Lala PK, Osmond DG (eds): Stem cells of Renewing Cell Populations. New York, Academic Press, 1976

ANDREW A: The APUD concept: Where has it led us? Brit Med Bull 38:221, 1982

BEAVEN MA: Histamine (second of two parts). N Engl J Med 294:320, 1976

BERTALANFFY FD: Cell renewal in the gastrointestinal tract of man. Gastroenterology 43:472, 1962

BERTALANFFY FD, NAGY KP: Mitotic activity and renewal rate of the epithelial cells of human duodenum. Acta Anat 45:362, 1961

BLOOM SR (ed): Gut Hormones. Edinburgh, Churchill Livingstone, 1978

CARDELL RR, Jr, BADENHAUSEN S, PORTER KR: Intestinal triglyceride absorption in the rat. J Cell Biol 34:123, 1967

CARTER DC: Cytoprotection and its possible role in the pharmacology of gastric mucosa. In Konturek SJ, Domschke W (eds): Gastric Secretion—Basic and Clinical Aspects, p 97. Stuttgart, Georg Thieme Verlag/New York, Thieme-Stratton, 1981

CHANG WWL, LEBLOND CP: Renewal of the epithelium in the descending colon of the mouse. I. Presence of three cell populations: Vacuolated-columnar, mucous, and argentaffin. Am J Anat 131:73, 1971

CHENG H, LEBLOND CP: Origin, differentiation and renewal of the four main epithelial cell types in the mouse small intestine. I. Columnar cells. Am J Anat 141:461, 1974 (*and the 4 next papers*)

CRANE RK (ed): Gastrointestinal Physiology II. International Review of Physiology. Vol 12. Baltimore, University Park Press, 1977

FERREIRA MN, LEBLOND CP: Argentaffin and other "endocrine" cells of the small intestine in the adult mouse. II. Renewal. Am J Anat 131:331, 1971

FRIEDMAN MHF (ed): Functions of the Stomach and Intestine. Baltimore, University Park Press, 1975

ITO S: Anatomic structure of the gastric mucosa. In American Physiological Society: Handbook of Physiology. Section 6 (Cole CF, ed): Alimentary Canal. Vol 2, p 705. Baltimore, Williams & Wilkins, 1967

ITO S: The fine structure of the gastric mucosa. In Proc Symp Gastric Secretion: Mechanisms and Control, p 3. Oxford, Pergamon Press, 1967

ITO S, LACY ER: Morphology of gastric mucosal damage, defenses and restitution in the presence of luminal ethanol. Gastroenterology 88:250, 1985

ITO S, WINCHESTER RJ: The fine structure of the gastric mucosa in the bat. J Cell Biol 16:541, 1963

JOHNSON LR (ed): Gastrointestinal Physiology. St. Louis, CV Mosby, 1977

LEBLOND CP, CHENG H: Identification of stem cells in the small intestine of the mouse. In Cairnie AB, Lala PK, Osmond DG (eds): Stem Cells in Renewing Cell Populations. New York, Academic Press, 1976

LEE ER: Dynamic histology of the antral epithelium in the mouse stomach: III. Ultrastructure and renewal of pit cells. Am J Anat 172:225, 1985

LEE ER, LEBLOND CP: Dynamic histology of the antral epithelium in the mouse stomach: II. Ultrastructure and renewal of isthmal cells. Am J Anat 172:205, 1985

LEE ER, LEBLOND CP: Dynamic histology of the antral epithelium in the mouse stomach: IV. Ultrastructure and renewal of gland cells. Am J Anat 172:241, 1985

LEE FD, TONER PG: Biopsy Pathology of the Small Intestine. London, Chapman & Hall, 1980

LEE ER, TRASLER J, DWIVEDI S, LEBLOND CP: Division of the mouse gastric mucosa into zymogenic and mucous regions on the basis of gland features. Am J Anat 164:187, 1982

LIPKIN M, SHERLOCK P, BELL B: Cell proliferation kinetics in the gastrointestinal tract of man. II. Cell renewal in stomach, ileum, colon, and rectum. Gastroenterology 45:721, 1963

MARQUES–PEREIRA JP, LEBLOND CP: Mitosis and differentiation in the stratified squamous epithelium of the rat esophagus. Am J Anat 117:73, 1965

MERZEL J, LEBLOND CP: Origin and renewal of goblet cells in the epithelium of the mouse small intestine. Am J Anat 124:281, 1969

MIYOSHI A (ed): Gut Peptides—Secretion, Function and Clinical Aspects. Tokyo, Kodansha Ltd/Amsterdam, Elsevier North-Holland Biomedical Press, 1979

MOE H: The goblet cells, Paneth cells and basal granular cells of the epithelium of the intestine. Int Rev Gen Exp Zool 3:241, 1968

MOOG F: The lining of the small intestine. Sci Am 245 No 5:154, 1981

NABEYAMA A, LEBLOND CP: "Caveolated cells" characterized by deep surface invaginations and abundant filaments in mouse gastrointestinal epithelia. Am J Anat 140:147, 1974

PALAY SL, REVEL JP: The morphology of fat absorption. In Meng HC: Lipid transport, p 1. Springfield, IL, Charles C Thomas, 1964

POTTEN CS, HENDRY JH: Stem cells in murine small intestine. In Potten CS (ed): Stem Cells: Their Identification and Characterization, p 155. Edinburgh, Churchill Livingstone, 1983

RICHARDSON KC: Electron microscopic observations on Auerbach's plexus in the rabbit, with special reference to the problem of smooth muscle innervation. Am J Anat 103:99, 1958

SEDAR AW: The fine structure of the oxyntic cell in relation to functional activity of the stomach. Ann NY Acad Sci 99:9, 1962

SEDAR AW: Stomach and intestinal mucosa. In Electron Microscope Anatomy, p 123. New York, Academic Press, 1964

SILEN W, ITO S: Mechanisms for rapid epithelialization of the gastric mucosal surface. Annu Rev Physiol 47:217, 1985

SPENCER RP: The Intestinal Tract: Structure, Function and Pathology in Terms of the Basic Sciences. Springfield, IL, Charles C Thomas, 1960

STRAUSS EW: Morphological Aspects of Triglyceride Absorption. In Codel CF, Heidel W (eds): Handbook of Physiology. Vol 3, sec 6, chap 71. Washington, American Physiological Society, 1968

TRIER JS: Studies on small intestinal crypt epithelium of the proximal small intestine of fasting humans. J Cell Biol 18:599, 1963

WALSH JH, GROSSMAN MI: Gastrin. N Engl J Med 292:1324, 1975

WEIRNIK G, SHROTER RG, CREAMER B: The arrest of intestinal epithelial "turnover" by the use of x-irradiation. Gut 3:26, 1962

ZEITOUN P, DUCLERT N, LIAUTAUD F ET AL: Intracellular localization of pepsinogen in guinea pig pyloric mucosa by immunohistochemistry. Histochemical and electron microscopic correlated structures. Lab Invest 27:218, 1972

19

Pancreas, Liver, and Gallbladder

PANCREAS

The pancreas is situated in the abdominal cavity with its head nestling in the concavity of the duodenum and its body extending toward the spleen (see Fig. 18-1). In the living state, it appears whitish with a tinge of pink, and it has a lobulated appearance because its capsule is thin enough to allow the underlying tissue to show through. The pancreas is both an exocrine and an endocrine gland, but most of its secretory cells are exocrine. Known as *acinar cells,* they produce *pancreatic juice,* which is delivered to the duodenum by way of the *pancreatic duct.* The pancreatic *hormones* are secreted by cells located in small pale-staining islands called *pancreatic islets* or *islets of Langerhans* (Fig. 19-1); these cells and the hormones they produce will be described in Chapter 22.

Covering the pancreas is a layer of connective tissue so thin that it scarcely merits being called a capsule. This layer is, in turn, covered by peritoneal mesothelium. From the capsule, connective tissue extends into the gland as septa that subdivide its parenchyma into *lobules.* The septa, too, are very thin (Fig. 19-1), but their positions are commonly accentuated by shrinkage artifact. Condensations of dense ordinary connective tissue surround the large ducts and their main branches, providing the pancreas with a certain amount of internal support.

Within each lobule, the secretory acini are tightly packed together with very little connective tissue between them (Figs. 19-1, 19-2, and 19-3A). Their constituent acinar cells appear roughly triangular in outline (Fig. 19-2). The cytoplasm in the broad base

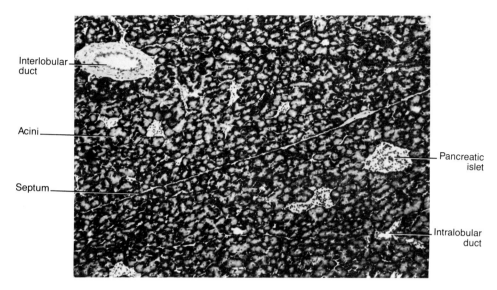

Interlobular duct

Acini

Septum

Pancreatic islet

Intralobular duct

Fig. 19-1. Photomicrograph of the pancreas (very low power). Septa are very thin and intralobular ducts are inconspicuous; pancreatic islets are also present.

of each acinar cell is intensely basophilic (Fig. 19-2) because of the presence of an extensive rough-surfaced endoplasmic reticulum (rER) (Fig. 19-4). The zymogen granules in the apical part of the cell (Figs. 19-3A and 19-4) are acidophilic, and the basal nucleus is spherical (Figs. 19-2, 19-3, and 19-4). Pancreatic acinar cells were described in detail in connection with protein secretion in Chapter 4, and their fine structure is summarized in the caption to Figure 19-4. Close to the luminal border of these cells, which bears a few short microvilli, the lateral borders exhibit junctional complexes (Fig. 19-5) similar to those described for intestinal lining cells (see Chap. 6 under Cell Junctions). The continuous tight junction (zonula occludens) of a pancreatic junctional complex impedes access of digestive enzymes (or their precursors) to the intercellular spaces following the release of zymogen granules into the acinar lumen. The adhering junctions of the complex reduce the risk of separation of acinar cells under conditions that increase the intraluminal hydrostatic pressure in the acinus. Each acinus is surrounded by a basement membrane, and the small spaces between acini are occupied by a delicate connective tissue that contains capillaries and autonomic nerve fibers. Adipocytes may also be present in this connective tissue.

A characteristic of the pancreas is that a nucleus can often be seen in the middle of an acinus (Figs. 19-2 and 19-3). Such nuclei belong to cells known as *centro-acinar cells.* Where an acinus has been cut centrally, it can be seen that these cells represent terminal cells of the duct system that are invaginated into the lumen of the acinus (Fig. 19-3), an arrangement that is unique to the pancreas. The narrow duct that leads from the acinus is known as an *intercalated duct;* it is lined with flattened cuboidal epithelium. Intercalated ducts open into inconspicuous *intralob-*

ular ducts that are lined with low columnar or simple cuboidal epithelium (Fig. 19-1). These intralobular ducts, which are also fairly narrow, constitute the tributaries of more prominent *interlobular ducts* extending between lobules and lined with low columnar epithelium (Fig. 19-1). The *main pancreatic duct* and *accessory pancreatic duct,* from which the interlobular ducts extend on all sides as lateral branches, are ensheathed with relatively large amounts of dense ordinary connective tissue, and they are lined with simple columnar epithelium containing some goblet cells. Small mucous glands may be present in the walls of the main duct near the duodenum. It should be noted that intralobular ducts are much less prominent in the pancreas than in the parotid (compare Fig. 19-1 with Fig. 18-13). Also, the presence of islets is a distinguishing feature of

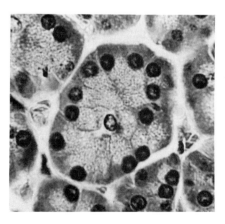

Fig. 19-2. Photomicrograph of a pancreatic acinus that exhibits the nucleus of a centro-acinar cell at its center.

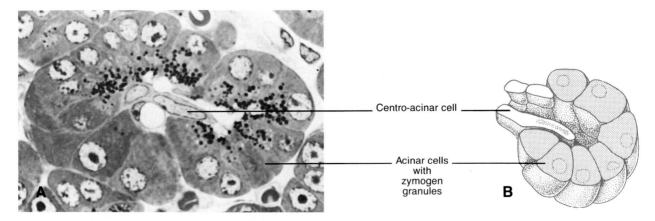

Fig. 19-3.   (A). Photomicrograph of a pancreatic acinus showing a centro-acinar cell at the origin of its intercalated duct (semithin section stained with toluidine blue). (B) Interpretive diagram.

the pancreas. These criteria, together with the presence of centro-acinar cells, make microscopic recognition of the pancreas a relatively simple matter.

The Secretion of Pancreatic Juice Is Regulated Primarily by Two Gastrointestinal Hormones.   Pancreatic juice is an alkaline digestive juice that contains many important enzymes needed to carry out further digestion of the food that leaves the stomach. These are trypsin, chymotrypsin, lipase, esterase, deoxyribonuclease, ribonuclease, phospholipase A, amylase, carboxypeptidases A and B, and elastase. The secretory activity of the pancreas therefore needs to be regulated to coincide with the delivery of stomach contents to the duodenum. The regulatory mechanism involves two gastrointestinal peptide hormones that are released by enteroendocrine cells of the intestinal mucosa when this is stimulated by acidic stomach contents. The two hormones pass into the circulating blood and reach the pancreatic acinar cells by way of pancreatic capillaries. One of these hormones, *secretin,* stimulates the release of *bicarbonate* ions and other nonenzymatic constituents of pancreatic juice. These constituents seem to be released by the *duct cells* of the pancreas. The other enzyme, *cholecystokinin-pancreozymin* (CCK-PZ), stimulates the release of *enzymes* from the pancreatic *acinar cells.* It has been established that stimulation of the vagus nerve will also elicit some pancreatic secretion, but regulation of the secretory activity of the pancreas is primarily hormonal.

LIVER

The liver, which appears reddish-brown in the living state, is the main metabolic organ of the body and also its largest compound gland, weighing approximately 3 pounds in the adult. Its thin but strong connective tissue *capsule* (Glisson's

capsule) is covered by peritoneal mesothelium. Most of this organ lies on the right-hand side of the body, with its smooth superior surface fitting the dome-shaped undersurface of the diaphragm (see Fig. 18-1). It possesses two main lobes, the right lobe being much larger than the left (see Fig. 18-1). Its inferior surface, which is shown exposed in Figure 18-1, is indented where it lies against other abdominal viscera; hence it is called the *visceral surface* of the liver. A short deep transverse fissure of this surface termed the *porta hepatis* (L. *porta,* gate) is the site where the major blood vessels, ducts, and lymphatics enter or leave the liver. As in other compound glands, the liver is made up of a parenchyma and a stroma. The parenchyma consists of epithelial cells of endodermal origin known as *hepatocytes,* whereas the stroma consists of ordinary connective tissue of mesenchymal origin. *Bile,* the exocrine secretion of the liver parenchymal cells, empties into the duodenum by way of the bile duct.

An important feature of the liver is that it has a *dual blood supply.* Approximately 75% of the blood it receives is *venous blood* laden with products of digestion that arrives by way of the *portal vein* from the small intestine. The remainder is arterial blood that reaches the liver by way of the hepatic artery. Both the portal vein and the hepatic artery enter the liver at the porta hepatis, and the *right* and *left hepatic ducts* and hepatic *lymphatics* leave the organ at the same site.

Whereas the exocrine secretory products of hepatocytes (*i.e.,* the *bile* constituents) are elaborated into tiny intercellular passageways called *bile canaliculi,* the internal secretions made by these cells (namely *glucose, plasma proteins,* and *lipoproteins*) are liberated into the bloodstream. The liver is therefore occasionally described as being partly exocrine and partly endocrine. Part of the surface of each hepatocyte accordingly borders on a *bile canaliculus,* and part of it borders on a *blood sinusoid.* Before explaining this further, it is necessary to consider the way in which the parenchyma of the liver is arranged.

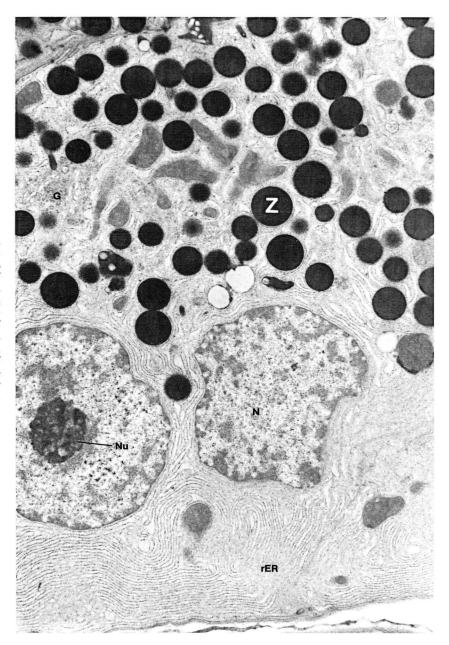

Fig. 19-4. Electron micrograph of an acinar cell of the pancreas (biopsy of human pancreas). Two parts of the nucleus (*N*) seem to be present in this plane of section. A prominent nucleolus (*Nu*) is visible at left. Electron-dense zymogen granules (*Z*) are packed into the apical region of the cytoplasm. Part of a stack of Golgi saccules (*G*) lies between the nucleus and the lumen of the acinus (which would be situated just above the top border of the micrograph). The basal region of the cytoplasm is filled with characteristically prominent parallel cisternae of rER. (Courtesy of K. Kovacs and E. Horvath)

INTERNAL ORGANIZATION OF THE LIVER

Three major interpretations now exist regarding the internal structure of the liver, each of which is based on a different structural or functional aspect of the organ. We shall begin by describing the so-called *classic lobule*, which is the type of organization implied when the term *liver lobule* is employed without qualification. The classic lobule was the first conceptual model to emerge from studies of the liver and its main usefulness today is to facilitate understanding of a newer, functionally based concept, that of the *liver acinus* (which will be described later in this chapter). A third conceptual model, the *portal lobule*, has not proved as useful as the other two, but a short description will be included for students who may be interested in plumbing.

Classic Liver Lobule

In most compound exocrine glands, lobules are parenchymal segments that are demarcated by interlobular septa, and this was the criterion initially adopted for recognizing

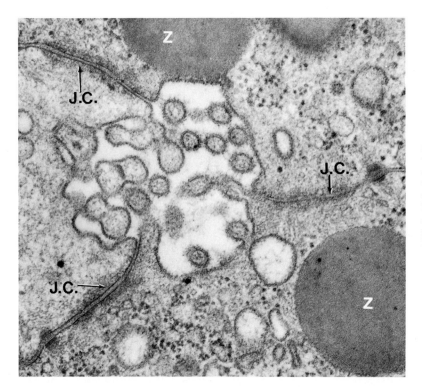

Fig. 19-5. Electron micrograph (×50,000) of the luminal region of a pancreatic acinus (guinea pig). At center, microvilli project into the lumen. The cell at left is a centro-acinar cell. At top, a zymogen granule (Z) is about to be secreted from an acinar cell. Another acinar cell is seen at lower right. Junctional complexes (*J.C.*) are present close to the lumen. (Farquhar MG, Palade GE: J Cell Biol 17:375, 1963)

liver lobules. However, some difficulty was encountered because in normal human liver (and also in the kidneys), no interlobular septa could be found. Septa were nevertheless found to demarcate lobules in the liver of pigs (Fig. 19-6; see also Fig. 1-9) and also in the liver of certain other animals. As seen in a cross section of pig liver, a typical classic lobule is hexagonal in outline, and the connective tissue in at least some of its corners contains branches of the portal vein, hepatic artery, and bile duct system, together with one or more lymphatics (see Fig. 1-9C). This characteristic grouping of the four tubes and the connective tissue that surrounds them is known as a *portal tract, area,* or *radicle.* Two such areas can be seen in Figure 19-6. Portal tracts are also present in human liver (Fig. 19-7, indicated by *arrows*), but normally they are *not connected with one another by connective tissue septa.* They nevertheless serve as landmarks that, if connected by imaginary lines, permit the outlines of classic lobules to be visualized. In addition, there is a landmark that indicates the central axis of the classic liver lobule; this is the *central vein* that drains blood from the lobule (Figs. 19-6 and 19-7). Nevertheless, classic lobules are not easy to recognize in human liver because they are not demarcated by septa and are therefore not really discrete units, as they are sometimes described. To visualize where their respective boundaries would lie, it is necessary to find their associated portal tracts arranged around their central veins.

Portal Tracts and Central Veins. Connective tissue extends into the liver at the porta hepatis in the form of a tree trunk that branches very extensively. The widest tube in every ramification of this tree is a thin-walled branch of the *portal vein.* This vessel is easily recognized because it is the tube with the widest lumen (Fig. 19-8). The branches of the *hepatic artery* that are also conveyed in the portal tracts have a much smaller lumen (Fig. 19-8C). The other tubes conveyed by branches of the connective tissue tree enable fluids to leave the liver. One is a branch of a *bile duct* and the other is a *lymphatic* (Fig. 19-8C). Portal tracts can also be sectioned at levels where one or more of these tubes has branched, in which case there can be more than four tubes in a portal tract.

Blood arriving by way of portal tract branches of the portal vein and hepatic artery enters relatively wide anastomosing and thin-walled *sinusoids* that extend from the periphery of the classic lobule to its *central vein* (Figs. 19-7 and 19-8). The central vein lacks a well-developed wall structure and has only minimal amounts of associated adventitial connective tissue (Fig. 19-8B). If it were not for its fairly large lumen, this vein would be more accurately described as a central venule, and in the terminology devised for the liver acinus, it is described as a *terminal hepatic venule.* The central veins of classic liver lobules open into larger *sublobular veins.* These, in turn, drain into *hepatic veins* that leave the liver posteriorly, emptying their blood

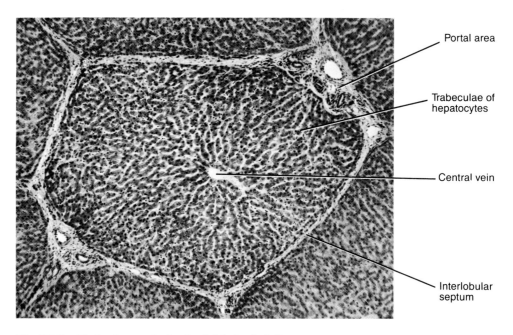

Portal area

Trabeculae of hepatocytes

Central vein

Interlobular septum

Fig. 19-6. Photomicrograph of a classic lobule of pig liver.

into the inferior vena cava. The system of veins that drains blood from the liver is not conveyed in any substantial tree of connective tissue as are the portal venous and hepatic arterial branches that supply blood to the liver. Furthermore, throughout the liver these two systems of blood vessels, although interconnected by sinusoids, remain separate. Accordingly, sinusoids and their associated hepatocytes are normally interpolated between (1) the portal venous and hepatic arterial circulations on the one hand, and (2) the hepatic venous drainage on the other (see Fig. 19-10*A*).

Liver Trabeculae Converge on Central Veins. In contrast to the regular arrangement of lobules that is seen in pig liver, human liver lobules are fitted together in a somewhat haphazard manner. Each lobule is nevertheless basically low columnar in shape and appears more or less hexagonal in cross section. In this plane of section, the classic lobule can be recognized by (1) a *radiating pattern* of hepatocytes that converges on the *central vein*, and (2) a peripheral *incomplete ring of two to four portal tracts* that are equidistant from the central vein (Fig. 19-7). As already

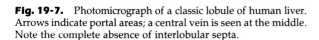

Fig. 19-7. Photomicrograph of a classic lobule of human liver. Arrows indicate portal areas; a central vein is seen at the middle. Note the complete absence of interlobular septa.

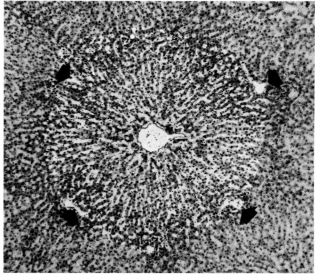

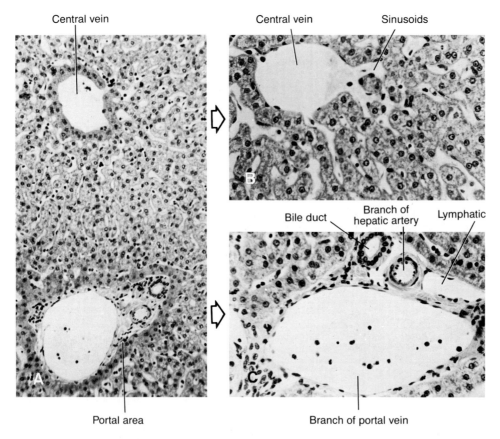

Fig. 19-8. Photomicrographs of the major landmarks of a classic liver lobule: its central vein and portal tracts. (A) Low power, showing center of lobule above and periphery of lobule below. (B) Central vein (medium power). (C) Portal area (medium power).

noted, the boundaries of the lobule must be construed by mentally connecting the existing portal tracts with imaginary ones so as to create a hexagonal outline.

In a lobule that has been cut in cross section, then, anastomosing rows of polyhedral hepatocytes separated by slitlike sinusoids converge on the central vein. Hepatocytes have been variously described as constituting irregular anastomosing *trabeculae* or *curved perforated plates.* Whichever way one chooses to think of them, they comprise an anastomosing three-dimensional spongework with blood-filled sinusoids in its interstices. In most places, the liver trabeculae (or plates) have the thickness of only a single hepatocyte. Hence the majority of hepatocytes have two of their surfaces bordering on sinusoids (see Fig. 19-10). Each of these surfaces is bathed with blood plasma from which substances are absorbed and into which internal secretions are liberated. In addition, every hepatocyte possesses strip-shaped surface recesses that border on *bile canaliculi.* These are the surfaces through which the cell elaborates the bile constituents that make up its exocrine secretion. Microvilli are present on both kinds of surfaces (see Figs. 19-10B and 19-15). The bile canaliculi are narrow

tubular channels, 1 μm to 2 μm in diameter, that lie *between* the cell membranes of adjacent hepatocytes (Figs. 19-9B and 19-10B). Continuous tight junctions seal off their lumina from the other intercellular spaces (Fig. 19-10B, see also Fig. 19-18). These zonula occludens junctions are generally associated with junctions of other types (desmosomes, gap junctions, or zonula adherens junctions) as junctional complexes (see Fig. 19-18).

Blood and Bile Flow in Opposite Directions in the Classic Lobule. It will be recalled that (1) liver sinusoids receive venous blood that comes from small branches of the portal vein and also arterial blood that comes from similar branches of the hepatic artery; and (2) branches of both types of vessels are situated in the portal tracts at the periphery of the lobule (Fig. 19-10A). The direction of blood flow along the sinusoids is therefore away from the portal tracts and toward the central vein. In contrast, the direction of bile flow along the bile canaliculi is toward the bile ducts in the portal tracts and away from the middle of the lobule (Fig. 19-10A). Hence in the classic lobule, *blood and bile flow in opposite directions.*

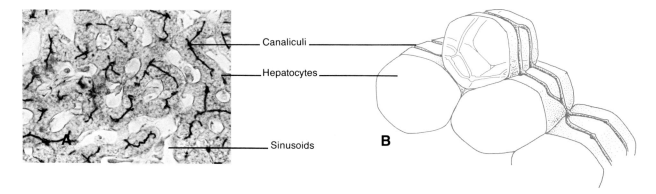

Fig. 19-9. (*A*) Photomicrograph of bile canaliculi between hepatocytes (stained histochemically for alkaline phosphatase), with (*B*) interpretive drawing. (*A*, courtesy of M. Phillips and J. Steiner)

Portal Lobule

The term *lobule* is also commonly employed to indicate a group of parenchymal exocrine secretory units that discharge their secretory product or products into branches of the same duct (*i.e.,* an intralobular duct). It is in this sense that the term is used with respect to the kidney, for example. A conceptual model that is based on *bile drainage* instead of microscopically recognizable units is the *portal lobule*. In this case, the exocrine secretory units are the liver trabeculae that secrete into the bile duct of a portal tract. Seen in cross section, these trabeculae would occupy a triangular area (indicated as a portal lobule in Fig. 19-11*B*). The portal lobule clearly does not correspond to the classic lobule because (1) its central axis is a bile duct in a portal tract instead of a central vein, and (2) the direction of bile flow is toward its center.

Although still adhered to by a few devotees, neither of the conceptual models considered thus far provides much insight into how hepatocytes carry out their various metabolic duties, an aspect of the liver with potentially more clinical significance than the direction of bile flow or microscopic parallels between human and pig liver.

Liver Acinus

Hepatocytes Play a Key Role in Body Metabolism. As well as having the important role of producing bile, hepatocytes carry out a broad range of metabolic duties that are of immense importance to the body as a whole. Thus after meals have been digested, hepatocytes convert the excess absorbed glucose into glycogen and subsequently convert it back into glucose as required to sustain the blood sugar level. They also perform well over 500 other useful metabolic functions that include (1) the detoxification of drugs and toxic substances, (2) the degradation of steroid hormones, and (3) the utilization of lipids in lipoprotein synthesis. The efficiency with which hepatocytes are able to perform such metabolic functions depends, to a consid-

erable extent, on where they lie relative to the incoming blood. In particular, it is influenced by the availability of oxygen and nutrients, and it is greatly affected by the presence and local concentration of any toxic substances that may be present in the blood that bathes each hepatocyte. Hence it is important to know each hepatocyte's position relative to its immediate blood supply, which constitutes the basis of the third conceptual model of liver organization that we shall now describe.

What Is a Liver Acinus? It is important to realize that when used in connection with the liver, the term *acinus* has the special meaning of a unit of parenchyma that is defined *in relation to its blood supply* (see references cited for Rappaport and also Rappaport et al). Thus the *liver acinus* is not a secretory unit that is exactly equivalent to the acini of other exocrine glands. It is, in fact, a partially undelineated and roughly ovoid mass of liver parenchyma that incorporates the contiguous parts of two neighboring classic lobules (Fig. 19-11*A*).

However, instead of viewing the liver acinus merely as a subdivision of adjacent classic lobules, the key to understanding what comprises this unit is to appreciate what constitutes its *vascular backbone*. It will be recalled that the blood reaching the liver sinusoids comes from the small portal venous and hepatic arterial vessels conveyed in the portal tracts. However, this blood is delivered by tiny terminal branches of such vessels and not by the portal tract vessels themselves (Fig. 19-10*A*). These terminal branches are fed by portal tract vessel side branches that branch from the portal tract vessels at intervals in any of the three directions indicated in Figure 19-11*A* (Rappaport). Moreover, side branches of the hepatic artery accompany side branches of the portal vein and, together with a bile ductule and one or more small lymphatics and peripheral nerves, the two vessels run side by side along the morphological axis of the acinus in such a way as to constitute its vascular backbone (Fig. 19-11*A*). From Figure 19-11 it can also be seen that the peripheral landmarks of the liver acinus are *two neighboring central veins* (which, in the terminology

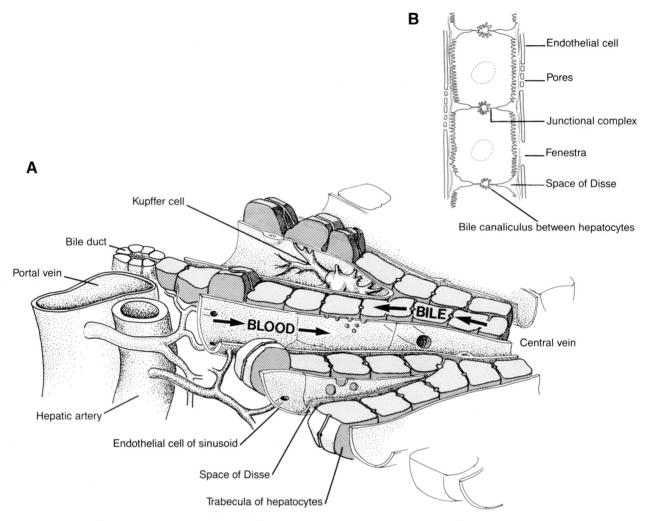

Fig. 19-10. (*A*) Schematic representation of part of a liver lobule, indicating the directions of blood and bile flow with respect to the portal area depicted at left. (*B*) Diagram showing the spatial arrangement of the endothelium of liver sinusoids, hepatocytes, and the space of Disse.

used for the liver acinus, are known as *terminal hepatic venules*) and usually *one associated portal tract* (allowing for the fact that in human liver some of these tracts are generally "missing").

Hepatocytes in Zone 3 of the Acinus Are at a Relative Disadvantage. Once the liver is thought of as being composed of acini instead of lobules, it becomes obvious that hepatocytes situated close to the vascular backbone of an acinus would be bathed with blood that is comparatively rich in nutrients and oxygen. On the other hand, hepatocytes situated farther away from such axial vessels would be relatively deprived of such essentials. Furthermore, they would be exposed to significantly higher concentrations of metabolic waste products. Such advantageous or disadvantageous positioning of hepatocytes within the acinus constitutes the basis for its *zonation*, which will now be described.

In *zone 1*, which is the spindle-shaped region immediately surrounding the axial vessels of the acinus (Fig. 19-11*A*), the hepatocytes obtain an excellent supply of nutrients and oxygen and are only minimally exposed to metabolic waste products. Such cells are able to synthesize glycogen and plasma proteins very actively. In *zone 2*, which is an ill-defined intermediate zone (Fig. 19-11*A*) that receives only second-class blood in terms of nutrients and oxygen, the cells are in a somewhat less privileged position. Then in *zone 3*, which extends from zone 2 to the nearest two central veins (Fig. 19-11*A*), the hepatocytes have to depend on a blood supply that is almost exhausted of nutrients and oxygen and that is highly charged with metabolites. Zone 3 constitutes the main site of alcohol and drug detoxification, and its hepatocytes are much more vulnerable to toxic damage than are those of zone 1.

There are at least three reasons why zone 3 is so sus-

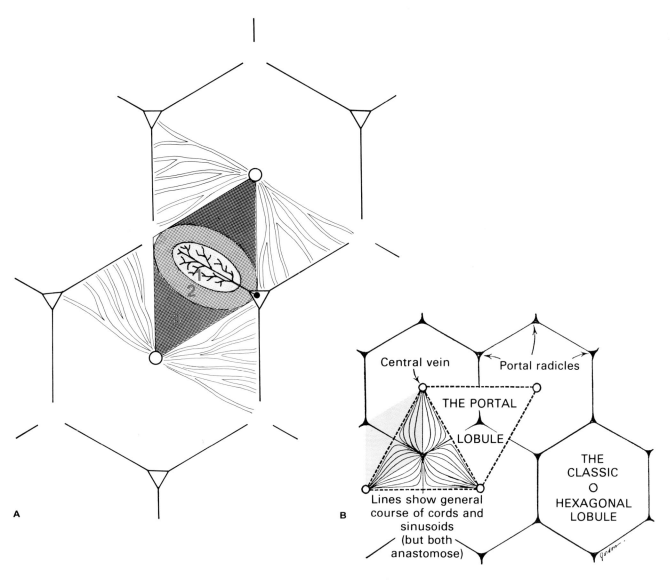

Fig. 19-11. Diagrammatic representations of (A) the liver acinus and (B) the classic lobule and portal lobule. In A, the three possible directions in which the vascular backbone of an acinus can extend from portal tract vessels are indicated by solid lines. (For details, see text.) In B, a liver acinus is indicated in blue to show its relationship to classic and portal lobules.

ceptible to damage. First, it is the last zone to receive nutrients from the incoming blood and is therefore the zone most deprived under conditions of malnutrition. Second, the hepatocytes in zone 3 are the most vulnerable to hypoxic damage and are in a critical predicament in the case of chronic alcoholism. Lastly, the hepatocytes in this zone are highly susceptible to cytotoxic damage by reactive or toxic metabolites that are produced during the course of detoxification reactions involving enzymes of the smooth-surfaced endoplasmic reticulum (sER).

Microscopic evidence of hepatocyte necrosis is more likely to be encountered in zone 3 than in zone 1. Fur-

thermore, because zone 3 is situated adjacent to central veins, evidence of necrosis is often seen in the vicinity of central veins. Finally, in the serious and virtually irreversible liver disease *cirrhosis*—the causes of which include chronic alcoholism, viral hepatitis, bile duct obstruction, and drug cytotoxicity—parenchymal necrosis can be so extensive that most of the liver acinus becomes replaced with fibrovascular scar tissue, eventually leaving only the isolated viable cores of acini (which generally represent zone 1) to carry out regeneration. The process of regeneration then leads to the development of *pseudolobules* that lack the vascular and canalicular connections necessary for them to function ef-

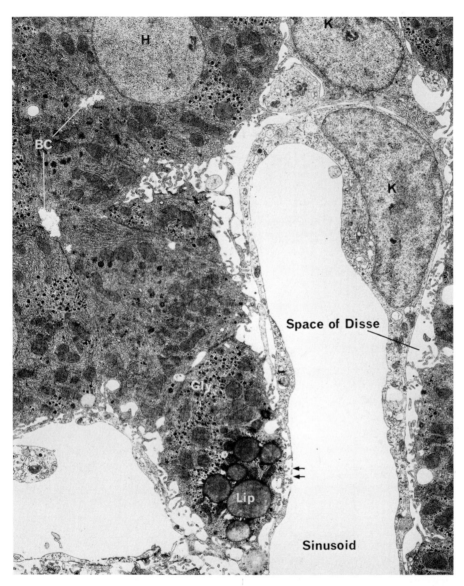

Fig. 19-12. Electron micrograph (×5000) of liver (rat), showing the space of Disse between the lining cells of sinusoids and hepatocytes (*H*). Between hepatocytes, bile canaliculi (*BC*) can be seen. Within the hepatocytes, glycogen areas (*Gly*) alternate with regions containing rER and mitochondria. Lipid droplets are labeled Lip. Two Kupffer cells (*K*) are seen at top right. Arrows indicate large endothelial cell fenestrae. (Courtesy of E. Rau)

fectively, with the result that liver function becomes greatly impaired. Further information about liver acinar involvement in toxic liver damage and cirrhosis can be found in the references cited for Rappaport, also Rappaport et al. Liver regeneration in general was briefly considered in connection with Growth Regulators in Chapter 5.

LIVER SINUSOIDS AND THE SPACE OF DISSE

A narrow space known as the *perisinusoidal space* or the *space of Disse* exists between the endothelial lining of the liver sinusoids and the hepatocytes that border on it (Figs. 19-10 and 19-12; see also Fig. 19-15). This space contains blood plasma, but in postnatal life, blood cells and platelets

are excluded from it. The electron microscope (EM) shows that it also contains vast numbers of microvilli; these project from the sinusoidal surface of the hepatocytes that border on the space (see Fig. 19-15).

Liver Sinusoids Are Provided with Macrophages Called Kupffer Cells. Two different cell types are found in the lining of liver sinusoids. In addition to *endothelial cells*, there are large stellate *Kupffer cells* representing macrophages derived from monocytes. In contrast to the macrophages in myeloid tissue, which although closely associated with sinusoids do not constitute an integral part of their lining, some of the Kupffer cells of the liver become incorporated into the sinusoidal lining by becoming interposed between endothelial cells (Figs. 19-12 and 19-13). Other Kupffer cells lie mainly in the space of Disse or assume a more imposing stance with their cell body extending

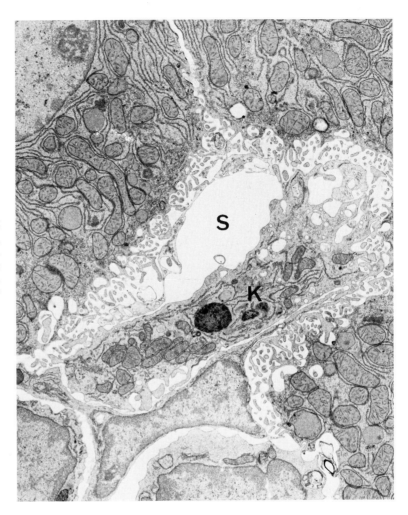

Fig. 19-13. Electron micrograph (×9700) of a Kupffer cell (*K*) in the lumen of a sinusoid (*S*) of rat liver. Dense bodies (secondary lysosomes) are evident near the middle of the cell. Note the numerous pseudopodia on this type of macrophage; they are readily seen at right. Some mitochondria are also present, especially in the left half of the cell. (Courtesy of A. Blouin)

across the sinusoidal lumen (Fig. 19-14). Being motile and capable of extensive phagocytosis, Kupffer cells guard against potential obstruction of the sinusoids by debris. They are also believed to play an important role in removing bacteria from the portal blood arriving from the intestine.

From Figure 19-13 it can be seen that Kupffer cells typically have an irregular outline. Their cytoplasm projects in the form of long thin pseudopods and microvilli, and clefts extend into the cell between these projections. Another feature of the Kupffer cell cytoplasm is that it contains distinctive wormlike structures, 140 nm across, with a midline that appears moderately electron dense. These structures are believed to represent intracellular reserves of cell membrane that are available for rapid phagocytic responses to particulate matter. They have been described in other types of macrophages as well. In addition, there are similarities between the nucleus of a Kupffer cell and that of a macrophage. The cytoplasm contains numerous endocytotic vesicles, and membrane-enclosed remnants of phagocytosed material (including hemosiderin from phagocytosed erythrocytes) are also commonly present.

From Figure 19-13 it can be seen that these cells have a fairly substantial complement of mitochondria and some rER, but their Golgi apparatus is not very prominent. Various types of dense bodies (secondary lysosomes) are also seen (Fig. 19-13). Like monocytes, Kupffer cells are peroxidase positive because they possess inconspicuous granules that contain this enzyme.

The Endothelial Lining of Sinusoids Is Fenestrated. Blood plasma that is free of suspended blood cells and platelets enters the space of Disse through large open fenestrae and smaller open pores that traverse the attenuated endothelial lining of the sinusoids (Figs. 19-10*B* and 19-15). The smaller pores are mostly localized in sites known as *sieve plates* (these can be seen to advantage in Fig. 19-14). The open pores in the sieve plates have an average diameter of approximately 100 nm (Wisse). Because the smallest chylomicrons are roughly comparable in size, they can probably gain access to the space of Disse through these pores as well as through the larger fenestrae, which have an average diameter of approximately 1 μm. Such larger fenestrations can also admit particulate material to

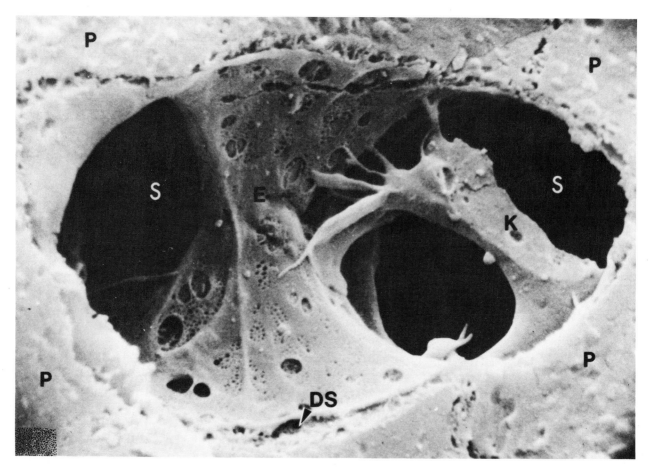

Fig. 19-14. Scanning electron micrograph (×7000) of a Kupffer cell (*K*) extending across the lumen of a liver sinusoid (*S*). This phagocytic cell is situated at a bifurcation of the sinusoid. At center, its cytoplasmic processes are seen adhering to endothelial lining cells (*E*) that are surrounded by parenchymal cells (hepatocytes) labeled P. The space of Disse (*DS*) can be discerned between the endothelium and the hepatocytes. Note also the open fenestrae and smaller sieve-plate pores that traverse the endothelial cells. Microvilli of underlying hepatocytes are visible through the large fenestrae at left. (Jones AL, Schmucker DL: Gastroenterology 73:833, 1977)

be disposed of by Kupffer cells. Because the open fenestrae and sieve plate pores lack diaphragms and do not impede the passage of plasma into the space of Disse, the hydrostatic pressure in the perisinusoidal space would approximate the intraluminal pressure in the sinusoid.

The space of Disse contains two kinds of supporting structures. First, there are enough collagen bundles (in the form of reticular fibers) and laminin (see Fig. 7-8*B*) to indicate the presence of a fairly extensive reticular scaffolding, and at least a minor amount of associated basement membrane material, arranged as a nonobstructing discontinuous supporting element that appears to be lacking beneath fenestrae and sieve plate pores (Fig. 19-14). Second, the endothelial layer is supported at some sites by cytoplasmic extensions of fat-storing cells known as *lipocytes*. As well as being associated with the space of Disse, these perisinusoidal storage cells lie interposed between hepatocytes

and are therefore considered to be an interstitial cell type of the parenchyma (Ito). A lipocyte containing fat storage droplets is illustrated in Figure 19-16; one of its supporting extensions is marked with an *arrow*. Besides storing fat and providing support, lipocytes store substantial quantities of vitamin A, the fat-soluble precursor of the visual pigment rhodopsin.

HEPATOCYTES

Hepatocytes have been used fairly extensively in this book to illustrate some of the basic features of cells, so all that is necessary at this stage is to review a few main points of interest. The fine structure of the hepatocyte nucleus, for example, is shown in Figure 2-2; nuclei of polyploid he-

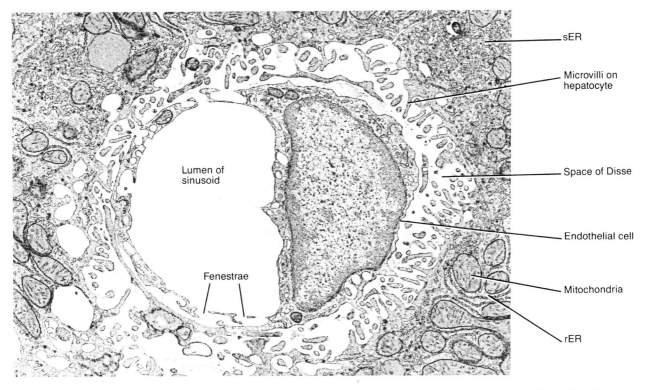

sER

Microvilli on hepatocyte

Space of Disse

Endothelial cell

Mitochondria

rER

Lumen of sinusoid

Fenestrae

Fig. 19-15.   Electron micrograph ($\times$14,300) of a liver sinusoid in cross section (rat liver). Open fenestrae are evident in the endothelial cell cytoplasm. Some of the longer structures in the space of Disse are cytoplasmic extensions of lipocytes; the remainder are microvilli of hepatocytes. (Courtesy of A. Blouin)

patocytes are illustrated in Figures 3-22 and 3-23. The storage of glycogen (Fig. 1-12) and fat (Fig. 1-13) in these cells was considered in Chapter 1.

It is no exaggeration to say that the cytoplasm of hepatocytes literally abounds with organelles and inclusions. Mitochondria are particularly numerous (Figs. 19-15 and 19-16); it has been estimated that there are approximately 800 in each hepatocyte. Hepatocytes require a substantial complement of these organelles to provide enough energy for their numerous metabolic duties. Free and membrane-bound polysomes are fairly abundant in hepatocytes. Both rER and sER are also prominent; the significance of this will be appreciated when we describe the functions of hepatocytes. Many Golgi stacks are scattered throughout the cytoplasm, some lying close to the nucleus and others lying near the bile canaliculi (Fig. 19-17). Lysosomes of all kinds are present, some of which are associated with bile canaliculi (Fig. 19-18).

Hepatocytes also contain a number of *peroxisomes (microbodies)* that are seen to advantage in Figure 19-18. In most species other than man, peroxisomes possess a semicrystalline core (nucleoid) that is probably urate oxidase (Fig. 19-18). Urate oxidase is required for urates to be metabolized in the body. Because humans lack this enzyme, they have to excrete uric acid along with urea in their urine.

Elevated uric acid levels in the body can lead to the development of acute gouty arthritis, a joint condition that was discussed in Chapter 8 in connection with Neutrophils. Other enzymes in peroxisomes can break down fatty acids by β-oxidation. This is thought to be the reason why hepatocyte peroxisome numbers increase when certain drugs are given to reduce plasma lipid and cholesterol levels. Further information may be found in the section on Peroxisomes in Chapter 4.

Hepatocytes possess three different kinds of surfaces, the first two of which have already been mentioned. Hepatocyte surfaces that border on the space of Disse, as stated, are covered with microvilli (Fig. 19-15), providing a large surface area that facilitates the absorption of substances from the bloodstream. Secretory products are discharged by exocytosis from the deeper regions of such surfaces (*i.e.*, from the areas that lie between the bases of microvilli). Hepatocyte surfaces that border on bile canaliculi are essentially secretory, but they still possess some microvilli (Fig. 19-17). The third kind of hepatocyte surface constitutes the lateral borders of the cell. Whereas in many species these lateral borders interdigitate fairly extensively, they do so hardly at all in man.

Without discussing liver function in great detail, we shall next comment on some of the more important functional

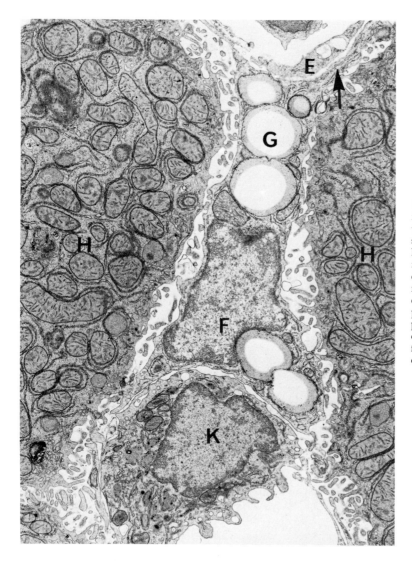

Fig. 19-16. Electron micrograph (×11,500) of a fat-storing cell (lipocyte), labeled F, lying between two hepatocytes (*H*) of rat liver. It also lies in association with a Kupffer cell (*K*) in a sinusoid (the lumen of which is seen as a clear space at *bottom right*). The lumen of another sinusoid, with an endothelial lining cell (*E*), is seen at top right. The fat-storage globules (*G*) of the lipocyte are partly extracted by fixative. The arrow indicates a cytoplasmic process extending from the lipocyte; such processes provide support for the endothelial lining cells (*E*) of sinusoids, as seen at top right, and also for Kupffer cells in the walls of sinusoids. (Courtesy of A. Blouin)

roles of hepatocytes and relate these functions to the organelles involved.

Detoxifying Role of Hepatocytes

Hepatocytes are responsible for carrying out a number of important transformation and conjugation reactions that play a key role in detoxifying certain endogenous and exogenous compounds that are deleterious to the body. For example, the ammonia that is formed during the course of amino acid deamination becomes highly toxic if it is allowed to reach a certain concentration. Hepatocytes normally keep toxic concentrations from being attained by using this ammonia to form urea, which is not as toxic and is efficiently eliminated from the body by the kidneys.

In addition, many exogenous substances, ranging from prescribed lipid-soluble drugs to pesticides and other toxic chemicals absorbed from external sources, are metabolized

and detoxified by hepatocytes. In some instances, the metabolites are more damaging than the substances themselves. Steroids and alcohol are also metabolized in hepatocytes. Sustained high levels of certain drugs or alcohol can lead to a marked increase in the amount of sER that is present in these cells because the enzymes responsible for detoxification are intimately associated with the sER.

Secretory Role of Hepatocytes

As well as secreting bile constituents, hepatocytes synthesize and liberate a number of important *internal secretions* into the bloodstream. We will discuss these first.

Glycogen Synthesis and Glucose Secretion. The blood sugar levels after dietary intake of carbohydrates would escalate uncontrollably if it were not for the fact that hepatocytes absorb excess glucose from the blood and, under

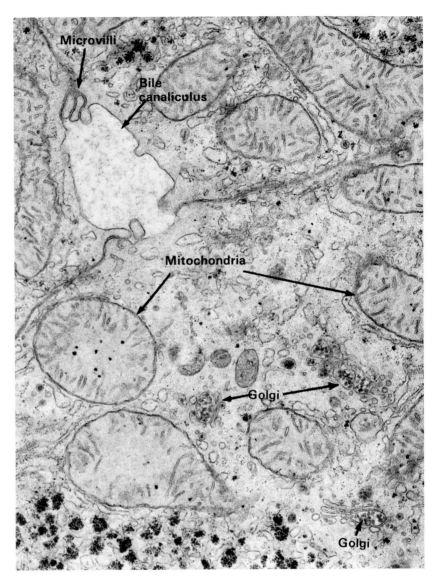

Fig. 19-17. Electron micrograph (×30,000) of hepatocytes (mouse liver). A bile canaliculus is seen at upper left, with microvilli projecting into its lumen. The abundant large mitochondria have numerous cristae. Within the Golgi saccules that are present below center, there are electron-dense lipoprotein particles. These represent precursors of the lipoproteins released to the plasma. Glycogen granules, arranged in rosettes (α-particles), are seen at bottom left, with tubules of sER between the rosettes. (Courtesy of A. Jézéquel)

the influence of *insulin* from the pancreas, convert this glucose into glycogen. Conversely, when the blood sugar level falls, they convert glycogen back into glucose and release this into the blood. In the EM, hepatocyte glycogen deposits appear as aggregates of electron-dense particles that are closely associated with tubules of the sER (see Figs. 4-27 and 19-17). Probable reasons for this characteristic association with the sER were discussed in Chapter 4 in the section dealing with the Smooth-Surfaced Endoplasmic Reticulum.

The hormone *cortisol*, which is produced by the adrenal cortex, can also bring about the formation of glycogen in hepatocytes. However, in this case, the glycogen is formed as a result of protein catabolism and its formation is accompanied by the release, not the removal, of blood glu-

cose. This effect of cortisol will be discussed more fully in the section on the Adrenal Cortex in Chapter 22.

Blood Protein Secretion. Hepatocytes secrete the albumins, fibrinogen, and most of the globulins of blood plasma. Together with several other proteins that participate in blood coagulation, these plasma proteins are secreted into the sinusoids. However, immunoglobulins are produced by plasma cells and not by hepatocytes. Secretory proteins synthesized by the rER pass through the Golgi complex and are released by exocytosis from the sinusoidal surfaces that are bathed with blood plasma.

Lipoprotein Secretion. Hepatocytes are also involved in the regulation of plasma lipid levels. Some of this lipid is

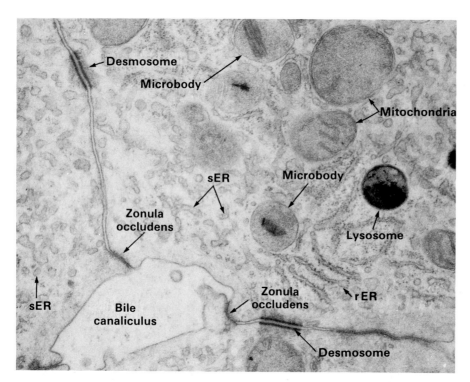

Fig. 19-18. Electron micrograph (×13,000) of three hepatocytes bordering on a bile canaliculus (liver of groundhog). The cells are joined by junctional complexes. In the hepatocyte at upper right, some rER can be seen (*right of center*). Note also a lysosome and two peroxisomes (labeled *microbody*) with characteristic crystalline nucleoids. Some sER is also present. (Courtesy of J. Steiner)

in the form of a loose complex of fatty acids and albumin. However, most of it is present as small particles in which triglycerides and cholesteryl esters are combined with protein. Such particles are described as blood *lipoproteins.* Lipid-containing particles on their own would be hydrophobic and therefore would be unable to remain in suspension. However, the protein with which the lipid-containing particles is associated renders them sufficiently hydrophilic to remain suspended in the plasma.

The blood contains five major classes of lipoprotein particles. *Chylomicrons* (described in Chap. 7 under Adipocytes and Adipose Tissue) are the largest of these particles. They are formed by intestinal absorptive cells mainly from triglycerides and cholesteryl ester, as outlined in the section on the Small Intestine in Chapter 18. Hepatocytes participate with other cells in removing chylomicrons from the blood following a fatty meal. Because chylomicrons are suspended in blood plasma, they readily enter the space of Disse and are probably absorbed as such by hepatocytes that then utilize their constituents. The other lipoproteins are known as *very low-density* or *pre-β lipoproteins* (VLDL), *remnants* or *slow pre-β lipoproteins, low-density* or *β lipoproteins* (LDL), and *high-density* or *α lipoproteins* (HDL). VLDL particles are somewhat smaller than chylomicrons and are relatively rich in triglycerides. They are synthesized by hepatocytes as described below. Slow pre-β lipoproteins (remnant particles) have an intermediate size range and intermediate density, and are derived from chylomicrons and VLDL. LDL particles are even smaller and denser because they contain less lipid. They are also the chief means by which cholesterol is transported throughout the body. HDL particles are the smallest and also the densest of the lipoprotein particles.

The VLDL released by hepatocytes is assembled in a stepwise manner. The sER in which its lipid component is synthesized is continuous with the rER in which its protein component is synthesized. From the ER, most if not all of the synthesized lipoprotein passes to the Golgi complex. Secretory vesicles that contain characteristic spherical electron-dense *lipoprotein particles,* approximately 30 nm to 60 nm in diameter, then bud from the Golgi stacks (Fig. 19-17) and move to the sinusoidal surfaces where their contents are released into the blood plasma.

IgA Secretion. Secretory IgA and *secretory component* (SC) involvement in its secretion were described in Chapter 10 in the section on Lymph Nodes. It will be recalled that IgA dimers (and to a lesser extent IgM pentamers) are secreted by mucosal epithelial cells as a result of becoming complexed with SC. This SC is a glycoprotein cell-surface receptor for IgA (and IgM). After IgA or IgM has complexed with its receptor, the ligand–receptor complex is internalized by receptor-mediated endocytosis. It is then transported across the cell, and, still in the form of the undissociated covalent complex, the dimeric IgA–SC complex is discharged by exocytosis from the luminal border of the cell. In similar fashion, hepatocytes take up IgA dimers and other polymeric forms of IgA that enter the bloodstream by way of the lymph that drains from the lamina propria of mucous membranes. This IgA is internalized from the plasma in the space of Disse, is transported across the cell, and then is discharged from a part of the cell surface that borders on a *bile canaliculus.* By this means, relatively large quantities of IgA reach the lumen of the small intestine through the bile. For further information, see Hall and Andrew.

Bile Secretion. *Bile,* the exocrine secretion of hepatocytes that enters the bile canaliculi, contains the bile pigment bilirubin, bile salts, cholesterol, lecithin, and fatty acids, together with ions and water. *Bilirubin* is a waste product that arises from the breakdown of hemoglobin primarily in macrophages of the spleen. This non–iron-containing waste product passes from macrophages into the bloodstream and is then absorbed by hepatocytes from the blood plasma that enters the space of Disse. Bilirubin is of no further use to the body. Hepatocytes carry out an important conjugation reaction that converts it into a more water-soluble conjugated form that then passes into the bile.

This reaction, in which bilirubin becomes conjugated with glucuronic acid to form *bilirubin glucuronide,* requires an enzyme called *glucuronyl transferase* that is associated with the sER of hepatocytes. Bilirubin glucuronide (the form of bilirubin that enters the bile from the blood) is generally referred to as *conjugated bilirubin.*

Bile salts, unlike bile pigment, are useful substances that are able to facilitate the digestion of fats after they reach the intestinal lumen. They are the sodium and potassium salts of cholesterol-derived bile acids (cholic and chenodeoxycholic acid and their derivatives) conjugated to either glycine or taurine by hepatocytes. As mentioned in Chapter 18, these salts participate in the formation of tiny particulate complexes known as *micelles* that, by incorporating lipids and products of lipid digestion, facilitate the absorption of monoglycerides and free fatty acids into intestinal absorptive cells. In the presence of monoglycerides and lecithin, the bile salts also possess substantial surfactant (detergentlike) activity and are largely responsible for emulsifying fats in preparation for their digestion by pancreatic lipase. Like bilirubin and cholesterol (which represents a third major constituent of bile), the bile salts are exocrine secretory products of hepatocytes.

Another important aspect of bile secretion relates to steroid hormones that are produced by the adrenal cortex and sex glands. Hepatocytes continuously absorb such hormones from the bloodstream and metabolize them to varying extents. The resulting metabolites, and to some extent the unchanged hormones themselves, become partly secreted into the bile. When the bile is delivered to the intestine, these steroid hormones are absorbed and reenter the bloodstream. There is therefore an enterohepatic circulation of steroid hormones.

There is also an enterohepatic circulation of bile pigments because when bilirubin reaches the intestine, it becomes changed into urobilinogen and stercobilinogen by the action of bacteria in the intestinal flora. Some of the urobilinogen is subsequently absorbed and thereupon enters the portal blood. Hepatocytes then extract it, convert it into conjugated bilirubin, and secrete it again into the bile.

Although hepatocytes secrete bile at a more or less constant rate, it is delivered to the intestine only when it will be of most use, which is when partly digested food is leaving the stomach. In the meantime, it collects in the gallbladder and becomes concentrated there, as will be described later in this chapter.

Jaundice (Icterus). The word *jaundice* is derived from the Fr. *jaune,* meaning yellow. Under normal conditions, the total blood level of bilirubin (conjugated and unconjugated) is insufficient to impart any noticeable yellow color to the skin. However, elevated blood levels of bilirubin (*hyperbilirubinemia*) can cause the skin, mucous membranes, and sclerae (the whites of the eyes) to take on a distinctly yellow color. A person with such an appearance is described as *jaundiced.*

There are three different underlying causes of this condition, which are described in the following section.

1. Normally, hepatocytes are able to extract bilirubin from the blood at a rate that is comparable with its rate of production by macrophages. However, if erythrocyte destruction is greatly accelerated, the rate of disposal may lag behind the rate of production. The resulting accumulation of bilirubin in the blood is manifested as jaundice. This is often referred to as *hemolytic jaundice* because it is due to increased destruction of erythrocytes.
2. The liver's capacity for absorbing, conjugating, or secreting bilirubin can be impaired in a number of ways. First, bilirubin may not be taken up from the blood as readily as it should. Second, there are specific genetic enzyme defects that do not allow hepatocytes to process bilirubin adequately. Third, liver damage can leave an insufficient number of fully functional hepatocytes to cope with all the bilirubin coming to them in the blood. Lastly, hepatocytes may become damaged in such a way that the bilirubin they absorb is inadequately secreted into their canaliculi and leaks back into the sinusoids.
3. The bile secreted into the duct system may be unable to flow into the intestine because of some obstruction in the bile duct system (*obstructive jaundice*). The most common kind of obstruction is a stone in one of the main drainage ducts. However, obstruction can be due to a malignancy of the head of the pancreas blocking the hepatopancreatic ampulla that opens into the duodenum. Under such conditions, bile is dammed back through the hepatocytes into the sinusoids.

BILE DUCTS AND LYMPHATICS

Bile canaliculi can be discerned in the light microscope following histochemical staining for the enzyme alkaline phosphatase, which is present in bile (Fig. 19-9A). Alternatively, they can be filled with an appropriate opaque material that is injected through the bile duct system and then is observed in cleared sections. They begin blindly within the liver trabeculae in the regions around central veins, and they anastomose freely as they extend along trabeculae toward the periphery of classic lobules (Fig. 19-10).

In the EM, it can be seen that bile canaliculi are bounded by two (occasionally three) hepatocytes (Fig. 19-18). At sites where the liver trabeculae reach portal tracts, canaliculi empty into short *canals of Hering,* which are bordered partly by hepatocytes and partly by duct cells. These canals connect with fine branches of the bile duct system called *bile ductules* that lie in the portal tracts. However, canals of

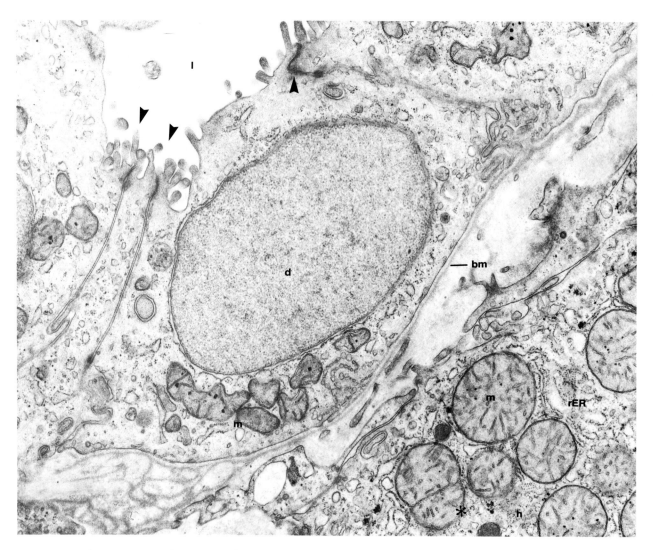

Fig. 19-19.   Electron micrograph (×16,400) of a part of a bile duct wall (rat liver). A few microvilli project from the duct cells (*d*) into the lumen (*l*). These duct cells contain very little rER and relatively few mitochondria (*m*). Arrowheads indicate junctional complexes between their lateral borders. The duct has a surrounding basement membrane (*bm*). Mitochondria (*m*) and rER can be distinguished in the hepatocyte (*h*) at lower right. The appearance of the mitochondrion marked with an asterisk suggests that it may be in the process of dividing. (Courtesy of M. J. Phillips)

Hering are not the only channels by which bile reaches the ductules, because leading out from the canals of Hering, there are narrow bypasses known as *preductules* or *chol-angioles,* and these, too, drain into the bile ductules. Preductules differ from canals of Hering in that they have no hepatocytes along their course; their walls are made up entirely of duct cells.

The cytoplasm of duct cells contains a moderate number of ribosomes but little rER. The Golgi apparatus is not prominent and the mitochondria are smaller than in hepatocytes (Fig. 19-19). Whereas the various branches of the bile duct system are surrounded by a prominent and continuous basement membrane, a prominent basement

membrane is not seen in association with hepatocytes (Fig. 19-19). Junctional complexes hold the lateral borders of contiguous duct cells together close to the lumen (Fig. 19-19, *arrowheads*). Microvilli project into the lumen of bile ducts (Fig. 19-19) and ductules.

Bile ductules, the smallest tributaries in the bile duct system, have walls of low cuboidal epithelium. The slightly larger ducts seen in portal areas have walls of typical simple cuboidal epithelium (Fig. 19-8C). Still larger bile ducts are lined by simple columnar epithelium. The *right* and *left hepatic ducts* leave the liver at the porta hepatis and unite to form the *common hepatic duct.* The walls of these comparatively wide extrahepatic ducts are strengthened with

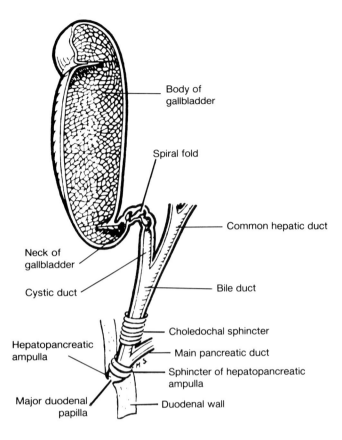

Fig. 19-20. Diagram of the gallbladder (cut open to show the folds on its inner surface), cystic duct, and bile duct. (After Grant JCB, Basmajian JV: Grant's Method of Anatomy, 7th ed. Baltimore, Williams & Wilkins, 1965)

Labels on figure:
Body of gallbladder
Spiral fold
Common hepatic duct
Neck of gallbladder
Cystic duct
Bile duct
Choledochal sphincter
Hepatopancreatic ampulla
Main pancreatic duct
Sphincter of hepatopancreatic ampulla
Major duodenal papilla
Duodenal wall

dense ordinary connective tissue, and they also contain some smooth muscle.

Lymphatics. Lymphatics have not been demonstrated in or around the liver trabeculae or sinusoids, but they are present in the various stromal components of the liver, that is, (1) in the connective tissue capsule, (2) in the connective tissue in the portal tracts, and (3) in the sparse connective tissue associated with the hepatic veins. The liver produces a great deal of lymph that is relatively rich in protein. The sites where this lymph is formed are not known with certainty, but is widely believed that most of the hepatic lymph originates as plasma from the space of Disse, and that this plasma infiltrates the connective tissue in the portal tracts and accumulates there as a protein-rich tissue fluid that drains away as lymph.

GALLBLADDER

A side branch called the *cystic duct* extends from the *common hepatic duct* to the *gallbladder,* which is an elongated thin-walled reservoir in which the bile is stored and concentrated (see Figs. 18-1 and 19-20). When the gallbladder

is not distended with bile, its mucous membrane shows an extensive pattern of small folds (Figs. 19-20 and 19-21). The neck of the gallbladder is twisted in such a way that its mucous membrane forms a supporting spiral fold (Fig. 19-20). Mucosal glands are confined to the vicinity of the neck region. The *epithelial lining* is made up of high columnar absorptive cells with microvilli (Fig. 19-21).

Beneath the epithelium is a *lamina propria* that is made of loose connective tissue (Fig. 19-21). The gallbladder has *no muscularis mucosae;* hence its mucous membrane borders on a *smooth muscle coat* that represents the *muscularis externa* (Fig. 19-21). Some of the muscle fibers in this coat are circularly arranged and some are longitudinal, but most are oblique. Connective tissue containing many elastic fibers fills the interstices between the bundles of smooth muscle fibers that constitute this coat.

External to the muscle coat is a thick *perimuscular (subserosal) coat* (Fig. 19-21A). This coat consists of loose connective tissue that may contain groups of fat cells. It conveys blood vessels, nerves, and lymphatics to the organ. Where the gallbladder is attached to the liver, the connective tissue of its perimuscular coat merges with that of the liver.

Bile Duct and Choledochal Sphincter. The duct that extends from the junction between the *cystic duct* and the *common hepatic duct* to the duodenum is called the *bile duct* (Fig. 19-20).

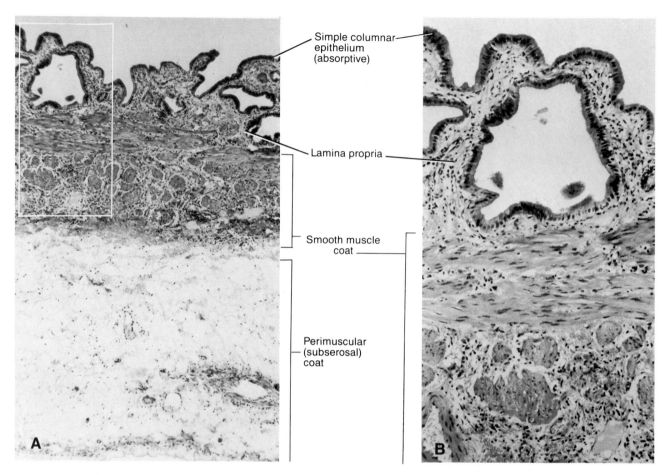

Simple columnar epithelium (absorptive)

Lamina propria

Smooth muscle coat

Perimuscular (subserosal) coat

A

B

Fig. 19-21. Photomicrographs illustrating the wall structure of the gallbladder. (*A*) Low power. (*B*) Boxed-in area in *A* under higher magnification. For details, see text.

Partway through the wall of the duodenum, the bile duct and the pancreatic duct generally unite, and the expanded lumen of the common duct is termed the *hepatopancreatic ampulla* (Fig. 19-20). This ampulla follows an oblique course through the duodenal wall and opens on the *major duodenal papilla* that projects into the duodenal lumen. The hepatopancreatic ampulla is provided with a sphincter that develops independently of the intestinal wall. The muscle that surrounds the preampullary part of the bile duct serves as the sphincter of that duct; it is called the *choledochal sphincter* (Fig. 19-20). Closure of the choledochal sphincter prevents bile from entering the duodenum, with the result that the bile passes, by way of the cystic duct, to the gallbladder, where it collects and becomes concentrated.

Cholecystography.   Water and ions become absorbed through the epithelium of the gallbladder into capillaries of the lamina propria, effecting at least a fivefold increase in the biliary concentration of bile pigment, bile salts, and cholesterol. If the gallbladder is concentrating bile normally, radiopaque substances (*e.g.*, iodine-containing tracer dyes) excreted into the bile become sufficiently concentrated for the gallbladder to be visualized radiographically (*cholecystography*). This permits gallbladder function to be checked by means of an x-ray series.

Emptying of the Gallbladder Is Elicited by a Gastrointestinal Hormone.   Dietary fats (even those in milk) are known to be particularly effective in causing the gallbladder to contract. The gastrointestinal hormone *cholecystokinin-pancreozymin* (CCK-PZ) is released by enteroendocrine cells of the intestinal mucosa in response to the presence of free fatty acids, peptides, or amino acids in the partly digested food reaching the intestine. This peptide hormone travels through the bloodstream to the gallbladder and thereupon elicits contraction of its smooth muscle, causing bile to enter the intestine.

SELECTED REFERENCES

Exocrine Pancreas*

BROOKS F: Diseases of the Exocrine Pancreas. Philadelphia, WB Saunders, 1980

_____

*For references on Endocrine Pancreas, see Selected References, Chapter 22.

CARO LG, PALADE GE: Protein synthesis, storage and discharge in the pancreatic exocrine cell. An autoradiographic study. J Cell Biol 20:473, 1964

EKHOLM R, EDLUND Y: Ultrastructure of the human exocrine pancreas. J Ultrastruct Res 2:453, 1959

HOWAT HT, SEARLES H (eds): The Exocrine Pancreas. Philadelphia, WB Saunders, 1979

JAMIESON JD, PALADE GE: Condensing vacuole conversion and zymogen granule discharge in pancreatic exocrine cells: Metabolic studies. J Cell Biol 48:503, 1971

PALADE GE, SIEKEVITZ P, CARO LG: Structure, chemistry, and function of the pancreatic exocrine cell. In de Reuch AVS, Cameron MP (eds): The Exocrine Pancreas. Ciba Foundation Symposium. Boston, Little, Brown, 1962

de REUCH AVS, CAMERON MP (eds): The Exocrine Pancreas. Ciba Foundation Symposium. Boston, Little, Brown, 1962

SARLES H: The exocrine pancreas. Int Rev Physiol 12:173, 1977

Liver

BLOUIN A, BOLENDER RP, WEIBEL ER: Distribution of organelles and membranes between hepatocytes and nonhepatocytes in the rat liver parenchyma. A stereological study. J Cell Biol 72:441, 1977

BROOKS SEH, HAGGIS GH: Scanning electon microscopy of rat's liver. Lab Invest 29:60, 1973

BRUNI C, PORTER KR: The fine structure of the parenchymal cell of the normal rat liver. 1. General Observations. Am J Pathol 46: 691, 1965

BURKEL WE: The fine structure of the terminal branches of the hepatic arterial system of the rat. Anat Rec 167:329, 1970

CARDELL RR, Jr: Action of metabolic hormones on the fine structure of liver cells III. Effects of adrenalectomy and administration of cortisone. Anat Rec 180:309, 1974

CARDELL RR, Jr: Smooth endoplasmic reticulum in rat hepatocytes during glycogen deposition and depletion. Int Rev Cytol 48: 221, 1977

CARRUTHERS JS, STEINER JW: Fine structure of terminal branches of the biliary tree. Arch Pathol 74:117, 1962

ELIAS H: A re-examination of the structure of the mammalian liver: I. Parenchymal architecture. Am J Anat 84:311, 1949

ELIAS H: A re-examination of the structure of the mammalian liver: II. Hepatic lobule and its relation to vascular and biliary systems. Am J Anat 85:379, 1949

FORKER EL: Mechanisms of hepatic bile formation. Annu Rev Physiol 39:323, 1977

FRANK BW, KERN F: Intestinal and liver lymph and lymphatics. Gastroenterology 55:408, 1967

HALL JG, ANDREW E: Biliglobulin: A new look at IgA. Immunology Today 1 No 5:100, 1980

HAMILTON RL, REGEN DM, GRAY ME, LEQUIRE VS: Lipid transport in liver. I. Electron microscopic identification of very low density lipoprotein in perfused rat liver. Lab Invest 16:305, 1967

HOWARD JG: The origin and immunological significance of Kupffer cells. In van Furth R (ed): Mononuclear Phagocytes. Oxford, Blackwell Scientific Publications, 1970

HRUBAN Z, SWIFT H: Uricase, localization in hepatic microbodies. Science 146:1316, 1964

ITO T: Recent advances in the study of the fine structure of the hepatic sinusoidal wall: A review. Gunma Rep Med Sci 6:119, 1973

ITO T: Structure and function of the fat-storing cell (FSC) in the liver—A review. Acta Anat Nippon 53:393, 1978

JONES AL, FAWCETT DW: Hypertrophy of the agranular endoplasmic reticulum in hamster liver induced by phenobarbital. J Histochem Cytochem 14:215, 1966

JONES AL, SCHMUCKER DL: Current concepts of liver structure as related to function. Gastroenterology 73:833, 1977

LEBOUTON AV, MARCHAND R: Changes in the distribution of thymidine-^{3}H labeled cells in the growing liver acinus of neonatal rats. Dev Biol 23:524, 1970

MA MH, BIEMPICA L: The normal human liver cell. Am J Pathol 62: 353, 1971

MOTTA P: Three-dimensional architecture of the mammalian liver. A scanning electron microscopic review. In Allen DJ, Motta PM, DiDio JA (eds): Three-Dimensional Microanatomy of Cells and Tissue Surfaces. New York, Elsevier North-Holland, 1981

MOTTA P, MUTO M, FUJITA T: The Liver. An Atlas of Scanning Electron Microscopy. Tokyo, Igaku-Shoin, 1978

NOVIKOFF AB, ESSNER E: The liver cell. Am J Med 29:102, 1960

RAPPAPORT AM: Acinar units and the pathophysiology of the liver. In Rouiller C (ed): The Liver: Morphology, Biochemistry, Physiology. Vol 1. New York, Academic Press, 1963

RAPPAPORT AM: The microcirculatory hepatic unit. Microvasc Res 6:212, 1973

RAPPAPORT AM: The microcirculatory acinar concept of normal and pathological hepatic structure. Beitr Pathol Bd 157:215, 1976

RAPPAPORT AM: Physioanatomical basis of toxic liver injury. In Farber E, Fisher MM (eds): Toxic Injury of the Liver, Part A, p 1. New York, Marcel Dekker, 1979

RAPPAPORT AM, MACPHEE PJ, FISHER MM, PHILLIPS MJ: The scarring of the liver acini (cirrhosis)—Tridimensional and microcirculatory considerations. Virchows Arch [A] 402:107, 1983

REICHEN J, PAUMGARTNER G: Excretory function of the liver. In Javitt NB (ed): International Review of Physiology: Liver and Biliary Tract Physiology I, Vol 21, p 103. Baltimore, University Park Press, 1980

RHODIN, JAG: Ultrastructure and function of liver sinusoids. Proceedings IVth International Symposium of RES, May 29–June 1, 1964, Kyoto, Japan

ROUILLER C (ed): The Liver: Morphology, Biochemistry, Physiology. 2 vols. New York, Academic Press, 1963–64

SASSE D, SCHENK A: A three-dimensional presentation of the functional liver unit. Acta Anat 93:78, 1975

SCHMID R: Bilirubin metabolism in man. N Engl J Med 287:703, 1972

STEIN O, STEIN Y: The role of the liver in the metabolism of chylomicrons, studied by electron microscope autoradiograhy. Lab Invest 17:436, 1967

STEINER JW, CARRUTHERS JS: Studies on the fine structure of the terminal branches of the biliary tree. I. The morphology of normal bile canaliculi, bile pre-ductules (ducts of Hering) and bile duct-ules. Am J Pathol 38:639, 1961

TANIKAWA K: Ultrastructural Aspects of the Liver and Its Disorders, 2nd ed. Tokyo, Igaku-Shoin, 1979

WISSE E: An electron microscope study of the fenestrated endothelial lining of rat liver sinusoids. J Ultrastruct Res 31:125, 1970

WISSE E: An ultrastructural characterization of the endothelial cell in the rat liver sinusoid under normal and various experimental conditions, as a contribution to the distinction between endo-thelial and Kupffer cells. J Ultrastr Res 38:528, 1972

WISSE E: Observations on the fine structure and peroxidase cyto-chemistry of normal rat liver Kupffer cells. J Ultrastruct Res 46: 393, 1974

WISSE E, DAEMS WT: Fine structural study on the sinusoidal lining cells of rat liver. In van Furth R (ed): Mononuclear Phagocytes. Oxford, Blackwell Scientific Publications, 1970

Gallbladder

CHAPMAN GB, CHIARDO AJ, COFFEY RJ, WEINEKE K: The fine structure of the human gallbladder. Anat Rec 154:579, 1966

FRIZZELL RA, HEINTZE K: Transport functions of the gallbladder. In Javitt NB (ed): International Review of Physiology: Liver and Biliary Tract Physiology I, Vol 21, p 221. Baltimore, University Park Press, 1980

HAYWARD AF: Aspects of the fine structure of gallbladder epithelium of the mouse. J Anat 96:227, 1962

HAYWARD AF: The structure of gallbladder epithelium. Int Rev Gen Exp Zool 3:205, 1968

KAY GI, WHEELER HO, WHITLOCK RT, LANE N: Fluid transport in rabbit gallbladder. A combined physiological and electron microscope study. J Cell Biol 30:237, 1966

MUELLER JC, JONES AL, LONG JA: Topographical and subcellular anat-omy of the guinea pig gallbladder. Gastroenterology 63:856, 1972

20

The Respiratory System

The blood that returns to the heart in the systemic circulation has a diminished content of oxygen and a correspondingly increased content of carbon dioxide. This blood is thereupon pumped by the right heart to the lungs, which are provided with a multitude of air-filled sacs termed *alveoli* and vast numbers of alveolar capillaries that bring the blood in the pulmonary circulation extremely close to the alveolar air. Oxygen diffuses from the alveolar air to the blood, and carbon dioxide diffuses in the reverse direction. The alveolar air is changed 12 to 15 times per minute (at rest) through respiratory movements, *inspiration* drawing air into the lungs and *expiration* expelling it.

The *lungs* are situated within a skeletal framework described as the *thoracic cage* that is made up of the vertebral column, ribs, costal cartilages, and sternum. At the bottom of this cage is a dome-shaped musculotendinous sheet, the *diaphragm*. The large compartment of the thoracic cavity occupied by each lung has a fibroelastic membranous lining called the *parietal pleura* (Fig. 20-1), the free serosal surface of which is covered with squamous mesothelial cells. Likewise, each lung is covered with *visceral pleura* (Fig. 20-1), the free serosal surface of which is similarly covered with squamous mesothelial cells. A thin film of tissue fluid between the parietal pleura and the visceral pleura reduces frictional rub between their apposed serosal surfaces during respiratory movements.

Except at the hilum (root) of the lung, which is the site where its extrapulmonary bronchus and major blood vessels, lymphatics, and nerves enter or leave (Fig. 20-1), each lung can move freely within the cavity that it occupies. At the hilum, the visceral pleural covering of each lung is continuous with the parietal pleural lining of each cavity (Fig. 20-1). The potential space jointly enclosed by the visceral and parietal pleura is called the *pleural cavity*. It should be understood that although a lung occupies

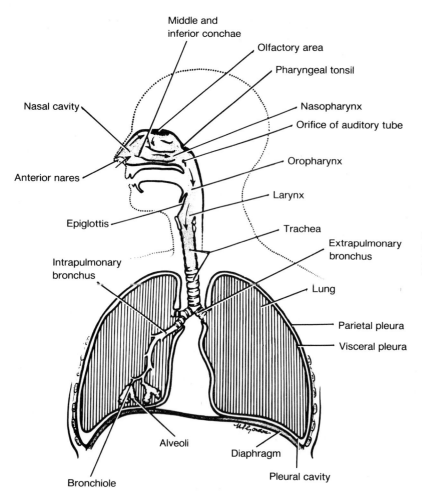

Middle and
inferior conchae

Olfactory area

Pharyngeal tonsil

Nasal cavity

Nasopharynx

Orifice of auditory tube

Anterior nares

Oropharynx

Larynx

Epiglottis

Trachea

Extrapulmonary
bronchus

Intrapulmonary
bronchus

Lung

Parietal pleura

Visceral pleura

Alveoli

Diaphragm

Bronchiole

Pleural cavity

Fig. 20-1. Schematic diagram of the parts of the respiratory system. (After Grant JCB: A Method of Anatomy, 4th ed. Baltimore, Williams & Wilkins, 1948)

a cavity in the thorax, it does not lie inside the pleural cavity but outside it, just as the intestines occupy the abdominal cavity but lie outside the peritoneal cavity.

Inspiration.   The arrangement of the ribs with respect to the vertebral column and sternum is such that contraction of the muscles attached to the ribs not only deepens the thoracic cage in the anteroposterior plane but also widens it. Moreover, contraction of the diaphragm (with simultaneous relaxation of the muscles of the abdominal wall, permitting the diaphragm to descend) elongates the cage. Hence by the contraction of certain muscles and the relaxation of others, the thoracic cage can be made larger by becoming deeper, wider, and longer, and this draws air into the lungs. It also draws extra blood into the pulmonary and extrapulmonary vessels of the thorax. During inspiration, air is drawn through the nose or mouth, down the trachea, and into the bronchial tree to its end branches. From there it reaches the passageways and air-filled sacs of the spongy, capillary-rich respiratory tissue where gas exchange occurs.

Expiration.   The very large size of the inflated lung compared with the size of its surrounding pleural cavity is a result of its being *stretched* in all directions. A large amount of *elastin* is present in the visceral pleura, in the partitions between the air sacs, and in the walls of the bronchial tree. When the lung grows, it becomes increasingly stretched as the thoracic cavity increases in size. As a consequence, the elastin in the lungs is always stretched, even at the end of expiration. Hence, if a hollow needle is inserted through the thoracic wall into the pleural cavity, air passes into this cavity and the lung collapses toward its hilum. The pleural cavity is thereby converted into a real (air-filled) cavity instead of a potential cavity. The condition in which there is air in the pleural cavity is called a *pneumothorax*, and it can develop as a complication of a penetrating injury to the thoracic wall (*e.g.*, when ribs are fractured). In certain diseases, the fluid in the pleural cavity, which normally constitutes no more than a film, becomes greatly increased in amount. This, too, permits the lung to retract. This condition is known as a *hydrothorax.*

Because the elastic tissue of the lungs remains stretched

even at the end of expiration, and becomes still more stretched on inspiration, it is scarcely necessary for an individual at rest to exert muscular contractions to expel air. The elastic recoil of the lungs in itself is almost enough to expel air through the bronchial tree. But during exercise—and probably also to some extent even in quiet breathing—expiration is facilitated by contractions of the abdominal muscles, which force the abdominal viscera against the undersurface of the diaphragm and so push it up into the thorax.

The descent and expansion of the lungs on inspiration require that the bronchial tree itself be elastic. Bronchi, for example, become longer and wider on inspiration. The root of the lung also descends on inspiration. On expiration, the various parts of the lung return to their original positions because of the recoil of the elastin in the bronchial tree.

The Respiratory System Consists of Conducting and Respiratory Portions. The system of interconnecting cavities and tubes that conducts air from outside the body to all parts of the lungs constitutes the *conducting portion* of the respiratory system; the pockets and passageways of the respiratory tissue of the lung (the only sites where gaseous exchange occurs) constitute the *respiratory portion* of the system. The conducting part of the system consists of the nose, nasopharynx, larynx, trachea, bronchi, and bronchioles (Fig. 20-1). Some of these structures are situated outside the lung and others (the intrapulmonary bronchi and the bronchioles) lie within it. The parts of the conducting system that lie outside the lung require fairly rigid walls; otherwise, strong inspiratory movements might cause them to collapse, as in sucking a drink through a wet straw. Rigidity is provided by cartilage or by bone.

The conducting portion of the respiratory system has other roles in addition to conducting air to and from the lungs. Its mucous membrane warms or cools and humidifies the incoming air and clears it of suspended particles. *Ciliary action* and *mucus* both play a key role in the trapping and disposal of potentially infectious microorganisms and other types of particles that enter the airways in the inhaled air. The mucus is normally of a consistency that allows it to be cleared continuously from the airways at a rate of about 4 mm per minute (the rate of tracheal mucociliary clearance). It moves in the form of a continuous *mucous blanket* (see Fig. 20-7B) that is propelled by ciliary activity toward the pharynx, an arrangement that is often referred to as a *mucociliary escalator.* The importance of a normal rate of tracheobronchial mucociliary clearance is well illustrated in the pediatric disorder *cystic fibrosis,* a characteristic symptom of which is that the airway mucus is excessively thick and viscid and is much more inclined to obstruct the airways than to keep them clear of inhaled particles. As a consequence, chronic pulmonary infections commonly occur in patients with this condition.

Hence under normal circumstances, the conducting portion of the respiratory system is an efficient air conditioner. Its component parts are described in the following section.

CONDUCTING PORTION OF THE RESPIRATORY SYSTEM

Nasal Cavities

The nose contains two *nasal cavities* separated by the *nasal septum.* Each cavity opens anteriorly at a *naris* or *nostril* and posteriorly into the *nasopharynx* (Fig. 20-1).

Bone, cartilage, and also dense connective tissue provide rigidity to the walls, floor, and roof of the nasal cavities and prevent their collapse on inspiration.

Each nasal cavity is divided into (1) a *vestibule,* the widened part just behind the naris; and (2) the remainder of the cavity, called its *respiratory portion.*

The *epidermis* covering the nose extends into each naris to line the anterior part of each vestibule. It is provided with many hair follicles and some sebaceous and sweat glands. Conceivably, the hairs strain very coarse particles from air being drawn through the nostrils. Farther back in the vestibule the *stratified squamous epithelium* is not keratinized, and still farther back it becomes *pseudostratified ciliated columnar* with goblet cells. From here on, the epithelium becomes part of a mucous membrane that lines the remainder of each nasal cavity (its respiratory portion). The epithelial component of this mucous membrane is pseudostratified columnar ciliated epithelium with goblet cells. The lamina propria contains mucous and serous glands and is adherent to the periosteum of the bone, or the perichondrium of the cartilage, beneath it. The basement membrane attaching the respiratory epithelium to the lamina propria is thicker than that of most epithelia.

The epithelial surface is covered with mucus that is produced by goblet cells and glands of the lamina propria. This mucus, together with any particles that it may have trapped, is moved posteriorly through the nasopharynx to the oropharynx by ciliary activity. Drainage of the nasal cavities is very dependent on normal ciliary motility, and loss of cilia as a result of disease or trauma can impair nasal drainage. The nature of *allergic rhinitis* (hay fever) and the way it can be treated with *antihistamines* were considered in Chapter 7 in the section on Mast Cells.

The *lamina propria* is relatively rich in elastin and is also highly vascular. Its great vascularity contributes warmth to the incoming air in cold weather. Lymphocytes, plasma cells, macrophages, and even granular leukocytes may be seen in this layer. Lymphatic nodules are most numerous near the entrance to the nasopharynx.

Nasal Conchae

Projecting medially from the lateral wall of each nasal cavity are three curved shelves, each supported by cancellous bone and covered by a mucous membrane (Fig. 20-2). Due to their shell-like appearance, these shelves have become known as the *superior, middle,* and *inferior conchae* (L. concha, shell) or *turbinates* (Fig. 20-1). In the middle and inferior

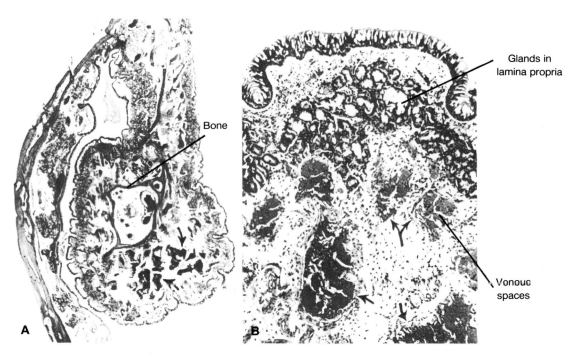

Fig. 20-2.   (*A*) Photomicrograph of a nasal concha cut in cross section (very low power). Arrows at lower right indicate large venous spaces distended with blood. (*B*) Photomicrograph of the mucous membrane covering a nasal concha. Arrows at lower right indicate venous spaces similar to those in *A*.

conchae, the lamina propria is extremely vascular with many thin-walled veins (Fig. 20-2). Most of the time these vessels are not fully distended, but under certain circumstances, they can become congested with blood. The two lower pairs of conchae can become sufficiently distended with blood to make the passage of air through the nasal cavities very difficult. This is the cause of the "stuffed-up nose" that some people suffer when they enter an overheated room or develop an upper respiratory-tract infection such as the common cold.

The mucous membrane of the roof and of the upper part of the lateral wall of the posterior region of each nasal cavity, including its superior concha, constitutes one half of the *olfactory organ*, the organ of smell, which is described below.

Olfactory Areas

The first neurons are believed to have evolved as a result of specialization of surface ectodermal cells. During the course of evolution, the cell bodies of most afferent neurons shifted to a more central and better protected location within the intervertebral foramina. However, olfactory chemoreceptor neurons are an exception because their cell bodies remain exposed at the body surface in the *olfactory areas*. There is one such area in each nasal cavity. Superficial positioning of neuronal cell bodies in an epithelium on the body surface is a much more hazardous arrangement than

having them more deeply situated with afferent fibers extending to the surface. Virtually all function of olfactory receptors can be lost as a result of destruction of the olfactory epithelium by the infections to which the nasal mucous membrane is so susceptible.

The olfactory area lines most of the roof of a nasal cavity (Fig. 20-1). It begins in front of the anterior end of the superior concha. From here, the olfactory area extends posteriorly for approximately 1 cm. From the roof, it also extends down both sides of each nasal cavity; on the lateral side, it extends over most of the superior concha, and on the medial side, it extends approximately 1 cm down the nasal septum.

The mucous membrane of the olfactory area consists of a thick *pseudostratified epithelium* (Fig. 20-3*A*) and a thick *lamina propria*.

The *epithelium* consists of three kinds of cells: (1) olfactory receptor cells, (2) sustentacular (supporting) cells, and (3) basal cells.

Olfactory Receptor Cells.   These are modified bipolar nerve cells; each has a cell body with a dendrite extending from its superficial end to the surface of the epithelium and an axon extending from its deeper end into the lamina propria (Fig. 20-3*A*). Like the sustentacular cells supporting them, the receptor cells lie perpendicular to the surface of the membrane, with their cell bodies fitted between the sustentacular cells so that their nuclei constitute a broad

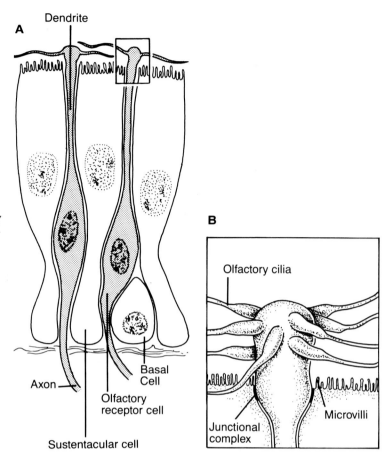

Fig. 20-3. Diagrammatic representation of olfactory epithelium. *B* shows details of the boxed-in area in *A*. See text for details.

zone of nuclei in the lower half of the membrane (Fig. 20-3A). The dendritic process of each bipolar cell ascends in a crevice between sustentacular cells toward the surface, where it terminates as a swelling termed an *olfactory vesicle*, which is shown within a box in Figure 20-2. This vesicle is a bulblike mass of cytoplasm that bulges out through the surface. Just below the surface, the olfactory vesicle is connected to the adjacent sustentacular cells by a junctional complex (Fig. 20-3B), and at the level of the zonula adherens of the complex, which lies just deep to a very tight zonula occludens, the sustentacular cells possess a prominent terminal web. The olfactory vesicle bears a cluster of long *olfactory cilia* (Fig. 20-3B), and its cytoplasm contains mitochondria, microtubules, some smooth-surfaced endoplasmic reticulum (sER), and the basal bodies of the olfactory cilia. The proximal portion of each olfactory cilium has the usual arrangement of microtubules, but generally only two microtubules extend into its narrower distal portion. Olfactory cilia lie parallel to the surface of the membrane, forming a tousled layer over the microvilli on the luminal border of the sustentacular cells (Fig. 20-3). This layer is kept moist by the secretion of underlying glands.

The unmyelinated axon of each receptor cell extends into the underlying lamina propria, where it combines with others to constitute bundles of *olfactory nerve fibers*. These fibers reach the *olfactory bulbs* (ovoid structures developing as anterior extensions of the olfactory area of the brain) by way of foramina in the cribriform plate of the ethmoid bone.

Sustentacular Cells.   The supporting cells of olfactory epithelium are tall and cylindrical, tapering toward their bases (Fig. 20-3A). Their luminal border is covered with microvilli (Fig. 20-3B). A brownish-yellow pigment similar to lipofuscin is present in their cytoplasm. This pigment imparts a yellow color to the olfactory areas. Sustentacular cell nuclei stain lightly and are ovoid; they lie superficial to the nuclei of the receptor cells (Fig. 20-3A).

Basal Cells.   Conical *basal cells* are scattered along the basement membrane (Fig. 20-3A). These cells are believed to be undifferentiated stem cells because in the mouse, they can give rise to new olfactory chemoreceptor neurons, the axons of which are evidently able to establish synaptic connections within the olfactory bulbs (Harding et al; also Graziadei). Their potential for producing such cells is suggestive of a replacement mechanism for the olfactory receptor cells, and such a mechanism is warranted in view of the vulnerable location of these receptors at the body surface. However, no other examples of postnatal replacement of neurons through a stem cell mechanism are known, so this seems to be a unique exception to the general rule that neurons are not replaced in postnatal life.

Lamina Propria. The underlying lamina propria contains many veins and also distinctive tubuloalveolar glands called the *glands of Bowman* that are apparently confined to olfactory areas. The chief kind of secretory cell in these glands contains abundant sER in its cytoplasm. The thin, watery secretion that reaches the surface of olfactory epithelium through their ducts has some of the characteristics of watery mucus. Its role seems to be to freshen the thin layer of fluid bathing the olfactory cilia; because these cilia are chemoreceptive, the substances responsible for odors have to dissolve in this surface layer.

The way odors are perceived is not understood. Individual olfactory receptors respond to a wide range of odoriferous substances. Odor discrimination undoubtedly requires recognition by the central nervous system of particular patterns of afferent impulses, relayed through the olfactory bulbs, from very large numbers of olfactory receptors.

Paranasal Sinuses

The *paranasal sinuses* are air-filled spaces within bones of the skull. Four of these spaces are associated with each nasal cavity. Named after the bones that contain them, they are the *frontal, ethmoidal, sphenoidal,* and *maxillary* sinuses. The maxillary sinus is the largest. The four sinuses on each side communicate with the nasal cavity on that side, and their mucosal lining is continuous with the mucosal lining of the nasal cavity. The ciliated epithelium of the sinuses is not as thick as that of the nasal cavity itself, nor does it contain as many goblet cells. The lamina propria is relatively thin and is continuous with the periosteum of the underlying bone. It consists chiefly of collagen fibers and contains eosinophils, plasma cells, and many lymphocytes, as well as fibroblasts. It possesses relatively few glands.

The apertures by which the paranasal sinuses communicate with the nasal cavities are so small that they can become obstructed when the surrounding mucosa becomes edematous as a result of inflammation. Normally, ciliary activity carries the mucus that is formed in the sinuses out of these spaces and into the nasal cavities. However, obstruction of the sinus openings can cause the sinuses to fill with mucus or, in the case of an infection, to fill with pus. Selective sympathomimetic drugs (designed to elicit an α_1-adrenergic response) are commonly employed as local vasoconstrictors to lessen the congestion around the orifices of inflamed sinuses and thereby promote sinus drainage.

Pharyngeal Tonsil

The *pharyngeal tonsil* consists of an unpaired median mass of lymphatic tissue in the lamina propria of the mucous membrane lining the roof and posterior wall of the nasopharynx (Fig. 20-1). Enlargement of the pharyngeal tonsil is described as *adenoids* (Gr. *aden,* gland) because the enlarged lymphatic follicles of the tonsil give it a glandlike appearance. Adenoids may obstruct the respiratory passageway and lead to persistent mouth breathing. The muscular actions involved in keeping the mouth always open, by changing the lines of force to which the facial bones are normally subjected, may prevent these bones from developing as they should. For this reason, and also because an enlarged pharyngeal tonsil is usually more or less persistently infected, surgical removal of adenoids is a relatively common operation.

The pharyngeal tonsil resembles the palatine tonsil in microscopic structure except that (1) it is more diffuse, (2) its covering epithelium dips down into it as folds rather than crypts, and (3) its epithelium may be pseudostratified, at least in some areas, instead of being stratified squamous nonkeratinizing epithelium.

Larynx and Epiglottis

The larynx is the sound-producing organ of the human voice; it lies between the pharynx and the trachea (Fig. 20-1). Its walls are kept from collapsing on inspiration by a number of cartilages that are interconnected by ligaments and extrinsic and intrinsic voluntary muscles. The larynx has two major functions. Its role in phonation (voice production) is well known, but phylogenetically this is a late development. A more fundamental function of the organ is that of preventing anything other than air from gaining access to the lower respiratory passages. If something else (*e.g.,* food, liquids, or inhaled foreign objects) enters the larynx, the cough reflex is set in motion to blow it out again. In this connection, it is of interest that some apparent drownings are, in fact, due to asphyxiation (choking) as a result of laryngeal spasm induced by water gaining access to the larynx.

Two pairs of mucosal folds project medially from the lateral walls of the larynx, one pair lying above the other. The upper pair of folds, termed the *vestibular folds* (Fig. 20-4), have a protective role. The lower pair of folds have cordlike free margins and are termed the *vocal folds* (Fig. 20-4) because their vibration is required in producing vocal sounds. They narrow the lumen into an anteroposterior slitlike aperture known as the *rima glottides* that is somewhat triangular in shape, with the apex of the triangle directed anteriorly. Between the two sets of folds the lumen widens, constituting a small chamber called the *ventricle* of the larynx (Fig. 20-4). Each lateral extension of the ventricle, bounded by a vestibular fold above and a vocal fold below, is known as a *sinus* of the larynx. Anteriorly, the sinus on each side extends upward as a *saccule* (Fig. 20-4).

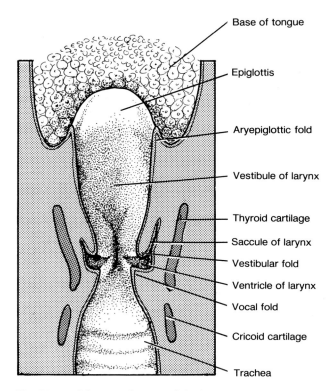

Base of tongue

Epiglottis

Aryepiglottic fold

Vestibule of larynx

Thyroid cartilage

Saccule of larynx

Vestibular fold

Ventricle of larynx

Vocal fold

Cricoid cartilage

Trachea

Fig. 20-4. Schematic diagram of the larynx and upper end of the trachea (posterior aspect of anterior half, cut in coronal section). The plane of section on the right side of the diagram is more anterior than that on the left, disclosing the saccule on that side of the larynx (tracheal cartilages omitted). (After Schaeffer)

Whereas the cores of the vestibular folds contain lamina propria and glands, the cores of the vocal folds are made up of elastic connective tissue and muscle; the region nearest their free margins is composed chiefly of elastic fibers. The shape and width of the aperture between the vocal folds and also the tension in these folds are regulated by (1) muscles that pull directly on the folds and (2) muscles that shift the parts to which they are attached.

The covering epithelium of the vocal folds, which are subject to considerable wear, is stratified squamous nonkeratinizing epithelium. All the epithelial lining of the larynx below the vocal folds is pseudostratified ciliated columnar epithelium with goblet cells. Above the vocal folds, most of the lining epithelium is of the same type, but patches of stratified squamous nonkeratinizing epithelium may be present. The cilia beat toward the pharynx. Except over the vocal folds, the lamina propria contains mucous glands. Lymphatic nodules, too, are found in this layer, particularly in the region of the ventricle and the vestibular folds.

The larynx is responsible for *phonation*, which means the utterance of sounds. This is due to the setting up of appropriate vibrations of the vocal folds as a result of the passage of air past their free margins. The pitch of each

sound is determined by the tension in these folds and the conformation of their free borders. *Vocalization* is an even more complex matter, requiring the additional participation of the lips, tongue, soft palate, and the cavities with which these various structures are associated.

Epiglottis. The *epiglottis* is a flaplike structure that projects upward and slightly posteriorly from the top of the larynx, to which it is attached anteriorly (Fig. 20-1). The epiglottis plays a passive role in keeping food and fluids out of the larynx during swallowing; when the larynx is brought upward and forward during the act of swallowing, the upper end of its tubular part becomes pressed against the posterior aspect of the epiglottis.

The epiglottis is supported internally by a plate of *elastic cartilage*. The perichondrium of this supporting plate is continuous with the lamina propria of the mucous membrane that covers both surfaces of the epiglottis. On the anterior surface, where the epiglottis comes into contact with the base of the tongue during swallowing, the epithelium is *stratified squamous nonkeratinizing epithelium* (Fig. 20-5). The epithelium covering the upper part of the posterior surface comes into contact with whatever is being swallowed and is therefore also subject to wear and tear. It, too, is stratified squamous nonkeratinizing epithelium. However, the epithelium covering the lower part of the posterior surface constitutes a part of the lining of the respiratory tube and hence is lined with *pseudostratified ciliated columnar epithelium with goblet cells* (Fig. 20-5). The cilia move mucus toward the pharynx. Mucous glands with some serous secretory units are present in the lamina propria under the posterior surface. They can also be present under the anterior surface (Fig. 20-5A).

Trachea

The trachea extends from the larynx, and it bifurcates at its lower end into two main (primary) bronchi (Fig. 20-1). Its walls are strongly supported by a series of 16 to 20 horseshoe-shaped cartilages that almost encircle the lumen. The open ends of these incomplete cartilaginous rings are directed posteriorly, and the gap between their ends is bridged by fibroelastic connective tissue and smooth muscle (Fig. 20-6). The spaces between the neighboring rings are filled with a dense fibroelastic connective tissue that is continuous with their perichondrium. This is a strong arrangement that enables the trachea to be extended when the head is tilted back, and it enables the trachea to elongate during inspiration.

Tracheobronchial Epithelium. The trachea and bronchi are lined by *pseudostratified ciliated epithelium* with goblet cells. In a hematoxylin and eosin (H & E) section, this epithelium appears as shown in Figure 4-31. Its appearance in the scanning electron microscope is shown in Figure 20-7, and its fine structure is illustrated in Figure 20-8.

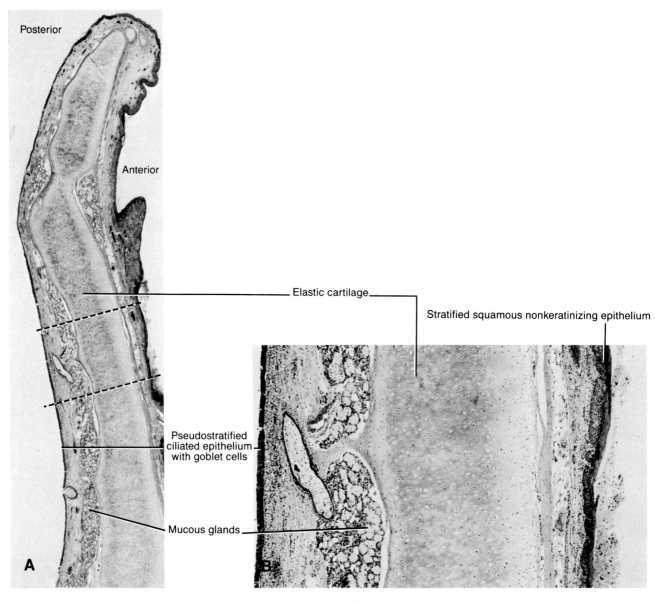

Fig. 20-5. (A) Photomicrograph of the epiglottis (low power). (B) Photomicrograph showing the area between the two dotted lines in A under higher magnification.

The *ciliated cells* possess at least 200 cilia; these are approximately 6 μm long and are arranged in rows on their luminal surface. The fine structure of their cilia and basal bodies was described in Chapter 4 and is illustrated in Figures 4-32 to 4-34.

In recent years, a number of *immotile cilia syndromes,* characterized by genetically determined defects in cilia, have come to light. Such specific ciliary defects include the lack of functional dynein, anomalies of the radial spoke linkages, and transposition of outer doublet microtubules to a central position. Such functional defects greatly impair

mucociliary clearance and lead to chronic respiratory diseases. For further information, see Sturgess and Turner.

The *goblet cells,* also called *mucous cells,* were described in Chapter 6 in connection with this type of epithelium. They secrete their mucus in a cyclical manner. The tracheobronchial epithelium also contains another type of cell known as the *brush cell* (Fig. 20-9) that has a tuft of microvilli extending from its luminal border like the bristles of a brush. The functions of brush cells, which in some species can also be found in very low numbers in the interalveolar walls, have never been satisfactorily elucidated.

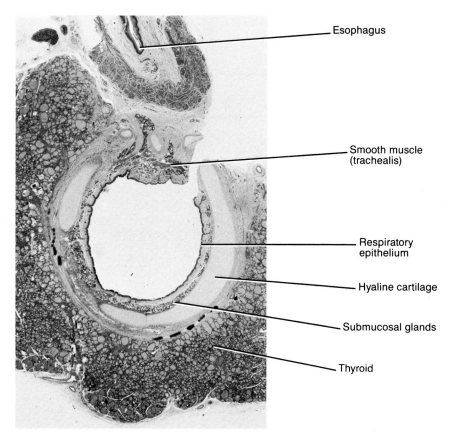

Fig. 20-6. Photomicrograph of a child's trachea (very low power).

Esophagus

Smooth muscle (trachealis)

Respiratory epithelium

Hyaline cartilage

Submucosal glands

Thyroid

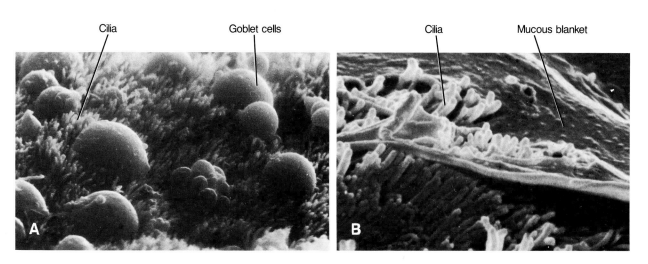

Cilia   Goblet cells   Cilia   Mucous blanket

A   B

Fig. 20-7. Scanning electron micrographs of the lining epithelium of the human trachea. (*A*) General view of surface with mucous blanket removed. (*B*) Area similar to *A* under higher magnification, showing its coating of sticky mucus. (*A,* courtesy of J. Sturgess; *B,* Sturgess JM: Am Rev Respir Dis 115:819, 1977)

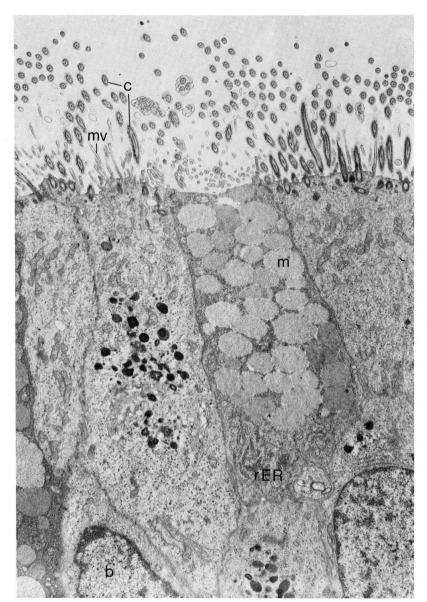

Fig. 20-8. Electron micrograph (×7500) of pseudostratified ciliated columnar epithelium with mucous (goblet) cells. This type of epithelium lines the trachea and bronchi. Illustrated here is the lining of a bronchus. A slightly darker staining mucous cell can be seen among the pale-staining ciliated columnar cells. Its apical cytoplasm contains large spherical secretory vesicles of mucus (*m*), and below these some rER is visible. On the apical surface of the columnar cells, there are cilia (*c*) and microvilli (*mv*). Note also the nuclei of basal cells (*b*) deeper in the membrane. (Courtesy of J. Sturgess)

One theory, still far from being substantiated, is that they have chemoreceptor function. A fourth type of cell seen in the tracheobronchial epithelium is the *basal cell* (Fig. 20-8, *bottom*). It is generally believed that these are stem cells that can produce new ciliated and mucous (goblet) cells. However, a certain amount of day-to-day replacement of mucous cells seems to be due to the fact that at least some of the mucus-secreting cells retain the capacity for mitosis (Ayers and Jeffery).

Afferent nerve fibers appear to end on and synapse with the base of some of the epithelial cells. *Neuroendocrine cells* analogous to enteroendocrine cells of the gastrointestinal tract are also present in the epithelium. Known also as *Kulchitsky* or *K cells*, they are scattered either singly or in small groups throughout the epithelium of the conducting airways, including the bronchioles. They are particularly numerous during fetal life. Typically, they have dense-cored secretory vesicles in the basal part of their cytoplasm lying next to the basement membrane. Some of these cells are thought to produce serotonin, and others evidently produce polypeptide hormones such as calcitonin. A third type produces the gastrin-releasing peptide bombesin. Like enteroendocrine cells, these cells can give rise to serotonin- or hormone-producing *carcinoid tumors.*

In addition to the various constitutive cells of the tracheobronchial epithelium, there are several different kinds of migratory cells, including intraepithelial lymphocytes and mast cells.

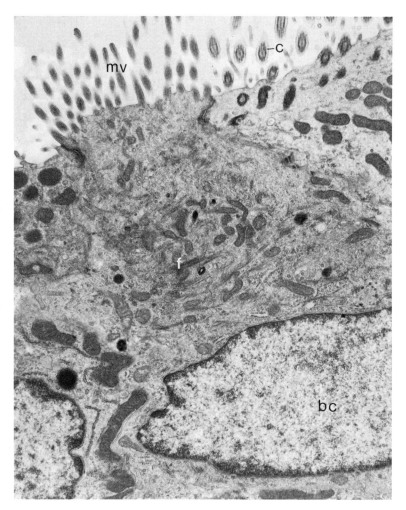

Fig. 20-9. Electron micrograph (×12,000) of a brush cell (*bc*) of pseudostratified ciliated columnar epithelium. This is a cell type found in tracheobronchial epithelium; the cell illustrated here is in a rat bronchiole. There are microvilli (*mv*) on its apical surface instead of cilia. In its cytoplasm, filaments (*f*), a few small round apical vesicles, mitochondria, and some rER (just above the nucleus) may be seen. The portion of the pale-staining ciliated cell at top right has cilia (*c*) and prominent mitochondria. (Courtesy of B. Meyrick and L. Reid)

Other Layers of the Tracheal Wall. The *lamina propria* of the tracheal mucosa is rich in elastic fibers; lymphocytes and lymphatic nodules are also present. Along the deep border of the lamina propria, there is a dense lamina of elastin. The secretory portions of many *mucous glands,* with some serous secretory units, are embedded in the *submucosa*. The ducts of these glands extend through the elastic lamina of the lamina propria and open onto the epithelial surface. Some secretory units may also be present in the lamina propria. The posterior wall of the trachea contains interlacing bundles of smooth muscle that comprise the *trachealis muscle* (Fig. 20-6). These muscle bundles are arranged chiefly in the transverse plane, and they are bound together by connective tissue that contains glands.

Bronchi

Extending from the lower end of the trachea to the roots of the lungs are the extrapulmonary portions of the two *main (primary) bronchi* (Fig. 20-1). The microscopic structure of the main bronchi is similar to that of the trachea.

Usually, the right lung is made up of three lobes and the left lung is made up of two. Each primary bronchus, in a sense, continues into the lower lobe of the particular lung to which it passes. The right primary bronchus, before doing so, gives off two branches to supply the middle and the upper lobes, respectively, of that lung. Likewise, the left primary bronchus, before continuing into the lower lobe of the left lung, gives off a branch to supply the upper lobe of that lung. At the hilum of each lung, the primary bronchus and its main branches become closely associated with the arteries that also enter the lung at this site and the veins and lymphatics that leave the lung, and all these tubular structures become invested in dense connective tissue. This complex of tubes invested in dense connective tissue is termed the *root* of the lung.

The microscopic structure of the *intrapulmonary bronchi* differs from that of the trachea and extrapulmonary portions of the primary bronchi in the following four ways.

1. In place of the horseshoe-shaped cartilages that characterize the trachea and extrapulmonary bronchi,

Mucous submucosal glands

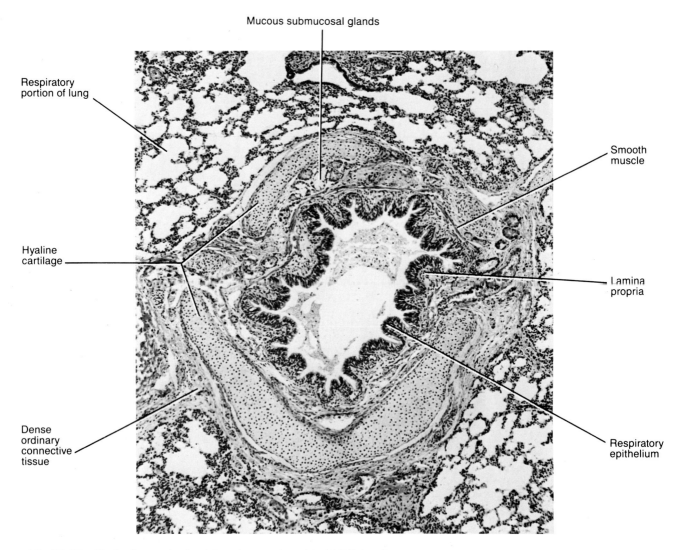

Respiratory portion of lung

Smooth muscle

Hyaline cartilage

Lamina propria

Dense ordinary connective tissue

Respiratory epithelium

Fig. 20-10.   Photomicrograph of an intrapulmonary bronchus (child's lung).

there are irregular plates of cartilage. Thus what appear as several cartilages in a section are commonly parts of a single cartilage of irregular shape (Fig. 20-10). The dense ordinary connective tissue in the spaces between them is continuous with their perichondrium.

2. Whereas smooth muscle is present only posteriorly in the trachea and extrapulmonary bronchi, in intrapulmonary bronchi, it encircles the entire lumen between the mucosa and the cartilage (Fig. 20-10). However, it is only rarely seen as a complete layer in sections because it is composed of two crisscrossing helical bundles that wind in opposite directions.

3. As seen in sections, the mucous membrane of intrapulmonary bronchi exhibits characteristic longitudinal folds caused by contracture of the smooth muscle bundles on fixation.

4. In place of the elastic lamina that demarcates the outer limit of the lamina propria of the trachea and extra-

pulmonary bronchi, there are longitudinal tracts of elastic tissue in the lamina propria. However, these tracts are not readily distinguished in routine H & E sections.

The intrapulmonary bronchi are lined with the pseudostratified ciliated columnar epithelium described above under Tracheobronchial Epithelium. Mucus secretion by the goblet cells in this membrane is again supplemented by that of submucosal mucous glands. The secretory portions of these glands lie mainly external to the muscle layer, between the cartilages (Fig. 20-10). Among their mucous secretory units, there are some serous secretory units and mucous units with serous demilunes. Myoepithelial cells, too, are present. The mixed secretion passes by way of a nonciliated collecting duct to a short and slightly funnel-shaped ciliated duct that opens onto the luminal surface of the bronchus. Bronchial submucosal glands are inner-

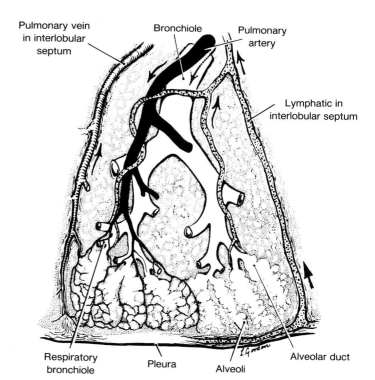

Fig. 20-11. Schematic diagram of a peripheral lobule of the lung. The sizes of the bronchioles, air passages, blood vessels, and lymphatics have been exaggerated for clarity. To make it easier to follow the course of the blood vessels and lymphatics, the former have been omitted from the right side of the diagram, and the latter have been omitted from the left side.

vated by both divisions of the autonomic nervous system. There is experimental evidence that sympathetic stimulation elicits mucus secretion (a *β*-adrenergic response). *α*-Adrenergic stimulation evidently elicits serous secretion instead. Parasympathetic stimulation through acetylcholine probably elicits both types of secretion nonselectively. Mucus secretion by the goblet cells in the surface epithelium appears to be a nonselective response to lung irritants. For further information, see Nadel.

We should also mention that lymph nodes are distributed along the course of bronchi in the outermost fibrous region of their walls.

The Bronchial Tract Branches Dichotomously. The pattern of branching in the bronchial tree is *dichotomous* (Gr. *dicha,* in two; *tome,* a cutting). It is also somewhat asymmetrical with respect to the length of the branches. Moreover, the summed cross-sectional area of each pair of branches becomes *greater* than the cross-sectional area of the parent tube. This is reflected in the velocity of air flow through the various-sized branches of the bronchial tree. For the same volume of air to flow through the parent tube as through its two branches, which contribute a greater combined surface area, it needs to move faster along the parent tube. It follows that the widest airways have the greatest velocity of air flow, and this should be kept in mind when interpreting breath sounds heard through a stethoscope.

Continued branching of the bronchial tract gives rise to a whole series of successively narrower bronchi and bronchioles. It is estimated that there are between 10 and 32 orders of branching, with a mean of approximately 18

branchings between the trachea and the narrowest bronchioles (Horsfield). A widely accepted model assumes an average of approximately 24 orders of branching (Weibel), but the actual number probably varies in relation to the distance between the hilum and the terminal branches of the bronchial tree in any given region of the lung.

The Lung Is Made up of Lobes, Segments, and Lobules. Anatomically, fissures subdivide the left lung into an *upper* (*superior*) and a *lower* (*inferior*) lobe. The right lung is similarly subdivided, but it has a *middle lobe* as well. On entering the lungs, the two *main* (*principal or primary*) *bronchi* branch to supply five large *lobar* (*secondary*) *bronchi,* one for each lobe. The lobes are further subdivided by connective tissue into *segments;* there are ten of these. Termed *bronchopulmonary segments,* these subdivisions of the lung are sufficiently well demarcated anatomically for the surgeon to be able to resect individual segments in the event that this becomes necessary. The lobar bronchi branch to supply *segmental* (*tertiary*) *bronchi,* one for each segment.

Because the lung develops in the same way as an exocrine gland, it also has a *lobular* organization. The bronchi are equivalent to extralobular ducts because they lie outside lobules. The smallest bronchi give rise to numerous generations of branches known as *bronchioles,* and the fine bronchioles enter the lung lobules at their apices (Fig. 20-11). These fine bronchioles are accordingly the counterparts of intralobular ducts. Lung *lobules* have a recognizable apex and base, but their shape and size are variable. The diameter of their base ranges from less than 1 cm to more than 2 cm, and their height varies even more. Bronchioles entering lobules mostly point outward toward the periphery of a

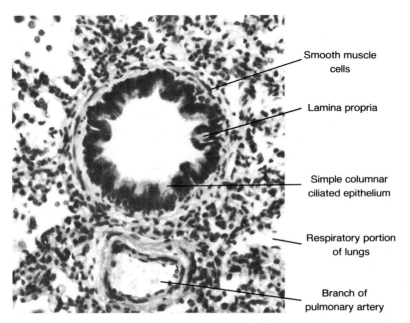

Smooth muscle cells

Lamina propria

Simple columnar ciliated epithelium

Respiratory portion of lungs

Branch of pulmonary artery

Fig. 20-12. Photomicrograph of a bronchiole along with a branch of the pulmonary artery. Cartilages and submucosal glands are lacking from the walls of bronchioles. Arteries of the pulmonary circulation have a thinner wall than do those of the systemic circulation.

lobe, and the peripheral lobules tend to have the elongated pyramidal shape depicted in Figure 20-11. Their bases are distinguishable as polygonal areas beneath the pleura. Lobules are separated from one another by fibrous septa, but in the human lung, these septa are incomplete and do not extend far into the lung.

Bronchioles

As a result of continued dichotomous branching, bronchi give rise to conducting passageways that have a somewhat simpler wall structure and a diameter of 1 mm or less. There are several differences between these narrower branches, which are termed *bronchioles,* and the generations of bronchi from which they originate. For example, bronchioles are lined by a *simple epithelium* instead of pseudostratified epithelium. In larger bronchioles, this is simple columnar ciliated epithelium (Fig. 20-12), whereas in smaller bronchioles, it is simple cuboidal nonciliated epithelium. The goblet cell population in the lining epithelium dwindles at a level that is slightly above the region where a gradual changeover occurs between ciliated and nonciliated cells, a region that is characterized by a mixture of both of these kinds of cells. Other distinguishing features of bronchioles are that they *do not have cartilages or glands* in their walls (Fig. 20-12).

On entering a lobule, a so-called *preterminal bronchiole* gives rise to other orders of bronchioles that extend in a treelike manner to all parts of the lobule. Bronchioles that lie within lobules are attached on all sides to the elastic spongework of tissue that contains the air spaces where gas exchanges occur (see Fig. 20-14). Cartilages are not needed in their walls because unlike bronchi and the tra-

chea, they show no tendency to collapse on inspiration. When the surrounding respiratory spongework becomes stretched during inspiration, bronchioles are, in fact, pulled open by expansion of the tissue attached to their circumference (Fig. 20-12).

The epithelial lining of bronchioles is not as thick as that of bronchi. In larger bronchioles, ciliated columnar cells predominate but tall nonciliated cells called *Clara cells* are scattered between them (Fig. 20-13). Clara cells possess numerous mitochondria, and in most species, there is also a relative abundance of sER. In man, however, the sER is not prominent. These cells also contain electron-dense secretory granules that are approximately 600 nm in diameter. Clara cells are metabolically very active and produce a serous secretion containing some protein, but the nature and functions of their secretion are not known with certainty. Furthermore, despite the fairly well-differentiated appearance of these cells, there are indications that they can serve as progenitor cells for other types of bronchiolar epithelial cells (Evans et al).

Next to the epithelial lining of bronchioles, there is a thin but elastic *lamina propria.* External to this lies a prominent coat of *smooth muscle* arranged as described for bronchi, and this, in turn, is surrounded by an external supporting layer of connective tissue (Fig. 20-12).

There Are Three Orders of Bronchioles. The *preterminal bronchiole* that supplies each lobule gives off branches known as *terminal bronchioles,* the number of which varies according to the size of the lobule. There are three to five (usually four) terminal bronchioles, with a diameter of approximately 0.2 mm. Each *preterminal bronchiole* supplies a *lobule* of the lung, and each *terminal bronchiole* supplies a unit of lung structure that is known as an *acinus.* The

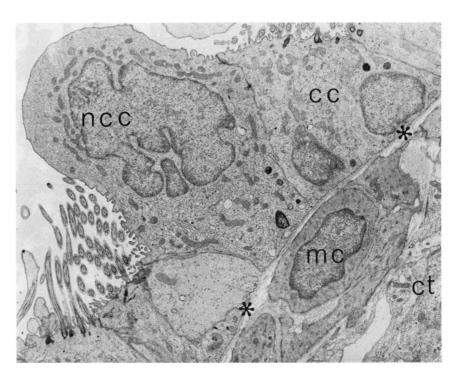

Fig. 20-13. Electron micrograph (×6000) of cells in the mucous membrane of a small bronchiole (mouse). Among the ciliated epithelial cells (*cc*), there is a nonciliated Clara cell (*ncc*), which has numerous mitochondria and abundant sER, especially under its apical surface. Asterisks indicate the basement membrane of the epithelium. Smooth muscle cells (*mc*) and fibroblasts of connective tissue (*ct*) are present in the underlying lamina propria. (Courtesy of A. Collet)

last three or so orders of bronchioles originating from terminal bronchioles are called *respiratory bronchioles* (Figs. 20-11, 20-14, and 20-15). These bronchioles possess alveoli in their walls.

RESPIRATORY PORTION OF THE RESPIRATORY SYSTEM

Gas exchanges between blood and air begin in the smallest bronchioles, which is why they are known as *respiratory bronchioles*. Whereas the trachea, bronchi, and bronchioles are tubes with walls of their own, the intralobular structures to which they lead (alveolar ducts, alveolar sacs, and alveoli) are *air spaces*. The air in these spaces is in close contact with capillaries to facilitate gas exchanges.

There Are Three Orders of Air Spaces. The respiratory bronchioles continue on as long branching hallways along which there are many open doors of two general sizes. The hallways are termed *alveolar ducts* (Figs. 20-14 and 20-15). The larger open doors open into rotunda-like spaces called *alveolar sacs* (marked with asterisks in Fig. 20-14*B*) and the smaller open doors open directly into *alveoli* (Fig. 20-14). Also, partitions subdivide the periphery of each alveolar sac into *alveoli*.

Alveoli and Pulmonary Surfactant

The basic structural and functional unit of respiratory gas exchange is the *alveolus*. This term is used to denote an *air space* (L. *alveolus*, small hollow space); hence the thin partitions between alveoli are known as *interalveolar walls* (*septa*). A lung alveolus can open directly into an alveolar sac, an alveolar duct, or a respiratory bronchiole (Figs. 20-14 and 20-15). Furthermore, in thick sections, it can be seen that the interalveolar walls are provided with apertures that are 7 μm to 8 μm in diameter (Fig. 20-16). Known as *alveolar pores*, these openings permit air to pass from one alveolus to another and hence facilitate the exchange of air between alveolar sacs if the usual supply routes become obstructed. It is estimated that the adult lungs have a total complement of approximately 300 million alveoli, representing a total surface area of approximately 80 square meters.

Interalveolar Walls. The delicate interalveolar walls are provided with very extensive capillary networks. The walls are internally supported by *elastic fibers* and fine *reticular fibers*, as well as by *basement membranes* (Fig. 20-17). At sites where alveoli and alveolar sacs extend from alveolar ducts, the duct walls contain smooth muscle cells and the mouths of the saccular structures are reinforced with rings of collagen fibers. The free surfaces of the interalveolar walls are covered with a continuous epithelium that is made up mainly of very flat *squamous epithelial cells* that are known as *type I pneumocytes* (Figs. 20-17 to 20-19). These cells are so thin that their attenuated cytoplasm cannot be resolved in the light microscope (LM). Indeed, the presence of such cells was a matter of some controversy that was not settled until their existence was confirmed in the electron microscope (EM).

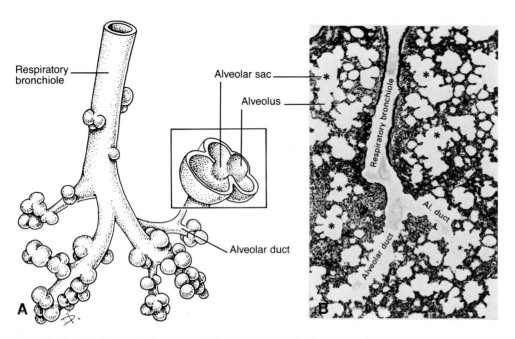

Fig. 20-14. (A) Schematic diagram and (B) photomicrograph of a respiratory bronchiole and alveolar ducts (child's lung). Asterisks in B indicate alveolar sacs.

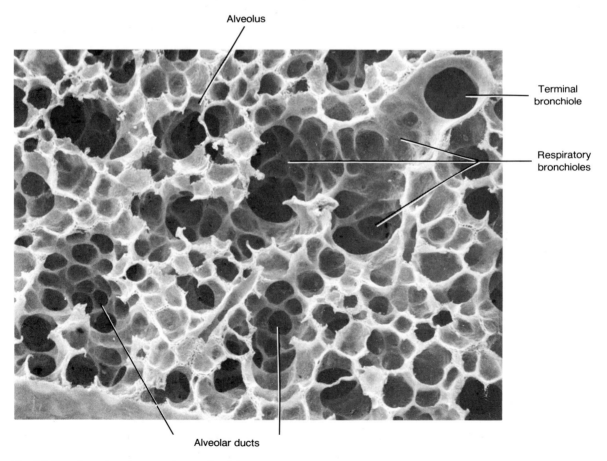

Fig. 20-15. Scanning electron micrograph of the respiratory portion of a lung (rabbit). A terminal bronchiole, respiratory bronchioles, alveolar ducts, and alveoli can be discerned in this micrograph. (Weibel ER: Design and structure of the human lung. In Fishman AP (ed): Pulmonary Diseases and Disorders, p 224. New York, McGraw-Hill, 1979)

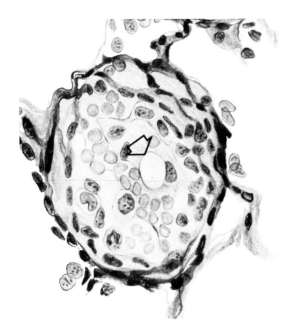

Fig. 20-16. Diagrammatic representation of an alveolar pore (indicated by *arrow*) opening into an alveolus, as seen in a thick section of lung.

As may be seen in Figures 20-17 and 20-18, air in the alveoli is separated from blood in the capillaries by (1) the cytoplasm of the type I pneumocytes that line alveoli; (2) the basement membrane of the alveolar epithelium, which at sites where it is apposed to the third component fuses with it; (3) the basement membrane of the capillary endothelial cells; and (4) the cytoplasm of these endothelial cells. This *alveolar–capillary barrier*, which mostly consists of only three layers because of fusion of the basement membranes, is only 0.2 μm to 2.5 μm thick. In certain sites, there are interstitial spaces between the basement membrane of the epithelium and that of the capillaries; reticular fibers, elastic fibers, and even cells can sometimes be found within such spaces (Fig. 20-17).

The alveolar epithelium is a continuous membrane that is made up of two types of epithelial cells that are interconnected by tight junctions. The majority of the cells are *type I pneumocytes*. Interspersed among them are rounded secretory cells known as *type II pneumocytes*. The squamous type I cells readily permit gases to diffuse through their cytoplasm whereas the rounded type II cells are essentially secretory cells. The type I cells are terminally differentiated and do not divide, but the type II cells retain the capacity

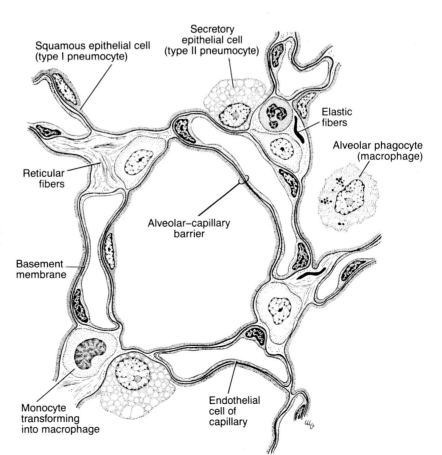

Fig. 20-17. Diagrammatic representation of the components of the interalveolar wall. See text for details. (After Bertalanffy and Leblond)

Squamous epithelial cell (type I pneumocyte)

Secretory epithelial cell (type II pneumocyte)

Elastic fibers

Alveolar phagocyte (macrophage)

Reticular fibers

Alveolar–capillary barrier

Basement membrane

Monocyte transforming into macrophage

Endothelial cell of capillary

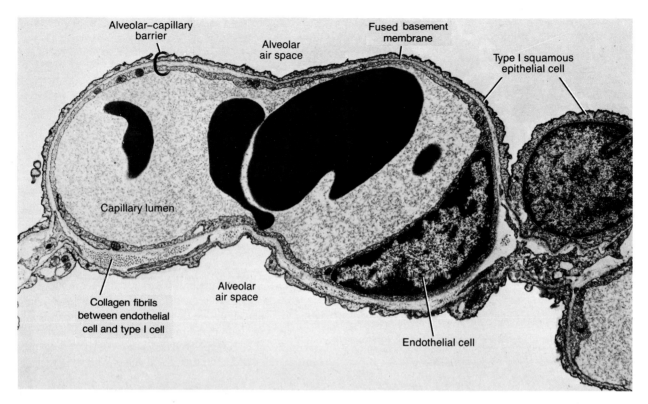

Fig. 20-18.   Electron micrograph of an alveolar capillary and a type I (squamous) pneumocyte in an interalveolar wall of the lung. The three components of the alveolar–capillary barrier are the cytoplasm of the type I pneumocyte, the endothelial cell cytoplasm, and the fused basement membrane between them. (Weibel ER: Physiol Rev 53:419, 1973)

for mitosis and are believed to serve as progenitor cells for type I cells as well as for type II cells.

As may be seen in Figure 20-19, the cytoplasm of the type I pneumocyte, across which gas exchanges occur, extends from its perinuclear region in many different directions in the form of extremely thin sheets that are sometimes described as apical plates. Although the cytoplasmic organelles are largely confined to the perinuclear region, microfilaments and microtubules can be distinguished within these sheetlike expansions.

The type II pneumocytes appear as rounded cells that bulge slightly from the alveolar surface (Figs. 20-17 and 20-20). With the EM, it can be seen that these cells are an integral part of the membrane because they are connected to the adjacent type I cells by tight junctions (Fig. 20-20). Type II pneumocytes possess some surface microvilli, and their cytoplasm has an extensive rough-surfaced endoplasmic reticulum (rER) and many mitochondria (Fig. 20-20). It also contains a prominent Golgi region and associated GERL and a variety of multivesicular bodies. However, the most distinctive feature of the type II cells is their content of *lamellar bodies* (Fig. 20-20). These are granules of electron-dense lamellar material that is rich in phospholipid

and is surrounded by a membrane. In human type II cells, the lamellae are concentrically arranged in whorls.

Lamellar bodies seem to be formed in the same way that other secretory vesicles are, but the sequence in which the protein, phospholipid, and carbohydrate constituents of the lamellar bodies are assembled is not very clear. Multivesicular bodies (which are believed to represent a type of secondary lysosome) have been implicated in the formation of lamellar bodies, but the relation between these relatively obscure structures and the production, intracellular degradation, or recycling of the secretory product of type II cells has not been elucidated.

The type II cell extrudes the contents of its lamellar bodies by exocytosis (Fig. 20-21). The liberated secretory product, chiefly phospholipid, then spreads across the surface of the film of tissue fluid that covers the alveolar epithelium. The functional role of this secretory product will now be described.

Pulmonary Surfactant.   The strong attractive forces between the water molecules in thin films of aqueous solutions are manifested as *surface tension*. The thin film of tissue fluid that is present on alveolar surfaces would exert sufficient surface tension to cause apposed surfaces of small alveoli to adhere to each other during inspiration if it were not for the presence of the secretory product of type II epithelial cells, which possesses detergentlike *surfactant* activity. The effect of this surfactant, which is chiefly *dipalmitoyl phosphatidylcholine,* is to diminish the attractive intermolecular forces between the water molecules at the surface of the film, reducing the surface tension and thereby making it easier for the inhaled air to spread adherent interalveolar walls apart. This, in turn, facilitates inflation of the alveoli. As we shall see, it is imperative for the lungs to have developed an adequate surfactant content by the time a newborn baby draws his first breath of air.

Pulmonary surfactant is a complex mixture of phospholipids, mainly dipalmitoyl phosphatidylcholine, complexed with proteins and carbohydrates. Once released from type II pneumocytes, the phospholipids become part of a *lipoprotein complex* that is called *tubular myelin* because it forms a highly distinctive tubular lattice. The presence of this lattice in the alveolar tissue fluid subphase is easily recognized in EM sections because of its electron density and because the majority of the tubules are square in cross section (Fig. 20-21). This subphase lattice is associated with a thin surface film of phospholipid on the alveolar tissue fluid that can just be discerned in Figure 20-21. The subphase lipoprotein complex supplies as much surfactant phospholipid and protein as is necessary to maintain a monomolecular film at the fluid–air interface.

Alveolar Macrophages. In LM sections, fairly large rounded cells that are different from type II pneumocytes can also be found bulging from interalveolar walls. Such cells occasionally appear to lie free in the alveolar air space (Fig. 20-17, *upper right,* and Fig. 20-22), but in life, they are loosely attached to surface epithelial cells and are immersed in little pools of alveolar tissue fluid. These cells commonly contain phagocytosed particles (Fig. 20-22) that include carbon particles derived from inhaled tobacco smoke. Indeed, the lungs of heavy smokers appear blackened because carbon-laden alveolar macrophages become more or less permanently incorporated into their interalveolar walls. Because of the marked phagocytic activity of such cells, they have long been known as *alveolar phagocytes.* They represent macrophages derived from monocytes that arrive by way of the bloodstream. Under some circumstances, the monocytes leave a capillary (Fig. 20-17), migrate through the epithelial lining, and enter the lumen of an alveolus where they transform into macrophages. However, alveolar macrophages can divide to form other macrophages, and there is evidence to suggest that the resident macrophage population in the lungs is, to some extent, self-propagating.

Alveolar macrophages remove dust particles and other kinds of debris that gain access to the alveolar air spaces. They are also believed to engulf and perhaps degrade pulmonary surfactant. Eventually, they move along the air passageways and reach bronchioles and then bronchi, whereupon they are carried to the pharynx by way of the mucociliary escalator and are discarded in sputum or swallowed.

If the lungs are congested with blood as a consequence of the heart becoming incompetent, blood commonly extravasates into the alveoli, whereupon alveolar phagocytes engulf erythrocytes and produce hemosiderin from the hemoglobin. Under such conditions, enough hemosiderin-containing macrophages can be coughed up with the sputum for it to give a positive histochemical reaction for iron. Such cells are called *heart-failure cells.*

DEVELOPMENT AND GROWTH OF THE LUNGS

Early development of the lungs (from week 5 to week 16) is comparable with that of exocrine acinar glands and is therefore described as the *pseudoglandular stage* of lung development. The lungs are derived from a longitudinal bulge in the endoderm-derived epithelium of the anterior wall of the foregut. The bulge pinches off as a tube that remains attached by its cephalic end to the foregut; this tube gives rise to the larynx and trachea. The caudal end of the tube bifurcates and forms the primary bronchial buds from which the two primary bronchi will develop. These tubular sprouts then give rise to secondary bronchi that branch dichotomously to form the tertiary bronchi. The branching then becomes less regular but continues on, giving rise to the various orders of bronchioles. In this manner, the epithelial tube gives rise to the epithelial lining and glands of the tracheobronchial tree. The associated connective tissue, smooth muscle, and cartilage arise from the mesenchyme into which it grows.

Virtually all orders of bronchi and bronchioles have developed by the end of the 16th week. During the ensuing *canalicular stage* of lung development, which lasts until the 24th week, the bronchiolar epithelium grows into the mesenchyme and begins forming the equivalent of secretory units (if we pursue the analogy between lungs and exocrine glands to its logical conclusion). Peripheral tubular branches of the developing tracheobronchial tree that until now have been lined with cuboidal epithelium start giving rise to so-called *canaliculi* that are characterized by having a flattened epithelial lining instead. These canaliculi subsequently widen as they lengthen. Toward the end of the canalicular stage, surfactant production commences.

The last prenatal stage of lung development does not occur until the last trimester (3-month period) of gestation. It is described as the *saccular stage* of development because it is characterized by the appearance of irregularly shaped, thin-walled structures known as *terminal sacs.* These sacs give rise to further generations of peripheral air spaces, serving as various kinds of transitional air passages until the final pattern of alveolar ducts and alveolar sacs emerges. In this last prenatal stage of lung development, elastic fibers

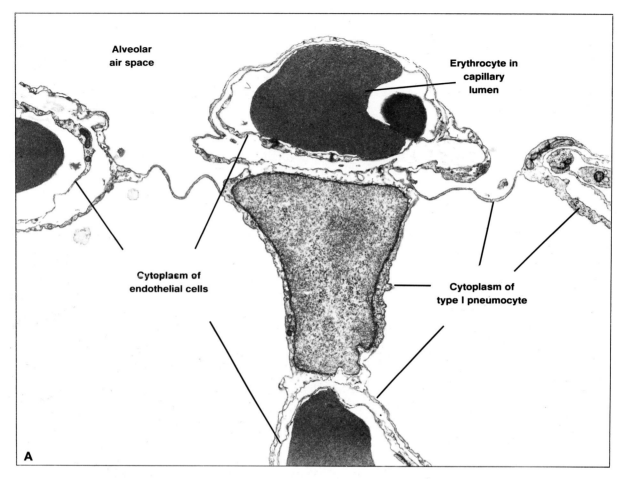

Fig. 20-19. (*A*) Electron micrograph of alveolar capillaries (*top, left,* and *bottom*) with an associated type I (squamous) pneumocyte (*center*) in the respiratory portion of a lung of the Etruscan shrew (*Suncus Etruscus,* a tiny mammal that has a body mass of only 2 g). (*B*) Interpretive schematic representation of *A.* (*Inset*) Low-power schematic representation indicating the positions of these cells and capillaries. (*A,* courtesy of E. R. Weibel)

and reticular fibers begin to form in the interstitial spaces and macrophages begin to appear within the air spaces. For further details of lung development, see Burri.

The number of true alveoli developing before birth is subject to interpretation, but it is estimated that at least *95% develop after birth.* Throughout prenatal life, the lungs are filled with fluid that appears to be produced primarily by the fetal lung tissue itself. Respiratory movements commence *in utero* in the second trimester, but for some unknown reason, they discontinue in the third trimester. Nevertheless, the capillary beds in the interalveolar walls become very extensive in the third trimester. The establishment of a sufficiently extensive capillary circulation through these walls is a prerequisite for viability in cases of premature birth. Lung alveoli are mostly formed during the first 8 years or so of postnatal life; the majority form within the first 3 years.

Adequate Amounts of Surfactant Are Required at Birth. It is very important for adequate numbers of well-differentiated type II pneumocytes to be present in the lungs by the time a baby is born because the surfactant they produce is essential for normal neonatal lung function. Surfactant secretion begins toward the end of the sixth month of fetal life, coinciding with maturation of type II cells and formation of the enzymes necessary for phospholipid synthesis. The extent of prenatal maturation can be assessed by physiochemical methods that estimate surfactant levels in the amniotic fluid.

Maturation of type II pneumocytes is accelerated by glucocorticoids such as cortisol. Endogenous thyroid hormone also plays a role. Furthermore, normal pituitary and adrenal function are both required for adequate maturation and surfactant secretion. For further information, see Burri.

For an infant to take in his first lungfull of air at birth, he has to overcome strong surface-tension forces. Premature infants, and even some full-term babies, can suffer from a condition known as the *respiratory distress syndrome* (RDS) that is characterized by respiratory difficulty and consequent cyanosis. This condition is due to a widespread failure of alveoli to open or to remain open.

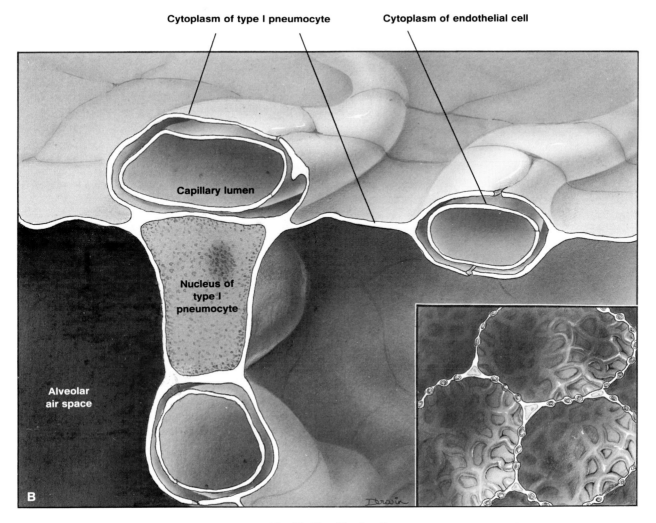

Fig. 20-19. (*Continued*)

It is a result of inadequate amounts of surfactant being produced in the lungs. When a newborn baby takes his first strong breath of air, the alveoli expand and normally do not collapse during expiration because of the influence of pulmonary surfactant. However, if a preterm infant is born before sufficient surfactant has been formed, the alveoli can collapse again on expiration, and respiratory movements may prove so inefficient that the infant may die within the first 2 days of life. This can now be avoided by administering a glucocorticoid to the mother from the middle of the sixth to the eighth month of pregnancy. Babies born after 37 weeks of gestation seldom develop RDS.

BLOOD SUPPLY, LYMPHATICS, AND SMOOTH MUSCLE INNERVATION OF THE LUNGS

The *pulmonary artery* delivers blood from the right ventricle to the alveolar capillary beds where it becomes oxygenated. The oxygenated blood then passes through the *pulmonary vein* to the left heart and is pumped through the systemic circulation. Hence the arteries of the pulmonary circulation carry the equivalent of venous blood, and the veins carry the equivalent of arterial blood.

The pulmonary artery enters the root of each lung and branches along with the bronchial tree. The small arterial branches reaching the respiratory bronchioles supply blood to the pulmonary capillaries, as shown at left in Figure 20-11. Because the blood pressure in the pulmonary artery and its branches is relatively low, these arterial branches are rather thin-walled compared with arteries of the systemic circulation (Fig. 20-12).

Blood from the pulmonary capillaries collects in branches of the thin-walled pulmonary vein. These branches begin within the substance of lobules and enter interlobular septa, where they empty into the interlobular veins (Fig. 20-11, *left*). At the apex of the lobule, the veins become associated with the bronchial tree and extend along it toward the hilum.

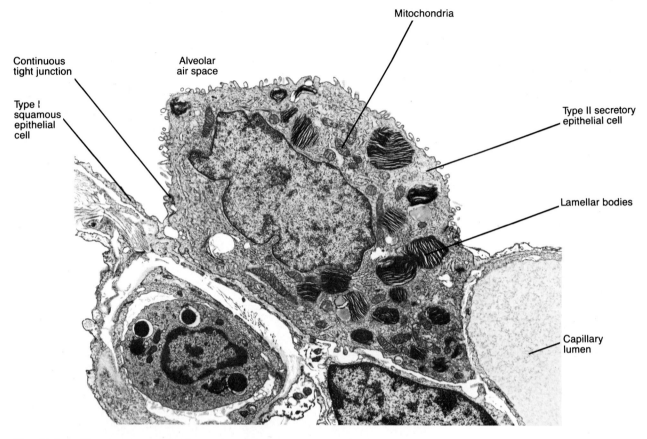

Fig. 20-20.   Electron micrograph of a type II pneumocyte in an interalveolar wall (dog lung). For details, see text. (Courtesy of E. R. Weibel)

Oxygenated blood is supplied under high pressure to the more central parts of the lung by the *bronchial arteries.* These arteries also travel with the bronchial tree, supplying the capillaries in its walls. In addition, they supply the lymph nodes that are associated with the bronchial tract. Also, branches of the bronchial arteries pass down the interlobular septa and provide the visceral pleura with oxygenated blood. The blood pressure and the oxygen content in the arterial part of the pulmonary circulation are low in comparison with the arterial part of the systemic circulation. Bronchopulmonary anastomoses nevertheless exist between arteries of these two circulations. Anastomoses also exist between veins of the two circulations.

Pulmonary Lymphatics.   Pulmonary *lymphatics* are largely confined to the dense ordinary connective tissue in the lung. Hence they are present in the visceral pleura and the interlobular septa (Figs. 20-11 and 20-23) and also in the dense connective tissue wrappings of the bronchi, bronchioles, arteries, and veins. The interalveolar walls do not contain lymphatics, but they are present in the connective tissue bordering on the alveolar ducts, and they are found at sites where interalveolar walls border on (1) the connective tissue wrappings of bronchioles or blood vessels, (2) interlobular septa, or (3) the visceral pleura.

The lung is conventionally regarded as having a *superficial* and a *deep* set of lymphatics. The superficial lymphatics are situated in the visceral pleura (Fig. 20-11, *bottom*). In smokers and city dwellers, these lymphatics are usually blackened with carbon particles. The larger superficial lymphatics are seen along the lines where interlobular septa join the pleura. The pleural lymphatics drain toward the hilar lymph nodes. The deep lymphatics are associated with branches of the pulmonary artery in the outer layers of the bronchial and bronchiolar walls and are also present in the interlobular septa (Fig. 20-11, *right*). They, too, drain toward the hilar lymph nodes. Those of the visceral pleura join those of the interlobular septa (Fig. 20-11, *bottom right corner*).

Innervation of Bronchial and Bronchiolar Smooth Muscle.   The bronchial tree is supplied with nerve fibers from both divisions of the autonomic nervous system. Parasympathetic stimulation by way of the vagus causes the bronchial and bronchiolar smooth muscle to contract.

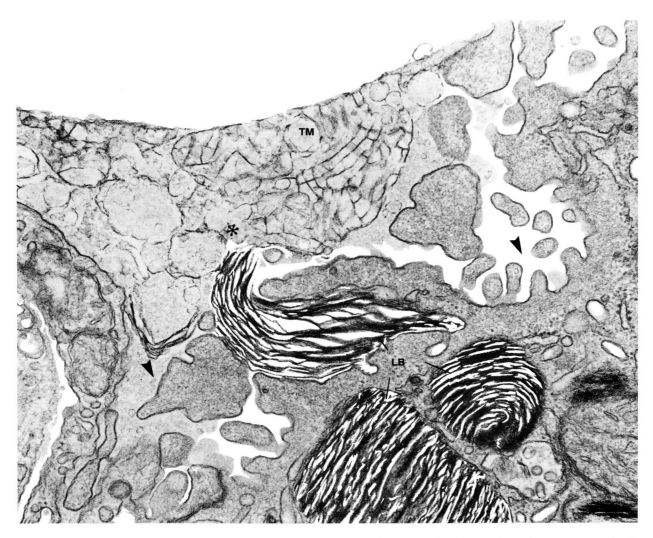

Fig. 20-21. Electron micrograph (×58,700) of lung tissue fixed by vascular perfusion (rat). Arrowheads indicate the true surface of the underlying type II pneumocyte. Above this lies a pool of alveolar tissue fluid that contains an electron-dense incomplete lattice structure (a liquid crystal) of so-called tubular myelin (*TM*). This component represents surfactant phospholipids that are present in the form of lipoproteins. It is released from lamellar bodies (*LB*) of the type II pneumocyte below. At the site marked with an asterisk, the contents of one of the lamellar bodies are being extruded by exocytosis. (Weibel ER, Gil J: Structure-function relationships at the alveolar level. In West JB (ed): Bioengineering Aspects of the Lung, p 1. New York, Marcel Dekker, 1977)

Conversely, sympathetic stimulation causes this muscle to relax.

Asthma. In the respiratory condition *asthma*, the smooth muscle in the walls of the smaller bronchioles contracts and the mucous membrane becomes edematous. This obstructs their lumen and makes breathing difficult. However, selective sympathomimetic drugs (that elicit a β_2-adrenergic response) can be inhaled as an aerosol to relax the bronchial smooth muscle during an asthmatic attack. During an asthmatic attack, an individual generally experiences more difficulty in *expelling* air from his lungs than in drawing it in. This is because expiration depends on the expulsion of air through elastic recoil of the lung tissue, and unobstructed bronchioles constitute an essential part of the conducting path through which this air must pass. Inspiratory movements can widen such airways, but forced expiratory movements serve only to compress them further.

NONRESPIRATORY FUNCTIONS OF THE LUNGS

In addition to their long-established role of being the sites of essential gas exchanges between the blood and air, the

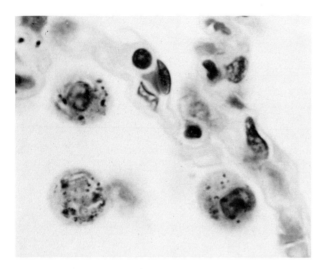

Fig. 20-22. Photomicrograph of three alveolar phagocytes in an alveolar space. Each contains phagocytosed carbon in its cytoplasm. (Courtesy of Y. Clermont)

lungs have a number of ancillary *nonrespiratory functions.* The presence of serotonin- and hormone-producing neuroendocrine (K) cells in the airway epithelium has already been mentioned. In addition, a number of vasoactive chemical mediators are either inactivated or added to the bloodstream in the pulmonary circulation. Bradykinin, norepinephrine, and serotonin are among the substances that are partly degraded (epinephrine is not affected). Also, at least one important chemical conversion into a more active form occurs primarily in the pulmonary circulation. In passing through the lung capillaries, the inactive precursor *angiotensin I,* which will be described in Chapter 21, is converted into its active form, *angiotensin II.* This conversion is brought about by the same enzyme that inactivates bradykinin (which is a vasoactive inflammatory mediator with histaminelike effects). The enzyme responsible (*converting enzyme* or *peptidyl dipeptidase*) is present on the luminal surface of the endothelial cells that line pulmonary, renal, and certain other capillaries and venules, and is preferentially distributed in surface-connecting caveolae beneath the luminal surface of these cells. It is similarly associated with the luminal surface of the aortic endothelium.

The last nonrespiratory function of the lungs that remains to be considered is the role played by their associated lymphoid tissue in the acquisition and maintenance of pulmonary mucosal immunity.

Bronchus-Associated Lymphoid Tissue

The gut-associated lymphoid tissue (GALT) and the bronchus-associated lymphoid tissue (BALT) are the two important components of the *mucosal immune system* (considered in connection with Lymphatic Nodules in Chap.

10). The lymphoid tissue associated with the tracheobronchial tract consists of solitary and aggregated unencapsulated lymphatic nodules, disorganized lymphocyte aggregates, and large numbers of individual lymphocytes. The latter include (1) lymphocytes scattered throughout the lamina propria of the bronchi and (2) intraepithelial lymphocytes. Many of the lymphocytes in the lamina propria are B cells, primarily of the IgA class. However, some of these cells are of the IgE class, and this is of relevance to immediate hypersensitivity reactions that occur in association with the airways (see Chap. 7). IgA-secreting plasma cells are commonly found in the lamina propria, and also in the submucosa in association with mucous glands. The serous secretory cells in these glands are known to produce the secretory component of secretory IgA and to participate in the secretion of this class of immunoglobulin.

Unencapsulated lymphatic nodules begin to develop in the lamina propria of bronchi a few days after birth, but probably at predetermined sites rather than at sites of antigenic stimulation. However, subsequent expansion of such nodules is antigen-dependent. The total amount of BALT tends to increase with age. Experimental studies indicate that it becomes concentrated mostly at bronchial bifurcations and in the regions between bronchi and accompanying branches of the pulmonary artery.

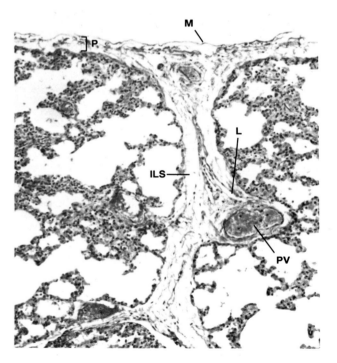

Fig. 20-23. Photomicrograph of the pleural border of a child's lung, showing the visceral pleura (*P*) and an interlobular septum (*ILS*) extending from the pleura into the substance of the lung. Squamous mesothelium (*M*) covers the pleural surface. Within the connective tissue septum, a branch of a pulmonary vein (*PV*) and lymphatics (*L*) can be distinguished.

As in Peyer's patches of the small intestine (see Chap. 10), the lymphatic nodules in BALT are provided with high endothelial venules, an access route for recirculating small lymphocytes. Furthermore, the overlying epithelial cells are nonciliated and flattened. Intraepithelial lymphocytes can become intimately associated with these cells in an arrangement that is closely similar to that described for M cells (see Fig. 10-6). Such follicle-associated epithelium is sometimes referred to as *lymphoepithelium.*

In addition, the lymphatic nodules of BALT are supplied with nerve fibers and efferent lymphatics, but they lack an afferent lymphatic supply. Germinal centers are seldom seen in these nodules. Studies in rabbits indicate that these nodules contain mostly B-cells, primarily of the IgA or IgM class, and that macrophages, too, are present. Dividing cells, if present, are found in the peripheral zone of the nodule.

The obvious similarities between the lymphatic nodules in BALT and GALT suggest that as in Peyer's patches, the thin covering epithelial cells (equivalent to M cells) are involved in antigen sampling, in this case from the lumen of the tracheobronchial tract. This facilitates the acquisition of pulmonary mucosal immunity to infective viruses and bacteria that reach the major extra- and intrapulmonary airways by way of the inhaled air. However, under normal circumstances, there is a general absence of both dividing cells and germinal centers in the lymphatic nodules of BALT, suggesting that antigenic stimulation is only minimal. Mucosal macrophages or other kinds of antigen-presenting cells could also transport microbial antigens through the efferent lymphatics of BALT to the draining hilar and mediastinal lymph nodes, facilitating the development of immune responses to such antigens within the draining nodes. For further information, see Bienenstock.

SELECTED REFERENCES

Upper Respiratory Tract and Conducting Airways

AYERS M, JEFFERY PK: Cell division and differentiation in bronchial epithelium. In Cumming G, Bonsignore G (eds): Cellular Biology of the Lung. Life Sciences Series, Vol 10. New York, Plenum, 1982

BREEZE RG, WHEELDON EB: The cells of the pulmonary airways. Am Rev Respir Dis 116:705, 1977

CASTLEMAN WL, DUNGWORTH DL, TYLER WS: Intrapulmonary airway morphology in three species of monkey: A correlated scanning and transmission electron microscopic study. Am J Anat 142: 107, 1974

COHEN AB, GOLD WM: Defense mechanisms of the lungs. Ann Rev Physiol 37:325, 1975

EVANS MJ, CABRAL–ANDERSON LJ, FREEMAN G: Role of the Clara cell in renewal of the bronchiolar epithelium. Lab Invest 38:648, 1978

FINK BR: The Human Larynx: A Functional Study. New York, Raven Press, 1975

GRAZIADEI, PPC: Cell dynamics in the olfactory mucosa. Tissue Cell 5:113, 1973

GRAZIADEI PPC, MONTI GRAZIADEI GA: Continuous nerve cell renewal in the olfactory system. In Jacobson M (ed): Handbook of Sensory Physiology, Vol IX. Development of Sensory Systems, p 55, New York, Springer-Verlag, 1978

HANCE AJ, CRYSTAL RG: The connective tissue of the lung. Am Rev Respir Dis 112:657, 1975

HARDING J, GRAZIADEI PPC, MONTI GRAZIADEI GA, MARGOLIS FL: Denervation in the primary olfactory pathway of mice. IV. Biochemical and morphological evidence for neuronal replacement following nerve section. Brain Res 132:11, 1977

HORSFIELD K: Lung morphology. In Stretton TB (ed): Recent Advances in Respiratory Medicine, No 1, p 123. Edinburgh, Churchill Livingstone, 1976

JEFFERY PK, CORRIN B: Structural analysis of the respiratory tract. In Bienenstock J (ed): Immunology of the Lung and Upper Respiratory Tract, p 1. New York, McGraw-Hill, 1984

KRAHL VE: Anatomy of the mammalian lung. In American Physiological Society: Handbook of Physiology. Section 3 (Fenn WO, Rahn H, eds), Respiration. Vol 1, p 213. Baltimore, Williams & Wilkins, 1964

KUHN C: The cells of the lung and their organelles. In Crystal RG (ed): The Biochemical Basis of Pulmonary Function, p 3. New York, Marcel Dekker, 1976

MACKLIN CC: The musculature of the bronchi and lungs. Physiol Rev 9:1, 1929

NADEL JA: Regulation of bronchial secretions. In Newball HH (ed): Immunopharmacology of the Lung. Lung Biology in Health and Disease, Vol 19, p 109. New York, Marcel Dekker, 1983

POLYZONIS BM, KAFANDARIS PM, GIGIS PI, DEMETRIOU T: An electron microscopic study of human olfactory mucosa. J Anat 128:77, 1979

STURGESS JM, TURNER JAP: Transposition of ciliary microtubules: Another cause of impaired ciliary motility. N Engl J Med 303: 318, 1980

STURGESS JM, TURNER JAP: Ultrastructural pathology of cilia in the immotile cilia syndrome. Perspectives in Pediatric Pathology 8: 133, 1984

WANG N, THURLBECK WM: Scanning electron microscopy of the lung. Hum Pathol 1:227, 1970

WEIBEL ER: Design and structure of the human lung. In Fishman AP (ed): Pulmonary Diseases and Disorders. New York, McGraw-Hill, 1979

WEIBEL ER: Looking into the lung: What can it tell us? AJR 133: 1021, 1979

WEIBEL ER: Lung cell biology. In Fishman AP (ed): Handbook of Physiology, Section 3: The Respiratory System, Vol 1. Circulation and Nonrespiratory Functions, p 47. Bethesda, MD, American Physiological Society, 1985

Interalveolar Walls, Pulmonary Surfactant, and Alveolar Macrophages

AVERY ME, FLETCHER BD: The lung and its disorders in the newborn infant. In Schaffer AJ (ed): Major Problems in Clinical Pediatrics, 3rd ed, Vol 1. Philadelphia, WB Saunders, 1974

AVERY ME, WANG NS, TAEUSCH HW, Jr: The lung of the newborn infant. Sci Am 228:74, April, 1973

BARTELS H: The air–blood barrier in the human lung: A freeze-fracture study. Cell Tissue Res 198:269, 1979

BERTALANFFY FD: Dynamics of cellular populations in the lung. In The Lung: Int Acad Pathol Monograph No 8, p 30. Baltimore, Williams & Wilkins, 1967

CHEVALIER G, COLLET AJ: In vivo incorporation of choline-^{3}H, leucine-^{3}H and galactose-^{3}H in alveolar Type II pneumocytes in relation to surfactant synthesis. A quantitative radioautographic study in mouse by electron microscopy. Anat Rec 174:289, 1972

VAN FURTH R: Cellular biology of pulmonary macrophages. Int Arch Allergy Appl Immunol (Suppl 76) 1:21, 1985

GODLESKI JJ, BRAIN JD: The origin of alveolar macrophages in mouse radiation chimeras. J Exp Med 136:630, 1972

LAMBERT MW: Accessory bronchiolo-alveolar channels. Anat Rec 127:472, 1957

LAMBERT MW: Accessory bronchiolo-alveolar communications. J Pathol Bact 70:311, 1955

MACKLIN CC: Alveolar pores and their significance in the human lung. Arch Pathol 21:202,1936

SOROKIN S: The cells of the lungs. In Nettesheim P, Hanna MG, Jr, Deatherage JW, Jr (eds): Morphology of Experimental Carcinogenesis, p 3. CONF 700501, Atomic Energy Commission, Oak Ridge, TN. 1970

STERN L (ed): Hyaline Membrane Disease: Pathogenesis and Pathophysiology. Orlando, Grune & Stratton, 1984

STRATTON JC: The ultrastructure of multilamellar bodies and surfactant in the human lung. Cell Tissue Res 193:219, 1978

TAKARO T, PRICE HP, PARRA SC: Ultrastructural studies of apertures in the interalveolar septum of the adult human lung. Am Rev Respir Dis 119:425, 1979

WEIBEL ER, GIL J: Structure-function relationships at the alveolar level. In West JB (ed): Bioengineering Aspects of the Lung, p 1. New York, Marcel Dekker, 1977

Lung Development

BOYDEN EA: Development of the human lung. In Kelley VC (ed): Brennemann's Practice of Pediatrics, Vol 4, chap 64. New York, Harper & Row, 1971

BURRI PH: Development and growth of the human lung. In Fishman AP (ed): Handbook of Physiology, Section 3: The Respiratory System, Vol 1. Circulation and Nonrespiratory Functions, p 1. Bethesda, MD American Physiological Society, 1985

COLLET AJ, DES BIENS G: Fine structure of myogenesis and elastogenesis in the developing rat lung. Anat Rec 179:343, 1974

HODSON W (ed): Development of the Lung. Lung Biology in Health and Disease, Vol 6. New York, Marcel Dekker, 1977

Pulmonary Blood Supply, Lymphatics, and Smooth Muscle Innervation

HUNG KS, HERTWECK MS, HARDY JD, LOOSLI CG: Innervation of pulmonary alveoli of the mouse lung: An electron microscopic study. Am J Anat 135:477, 1972

LAUWERYNS J: The blood and lymphatic microcirculation of the lung. Pathol Annu 6:363, 1971

Bronchus-Associated Lymphoid Tissue and Metabolic Functions of the Lungs

BIENENSTOCK J: Bronchus-associated lymphoid tissue. In Bienenstock J (ed): Immunology of the Lung and Upper Respiratory Tract, p 96. New York, McGraw-Hill, 1984

BIENENSTOCK J (ed): Immunology of the Lung and Upper Respiratory Tract. New York, McGraw-Hill, 1984

BRANDTZAEG P: Immune functions of human nasal mucosa and tonsils in health and disease. In Bienenstock J (ed): Immunology of the Lung and Upper Respiratory Tract, p 28. New York, McGraw-Hill, 1984

HEINEMANN HO: The lung as a metabolic organ: An overview. Fed Proc 32:1955, 1973

HEINEMANN HO, FISHMAN AP: Nonrespiratory functions of mammalian lung. Physiol Rev 49:1, 1969

RYAN JW, NIEMEYER RS, GOODWIN DW: Metabolic fates of bradykinin, angiotensin I, adenine nucleotidase and prostaglandins E1 and F1 alpha in the pulmonary circulation. Adv Exp Med Biol 21: 259, 1972

21

The Urinary System

In addition to producing energy and resulting in the formation of cell products that are of value to the body, the various metabolic activities of cells result in the production of waste substances that pass through tissue fluid into the bloodstream. One such by-product of metabolism, carbon dioxide, is eliminated in the lungs. Nitrogenous breakdown products of protein catabolism and a variety of other toxic waste substances are eliminated from the bloodstream by the kidneys. The combined capacity of both kidneys is such that they are able to purify almost one quarter of the total amount of blood leaving the heart on a moment-to-moment basis. The first step in such purification is that their fenestrated *glomerular capillaries* permit water and substances in simple solution to pass into the beginning of long *kidney (renal) tubules*. Although certain of these dissolved substances are waste substances, others are still potentially useful to the body and are therefore conserved. Hence most of the water and the other useful substances in the *urinary filtrate* are resorbed as this fluid moves along the tubules. In contrast, the waste substances are allowed to continue on their way along the renal tubules. They subsequently leave the kidneys as constituents of the *urine* that drains into the *urinary bladder* by way of the *ureters*.

The tubular organization that enables the kidneys to remove waste products from the blood permits them to perform other useful functions as well. By regulating the amount of water that is lost in the urine, the kidneys play a major role in maintaining the *fluid balance* of the body. They also regulate differential *electrolyte loss* in the urine. An additional important function of the kidneys is that they produce *erythropoietin*, the hormone that regulates erythropoiesis in myeloid tissue.

A distinctive spherical arrangement of fenestrated capillaries termed a *glomerulus* (L. for small ball) is invaginated into the proximal blind end of each kidney tubule, forming a spherical-to-ovoid filtration unit known as a *renal corpuscle*. The fluid that passes through the walls of these *glomerular capillaries* is known as the *glomerular filtrate*. Because it takes some time for the glomerular filtrate to reach the distal end of the tubules, which have a total length of up to 6.5 cm, there is ample opportunity for

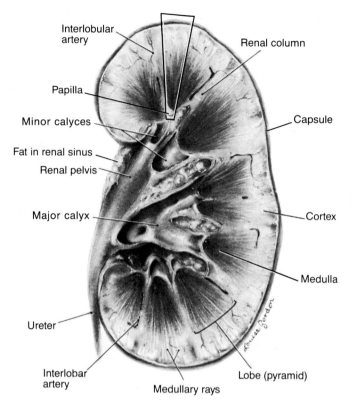

Interlobular artery

Renal column

Papilla

Minor calyces

Fat in renal sinus

Renal pelvis

Major calyx

Capsule

Cortex

Medulla

Ureter

Interlobar artery

Medullary rays

Lobe (pyramid)

Fig. 21-1. Diagrammatic representation of a kidney cut through its hilum, as seen with the unaided eye (cut surface).

their lining cells (1) to resorb useful constituents from the filtrate and (2) to excrete unwanted substances into the tubules.

A kidney tubule and its associated glomerulus constitute a *nephron,* the structural and functional unit of the kidney. There are approximately 1.3 million nephrons in each human kidney. These drain by way of a branching system of *collecting ducts* into the *renal pelvis,* which is the expanded funnel-like proximal end of the associated ureter (Fig. 21-1).

The hemodynamic arrangement in the renal glomeruli is not unlike that found in ordinary capillaries when their venous outflow is obstructed. Such conditions cause the hydrostatic pressure to remain high along the entire length of each capillary. Hence glomerular capillaries produce glomerular filtrate but do not resorb it. In other sites, this would cause edema, but in the renal glomeruli, it results in a continuous production of glomerular filtrate. Another factor that facilitates the production of copious volumes of glomerular filtrate is that the endothelial cells of glomerular capillaries are provided with fenestrae that *lack occluding diaphragms;* in other words, their cytoplasm is traversed by open apertures through which filtrate (but not blood cells) can easily pass. The filtrate that leaves these capillaries gains access to the lumen of kidney tubules across a special kind of epithelium that will be described later in this chapter.

KIDNEYS

Each kidney has the general shape of a lima bean, with an extensive convex surface and a smaller concave border (Fig. 21-1). In the concavity of the kidney, which is known as its *hilum,* a variable amount of adipose tissue is present. The drainage tube of the kidney, called its *ureter,* together with the renal artery, vein, and lymphatics and their surrounding nerve plexus, reach the kidney through the hilar fat tissue (Fig. 21-1). The kidney is enclosed by a tough *capsule* of dense ordinary connective tissue. The outer region of the kidney is known as its *cortex* (L. for bark or shell) and its inner region is called its *medulla* (L. for marrow, meaning the middle). In contrast to the cortex, the medulla has a striated appearance caused by striations that fan out from the hilum (Fig. 21-1).

The Human Kidney Is Multilobar. The unit of gross kidney structure is the *lobe.* In contrast to the unilobar kidney of laboratory rodents, which consists of only one lobe, the human kidney is composed of up to 18 lobes. Each lobe is made up of a conical medullary pyramid and a cap of cortical tissue, so each pyramid of the kidney corresponds to the medullary portion of one kidney *lobe* (Fig. 21-1). During fetal life and for the first few months after birth, lobes can be discerned at the kidney surface. In a few cases, they can even be distinguished in adult life; this is termed

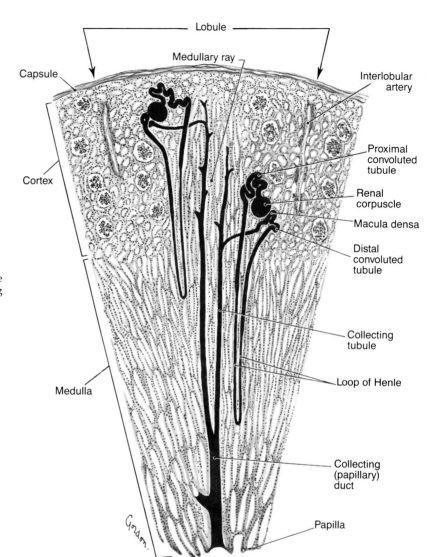

Lobule

Medullary ray

Capsule

Cortex

Medulla

Gordon.

Interlobular artery

Proximal convoluted tubule

Renal corpuscle

Macula densa

Distal convoluted tubule

Collecting tubule

Loop of Henle

Collecting (papillary) duct

Papilla

Fig. 21-2. Schematic representation of the basic arrangement of nephrons and collecting tubules in a lobule of the kidney.

fetal lobulation, which is a misnomer because lobes and not lobules are seen. In most cases, however, this delineation between lobes becomes blurred in early childhood, and the cortical tissue that caps each medullary pyramid merges with that of its neighbors. A lobed appearance is nevertheless retained in the medulla, because although some pyramids fuse during development, most remain as recognizable entities. Individual medullary pyramids are also separated from one another by substantial partitions of cortical substance that extend for some distance into the medulla. These partitions are known as *renal columns* or *columns of Bertin* (Fig. 21-1).

The apex of each medullary pyramid forms a rounded *papilla* that projects into the renal pelvis (Fig. 21-1). Because the human kidney has many papillae, the proximal end of the ureter consists of a number of *major calyces,* each sub-

divided into *minor calyces.* A minor calyx is a funnel-shaped structure that fits over a papilla (Fig. 21-1). The epithelial covering of the papilla is continuous with the epithelial lining of its associated calyx. Whereas the papilla is largely covered with simple columnar epithelium, the calyx is lined with transitional epithelium as is the rest of the ureter.

Kidney Lobules. Each lobe of the kidney consists of a number of *lobules* (Fig. 21-2) that are less obviously demarcated than lobes. However, *interlobular arteries* (which will be considered later in this chapter) ascend into the cortex between lobules, and where present in sections, they serve as useful landmarks that delineate lobules (Figs. 21-2 and 21-3). A lobule can be defined as a small part of an organ that is separated from other parts by connective tissue partitions or by some other means. However, in glandular

Interlobular artery

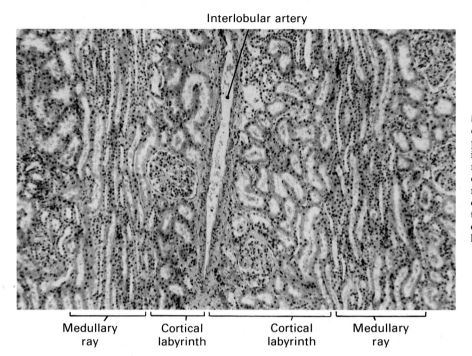

Medullary ray   Cortical labyrinth   Cortical labyrinth   Medullary ray

Fig. 21-3. Low-power photomicrograph of kidney cortex, showing parts of two lobules separated by an interlobular artery. Each of the two medullary rays that form the central cores of the two lobules is surrounded by the renal corpuscles and convoluted tubules of the nephrons that empty into the collecting ducts of the ray; they comprise the cortical labyrinth.

tissue, the small parts separated from one another by partitions are generally constituted of secretory units that drain into a single common duct that leaves the lobule. Hence the parts that drain into a single common duct became called *lobules* in the kidney even though these parts are not separated from one another by partitions. So in the kidney, lobules correspond to the parts of the organ in which all the nephrons drain into the same collecting tubule. Because these areas of tissue (lobules) are not separated from one another by other tissues, it is not easy to find them; it is much easier to recognize their central cores, which are known as *medullary rays.*

Medullary Rays. Medullary rays are raylike extensions of medullary tissue that project into the renal cortex from each medullary pyramid (Figs. 21-1, 21-2, and 21-3). In the middle of each medullary ray, there is a branched collecting tubule that drains the surrounding nephrons (Fig. 21-2). This collecting tubule is the counterpart of a branched *intralobular duct* of a compound exocrine gland, and the group of nephrons that open into it are equivalent to a *lobule* of such a gland (Fig. 21-2). Each nephron descends toward the medulla and then loops back into the cortex before emptying into the branched collecting tubule (Fig. 21-2). The collecting tubule then descends through the medulla and opens onto a papilla at the renal pelvis (Fig. 21-2).

When seen in sections, medullary rays are flanked by cortical tissue that contains the tortuous parts of nephrons (Fig. 21-2). This cortical tissue is often referred to as the

cortical labyrinth to distinguish it from medullary rays (Fig. 21-3). Medullary rays are narrowest at sites where they approach the kidney surface because in the outer region of the cortex, they only contain collecting tubules and the looped parts of nephrons whose glomeruli lie in the outermost region of the cortex. However, as medullary rays descend toward the medulla, they also incorporate the looped parts of nephrons whose glomeruli lie in the deeper region of the cortex, and this makes them broader (Fig. 22-2). On entering the medulla, a medullary ray is no longer called a ray because it does not stand out like a ray against a background of different character.

Nephrons and Their Course Within the Kidney Lobule. As may be seen in Figures 21-2 and 21-4, a thick-walled tubule called the *proximal convoluted tubule* leads from the *renal corpuscle* and pursues a tortuous course in the cortical tissue close to the site from which it started. It then extends straight down into the medulla as the *descending limb of the loop of Henle.* The proximal portion of the descending limb of the loop of Henle is thick-walled like the proximal convoluted tubule, but the distal portion is thin-walled (Fig. 21-4). The descending limb of the loop of Henle extends for some distance into the medulla and then loops back into the cortex as the straight *ascending limb of the loop of Henle.* The ascending limb is thin-walled deep in the medulla but becomes thick-walled before it enters the cortex, where it leads into the tortuous thick-walled *distal convoluted tubule* (Figs. 21-2 and 21-4). Nephrons with glomeruli that are situated near the corticomedullary border (*juxta-*

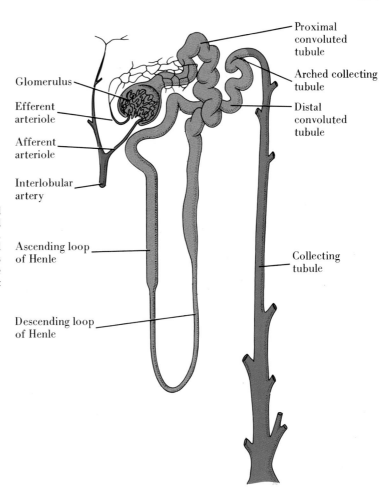

Fig. 21-4. Diagrammatic representation of a typical nephron, with its glomerulus at its blind end, and connecting at its distal end with a collecting tubule. The normal anatomical relation between the distal convoluted tubule and the root of the glomerulus is not shown. Actually, the tubule returns closer to the glomerulus, fitting into the space between the afferent and efferent arterioles.

medullary glomeruli) have longer loops of Henle than those with glomeruli that are situated more peripherally (Fig. 21-2).

Close to the renal corpuscle from which the course of the nephron began, the ascending limb of the loop of Henle approaches the *vascular pole* of the renal corpuscle, which is the site where afferent and efferent blood vessels join the glomerulus. From this point on, the tubule is called the *distal convoluted tubule*. A distinctive feature of the very beginning of the distal convoluted tubule where it lies in contact with the vascular pole is that it is densely nucleated; this site is accordingly known as the *macula densa* (Figs. 21-2 and 21-5). The far end of the distal convoluted tubule opens into the branched system of straight *collecting tubules* that extends down through the medulla and opens through a *main collecting duct* (*papillary duct* or *duct of Bellini*) onto a papilla (Fig. 21-2).

Collecting ducts are not considered parts of nephrons because they develop independently. Thus nephrons arise from kidney mesoderm that becomes organized as renal tubules. Collecting tubules, on the other hand, are deriv-

atives of the developing ureters. When the forerunner of each ureter grows out from the developing urinary bladder and enters a kidney, it forms the renal pelvis and branches extensively so as to produce a branching system of collecting tubules. These tubules manage to interconnect with the nephrons in such a way that direct continuity of their respective lumina is established.

The various parts of the nephron will now be considered separately.

Renal Corpuscle and Juxtaglomerular Complex

The *renal corpuscle* is generally ovoid, with a diameter of 150 µm to 250 µm. It is a somewhat complex structure consisting of glomerular capillaries, their afferent and efferent vessels (arterioles), supporting mesangial cells, a special covering epithelium, and the remainder of the expanded proximal blind end of a nephron. The epithelial covering of each glomerular capillary constitutes the *glomerular epithelium*, which is also known as the *visceral layer*

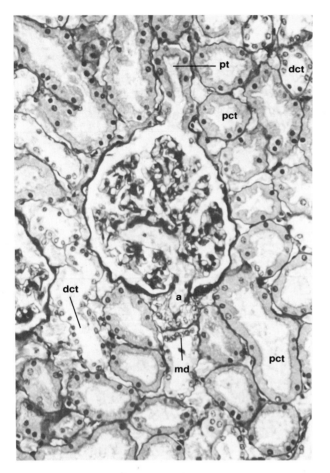

Fig. 21-5. Photomicrograph of kidney cortex, showing a renal corpuscle and the surrounding proximal and distal convoluted tubules (PAS and hematoxylin). This plane of section includes both the vascular pole and the tubular pole of the renal corpuscle. At the vascular pole, the lumen of an ateriole (*a*) and the macula densa (*md*) in the wall of the distal tubule can be distinguished. Some lacis cells can also be seen between the arteriole and the macula densa. At the tubular pole, the capsular space is continuous with the lumen of the proximal convoluted tubule (*pt*); this and other sections of the proximal convoluted tubule (*pct*) exhibit a distinct PAS-positive striated border. In contrast, cross sections of the distal convoluted tubule (*dct*) exhibit more nuclei in their paler staining walls and lack a distinct striated border. The basement membranes of the tubules and renal corpuscle appear distinctly following PAS staining.

of Bowman's capsule (Figs. 21-6 and 21-7). The epithelium that constitutes the outer wall of the renal corpuscle is called the *capsular epithelium* or the *parietal layer of Bowman's capsule* (Figs. 21-6 and 21-7). It is continuous with the glomerular epithelium. The lumen of the renal corpuscle is known as the *capsular (Bowman's) space.*

A special vascular arrangement enables the glomerular capillaries of the renal corpuscle to produce large quantities of glomerular filtrate. Whereas capillaries generally open into venules, the glomerular capillaries open into an *efferent*

arteriole of a construction similar to that of the *afferent arteriole* that supplies them (Figs. 21-6 and 21-7). Both of these arterioles possess smooth muscle cells in their media, and it is the differential in their respective tonus that maintains a high hydrostatic pressure along the entire length of the glomerular capillaries. The overall diameter of the afferent arteriole is larger than that of the efferent arteriole, but the luminal diameter is more or less comparable in both vessels (see Fig. 21-9) because the afferent arteriole has a thicker media.

Vascular Pole and Juxtaglomerular Cells. At the vascular pole of the renal corpuscle, the distal convoluted tubule fits between the afferent and the efferent arterioles (Fig. 21-7). At this site, as already noted, there is a specialized region in the wall of the distal tubule. The side of the tubule facing the glomerulus is characterized by the presence of a densely nucleated spot termed the *macula densa.* Here the epithelial cells are narrower than usual; hence their nuclei lie closer together (Figs. 21-7 and 21-8). This heavily nucleated site is generally considered to indicate the very beginning of the distal convoluted tubule. Between the macula densa and the glomerulus, and lying in the notch between the afferent and the efferent arterioles, there is a group of small cells with pale-staining nuclei. These cells are known as *lacis (Goormaghtigh's) cells* (Figs. 21-7 and 21-8). They are believed to be supporting mesangial cells (which will be described later in this chapter), so they are also often referred to collectively as the *extraglomerular mesangium.*

An even more significant feature of the vascular pole of the renal corpuscle is the presence of special modified smooth muscle cells in the media of the afferent arteriole. Because these cells lie close to the glomerulus, they are known as *juxtaglomerular (JG) cells.* Unlike ordinary smooth muscle cells, their nucleus is rounded instead of elongated and their cytoplasm contains numerous large secretory granules (Figs. 21-7 and 21-8). Although these granules are not evident in hematoxylin and eosin (H & E) sections, they are PAS-positive and they can be demonstrated very clearly by appropriate special staining methods (Fig. 21-8). The term *juxtaglomerular complex* is used to describe the closely associated macula densa, lacis cells, and JG cells. There are a number of features of this complex that are unique. (1) Although JG cells are present in the walls of the afferent arteriole, they are seldom found in the efferent arteriole. (2) The internal elastic lamina of the arteriole is missing where JG cells are present. These cells therefore lie in close contact with the endothelial lining of the arteriole and hence with the blood in its lumen. (3) JG cells also lie in close contact with the macula densa (Figs. 21-7 and 21-8), nestling in the crevice between the afferent and efferent arterioles. (4) The basement membrane that otherwise surrounds the nephron along its entire length is absent at the macula densa (McManus). Hence the JG cells are in close contact with the epithelial lining cells of the distal tubule

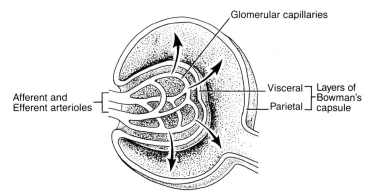

Fig. 21-6. Simplified schematic representation of the basic organization of a renal corpuscle. See text for details.

Glomerular capillaries

Afferent and
Efferent arterioles

Visceral ⎤ Layers of
⎦ Bowman's
Parietal ⎦ capsule

at this site. (5) JG cells are innervated by adrenergic nerve fibers, and sympathetic stimulation increases their rate of secretion. (6) Whereas in the other renal tubular cells the Golgi apparatus is situated between the nucleus and the luminal border of the cell, in most cells of the macula densa it is situated on the side that faces the JG cells (McManus). Finally, the lacis cells show extensive interdigitations and are interconnected not only with one another but also with JG cells by means of gap junctions. This is regarded as being suggestive of some functional cooperation between these two types of cells (Gorgas).

JG Cells Play a Key Role in the Regulation of Blood Pressure. It is now firmly established that JG cells are involved in the maintenance of normal blood pressure. The student is probably aware that *high blood pressure (hypertension)* is by no means uncommon in individuals who have passed the prime of life, and that it can also occur in younger people. Hypertension results when the *arterioles* of the body become *constricted;* this raises the pressure within the arterial system. This, of course, puts more work on the heart, which therefore tends to become hypertrophied. The arteriolar constriction may be due, at least for a time, to increased tonus or hypertrophy of the muscle cells of the arteriolar walls, with the cells of the wall remaining healthy. But, in many instances, the arteriolar walls become diseased, and deposits of abnormal materials accumulate in them; these deposits encroach on the lumen of the vessel and narrow it further. This type of hypertension is almost always associated with kidney disease.

An important cell type that is known to participate directly in a homeostatic mechanism that normally keeps the systemic blood pressure within appropriate limits is the JG cell of the kidney. JG cells are involved because their secretory granules contain an enzyme called *renin* (L. *renis,* kidney) that is liberated into the bloodstream whenever there is a decrease in the blood pressure. In this case, the JG cells are, in fact, responding to a decrease in the rate of blood flow through the kidneys (*renal ischemia*), and under conditions in which the renal blood flow is chronically impaired due to kidney disease, consistently elevated levels of renin can be present in the bloodstream. This, in turn,

can lead to elevation of the systemic blood pressure because renin acts to *raise the blood pressure.* The steps involved are described in the following paragraphs.

Once renin becomes liberated into the bloodstream, it acts on the plasma globulin *angiotensinogen* and converts it into a decapeptide called *angiotensin I.* This peptide is inactive, but it is acted upon by an endothelium-associated enzyme (*converting enzyme* or *peptidyl dipeptidase*) that changes it to an octopeptide, *angiotensin II,* that brings about *arteriolar vasoconstriction* and thereby *raises the blood pressure.* However, the effect of angiotensin II is only transitory; hence it does not cause sustained hypertension unless it is formed on a continuous basis.

JG cells are able to respond to a fall in blood pressure in two different ways. The first way is that they respond to the *degree of stretch* in the wall of the afferent arteriole, releasing renin whenever the wall of this vessel is not being stretched to the customary extent. This results in more angiotensin II being formed in the blood, which, in turn, has two effects, both of which can raise the blood pressure. First, angiotensin II has a direct effect on the smooth muscle cells in the walls of *arterioles.* By stimulating these cells to contract, it decreases the luminal diameter of all the arterioles in the body and thereby raises the blood pressure in the circulatory system as a whole. Second, angiotensin II stimulates the *adrenal cortex* to secrete increased amounts of the hormone *aldosterone* (which will be described in Chap. 22). Aldosterone acts on the distal convoluted tubules and the collecting tubules, causing them to resorb more sodium and water. This has the effect of increasing the fluid content of the circulatory system and thereby raising the pressure within the system.

The second way in which JG cells are involved in the regulation of blood pressure is that they monitor the *chloride concentration* of the urinary filtrate reaching the distal tubule. This concentration is a function of the glomerular filtration rate, and it drops when there is a decrease in the blood pressure. The information again seems to be utilized by the JG cells to help determine the amount of renin that they should release in order to restore the blood pressure to its normal limits. JG cells also release renin in response

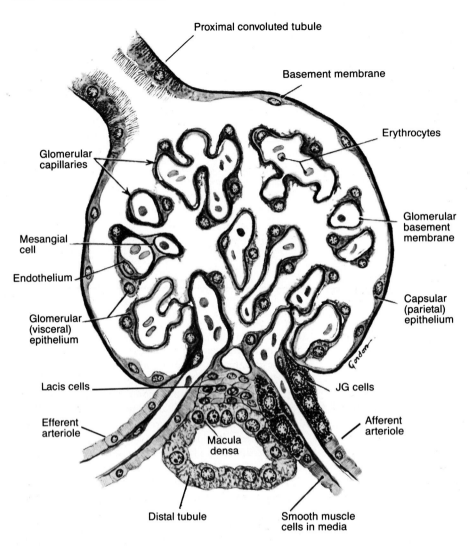

Proximal convoluted tubule

Basement membrane

Erythrocytes

Glomerular
capillaries

Glomerular
basement
membrane

Mesangial
cell

Endothelium

Glomerular
(visceral)
epithelium

Capsular
(parietal)
epithelium

Lacis cells

JG cells

Efferent
arteriole

Afferent
arteriole

Macula
densa

Distal tubule

Smooth muscle
cells in media

Fig. 21-7. Diagrammatic representation of a renal corpuscle, showing its juxtaglomerular apparatus (stained by the PAS technique). Its tubular pole is at the top, and its vascular pole is at the bottom. See text for details.

to sympathetic (adrenergic) stimulation. Moreover, the amount of renin that they release is subject to local regulation because of a parallel direct mechanism that causes the afferent arteriole to dilate following a fall in blood pressure.

Hence JG cells respond to a fall in blood pressure by releasing an appropriate quantity of their renin, which, by producing angiotensin II (and also another peptide called *angiotensin III*), acts to restore the blood pressure to its normal limits. This effect is normally self-limiting because extra chloride in the filtrate reaching the macula densa and regained stretch in the wall of the afferent arteriole slow down the secretory activity of the JG cells. Finally, we should add that although chronically impaired renal circulation can be manifested as persistent hypertension, the basis for development and continuation of the common type of hypertension is a relatively complex matter because electrolyte and water retention, aldosterone secretion, kid-

ney disease, and even emotional factors seem to be involved.

Glomerular Capillary Loops Are Supported by Basement Membranes and Mesangial Matrix. The afferent arteriole supplies blood to a spherical arrangement of anastomosing glomerular capillary loops that is attached to the vascular pole of the renal corpuscle (Fig. 21-9). The sites where these capillary loops join the afferent and efferent arterioles are often referred to as the stalks from which the capillary loops hang. The delicate axial stalks are made up of stellate *mesangial cells* and an amorphous intercellular matrix that these cells produce (Fig. 21-10). From Figure 21-10 it can be seen that the glomerular epithelium does not necessarily cover the entire surface of every capillary loop. In some cases, it surrounds two crisscrossing or adjacent capillary loops and their common mesangial stalk *as a whole* (Fig. 21-10).

In such cases, the substantial basement membrane pro-

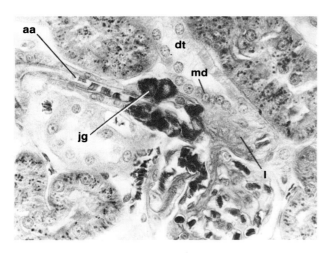

Fig. 21-8. Photomicrograph of a juxtaglomerular complex (rat kidney stained with Biebrich scarlet and ethyl violet). Juxtaglomerular cells (*jg*) are seen here in the walls of the afferent arteriole (*aa*); JG cells become specifically stained with this method. Nuclei of lacis cells (*l*) can just be discerned in the region between the juxtaglomerular cells and the macula densa (*md*), which is a part of the wall of the distal tube (*dt*). (Mujović S: Acta Anat 118:181, 1984)

duced by the glomerular epithelium does not extend around the entire perimeter of each capillary (Fig. 21-10). The necessary additional support is provided by glomerular mesangial cells. These cells produce collagens of several different types along with chondroitin sulfate proteoglycan and fibronectin, and they are responsible for secreting the intercellular *mesangial matrix* (Fig. 21-10) that covers the glomerular capillaries where they lack epithelium-derived basement membrane.

The endothelial cells of the glomerular capillaries also lay down a thinner basement membrane of their own that fuses with the epithelial basement membrane (Fig. 21-10). At sites where the thick epithelial basement membrane is lacking, the endothelial basement membrane becomes continuous with the mesangial matrix instead (Fig. 21-10).

Mesangial Cells. The cells that produce the extracellular matrix in the stalk regions of the glomerular capillaries have a fairly small and dark-staining nucleus and are more or less stellate in shape. They are able to extend their cytoplasmic processes between endothelial cells so as to reach into the capillary lumen, and they can phagocytose macromolecular materials from intercapillary spaces. Lysosomes and lipofuscin granules are recognizable in their cytoplasm. Mesangial cells have two important roles: (1) that of keeping the glomerular filter free of debris, and (2) that of providing additional support at sites where the epithelial basement membrane is lacking.

Glomerular Filtration Barrier

To pass through the filtration barrier in the kidney, a blood-borne molecule needs to negotiate (1) the endothelium of the glomerular capillaries, (2) the glomerular basement membrane, and (3) the epithelial covering of the capillaries (the glomerular epithelium or visceral layer of Bowman's capsule). Because the endothelium is fenestrated with open pores that are up to 100 nm in diameter, it poses no obstacle; this layer is unable to hold back anything smaller than blood cells and platelets. The glomerular basement membrane, on the other hand, is of central importance in the filtration process because it behaves as a molecular sieve, permitting the passage of only relatively small molecules that lack a high net negative charge. At present it seems doubtful that any part of the glomerular epithelium manifests selectivity during normal glomerular filtration. Earlier findings that seemed to suggest some importance in this respect have now been reinterpreted, making it seem more likely that the epithelial layer plays a totally nonselective role in the filtration process.

Glomerular Basement Membrane. The glomerular basement membrane (GBM) is noticeably thicker than other basement membranes because, as just explained, it mostly represents a *fused basement membrane* that is made up of both the epithelial and the endothelial basement membrane. In electron micrographs, it exhibits a three-layered appearance. The electron-lucent layer next to the endothelium is known as the *lamina lucida* (or *rara*) *interna* (Fig. 21-11*A*). The middle layer, which is comparatively electron dense, is called the *lamina densa* (Fig. 21-11*A*). The electron-lucent layer adjacent to the visceral (glomerular) epithelium is termed the *lamina lucida* (or *rara*) *externa* (Fig. 21-11*A*). The reason for special terminology in the case of the GBM is that when the epithelial and the endothelial basement membranes fuse, the lamina fibroreticularis (the third layer present in other basement membranes) becomes excluded. Hence each electron-lucent layer of the GBM represents a cell membrane–associated *lamina lucida,* the thick *lamina densa* of the GBM represents a fusion product of the corresponding layer of the epithelial and the endothelial basement membrane, and the *lamina fibroreticularis* of these two basement membranes is missing. It is possible to discern the type IV collagen-containing meshwork of the lamina densa in Figure 21-11*A*. Additional loosely arranged wispy cords extend across the laminae lucidae to the cells on either side of the GBM (Fig. 21-11*A*). A description of the molecular organization of basement membranes may be found in the section on Basement Membranes in Chapter 7; this organization is depicted in Figure 7-9. For further details about the fine structure of the GBM, see Laurie et al.

Experimental studies indicate that new basement membrane material is always being added to the GBM, mainly on its epithelial side. Where mesangial cells are present,

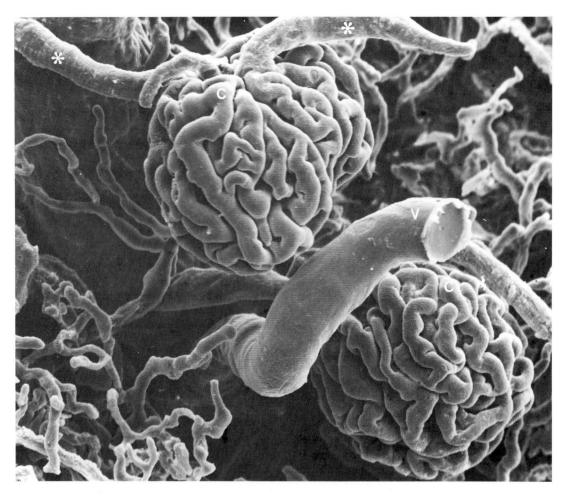

Fig. 21-9. Scanning electron micrograph of renal glomeruli and other cortical vessels of the kidney (corrosion cast of kidney cortex). At top, afferent and efferent arterioles (indicated by *asterisks*) can be recognized. The wider vessel at *center* (*v*) is probably a stellate vein. At lower left and upper right, capillary beds of the cortex are present. The capillary loops of the glomeruli (*c*) show numerous anastomoses. (Courtesy of L. Arsenault)

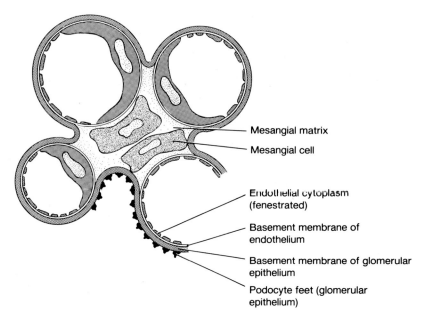

Mesangial matrix

Mesangial cell

Endothelial cytoplasm (fenestrated)

Basement membrane of endothelium

Basement membrane of glomerular epithelium

Podocyte feet (glomerular epithelium)

Fig. 21-10. Diagram illustrating the position of mesangial cells in relation to capillaries in a glomerular tuft. Whereas the basement membrane of the endothelial cells surrounds each capillary, the basement membrane beneath the podocyte feet does *not* surround each capillary completely. It is present only where the capillaries are covered with epithelium (in the form of podocyte feet), as shown at lower right. The podocyte feet would extend all over the capillary tuft shown in this diagram. The mesangial cells and their matrix form the core of the tuft.

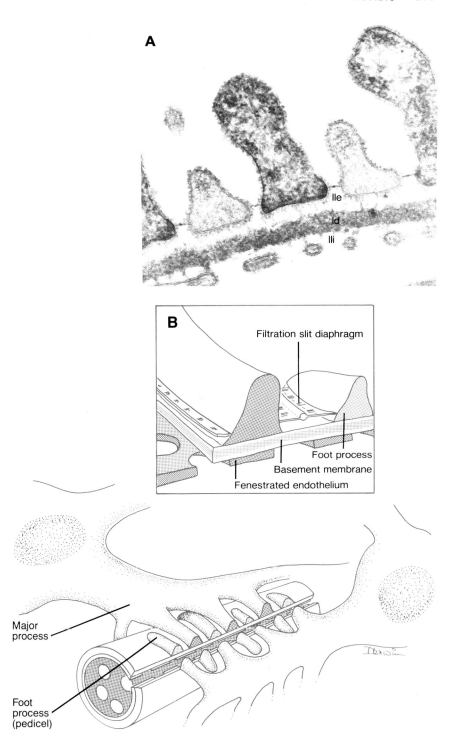

Fig. 21-11. (A) Electron micrograph (×60,000) of the glomerular filtration barrier (rat kidney, fixed in the presence of tannic acid). Glomerular filtrate passes from the lumen of a glomerular capillary (*lower right*), through the fenestrated endothelium extending across the bottom of the micrograph, and then across the lamina lucida interna (*lli*), lamina densa (*ld*), and lamina lucida externa (*lle*) of the glomerular basement membrane. Interdigitating podocyte foot processes interconnected by filtration-slit diaphragms can be seen on the epithelial side of the basement membrane, and the space above these is part of the capsular space (*upper left*). (B) Interpretive schematic drawings. (*A*, Tisher CC: Anatomy of the kidney. In Brenner BM, Rector FC (eds): The Kidney, Vol 1. Philadelphia, WB Saunders, 1976)

they probably aid in disposing of the basement membrane material on the endothelial side of the GBM by removing accumulations of debris or old altered GBM through phagocytosis. Studies in rats indicate that the turnover time of the GBM is approximately 1 year.

Glomerular Epithelial Cells Are Known as Podocytes.

Scanning electron micrographs show very clearly that the component cells of the *glomerular epithelium* (*visceral layer* of Bowman's capsule) are of a unique shape that appears to be designed to facilitate access of the glomerular filtrate to the capsular space. The distinctive shape of these cells earned them the name *podocytes* (Fig. 21-12). Projecting

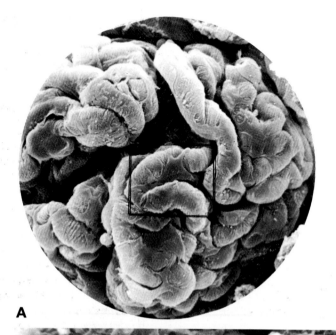

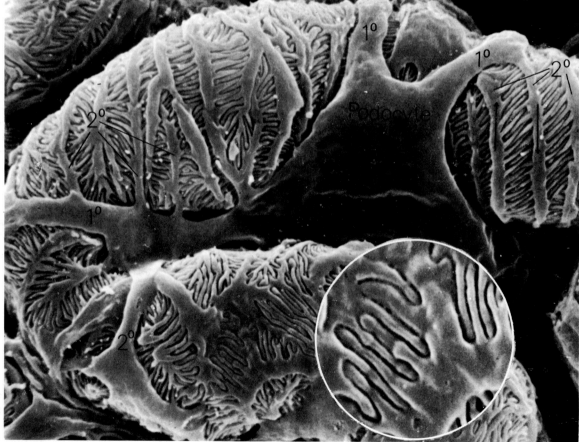

Fig. 21-12. Scanning electron micrographs of glomerular capillary loops, showing the glomerular epithelium that constitutes the visceral layer of Bowman's capsule. (*A*) Under low magnification (X700). (*B*) Boxed-in area in *A* seen under higher magnification (×4000). The primary extensions (1°) of the podocytes that constitute this epithelium give rise to secondary processes (2°) from which podocyte feet (pedicels) extend as side branches. Arrows indicate interdigitating secondary processes of two neighboring podocytes. (*Inset*) Parts of two adjacent secondary podocyte processes, showing their associated lateral foot processes with the intervening filtration slits between these processes, seen under higher magnification (×6000). (Ross MH, Reith EJ: Histology. A Text and Atlas. New York, Harper & Row/JB Lippincott, 1985)

from the surface of the glomerular capillaries into the capsular space are the cell bodies of podocytes (Figs. 21-11, *bottom,* and 21-12). Each podocyte adheres to the outer surface of a capillary by means of several long cytoplasmic processes (Fig. 21-12*B*). The *primary (major) processes* that extend from its cell body bear numerous *secondary processes,* from which side branches called *podocyte feet* or *pedicels* (Gr. *podos,* foot) extend to the outer surface of the GBM (Figs. 21-11, *bottom,* and 21-12*B*). The closely spaced array of foot processes extending from a secondary process of one podocyte interdigitate with a corresponding array extending from another podocyte, leaving only narrow clefts between neighboring podocyte feet. Hence the entire outer surface of the glomerular capillaries projecting into the capsular space is covered with closely approximated interdigitating foot processes of podocytes, with only narrow slitlike spaces between them (Fig. 21-12). These slits are 20 nm to 30 nm wide and are termed *filtration slits.* With special fixation, it can be seen that each filtration slit is spanned by a shelflike *filtration-slit diaphragm* that is 5 nm to 7 nm thick (Fig. 21-11*A* and B). This diaphragm possesses a central electron-dense rib (Fig. 21-11*A*) that represents an axial thickening that extends along its middle (Fig. 21-11*B*). Seen in face view, the filtration-slit diaphragm has a zipperlike appearance with a regular periodicity (Fig. 21-11*B*). The glomerular filtrate is required to pass through this diaphragm in order to enter the capsular space.

The Glomerular Basement Membrane Is Responsible for Filtration Selectivity. The results of electron microscope (EM) tracer studies indicate that the GBM can impede the passage of macromolecular substances over a wide range of molecular weights; its filtering action depends not only on *molecular size* but also on *molecular charge.* Molecules with a molecular weight that is in excess of 69,000 daltons or that have a high net negative charge (*i.e.,* polyanionic molecules) are unable to cross the glomerular filtration barrier. As a consequence, the plasma protein content of the glomerular filtrate is normally very low (0.03%). It is now evident that the GBM constituent that is chiefly responsible for this effect is heparan sulfate proteoglycan. Enzymatic removal of the heparan sulfate from the GBM causes a dramatic increase in the permeability of this structure to the negatively charged macromolecules that it normally excludes (Kanwar et al).

The functional role of the filtration-slit diaphragm that is present between adjacent foot processes of podocytes, previously believed to represent an ancillary molecular sieve capable of holding back macromolecules of intermediate molecular weight, is now an open question. The fine filtering function formerly ascribed to this structure is now more readily explained in terms of the molecular composition and size- and charge-selective properties of the GBM, and pathological changes in the GBM that lead to proteinuria corroborate this view. For further information on the filtering function and permeability properties of the GBM, see Farquhar.

The precise size limit of the molecules that pass the glomerular filter has proved difficult to establish. Plasma albumin, which represents a substantial proportion of the total plasma protein, has a molecular weight of 69,000 daltons and an effective molecular diameter of approximately 7 nm. Whereas molecules of this protein appear to have dimensions just small enough to pass through the intermolecular spaces in the GBM, these spaces are probably occupied by other macromolecules under conditions of normal blood flow. Probably of more significance is the fact that because albumin molecules are anionic, they are held back by negative charges in the filter.

Immune Complexes Can Become Lodged in the Glomerular Basement Membrane. It might be thought that the GBM would be in imminent danger of becoming plugged up with the macromolecules that it has strained out. Continual turnover of basement membrane material, continual blood flow in the glomerular capillaries, and vigilant phagocytic activity on the part of the glomerular mesangial cells presumably help to prevent this from happening. However, under certain circumstances, such obstruction does occur. *Antigen–antibody complexes* forming in the bloodstream, or gaining access to it from elsewhere, can become localized in the GBM as irregularly shaped deposits beneath the podocyte feet. It is relatively uncommon for the antibody component of such complexes to be directed against a component of the basement membrane itself. More generally, soluble immune complexes are formed elsewhere under conditions of antigen excess and then become trapped on their way through the filter. Such complexes can activate the complement system, which, in turn, tends to attract neutrophils to the site. Lysosomal enzymes escaping from these cells may then damage the glomerulus. There is also a less common form of glomerular damage that is due to the formation of antibody directed against some antigenic component of the GBM itself. This second form of glomerular damage represents an example of autoimmunity. Here again, the complement system may become activated, resulting in inflammatory destruction of the glomerular filtration barrier.

Proximal Convoluted Tubule

The *proximal convoluted tubule* is the longest segment of the nephron. On leaving the tubular pole of the renal corpuscle, it winds its way through the renal cortex and then enters a medullary ray. Here it descends into the medulla as the thick descending portion of the loop of Henle, which is not convoluted but has a similar general microscopic appearance. These two parts of the nephron are therefore often described as the *convoluted part* and the *straight part* of the proximal tubule. There are several microscopic features that allow proximal convoluted tubules to be distinguished from distal convoluted tubules, which are also present in the renal cortex. Because the proximal tubule is longer, more sections of it are present than of the distal tubule. The cells of the proximal tubule are also larger (Figs.

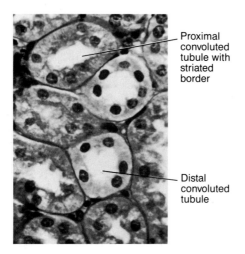

Proximal
convoluted
tubule with
striated
border

Distal
convoluted
tubule

Fig. 21-13. Photomicrograph comparing proximal and distal convoluted tubules of the kidney cortex (PAS and hematoxylin). For details, see text.

21-5 and 21-13) and more acidophilic. In cross section, they appear wide and triangular with a basal spherical nucleus. The lateral borders of these cells interdigitate very extensively, which makes them indistinct in light microscope (LM) sections. The luminal border of these cells is covered with many microvilli (Fig. 21-14) that, at the LM level, appear as a *striated (brush) border* (Figs. 21-5 and 21-13). This resorptive border is seen to advantage following PAS staining because of the abundant glycoproteins in its cell coat (Figs. 21-5 and 21-13).

The proximal convoluted tubule actively *resorbs* a number of constituents. These include water and many different ions, notably sodium, chloride, calcium, and phosphate. Glucose and amino acids, too, are resorbed by this part of the nephron. In addition, small quantities of plasma proteins of sufficiently low molecular weight to pass through the filtration barrier are retrieved through pinocytosis and are subsequently released into the interstitial spaces in the form of amino acids. The proximal convoluted tubule also *excretes* certain metabolites, dyes, and drugs, including penicillin. These substances are added to the filtrate as it passes along the lumen.

Between 60% and 70% of the water and the sodium passing along the nephron are resorbed by the proximal convoluted tubule. One of the pumps involved in the retrieval of sodium is Na^+-K^+-ATPase, the activity of which is highest along the lateral regions of the cell membrane of the lining cells. The sodium pumps move sodium ions out into the interstitial spaces around the sides and bases of the epithelial cells. Due to osmosis, the accumulated sodium ions, together with chloride ions that accompany them passively, withdraw water from the filtrate by way of the epithelial cells. The absorbed water does not accumulate in the interstitial spaces because it passes into the extensive capillary network in this region. Hence resorption

of sodium and water in this portion of the nephron are both attributable to the action of the sodium pumps.

Operation of the sodium pumps requires a considerable expenditure of energy. It is therefore not surprising that abundant large mitochondria are present in the bases of these cells (Figs. 21-14 and 21-15). To provide the expanse of cell membrane necessary for effective ion transport, there are also numerous basal infoldings of the cell membrane (Fig. 21-15). However, in both the proximal and the distal tubules, much of this apparent infolding is due to extensive interdigitation of the lateral borders of adjacent cells. Moreover, the epithelial cells possess numerous basal processes that also interdigitate very extensively.

Because the proximal convoluted tubule resorbs water at the same rate that it resorbs sodium and chloride, the filtrate reaching the loop of Henle has the same osmotic pressure as the filtrate that entered the proximal convoluted tubule. Hence the fluid in the proximal convoluted tubule remains isosmotic (*isotonic*) with blood plasma.

Loop of Henle

The *loop of Henle* consists of (1) an initial *thick descending portion* that represents a continuation of the proximal convoluted tubule and that is therefore also often referred to as the *pars recta* (straight part) of the proximal tubule; (2) a *thin descending portion*; (3) a *thin ascending portion*; and (4) a *thick ascending portion* (Fig. 21-4) that, because it represents the beginning of the distal tubule and resembles this tubule in microscopic structure, is similarly known as its *pars recta*. The ascending limb of the loop is situated alongside the descending limb, which extends for a variable distance into the medulla. As mentioned earlier in connection with Figure 21-2, nephrons with glomeruli that are situated near the corticomedullary border (*i.e., juxtamedullary nephrons*) have a longer loop of Henle that extends farther into the medulla than that of nephrons whose glomeruli are situated in the outer region of the cortex. In contrast, most of the loop of Henle of a superficial nephron can be situated within a medullary ray (Fig. 21-2). The thin segment of the loop of Henle has a narrow lumen with a thin wall that is composed of squamous epithelial cells (Fig. 21-16). However, apart from the absence of blood cells in its lumen, there are no reliable microscopic criteria that allow a distinction to be made between this part of the loop of Henle and the many straight thin-walled blood vessels that are also present in the medulla.

Distal Convoluted Tubule

Representing the most distal portion of the nephron is the *distal convoluted tubule*, which, like the proximal convoluted tubule, is situated in the renal cortex. Beginning at the *macula densa*, which, as noted, lies in close association with the vascular pole of the renal corpuscle of the same neph-

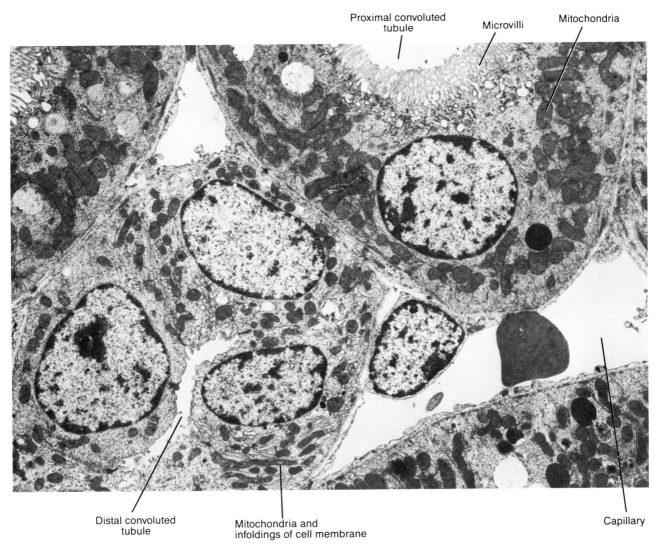

Proximal convoluted tubule   Microvilli   Mitochondria

Distal convoluted tubule   Mitochondria and infoldings of cell membrane   Capillary

Fig. 21-14. Electron micrograph (×10,000) comparing proximal and distal convoluted tubules of the kidney cortex. For details, see text. (Courtesy of E. Rau)

ron, the distal convoluted tubule pursues a tortuous course until it reaches the proximal end of the collecting tubule into which it drains. Because the distal convoluted tubule is shorter than the proximal convoluted tubule, sections of it are somewhat less numerous (Fig. 21-5). Furthermore, the cells that line this portion of the nephron are not as large or as acidophilic as those that line the proximal convoluted tubule. Hence this part of the nephron has a larger number of spherical nuclei in its wall, and its lumen appears wider (Figs. 21-5 and 21-13). The luminal border of its lining cells does not have a sufficient number of microvilli for it to exhibit a distinct striated border (Figs. 21-5, 21-13, and 21-14). Their lateral borders are slightly more distinct than those of the proximal tubule (Fig. 21-13). As in the

proximal tubule, deep basal infoldings and interdigitations of the cell membrane are associated with relatively numerous mitochondria that, in this case, can be markedly elongated (Fig. 21-14).

The mineralocorticoid *aldosterone*, the chief steroid hormone produced by cells of the zona glomerulosa of the adrenal cortex, promotes *sodium resorption* in this last part of the nephron. *Atrial natriuretic factor* (ANF), a peptide hormone liberated by atrial cardiac muscle cells in response to atrial distention, promotes renal *sodium* (and potassium) *excretion*. The various ways in which ANF participates in the regulation of blood pressure, including its effects on renin secretion and aldosterone secretion, were considered in Chapter 15 under Cardiac Muscle.

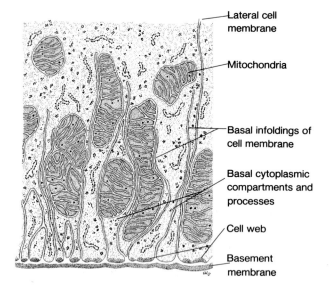

Lateral cell membrane

Mitochondria

Basal infoldings of cell membrane

Basal cytoplasmic compartments and processes

Cell web

Basement membrane

Fig. 21-15. Drawing illustrating the basal portion of the cells of a proximal convoluted tubule as seen in the EM. (Courtesy of E. Rau)

Collecting Tubule

The *collecting tubules* of the kidney, which represent the small tributaries of its branched collecting ducts, lie, for the most part, within its medulla and medullary rays. They are readily distinguishable from parts of nephrons and medullary blood vessels by the fact that they are made up of cuboidal or columnar cells, the lateral borders of which appear *distinct* because they are not markedly interdigitated (Fig. 21-16). The branching systems of collecting ducts that drain urine into the renal pelvis open onto the renal papillae. The main collecting ducts (*papillary ducts* or *ducts of Bellini*) are readily distinguishable by their wide lumen and their pale-staining simple columnar lining (Fig. 21-16). The essential function of collecting tubules and ducts is to *resorb water,* as will be explained in the following section.

A Countercurrent Mechanism Is Responsible for Concentrating Urine. Each of the various parts of the kidney tubule (and here we are referring to the collecting tubule as well as the nephron) has its own distinctive permeability characteristics for water, ions, and waste substances such as urea. In particular, the thick-walled portion of the ascending limb of the loop of Henle is (1) virtually impermeable to water and (2) very active in pumping out chloride ions, accompanied by sodium ions, from the filtrate within its lumen. As a result, these ions become transferred to the medullary interstitial spaces and the filtrate becomes increasingly hypotonic as it approaches the distal convoluted tubule. Chloride and sodium ions also pass passively from the thin-walled portion of the ascending limb of the loop of Henle into the medullary interstitial spaces. The combined result is that sodium, chloride, and urea build up in the medullary interstitial spaces as an *interstitial concentration gradient,* the concentration of which increases with proximity to the renal papillae.

The significance of this increasingly hypertonic environment is that the filtrate is required to traverse it before draining from a collecting duct. In the presence of *vasopressin,* which is the *antidiuretic hormone* (ADH) released from the posterior lobe of the pituitary, water is osmotically withdrawn from the filtrate while this is passing to the papillae by way of the collecting tubules. The thin wall of the capillarylike blood vessels of the medulla, which, because they extend straight down into the medulla, are known as *vasa recta,* is freely permeable to water and ions. These vessels participate passively in maintaining the medullary interstitial concentration gradient by (1) carrying away extra water withdrawn from the collecting tubules and (2) leaving undisturbed the concentration gradient of solutes and urea that exists in the medullary interstitial spaces. The effect of ADH is to *increase the permeability of the collecting tubules to water* so that the urine becomes hypertonic. In the absence of adequate levels of this hormone, the urine remains voluminous and hypotonic. The condition in which there is excessive production of dilute urine caused by an ADH deficiency is called *diabetes insipidus* (see Chap. 22).

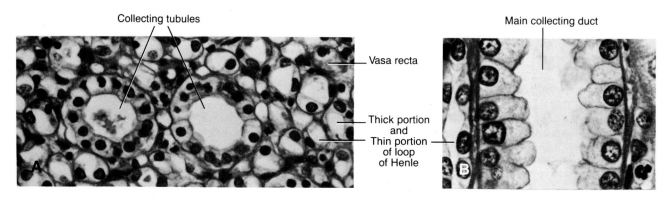

Collecting tubules

Main collecting duct

Vasa recta

Thick portion and Thin portion of loop of Henle

Fig. 21-16. Photomicrographs of collecting tubules in medulla of kidney. (*A*) Transverse section through two collecting tubules. (*B*) Longitudinal section through a main collecting duct.

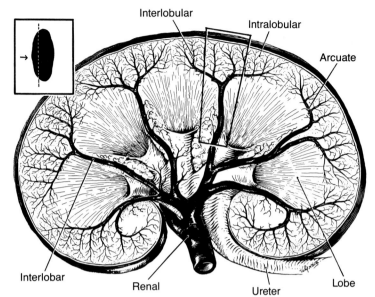

Fig. 21-17. Schematic diagram of the blood supply of the kidney, cut as shown in the inset to disclose its arterial supply.

More detailed accounts of the countercurrent mechanism can be found in textbooks of physiology.

Connective Tissue Component of the Kidney

The kidney has a thin but tough fibrous capsule and some loose connective tissue accompanies its large blood vessels, but unless diseased, the kidney is otherwise remarkably free of connective tissue. Its component nephrons and small collecting tubules are surrounded by only minimal amounts of loose connective tissue. In addition, each kidney tubule is surrounded by a well-developed basement membrane that is seen to advantage with PAS staining (Fig. 21-5).

The capsule of a healthy kidney is smooth and glistening. At autopsy, it can readily be stripped from the cortex, but in certain kinds of kidney disease, fibrous tissue forms in the cortical parenchyma and extends into the capsule, binding the capsule firmly to the kidney. In this case, the capsule cannot be easily stripped from the organ at autopsy, and this finding is noted by the pathologist as an indication that the kidney was diseased.

Blood Supply and Lymphatics of the Kidney

Each kidney is supplied by a large *renal artery* that arises from the abdominal aorta. Close to the hilum of the kidney, the renal artery divides into two large branches (Fig. 21-17). From these two branches, five end arteries originate. Called *segmental arteries,* each of these vessels supplies a particular region of the kidney. The segmental arteries give off branches that ascend toward the cortex as *interlobar arteries* (Figs. 21-17 and 21-18). Some of the interlobar arteries divide into main branches within the renal columns, but most branch at the corticomedullary border. Their

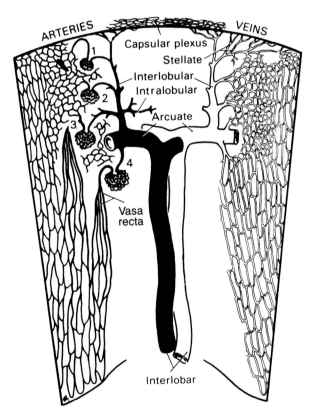

Fig. 21-18. Schematic diagram of the blood vessels within the boxed-in area in Figure 21-17, shown in more detail. (After Morison)

branches arch along this border and are consequently known as *arcuate* (L. *arcuatus,* arched) *arteries* (Figs. 21-17 and 21-18). There are no anastomoses between interlobar arteries or between their arcuate arteries. Hence the occlusion of an interlobar artery by a thrombus leads to death of a pyramid-shaped zone of kidney tissue that corresponds to the region supplied by its arcuate arteries. Such a region of dead tissue is described as a kidney *infarct.*

The arcuate arteries give off branches that ascend into the cortex (Figs. 21-17, 21-18, and 21-19). These vessels run between lobules, so they are called *interlobular arteries.* They mark the boundaries of lobules and therefore alternate with medullary rays, which constitute the central cores of lobules (Fig. 21-3). The interlobular arteries give off branches on all sides (Fig. 21-19). These branches enter the surrounding lobules; hence they are known as *intralobular arteries* (Figs. 21-17 and 21-18). They give rise to the afferent arterioles of glomeruli (Fig. 21-19). Terminal branches of the interlobular arteries also continue on and supply the capillary beds of the capsule (Fig. 21-18). Whereas extensive arterial trees supply all parts of the cortex, the medulla has no direct arterial supply (Fig. 21-17).

The efferent arterioles from the glomeruli in the outer region of the cortex empty their blood into the capillary beds that surround the proximal and distal convoluted tubules (Fig. 21-18). Deeper in the cortex, the equivalent vessels supply blood not only to cortical capillaries but also to long straight thin-walled vessels that descend into the medulla (Fig. 21-18). These vessels are often referred to as the *arterial vasa recta.* The efferent vessels from the deepest glomeruli, some of which lie below the level of the arcuate arteries, deliver blood chiefly to the arterial vasa recta (Fig. 21-18). Because the arterial vasa recta supplying the capillary beds of the medulla receive blood from the efferent vessels of glomeruli, the blood reaching the medulla has already passed through glomeruli.

The *renal capillaries* and the *venous vasa recta* into which these capillaries empty are provided with a fenestrated endothelium, the fenestrae of which are covered by diaphragms. Blood returns from the cortical and the medullary capillaries by way of the system of vessels depicted on the right side of Figure 21-18. In general, the venous vasa recta and the veins correspond to the arterial vasa recta and the arteries just described. At the kidney surface, small veins arise from the capillary beds in the capsule and from the superficial region of the cortex and converge on *interlobular veins.* These end branches radiate out from the ends of the interlobular veins in a starlike pattern, so they are known as *stellate veins* (Fig. 21-18). For further details of the renal vasculature, see Kriz et al.

Renal Lymphatics. The main lymphatic drainage system of the kidney begins with *intralobular lymphatics.* From these beginning branches, the renal lymphatics accompany the main blood vessels of the vascular tree. They lead through *interlobular* and *arcuate lymphatics* to *interlobar lymphatics* that extend down through the medulla. Lymph then drains by way of hilar collecting lymphatics to lymph nodes that border on the abdominal aorta. Anastomosing with this main lymphatic drainage system is a subsidiary capsular drainage system. The fine structure of a renal lymphatic capillary, the type of vessel in which the lymph first collects, is illustrated in Figure 16-28. In contrast to the renal cortex, the renal medulla appears to lack a rich network of lymphatic capillaries. For further information, see O'Morchoe.

Development and Growth of Nephrons

Human kidney development is finished by the time of birth, so any evidence that nephrons are still developing is considered a sign that the baby was born prematurely. However, glomerular differentiation continues for a few months after birth in the rat. The first-formed glomeruli, which are also the largest, lie near the arcuate vessels, whereas the last-formed glomeruli lie in the outer cortex immediately under the capsule; these outermost glomeruli are the smallest in the kidney.

Experimental excision of one of the kidneys during adult life leads to compensatory growth of the other kidney. This increase in size results because the nephrons become larger (*i.e.,* compensatory hypertrophy) and not more numerous. However, there is an increase in the total number of cells in each nephron. The kidneys also enlarge during pregnancy, at which time it is possible to find mitotic figures in some of their nephrons. Such enlargement of the kidneys is described as *physiological hypertrophy.*

URETERS

The *ureters* are essentially long straight excretory ducts with fairly thick muscular walls that are lined with *transitional epithelium* (Fig. 21-20). The dense connective tissue in the underlying *lamina propria* becomes looser at sites where it approaches the adjacent layer of smooth muscle. Except at the renal pelvis, prominent longitudinal folds of the mucous membrane give the lumen of the ureter a characteristic stellate appearance (Fig. 21-20). The combination of transitional epithelium (which can withstand being stretched without rupturing) and extensive longitudinal folds allows the ureter to become distended so that small kidney stones (*renal calculi,* from the L. for pebble) can be voided in the urine.

The upper two thirds of the ureter has two layers of *smooth muscle;* the inner layer is longitudinal and the outer layer is circular, which is the reverse arrangement of that seen in the intestine. Furthermore, the connective tissue in the two muscle layers merges with that of the lamina propria and the adventitia, making the layers of smooth muscle in the ureter less distinct than those of the intestine. In the lower third of the ureter, an additional outer longitudinal layer of smooth muscle is present. Fortunately for astronauts traveling in space, gravity is not required for the urine to drain into the bladder. Instead, peristaltic con-

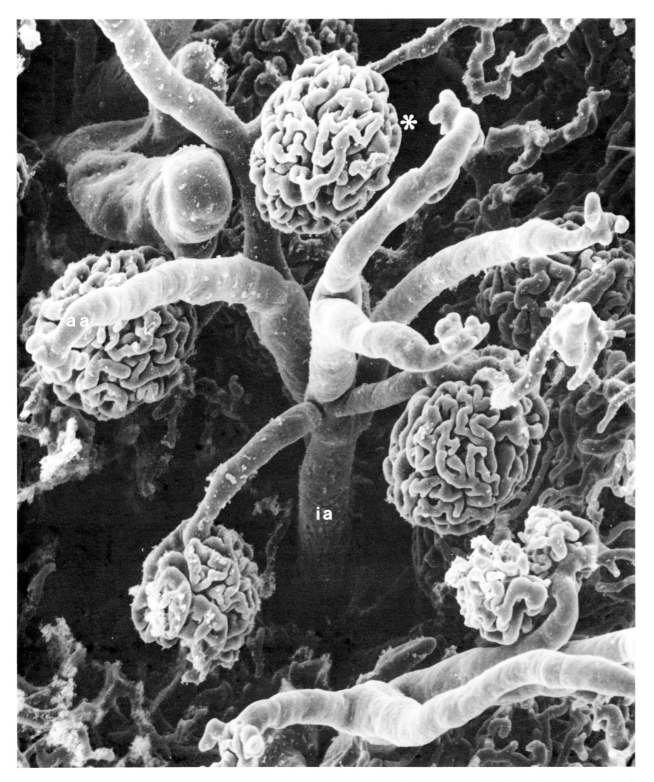

Fig. 21-19. Scanning electron micrograph (×450) of the arterial blood supply to renal glomeruli (vascular cast of rat kidney cortex). The afferent arterioles (*aa*) that supply the glomeruli (*asterisk*) receive blood from an interlobular artery (*ia*). (Courtesy of S. Erlandsen)

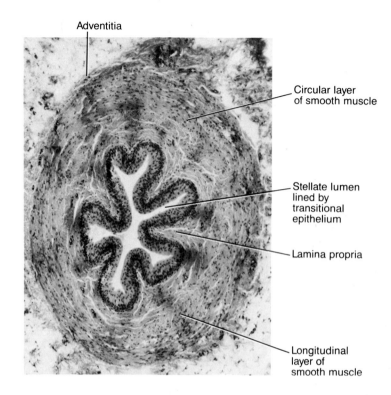

Adventitia

Circular layer
of smooth muscle

Stellate lumen
lined by
transitional
epithelium

Lamina propria

Longitudinal
layer of
smooth muscle

Fig. 21-20. Photomicrograph of a ureter (low power). See text for details.

tractions of the smooth muscle in the walls of the ureters gently squeeze the urine toward the bladder.

The outermost coat of the ureter, its *adventitia*, consists of fibroelastic connective tissue with associated blood vessels, lymphatics, and nerves.

The ureters follow an oblique course through the bladder wall. In conjunction with small folds of the bladder mucosa that serve as flap valves and guard the openings of the ureters into the bladder, this arrangement prevents urine from refluxing into the ureters when the bladder contracts.

URINARY BLADDER

The *urinary bladder* is a muscular-walled reservoir in which the urine is stored until it is voided. Because the bladder is a sac and not a tube, the three layers of smooth muscle that comprise its muscular coat are not very distinct. In many respects, however, its wall structure resembles that of the ureters.

The bladder is lined with *transitional epithelium* (Fig. 21-21). Stretching of the bladder wall as a result of distension with urine is accommodated by flattening of its numerous mucosal folds and expansion of its thick transitional epithelium until this eventually resembles a stratified squamous epithelium. The EM has disclosed a further feature of the surface cells in this epithelium that appears to help them withstand being stretched and may also help to restrict fluid movement across their luminal border. The luminal part of their cell membrane, which in the nondistended state shows uneven contours and recesses (Fig.

21-22), is reinforced by surface structures known as *plaques* (Figs. 21-22 and 21-23). These are areas where the cell membrane has a special thickening on its external (luminal) surface (Staehelin et al). Plaques occupy approximately 75% of the surface area of this region of the cell membrane and are characterized by the presence of closely packed hexagonal subunits that are arranged along the membrane surface. The narrow regions of cell membrane between the plaques do not have an unusual appearance. Associated with the plaques, there are cytoplasmic filaments that are believed to bear and distribute some of the strain when the epithelium is stretched out flat (Fig. 21-23A). When the bladder is not distended, the hingelike regions of cell membrane between the more rigid plaques allow the luminal part of the cell membrane to become infolded as illustrated in Figures 21-22 and 21-23B. In addition, *desmosomes* help to maintain strong cohesion between these epithelial cells, and *tight junctions* between the lateral borders of the superficial cells help to reduce the leakage that tends to occur across the epithelium as a result of hydrostatic and osmotic pressure differences.

The fibroelastic *lamina propria* beneath the bladder epithelium also constitutes the cores of the mucosal folds. Its deepest layer is somewhat looser in texture and contains a higher proportion of elastic fibers; this deep layer is sometimes referred to as the *submucosal layer* of the bladder. The *muscular coat* of the bladder is made up of three layers (Fig. 21-21) that cannot readily be distinguished from one another. Their respective thicknesses vary in different parts of the bladder. In general, the middle circular coat is the most prominent (Fig. 21-21). The *adventitia* of the bladder

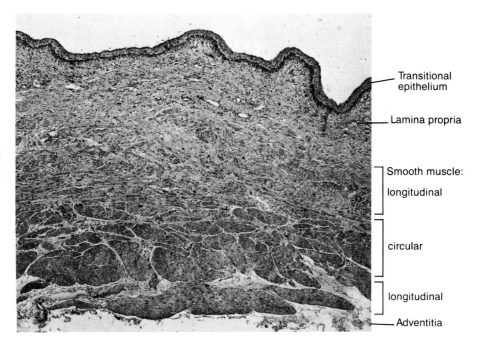

Fig. 21-21. Photomicrograph of urinary bladder of monkey (low power). See text for details. (Courtesy of C. P. Leblond)

Labels on figure:
- Transitional epithelium
- Lamina propria
- Smooth muscle: longitudinal
- circular
- longitudinal
- Adventitia

is fibroelastic in nature. Over the superior surface of the bladder, this external connective tissue layer is covered with peritoneum, forming a *serosa*. Over the remainder of the organ, it merges with the adjacent connective tissue.

URETHRA

The *urethra* is the unpaired tubular passageway that conveys the urine from the bladder to the exterior of the body. In males, it also belongs to the reproductive system, so rather than dealing with it here, we shall describe it in Chapter 24. Because this is not true in females, we shall describe the female urethra here.

The female *urethra* is a fairly straight muscular-walled tube, the lumen of which appears crescent-shaped in transverse section. Over most of its course, the lining *epithelium* is stratified (or pseudostratified) columnar epithelium, with small associated mucus-secreting mucosal glands. However, the proximal end of the urethra is lined with transitional epithelium, and at the distal end of the urethra, the lining changes to stratified squamous nonkeratinizing epithelium where it approaches the external urethral orifice. The *lamina propria* of the urethra is thick and fibroelastic and contains a plexus of thin-walled veins. Adjacent to this layer is a rather indistinct *muscular coat* that is made up of an inner longitudinal layer and an outer circular layer of smooth muscle. Encircling the urethra at the external urethral orifice is the *sphincter urethrae*, a voluntary sphincter consisting of skeletal muscle fibers.

INNERVATION OF THE URINARY SYSTEM

Nerve fibers reach the kidney by way of the renal plexus. This is a network of nerve fibers that extends along the renal artery from the aorta to the kidney. The bodies of ganglion cells may also be present in the renal plexus; if so, they are regarded as outlying cells of diffuse celiac and aortic ganglia. Most of the fibers in the renal plexus belong to the *sympathetic* division of the autonomic system and are derived from the cells of the celiac and aortic ganglia. *Parasympathetic* fibers are present in the renal plexus in smaller numbers. These are derived from the vagus nerve, whose fibers course through the celiac plexus without interruption and reach the renal plexus.

The nerve fibers from the renal plexus, as noted, follow the arteries into the substance of the kidney. They form extensive perivascular networks and supply the epithelium of convoluted tubules, the transitional epithelium of the renal pelvis, and the walls of arteries and veins.

Kidneys that have been transplanted or that have been experimentally denervated can still function, so kidney function is not entirely dependent on nervous control. However, nervous mechanisms do regulate kidney function to a certain extent. It seems likely much of this control occurs through the sympathetic innervation of blood vessels. Some of the impulses conveyed by the nerve fibers in the renal plexus are afferent, because transection of these fibers abolishes pain of renal origin.

The urinary bladder is supplied by both sympathetic and parasympathetic fibers, the latter being derived from the sacral outflow.

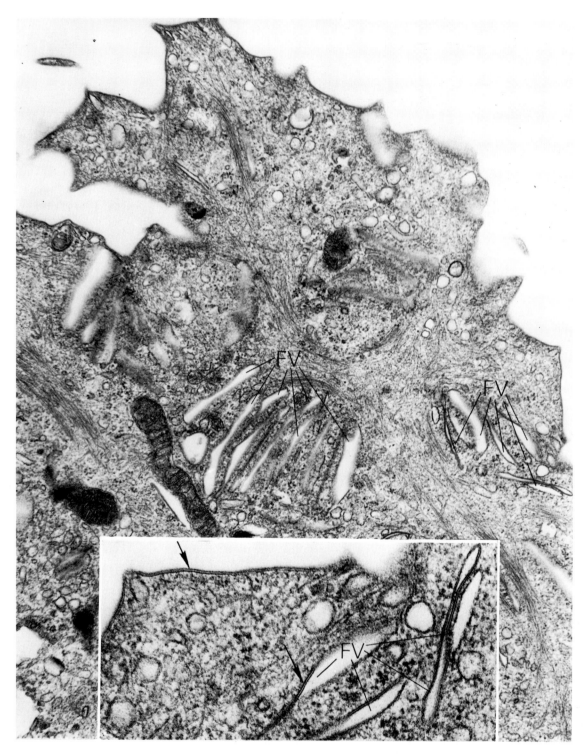

Fig. 21-22. Electron micrograph (×27,000) of part of the luminal border of a superficial epithelial cell of the urinary bladder, showing its appearance in the nondistended state. Rigid plaques on the cell membrane, with hinge regions between them, give the luminal surface a spiky appearance and enable this part of the cell membrane to fold up into the cell as depicted in Figure 21-23. Bundles of filaments and fusiform vesicles (*FV*), which represent temporary infoldings of the cell membrane, are readily discernible in the cytoplasm. (*Inset*) Electron micrograph of part of the luminal border of such a cell, showing the cell membrane and its temporary infoldings under higher magnification (×60,000). Arrows indicate rigid plaques. (Ross MH, Reith EJ: Histology. A Text and Atlas. New York, Harper & Row/JB Lippincott, 1985)

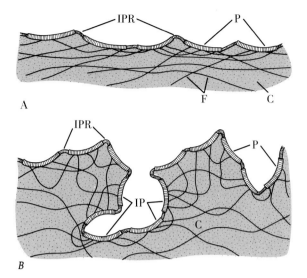

A

B

Fig. 21-23. Schematic representation of part of the luminal border of a superficial epithelial cell of the urinary bladder, showing its appearance (*A*) in the distended state and (*B*) in the nondistended state. In the distended state, the plaques (*P*) and the interplaque regions (*IPR*) between them are pulled taut, the strain being borne by cytoplasmic filaments (*F*) associated with the cytoplasmic aspect of the plaques. In the nondistended state, plaques fold into the cytoplasm (*C*) as invaginated plaques (*IP*) and give the luminal border the characteristic spiky outline depicted in *B*. (Staehelin LA, Chlapowski FJ, Bonneville MA: J Cell Biol 53:73, 1972)

SELECTED REFERENCES

General

BRENNER BM, RECTOR FC (eds): The Kidney, Vol 1. Philadelphia, WB Saunders, 1976

CHAPMAN WH, BULGER RE, CUTLER RE, STRIKER GE: The Urinary System—an Integrated Approach. Philadephia, WB Saunders, 1973

DALTON AJ, HAGUENAU F (eds): Ultrastructure of the Kidney. New York, Academic Press, 1967

GOLDEN A, MAHER JF: The Kidney, 2nd ed. Baltimore, Williams & Wilkins, 1977

GOSLING JA, DIXON JS, HUMPHERSON JR: Functional Anatomy of the Urinary Tract: An Integrated Text and Color Atlas. London, Gower Medical Publishing, 1983

MOFFAT DB: The Mammalian Kidney. London, Cambridge University Press, 1975

ROUILLER C, MULLER AF (eds): The Kidney: Morphology, Biochemistry, Physiology. Vols 1 and 2, New York. Academic Press, 1969

Juxtaglomerular Complex and Vascular Pole of Renal Corpuscle

BARAJAS L: Anatomy of the juxtaglomerular apparatus. Am J Physiol 237:F333, 1979

BARAJAS L: The ultrastructure of the juxtaglomerular apparatus as disclosed by three-dimensional reconstructions from serial sections. The anatomical relationship between the tubular and vascular components. J Ultrastruct Res 33:116, 1970

CHRISTENSEN JA, MEYER DS, BOHLE A: The structure of the human juxtaglomerular apparatus. Arch Pathol Anat Histol 367:83, 1975

EVAN AP, DAIL WG: Efferent arterioles in the cortex of the rat kidney. Am J Anat 187:135, 1977

GORGAS K: Struktur und innervation des juxtaglomerulären apparates der ratte. Advances in Anatomy, Embryology, and Cell Biology, Vol 54, Fasc 2. Berlin, Springer-Verlag, 1978

HARTROFT PM: The juxtaglomerular complex as an endocrine gland. In Bloodworth JB (ed): Endocrine Pathology, p 641. Baltimore, Williams & Wilkins, 1968

KOMADINOVIĆ D, KRSTIĆ R, BUCHER O: Ultrastructural and morphometric aspects of the juxtaglomerular apparatus in the monkey kidney. Cell Tissue Res 192:503, 1978

MCMANUS JFA: Further observations on the glomerular root of the vertebrate kidney. Quart J Micr Sci 88:39, 1947

PITCOCK JA, HARTROFT PM, NEWMARK LN: Increased renal pressor activity (renin) in sodium deficient rats and correlation with juxtaglomerular cell granulation. Proc Soc Exp Biol Med 100:868, 1959

SCHILLER A, TAUGNER R: Are there specialized junctions in the pars maculata of the distal tubule? Cell Tissue Res 200:337, 1979

TOBIAN L, JANECEK J, TOMBOULIAN A: Correlation between granulation of juxtaglomerular cells and extractable renin in rats with experimental hypertension. Proc Soc Exp Biol Med 100:94, 1959

Glomerular Filtration Barrier and Mesangium

BRENNER BM, BAYLIS C, DEEN WM: Transport of molecules across renal glomerular capillaries. Physiol Rev 56:502, 1976

FARQUHAR MG: The glomerular basement membrane: A selective macromolecular filter. In Hay ED (ed): Cell Biology of Extracellular Matrix, p 335. New York, Plenum, 1981

FARQUHAR MG, PALADE GE: Functional evidence for the existence of a third cell type in the renal glomerulus. Phagocytosis of filtration residues by a distinctive third cell. J Cell Biol 13:55, 1962

FARQUHAR MG, PALADE GE: Glomerular permeability. II. Ferritin transfer across the glomerular capillary wall in nephrotic rats. J Exp Med 114:699, 1961

FARQUHAR MG, WISSIG SL, PALADE GE: Glomerular permeability. I. Ferritin transfer across the normal glomerular capillary wall. J Exp Med 113:47, 1961

FUJITA T, TOKUNAGA J, EDANAGA M: Scanning electron microscopy of the glomerular filtration membrane in the rat kidney. Cell Tissue Res 166:299, 1976

GRAHAM RC, KARNOVSKY MJ: Glomerular permeability: Ultrastructural cytochemical studies using peroxidases as protein tracers. J Exp Med 124:1123, 1966

HALL BV: Further studies of the normal structure of the renal glomerulus. Proc Sixth Ann Conf Nephrotic Syndrome, p 1. New york, National Nephrosis Foundation, 1964

KANWAR YS, LINKER A, FARQUHAR MG: Increased permeability of the glomerular basement membrane to ferritin after removal of glycosaminoglycans (heparan sulfate) by enzyme digestion. J Cell Biol 86:688, 1980

KARNOVSKY MJ, RYAN GB: Substructure of the glomerular slit diaphragm in freeze-fractured normal rat kidney. J Cell Biol 65:233, 1975

LATTA H, JOHNSTON WH, STANLEY TM: Sialoglycoproteins and filtration barriers in the glomerular capillary wall. J Ultrastruct Res 51: 354, 1975

LAURIE GW, LEBLOND CP, INOUÉ S ET AL: Fine structure of the glomerular basement membrane and immunolocalization of five basement membrane components to the lamina densa (basal lamina) and its extensions in both glomeruli and tubules of the rat kidney. Am J Anat 169:463, 1984

MENEFEE MG, MUELLER CB: Some morphological considerations of transport in the glomerulus. In Dalton AJ, Haguenau F (eds): Ultrastructure of the Kidney, p 73. New York, Academic Press, 1967

MICHIELSEN P, CREEMERS J: The structure and function of the glomerular mesangium. In Dalton AJ, Haguenau F (eds): Ultrastructure of the Kidney, p 57. New York, Academic Press, 1967

RYAN GB, HEIN SJ, KARNOVSKY MJ: Glomerular permeability to proteins. Lab Invest 34:415, 1976

SUZUKI Y, CHURG J, GRISHMAN E ET AL: The mesangium of the renal glomerulus. Electron microscope studies of pathologic alterations. Am J Pathol 43:555, 1963

TRUMP BF, BENDITT EP: Electron microscopic studies of human renal disease. Observations on normal visceral glomerular epithelium and its modifications in disease. Lab Invest 11:753, 1962

VENKATACHALAM MA, KARNOVSKY MJ, FAHIMI HD, COTRAN RS: An ultrastructural study of glomerular permeability using catalase and peroxidase as tracer proteins. J Exp Med 132:1153, 1970

WALKER F: The origin, turnover, and removal of glomerular basement membrane. J Pathol 110:233, 1973

Kidney Tubular Development, Growth, Structure, and Functions

ANDREWS PM, PORTER KR: A scanning electron microscopic study of the nephron. Am J Anat 140:81, 1974

CLARK SL Jr: Cellular differentiation in the kidneys of newborn mice studied with the electron microscope. J Biophys Biochem Cytol 3:349, 1957

KURTZ SM: The electron microscopy of the developing human renal glomerulus. Exp Cell Res 14:355, 1958

LATTA H, MAUNSBACH AB, OSVALDO L: The fine structure of renal tubules in cortex and medulla. In Dalton AJ, Haguenau F (eds): Ultrastructure of the Kidney, p 2. New York, Academic Press, 1967

LEESON TS: Electron microscopy of the developing kidney: An investigation into the fine structure of the mesonephros and metanephros of the rabbit. J Anat 94:100, 1960

MACDONALD MS, EMERY JL: The late intrauterine and postnatal development of human renal glomeruli. J Anat 93:331, 1959

RHODIN J: Anatomy of the kidney tubules. Int Rev Cytol 7:485, 1958

RUSKA H, MOORE DH, WEINSTOCK J: The base of the proximal convoluted tubule cells of rat kidney. J Biophys Biochem Cytol 3: 249, 1957

SULKIN NN: Cytologic study of the remaining kidney following unilateral nephrectomy in the rat. Anat Rec 105:95, 1949

TISHER CG: Functional anatomy of the kidney. Hosp Prac, p 53, May, 1978

TRUMP BF, TISHER CC, SALADINO AJ: The nephron in health and dis-

ease. In Bittar EE (ed): The Biological Basis of Medicine, Vol 6, p 387. London, Academic Press, 1969

WIRZ H: Introduction—Tubular transport mechanism with special reference to the hairpin countercurrent. In Duyff JW et al (eds): XXII International Congress of Physiological Sciences, Symposium VII. Vol 1, p 359. New York, Excerpta Medica Foundation, 1962

Connective Tissue, Blood Supply, Lymphatics, and Innervation of the Kidney

BARINGER JR: The dynamic anatomy of the microcirculation in the amphibian and mammalian kidney. Anat Rec 130:266, 1958

BIALESTOCK D: The extra-glomerular arterial circulation of the renal tubules. Anat Rec 129:53, 1957

BRENNER BM, BEEUWKES R: The renal circulations. Hosp Prac, p 35, July, 1978

GRAVES FT: The anatomy of the intrarenal arteries in health and disease. Br J Surg 43:605, 1956

GRAVES FT: The anatomy of the intrarenal arteries and its application to segmental resection of the kidney. Br J Surg 42:132, 1954

GRUBER CM: The autonomic innervation of the genitourinary system. Physiol Rev 13:497, 1933

KRIZ W, BARRETT JM, PETER S: The renal vasculature: Anatomical–functional aspects. In Thurau K (ed): International Review of Physiology, Vol 11. Kidney and Urinary Tract Physiology II, p 1. Baltimore, University Park Press, 1976

LEESON TS: An electron microscopic study of the postnatal development of the hamster kidney, with particular reference to intertubular tissue. Lab Invest 10:466, 1961

MORE RH, DUFF GL: The renal arterial vasculature in man. Am J Pathol 27:95, 1950

MORISON DM: A study of the renal circulation, with special reference to its finer distribution. Am J Anat 37:53, 1926

O'MORCHOE CCC: Lymphatic drainage of the kidney. In Johnston MG (ed): Experimental Biology of the Lymphatic Circulation, p 261. Amsterdam, Elsevier Biomedical Press, 1985

PEASE DC: Electron microscopy of the vascular bed of the kidney cortex. Anat Rec 121:701, 1955

PEIRCE EC: Renal lymphatics. Anat Rec 90:315, 1944

SYKES D: The correlation between renal vascularization and lobulation of the kidney. Br J Urol 36:549, 1964

SYKES D: Some aspects of the blood supply of the human kidney. Symp Zool Soc London 11:49, 1964

TRUETA J, BARCLAY AE, DANIEL P ET AL: Studies of the Renal Circulation. Oxford, Blackwell Scientific Publications, 1947

Urinary Bladder

HICKS RM, KETTERER B: Isolation of the plasma membrane of the luminal surface of rat bladder epithelium, and the occurrence of a hexagonal lattice of subunits both in negatively stained whole mounts and in sectional membranes. J Cell Biol 45:542, 1970

STAEHELIN A, CHLAPOWSKI FJ, BONNEVILLE MA: Lumenal plasma membrane of the urinary bladder. I. Three-dimensional reconstruction from freeze-etch images. J Cell Biol 53:73, 1972

22

The Endocrine System

Whereas exocrine glands characteristically release their secretions onto body surfaces, *endocrine glands* deliver *hormones* into the bloodstream. In addition, certain hormones are secreted by cells that are not conventionally regarded as belonging to the endocrine system. Such hormones include erythropoietin, thymic hormones, and the gastrointestinal peptides, all of which have been discussed in preceding chapters. Also, the sex glands (the ovaries and testes) produce reproductive hormones that will be considered in relation to their reproductive functions in Chapters 23 and 24.

Some of the earliest knowledge about classical endocrinology was gained from observations made at autopsy that linked previously recognized clinical conditions to gross or microscopic changes in what we now know to be endocrine glands. As matters turned out, however, this led to a rather narrow view of what constitutes the *endocrine system*, with the result that a group of only six *endocrine organs* (excluding the gonads, which were considered primarily reproductive in function) became recognized as components of the *endocrine system*. These organs are the *pituitary* (*hypophysis*), *thyroid*, *parathyroids*, *adrenals*, *pancreatic islets* (*islets of Langerhans*), and *pineal*. The gonads (*i.e.*, the *ovaries* and *testes*) really belong to the endocrine system as well, but, for the most part, they will be dealt with separately in connection with the female and male reproductive systems.

Hormonal Communication Can Be Thought of as a Humoral Extension of Neural Transmission. In recent years it has become evident that there are some close similarities between (1) the short-range chemical *synaptic* transmission that characterizes the nervous system and (2) the long-range *humoral* (hormonal) or shorter range *paracrine* (lateral) chemical signaling that characterizes endocrine communication between cells. The distinction formerly drawn between these two forms of intercellular communication no longer seems useful because, in some cases, the same messenger molecules are known to be capable of both short-range and long-range signaling. In other words, they are equally effective as neurotransmitters or hormones. Some examples of this dual role were mentioned in connection with enteroendocrine cells in Chapter 18 (in the section on the Stomach). Hence although it expedites learning about hormones to treat the endocrine organs as a separate system, it should always be borne in mind that their hormones act in conjunction with the central, peripheral, and autonomic divisions of the nervous system and also with the hormones that are produced elsewhere in the body. Hence it is better to think of endocrine functions as representing the endocrine activities of an integrated *neuroendocrine system.*

Some Hormone Receptors Are Intracellular Whereas Others Are Present on the Cell Surface. The many different hormones are all either (1) cholesterol derivatives (steroids) or (2) amino acid derivatives (proteins, glycoproteins, peptides, or modified amino acids, *e.g.,* catecholamines). Because the *steroid hormones* and *thyroid hormone* are lipid soluble, they are able to diffuse through the cell membrane. They then bind to specific *intracellular receptor proteins* that are present in the cytoplasm of their target cells, which is the term employed for the cells on which they act. In contrast, all the *amino acid–derived hormones* except thyroid hormone are hydrophilic, and instead of passing through the cell membrane, they bind to specific *hormone receptors* in the *cell membrane* of their target cells. The great majority of hormones interact with their target cells in this manner. Individual cells can be target cells for more than one hormone, and individual hormones can have more than one kind of target cell.

When a steroid hormone enters the cell and complexes with its intracellular receptor protein, the hormone–receptor complex undergoes an activation process and then becomes bound to chromatin, where it brings about a change in the rate at which specific genes are being transcribed. Thyroid hormone is believed to act in a similar way, but the details of how this is achieved are not as clearly established.

All the other hormones, as noted, interact with specific receptors in the cell membrane. In most cases, formation of the hormone–receptor complex at the cell surface elicits the intracellular mobilization of a *second messenger,* the best characterized example of which is *cyclic adenosine monophosphate* (cAMP). This second messenger then mediates the effects of the hormone. In a few cases, the second messenger is believed to consist of intracellular *calcium ions* that appear to act in conjunction with derivatives of cell membrane lipids. In certain cases (*e.g.,* insulin), the cell internalizes the hormone itself in the form of its hormone–receptor complex. For further introductory comment on hormones and their second messengers, see Snyder and also Berridge.

The remainder of this chapter deals with the various endocrine organs. We shall begin with the pituitary and the closely related parts of the hypothalamus because some of the hormones produced and released by these two important structures influence the secretory activities of certain other endocrine glands.

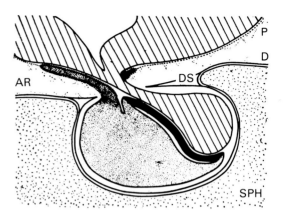

Fig. 22-1. Schematic diagram of the pituitary gland, in sagittal section, showing the relation of the pars tuberalis to the meninges. (*Crosshatched,* hypothalamus floor and pars nervosa; *fine stipple,* pars anterior; *coarse stipple,* pars tuberalis; *solid black,* pars intermedia; *SPH,* sphenoid bone; *P,* pia mater; *D,* dura mater; *DS,* diaphragma sellae; *AR,* arachnoid spaces) (Atwell WJ: Am J Anat 37: 159, 1926)

PITUITARY (HYPOPHYSIS)

The pituitary gland is roughly ovoid, measuring approximately 1.5 cm in the transverse plane and 1 cm in the sagittal plane but becoming a little larger during pregnancy. It is attached by its *infundibular stalk* to the median eminence of the tuber cinereum, which is the part of the hypothalamus that constitutes the floor of the third ventricle of the brain. The pituitary is protected by a bony prominence on the upper surface of the sphenoid bone (Fig. 22-1). Here it lies in a depression known as the *sella turcica* that has a high back and a high front like a Turkish saddle. The dura mater dips down into this depression, enveloping the pituitary in a fibrous *capsule* and covering it superiorly with a fibrous shelf called the *diaphragma sellae* (Fig. 22-1).

The pituitary is made up of four parts. (1) The main part, which lies anterior to a row of follicles, is termed its *pars anterior* (Fig. 22-1, *fine stipple*) or *pars distalis.* (2) A projection from this, the *pars tuberalis* (Fig. 22-1, *coarse stipple*), extends up along the anterior and lateral aspects of the infundibular stalk. (3) A narrow band of poorly developed glandular tissue along the posterior border of the row of follicles comprises the *pars intermedia* (Fig. 22-1, *solid black*). (4) The part that is posterior to the pars intermedia is called the *pars posterior* or *pars nervosa* (Fig. 22-1, *crosshatched*). The pars nervosa fits into a concavity on the posterior aspect of the pars anterior, from which it is separated by the pars intermedia.

The pars nervosa develops as a downgrowth from the base of the brain (Fig. 22-2). The other three parts of the gland are epithelial in origin and develop as an upgrowth of the oral ectoderm from the roof of the oral cavity (Fig. 22-2). The part of the pituitary that is derived from the

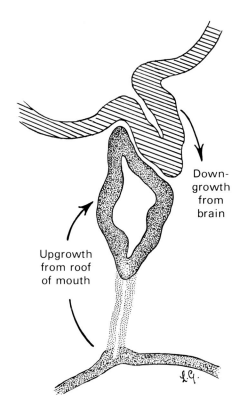

Fig. 22-2. Schematic diagram illustrating the development of the pituitary gland from its two main sources.

brain is sometimes referred to as the *neurohypophysis*, and the parts that develop from oral ectoderm are often collectively referred to as the *adenohypophysis*.

In the human pituitary, the pars intermedia is rudimentary and ill-defined; however, its general position is indicated by the presence of nearby vestigial colloid-filled follicles (Fig. 22-3), the lumina of which represent remnants of a deep cleft that forms during development. Soon after the pars intermedia develops, its cells invade the pars anterior and become diffusely distributed in it, with the result that the anterior boundary of the pars intermedia becomes rather difficult to discern (Fig. 22-3).

Anterior Lobe and Its Relation to the Hypothalamus

Now more commonly referred to as the *anterior pituitary*, the *pars anterior* (*pars distalis*) is composed of thick branching cords of secretory epithelial cells with supporting reticular fibers and wide fenestrated capillaries lying between these cords (Fig. 22-4). Many of these cells stain intensely because of their abundant content of hormone-containing secretory granules and have therefore become known as *chromophils*. Other cells contain less stored hormone, appear smaller, and show very little or no staining and are

therefore known as *chromophobes* (Fig. 22-4). When seen in the electron microscope (EM), these cells lack distinguishing features, so they are often described as *null cells* (see Fig. 22-6). They seem to be the same cells as chromophils, but in a quiescent or more or less degranulated phase of secretion. Chromophils are conventionally subdivided into pituitary *acidophils* and *basophils* according to the affinity with which their specific granules take up acid or basic stains (Fig. 22-4). However, in hematoxylin and eosin (H & E) sections, the difference between acidophils and basophils is not very noticeable and special staining methods are necessary to make the difference obvious. An additional staining characteristic of two of the three kinds of basophils (Table 22-1) is that they are PAS-positive because the hormones they produce (in one case TSH and in the other case FSH and LH; see Table 22-1) are glycoproteins. These three hormones, together with ACTH, are called *trophic hormones* (Gr. *trophein,* to nourish) because they promote the growth and secretory activity of other endocrine glands. (The less appropriate spelling *tropic* is sometimes substituted for *trophic;* hence *corticotrope, somatotrope,* etc.) Most of the discussion on the two gonadotrophins FSH and LH, produced in both females and males, will be found in Chapters 23 and 24.

In the EM, the various kinds of chromophils exhibit features that are typical of cells that actively produce secretory proteins, polypeptides, or glycoproteins, and to a certain extent the various cell types can be discerned on the basis of the size and uniformity of staining of their stored secretory granules. However, to identify them with certainty, it is necessary to use immunofluorescent or immunocytochemical staining at the light microscope (LM) level or, more reliably, immunocytochemical staining at the EM level. It is now established that the anterior pituitary contains two distinct types of acidophils and at least three distinct types of basophils. The names of these five cell types and the hormones that they produce are given in Table 22-1.

Each of these various kinds of chromophils has its own characteristic distribution. Typically, about half the chromophils seen in the lateral wings of a horizontal section of the anterior lobe are somatotrophs. The anteromedial region between these wings is rich in corticotrophs and, to a certain extent, corticotrophs invade the posterior lobe as well. Thyrotrophs are fairly abundant toward the anteromedial border, whereas mammotrophs and gonadotrophs are more random in their distribution.

The Anterior Pituitary Is Connected to the Hypothalamus by a Neuroendocrine Link. An important vascular and hormonal link exists between (1) the neural tissue of the infundibular stalk and neighboring part of the hypothalamus (the median eminence) and (2) the glandular epithelial tissue of the anterior pituitary. This neural tissue and the glandular epithelial tissue are both provided with plexuses of fenestrated capillaries, and the two plexuses

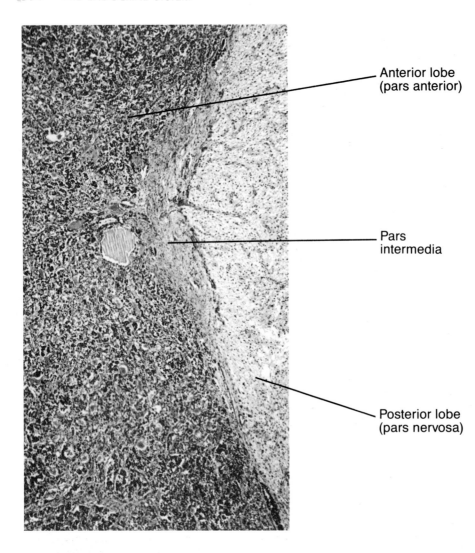

Anterior lobe
(pars anterior)

Pars
intermedia

Posterior lobe
(pars nervosa)

Fig. 22-3. Photomicrograph of a transverse section through the pituitary, showing its three parts (low-power view of horizontal section). The anterior boundary of the pars intermedia is marked by the presence of colloid-filled follicles, one of which is seen at middle left.

are interconnected by portal vessels that extend down the infundibular stalk (Fig. 22-5, shown at *left*). These portal vessels convey venous blood from the capillary plexuses of the hypothalamus and infundibular stalk (which lie outside the blood–brain barrier) to the capillary plexuses in the epithelial glandular tissue, a vascular arrangement referred to as the *hypophysioportal circulation*. The significance of this special vascular connection is that it enables regulatory hormones that are produced by certain hypothalamic neurons to reach their target secretory epithelial cells in the anterior pituitary, as we shall now explain.

The hypothalamus has an essential neuroendocrine-integrating role. It contains fairly diffuse groups of neurosecretory cells (*i.e.*, secretory neurons) that secrete peptide hormones through their axons into the circulation. All but two of these hormones are directed to the anterior pituitary by the hypophysioportal circulation. Here they regulate the secretory activities of the various types of hormone-

secreting cells in this part of the pituitary. Two other peptide hormones, vasopressin and oxytocin (which will be described subsequently), enter blood capillaries in the posterior lobe (Fig. 22-5, shown at *right*).

Hypothalamic Hormone-Releasing and Hormone-Inhibiting Hormones Regulate Anterior Pituitary Secretion. The so-called *hypophysiotrophic hormones* and *factors* that regulate the output of the anterior pituitary hormones are listed in Table 22-2. From this table it can be seen that three cases of dual regulation by releasing and inhibiting hormones (or factors) are now recognized. In the other three cases, only the releasing hormone has been identified so far.

The cell bodies of the so-called *tuberohypophyseal neurons* that produce these regulating hormones are situated in a number of different and, in some cases, overlapping locations in the hypothalamus. The term *hypophysiotrophic area* is used to denote the diffuse area over which their cell

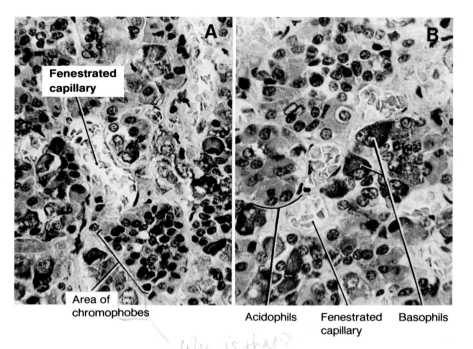

Fig. 22-4. Photomicrographs of the anterior lobe of the pituitary gland. (*A*) An area of chromophobes, with their nuclei close together. A fenestrated capillary and some chromophils can be seen also. (*B*) Acidophils, basophils and fenestrated capillaries.

bodies are distributed. Their axons extend down to the infundibular region and median eminence as the *tuberoinfundibular tract.* Many of these axons terminate in close association with the fenestrated capillary plexuses of the median eminence and infundibular stalk (as shown at *left* in Fig. 22-5).

Some of the other tuberohypophyseal axon terminals are believed to liberate regulating hormones into the cerebrospinal fluid (CSF) contained in the third ventricle. Stretching through the floor of this ventricle, there are modified ependymal cells known as *tanycytes* (Gr. *tanyō*, to stretch). These distinctive glial cells possess active trans-

port mechanisms for a number of different hormones and are believed to play a key role in transferring hormones from the CSF in the third ventricle to the blood in the hypophysioportal circulation. Moreover, they possess long basal processes and therefore span the full thickness of the wall of the median eminence. As a consequence, their luminal border is bathed by the CSF in the third ventricle and their basal processes extend to the outer limit (pia mater) of the median eminence. In many instances, these processes terminate in close association with the fenestrated capillaries of the median eminence and infundibular stalk. Such cells possess the requisite transport mechanisms and

Table 22-1   The Cell Types and Hormones of the Anterior Pituitary

Cell Class	Cell Type	Hormones Produced
Acidophil	Somatotroph	Growth hormone (GH) or somatotrophin (STH) (protein)
Acidophil	Mammotroph	Prolactin (PRL) or lactogenic hormone (LTH) (protein)
Basophil	Thyrotroph	Thyroid-stimulating hormone or thyrotrophin (TSH) (glycoprotein)
Basophil	Gonadotroph	Follicle-stimulating hormone (FSH) and luteinizing hormone (LH) (glycoproteins)
Basophil	Corticotroph	Adrenocorticotrophic hormone or corticotrophin (ACTH) (polypeptide) and melanocyte-stimulating hormone (MSH) (peptide)

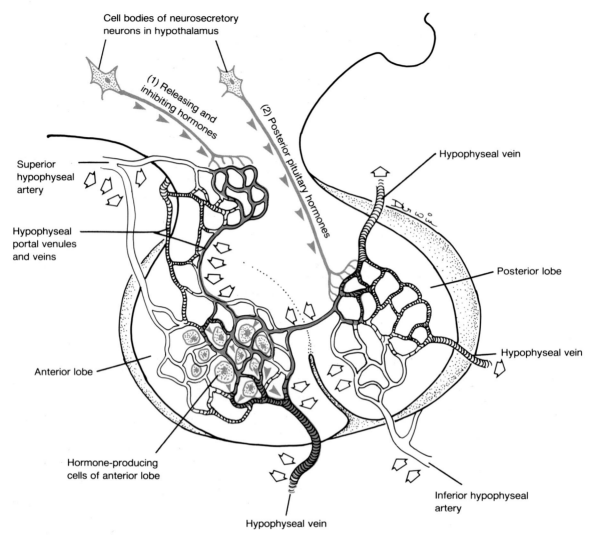

Fig. 22-5. Schematic representation of the pituitary, illustrating (1) the hypophysioportal circulation and the pathway followed by the hypothalamic hypophysiotrophic hormones (releasing and inhibiting hormones) in reaching the anterior pituitary by way of this circulation (*left*); and (2) the pathway by which the posterior pituitary hormones oxytocin and vasopressin (ADH) reach the capillaries of the posterior lobe (*right*). Hormone-containing blood leaves each lobe of the pituitary through a number of hypophyseal veins, only one of which is shown in detail. Open arrows indicate the direction of blood flow, and blue arrowheads indicate the path taken by the hormones involved.

are appropriately situated to facilitate the passage of hypothalamic-regulating hormones from the CSF to the hypophysioportal circulation.

We shall now consider in more detail the various types of chromophils and the hormones that they secrete.

Somatotrophs and Growth Hormone (Somatotrophin). The cells that secrete *growth hormone* (*somatotrophin*) are known as *somatotrophs*. These are spherical to ovoid cells with a fairly well-developed rough-surfaced endoplasmic reticulum (rER) and abundant relatively large secretory

granules that are approximately 350 nm in diameter (Fig. 22-6, *lower left*).

Normal levels of growth hormone are essential if adequate growth of chondrocytes and adequate secretion of cartilage matrix are to occur in the epiphyseal plates of long bones. Under conditions of growth hormone deficiency, relatively small numbers of new chondrocytes are generated in the epiphyseal plates as they ossify and relatively small amounts of cartilage matrix are produced. Calcification, on the other hand, is not affected, and as a result, the zone of maturing cartilage becomes very thin

Table 22-2   The Releasing and Inhibiting Hormones and Factors Produced by the Hypothalamus

Anterior Pituitary Hormone	Hypothalamic Releasing Hormone	Hypothalamic Inhibiting Hormone
Growth hormone (GH) or somatotrophin (STH)	Growth hormone-releasing hormone (GRH) or somatotrophin-releasing hormone (SRH)	Growth hormone-inhibiting hormone (GIH), somatotrophin–release-inhibiting hormone (SRIH), or somatostatin
Prolactin (PRL) or lactogenic hormone (LTH)	Prolactin-releasing hormone (PRH)	Prolactin-inhibiting hormone (PIH)
Thyroid-stimulating hormone or thyrotrophin (TSH)	Thyroid-stimulating hormone-releasing hormone or thyrotrophin-releasing hormone (TRH)	
Follicle-stimulating hormone (FSH)	Gonadotrophin-releasing hormone (GnRH, sometimes called LHRH)	
Luteinizing hormone (LH)	Gonadotrophin-releasing hormone (GnRH, sometimes called LHRH)	
Adrenocorticotrophic hormone or corticotrophin (ACTH)	Corticotrophin-releasing hormone (CRH)	
Melanocyte-stimulating hormone (MSH)	Melanocyte-stimulating hormone-releasing factor (MRF)	Melanocyte-stimulating hormone-inhibiting factor (MIF)

(Fig. 22-7B) compared with normal (Fig. 22-7A). Short stature due to growth hormone deficiency is often referred to as *pituitary dwarfism.*

Toward the end of adolescence, the body normally stops growing. However, the development of a *somatotroph adenoma* (*i.e.*, a secreting tumor of somatotrophin-producing cells) can result in continuous unregulated production of growth hormone, with the result that body growth does not cease. Such acquisition of excessive stature is described as *pituitary gigantism.*

If a somatotrophin-producing tumor develops after the epiphyseal plates have become replaced by bone (*i.e.*, after normal growth is over), no further growth in stature occurs. In this case, however, bone growth is stimulated. The bones of the hands and feet thicken and there is overgrowth of the mandible and other facial bones, and the skin and other tissues are affected as well. This condition is known as *acromegaly* (Gr. *akron*, extremity; *megas*, large) because growth of the bones in the hands and feet makes these extremities large.

Although the primary clinical manifestations of growth hormone deficiency or excess are seen in the skeletal tissues, this hormone is known to promote the growth of many other kinds of cells as well. Its growth-promoting effects are mediated at least in part by two insulinlike growth factors called *IGF-I* and *IGF-II*. These two proteins are similar to the proinsulin molecule and are often referred to as the *somatomedins*. They are produced by the liver when

growth hormone reaches this organ. For further information, see Rogol and Blizzard.

Growth hormone is believed to exert a negative feedback effect on its own secretion at the hypothalamic level by promoting somatostatin secretion in the hypothalamus. There are indications that insulinlike growth factors may be involved in the negative feedback regulation of growth hormone secretion through somatostatin.

Mammotrophs and Prolactin.   In males and in females who are not pregnant or lactating, mammotrophs (which are also known as *lactotrophs* or *lactotropes*) are commonly rather small and spindle-shaped, with only a few fairly small granules that are approximately 200 nm in diameter (Fig. 22-6, *top right* and *lower right*). During pregnancy and lactation, however, these granules can triple in size.

There is evidence in the case of mammotrophs and somatotrophs that when the secretory activity of hormone-secreting cells becomes acutely suppressed as a result of negative feedback, excess hormone-containing secretory granules are disposed of by becoming subjected to intracellular lysosomal degradation.

Hyperplasia of pituitary mammotrophs occurs during pregnancy in response to high estrogen levels. Similar estrogen-induced hyperplasia of these cells can also occur in the pituitary of the newborn.

A number of different hormones are necessary for maternal breast development during pregnancy (see Chap.

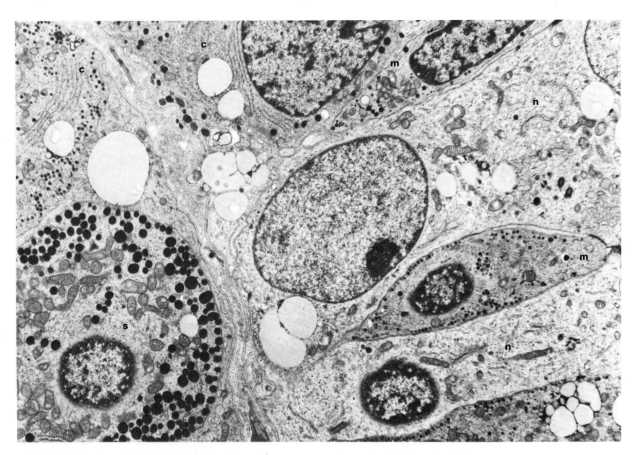

Fig. 22-6. Electron micrograph of four of the cell types that are present in the anterior pituitary (biopsy of human pituitary). At lower left, a rounded somatotroph (*s*) with abundant, relatively large granules (together with prominent mitochondria) is seen. At top left and top center, there are corticotrophs (*c*), which are characterized by having granules of variable electron density and size. At top right and lower right, there are spindle-shaped mammotrophs (*m*); these contain relatively small granules. Between the two mammotrophs, and also at bottom right, there are pale-staining cells that lack distinguishing features; these are described as null cells (*n*). (Courtesy of K. Kovacs and E. Horvath)

23). By the time her baby is born, the mother's breasts are large enough to produce adequate amounts of milk, but for them to do so requires the specific stimulus of *prolactin* (*lactogenic hormone*), which by the end of pregnancy is being secreted in fairly large quantities. Mammotrophs will continue to secrete this hormone as long as an infant is being breast-fed. The smaller quantities of prolactin secreted earlier in pregnancy probably promote breast development.

Prolactin, like growth hormone, can inhibit its own secretion by feedback inhibition at the hypothalamic level. Prolactin (PRL) and thyroid-stimulating hormone (TSH) have their own releasing hormones, PRH and TRH. However, thyrotrophin-releasing hormone (TRH) is equally effective in releasing TSH and PRL. Hence, in a sense, PRL is provided with two releasing hormones. Even so, hypothalamic control of prolactin secretion is believed to be mediated primarily through inhibition because if the infundibular stalk is damaged to the extent that the hypo-

physioportal circulation is impaired, PRL secretion is augmented.

PIH, the hormone that inhibits PRL release, was formerly believed to be dopamine, but it would seem that the effect of the high concentration of this neurotransmitter present in the median eminence may have been confused with that of the inhibitory hormone itself. In this case, it is conceivable that PIH, like the other hypophysiotrophic hormones, may turn out to be another small peptide.

Thyrotrophs and Thyroid-Stimulating Hormone. Thyrotrophs can appear somewhat angular in outline, and their secretory granules are comparatively small (up to 150 nm in diameter). They produce the glycoprotein hormone TSH, which exerts a trophic influence on thyroid follicular cells. The various actions of TSH on these cells will be considered later in this chapter when we deal with the thyroid gland.

The secretory activity of thyrotrophs is regulated through negative feedback by the level of thyroid hormone in the

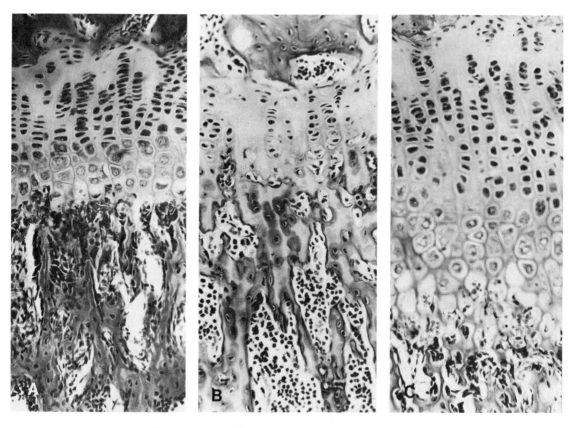

Fig. 22-7. Photomicrographs illustrating the effects of (*B*) suppression and (*C*) administration of growth hormone on growth of the epiphyseal plate, as compared with (*A*) an untreated control. (*A*) Metaphysis of tibia of a rat nearing full growth. (*B*) Metaphysis of a rat of the same age after suppression of secretion of growth hormone. The epiphyseal disk is thinner and lacks a zone of maturing cells. (*C*) Metaphysis of a rat of the same age after injections of growth hormone. The epiphyseal disk here is thicker than in *A*.

bloodstream. When this level rises above its normal limits, no further release of TSH occurs in response to the hypothalamic releasing hormone TRH. Hence regulation of TSH secretion occurs primarily at the pituitary level. The extent to which the hypothalamus participates in this regulation has not been elucidated.

Gonadotrophs and the Gonadotrophins. Gonadotrophs are mainly fusiform cells that have an eccentric nucleus and generally a rather heterogeneous content of secretory granules with a medium size range (200 nm to 400 nm) and variable electron density (Fig. 22-8). Although the possibility of the existence of two subtypes of gonadotrophs (one secreting FSH and the other secreting LH) is not entirely ruled out, the fact that there are individual gonadotrophs that contain granules with affinities for specific antibodies to both of these hormones makes it seem more likely that these cells can produce either or both of these hormones, depending on which ones are required. Also, only one releasing hormone, GnRH, is necessary to bring about the release of either FSH or LH.

The functions of the gonadotrophins (FSH and LH) are to stimulate the gonads so as to bring about the development and maturation of germ cells and the secretion of sex hormones. Under ordinary circumstances, there is a negative feedback arrangement whereby increased levels of sex hormones in the blood prevent the gonadotrophs from oversecreting. However, if the gonads are removed, this inhibitory effect on gonadotrophs is lost and, as a consequence, they oversecrete.

The feedback arrangements that exist between the sex hormones and gonadotrophs are complex and are best dealt with in the context of the reproductive system, so they will be considered in Chapters 23 and 24. Feedback is believed to occur at both the pituitary and the hypothalamic levels. However, the feedback arrangements are fairly complex because in at least one case, namely that of estrogen, feedback is *positive* (*i.e.*, an increase in estrogen levels stimulates further production of estrogen). Furthermore, these feedback arrangements somehow result in the independent regulation of FSH and LH secretion by gonadotrophs even though there is only a single releasing factor and an ap-

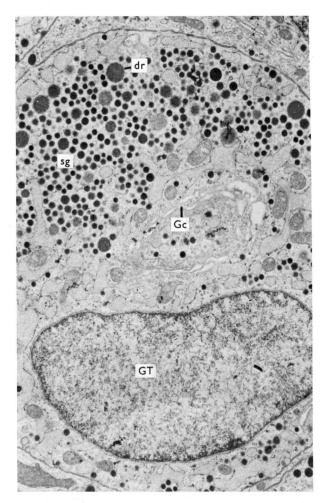

Fig. 22-8. Electron micrograph (×5400) of a portion of a gonadotroph (*GT*) in the anterior pituitary of a female rat. Note its rounded contours, rER, Golgi complex (*Gc*), and content of secretory granules. The cell also contains a few dense droplets (*dr*). (Farquhar MG: Mem Soc Endocrinol 19:101, 1971)

parent absence of inhibiting hormones for these gonadotrophins (see Table 22-2).

Corticotrophs, Adrenocorticotrophic Hormone, and Melanocyte-Stimulating Hormone. Corticotrophs, which are typically spherical to ovoid, contain granules that are only approximately 100 nm to 200 nm in diameter and that show noticeable variation both in their electron density and in their size (Fig. 22-6, *top left* and *top center*). The chief hormone produced by corticotrophs is *adrenocorticotrophic hormone* (ACTH). However, this hormone is synthesized in the form of a large precursor protein called *pro-opiomelanocortin* or *pro-ACTH/endorphin*, from which a number of other secretory peptides are also derived. These additional peptides include (1) *β*-lipotropin (*β*LPH), the functional role of which is still being elucidated; and (2) *β*-endorphin, which is a potent opioid peptide.

In some mammalian species, corticotrophs situated in the less well-defined pars intermedia appear to be capable of processing the same precursor protein in a slightly different manner, producing primarily *β*-endorphin and *α*-MSH, which has melanocyte-stimulating activity. However, because the human pars intermedia is so poorly developed, it seems very doubtful that it produces *α*-MSH under normal conditions. *γ*-MSH, which also has melanocyte-stimulating activity, is an additional cleavage product of pro-opiomelanocortin that, at least under certain conditions, can be released from corticotrophs during ACTH formation. However, the most likely reason for hyperpigmentation of endocrine origin occurring in humans (*e.g.*, in primary adrenocortical insufficiency), is that the ACTH molecule incorporates an amino acid sequence identical to a portion of the *β*-MSH sequence, and as a consequence, ACTH has demonstrable *β*-MSH activity. *β*-MSH itself is not detectable in the circulation. The effect of MSH on melanocytes is that it promotes melanin synthesis and enhances dispersion of this pigment throughout these cells.

The secretion of ACTH is inhibited by negative feedback arrangements that operate at both the pituitary and the hypothalamic levels. Thus the glucocorticoid cortisol, which is released by the adrenal cortex in response to ACTH, can suppress the secretion of ACTH by acting (1) on corticotrophs and (2) on the hypothalamus.

Posterior Lobe

The *pars nervosa (neurohypophysis)* constitutes the *posterior lobe* of the pituitary (Fig. 22-3). *Hypothalamohypophyseal tracts* of unmyelinated axons extend down into the posterior lobe from the hypothalamus (Fig. 22-9). The cell bodies to which most of these axons belong are located in the *paraventricular nucleus* and the *supraoptic nucleus* of the hypothalamus (in this context the term *nucleus* is employed to designate a particular group of nerve cell bodies). Two peptide hormones are synthesized by the nerve cell bodies in these nuclei, and because they are secreted from axon terminals in the posterior lobe they are often referred to as the *posterior pituitary hormones*. The two kinds of neurosecretory cells that produce them exhibit all the usual features of neurons, including Nissl bodies in their cytoplasm (Fig. 22-10).

The hormone *oxytocin* is synthesized primarily in the *paraventricular nucleus*. *Vasopressin*, an alternative name for which is *antidiuretic hormone* (ADH), is synthesized primarily in the *supraoptic nucleus*. In each case, the hormone is transported down the axon in the form of a noncovalent complex with a carrier protein known as a *neurophysin*. Such complexing is thought to reduce the likelihood of leakage of the peptide through the limiting membrane of the neurosecretory granules. These granules appear to be stored in the axon terminals until their contents are discharged by exocytosis. Accumulations of granular secretory material sometimes appear as irregular basophilic masses

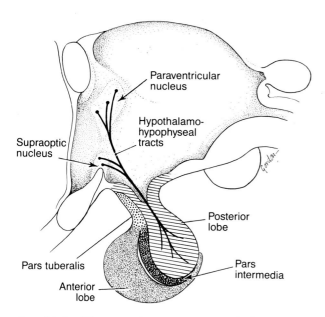

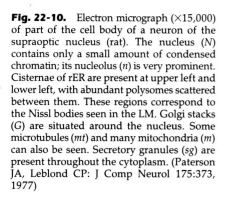

Fig. 22-9. Diagrammatic representation of the hypothalamohypophyseal tracts. See text for details.

in axon terminals or within local swellings of the axon; such accumulations are known as *Herring bodies.* An intimate association between the neurosecretory axon terminals and fenestrated capillaries in the posterior lobe facilitates passage of these two hormones into the bloodstream. The posterior lobe also contains a population of glial cells known as *pituicytes* that are generally assumed to serve some supporting function.

At term, *oxytocin* (Gr. *oxys,* swift; *tokos,* birth) induces peristaltic contractions of uterine smooth muscle that facilitate parturition (childbirth). Its main clinical applications are to induce labor and to control postpartum bleeding. This hormone is also responsible for causing myoepithelial cells of the mammary glands to contract during breast-feeding, with resulting milk ejection from the secretory alveoli. It will be appreciated that milk letdown (ejection) is not the same process as milk secretion, which is stimulated by prolactin, not oxytocin. Lactation will be described in more detail in Chapter 23.

Vasopressin (ADH) promotes water resorption through the walls of the collecting tubules of the kidneys. This role of vasopressin was considered in Chapter 21 in the section

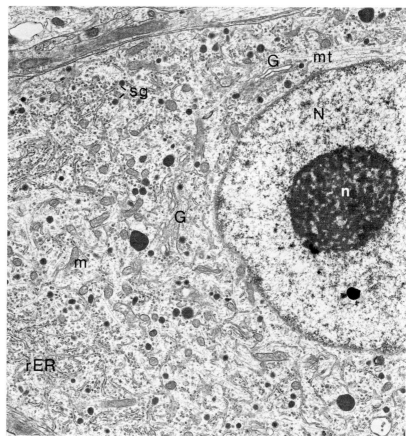

Fig. 22-10. Electron micrograph (×15,000) of part of the cell body of a neuron of the supraoptic nucleus (rat). The nucleus (*N*) contains only a small amount of condensed chromatin; its nucleolus (*n*) is very prominent. Cisternae of rER are present at upper left and lower left, with abundant polysomes scattered between them. These regions correspond to the Nissl bodies seen in the LM. Golgi stacks (*G*) are situated around the nucleus. Some microtubules (*mt*) and many mitochondria (*m*) can also be seen. Secretory granules (*sg*) are present throughout the cytoplasm. (Paterson JA, Leblond CP: J Comp Neurol 175:373, 1977)

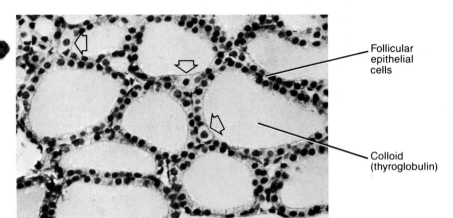

Follicular
epithelial
cells

Colloid
(thyroglobulin)

Fig. 22-11. Photomicrograph of thyroid gland of dog (low power). Arrows indicate parafollicular (C) cells; the remainder are follicular cells.

on the Collecting Tubule. The condition *diabetes insipidus,* which is different from "sugar" diabetes (*diabetes mellitus,* which will be described later in this chapter), is characterized by the production of copious urine of low specific gravity. It is due to insufficient release of ADH by the posterior lobe. Because this hormone is not available in the necessary quantities, the collecting tubules in the kidneys do not resorb enough water from the urinary filtrate and the volume of urine remains many times greater than normal. A second noteworthy effect of vasopressin is that when present in relatively high concentration, it can act as a potent vasoconstrictor. This property enables it to play an important role in the restoration of arterial blood pressure when this drops in an emergency situation.

THYROID

The *thyroid* is a highly vascular bilobed bland, the lobes of which lie, for the most part, in either side of the trachea, inferior to and around the base of the larynx. Its delicate fibroelastic connective tissue capsule is surrounded by an outer fascial sheath that is part of the pretracheal fascia. Fine fibrous septa convey blood vessels, lymphatics, and nerves into the thyroid and subdivide its parenchyma into poorly delimited lobules that are composed of spherical structural units called thyroid *follicles* (Fig. 22-11). These are essentially storage compartments with walls that are made up of simple cuboidal *follicular epithelial cells.* Each thyroid follicle stores a PAS-positive acidophilic secretory glycoprotein known as *thyroglobulin* in its lumen; this stored secretion is often referred to as the *colloid* component of the gland. The thyroid follicle is both the structural unit and the functional unit of the thyroid gland; there are no trabeculae of secretory cells as in most other endocrine glands. The follicles are tightly packed within a delicate network of reticular fibers that incorporates an extensive capillary bed. However, this capillary plexus is seldom evident in routine LM sections because blood becomes squeezed out of most of the capillaries. Sections of thyroid

that have been obtained from young individuals have follicles that are fairly uniform in appearance, but these become increasingly irregular and variable in shape with advancing age.

Whereas the vast majority of hormone-producing cells in the thyroid are *follicular epithelial cells,* a few of the cells that are present in the walls of its follicles are known as *parafollicular (C) cells.* The endoderm-derived *follicular epithelial cells* produce *thyroid hormone,* the circulating forms of which are *thyroxine* (tetraiodothyronine, which is abbreviated as T4) together with some *triiodothyronine* (T3). Circulating T4 becomes largely converted into T3, but both forms of the hormone exert an effect on target cells. The *parafollicular cells* or *C cells* of the thyroid (C for *calcitonin*), which are believed to be derived from the neural crest, produce the polypeptide hormone *calcitonin.*

In the next section, we shall consider both the production of thyroglobulin and its *extracellular iodination,* which is achieved through the combination of oxidized iodine radicals with its tyrosyl residues. After the stored thyroglobulin has become iodinated, it is then available for breakdown so as to form thyroid hormone.

Thyroid Follicular Cells

In the EM it can be seen that the follicular epithelial cells have apical microvilli on their luminal surface (Fig. 22-12A). They also exhibit obvious signs of active glycoprotein synthesis and secretion. These indications include the presence of widely dilated cisternae of rER and distended Golgi saccules (Fig. 22-12B) and the accumulation of apical secretory vesicles (Fig. 22-12A) that discharge their glycoprotein content by exocytosis into the follicular lumen. Besides producing thyroglobulin, these cells are able to trap iodide from the bloodstream by means of an active transport mechanism. Furthermore, they produce a peroxidase that is employed to oxidize this iodide. The oxidized iodine thus produced is utilized to iodinate the tyrosyl groups of the noniodinated thyroglobulin. Radioautographic studies using radioactive iodine have disclosed that iodination occurs

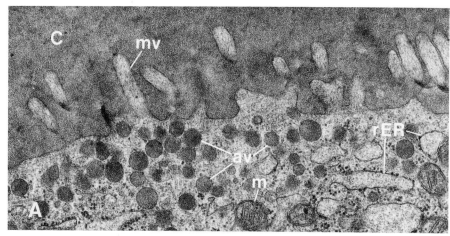

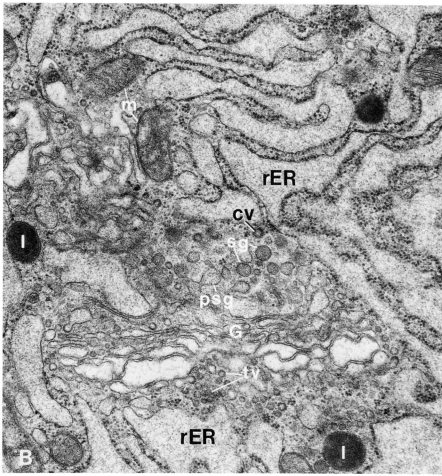

Fig. 22-12. Electron micrographs of representative regions of a follicular cell of the thyroid. (*A*) The apical surface bordering on the colloid (*C*) has microvilli (*mv*) on it. The apical vesicles (*av*) contain material with the same electron density as the colloid. (*B*) The organelles involved in the secretion of thyroglobulin. Distended cisternae of rER are prominent. Protein is being transported by transfer vesicles (*tv*) to the Golgi (*G*), where most of the carbohydrate groups are being added. Prosecretory granules (*psg*) that bud from the Golgi become secretory granules (*sg*) and eventually apical vesicles (*av* in part *A*). A coated vesicle (*cv*), some dense bodies that are probably lysosomes (*l*), and mitochondria (*m*) are also present. (Haddad A, Smith MD, Herscovics A: J Cell Biol 49:856, 1971)

intraluminally within 1 μm of the region of cell membrane that lies along the luminal border of the follicular epithelial cells. For further details, see Nadler.

Secretion of thyroglobulin, its extracellular iodination, and its subsequent intracellular degradation to produce thyroid hormone, all proceed concurrently within or in close association with the same cells. These three concurrent activities are manifested as a continuous turnover of the thyroglobulin in the lumen. The steps involved in producing the hormone are as follows. Under the influence of FSH, the follicular cells actively take up iodinated thyroglobulin by endocytosis from the lumen of each thyroid follicle and

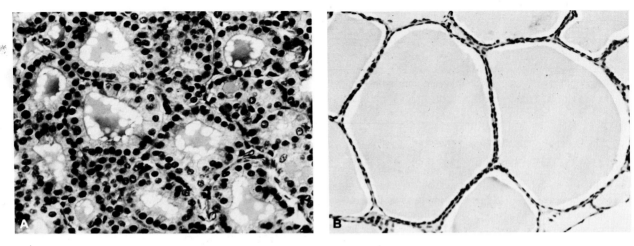

Fig. 22-13. Photomicrographs of two abnormal thyroid glands, showing the appearance of (*A*) a parenchymatous goiter developing in response to the administration of TSH (dog), and (*B*) a simple colloid goiter. See text for details.

then submit it to lysosomal digestion. Two products liberated as a result of intracellular proteolysis are T3 and T4. These iodinated amino acid derivatives are small enough to diffuse out of the cells, whereupon they enter the circulation by way of the numerous fenestrated capillaries that are closely associated with these cells. The T3 and T4, which are both components of thyroid hormone, have been shown to play a key role in maintaining the normal development, growth, and function of a broad range of body tissues and organ systems. It would appear that thyroid hormone is almost universally necessary for the basic metabolic activities of the body cells to proceed at their normal rate.

TSH Affects the Functional Activity and Microscopic Appearance of Thyroid Follicular Cells. The histological appearance of thyroid follicles and their component cells closely reflects the state of functional activity of the gland. The trophic influence of TSH secreted by the thyrotrophs of the anterior pituitary causes the follicular cells to increase in height as a result of hypertrophy. It also brings about an increase in the number of follicular cells in the walls of each follicle by inducing hyperplasia. Other effects of stimulation by TSH include (1) acceleration of the relative rates of synthesis, exocytosis, and iodination of thyroglobulin; and (2) accelerated endocytosis and intracellular breakdown of colloid, resulting in an increase in the number of intracellular endocytotic vesicles containing iodinated thyroglobulin. These effects result in an increased production of thyroid hormone, and the net result is a reduction in volume, rather than expansion, of the intraluminal colloid. The additional amounts of membrane added to the luminal cell border of the follicular cells as a result of augmented exocytosis are retrieved through augmented endocytosis. Some coated pits and coated vesicles seem to be involved in this process of endocytosis and membrane retrieval.

Without the stimulus of TSH, the follicular cells become squamous instead of cuboidal. If, on the other hand, there is a deficiency of *iodide* in the diet (which nowadays can be avoided by incorporating iodide into table salt), thyroid hormone is not secreted in adequate amounts. This leads to a reduction in the level of negative feedback being exerted on the pituitary thyrotrophs, which in turn results in an overproduction of TSH. The elevated TSH levels lead to a marked hypertrophy and hyperplasia of the thyroid follicular cells, which becomes manifested externally as an obvious enlargement of the thyroid. An enlarged thyroid is called a *goiter*. In this case, the enlargement is due to an increase in the number and size of the parenchymal (follicular) cells of the gland, so this type of goiter is described as a *parenchymatous goiter* to distinguish it from a *colloid goiter* in which enlargement of the gland is due to the production of excessive amounts of colloid (compare parts *A* and *B* of Fig. 22-13).

Marked protrusion of the eyeballs (termed *exophthalmos*) can be a sign of overproduction of thyroid hormone (*hyperthyroidism*). In most cases of exophthalmic goiter, which has the histological appearance of a parenchymatous goiter, the stimulus for hypertrophy and hyperplasia of the follicular cells is not FSH but a circulating factor that was formerly known as LATS (*long-acting thyroid stimulator*) but that is now more commonly referred to as TSI (*thyroid-stimulating immunoglobulin*) because it is known to be an antibody of the IgG class. Actually, there are several different TSIs that seem to be directed against the TSH receptor or some cell-surface molecule that is closely associated with it. When a TSI binds to thyroid follicular cells, it activates the TSH receptor and stimulates the cells, mimicking the effect of TSH. Hyperthyroidism can also be due to unregulated output of thyroid hormone by a thyroid adenoma.

Finally, we should add that autoimmunity to thyroglobulin can develop as a result of increased exposure of this normally secluded antigen to the body's immune system. The resulting hypothyroid condition is known as *chronic autoimmune thyroiditis (Hashimoto's disease)*. Insufficient production of thyroid hormone during fetal life and infancy can result in severe mental retardation and stunting of body growth; this condition is known as *cretinism*. However, although hypothyroidism has profound consequences if it develops early in life, its effects are less serious when it is later in onset.

Thyroid Parafollicular Cells (C Cells)

The thyroid gland contains a widely dispersed population of large, rounded pale-staining cells that have a central spherical nucleus (Fig. 22-11, indicated by *arrows*, and Fig. 22-14). With the EM, it can be seen that these cells lie enclosed within the same basement membrane as the follicular epithelial cells. However, because there are attenuated parts of follicular cells interposed between them and the colloid, they do not border directly on the colloid (Fig. 22-14). They therefore lie *beside* follicles and are accordingly known as *parafollicular cells* (Gr. *para*, beside). In their cytoplasm, there are abundant spherical secretory granules, 100 nm to 200 nm in diameter, that contain the polypeptide hormone *calcitonin*, which is why these cells are also known as *C cells*. The electron density of these granules is characteristically rather variable (Fig. 22-15).

Calcitonin (CT) is a blood calcium-lowering hormone that has an antagonistic action to parathyroid hormone (PTH). When plasma calcium ion concentrations exceed their normal limit, parafollicular cells release their CT by exocytosis. The available evidence indicates that the principal target cell of CT in bone tissue is the osteoclast. After resorption of bone tissue has been stimulated by PTH, both the area and the resorptive activity of the ruffled border, which is the part of the osteoclast surface that is specialized for bone resorption (see Chap. 12 under Osteoclasts), become in-

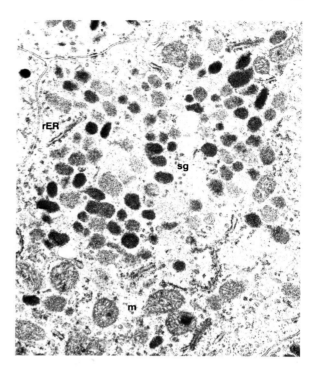

Fig. 22-15. Electron micrograph of part of the cytoplasm of a parafollicular (C) cell of the thyroid (C-cell hyperplasia in biopsy of human thyroid). Characteristic secretory granules (*sg*) with variable electron density, a few mitochondria (*m*), and occasional isolated cisternae of rER can be discerned in the pale-staining cytoplasm. (Courtesy of K. Kovacs and E. Horvath)

creased (King et al). Calcitonin has the effect of reducing the number and extent of the ruffled borders in the stimulated cells, thereby diminishing preexisting bone resorption and consequent liberation of calcium ions from bone matrix (Holtrop et al). In addition, CT reduces osteoclast numbers. The possibility that CT promotes the formation of new bone has also been suggested, but there is little evidence to support this idea. Finally, CT promotes the excretion of calcium and phosphate from the kidneys.

No serious clinical consequences appear to result from excessively high or abnormally low levels of CT, and this has created some doubt about whether this hormone has much physiological importance in man.

For a fuller discussion of the effects of CT on bone resorption and for further details of the systemic regulation of blood calcium levels, see Chapter 12 under Osteoclasts.

PARATHYROIDS

There are usually four parathyroid glands, but there can be more. They are so named because they lie *beside* the thyroid. More precisely, they are usually arranged two on each side, on the posterior side of the lobes of the thyroid gland, immediately outside the true capsule of the thyroid

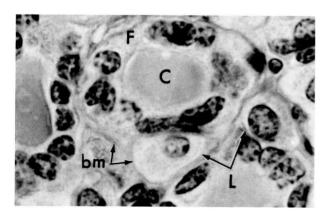

Fig. 22-14. Photomicrograph of a thyroid follicle (rat) with two light-staining parafollicular cells (*L*), one just below center and the other right of center. The basement membrane (*bm*) of the follicle extends around the outside of the parafollicular cell below center so as to include this cell in the same follicle. The parafollicular cells are effectively separated from the colloid (*C*) by adjacent follicular cells. Follicular cells are labeled F. Masson's trichrome stain. (Young BA, Leblond CP: Endocrinology 73:669, 1963)

but inside its outer fascia. The upper parathyroids lie about midway along the lobes, whereas the lower ones lie near the lower ends of the lobes. The upper ones are of a flattened ovoid shape, the lower ones roughly that of a flattened sphere. Their greatest diameter is slightly more than 0.5 cm, and they are yellow-brown when seen in the fresh state. Both the upper and the lower parathyroids are supplied with blood from the inferior thyroid artery, so these small glands can sometimes be found by tracing the arterial branches arising from the inferior thyroid artery to their terminations.

The numbers and sites of parathyroid glands vary with species. In the rat, there are only two, and these lie buried in the substance of the thyroid gland, one in each lobe. In the dog, parathyroid glands may sometimes be found as far down as the bifurcation of the trachea. Even in man, aberrant parathyroid glands are not uncommon, and if a tumor develops in one of these, it may be difficult to find.

Each endoderm-derived parathyroid gland is covered by a delicate connective tissue *capsule*. Septa penetrate the gland, carrying blood vessels and a few vasomotor nerve fibers into its substance. The septa do not divide the gland into distinct lobules. Until a few years before puberty, only one type of secretory cell is found in the gland. This is termed the *chief (principal)* cell. It is smaller than the secretory cells of most endocrine glands; hence in the parathyroid glands the nuclei of the parenchymal cells lie very close to one another (as seen at *right* in Fig. 22-16). The chief cells do not exhibit any granules in H & E sections, but the presence of granules in these cells can be demonstrated at the LM level by special staining. In the parathyroids, the parenchymal cells are arranged as large clumps and unusually wide irregular cords supported by reticular fibers. Wide capillaries, too, are present in the the parathyroids but they are seldom obvious.

A few years before puberty, clumps of cells with noticeably more cytoplasm than the chief cells make their appearance in the parathyroid glands. Unlike the chief cells, these cells have an acidophilic cytoplasm and are accordingly known as *oxyphil* (Gr. *oxys,* acid) cells (seen at *left* in Fig. 22-16). Oxyphil cells are not as numerous as chief cells. Because transitional forms exist between chief cells and oxyphil cells and the chief cells are the first to appear, chief cells are believed to transform into oxyphil cells. However, the functional significance of the oxyphil cells is unknown. One of their interesting features is that they contain very large numbers of mitochondria (Fig. 22-17).

Althought the chief cells possess a fairly prominent Golgi complex, they characteristically contain only a few stored hormone-containing secretory granules (Fig. 22-17). However, they store relatively large amounts of glycogen and lipid (Fig. 22-17), the presence of which largely accounts for their pale appearance in H & E sections.

Parathyroid hormone (PTH) is a blood calcium–raising hormone, the effects of which are antagonistic to those of calcitonin. The chief cells release PTH whenever the plasma

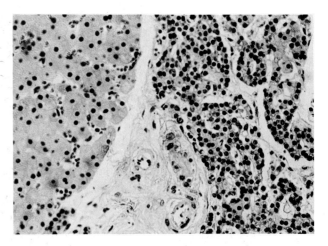

Fig. 22-16. Photomicrograph of a part of a parathyroid gland, showing its two cell types. An area of larger oxyphil cells is seen at left and an area of smaller chief cells is seen at right.

calcium level drops below its normal limits. One of the primary target cells for this hormone in bone tissue is again the osteoclast, which responds to PTH by increasing both the area and the resorptive activity of its ruffled border. PTH also brings about an increase in the number of osteoclasts that are present on resorbing bone surfaces. As discussed in Chapter 12 in the section on Osteoclasts, the question of how PTH affects osteocytes is still unsettled and requires further elucidation. However, there is now fairly general agreement that the liberation of calcium ions from bone matrix as a result of increased resorptive activity of osteoclasts is a major factor in restoring diminished blood calcium levels to normal. In addition there are two other important mechanisms by which PTH is able to bring a low blood calcium level up to normal. First, it promotes calcium resorption by the distal convoluted tubules of the kidneys, at the same time decreasing the rate of phosphate resorption by the proximal convoluted tubes. Second, it promotes the synthesis of a vitamin D_3 derivative that enhances calcium absorption by the gut. For a fuller and more detailed discussion of these actions of PTH, refer to the section on The Systemic Regulation of Blood Calcium Levels under Osteoclasts in Chapter 12. The clinical repercussions of PTH deficiency and PTH excess are also dealt with in that section.

ADRENALS

The *adrenal (suprarenal) glands* are paired, flattened yellow masses that lie, as their name implies, in contact with the superomedial border of the kidneys. The right adrenal gland, which is sometimes described as having the shape of a cocked hat, occupies the space between the right kidney and the inferior vena cava. The left adrenal gland, which

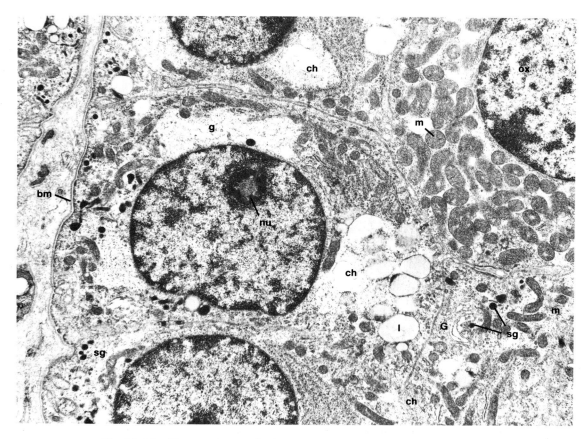

Fig. 22-17. Electron micrograph of three chief cells and an oxyphil cell of the parathyroid (biopsy of human parathyroid). At left, three chief cells (*ch*) are seen bordering on the interstitial connective tissue; their basement membrane (*bm*) is clearly visible. These cells typically contain only a few electron-dense secretory granules (*sg*) packaged in the Golgi region (*G*). Their spherical nucleus has a prominent nucleolus (*nu*). Lipid droplets (*l*) and regions where glycogen was present (*g*) are also recognizable. Mitochondria (*m*) are rod-shaped. At upper right, a rounded oxyphil cell (*ox*) is present. It has a spherical central nucleus and is characterized by having an abundance of mitochondria (*m*) in its cytoplasm. (Courtesy of K. Kovacs and E. Horvath)

is roughly crescent-shaped, covers the upper part of the medial border of the left kidney. Each adrenal gland is approximately 5 cm long, 3 cm to 4 cm wide, and somewhat less than 1 cm thick. It is made up of an *adrenal cortex* and an *adrenal medulla* that have entirely different developmental origins, structural characteristics, and functions. The first fundamental difference between the cortex and the medulla is the way it develops.

Development of the Adrenals. The first sign of the developing adrenals is a thickening of the mesoderm near the root of the dorsal mesentery. Bilateral masses of mesoderm form in this region, close to the developing kidneys. As development proceeds, the original mass of cells comprising the cortex becomes surrounded by a second mass of cells that are derived approximately from the same site as the first. The original (inner) mass forms what is called the *provisional* or *fetal cortex of the gland,* and the second (outer) mass that covers it forms the *permanent cortex.*

In the meantime, neuroectodermal cells have migrated from the neural crest to form the celiac ganglia. However, some of the cells, instead of developing into ganglion cells at this site, migrate into the cortical tissue to take up a position in its central part. A continuous migration of cells from the developing celiac ganglia proceeds until approximately the time of birth, so that substantial numbers of cells come to occupy the central part of the adrenal gland to comprise its *medulla.* Thus the cells of the adrenal medulla are the same kind as those that become ganglion cells of the sympathetic nervous system.

The provisional or fetal cortex—derived from the first group of mesodermal cells to separate from the coelomic epithelium—becomes arranged into cords separated by blood vessels, and the structure as a whole reaches a high state of development during fetal life. Not only do the cells of the provisional cortex comprise the bulk of cortical tissue that exists at this time, they are so numerous that they make each adrenal cortex of the human fetus an organ of

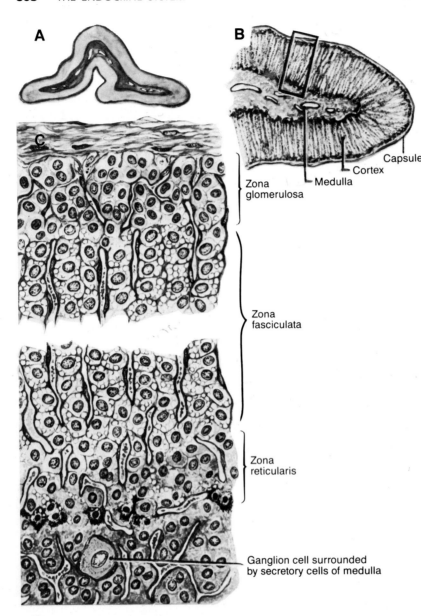

A

B

Capsule
Cortex
Medulla

Zona
glomerulosa

Zona
fasciculata

C

Zona
reticularis

Ganglion cell surrounded
by secretory cells of medulla

Fig. 22-18. Diagrammatic representation of the adrenal gland. (*A*) Scanning power. (*B*) Very low power. (*C*) Boxed-in area in *B* under higher magnification.

impressive size. The cells of the permanent cortex do not develop to any great extent during this time. However, after birth the provisional cortex, so highly developed during fetal life, undergoes rapid involution. As this occurs, the cells of the permanent cortex begin to differentiate, but for a few years they do not become organized into the three zones that are characteristic of the adult cortex.

The fact that the provisional cortex is so highly developed in fetal life and then involutes after birth is a clear indication that, like the placenta, it serves a special purpose in fetal life. It is now known that the adrenal cortex becomes very active in producing corticosteroids during fetal life. Furthermore, throughout this period, it cooperates functionally with the placenta in producing estrogen.

Acquisition of a permanent cortex gives each adrenal gland a distinctive microscopic appearance that greatly facilitates its histological recognition. In cross section, the outline of the gland is characteristically triangular (Fig. 22-18*A*). The thick fibroelastic connective tissue *capsule*, the *cortex*, and the central *medulla* are readily recognizable under low power (Figs. 22-18*B* and 22-19). Wide fenestrated capillaries supply both the cortex and the medulla. Hormones readily pass into these capillaries from the mesoderm-derived secretory epithelial cells that lie in close association with them. The adrenal medulla is supplied both with arterial blood and with blood that has already passed through the cortical capillaries. This arrangement brings hormones that are made in the adrenal cortex into contact

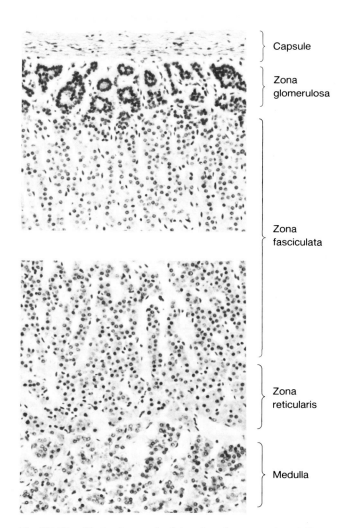

Capsule

Zona
glomerulosa

Zona
fasciculata

Zona
reticularis

Medulla

Fig. 22-19. Photomicrograph of the adrenal cortex and medulla at a magnification similar to that in Figure 22-18C.

with the cells in the adrenal medulla. Venules draining the medullary capillaries empty into a large central vein, the tributaries of which are large enough to be quite conspicuous in sections (Fig. 22-18A and B).

Adrenal Cortex

The unique histological organization of the adrenal cortex (Figs. 22-18 and 22-19) makes its microscopic recognition very easy. This part of the gland is made up of three zones known as the *zona glomerulosa,* the *zona fasciculata,* and the *zona reticularis.* These are descriptive terms that refer to the arrangement of the secretory epithelial cells. In the *zona glomerulosa,* which is the outermost zone, the cells are relatively small and they are arranged in more or less spherical groups (L. *glomerulus,* little ball). In the *zona fasciculata,* which is by far the thickest zone, the cells are

larger and vacuolated and they are arranged in the form of narrow radially oriented columns that are only one cell thick in some places. Between these columns, there are long, straight fenestrated capillaries. In the *zona reticularis,* which is an innermost zone of comparable thickness to the zona glomerulosa, cords of slightly smaller cells are arranged in the form of an irregular anastomosing network. Some of the cells in this inner zone have pyknotic nuclei. The secretory epithelial cells of all three zones are closely associated with fenestrated capillaries (Fig. 22-18C). Because they all produce steroid hormones, they all contain a prominent smooth-surfaced endoplasmic reticulum (sER; Fig. 22-20). Their vacuolated appearance in LM sections, most noticeable in the zona fasciculata, is due to their abundant content of lipid droplets (Fig. 22-20) containing cholesteryl esters, which are the precursors of the steroid hormones that are made by these cells. Zona fasciculata cells have also been shown to contain considerable quantities of ascorbic acid (vitamin C). ACTH, if given in sufficient amounts, rapidly depletes these cells of much of their cholesterol and ascorbic acid. Both effects—depletion of ascorbic acid or cholesterol—have been used in experimental animals to assay ACTH. The cells are rich in mitochondria; these differ from typical mitochondria in that their cristae are tubular instead of shelflike (Fig. 22-20).

The Adrenocortical Hormones (Corticosteroids)

A properly functioning adrenal cortex (or, failing this, replacement therapy using exogenous corticosteroids) is essential to life because several of the steroid hormones that it produces play key roles in regulating important metabolic activities of the body (the adrenal medullary hormones, on the other hand, are nonessential).

The adrenal cortex produces two major classes of steroid hormones known as the *glucocorticoids* and the *mineralocorticoids.* In addition, it produces minor quantities of *sex hormones.* We shall begin by considering the glucocorticoids and their main biological effects. The chief glucocorticoid is *cortisol,* also known as *hydrocortisone,* and the most important effects of cortisol in the body are described below.

Cortisol Has a Profound Effect on Protein and Carbohydrate Metabolism. With respect to protein metabolism, cortisol acts as a catabolic hormone. Thus in the liver it stimulates the conversion of proteins into carbohydrate. Because both cortisol and insulin cause hepatocytes to accumulate glycogen, it should be explained that the ways in which these two hormones exert this effect are quite different. Insulin causes hepatocytes to store glucose from the blood as glycogen; in other words, the glycogen that appears in hepatocytes as a result of insulin activity *lowers* the blood sugar level. On the other hand, cortisol causes production of carbohydrate from protein or protein precursors; hence cortisol promotes the synthesis of glycogen in hepatocytes without taking glucose from the blood

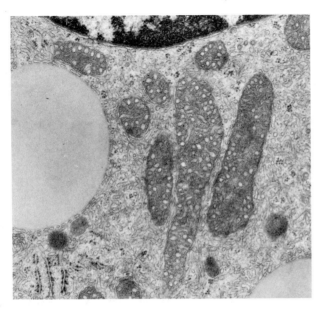

Fig. 22-20. Electron micrograph (×28,600) of a portion of a cell of the adrenal zona fasciculata. The large pale circular areas at left and bottom right are lipid droplets; these store cholesteryl esters that serve as precursors of steroid hormones. Three cisternae of rER can be seen at bottom left. The appearance of tiny holes in the large dark mitochondria at right is due to tubular cristae being cut in cross or oblique section. The cytoplasm is packed with tubules of sER, which is involved in the synthesis of steroid hormones. A small portion of the nucleus is seen at top. (Courtesy of J. Long)

and so lowering the blood sugar level; indeed, its action in causing formation of carbohydrate from protein provides extra sugar for the blood and tends to *raise* the level of blood sugar. Insulin, therefore, has an antidiabetogenic effect in that it tends to lower the blood sugar level, and cortisol has a diabetogenic effect in that it tends to raise the blood sugar level. Normally, of course, these two effects are balanced, but in the absence of either hormone, the effects of the other are manifested. Without cortisol, hypoglycemic (*i.e.,* low blood sugar–induced) death ensues because of inadequate output of glucose by the liver.

Cortisol Depletes Lymphatic Tissue and Suppresses Immune Responses. The catabolic effect of cortisol is manifested by its effect on lymphatic tissue also; the administration of pharmacological doses of this hormone leads to a rapid reduction in the size of the lymphocyte populations of the thymus, spleen, and other lymphatic tissue. Because cortisol can inhibit DNA synthesis and hence mitosis, such depletion of lymphocyte depots is believed to be in large part due to a decrease in the rapid turnover of lymphocyte populations in these depots. Because cortisol exerts inhibitory effects on both proliferation and protein synthesis, it can decrease the production of (1) cytotoxic T cells and (2) plasma cells and antibodies. Hence *cortisol has potent immunosuppressive activity.* In addition, there are indications that changing levels of cortisol oc-

curring within the physiological range can bring about a redistribution of circulating T lymphocytes within the body.

Cortisol Exerts Anti-inflammatory Effects. Cortisol also has a useful capacity for alleviating inflammatory reactions and for suppressing allergic responses. However, it acts on the symptoms and not on the cause. It can therefore be harmful to employ cortisol or synthetic steroids to allay acute inflammation in situations in which this is essential for overcoming an infection. An observable effect of administering cortisol is that it causes eosinophils to leave the circulation and enter loose connective tissue; hence it produces *eosinopenia.*

Two other important effects of cortisol are that (1) it affects the body's water distribution and clearance through a number of different mechanisms, and (2) it can retard the healing of wounds primarily because of a suppressive effect on fibroblast proliferation. Lastly, it should be remembered that cortisol constitutes the main feedback signal that suppresses pituitary ACTH secretion.

The Regulation of Cortisol Secretion. Cortisol is secreted mainly by the *zona fasciculata,* with a smaller contribution from the *zona reticularis.* Its secretion is regulated by a negative feedback arrangement involving the corticotrophs of the anterior pituitary. When the blood levels of cortisol decrease, the corticotrophs respond by secreting more ACTH, and this stimulates further output of cortisol by the adrenal cortex. The rising levels of cortisol then suppress further ACTH release by the corticotrophs. However, superimposed on this essential feedback loop is a marked diurnal variation of ACTH and cortisol secretion. Similar diurnal variation also occurs in the case of aldosterone. In most people, these hormones reach their highest levels early in the morning, just before awakening, and then decline to their lowest levels by the late evening. However, the cycle of secretory activity is related to the customary hours of sleeping and awakening and does not necessarily correspond to any particular hours of the day or night. In addition, it is clearly established that *stress stimulates the output of ACTH.* The feedback arrangements that regulate the secretion of ACTH and hence cortisol have been shown to operate at both the pituitary and the hypothalamic levels, with the diurnal variation and the effects of stress being mediated through the hypothalamus by the hypothalamic releasing hormone CRH. Furthermore, it has been shown that cortisol decreases the responsiveness of corticotrophs to this releasing hormone.

Mineralocorticoids. These corticosteroids are particularly important to the internal economy of the body because they help to maintain its electrolyte and water balance by promoting the resorption of sodium from the distal convoluted tubules and cortical collecting tubules of the kidneys. The most potent mineralocorticoid is *aldosterone.* The role of aldosterone is thus to conserve body sodium. In cases of adrenocortical insufficiency (Addison's disease), or following adrenalectomy (surgical removal of the adrenals), sodium is lost from the body into the urine, and potassium accumulates in the blood. Mineralocorticoids are secreted only by the cells of the *zona glomerulosa*. Aldosterone secretion is stimulated by the *angiotensins*, which are formed when *renin* is released from the juxtaglomerular (JG) cells of the kidneys (as described in Chap. 21 under Renal Corpuscle and Juxtaglomerular Complex). It is also stimulated, although only transiently, by high levels (*i.e.*, stress levels) of ACTH from the anterior pituitary. Secretion of the other mineralocorticoids is nevertheless stimulated on a more sustained basis by ACTH. The main sites at which sodium becomes resorbed into the body are the distal convoluted tubules and cortical collecting tubules of the kidneys, but aldosterone also promotes sodium resorption in the sweat glands and salivary glands and increases sodium absorption in the gut.

Sex Hormones. The third group of steroid hormones made by the adrenal cortex are sex hormones, chiefly weak *androgens.* In the adrenals, they are produced mainly by the cells of the zona reticularis, with some synthesis occurring in the zona fasciculata as well. This capacity of the adrenal cortex for producing sex hormones becomes important in understanding how certain disorders of the adrenal glands can lead to abnormal development of the fetal genitalia during pregnancy. For example, excessive levels of adrenal androgens have the potential to exert a masculinizing influence on developing female genitalia, which can result in a condition called *female pseudohermaphroditism.*

ACTH Maintains the Size and Functional Activity of the Adrenal Cortex and Promotes the Secretion of Cortisol. The effects of ACTH on the adrenal cortex are of two general kinds. First, ACTH is essential for maintaining the proper mass of the adrenal cortex. Thus following hypophysectomy (surgical removal of the pituitary), or in response to prolonged feedback inhibition by cortisol, the cortex becomes much smaller, mainly because of substantial depletion of the zona fasciculata. The administration of ACTH restores the usual size of this zone and also restores adequate function in terms of cortisol output.

Experimental regeneration studies suggest that the zona glomerulosa may represent the germinative zone of the adrenal cortex. Furthermore, *in vitro* studies have shown that the addition of ACTH to zona glomerulosa cells can cause them to acquire characteristics that are ordinarily manifested by cells of the zona fasciculata. Also, whereas the zona glomerulosa is not greatly changed by hypophysectomy and subsequent administration of ACTH, the zona fasciculata becomes much thicker. The most likely explanation for such observations is that ACTH not only promotes the growth of cells in the zona glomerulosa but also promotes maturation of the deepest cells in this zone into cells of the fasciculata type. In the human adrenal, it is nevertheless somewhat unclear whether this trophic re-

sponse of the zona glomerulosa to ACTH represents hypertrophy, hyperplasia, or a mixture of the two.

Thus it would seem that ACTH is responsible for maintaining the size of the secretory epithelial cell population of the adrenal cortex by regulating growth in the zona glomerulosa and differentiation or maturation of glomerulosa cells into those of the fasciculata type. Whether this hormone is similarly involved in bringing about further differentiation or maturation of fasciculata cells into cells of the reticularis type is unknown.

The status of the zona reticularis (other than its role in producing sex hormones and small amounts of glucocorticoids) is not clear. If the zona glomerulosa is indeed the germinative zone of the cortex and maintains the cortical cell population, it could be assumed that the zona reticularis represents a less active zone in which the cortical cells will eventually die. This hypothesis is often described as the "graveyard" concept of this zone.

However, this hypothesis is essentially only an extrapolation of results obtained from regeneration studies in experimental animals, and there is no direct evidence that, under normal conditions, human adrenal cortical cells arise exclusively in the zona glomerulosa and move down en masse to their deathbed in the zona reticularis. The results obtained from these regeneration studies are consistent with the existence of a renewing cell population, the earliest cells of which are present in the zona glomerulosa just beneath the capsule. As these cells and their progeny proliferate, it could be expected that the newer cells would slowly become displaced farther away from the capsule, and that by the time they or their progeny reached the zona fasciculata or zona reticularis they would take on the structural and functional characteristics of the secretory cells that are present in these layers. There seems to be little reason to believe that proliferation would be confined solely to the zona glomerulosa or that the cells would necessarily have to die after they reached the zona reticularis. It is therefore conceivable that ACTH promotes hypertrophy and hyperplasia in all three zones of the adrenal cortex, with its effect going unnoticed in the zona reticularis because this zone contains a high proportion of terminally differentiated or ACTH-unresponsive cells.

The second general effect of ACTH on the adrenal cortex is a stimulatory effect on hormone secretion. As already noted, ACTH produced in excess under conditions of undue stress elicits only a transient increase in aldosterone secretion. It nevertheless elicits a sustained increase in cortisol output by the zona fasciculata and zona reticularis. The somewhat lower levels of ACTH that reach the adrenal cortex under ordinary nonstressful circumstances are believed to have the effect of maintaining the responsiveness of the glomerulosa cells to the angiotensins instead of acting directly to elicit aldosterone secretion.

Adrenal Medulla

The *adrenal medulla* contains large, ovoid, pale-staining secretory cells arranged for the most part in the form of irregularly anastomosing cords and positioned so as to abut wide fenestrated capillaries and venules (Fig. 22-18). The

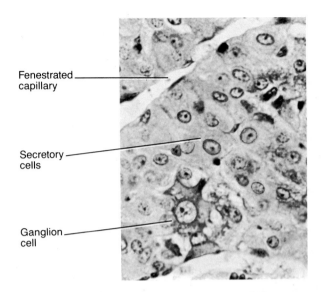

Fenestrated capillary

Secretory cells

Ganglion cell

Fig. 22-21. Photomicrograph of a part of the adrenal medulla (high power).

hormone-containing granules in these cells take on a yellowish-brown color if the tissue is treated with chromic acid or a reducible chromium salt. This coloration of the granules, referred to as the *chromaffin reaction*, is due to their content of *epinephrine* (alternatively known as *adrenaline*) and *norepinephrine* (*noradrenaline*), which become oxidized to the brown pigment melanin. The hormone-secreting cells of the adrenal medulla are accordingly known as *chromaffin cells* or *pheochromocytes* (Gr. *phaios*, dusky or dun brown). Scattered among the secretory cells, either singly or in small groups, lie a few cell bodies of postganglionic sympathetic ganglion cells (Figs. 22-18 and 22-21). The nucleus of both kinds of cells is large and spherical, with much extended chromatin and a prominent nucleolus (Fig. 22-18 and 22-21).

Relation Between the Adrenal Medulla and the Remainder of the Sympathetic Nervous System. The secretory (*chromaffin*) cells of the adrenal medulla are derived from the same group of neural crest cells that gives rise to the sympathetic ganglion cells in the celiac plexus. On migrating to the central region of the developing adrenal glands, most of these neuroectodermally derived cells differentiate into secretory cells that are distributed along blood vessels (Fig. 22-18). The secretory cells nevertheless maintain the same position in the two-neuron sympathetic chain as postganglionic sympathetic neurons and are therefore innervated by cholinergic *preganglionic fibers*, not by postganglionic fibers as are the other innervated secretory cells in the body. Hence the secretory cells of the adrenal medulla represent developmental and functional counterparts of postganglionic neurons of the sympathetic division of the autonomic nervous system.

The Adrenal Medullary Hormones (Epinephrine and Norepinephrine)

The neurotransmitter released at almost all postganglionic sympathetic endings is norepinephrine. Secretion of the adrenal medullary hormones (*primarily epinephrine* in man) into the bloodstream by the secretory cells of the adrenal medulla reinforces the action of the norepinephrine released at such endings, bringing about a broad-based sympathetic response. The minimal amounts of adrenal medullary hormone liberated under resting conditions are increased by physical exertion (*e.g.*, exercise), emotional states (*e.g.*, frustration, anger, or fright), and physical stress (*e.g.*, severe cold, pain, or hypoglycemia, and also during major surgery), and the blood levels of these two hormones can become markedly elevated in life-threatening or emergency situations (*e.g.*, anoxia or asphyxia). Epinephrine is somewhat more effective than norepinephrine in raising blood glucose levels, increasing cardiac output, and lowering peripheral resistance to blood flow, but it is less effective than norepinephrine in raising systolic and diastolic blood pressure. Both of these hormones also augment the metabolic activity of skeletal muscles and increase overall alertness through an effect on the nervous system.

Epinephrine and norepinephrine are both *catecholamines* (amines with a catechol group in their molecular structure) that are derived from the amino acid tyrosine. This amino acid becomes converted first to dihydroxyphenylalanine (dopa), then to dopamine, and then to norepinephrine. Epinephrine is produced by methylation of norepinephrine.

Chromaffin Granules. In the chromaffin reaction, norepinephrine yields a darker colored oxidation product than does epinephrine. The finding that the reaction product is darker in color in certain cells than in others led to the hypothesis, which has since been verified, that some cells produce epinephrine whereas others produce norepinephrine.

In electron micrographs, the hormone-containing granules of the adrenal medullary secretory cells appear electron dense and are round to oval with diameters in the range of 225 nm or 300 nm (Fig. 22-22). The oval appearance of granules is thought to indicate a tendency for their membranous walls to flatten as a result of fixation artifact. However, some of the oval profiles that are present in the general vicinity of the Golgi complex could represent oblique sections of developing secretory granules that are still more or less cylindrical. The secretory granules are each bounded by a limiting membrane, and their core can look more electron dense than their periphery. Such an appearance, with a dense core surrounded by a lighter halo, is again thought to represent a fixation artifact.

Except for the presence of these characteristic hormone-containing storage granules, the catecholamine-secreting cells of the adrenal medulla lack distinctive features at the EM level. In addition to possessing a moderate content of free ribosomes and a small amount of rER, they have a

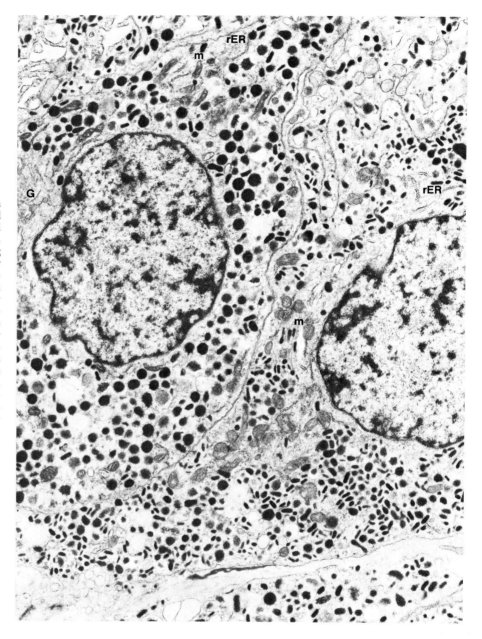

Fig. 22-22. Electron micrograph (×10,000) of the two secretory cell types that are present in the adrenal medulla (baboon). The cell at left, which is characterized by having larger and more rounded secretory granules (300 nm in diameter), secretes epinephrine. Mitochondria (*m*), a Golgi region (*G*), and a few cisternae of rER can also be discerned. The cell at right, which has smaller and more irregularly shaped or flattened secretory granules (225 nm in diameter), secretes norepinephrine. Flattening of the granules in these cells is a fixation artifact. Mitochondria (*m*) and cisternae of rER can again be discerned in the cytoplasm. (Courtesy of S. Carmichael)

fairly prominent Golgi complex, where their secretory granules are packaged. However, several of the substances that are present in these granules (catecholamines included) accumulate there after the granules have been formed, with the result that chromaffin granules attain a fairly complex chemical composition. In addition to epinephrine and norepinephrine, their contents include a number of enzymatic and nonenzymatic proteins as well as adenosine triphosphate (ATP), other nucleotides, and some phospholipids. It has recently been found that chromaffin granules also store several opioid peptides (*enkephalins*) and their precursors, suggesting that opioid peptides may participate in

the modulation and coordination of broad-based sympathetic responses. It also seems probable that the opioid peptides released from this source would be involved in mediating analgesic responses in long-lasting stress situations.

EM studies support the contention that the adrenal medulla contains two separate kinds of hormone-secreting cells that each release a different catecholamine. Epinephrine-containing granules can appear a little less electron dense than those storing norepinephrine if glutaraldehyde has been used for fixation, but in all other respects, the two cell types appear similar in the EM (Fig. 22-22).

Adrenal Blood Vessels, Lymphatics, and Nerve Supply.
The blood reaching the adrenal glands is supplied by the aorta and by the renal and inferior phrenic arteries. The arteries supplying each adrenal gland branch extensively as they reach the gland. Some of their branches supply the capillary bed in the capsule. Others penetrate directly into the medulla and supply the capillary bed of that region. However, the majority empty into cortical capillaries that course from the glomerulosa to the reticularis before draining into medullary venules. These cortical capillaries are generally collapsed and therefore inconspicuous in routine sections. Hence the adrenal medulla is provided with (1) capillaries that supply its cells with oxygenated blood, and (2) venules that receive the blood returning from cortical capillaries. Both the medullary capillaries and the medullary venules have fenestrae in their endothelium that facilitate hormonal entry into the circulation. From the medullary capillaries, blood drains through venules to the large central vein that emerges from the gland at its hilum. Other veins arise from the capsule. Lymphatics are also present in association with the larger veins and the capsule.

The adrenal cortex and capsule as well as the adrenal medulla have a sympathetic nerve supply. However, apart from the postganglionic sympathetic vasomotor fibers supplying their blood vessels, the functional significance of this innervation is unclear. As already noted, the functionally important innervation of the gland is the preganglionic cholinergic sympathetic fibers that extend directly to its medullary chromaffin cells.

Paraganglia

The catecholamine-secreting chromaffin cells of the adrenal medulla arise from sympathetic ganglion precursor cells that migrate from the developing celiac ganglia to the developing adrenal glands. Many additional clusters of chromaffin cells that also result from such migration can be found deep to the peritoneum, in the vicinity of the sympathetic ganglia. The secretory cells are arranged in little clumps or cords that are richly provided with small blood vessels. Because these small masses of secretory tissue are associated with ganglia, they are known as *paraganglia* (Gr. *para*, beside).

Secreting tumors of chromaffin cells are termed *pheochromocytomas*. They can arise from paraganglia or from the adrenal medulla. Although not common, these catecholamine-producing tumors can be of clinical importance because their unknown existence may lead to unforeseen complications during the course of surgery or parturition.

PANCREATIC ISLETS (ISLETS OF LANGERHANS)

The pancreas is made up of (1) an acinar *exocrine component*, which was described in Chapter 19; and (2) a diffuse *en-*

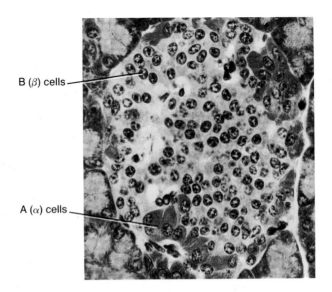

B (β) cells
A (α) cells

Fig. 22-23. Photomicrograph of a pancreatic islet of guinea pig (Gomori stain for A [α] and B [β] cells). See text for details. (Courtesy of W. Wilson)

docrine component, which is similarly of endodermal origin and constitutes the *pancreatic islets* (*islets of Langerhans*). This endocrine component of the gland consists of widely distributed clusters of hormone-secreting cells that produce the three hormones *insulin, glucagon,* and *somatostatin.*

The islets are most numerous in the tail of the pancreas. In H & E sections, they appear as pale, pink-staining irregularly shaped islands that are widely scattered among the much darker staining exocrine secretory acini. Special staining methods (*e.g.,* Gomori staining, which gives the colors cited) or, better still, immunofluorescent staining are necessary to distinguish islet cell types at the LM level. Most of these cells are relatively small blue-staining B (β) cells (Fig. 22-23). Larger pink-staining A (α) cells are distributed in small groups around B cells (two such groups can be recognized in Fig. 22-23). Islets also contain other types of secretory cells that cannot be identified without immunofluorescent staining; these are considered below. Between the hormone-secreting cells, which are arranged in the form of anastomosing cords, there are numerous fenestrated capillaries with minimal amounts of loose connective tissue containing a few autonomic nerve fibers. However, these stromal elements are not obvious in H & E sections. Each islet has a surrounding sheath of delicate loose connective tissue that is very scant and scarcely merits being called a capsule. From this sheath, reticular fibers extend into each islet and provide support for its cords of secretory cells and its numerous capillaries.

At least four different types of islet secretory cells have now been identified at the EM level on the basis of the size, electron density, and intracellular distribution of their respective secretory granules. However, these individual

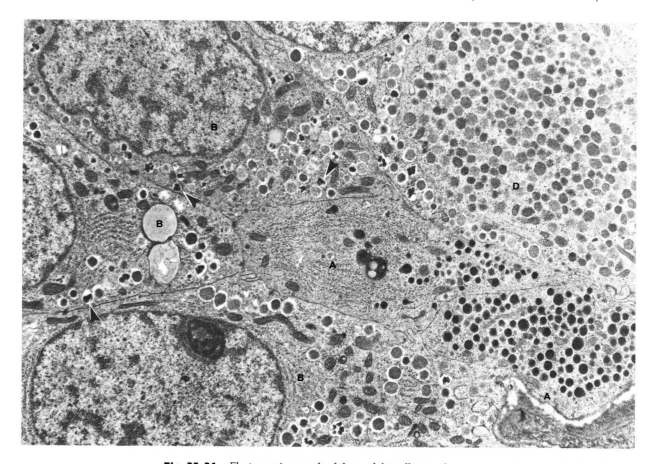

Fig. 22-24. Electron micrograph of three of the cell types that are present in pancreatic islets (biopsy of human pancreas). At left, three dark-staining B (β) cells with relatively large secretory granules, some of which exhibit irregularly shaped crystalline contents (indicated by arrowheads), along with dark-staining large mitochondria and some rER, are present. At center and lower right, parts of two dark-staining A (α) cells can be seen; these have abundant electron-dense granules, and the cell at center exhibits parallel cisternae of rER. At upper right, there is a lighter staining D (δ) cell with characteristically large paler staining granules of variable electron density. The left-hand side of the micrograph is toward the interior of the islet and the right-hand side is toward its periphery. (Courtesy of K. Kovacs and E. Horvath)

cell types can only be recognized with certainty by immunocytochemical staining at the EM level. Besides the A (α) *cells* and B (β) *cells* just described, they include D (δ) *cells* and F *cells*. The B cells are the most common and the F cells are the rarest. *A cells* produce the polypeptide hormone *glucagon,* B cells produce the polypeptide hormone *insulin,* D cells produce the peptide *somatostatin,* and F cells produce a polypeptide called *pancreatic polypeptide,* the function of which is unknown.

Because all these cell types secrete amino acid–derived hormones, they all exhibit the usual features of cells engaged in active protein synthesis. However, to some extent, they can be recognized on an individual basis by the EM appearance of their secretory granules, as described in the following section.

A (α) Cells and Glucagon. The glucagon-containing secretory granules of pancreatic A cells are characterized by having an electron-dense content that still fills the secretory vesicles after fixation. Furthermore, they possess a large and very electron-dense spherical core surrounded by a thin rim that is slightly less electron dense (Fig. 22-24, *lower right*). Their diameter, which is in the range of 250 nm to 300 nm, is roughly similar to that of pancreatic B cell granules (Fig. 22-24).

The actions of *glucagon* are antagonistic to those of insulin (see below). Glucagon *raises the blood glucose level* by promoting the formation of glucose from the glycogen being stored in hepatocytes. It also exerts effects on protein and fat metabolism. Glucagon release is inhibited by an increase in the blood glucose level.

B (β) Cells and Insulin.   The insulin-containing secretory granules of pancreatic B cells commonly exhibit an electron-dense crystalline core of irregular shape. Furthermore, their content is characteristically withdrawn from their limiting membrane following fixation (Fig. 22-24). Their overall diameter is not very different from that of pancreatic A cell granules (Fig. 22-24).

Insulin is synthesized in the rER as a polypeptide called *preproinsulin.* This has its signal sequence removed and becomes *proinsulin,* which has some hormonal activity but not as much as insulin. The prohormone proinsulin then becomes modified in the Golgi complex with the result that, under normal conditions, the secretory vesicles (granules) leaving the Golgi complex contain the hormone *insulin.* However, under conditions of prolonged stimulation, B cells secrete some proinsulin as such.

Insulin is secreted in response to an elevated blood sugar level such as that resulting from the consumption of a carbohydrate-containing meal. Its two principal actions are (1) to *promote glucose uptake* in a number of different cell types, and (2) to *lower the blood glucose level* whenever this level rises; insulin effects such a reduction by promoting the conversion of glucose into glycogen in hepatocytes and muscle cells and also by promoting lipid synthesis in adipose tissue. The release of insulin is elicited directly by elevated blood glucose levels; it is also elicited by several peptide hormones, including glucagon, cholecystokinin-pancreozymin, and secretin.

Under normal conditions, B cells store a 1- to 2-day's supply of insulin, almost a lethal quantity if it were ever to become discharged into the bloodstream all at once. An excessive dose of insulin can reduce the blood sugar level to the point of inducing convulsions or unconsciousness; this is called *insulin shock.* Indeed, too much insulin is fatal because the blood sugar level drops below the minimum necessary to sustain cellular viability. Occasionally, hormone-secreting islet tumors develop, and in cases in which B cells are secreting, this can lead to hyperinsulinism and even fatal hypoglycemia because in this instance insulin release is not regulated by the blood sugar level.

In the serious metabolic disease *diabetes mellitus* (L. *mellitus,* sweetened with honey), there is *insulin deficiency* leading to elevation of the blood glucose level (*i.e., hyperglycemia*). This condition is also characterized by the presence of glucose in the urine, (*i.e., glycosuria*). In nondiabetics all the glucose passing through the glomerular filtration barrier is resorbed from the glomerular filtrate as it passes along the kidney tubules. Hence it is not normal to find blood sugar in the urine. In untreated diabetics, however, the blood sugar level rises above the concentration at which all the glucose in the glomerular filtrate can be resorbed (a concentration called the *renal threshold for glucose*) and glucose appears in the urine.

D (δ) Cells, Somatostatin, and the Paracrine Regulation of Islet Hormone Secretion.   Compared with A and B cells, D cells have rather large secretory granules that are less electron dense (Fig. 22-24), and their other secretory organelles are less prominent. Also, these somatostatin-containing secretory granules are more variable in their electron density (Fig. 22-24).

Somatostatin is a peptide neurohormone and neurotransmitter (or neuromodulator) that owes its name to its first-discovered role as the hypothalamic hypophysiotrophic hormone that inhibits the release of growth hormone (as described above in the section dealing with the Pituitary). However, it is now known that somatostatin inhibits the release of a number of other hormones as well. Included among these are insulin, glucagon, and even somatostatin itself. Furthermore, insulin inhibits the release of glucagon, and glucagon stimulates the release of insulin and pancreatic somatostatin. The interactive mutual regulation of secretory activity occurring in A, B, and D cells, and the fact that these cells lie in close proximity to one another, is strongly suggestive of some special arrangement that facilitates side-by-side cell-to-cell regulation. This kind of close-range regulation, which is mediated through the lateral diffusion of signal molecules, is described as *paracrine* regulation. Gap junctions are also present between adjacent pancreatic A, B, and D cells and may also be significant in this connection. As noted earlier, the role of human *pancreatic polypeptide* released from pancreatic F cells has not been elucidated, so it is not known whether F cells, too, are involved in the paracrine regulation of islet hormone secretion. For further information relating to the many effects of somatostatin, see Reichlin.

Autonomic Regulation of Islet Hormone Secretion.   Finally, there are also indications that insulin and glucagon secretion are influenced by activity of the autonomic nervous system. The secretory activities of pancreatic A and B cells can be modulated by sympathetic stimulation. Insulin secretion, for example, decreases in response to sympathetic stimulation and is promoted by parasympathetic stimulation. Also, *neuroinsular complexes* have been found in which autonomic ganglion cells lie in intimate association with islet cells.

PINEAL (EPIPHYSIS)

The *pineal body* (*epiphysis*), a median appendage of the diencephalon that is approximately 7 mm long and 5 mm wide and that derives its name from the fact that it is shaped like a pine cone (L. *pineus,* relating to the pine), is an endocrine gland of neuroectodermal origin. A short *pineal stalk* attaches this gland to the roof of the third ventricle. Pia mater covers the pineal in the form of a thin connective tissue capsule from which irregular trabeculae and septa of connective tissue extend into the substance of the gland, subdividing its interior into poorly demarcated lobules. Within the lobules, there are clumps of large pale-staining secretory cells called *pinealocytes.* These cells are characterized by having a large ovoid nucleus with a prominent nucleolus and a deep indentation on one side, and also by the fact that they possess cytoplasmic processes with club-shaped tips (Fig. 22-25B). To a certain extent, pinealocytes resemble neurons. Between the secretory cells, there are

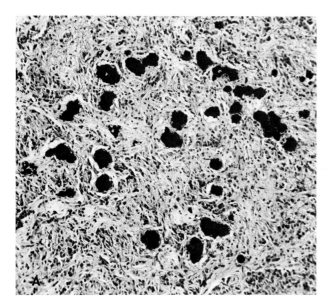
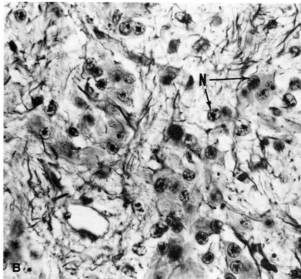

Fig. 22-25. (*A*) Photomicrograph of a portion of the pineal body, showing brain sand. (*B*) Photomicrograph of a representative part of the pineal body (stained with Heidenhain's iron hematoxylin). Pinealocytes have a relatively large nucleus (*N*) with a prominent nucleolus. (*A*, courtesy of E. Anderson; *B*, Anderson E: J Ultrastruct Res (Suppl 8), 1965)

abundant nonfenestrated capillaries and some glial cells that seem to be fibrous astrocytes. This gland characteristically contains small calcified concretions of unknown significance that can be seen in x-ray films and that are occasionally referred to as *brain sand* (Fig. 22-25*A*).

The primary nerve supply of the pineal body consists of postganglionic sympathetic fibers that extend to the pineal from the superior cervical ganglia of the sympathetic trunks. There is evidence that sympathetic nerve impulses play a major role in regulating the secretory activity of the pineal body in relation to the photoperiod of the light entering the eyes. The functional basis of pineal secretion will now be described.

The pinealocytes produce *melatonin*, which is an active derivative of serotonin with the capacity to exert a suppressive effect on gonadotrophin secretion. Pineal secretion therefore has the effect of retarding gonadal growth and function. Studies in experimental animals have demonstrated that melatonin is produced in the pineal only during periods when no light is entering the eyes. There is also a certain amount of clinical evidence suggesting that in man the functional role of the pineal is to prevent the onset of precocious gonadal function. Such an antigonadotrophic function would be consistent with the finding that the pineal is comparatively large during infancy and then begins to involute to a smaller size just before puberty.

At the hypothalamic level, the pineal hormone or hormones—which may turn out to include active peptides in addition to melatonin—appear to exert a suppressive effect on the release of GnRH. They may also act at the pituitary level by decreasing gonadotroph responsiveness to this hormone. At present, it is not

clear whether some of the antigonadotrophic effects of pineal extracts formerly attributed to melatonin are mediated, at least in part, by one or more peptides or small polypeptides that are also produced by this gland. Furthermore, the physiological importance of the antigonadotrophic influence of human pineal secretion has proved to be difficult to assess. For further information, see Wurtman; also Reiter.

SELECTED REFERENCES

General

BERRIDGE MJ: The molecular basis of communication within the cell. Sci Am 253 No. 4:142, 1985

DONALD RA (ed): Endocrine Disorders: A Guide to Diagnosis. New York, Marcel Dekker, 1984

FELIG P, BAXTER JD, BROADUS AE, FROHMAN LA (eds): Endocrinology and Metabolism. New York, McGraw-Hill, 1981

KAHN CR: Membrane receptors for hormones and neurotransmitters. J Cell Biol 70:261, 1976

MCEWEN, BS: Interactions between hormones and nerve tissue. Sci Am 235:48, July, 1976

MOTTA PM (ed): Ultrastructure of Endocrine Cells and Tissues. Boston. Martinus Nijhoff, 1984

O'MALLEY BW, SCHRADER WT: The receptors of steroid hormones. Sci Am 234:32, Feb, 1976

SNYDER SH: The molecular basis of communication between cells. Sci Am 253 No. 4:132, 1985

TEPPERMAN J: Metabolic and Endocrine Physiology: An Introductory Text, 4th ed. Chicago, Year Book Medical Publishers, 1980

Pituitary and Hypothalamus*

BAIN J, EZRIN C: Immunofluorescent localization of the LH cell of the human adenohypophysis. J Clin Endocrinol 30:181, 1970

BARGMANN W: Neurosecretion. Int Rev Cytol 19:183, 1966

BODIAN D: Herring bodies and neuroapocrine secretion in the monkey. An electron microscope study of the fate of the neurosecretory product. Bull Johns Hopkins Hosp 118:282, 1966

BROWNSTEIN MJ, RUSSEL JT, GAINER H: Synthesis, transport, and release of posterior pituitary hormones. Science 207:373, 1980

DANIEL PM: The anatomy of the hypothalamus and pituitary gland. In Martini L, Ganong WF (eds): Neuroendocrinology. Vol 1, p 15. New York, Academic Press, 1966

EIPPER BA, MAINS RE: Structure and biosynthesis of pro-adrenocorticotropin/endorphin and related peptides. Endocr Rev 1:1, 1980

EZRIN C: Chapters 1–4. In Ezrin C, Godden JO, Volpé R, Wilson R (eds): Systemic Endocrinology. Hagerstown, Harper & Row, 1973

FARQUHAR MG: Processing of secretory products by cells of the anterior pituitary gland. Mem Soc Endocrinol 19, Subcellular Organization and Function. In Heller H, Lederis K (eds): Endocrine Tissues. London, Cambridge University Press, 1971

GREEN JD: The comparative anatomy of the portal vascular system and of the innervation of the hypophysis. In Harris, GW, Donovan BT (eds): The Pituitary Gland. Vol 1, p 127. Berkeley, University of California Press, 1966

GUILLEMIN R, BURGUS R: The hormones of the hypothalamus. Sci Am 227:24, Nov, 1972

HOLMES RL, BALL, JN: The Pituitary Gland. A Comparative Account. Biological Structure and Function Series. Vol 4. London, Cambridge University Press, 1974

von LAWZEWITSCH I, DICKMANN GH, AMEZÚA L, PARDAL C: Cytological and ultrastructural characterization of the human pituitary. Acta Anat 81:286, 1972

von LAWZEWITSCH I, SARRAT R: Comparative anatomy and the evolution of the neurosecretory hypothalamic-hypophyseal system. Acta Anat 81:13, 1972

MCCANN SM: Luteinizing-hormone-releasing hormone. N Engl J Med 296:797, 1977

PAGE RB, MUNGER BL, BERGLAND RM: Scanning microscopy of pituitary vascular casts. Am J Anat 146:273, 1976

PATERSON JA, LEBLOND CP: Increased proliferation of neuroglia and endothelial cells in the supraoptic nucleus and hypophysial neural lobe of young rats drinking hypertonic sodium chloride solution. J Comp Neurol 175:373, 1977

PHILLIPS LS, VASSILOPOULOU-SELLIN R: Somatomedins. N Engl J Med 302:371, 1980

PURVES HD: Cytology of the adenohypophysis. In Harris GW, Donovan BT (eds): The Pituitary Gland. Vol 1, p 147. Berkeley, University of California Press, 1966

REICHLIN S: Somatostatin (First of two parts). N Engl J Med 309:1495, 1983

REICHLIN S: Somatostatin (Second of two parts). N Engl J Med 309:1556, 1983

ROGOL AD, BLIZZARD RM: Growth hormone physiology and pathophysiology: A review. Growth Genetics & Hormones 1:1, 1985

SAWYER, WH: Neurohypophyseal hormones. Pharmacol Rev 13:225, 1961

SLADEK JR, SLADEK CD: Localization of serotonin within tanycytes of the rat median eminence. Cell Tissue Res 186:465, 1978

TIXIER–VIDAL A, FARQUHAR MG (eds): The Anterior Pituitary. New York, Academic Press, 1975

VAZQUEZ R, AMAT P: The ultrastructure of the Herring bodies in rats subjected to different experimental conditions. Cell Tissue Res 189:41, 1978

Thyroid Gland and Thyroid Follicular Cells

BOWERS CY, SCHALLY AV, REYNOLDS GA, HAWLEY WD: Interactions of L-thyroxine of L-triiodothyronine and thyrotrophin-releasing factor on the release and synthesis of thyrotrophin from the anterior pituitary gland of mice. Endocrinology 81:741, 1967

FUJITA H: Fine structure of the thyroid cell. Int Rev Cytol 40:197, 1975

INGBAR SH, BRAVERMAN LE (eds): Werner's The Thyroid. A Fundamental and Clinical Text, 5th ed. Philadelphia, JB Lippincott, 1986

NADLER NJ: Secretory process in thyroid cells. In Cantin M (ed): Cell Biology of the Secretory Process, p 423. Basel, S Karger, 1984

NADLER NJ, YOUNG BA, LEBLOND CP, MITMAKER B: Elaboration of thyroglobulin in the thyroid follicle. Endocrinology 74:333, 1964

OPPENHEIMER JH: Thyroid hormone action at the cellular level. Science 203:971, 1979

STUDER H, GREER MA: The Regulation of Thyroid Function in Iodine Deficiency. Bern, Huber, 1968

Parathyroids and C Cells of the Thyroid*

AUSTIN LA, HEATH H: Calcitonin: Physiology and pathophysiology. N Engl J Med 304:269, 1981

BUSSOLATI G, PEARSE AGE: Immunofluorescent localization of calcitonin in the "C" cells of pig and dog thyroid. J Endocrinol 37:205, 1967

COPP DH: In Bourne GH (ed): The Biochemistry and Physiology of Bone. Vol 2, p 337. New York, Academic Press, 1972

COPP DH, COCKCROFT DW, KYETT Y: Ultimobranchial origin of calcitonin, hypocalcemic effect of extracts from chicken glands. Can J Physiol Pharmacol 45:1095, 1967

COPP DH, TALMAGE RV (eds): Endocrinology of calcium metabolism. Proc 6th Parathyroid Conf, 1977. Amsterdam, Excerpta Medica, 1978

FETTER AW, CAPEN CC: The ultrastructure of the parathyroid gland of young pigs. Acta Anat 75:359, 1970

GREEP RO, TALMAGE RV (eds): The Parathyroids. Springfield, Il, Charles C Thomas, 1961

HIRSCH PF, MUNSON PL: Thyrocalcitonin. Physiol Rev 49:548, 1968

HOLTROP ME, KING GJ, COX KA, REIT B: Time related changes in the ultrastructure of osteoclasts after injection of parathyroid hormone in young rats. Calcif Tissue Int 27:129, 1979

HOLTROP ME, RAISZ LG, SIMMONS H: The effects of parathyroid hormone, colchicine and calcitonin on the ultrastructure and activity of osteoclasts in organ culture. J Cell Biol 60:346, 1974

HOWARD JE, THOMAS WC: The biological mechanisms of transport and storage of calcium. Can Med Assoc J 104:699, 1971

---

* For references on Gonadotrophins, see Selected References, Chapters 23 and 24.

* For additional references on Parathyroid Hormone and Calcitonin, see Selected References, Chapter 12.

KING GJ, HOLTROP ME, RAISZ LG: The relation of ultrastructural changes in osteoclasts to resorption in bone cultures stimulated with parathyroid hormone. Metab Bone Dis Rel Res 1:67, 1978

MACINTYRE I: Calcitonin: A general review. Calcif Tissue Res 1: 173, 1967

MARKS SC: The thyroiid parafollicular cell as the source of a potent osteoblast-stimulating factor: evidence from osteopetrotic mice. J Bone Joint Surg 51A:875, 1969

MUNGER BL, ROTH SI: The cytology of the normal parathyroid glands of man and Virginia deer. A light and electron microscopic study with morphologic evidence of secretory activity. J Cell Biol 16: 379, 1963

NUNEZ EA, GERSHON MD: Cytophysiology of thyroid parafollicular cells. Int Rev Cytol 52:1, 1978

PEARSE AGE: The cytochemistry of the thyroid "C" cells and their relationship to calcitonin. Proc R Soc Biol 164:478, 1966

PEARSE AGE, CARVALHEIRA AF: Cytochemical evidence for an ultimobranchial origin of rodent thyroid C cells. Nature 214:929, 1967

RASMUSSEN H, PECHET MA: Calcitonin. Sci Am 223:42, Oct, 1970

TALMAGE RV: The physiological significance of calcitonin. In Peck WA (ed): Bone and Mineral Research Annual, 1, p 74. Amsterdam, Excerpta Medica, 1983

TALMAGE RV, OWENS M, PARSONS JA (eds): Calcium-regulating Hormones. Proc 5th Parathyroid Conf, Amsterdam, Excerpta Medica, 1975

TALYOR S (ed): Calcitonin. Proc Symp Thyrocalcitonin and the C Cells. London, Heinemann, 1968

YOUNG BA, LEBLOND CP: The light cells as compared to the follicular cell in the thyroid gland of the rat. Endocrinology 73:669, 1963

Adrenal Gland (General) and Adrenal Cortex

BLASCHKO H, SAYERS G, SMITH AD (eds): Adrenal Gland. In Handbook of Physiology, Section 7, Endocrinology. Washington, DC, American Physiological Society, 1975

CURRIE AR, SYMINGTON T, GRANT JK (eds): The Human Adrenal Cortex. Baltimore, Williams & Wilkins, 1962

EISENSTEIN AB (ed): The Adrenal Cortex. Boston, Little Brown & Co, 1967

KOTCHEN TA, GUTHRIE GP: Renin-angiotensin-aldosterone and hypertension. Endocr Rev 1:78, 1980

IDELMAN S: Ultrastructure of the mammalian adrenal cortex. Int Rev Cytol 27:181, 1970

LONG JA, JONES AL: Observations on the fine structure of the adrenal cortex of man. Lab Invest 17:355, 1967

MOON HD (ed): The Adrenal Cortex, New York, Hoeber, 1961

PRUNTY FTG (ed): The adrenal cortex. Br Med Bull 18:89, 1962

RYAN US, RYAN JW, SMITH DS, WINKLER H: Fenestrated endothelium of the adrenal gland: Freeze-fracture studies. Tissue Cell, 7:181, 1975

SYMINGTON T: Functional Pathology of the Human Adrenal Gland. Baltimore, Williams & Wilkins, 1969

Adrenal Medulla

BROWN WJ, BARAJAS L, LATTA H: The ultrastructure of the human adrenal medulla: With comparative studies of white rat. Anat Rec 169:173, 1971

CARMICHAEL SW: The Adrenal Medulla, Vols 1 to 3. Annual Research Reviews. Montreal, Eden Press, 1979–1984

CARMICHAEL SW, WINKLER H: The adrenal chromaffin cell. Sci Am 253 No 2:40, 1985

LIVETT BG: The secretory process in adrenal medullary cells. In Cantin M (ed): Cell Biology of the Secretory Process, p 309. Basel, S Karger, 1984

WINKLER H, CARMICHAEL SW: The chromaffin granule. In Poisner AM, Trifaró JM (eds): The Secretory Granule. Amsterdam, Elsevier Biomedical Press, 1982

Pancreatic Islets

COOPERSTEIN SJ, WATKINS D (eds): The Islets of Langerhans. Biochemistry, Physiology, and Pathology. New York, Academic Press, 1981

GOMEZ–ACEBO J, PARRILLA R, R-CANDELA JL: Fine structure of the A and D cells of the rabbit endocrine pancreas in vivo and incubated in vitro. I. Mechanism of secretion of the A cells. J Cell Biol 36:33, 1968

HELLERSTRÖM C: Growth pattern of pancreatic islets in animals. In Volk BW, Wellmann KF (eds): The Diabetic Pancreas. New York, Plenum, 1977

HELLERSTRÖM C, ANDERSSON A: Aspects of the structure and function of the pancreas B-cell in diabetes mellitus. Acta Paediatr Scand (Suppl 1) 270:7, 1977

LACY PE: The pancreatic beta cell: Structure and function. N Engl J Med 276:187, 1967

ORCI L, PERRELET A: The morphology of the A-cell. In Unger RH, Orci L (eds): Glucagon: Physiology, Pathophysiology, and Morphology of the Pancreatic A-Cells, p 3. New York, Elsevier North-Holland, 1981

UNGER RH, ORCI L: Control of glucagon secretion: Within-islet controls. In Unger RH, Orci L (eds): Glucagon: Physiology, Pathophysiology, and Morphology of the Pancreatic A-Cells, p 161. New York, Elsevier North-Holland, 1981

VOLK BW, WELLMANN KF (eds): The Diabetic Pancreas. New York, Plenum, 1977

Pineal

ANDERSON E: The anatomy of bovine and ovine pineals: Light and electron microscope studies. J Ultrastruct Res (Suppl 8) May, 1965

KELLY DE: Pineal organs: Photoreception, secretion and development. Am Sci 50:597, 1962

MØLLER M: Presence of a pineal nerve (nervus pinealis) in the human fetus: A light and electron microscopical study of the innervation of the pineal gland. Brain Res 154:1, 1978

MØLLER M: The ultrastructure of the human fetal pineal gland. Cell Tissue Res 151:13, 1974

REITER RJ: The pineal and its hormones in the control of reproduction in mammals. Endocr Rev 1:109, 1980

REITER RJ (ed): The Pineal and Its Hormones. Progress in Clinical and Biological Research, Vol 92. New York, Alan R Liss, 1982

SIZONENKO PC, AUBERT ML: Neuroendocrine changes characteristic of sexual maturation. J Neurol Transm [Suppl] 21:159, 1986

WOLSTENHOLME GEW, KNIGHT J (eds): The Pineal Gland. Ciba Foundation Symposium. Edinburgh, Churchill-Livingstone, 1971

WURTMAN RJ, AXELROD J: The pineal as a neuroendocrine transducer. Hosp Pract 15 No. 1:82, 1980

WURTMAN RJ, MOSKOWITZ MA: The pineal organ. N Engl J Med 296: 1329, 1977

23

The Female Reproductive System

The female reproductive system is made up of the paired *ovaries* and *uterine tubes* (*oviducts*); the *uterus, vagina,* and *external genitalia;* and the paired *mammary glands.*

Ovaries, Ovulation, and Corpus Luteum. The *ovaries* of a sexually mature woman are somewhat flattened ovoid organs that are 2.5 cm to 5 cm long and 1.5 cm to 3 cm wide (Fig. 23-1). A fold of peritoneum called the *mesovarium* connects the anterior aspect of each ovary to the broad ligament, and an *ovarian ligament* connects the medial aspect of each ovary to the uterus (Fig. 23-1). An unusual feature of the ovaries is that they are covered with a cuboidal epithelium instead of a typical squamous mesothelium. They are each made up of a cortex and a medulla; the medulla is well supplied with blood vessels. Numerous pits and scars are present on the surface of the ovaries as a result of the liberation of secondary oocytes, which are the immediate precursors of ova. These oocytes are produced on a cyclical basis in the ovarian cortex within spherical epithelial vesicles termed *ovarian follicles.* Until a woman reaches the age of menopause, one of the follicles that are ripening each month in either of the ovaries becomes fully mature and ruptures onto the ovarian surface approximately every 28 days; this results in the liberation of a secondary oocyte, an event termed *ovulation.* The remainder of the follicle then becomes transformed into a structure called a *corpus luteum,* the endocrine function of which will be considered later in this chapter.

Unless a pregnancy occurs, the corpus luteum ceases to function only 10 to 12 days after it is formed and then begins to degenerate, subsequently becoming replaced by scar tissue. The many scars that accumulate from monthly ovulations are what cause the ovarian surface to become wrinkled and pitted. Furthermore, because it is necessary for the covering epithelium to maintain a continuous lining for the various pits and

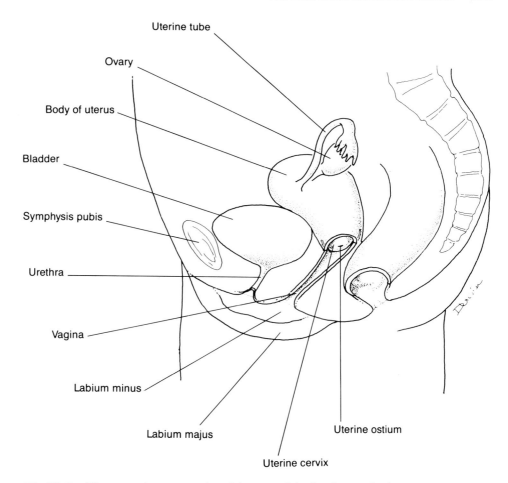

Fig. 23-1. Diagrammatic representation of the parts of the female reproductive system.

crevices, the bottom of such a crevice will occasionally become pinched off as an inclusion cyst. If pregnancy occurs, ovulation is interrupted—generally until the baby is born—and the corpus luteum that forms at the site of ovulation ordinarily continues to develop and function until approximately the middle of the third month of gestation, and by the time it degenerates, it has become large enough to leave a comparatively large scar on the ovary.

Path Taken by the Oocyte. When a mature follicle ruptures onto the ovarian surface, its secondary oocyte, together with some attached follicular cells, is extruded directly into the peritoneal cavity. As may be seen in Figure 23-1, the fimbriated, funnel-shaped proximal end of each uterine tube (L. *fimbriae*, fringe) is positioned very near its associated ovary. This expanded end of the uterine tube encompasses enough of the ovarian surface for the liberated oocyte to enter its lumen. Fluid currents created by ciliary activity and gentle waving of the fimbriae probably assist in drawing the oocyte into the uterine tube after it leaves the ovary.

The primary role of the *uterine tubes* is to convey liberated oocytes (usually only one per month) toward the uterus. Each uterine tube is provided with smooth muscle in its wall and ciliated cells in its epithelial lining. Peristaltic contractions of its muscular wall sweep toward the uterus and are mainly responsible for transporting the oocyte to the site where it will implant if fertilization occurs. Beating of cilia of the epithelial lining may also assist in transporting the oocyte, but this does not seem to be as important.

Fertilization Generally Occurs in a Uterine Tube. The mucosa of each uterine tube forms a complex arrangement of longitudinal folds with cores of lamina propria. These folds probably ensure that the oocyte remains in close contact with living cells and compatible fluids throughout its journey along the tube. They also provide similar protection for male gametes when these are introduced into the vagina, because spermatozoa can swim up the cervical canal into the body of the uterus (Fig. 23-1) and then enter uterine tubes. Indeed, it is in the maze created by the mucosal folds of a uterine tube that fertilization generally occurs (see Fig. 23-10).

Uterus, Endometrium, and Menstruation.   The *uterus* is a hollow organ with thick muscular walls. Occupying a central position in the pelvic cavity (Fig. 23-1), it has the shape of a somewhat flattened inverted pear. Its wide superior part is known as its *body*. The uppermost part of the body—the region above the level of the orifices of the uterine tubes—is known as the *fundus*. Because the body of the uterus is somewhat flattened, its central cavity is slitlike, with its anterior and posterior walls in apposition. Opening into this cavity is the canal of the *cervix*, which is the lowermost part of the uterus (Fig. 23-1). The distal end of the cervical canal opens into the *vagina* (Fig. 23-1).

The body of the uterus is lined by a mucous membrane that is provided with simple tubular glands and that is known as the *endometrium* (Gr. *metra*, womb). Approximately every 28 days, the part of the endometrium that borders on the uterine lumen breaks down and is exfoliated into the cavity of the uterus. During the process of exfoliation, which lasts approximately 4 days, the raw surface created by exfoliation bleeds. The resulting mixture of blood, glandular secretions, and degenerating endometrial tissue passes through the cervical canal and vagina as the *menstrual flow* (L. *mensis*, month). This manifestation of the exfoliation process is known as *menstruation*. Following menstruation, the endometrium regenerates. Ovulation, which is also repeated on a 28-day cycle, occurs approximately midway between menstrual periods. Menstruation becomes interrupted if fertilization and implantation occur; hence a "missed" menstrual period is a time-honored although inconclusive sign of pregnancy. Menstruation does not resume until some months after the baby is born.

Vagina, External Genitalia, and Mammary Glands.   The *vagina* (L. for sheath) is a flattened tube (Fig. 23-1) that serves as a sheath for the male organ in sexual intercourse and also constitutes the lower end of the birth canal. Its wall consists mainly of smooth muscle and fibroelastic connective tissue, and its mucous membrane is raised into transverse folds known as rugae. It is lined with a stratified squamous nonkeratinizing epithelium that also covers the portion of the uterine cervix that projects into the vagina.

The *external genitalia* are richly provided with afferent nerve endings. They consist of several structures. A mass of adipose tissue over the symphysis pubis raises the skin into a rounded eminence called the *mons pubis* or *mons veneris*, which after puberty is covered with hair. Two folds of skin, the *labia majora* (Fig. 23-1), extend posteriorly from just below the mons pubis, with the vagina opening into the cleft between them. The outer aspect of each of these folds tends to be pigmented and has many hair follicles and sebaceous glands. The inner surface also possesses hair follicles and sebaceous glands, but the hairs here are much finer. Sweat glands, too, are present. The cores of these folds contain adipose tissue and some smooth muscle.

Near the anterior end of the cleft between the labia majora lies a small body of erectile tissue called the *clitoris*,

which is the homologue of the penis. Two delicate folds of skin called the *labia minora* lie medial to the labia majora (Fig. 23-1), extending posteriorly from a point just anterior to the clitoris. The labia minora possess no hairs, but sebaceous glands and sweat glands are present on their surfaces. Although the inner surface of each fold is skin, it exhibits the pink color of a mucous membrane.

The labia minora enclose the vestibule of the vagina. In a virgin, an incomplete membranous fold called the *hymen* projects centrally from the rim of the vestibule and partly occludes the vaginal opening. A small tubuloalveolar mucus-secreting gland called a *gland of Bartholin* lies on either side of the vestibule, its duct opening into the groove between the hymen and a labium minus. Elongated masses of erectile tissue constituting the bulb of the vestibule lie beneath the surface along each side of the vestibule. Many mucous glands are present around the vestibule. The urethral orifice lies in the midline between the clitoris and the opening of the vagina.

Each of the *mammary glands* is composed of a number of compound alveolar glands that produce milk in readiness for breast-feeding. The breasts enlarge at puberty because of the deposition of adipose tissue, but they develop fully only if pregnancy occurs, as will be explained at the end of this chapter.

Some aspects of the female reproductive system that we shall consider require familiarity with the process by which female germ cells (gametes) are formed. In contrast to the early stages of spermatogenesis, the early stages of *oogenesis* (*i.e.*, the process by which ova are formed) take place *in utero*. Oogenesis nevertheless has a number of features in common with spermatogenesis, so we shall start with a general consideration of meiosis and the chromosomal basis of gametogenesis.

OOGENESIS

Typical somatic cells contain 23 pairs of chromosomes; their total of 46 chromosomes is known as the *diploid* (2n) chromosome number (see Chap. 3 under Chromosome Identification). Because germ cells receive only a single member of each chromosome pair, they have a total of 23 chromosomes, which is designated the *haploid* (n) chromosome number. Haploid germ cells are derived from diploid precursors by a two-staged division process called *meiosis* (Gr. for diminution). The *first meiotic division* (meiosis I) is a *reduction division* that results in each daughter cell having only the haploid chromosome number. The *second meiotic division* (meiosis II) is essentially a *mitotic division* that follows on from meiosis I *without intervening duplication of the nuclear DNA* (Fig. 23-2, stage 7). As will be explained in Chapter 24, in males all four of the daughter cells resulting from the first and second meiotic divisions become gametes (germ cells). In females, however, only *one ovum*

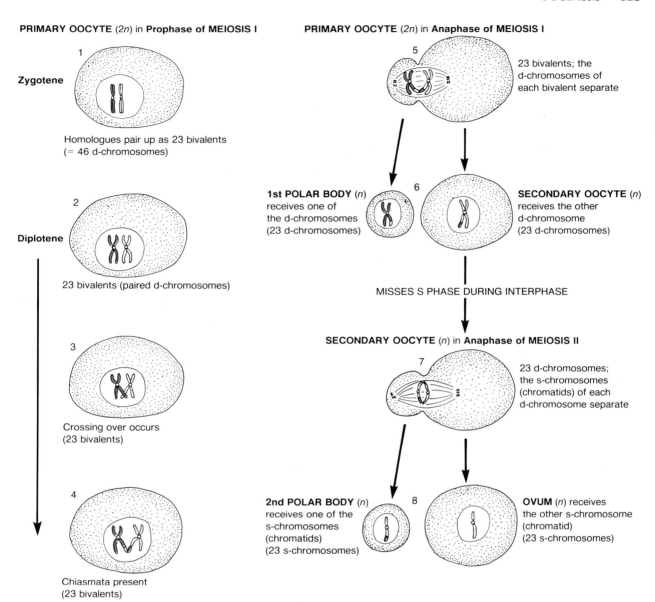

PRIMARY OOCYTE (*2n*) in **Prophase of MEIOSIS I**

1
Zygotene

Homologues pair up as 23 bivalents
(= 46 d-chromosomes)

2
Diplotene

23 bivalents (paired d-chromosomes)

3

Crossing over occurs
(23 bivalents)

4

Chiasmata present
(23 bivalents)

PRIMARY OOCYTE (*2n*) in **Anaphase of MEIOSIS I**

5

23 bivalents; the
d-chromosomes of
each bivalent separate

1st POLAR BODY (*n*)
receives one of
the d-chromosomes
(23 d-chromosomes)

6

SECONDARY OOCYTE (*n*)
receives the other
d-chromosome
(23 d-chromosomes)

MISSES S PHASE DURING INTERPHASE

SECONDARY OOCYTE (*n*) in **Anaphase of MEIOSIS II**

7

23 d-chromosomes;
the s-chromosomes
(chromatids) of each
d-chromosome separate

2nd POLAR BODY (*n*)
receives one of the
s-chromosomes
(chromatids)
(23 s-chromosomes)

8

OVUM (*n*) receives
the other s-chromosome
(chromatid)
(23 s-chromosomes)

Fig. 23-2. Schematic representation of some important stages of meiosis in females. These diagrams begin with the zygotene stage of meiosis I (stage 1). For clarity, only one representative pair of homologues is shown. During the diplotene stage of meiosis I, crossing over occurs (stage 3). The second maturation division, which produces the ovum (stages 7 and 8), is completed only if fertilization occurs. See text for details.

arises from these two consecutive divisions; the remainder of the daughter cells are much smaller cells known as *polar bodies* that rapidly degenerate (Fig. 23-2, stages 6 and 8).

Female *primordial germ cells* originate from yolk sac endoderm and migrate into the developing ovaries, where they differentiate into cells called *oogonia* (Gr. *oon,* egg; *gone,* generation). Early in fetal life, oogonia undergo a number of consecutive mitotic divisions, establishing

themselves in relatively large numbers, but most die during the course of subsequent development. The surviving population develops into larger cells called *primary oocytes.* Hence primary oocytes, which are diploid, are formed in prenatal life. At this time, primary oocytes also commence their first meiotic division (*meiosis I*). However, they do not complete this division until after puberty, and in each case, they resume the process of meiosis *on an individual basis* in any follicle that has matured to the extent that it is ready to rupture at the ovary surface.

Beginning of the First Meiotic Division. When a primary oocyte passes through S and G₂ of the cell cycle and enters the *prophase* of meiosis I, its 46 double (d-) chromosomes initially become visible at the light microscope level as long slender threads. (As explained in the Note on Terminology under Mitosis in Chapter 3, the designation *d-chromosome* has been introduced in this textbook only as a shorthand way of specifying a *double-threaded chromosome*, and *s-chromosome* is employed to specify a *single-threaded chromosome*.) The first stage of prophase is accordingly described as *leptotene* (Gr. *leptos*, slender; *tainia*, ribbon). Four other stages of prophase follow, making the prophase of meiosis I more complicated and more lengthy than its equivalent in mitosis. As noted, in females this prophase commences before birth and lasts until shortly before ovulation in each case. The second stage of prophase I is called *zygotene* (Gr. *zygon*, yoked). Unlike the process of mitosis, in zygotene the two homologues comprising each chromosome pair (and in males the X and Y chromosome combination as well) pair up and lie alongside each other (Fig. 23-2, stage 1). Each pair of chromosomes thus associated is described as a *bivalent*. Toward the end of zygotene, special ribbonlike structures called *synaptonemal complexes* develop between the paired chromosomes. These structures will be described in Chapter 24 in connection with Figure 24-5, in which they are illustrated. Their important functional role is to bring about and to maintain precise alignment between the homologous parts of the paired chromosomes so that genetic recombination can take place between them. In the third stage of prophase I, which is known as *pachytene* (Gr. *pachytes*, thickness), the two chromosomes comprising each bivalent become thicker and shorter because of further condensation of their chromatin. Furthermore, the fact that each chromosome consists of two s-chromosomes begins to become microscopically apparent. The double nature of these chromosomes is fairly obvious by the fourth stage (Fig. 23-2, stage 2), so this stage is known as *diplotene* (Gr. *diplous*, twofold). Hence, at this stage, each bivalent can be seen to consist of two d-chromosomes that will give rise to four chromatids.

Until diplotene, one homologue of each bivalent is still entirely of maternal origin and the other is still entirely of paternal origin. During diplotene, however, mutual exchange of genes between these two chromosomes occurs through the following mechanism. As shown in Figure 23-2, stage 3, part of a chromatid belonging to one chromosome of the bivalent can come to lie across a chromatid belonging to the other chromosome of the bivalent in such a way as to constitute a *chiasma* (X-shaped crossing). Where this configuration arises, it evidently predisposes both chromatids to breakage at the site where they cross each other. The broken ends thereupon rejoin, but when this happens, each broken chromatid just as readily rejoins with

the broken chromatid of the other homologue in the bivalent (Fig. 23-2, stage 4) instead of reconstituting the original (parental) arrangement. This process of *crossing over* that occurs between the homologues results in a mutual interchange of portions of their chromatids and therefore an interchange between some of the genes derived from the mother and the corresponding paternally derived genes, which achieves a recombination of the genes that are being passed on to the germ cells. Hence from the diplotene stage on, both chromosomes of a bivalent carry genes that are derived from both parents.

Prophase of meiosis I ends with a stage called *diakinesis*. At this final stage in its prenatal development, the primary oocyte enters a prolonged resting period termed the *dictyotene* stage. Dictyotene represents a suspension of the final stage of prophase until after the age of sexual maturity. For the duration of this resting period, which occurs only in oogenesis, the two chromosomes in each bivalent assume a partly extended appearance (Gr. *diktyon*, net) with the result that the nucleus, although still in prophase, now has the microscopic appearance of being in interphase.

A primary oocyte stays in suspended prophase from fetal life until just prior to ovulation, at which time it gives rise to a secondary oocyte. Women ovulate every month until menopause, which in most cases occurs at approximately the age of 45 to 55 years, so this resting period can represent a substantial length of time. As noted in connection with Chromosomal Anomalies in Chapter 3, this lengthy interruption in the time course of oogenesis is considered a contributing factor to the development of *Down syndrome* (*Trisomy 21*) because the risk of bearing a child with Down syndrome rises with an increase in maternal age at conception. Trisomy 21 is most likely to occur at the anaphase stage of meiosis I when, under ordinary circumstances, the two homologues of a bivalent would separate. Probably the bivalent of chromosome 21 never forms, and the two chromosomes remain as univalents. Univalents have an equal chance of segregating to either daughter cell; hence both chromosome 21s can finish up in the same daughter cell, giving it 24 chromosomes. Such a failure of any two homologous chromosomes to separate at anaphase and thereby segregate to both daughter cells is known as *nondisjunction*. If a secondary oocyte that possesses an extra chromosome 21 gives rise to a similar ovum that then becomes fertilized, the baby will have Down syndrome and possess 47 chromosomes (see Fig. 3-21). If an ovum that receives only 22 chromosomes becomes fertilized, it will not produce a viable fetus.

Down syndrome is not always a result of an entire extra chromosome 21; in approximately 4% of the cases, it results from the presence of only an *extra portion* of a chromosome 21. This is due to *translocation* of a segment of a chromosome 21 to another autosome, with the result that the infant receives not only the usual paired chromosome 21 but also an extra piece of a chromosome 21 attached to another chromosome (which is usually a chromosome 14 but is sometimes a chromosome 15 or, very occasionally, a chromosome 13).

Completion of the First Meiotic Division. Under the influence of pituitary gonadotrophins (which will be considered later in this chapter), the process of meiosis is resumed on an individual basis in primary oocytes that are about to give rise to a secondary oocyte in readiness for ovulation. At this time, the nuclear envelope fragments, a mitotic spindle is formed, and the cell enters metaphase I, during which all the bivalents become transversely aligned in the equatorial plane. However, another essential difference between meiosis I and mitosis now becomes apparent. The centromeres of the two chromatids that belong to each homologue of the bivalent *fail to dissociate* from each other. As a consequence, in the ensuing anaphase I the two *homologues* of each bivalent *dissociate* from each other but the two sister *chromatids* of each homologue *remain associated* (Fig. 23-2, stage 5). Hence the homologues segregate to different daughter cells, but they remain intact in the form of paired chromatids that are still attached to each other by means of their centromeres. In the case of male gametogenesis, the X and the Y chromosomes behave in the same way as a homologous pair of autosomes and likewise segregate to different cells. Segregation of a representative pair of homologues is depicted in Figure 23-2.

The net result of the *first maturation division* (Fig. 23-2, stage 5) is that each daughter cell of the primary oocyte receives an intact d-chromosome representing a pair of chromatids. This two-way allocation of the total chromosome complement results in each daughter cell receiving *23 d-chromosomes* and not the 46 s-chromosomes that would result from an ordinary mitotic division. Thus whereas the primary oocyte was *diploid*, the secondary oocyte is *haploid*. It is important to realize that the terms *haploid* and *diploid* describe the total number of chromosomes in the cell, regardless of whether they are d-chromosomes or s-chromosomes. Chromosomes that were originally of maternal or paternal origin have an equal chance of segregating to either daughter cell. A further unusual feature of the first maturation division is that the two resulting daughter cells are of unequal size. One cell, the *secondary oocyte*, is large and the other cell, the *first polar body*, is small (Fig. 23-2, stage 6). The polar body does not produce an ovum (Fig. 23-2, stage 6).

Second Meiotic Division. An important feature of the second meiotic division (meiosis II) is that the secondary oocyte enters its *second maturation division* without undergoing duplication of its nuclear DNA, that is, *in the absence of a preceding S phase* (Fig. 23-2). At metaphase II, the 23 d-chromosomes of the haploid secondary oocyte become aligned in the equatorial plane. At the ensuing anaphase II, the d-chromosomes become split at their centromeres and their two constituent chromatids separate as in ordinary mitosis (Fig. 23-2, stage 7). The net result of the second

maturation division is that each daughter cell of the secondary oocyte receives one chromatid of every d-chromosome. Thus the larger daughter cell, the *ovum*, receives 23 s-chromosomes and is again *haploid*. The smaller daughter cell, termed the *second polar body* and likewise haploid, is of no further importance to reproduction (Fig. 23-2, stage 8).

Some familiarity with the main stages of meiosis is necessary for thorough understanding of the microscopic structure of ovarian follicles and of the maturation process that occurs in these structures, as described in the following section.

OVARIES

The ovarian surface is covered with a simple cuboidal epithelium that becomes somewhat flatter in older women, although it remains cuboidal in the surface pits and crevices. The cortical connective tissue consists of spindle-shaped, fibroblastlike stromal cells, between which there are numerous fine collagen fibers. These cells and fibers are arranged in a characteristic "swirly" pattern. However, the layer of cortex immediately beneath the epithelium differs in that it has a higher proportion of intercellular substance, and its fiber bundles and cells are arranged more or less parallel to the surface. This layer is called the *tunica albuginea* (Fig. 23-3); the white appearance that its name suggests is due to its great content of intercellular substance and lack of vascularity. It becomes increasingly fibrous with age.

The medulla is small compared to the cortex, and its connective tissue is loosely arranged. It differs further in that it contains more elastic fibers, some smooth muscle cells, spiral arteries, and many convoluted veins (Fig. 23-3). Small blood vessels extend from the medulla into the cortex.

Each ovary develops from a ridge known as a *gonadal* (*genital*) *ridge* that bulges into the coelomic cavity. The surface mesodermal cells of the ridge give rise to the covering epithelium of the ovary, and cords of cells similar to the covering cells appear among the stromal cells. This is reminiscent of the development of epithelial glands, and one commonly held view is that the cords of cells appearing in the cortex at this time represent downgrowths of the surface epithelium. However, a number of alternative hypotheses have been advanced regarding their developmental origin, and these appear to be equally acceptable (see Zamboni). Primordial germ cells developing from yolk sac endoderm migrate into the cortex and become closely associated with these epithelial cords, the cells of which give rise to their investing follicular epithelial cells.

Ovarian Changes Occurring at Puberty. In girls, puberty occurs as a result of the secretion of substantial quantities of *estrogen*. This estrogen, which is the generic term for

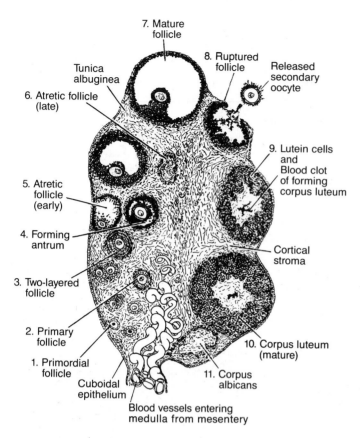

7. Mature follicle

8. Ruptured follicle

Released secondary oocyte

Tunica albuginea

6. Atretic follicle (late)

9. Lutein cells and Blood clot of forming corpus luteum

5. Atretic follicle (early)

4. Forming antrum

Cortical stroma

3. Two-layered follicle

2. Primary follicle

1. Primordial follicle

10. Corpus luteum (mature)

Cuboidal epithelium

11. Corpus albicans

Blood vessels entering medulla from mesentery

Fig. 23-3. Schematic diagram of an ovary, showing the sequence of events in the development, growth, and rupture of an ovarian follicle, and the formation and involution of a corpus luteum. (Patten BM: Human Embryology. New York, Blakiston Division of McGraw-Hill, 1946)

estradiol and other related female sex hormones, is responsible for development of the secondary female characteristics that appear at this time. Its secretion is a consequence of the ripening of a succession of ovarian follicles that, at puberty, begin to mature on a cyclical basis as a result of stimulation by *follicle-stimulating hormone* (FSH).

From the age of approximately 6 years until puberty, the FSH levels stay comparatively low; luteinizing hormone (LH) levels, which are pulsatile, are similarly of low amplitude. At this time, the main products of ovarian steroidogenesis (which will be considered later in this chapter) are estrogen precursors (androgens) rather than estrogen itself. Furthermore, the small amounts of estrogen that are produced during childhood exert a strong negative feedback on gonadotrophin secretion, acting primarily at the pituitary level and possibly at the hypothalamic level as well.

This strong inhibition by estrogen is believed to be due to a high sensitivity to estrogen negative feedback and an absence of the estrogen positive feedback mechanism that comes into effect at puberty (soon to be described). Although there is some release of gonadotrophin-releasing hormone (GnRH; see Chap. 22) during childhood, pituitary gonadotrophs remain only minimally responsive to GnRH at this time. Estrogen is thought to be only one of a number of different factors that inhibit GnRH secretion in prepubertal girls. This inhibition gradually declines as the age of puberty is approached, and follicles begin ripening to the secondary follicle stage (see below), after which they degenerate.

The onset of *puberty* is marked by a decreasing sensitivity to estrogen negative feedback, which becomes reduced to a low level from puberty onward, and the development of a positive estrogen feedback mechanism. At the same time, there is an increasing responsiveness of gonadotrophs to GnRH. Following puberty, the pulsatile secretory activity of GnRH neurons (and the resulting gonadotroph response) becomes greatly amplified and the effects of this secretory activity become much more obvious, constituting the basis for the 28-day *ovarian cycle*. For further information, see Judd; also Norman.

Ovarian Follicles

We shall now consider how the ovarian follicles develop, mature, and liberate their oocytes at ovulation.

Follicular Development. At the periphery of the ovary, just beneath its epithelial covering, there are some follicles that have not yet responded to FSH. Termed *primordial follicles* (Fig. 23-3), they contain a *primary oocyte*, approximately 25 μm to 30 μm in diameter, that is in its resting (dictyotene) stage of meiosis I. Surrounding the primary oocyte is a single layer of squamous *follicular epithelial cells*, which are alternatively known as *granulosa cells*, enclosed within their basement membrane (Fig. 23-4A).

Cyclic secretion of FSH by gonadotrophs commences at puberty. Its effect is to stimulate groups of follicles (1) to

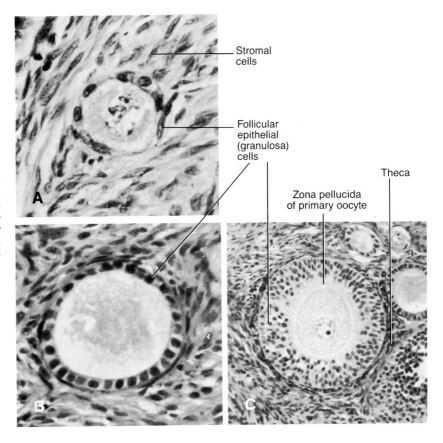

Fig. 23-4. Photomicrographs of developing ovarian follicles (dog ovary). (*A*) Primordial follicle with one layer of flattened cuboidal follicular cells. (*B*) Primary follicle with single layer of low columnar follicular cells. (*C*) Ripening follicle with stratified follicular epithelium, zona pellucida, and developing theca.

undergo further *development* and (2) to produce *estrogen* in sufficient quantity to support full female reproductive function. Every 28 days or so, approximately 20 to 50 primordial follicles respond to FSH. Their follicular cells acquire more FSH receptors and change from being flattened to having a cuboidal and then a more columnar shape (Figs. 23-3 and 23-4*B*). The primary oocytes lying within these ripening follicles enlarge and acquire a glycoprotein-containing covering of amorphous extracellular material known as the *zona pellucida* (Figs. 23-4*C* and 23-5). This outer layer is traversed by delicate cytoplasmic processes of follicular cells and also by microvilli projecting from the surface of the oocyte. Furthermore, the oocyte contains many coated vesicles, indicating macromolecular uptake from its microenvironment through receptor-mediated endocytosis (see Fig. 4-23*A*).

After a follicle has enlarged to some extent because of growth of its primary oocyte and follicular cells, it is known as a *primary follicle* (Figs. 23-3 and 23-4). The follicular cells now show evidence of a hyperplastic as well as a hypertrophic response to FSH. As the follicular epithelial cells proliferate, the walls of the follicles come to contain more than a single layer of these cells (Figs. 23-3 and 23-4*C*). In addition, the zona pellucida becomes more distinct (Fig. 23-4*C*), and the stromal cells surrounding the follicle differentiate into a capsulelike *theca* (Gr. *theke*, box; Fig.

23-4*C*). However, only one of the follicles that is beginning to mature in each cycle actually completes the process; the remainder undergo a degenerative process called *follicular atresia*. The microscopic criteria by which *atretic follicles* (Fig. 23-3) can be recognized will be considered later in this chapter. Maturation of the dominant follicle and of other follicles that have not yet become atretic continues as described below.

At the *secondary follicle* stage, tiny intercellular discontinuities filled with pools of *follicular fluid* appear among the follicular cells, which at this stage are more commonly referred to as *granulosa cells*. The spaces between the granulosa cells then coalesce until they become one space called an *antrum* that is filled with nutritive follicular fluid (Figs. 23-3 and 23-5). A *cumulus oophorus* (L. *cumulus*, heap; Gr. *oon*, egg, *phorus*, bearer) that is made up of granulosa cells supports the primary oocyte in the antrum (Figs. 23-3 and 23-5).

Which Cells Produce Estrogen? During the course of maturation of the follicle, the theca differentiates into (1) a cellular and well-vascularized inner region called the *theca interna* (Fig. 23-5*B*) that is made up of *thecal cells* with a prominent smooth-surfaced endoplasmic reticulum (sER) and mitochondria with tubular cristae, and (2) a more fibrous outer region termed the *theca externa*. These two regions of the theca blend imperceptibly with each other,

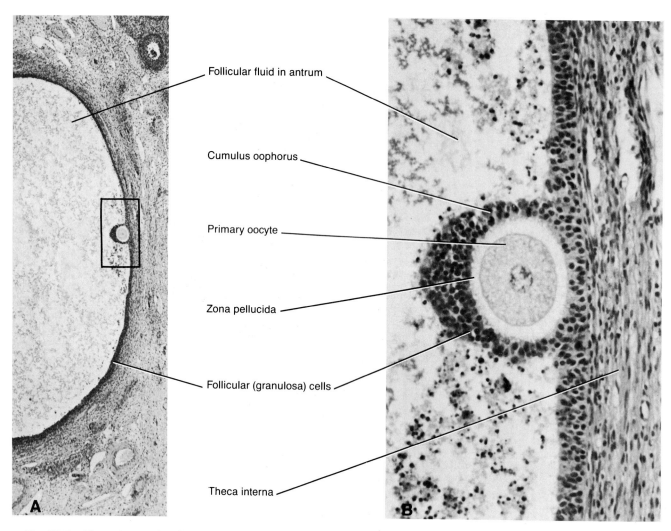

Fig. 23-5. Photomicrographs of maturing ovarian follicle. (A) Very low power. (B) Boxed-in area in A, seen under higher magnification.

making it difficult to distinguish them as distinct layers. The vascular theca interna produces the nutritive follicular fluid as a fluid exudate. Furthermore, the spindle-shaped *thecal cells* that are present in this part of the theca secrete fairly large quantities of androgen substrates. These intermediary compounds of steroid biosynthesis then pass through the follicular fluid to the nonvascularized granulosa cells, which convert them into estrogen. In addition to intrafollicular estrogen production as a result of cooperative steroidogenesis between the thecal and the granulosa cells, estrogen is produced directly by the thecal cells and passes into the numerous small blood vessels of the theca interna. Widely scattered groups of stromal secretory cells known as *interstitial cells* (sometimes referred to collectively as the *interstitial gland* of the ovary) probably also produce some of the androgen substrate that is utilized by the granulosa cells for conversion into estrogen. The interstitial cells also

synthesize some estrogen directly. For further information, see Brodie.

Follicular Maturation. The dominant follicle continues to develop until it approaches maturity, at which time it bulges from the ovarian surface as a *mature, tertiary,* or *Graafian follicle* (Figs. 23-3 and 23-5). Final maturation of the follicle is brought about by LH. *Ovulation* is triggered by a prior surge of LH, for which the preovulatory granulosa (follicular epithelial) cells and thecal cells possess receptors. The acquisition of LH receptors by the granulosa cells has been shown to be induced by FSH acting in conjunction with estrogen. The basis for the preovulatory midcycle surge of LH secretion (which is accompanied by a peak in FSH, the LH receptor inducer, as well) is described in the following section.

During the first half of the ovarian cycle (*i.e.*, the period in which the follicles are ripening under the influence of FSH; see Fig. 23-8), the GnRH neurons in the hypothalamus are producing low-amplitude pulses of GnRH with a relatively fast pulse frequency (one pulse every 1 to 2 hours). This causes the gonadotrophs to synthesize and accumulate gonadotrophins. Some FSH is released, and this brings about follicular development with resulting formation of estrogen. The rising estrogen levels in the bloodstream have the effect of promoting the accumulation of LH and FSH in the gonadotrophs. The estrogen levels rise and peak a day or so before the midcycle LH surge, and in so doing, they exceed the critical level at which estrogen begins to exert a positive feedback effect (operating primarily at the pituitary level) that induces the gonadotrophs to release their accumulated gonadotrophins. This release becomes manifested as the midcycle surge of LH that is responsible for ovulation.

During the second half of the ovarian cycle (*i.e.*, the period in which the follicles are secreting progesterone as well as estrogen), the rising progesterone levels decrease the pulse frequency but not the pulse amplitude of GnRH release. For further details, see Judd; also Norman.

Ovulation is preceded by substantial accumulation of the follicular fluid that is exuding from the theca interna, separation of the primary oocyte and its attached granulosa cells from the cumulus oophorus, and the completion of meiosis I. The secondary oocyte that is thereby produced is extruded through rupture of the mature follicle onto the ovarian surface. Still invested by attached granulosa cells that constitute a so-called *corona radiata*, the secondary oocyte enters the proximal end of the associated uterine tube (see Fig. 23-10). This cell then commences its second maturation division, which proceeds as far as metaphase II but *only reaches completion if fertilization occurs* (see Fig. 23-10).

Corpus Luteum

The next important effect of LH is that it brings about *luteinization* of the ruptured follicle. In response to LH, the remaining granulosa and thecal cells of the ruptured follicle transform into *lutein cells*. These cells constitute a relatively short-lived endocrine organ, approximately 1.5 cm to 2 cm in diameter, that is known as a *corpus luteum* because it has a yellow color due to the presence of a yellow *lutein pigment* in its lutein cells (L. *luteus*, yellow).

Development of the Corpus Luteum.   The minor bleeding that occurs during rupture and collapse of the mature follicle at ovulation results in its filling with a blood clot so as to form a so-called *corpus hemorrhagicum* (labeled *hf* in Fig. 23-6). The remains of this blood clot can later be found at the center of the corpus luteum (Fig. 23-3). In response to LH, the granulosa cells hypertrophy, acquire more sER, and become transformed into pale-staining, lipid-filled *granulosa lutein cells*. The thecal cells of the theca interna likewise become transformed into *theca lutein cells*, which have a similar microscopic appearance but are smaller and

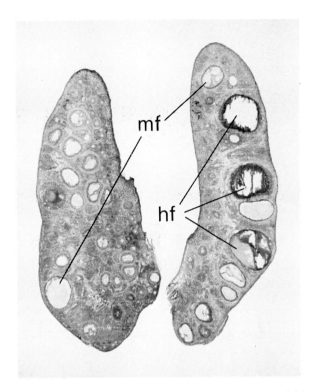

Fig. 23-6.   Photomicrograph showing mature unruptured follicles (*mf*) in the ovary at left and postovulatory hemorrhagic follicles (*hf*), known also as corpora hemorrhagica, in the ovary at right (rabbit ovaries from two different animals; very low power). In multiparous animals such as the rabbit, a number of follicles reach maturity in each ovarian cycle.

less numerous (Fig. 23-7B). Abundant capillaries and other stromal elements grow between the clumps and cords of lutein cells from the theca interna (Fig. 23-7B).

Which Cells Produce Progesterone?   The corpus luteum produces both *progesterone* and *estrogen* (Fig. 23-8) and, as was the case with estrogen secretion during follicular development, it is the *granulosa cells* (now called *granulosa lutein cells*) that produce most of the progesterone, which is the hormone that is responsible for preparing the uterine lining (endometrium) for implantation of a fertilized ovum. However, the thecal cells and the interstitial cells are also able to synthesize progesterone. Granulosa cells are also able to produce small amounts of progesterone from the androgen precursors that are supplied by the thecal cells during the preovulatory part of the ovarian cycle. The estrogen that is secreted in the postovulatory part of the cycle (Fig. 23-8) comes from the granulosa lutein cells, thecal cells, and interstitial cells. The granulosa cells continue to utilize androgen substrate from the thecal cells for the production of estrogen.

Fate of the Corpus Luteum.   The corpus luteum continues to enlarge because of hypertrophy of its lutein cells, but in the absence of fertilization, it has a lifespan of only ap-

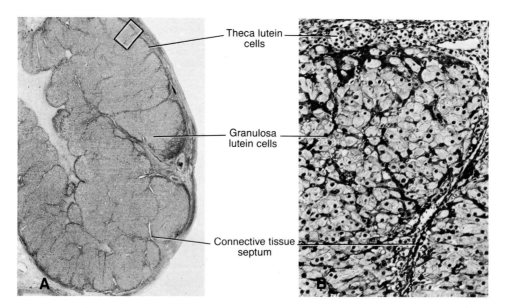

Fig. 23-7. Photomicrograph of a corpus luteum of pregnancy. (*A*) Very low power. (*B*) Boxed-in area in *A*, seen under higher magnification.

proximately 14 days (Fig. 23-8). The resulting decline in production of progesterone and estrogen (particularly the former) brings on the process of menstruation (Fig. 23-8). When the corpus luteum involutes, it is replaced by a small region of white scar tissue called a *corpus albicans* (Fig. 23-3).

If, on the other hand, *fertilization* and *implantation* both occur, the corpus luteum persists longer than 2 weeks. It grows to a diameter of approximately 5 cm and continues to secrete progesterone and estrogen in quantities that are sufficient to maintain the endometrium in a secretory condition until approximately the ninth or tenth week of gestation. After this, the placenta takes over full-scale production of progesterone and, by cooperating with the fetal adrenal cortex and fetal liver, forms the necessary amounts of estrogen as well. The extended luteal lifespan and luteal hormone secretion is brought about by the luteotrophic action of a glycoprotein hormone called *human chorionic gonadotrophin* (HCG) that is produced by the trophoblast cells of the implanted conceptus (the term used to describe the embryo and its various extraembryonic membranes). During pregnancy, the blood level of HCG rapidly rises to the level at which this hormone becomes detectable in the maternal urine, a manifestation that constitutes the basis of *pregnancy testing*. This important hormone soon takes over the role of LH in maintaining the corpus luteum of pregnancy. In approximately the third month of gestation, the large corpus luteum of pregnancy begins to involute and it eventually becomes replaced by a corpus albicans of substantial dimensions.

Summary of the Main Feedback Arrangements Relating to Ovarian Hormone Secretion.   In the *proliferative phase*

of the menstrual cycle (which will be described later in this chapter), *FSH* released from pituitary gonadotrophs brings about follicular recruitment and development (Fig. 23-8). However, estrogen production by the follicular cells of ripening follicles (with some help from thecal and interstitial cells) results in a rise in the blood *estrogen* level, and this estrogen exerts a negative feedback effect at the pituitary and hypothalamic levels on the further release of FSH. In addition, a polypeptide called *follicular inhibin (folliculostatin)* that is produced by the follicular cells is also believed to inhibit FSH release, probably by acting at the hypothalamic level as well as at the pituitary level.

Similarly, in the *secretory phase, LH* brings about *progesterone* secretion (Fig. 23-8), and in the presence of estrogen, the resulting rise in blood progesterone suppresses further LH secretion because of a negative feedback effect on the GnRH neurons in the hypothalamus. Indeed, this potent combination of progesterone and estrogen is so effective at inhibiting the secretion of GnRH that pharmacological doses of these two steroids are employed in *birth control pills* to suppress ovulation. Finally, the *midcycle surge of LH* that triggers ovulation results from *positive feedback* at the pituitary level by the high estrogen level attained at that time.

Follicular Atresia.   Ordinarily, only one of the many follicles that begin to develop in response to FSH in each cycle reaches maturity and liberates its oocyte. The remainder undergo a degenerative change known as *follicular atresia*. Such degeneration, which can happen at virtually any stage of follicular development, is believed to be a consequence of insufficient levels of FSH and LH at the time when the receptor numbers for these two gonadotro-

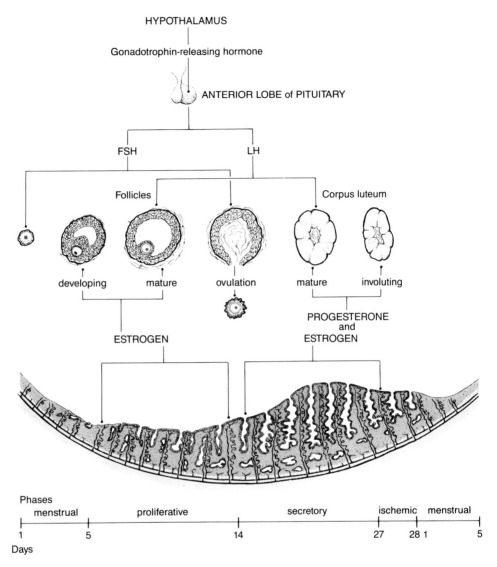

Fig. 23-8. Summary diagram of ovarian hormone secretion and its effects on the endometrium. See text for details. (After Moore KL: The Developing Human. Clinically Oriented Embryology, 3rd ed. Philadelphia, WB Saunders, 1982; modified with permission)

phins become maximal in the follicles and their associated thecae.

Although atretic follicles may at first sight look like primary, secondary, or tertiary follicles, there are also signs that their development has discontinued. The histological signs of early atresia are not as obvious as the later stages of this process in which fibroblasts invade the degenerating follicle and begin to replace it with connective tissue (Fig. 23-9). In atretic follicles, it is nevertheless often possible to recognize the absence of a blood clot (bleeding occurs only if the follicle reaches maturity and ruptures), disorganization of the normal arrangement of the follicular cells and pyknosis of their nuclei (a sign of necrosis), or shrinkage or other kinds of distortion of the oocyte or its nucleus.

Finally, we should note that the *interstitial cells* that comprise the *interstitial gland* of the ovary mentioned earlier in this chapter in connection with estrogen formation are believed to be derived from the theca interna cells of ripening follicles that have undergone atresia.

Ovarian Follicles Become Unresponsive to FSH at Menopause. After the ovaries have carried out their essential reproductive function for approximately 40 years, their function becomes sporadic. They then cease liberating oocytes and producing hormones. When ovulation is discontinued, no more corpora lutea are formed. The most obvious sign of ovarian failure is therefore that the *menses*

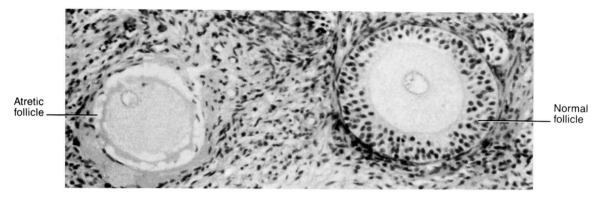

Fig. 23-9. Photomicrograph showing an atretic follicle compared with a normally developing follicle. Degeneration of the follicular cells has occurred in the atretic follicle.

(menstruations) cease, which is why this time in a woman's life is called *menopause* (Gr. *pausis,* cessation).

Menopause occurs at the average age of 51 years, and it marks the end of a woman's reproductive life. Actually, fertility declines over the decade preceding menopause. An artificial menopause occurs earlier if the ovaries are surgically removed or if their function is prematurely impaired (*e.g.,* as a result of disease or exposure to ionizing radiation).

Signs and symptoms of the onset of menopause include vasomotor disturbances that lead to the experiencing of "hot flashes." Some reduction in breast size and accelerated osteoporosis may also be noticed at this time. Particularly distressing symptoms can generally be ameliorated through the judicious administration of estrogen, generally in cyclic dosages and on the appropriate days in combination with progesterone.

The rationale for including progesterone in this regimen is as follows. Because the endometrium and breast tissue are both target tissues for estrogen, the risk exists that postmenopausal estrogen-replacement therapy will promote the growth of a developing or undetected endometrial or breast malignancy (carcinoma). In the case of endometrial cancer, progesterone has the potential to lessen this risk because one of its effects on endometrial cells is to *decrease the number of estrogen receptors* that they contain. In the normal menstrual cycle, which will be described subsequently, this action limits estrogen-induced endometrial growth by approximately the middle of the secretory phase and, some days later, withdrawal of both progesterone and estrogen starts to have functional repercussions that bring on menstruation (Fig. 23-8). Estrogen-replacement therapy is designed to mimic and perpetuate this cycle. The situation with regard to the hormone dependency of breast carcinomas is not as clear because a very high proportion and perhaps almost all of them have estrogen receptors, and some of them also possess (in various combinations) receptors for progesterone, androgens, prolactin, and other hormones as well.

It should be noted that the changes in hormone levels that occur at menopause are due to a functional exhaustion of the ovarian follicles (*ovarian failure*) and not failure of the anterior pituitary. Indeed, as the blood estrogen level falls after menopause, the negative feedback arrangements operating between FSH and estrogen result in a sufficiently increased blood level of FSH for relatively large amounts

of this hormone to appear in the urine. Histologically, postmenopausal ovaries can be recognized by their smaller size and the absence of developing or mature follicles or active corpora lutea.

Because of the lower blood level of estrogen following menopause, estrogen-dependent parts of the female reproductive tract tend to atrophy. For example, the vaginal lining can become thinner and therefore more susceptible to infections.

UTERINE TUBES

Each *uterine tube* (*Fallopian tube* or *oviduct*) has a total length of approximately 12 cm. At its proximal end, there is a fimbriated (fringed) flared region called its *infundibulum* that leads into a longer, thin-walled part called its *ampulla.* This, in turn, opens through a short and thicker walled *isthmus* into an *intramural portion* that traverses the uterine wall and opens onto its inner surface at a small uterine ostium (Fig. 23-10). A uterine tube is the usual site of both fertilization and early cleavage of the zygote (fertilized ovum). This normally reaches the blastocyst stage of development by approximately the time it enters the uterus roughly 5 days after ovulation (Fig. 23-10; see also Fig. 5-1*B*).

A labyrinth of primary, secondary, and tertiary longitudinal mucosal folds projects into the lumen of the ampulla. The isthmus has a more stellate lumen with a smaller number of simpler longitudinal folds (Fig. 23-11). The simple columnar epithelial lining of the uterine tube, the lamina propria of which is delicate and relatively vascular, is made up of ciliated cells with interspersed nonciliated secretory cells that are believed to produce a nutritive secretion. The relative and absolute heights of these cells vary in relation to cyclic variation in the levels of ovarian hormone secretion. Both kinds of cells begin to increase in height shortly after menstruation, and by the time of ovulation, they are both approximately 30 μm high. The ciliated cells then

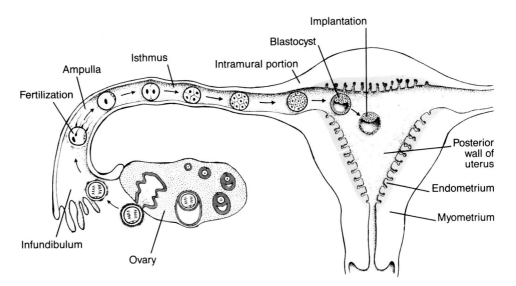

Fig. 23-10. Diagram showing the parts of a uterine tube and the transport of a cleaving zygote. (After Moore KL: The Developing Human. Clinically Oriented Embryology, 3rd ed. Philadelphia, WB Saunders, 1982; modified with permission)

become shorter than the nonciliated secretory cells, making the surface irregular. Experimental observations are at some variance with the earlier belief that the cilia of the isthmus always beat in the direction of the uterus, and it is possible that the ciliary activity of this region facilitates the transport of spermatozoa up through the isthmus as well as sweeping fluid with the liberated oocyte (or cleaving zygote) down through the ampulla.

It will be recalled that tubal peristalsis is primarily responsible for propelling the oocyte toward the uterus. Hence each uterine tube has muscular walls with a well-developed smooth muscle coat consisting of two indistinctly delineated layers of muscle, the inner one being arranged in a circular or spiral manner and the outer one being longitudinal (Fig. 23-11). The inner layer of the smooth muscle coat is particularly thick in the isthmus (Fig. 23-11*B*) and in the intramural portion of the tube. The outermost (serosal) layer of each uterine tube is a covering of peritoneal mesothelium with an underlying layer of loose connective tissue.

UTERUS

The body of the uterus has walls that are 1 cm to 1.5 cm thick and that consist mainly of smooth muscle arranged in the form of a thick muscle coat called the *myometrium.* This muscle coat is lined by a substantial mucous membrane called the *endometrium,* and it is covered by a thin serosa similar to that of the uterine tubes. The *myometrium* consists of three poorly defined layers of smooth muscle fibers; its thick middle layer is circular and the inner and outer layers are longitudinal or oblique. The middle layer of the myo-

metrium is often referred to as the *stratum vasculare* because it contains some comparatively large blood vessels.

During pregnancy, high blood levels of *estrogen* stimulate the smooth muscle fibers of the myometrium to undergo hypertrophy and hyperplasia, resulting in considerable growth of the uterus. Contraction of uterine smooth muscle is elicited by the peptide hormone *oxytocin* which is released by the posterior pituitary. Oxytocin is therefore administered clinically if it becomes necessary to induce labor to expedite childbirth.

Endometrium

The *endometrium* is the functionally important mucosal lining of the uterus. It consists of (1) a simple columnar *epithelial lining,* with (2) numerous associated simple tubular mucosal glands, the *endometrial glands,* that extend down almost to the myometrium, and (3) an *endometrial stroma* representing a substantial lamina propria. Some of the columnar surface epithelial cells are ciliated, and the remainder bear microvilli. The endometrium is functionally described as being made up of a relatively thick superficial region known as its *functional layer,* which exfoliates at menstruation, and a thin *basilar layer,* which is retained and subsequently regenerates a new functional layer.

The Endometrium Undergoes Cyclic Changes That Are Referred to as the Menstrual Cycle. The functional characteristics and microscopic appearance of the functional layer of the endometrium vary from one phase of the menstrual (uterine) cycle to the next. Like the ovarian cycle, the *menstrual cycle* is conventionally regarded as having a total duration of 28 days, but this can vary by a few days (Fig. 23-8). The length of menstrual cycles may not even

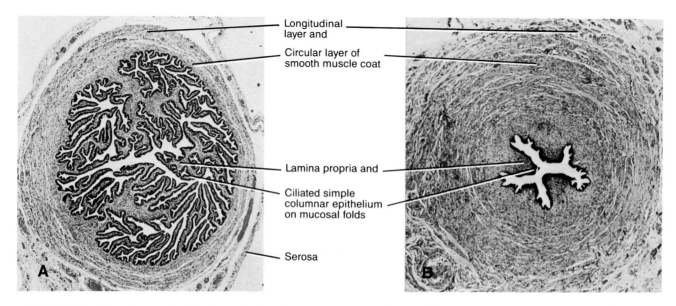

Fig. 23-11. Photomicrographs of uterine tube (very low power). (*A*) Ampulla. (*B*) Isthmus.

be consistent in the same woman. It is customary to number the days of the cycle from the *first day of menstruation;* this is a concession to medical practice because the first day of menstruation is generally a date that patients easily recall. The process of menstruation commonly lasts for 4 days, but it can be a day or so shorter or longer.

The first 4 or 5 days of the menstrual cycle constitute the *menstrual phase.* This is followed by the *proliferative (estrogenic, follicular) phase,* which lasts for approximately 9 days. At this time, the endometrium doubles or triples in thickness as a result of cellular *proliferation.* This regenerative phase is brought about by the *estrogen* being produced at this time by the ripening ovarian follicles (Fig. 23-8). The latter portion of the proliferative phase, although not easy to define in terms of duration or days of the cycle, is sometimes referred to as the *interval phase* because the endometrium is fully regenerated but its glands have still not begun to secrete. Ovulation occurs at some time in the second or third week of the cycle and is conventionally assigned to day 14 (Fig. 23-8).

Following ovulation is the *secretory (progestational or progravid) phase,* which lasts for approximately 13 days. During this phase, the endometrial glands begin to *secrete* and the endometrium continues to thicken (Fig. 23-8). In this phase, the endometrium comes under the influence of increased levels of *progesterone* (in combination with estrogen) from the corpus luteum (Fig. 23-8). When the corpus luteum begins to regress after approximately 12 days, there is a marked decline in these ovarian hormone levels. At this point, the endometrium enters the *ischemic phase,* which lasts for approximately a day (Fig. 23-8). During this phase, the functional layer of the endometrium undergoes sporadic episodes of cessation of its local blood supply that

result in periods of intermittent hypoxia. Resulting ischemic necrosis of the functional layer of the endometrium leads to its exfoliation during the ensuing *menstrual phase,* which signals the beginning of the next menstrual cycle (Fig. 23-8).

At any given phase of the menstrual cycle, the histological appearance of the endometrium closely reflects the pattern of hormone secretion that is occurring in the ovaries. Thus in the proliferative phase, when the endometrial cells are being acted upon mainly by estrogen, the epithelial cells and the stromal cells still present in the persisting basilar layer undergo hormone-induced proliferation, and the regenerating epithelial cells migrate from the tops of the regenerating glands to cover the denuded surface that is left at the end of menstruation. At this stage, *mitotic figures* can be found among the stromal cells as well as among the epithelial cells. A morphological characteristic of the proliferative phase is that the endometrial glands are relatively straight and narrow, and their cells are fairly dark staining (Fig. 23-12*A*); in addition, the stroma in which the glands are embedded is highly cellular.

In response to the substantial levels of progesterone that are secreted together with estrogen in the second half of the menstrual cycle (Fig. 23-8), the endometrial glands show evidence of active *secretion.* They also widen, take on a sacculated appearance, and become irregularly coiled or tortuous (Fig. 23-12*B*). This sacculation can give them a ladderlike appearance when they are seen cut in tangential section. The glandular secretory cells hypertrophy and become pale staining because of the accumulation of considerable amounts of *glycogen* (Fig. 23-13*A*). Eventually they become somewhat ragged in appearance because of their abundant content of this storage product (Fig. 23-13*B*). The

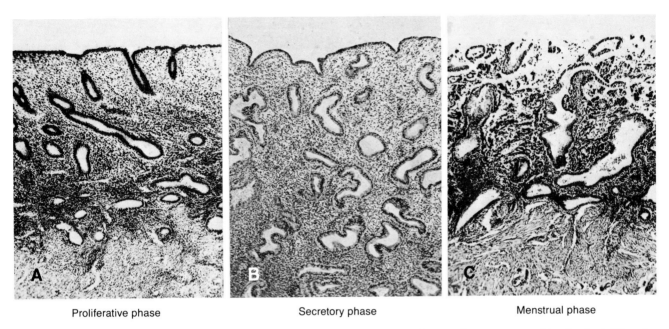

| Proliferative phase | Secretory phase | Menstrual phase |

Fig. 23-12. Photomicrographs of endometrium, showing the appearance of its glands at different phases of the menstrual cycle (very low power). See text for details.

copious viscid secretion that these cells produce is rich in glycogen; hence the endometrium provides a highly suitable nutritive environment when a blastocyst implants. Further characteristics of the secretory phase are that the stroma becomes increasingly vascular, its blood vessels elongate, and excess tissue fluid accumulates between the stromal cells.

The episodes of intermittent *ischemia* (Gr. *ischo*, to keep back; *haima*, blood—meaning reduced blood supply) that occur in the functional layer of the endometrium at the end of the secretory phase are due to falling levels of ovarian hormones and are primarily a response to the decline in the blood level of progesterone. Their occurrence is related to the distinctive vascular supply of the endometrium, which is as follows. Arterial blood is brought to the endometrium by small branches of the uterine artery. Near the border where the myometrium meets the endometrium, each of these branches gives rise to a few straight branches that supply the basilar layer of the endometrium. In addition, each small branch of the uterine artery gives rise to a *spiral (coiled) artery* that supplies the functional layer of the endometrium (Fig. 23-8, *bottom*). The spiral arteries lengthen as the endometrium doubles in thickness during the secretory phase (Fig. 23-8). However, once the endometrium regresses because of the subsequent decline in ovarian hormone levels, these elongated spiral arteries are now too long to fit into the tissue and they buckle and kink. The resulting deformation of these vessels induces episodes of sustained vasoconstriction that result in ischemic necrosis of the regions that they supply. Consequent

damage to the walls of the spiral arteries and other vessels in the functional layer also results in prolonged bleeding when these arteries open up again. This ischemic (premenstrual) phase is therefore characterized by the presence of small pools of extravasated blood in the stroma, and also by the invasion of already necrotic endometrial tissue by neutrophils. Exfoliation of the necrotic endometrial tissue (Fig. 23-12C) and endometrial bleeding onto the raw surface, which occurs without clotting of the blood, manifests itself as *menstrual bleeding*. The basilar layer remains unscathed by the process because it has its own independent and uninterrupted blood supply.

On occasion, women will experience bleeding from the endometrium at the usual time for menstruation *without ovulation having occurred*, that is, without development of a corpus luteum. At least some of these instances of *anovulatory menstruation* are due to declining blood levels of estrogen. The bleeding that occurs is believed to be a delayed response to the reduction in estrogen output from the ovaries that occurs after the dominant follicle has matured. Anovulatory cycles are probably not as uncommon as once thought; a healthy woman may have three or four such cycles a year, the proportion being higher near puberty and menopause.

If *implantation* occurs, the stromal cells of the endometrium enlarge and accumulate glycogen and lipid in response to increasing progesterone levels. This change is described as the *decidual reaction* (the L. word *deciduus*, meaning a falling off, refers to the membrane that forms from the functional layer of the endometrium during pregnancy and that is cast off at the time of birth).

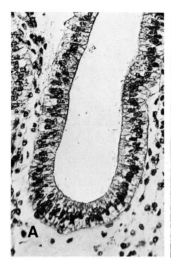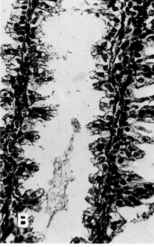

Fig. 23-13. Photomicrographs of the basal regions of endometrial glands (medium power). (*A*) Early secretory phase. Glycogen spaces are present, especially at the bases of the cells. (*B*) Late secretory phase. The gland has a sacculated, ladderlike appearance.

PLACENTA

The *placenta,* which is commonly described as having the form of a floppy flat cake (L. *placenta,* cake), is approximately 3 cm thick and reaches a diameter of approximately 20 cm. Although primarily fetal in origin, it also possesses a maternal component. The *fetal portion* of the placenta arises from the *chorion,* which is one of the extraembryonic membranes of the conceptus. The *maternal portion* is derived from the *decidua basalis,* which is the region of endometrium that underlies the site of implantation. The main functional importance of the placenta is that it is the site of interchange of blood-borne substances between the maternal and the fetal bloodstreams, for example, nutrients, blood gases (see Fig. 23-16), hormones, by-products of metabolism, humoral antibodies of the IgG class, and any drugs (alcohol, caffeine, etc.) or viruses that may be circulating in the maternal blood. In addition, the placenta itself serves as a major source of certain hormones during the course of pregnancy.

To be able to interpret what is seen in a section of the placenta, it is necessary to know something about the way in which the placenta develops.

Development of the Placenta. By the late blastocyst stage of development, the cells of the morula (Fig. 23-14*A*) have given rise to (1) an *inner cell mass* from which the embryo will develop and (2) an outer layer of *trophoblast cells* (Gr. *trophein,* to nourish; *blastos,* germ) that encloses the blastocyst cavity (Fig. 23-14*B*). In most cases, the blastocyst implants high on the posterior uterine wall (Fig. 23-10). The trophoblast cells are highly invasive and enable the conceptus to implant by eroding the endometrium (Fig. 23-14*C*). Their name is derived from their key role in obtaining nourishment for the developing embryo, that is, the fact that they enable the blastocyst to embed itself deeply in the progesterone-primed secretory endometrium and thereby to obtain an adequate supply of nutrients through the eroded glands and vessels of this layer. The endometrial defect caused by implantation is sealed by a temporary *closing coagulum* of fibrin and cellular debris that suffices until endometrial epithelium grows over the implantation site (Fig. 23-14*D*).

Continuing proliferation of the trophoblast cells leads to the development of two layers, an inner pale-staining layer of individual cells called the *cytotrophoblast* (Fig. 23-14*D*) and an outer, darker staining layer called the *syncytiotrophoblast* (Fig. 23-15). The syncytiotrophoblast constitutes a *syncytium* (Gr. *syn,* together; Fig. 23-14*D*), which means that all its cells fuse together as one continuous mass of multinucleated cytoplasm that lacks any cell boundaries. The cytotrophoblast, on the other hand, remains constituted of individual cells (Fig. 23-15*A*). The syncytiotrophoblast continues to grow and invade the endometrium as irregularly shaped protrusions. Between these protrusions, there are open spaces called *lacunae* (Fig. 23-14*D*) that are filled with maternal blood from the uterine veins and venous sinuses that the syncytiotrophoblast has eroded. Cytotrophoblast then begins to grow into these protrusions in the form of fingerlike extensions; the two layers form structures that are known as *primary placental villi.* Then mesenchyme also grows into their middle and gives rise to a core of loose connective tissue (Fig. 23-15), the blood capillaries of which become a part of the embryonic circulatory system.

Tufted invasive extensions grow from the part of the chorion that is associated with the decidua basalis. These extensions are known as *chorionic villi* (Figs. 23-16 and 23-17) because the trophoblast and its associated connective tissue (which arises from extraembryonic somatic mesoderm) comprise the *chorion.* They soon develop into numerous large and irregularly shaped branching outgrowths of what is termed the *villous chorion.* Some of the chorionic villi, which are all confined to a disklike area of the chorion known as the *chorionic plate* (Fig. 23-16), become anchored to the decidua. The expansive arrangement of chorionic villi is continually bathed with maternal blood that circulates through the *intervillous space* (Fig. 23-16), an extensive cavernous sinus that results from enlargement of the blood lacunae and their coalescence to form one continuous space. This blood is admitted to the intervillous space primarily from eroded spiral arteries; it leaves by way of eroded endometrial veins. At approximately the midpoint of the gestation period, the cytotrophoblast layer begins to disappear, and by term almost all its cells have fused with the syncytiotrophoblast.

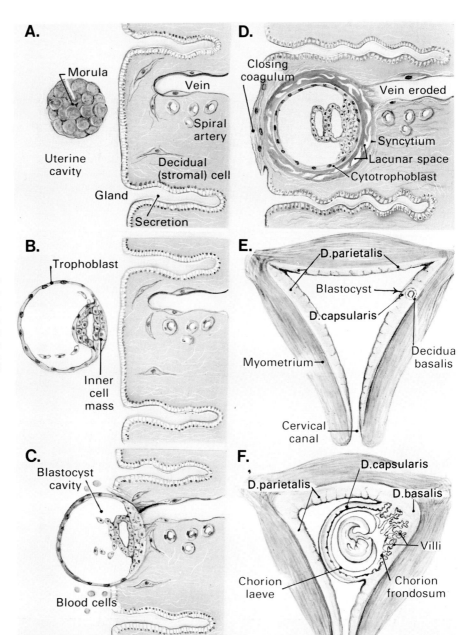

Fig. 23-14. Schematic diagram of implantation and development of the fertilized ovum. *A, B, C,* and *D* illustrate stages in formation of the blastocyst and embedding of the blastocyst in the uterine wall. The relation of the growing embryo to the deciduae of the uterus is shown in *E* and *F.*

The Deciduae. The functional layer of the endometrium is destined to be shed when a baby is born and in this context is referred to as the *decidua* (Fig. 23-14*E* and *F*). The names of the various areas of the decidua refer to their positions relative to the site of implantation.

The *decidua parietalis* (*parietal* means *forming,* or *situated on, a wall*) lines the entire pregnant uterus except where the placenta is forming (Fig. 23-14*F*).

The *decidua capsularis* is the portion of endometrium superficial to the developing embryo: it forms a *capsule* over it (Fig. 23-14*E* and *F*). As the embryo becomes larger, the decidua capsularis becomes thin and atrophic. The chorionic sac that contains the embryo becomes so large that the decidua capsularis comes into contact with the decidua parietalis at the opposite surface of the uterus; hence the uterine cavity is obliterated. The decidua capsularis thereupon blends with the decidua parietalis and disappears as a separate layer.

The *decidua basalis* is the zone of endometrium that lies between the chorionic sac and the basal layer of endometrium (Figs. 23-14*E* and *F,* 23-16, 23-17, and 23-18). The decidua basalis becomes the maternal part of the placenta. This is the only part of the placenta of maternal origin. After the placenta is delivered at term, this layer is visible only as poorly defined bits of membrane.

The entire surface of the chorionic sac is at first covered with

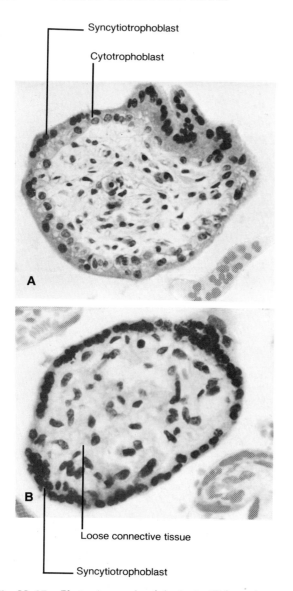

Syncytiotrophoblast

Cytotrophoblast

A

B

Loose connective tissue

Syncytiotrophoblast

Fig. 23-15.   Photomicrographs of chorionic villi from placentas obtained (*A*) in the second trimester of a pregnancy and (*B*) at full term. See text for details.

chorionic villi. As the sac enlarges, those villi associated with the decidua capsularis degenerate and disappear, so that by week 16, most of the surface of the sac is smooth. This large area is called the *chorion laeve* (L. *levis*, smooth) (Figs. 23-14*F*, 23-17, and 23-18). The remainder of the surface of the sac, that is, the part adjacent to the decidua basalis, continues to be covered with villi that keep growing and branching. This part, which constitutes the fetal part of the placenta, is called the *chorion frondosum* (Fig. 23-14*F*).

The Layers That Constitute the Placental Barrier. Throughout the first half of gestation, six components separate the fetal circulation from the maternal circulation. Comprising what is termed the *placental barrier,* these components are as follows. First, both the chorionic villi and the chorionic plate are entirely covered by (1) the *syncytiotrophoblast,* which is characterized by numerous comparatively small and dark-staining nuclei, and (2) an underlying layer of *cytotrophoblast cells* (Fig. 23-15*A*). Internal to these two outermost layers of the fetal portion of the placenta there are (3) the underlying trophoblastic *basement membrane,* and (4) the fetal *loose connective tissue* that constitutes the core of each villus. The two remaining components of the barrier are (5) the *endothelium* of the fetal capillaries (Fig. 23-15*A*) and (6) its surrounding *basement membrane.* At full term, however, the cytotrophoblast layer is reduced to small fragments, so by then the placental barrier really only consists of five fetal components instead of six (Fig. 23-15*B*).

In the EM, it can be seen that the *cytotrophoblast cells* contain abundant ribosomes and some mitochondria and glycogen, but they lack stored lipid (Fig. 23-19). These cells remain poorly differentiated in comparison with the syncytiotrophoblast. The underlying basement membrane is nevertheless well developed (Fig. 23-19). The syncytiotrophoblast has an irregular outer border that bears numerous microvilli (Fig. 23-19). Its fused mass of cytoplasm contains numerous lipid droplets (Fig. 23-19), a fairly extensive rough-surfaced endoplasmic reticulum, Golgi saccules, and mitochondria. These lipid droplets can be very large and abundant early in pregnancy, but later they become smaller and less numerous. Glycogen is either absent or present only in small amounts. When the cytotrophoblast layer is no longer present, the syncytiotrophoblast rests on a condensed network of reticular fibers.

A point of interest is that during pregnancy small protuberances of the syncytiotrophoblast known as *syncyctial sprouts* can break off from the placenta and enter the maternal circulation, whereupon they are inclined to lodge in the mother's lungs. Here they are rapidly destroyed by local enzyme action and consequently present no clinical problem.

Several Important Hormones Are Produced by the Placenta. The syncytiotrophoblast is thought to be the placental source of *human chorionic gonadotrophin* (HCG), which is the glycoprotein gonadotrophic hormone that maintains the corpus luteum of pregnancy by mimicking the luteotrophic action of LH during the first few months of gestation. The same layer of the placenta is also believed to be the site of production of *human chorionic somatomammotrophin* (HCS), a placental protein hormone that is primarily lactogenic in action but also has a minor amount of growth-promoting activity. In addition, the steroid hormones *progesterone* and *estrogen* are produced by the placenta, but placental formation of estrogen requires the cooperation of the fetal adrenal cortex and also the fetal liver.

UTERINE CERVIX

The comparatively narrow inferior portion of the uterus is known as the uterine *cervix* (L. for neck). It opens into the

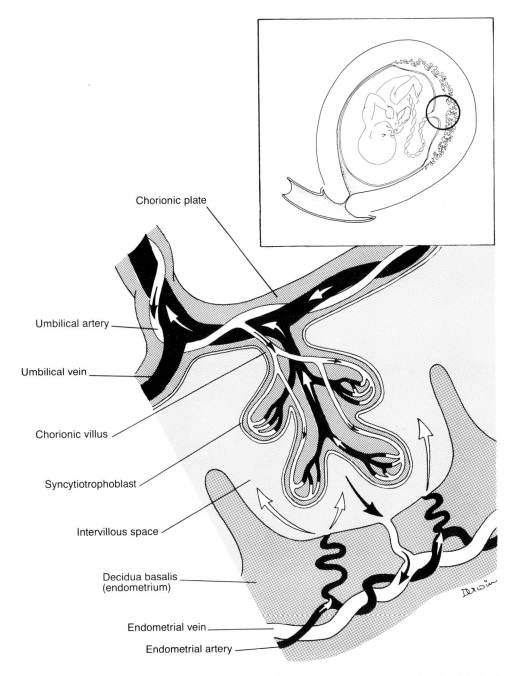

Chorionic plate

Umbilical artery

Umbilical vein

Chorionic villus

Syncytiotrophoblast

Intervillous space

Decidua basalis
(endometrium)

Endometrial vein

Endometrial artery

Fig. 23-16. Schematic representation of the general organization of the placenta, showing details of the area indicated in the inset. Oxygenated blood is indicated in black.

upper end of the vagina by way of the *uterine ostium* (Fig. 23-1). In addition to being the narrowest part of the uterus, the cervix undergoes little or no expansion during pregnancy; hence a considerable degree of cervical dilatation needs to occur during childbirth. Furthermore, the walls of the cervix consist chiefly of dense ordinary connective tissue, with comparatively little smooth muscle. In the later stages of pregnancy, this dense fibrous tissue undergoes a

softening-up process. Experimental evidence in other mammals suggests that this necessary change is brought about by a polypeptide hormone called *relaxin* that is believed to be secreted primarily by the corpus luteum of pregnancy, perhaps with lesser amounts coming from the decidua as well. Relaxin is also believed to expedite parturition by inducing some slackening of the pubic symphysis.

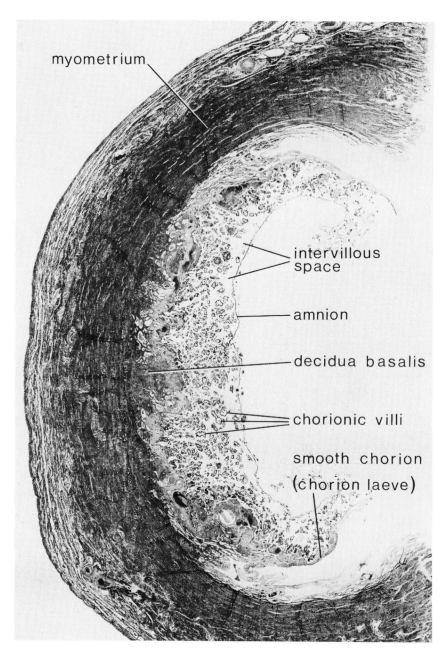

myometrium

intervillous
space

amnion

decidua basalis

chorionic villi

smooth chorion
(chorion laeve)

Fig. 23-17. Photomicrograph of part of the uterus, with placenta *in situ* (very low power). (Courtesy of J. Boyd and W. Hamilton)

However, the precise role of relaxin in facilitating childbirth is not clear. For example, relaxin levels seem to decline as term approaches, and pelvic relaxation is very variable from one pregnant woman to another. Experimental evidence suggests that both fibroblast and osteoclast function may be affected by this hormone and that its action may involve some change in the state of aggregation of collagen fibrils. There are indications that the fibrocartilage of the pubic symphysis becomes replaced by a more flexible type of connective tissue that is better adapted to accommodate the widening birth canal. Presumably, the dense fibrous tissue of the uterine cervix undergoes the same sort of change to facilitate childbirth. For further information, see Schwabe et al.

The flattened *cervical canal* (Fig. 23-20) is lined with a pale-staining simple columnar *mucus-secreting epithelium* that possesses some ciliated cells. Branched tubular mucous glands lined with the same type of epithelium extend into its fibrous lamina propria, and it possesses elaborate mucosal ridges and folds that account, at least in part, for its glandular appearance (Fig. 23-20). The cervical canal is filled with mucus that is produced by the epithelial lining

(Fig. 23-21). Stratified squamous nonkeratinizing epithelium also covers the part of the cervix that projects into the vagina (Fig. 23-1).

In some instances this squamocolumnar junction lies farther up the cervical canal, whereas in others the columnar epithelium of the canal continues out from uterine ostium and covers small areas of the vaginal surface of the cervix close to the ostium. In the latter case, the small areas of simple columnar epithelium are known as *physiologic erosions*. (The stratified squamous nonkeratinizing epithelium that generally covers the cervix gives it a pink-gray color whereas simple columnar epithelium makes it appear red, hence the misnomer *erosion*.) A contributing factor to the development of such "erosions" is the fact that the uterine ostium sometimes becomes somewhat everted as a result of childbearing, and this eversion tends to expose the columnar epithelium. The clinical relevance of the squamocolumnar junction is that it is the site where most precancerous lesions and carcinomas of the cervix develop.

VAGINA

The *vagina* is a sheathlike and fibromuscular-walled tube that opens onto the body surface (Fig. 23-1). Its lumen is flattened anteroposteriorly; hence under most circumstances its anterior and posterior mucosal surfaces lie in contact with each other. Also, except in the upper part of the vagina, a longitudinal ridge extends along the apposed anterior and posterior surfaces. Between these longitudinal ridges, there are numerous transverse mucosal ridges called *rugae*.

The lining epithelium of the vagina is stratified squamous nonkeratinizing epithelium, which in adult women is fairly thick. However, prior to puberty and after menopause, this epithelium is quite thin because of low levels of stimulation by estrogen, and as a consequence, vaginal infections are not uncommon during childhood. This part of the reproductive tract is not provided with any glands of its own, but it is kept moist by mucus that drains down from the cervical glands and cervix by way of the cervical canal. A plexus of small veins is present in the outer region of the fibroelastic lamina propria that underlies the epithelium, and this gives the layer a fairly vascular appearance (Fig. 23-22).

External to the lamina propria, there is a smooth muscle coat that has some circularly arranged bundles of muscle in its poorly defined inner region with more numerous longitudinally arranged bundles of muscle in its outer region (Fig. 23-22). There are also some circularly arranged skeletal muscle fibers encircling the vaginal orifice. The outermost layer of the vagina is a fibrous adventitia that attaches the vagina to the urethra and also to other adjacent organs. The superior part of the posterior wall of this organ is a serosal surface that is covered with peritoneal mesothelium.

When the vaginal epithelium is being acted upon by estrogen, it shows some tendency to thicken as a result of mitosis occurring in its basal layer and also in the adjacent

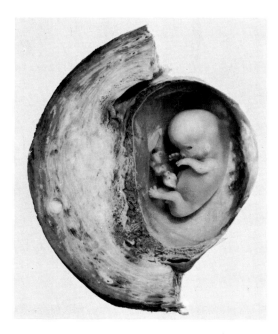

Fig. 23-18. Photograph of part of the uterine wall with attached placenta, fetus, and fetal membranes. At lower right, the wall of the chorionic sac (in which the fetus lies) is smooth. This is the chorion laeve. At center, the fetal part of the placenta is formed by the chorion frondosum. (Courtesy of J. Boyd and W. Hamilton)

and its associated glands. This mucus varies somewhat in viscosity and amount according to the cyclic changes in ovarian hormone levels that occur during the course of the menstrual cycle. Thus when secreted under the influence of the high levels of estrogen that are attained toward the time of ovulation, this mucus is copious and it has a fairly thin consistency that makes it relatively easy for spermatozoa to enter the cervical canal. Following ovulation, however, the cervical mucus becomes noticeably thicker and more viscid and hence more difficult to penetrate. This change in its consistency is a reflection of the influence of progesterone on its secretion.

Cervical glands occasionally become closed off, whereupon they can give rise to cysts called *nabothian follicles*. Such cysts may cause elevations on the surface of the part of the cervix that projects into the vagina, and these elevations may be seen or palpated on vaginal examination.

The mucosal layer of the uterine cervix is not exfoliated in the menstrual flow because its lamina propria is not provided with spiral arteries as in the body of the uterus. Hence the intermittent endometrial ischemia that characterizes the premenstrual part of the menstrual cycle does not affect the uterine cervix.

A short distance above the level of the uterine ostium (the external os of the cervix), the epithelium changes abruptly from the simple columnar mucus-secreting lining that is seen in the cervical canal to the stratified squamous nonkeratinizing epithelium lining that is seen in the vagina

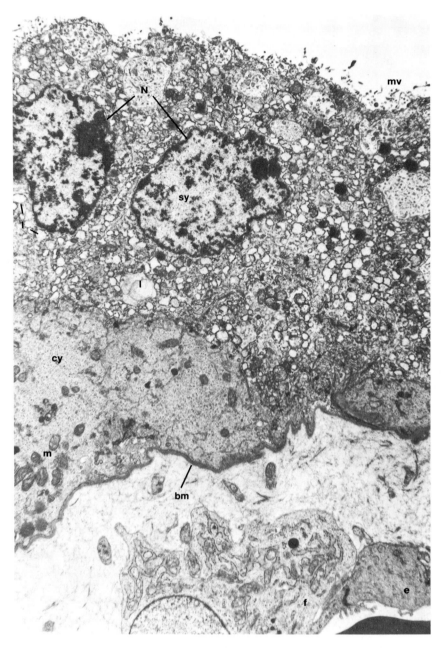

Fig. 23-19. Electron micrograph of the syncytiotrophoblast and underlying cytotrophoblast of the placenta (biopsy of human placenta, first trimester). The syncytiotrophoblast (*sy*) is a multinucleated mass of cytoplasm, two nuclei (*N*) of which are seen in this micrograph. It contains numerous lipid droplets (*l*) and has some microvilli (*mv*) on its free border. Beneath the syncytiotrophoblast, there is a less highly differentiated layer of individual cytotrophoblast cells (*cy*) with mitochondria (*m*) and numerous ribosomes. This inner layer is attached to the underlying connective tissue by a thick basement membrane (*bm*). Parts of a fibroblast (*f*) and of a capillary endothelial cell (*e*) are also present in the loose connective tissue at the bottom of the micrograph. (Courtesy of L. Asa and D. McComb)

layer (which is known as its parabasal layer). It also exhibits some relatively minor but characteristic cytological changes. Thus the more superficial cells, which in this type of epithelium are still nucleated, appear more acidophilic when the time of ovulation is approaching. This change in their appearance can be recognized on cytological examination of smears made of exfoliated vaginal cells. The increased acidophilia in these cells is believed to indicate that they are beginning to undergo keratinization, but under normal circumstances, this is as far as the process usually goes. There are also other criteria that can be employed. The

study of desquamated vaginal cells in smears can be helpful in determining the time of ovulation and the effectiveness of estrogen therapy, and in diagnosing atrophic conditions of the vaginal epithelium due to estrogen deficiency.

Advantage is taken of the ability of estrogen to thicken and even to keratinize the vaginal epithelium in the treatment of certain vaginal infections, particularly those that occur before puberty, because in young girls this epithelium is thin and vulnerable.

Another effect of estrogen on vaginal epithelial cells is that it promotes their storage of glycogen and lipid, which

Cervical glands

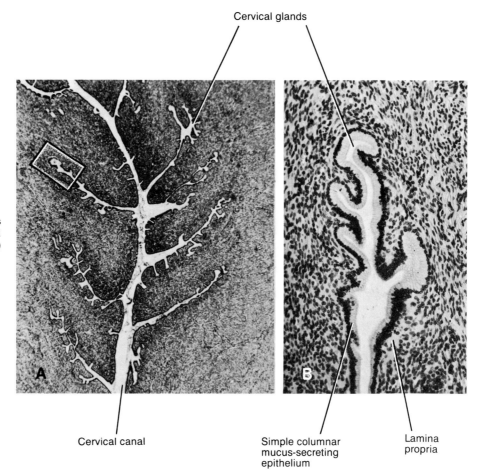

Fig. 23-20. Photomicrographs of uterine cervix. (*A*) Cervical canal and glands (very low power). (*B*) Cervical gland (medium power).

Cervical canal

Simple columnar mucus-secreting epithelium

Lamina propria

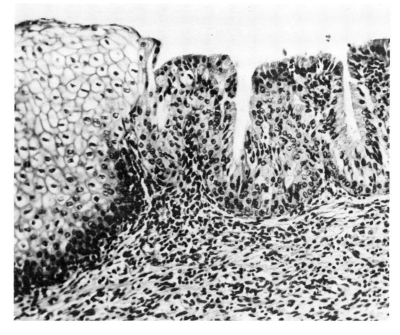

Fig. 23-21. Photomicrograph of a longitudinal section of the cervix, near the site where the cervical canal opens into the vagina. The stratified squamous nonkeratinizing epithelium that covers the vaginal portion of the cervix, and extends for a very short distance into the canal, is seen at left, and the columnar epithelium that lines the remainder of the canal is seen at right. The junction between the two types of epithelium is seen midway between left and center.

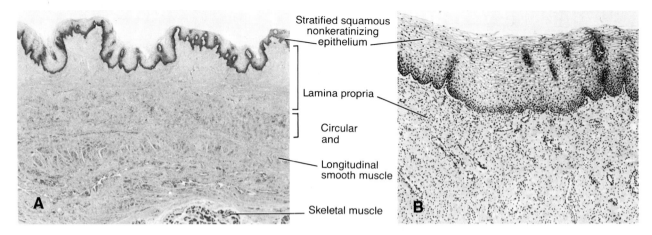

Fig. 23-22. (*A*) Photomicrograph of wall of the vagina (very low power). (*B*) Photomicrograph of glycogen-containing epithelium and vascular lamina propria of the vagina (higher magnification).

makes them appear swollen, empty, and pale in hematoxylin and eosin sections (Fig. 23-22). Their glycogen content becomes maximal at the time of ovulation. It is possible that this stored glycogen serves as a source of nutrients for spermatozoa when these have been introduced into the vagina, but its usual role is to give rise to lactic acid as a result of bacterial fermentation, and the acid conditions thus produced help to maintain a suitable microflora in the lumen.

Finally, a number of surface cells become desquamated from the vaginal epithelium during the secretory phase of the menstrual cycle, but not enough cells are lost to affect the appearance of this epithelium in sections.

Vaginal Smears. Cells for cytological evaluation can be obtained from the vagina fairly readily. Such cells may be derived from (1) the endometrium of the body of the uterus, (2) the cervical canal, or (3) the vaginal surface of the cervix or the lining of the vagina. Their study may be informative for two reasons. (1) Because the appearance of the cells of these various sites is affected by hormone levels, the cells in vaginal smears may give some information about the hormone balance of the woman at the time they are obtained; and (2) cells indicative of having desquamated from an early cancer, growing in the cervix or the body of the uterus, may sometimes be found during an otherwise routine check of a patient and so indicate the need for more detailed examination for cancer. For both reasons, it has become common practice to study cells obtained by gently wiping the lining of the vagina or the covering of the cervix and/or cells aspirated or otherwise obtained from the lower part of the cervical canal.

MAMMARY GLANDS

The paired *mammary glands* (*breasts*) each consist of up to 20 or so individual *compound alveolar glands* that have separate openings onto a conical surface elevation of the breast termed the *nipple*. By the time of birth, a *rudimentary duct*

system has formed in each breast, but breast development becomes arrested at this stage. Then, as the age of puberty approaches, a girl's breasts—which up until now have been flat—enlarge and become more or less hemispherical. Also, the nipples become more prominent. Most of this increase in breast size is due to the accumulation of adipocytes in the connective tissue between the lobes and lobules of the breast. At puberty, the epithelial duct system develops beyond a rudimentary stage, but this change is not as striking as the increase in the amount of fat tissue in the breasts. Secretory alveoli do not develop at this time; they form only during pregnancy.

In males, the mammary glands generally show no substantial change at puberty, remaining flat. Small masses of breast tissue nevertheless develop in approximately 50% of adolescent boys and may remain for a year or so before regressing. Similar physiological development of breast tissue occurs with an approximately similar incidence in aging men. Uncommonly, at either of these times, there is considerable breast enlargement of the type occurring in females. This condition is called *gynecomastia* (Gr. *gynaikos*, woman; *mastos*, breast).

Estrogen is primarily responsible for bringing about the changes that occur in the female breasts at puberty and also for physiological or pathological gynecomastia in men. Like the endometrium, then, breast tissue is an estrogen target tissue.

During pregnancy, the high *progesterone* levels that are attained act together with estrogen to stimulate the development of secretory alveoli in the mother's breasts. The added influence of high *prolactin* levels and *chorionic somatomammotrophin* then brings on the full development of these alveoli and elicits their secretory activity. Insulin, adrenal glucocorticoids, growth hormone, and thyroid hormone are also believed to be necessary for full mammary development and lactation, although their action may be a permissive one. The hormone dependency of *breast car-*

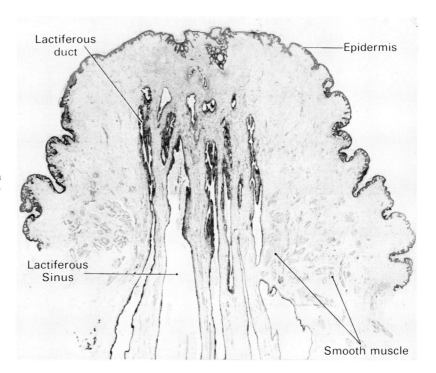

Lactiferous duct

Epidermis

Lactiferous Sinus

Smooth muscle

Fig. 23-23. Photomicrograph of a section of a nipple, cut perpendicular to the skin surface (very low power).

cinomas has already been mentioned in connection with estrogen replacement therapy in the section on Ovaries.

Nipples. The *nipples* and their surrounding skin (which is termed the *areola* of the nipple) are well supplied with afferent nerve endings and are commonly somewhat pigmented. Numerous irregularly shaped dermal papillae approach the epidermal surface closely; the overlying epidermis is very thin (Fig. 23-23). Opening at separate orifices onto the surface of each nipple are the main ducts of the many compound glands that comprise each breast. These main ducts are termed *lactiferous ducts*. Close to their external orifices, these ducts are lined with stratified squamous keratinizing epithelium. Deeper in the nipple, they are lined with two layers of columnar epithelial cells. The supporting dense connective tissue is provided with small bundles of smooth muscle (Fig. 23-23), some circularly arranged around the lactiferous ducts and others lying parallel with these ducts. Near the external orifice of each lactiferous duct, the duct dilates and forms a *lactiferous sinus* that is wide enough to store milk during milk ejection.

The epidermis of the nipple, like that of the vagina, is sensitive to estrogen. In connection with the problem of "sore nipples"—a condition that results when some women attempt to nurse their babies—it is interesting to note that estrogen may be in short supply in a woman for a while after she has given birth. The reason is that estrogen production during pregnancy involves the placenta; hence, when the placenta is delivered following birth, the mother is deprived of what has been her chief source of this hormone. Eventually, of course, her ovaries will produce a sufficiency, but there may be an interval during which the epidermis of the nipples

suffers lack of stimulation by estrogen. Indeed, one type of sore nipple is directly attributable to estrogen deficiency.

Resting Breast

The term *resting breast* is applied to the postpubertal female breast that has not yet been hormonally stimulated to secrete and that is therefore still in an *inactive* (*i.e.*, nonlactating) state. Histological sections show that, at this stage, the internal epithelial tissue of the breast is represented only by its *duct systems* (Figs. 23-24 and 23-25). The parenchyma (*i.e.*, ducts) and stroma of the resting breast have a characteristic organization that will now be described.

Each compound gland that opens into a *lactiferous sinus* constitutes a *lobe* that consists of many *lobules*. As in the case of other exocrine glands, it develops as a result of downgrowth of the surface epithelium into the underlying connective tissue (see Fig. 5-2). Together with the adjoining papillary layer of the dermis, a downgrowth of the epidermis invades the reticular layer of the dermis and begins to form the duct system. As a consequence, the connective tissue that invests the duct system closely resembles the papillary layer of the dermis in that it is relatively cellular (Figs. 23-24 and 23-25). Substantial partitions of coarser and less cellular *interlobular connective tissue* separate islands of this relatively cellular *intralobular connective tissue* (Fig. 23-25). The connective tissue of these relatively wide partitions closely resembles that of the overlying reticular layer of the dermis (Fig. 23-24). The largest of these supporting partitions are termed *suspensory ligaments* (*of*

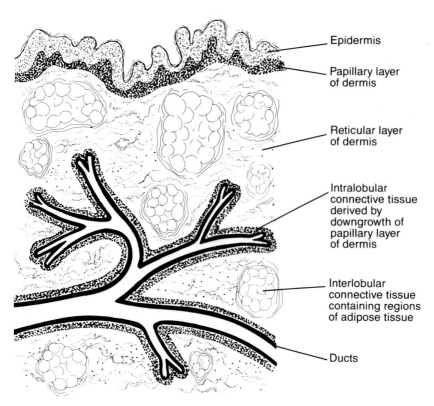

Epidermis

Papillary layer
of dermis

Reticular layer
of dermis

Intralobular
connective tissue
derived by
downgrowth of
papillary layer
of dermis

Interlobular
connective tissue
containing regions
of adipose tissue

Ducts

Fig. 23-24. Schematic diagram of the organization of the resting breast, illustrating how its intralobular connective tissue corresponds to the papillary layer of the dermis. Extensions of the reticular layer of dermis constitute interlobular suspensory ligaments and septa.

Cooper). In the postpubertal breast, fairly substantial deposits of adipose tissue are also present in the partitions of interlobular connective tissue (Fig. 23-24). The intralobular ducts are lined with cuboidal to low columnar epithelial cells; in the wider ducts these are arranged as a double layer, and in the narrower ducts they are arranged as a single layer.

Lactation

Further changes in the epithelial tissue of the breast ensue if pregnancy occurs. The duct system first completes its development and then secretory alveoli bud from its smallest intralobular branches. By the second half of pregnancy, well-established lobules that contain secretory alveoli in addition to intralobular ducts can be recognized in sections (Fig. 23-26). As a consequence of continuing growth of the lobules, the interlobular connective tissue between them becomes reduced to thin partitions (Fig. 23-26). At this stage, each secretory alveolus consists of a simple columnar epithelium, together with associated myoepithelial cells.

There is a subsequent substantial rise in the blood levels of (1) progesterone and (2) the maternal and placental lactogenic hormones. In conjunction with similarly escalating levels of estrogen, these three hormones elicit a *secretory* phase that follows the *proliferative* phase we have just de-

scribed. In the third trimester (3-month period) of pregnancy, the secretory cells begin to secrete a protein-containing serous fluid that also has a low fat content; this fluid is called *colostrum.* Such secretory activity causes further enlargement of the breasts, but milk is not produced until a few days after delivery. A characteristic microscopic feature of breast tissue that has reached this stage of development is that its secretory alveoli and ducts become more distended in some lobules than in others due to uneven rates of secretion (Fig. 23-26). This feature aids considerably in its identification.

This distended appearance of the lobules is further accentuated in the *lactating breast* of a nursing mother. The abundant alveoli become filled with secretion, and the interlobular connective tissue becomes reduced to comparatively thin septa. Many alveoli continue to appear distended whereas others appear almost empty. At the electron microscope level, the alveolar secretory cells show morphological evidence of active lipid and protein secretion. They contain prominent lipid droplets of all sizes; these lack a surrounding membrane and some of them are very large (Fig. 23-27). Very electron-dense secretory granules that contain milk protein are also present in the cytoplasm (Fig. 23-27). When these cells are actively secreting, they are columnar with a dome-shaped luminal end that bears a few microvilli (Fig. 23-27). The view is widely held that when these cells extrude their lipid droplets by exocytosis, the droplets take with them an investing layer of cell mem-

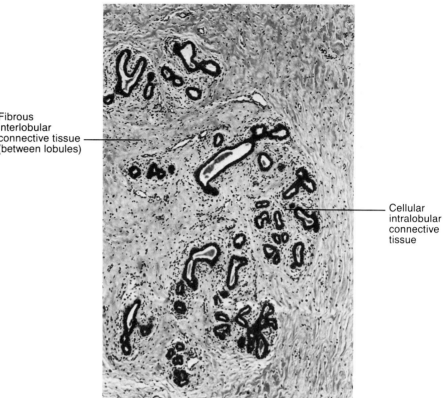

Fibrous
interlobular
connective tissue
(between lobules)

Cellular
intralobular
connective
tissue

Fig. 23-25. Photomicrograph of resting (inactive) breast. Intralobular ducts, but not secretory alveoli, can be seen within the lobules.

Interlobular septa (fibrous)

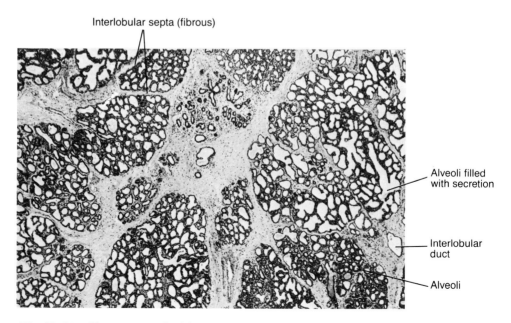

Alveoli filled
with secretion

Interlobular
duct

Alveoli

Fig. 23-26. Photomicrograph of fully developing breast. This tissue was obtained during the fifth month of pregnancy, when the secretory changes associated with lactation become manifest. Alveoli at upper right are distended with colostrum; many of those at bottom right have not yet begun to secrete.

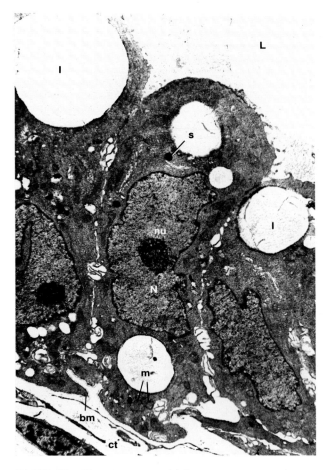

Fig. 23-27. Electron micrograph of alveolar secretory cells of a lactating breast (biopsy of human lactating breast). The nuclei (*N*) of these columnar secretory cells are centrally or basally situated and have a prominent nucleolus (*nu*). Lipid droplets (*l*), some of which are large, commonly accumulate in the domelike luminal end of the cell, which is seen bordering on the lumen (*L*). Between the basal end of these cells and the underlying connective tissue (*ct*), there is a basement membrane (*bm*). The dark staining of the cytoplasm is due to the presence of many ribosomes and polysomes and a moderate number of cisternae of rER, which are barely discernible at this magnification. Electron-dense secretory granules (*s*) containing milk proteins are also present in these cells. Mitochondria (*m*) are fairly numerous, but they are not easily discerned because of the dark staining of the cytoplasm. (Courtesy of D. Murray and I. Murray)

brane. Exocytosis of the milk proteins, however, is achieved in the usual manner.

Milk contains considerable quantities of fat as well as proteins, lactose, and vitamins. The main milk proteins are casein, lactalbumin, and secretory IgA. Transference of IgA antibodies to the newborn, initially by way of colostrum and then by way of breast milk, is an important way of conferring passive enteric immunity until the baby produces enough IgA and other classes of antibodies of its own.

Prolactin Secretion. Under ordinary circumstances, the secretory activity of mammotrophs is suppressed by the secretion of prolactin-inhibiting hormone (PIH). Prolactin (PRL) secretion is nevertheless increased by physical, surgical, and emotional stress, including such odd stimuli as parachute jumping and psychological testing of neurotic women.

As noted in Chapter 22, the chemical identity of PIH requires further elucidation. Dopamine has been shown to be an important inhibitor of PRL secretion, but at present, it is still unclear whether this neurotransmitter is solely responsible for the negative regulation of PRL secretion. Dopamine nevertheless constitutes an important link in the chain because PRL elicits the release of dopamine from tuberohypophyseal neurons of the hypothalamus, and the dopamine directly or indirectly inhibits further PRL secretion. Hence dopamine is part of a negative feedback loop whereby PRL inhibits its own secretion at the hypothalamic level. For further information, see Judd.

Lactation Begins Shortly After Delivery. As a consequence of the high levels of estrogen, progesterone, and PRL attained by the end of a full-term pregnancy, the breasts have undergone full development and have begun to secrete. However, the action of PRL in bringing about milk secretion is antagonized by high levels of estrogen. With expulsion of the placenta at delivery, the maternal blood levels of estrogen (and progesterone) show a rapid decline, and this allows the high levels of PRL to exert their full effect on milk secretion.

An odd side-effect of parturition is that PRL secretion by the pituitary mammotrophs of the newborn baby—which, as noted in Chapter 22, may have undergone a hyperplastic response to high maternal estrogen levels—occasionally manifests itself as transient milk secretion by the breast tissue of the infant. Such milk secretion by newborn babies, again elicited by estrogen withdrawal, is sometimes referred to by those without medical training as witch's milk.

Once maternal lactation begins 1 to 3 days after delivery, PRL secretion must continue for milk production to be maintained. Also, posterior pituitary function is involved, as will be explained in the following section dealing with milk ejection.

During the interval over which a new mother is enthusiastically breast-feeding her (or anyone else's) baby, ovulation and menstruation may be interrupted. However, this natural means of contraception is by no means universal, especially in developed countries, and some women become pregnant again during the nursing period. The basis for such interruption of ovulation and menstruation appears to be that the afferent stimuli from the nipple (1) inhibit the pulsatile secretion of GnRH, and (2) block the positive feedback loop whereby increasing estrogen levels elicit the LH surge that is responsible for ovulation. Also of interest is the fact that a new pregnancy does not interfere with already established lactation; hence a mother can continue to nurse one baby after she has conceived another.

Milk Ejection Is a Reflex Response to Suckling. Although milk is secreted on a continuous basis, it is expressed from the breast only during nursing. Such expression is termed *milk ejection* or *milk let-down*. Suckling gives rise to afferent impulses that are relayed to the hypothalamus, where they (1) stimulate oxytocin-producing neurons, the cell bodies of which are situated mainly in the paraventricular nucleus, to release this hormone from their axon terminals in the posterior lobe of the pituitary; and (2) suppress the release of PIH. The oxytocin thereupon stimulates contraction of the myoepithelial cells in the breast, which causes milk to be expressed through the nipple from the lactiferous ducts. This response is termed the *milk ejection reflex*. The suppressive effect exerted by the stimulus of suckling on the release of PIH maintains prolactin secretion so that lactation continues.

Regression of Breast Tissue. Following the discontinuation of breast-feeding, most of the secretory alveoli in the mother's breast become resorbed and the lobules shrink. The partitions of interlobular connective tissue become correspondingly thicker. Then at menopause, the decline in blood estrogen levels results in some atrophy of both the parenchymal and the stromal components of the breast. Irregular growth and secretory changes may also occur. As a consequence, the epithelium of some ducts may proliferate whereas that of other ducts may secrete and convert the ducts concerned into cysts.

SELECTED REFERENCES

Comprehensive

AUSTIN CR, SHORT RV (eds): Reproduction in Mammals. Books 1 to 6. London, Cambridge University Press, 1972 to 1976

GREEP RO: The female reproductive system. In Greep RO, Koblinsky MA, Jaffe FS (eds): Reproduction and Human Welfare: A Challenge to Research, p 81. Cambridge, MA, MIT Press, 1976

GREEP RO (ed): Handbook of Physiology, Section 7: Endocrinology. Vol II: Female Reproductive System. Washington, DC, American Physiological Society, 1975

JOHNSON MH, EVERITT BJ: Essential Reproduction. Oxford, Blackwell Scientific Publications, 1980

JUDD SJ: The neuroendocrinology of reproduction. In Shearman RP (ed): Clinical Reproductive Endocrinology, p 1. Edinburgh, Churchill Livingstone, 1985

NORMAN RL (ed): Neuroendocrine Aspects of Reproduction. New York, Academic Press, 1983

Ovaries, Oogenesis, Ovarian Follicles, Corpus Luteum, and Ovarian Steroidogenesis

ANDERSON E, BEAMS HW: Cytological observations on the fine structure of the guinea pig ovary with special reference to the oogonium, primary oocyte and associated follicle cells. J Ultrastruct Res 3:432, 1960

BALBONI GC: Histology of the ovary. In James VHT, Serio M, Giusti G (eds): The Endocrine Function of the Human Ovary. Proceedings of the Serono Symposia, Vol 7. London, Academic Press, 1976

BJERSING L: Maturation, morphology, and endocrine function of the ovarian follicle. In Channing CP, Segal SJ (eds): Intraovarian Control Mechanisms. Advances in Experimental Medicine and Biology, Vol 147, p 1. New York, Plenum, 1981

BRODIE AMH: Biosynthesis, metabolism, and secretion of ovarian steroid hormones. In Serra GB (ed): The Ovary, p 3. New York, Raven Press, 1983

CENTOLA GM: Structural changes: Follicular development and hormonal requirements. In Serra GB (ed): The Ovary, p 95. New York, Raven Press, 1983

COUTTS JRT (ed): Functional Morphology of the Human Ovary. Lancaster, England, MTP Press, 1981

COWELL CA, WILSON R: The Ovary. In Ezrin C, Godden JO, Volpé R, Wilson R (eds): Systemic Endocrinology. Hagerstown, Harper & Row, 1973

CRISP TM, DESSOUKY DA, DENYS FR: The fine structure of the human corpus luteum of early pregnancy and during the progestational phase of the menstrual cycle. Am J Anat 127:37, 1970

DORRINGTON JH, ARMSTRONG DT: Effects of FSH on gonadal functions. Recent Prog Horm Res 35:301, 1979

ENDERS AC: Observations on the fine structure of lutein cells. J Cell Biol 12:101, 1962

HERTIG AT, ADAMS EC: Studies on the human oocyte and its follicle. I. Ultrastructural and histochemical observations on the primordial follicle stage. J Cell Biol 34:647, 1967

JONES RE (ed): The Vertebrate Ovary: Comparative Biology and Evolution. New York, Plenum, 1978

MATHIEU P, RAHIER J, THOMAS K: Localization of relaxin in human gestational corpus luteum. Cell Tissue Res 219:213, 1981

MCEWEN BS: Interactions between hormones and nerve tissue. Sci Am 235:48, July, 1976

MOTTA PM, HAFEZ ESE (eds): Biology of the Ovary. Boston, Martinus Nijhoff, 1980

OHNO S, KLINGER HP, ATKIN NB: Human oogenesis. Cytogenet Cell Genet 1:42, 1962

OJEDA SR, ANDREWS WW, ADVIS JP, SMITH WHITE S: Recent advances in the endocrinology of puberty. Endocr Rev 1:228, 1980

RICHARDSON GS: Ovarian physiology. N Engl J Med 294: May 5, p 1008; May 12, p 1064; May 19, p 1121; and May 26, p 1183, 1966

RYAN KJ, PETERS Z, KAISER J: Steroid formation by isolated and recombined ovarian granulosa and thecal cells. J Clin Endocrinol Metab 28:355, 1968

SERRA GB (ed): The Ovary. New York, Raven Press, 1983

ZAMBONI L: Modulations of follicle cell-oocyte association in sequential stages of mammalian follicle development and maturation. In Crosignani PG, Mishell DR (eds): Ovulation in the Human, p 1. London, Academic Press, 1976

Uterus, Endometrium, Cervix, Uterine Tubes, and Vagina

BERTALANFFY FD, LAU C: Mitotic rates, renewal times, and cytodynamics of the female genital tract epithelia in the rat. Acta Anat 54:39, 1963

BLERKOM VAN J, MOTTA P: The Cellular Basis of Mammalian Reproduction. Baltimore, Urban & Schwarzenberg, 1979

HAFEZ ESE (ed): Scanning Electron Microscopic Atlas of Mammalian Reproduction. New York, Springer-Verlag, 1975

HAFEZ ESE, BLANDAU RJ: The Mammalian Oviduct: Comparative Biology and Methodology. Chicago, University of Chicago Press, 1969

KEMP BE, NIALL HD: Relaxin. Vitam Horm 41:79, 1984

LUDWIG H, METZGER H: The Human Female Reproductive Tract. A Scanning Electron Microscopic Atlas. New York, Springer-Verlag, 1976

MARKEE JE: The morphological and endocrine basis for menstrual bleeding. Prog Gynec 2:63, 1950

MARTEL D, MALET C, GAUTRAY JP, PSYCHOYOS A: Surface changes of the luminal uterine epithelium during the human menstrual cycle: A scanning electron microscopic study. In de Brux J, Mortel R, Gautray JP (eds): The Endometrium Hormonal Impacts, p 15. New York, Plenum, 1981

PAPANICOLAOU GN: The sexual cycle in the human female as revealed by vaginal smears. Am J Anat 52:519, 1933

SCHWABE C, STEINETZ B, WEISS G ET AL: Relaxin. In Greep RO (ed): Recent Progress in Hormone Research, Vol 34, p 123. New York, Academic Press, 1978

WYNN RM (ed): Biology of the Uterus. New York, Plenum, 1977

Ovulation, Implantation, and Placenta

AUSTIN CR: The Mammalian Egg. Oxford, Blackwell Scientific Publications, 1961

BEACONSFIELD P, BIRDWOOD G, BEACONSFIELD R: The placenta. Sci Am 243 No. 2:94, 1980

BEER AE, BILLINGHAM RE: The Immunobiology of Mammalian Reproduction. Englewood Cliffs, NJ, Prentice-Hall, 1976

BLANDAU RJ (ed): The Biology of the Blastocyst. Chicago, University of Chicago Press, 1971

BOYD JD, HAMILTON WJ: Development of the human placenta in the first three months of gestation. J Anat 94:297, 1960

BOYD JD, HAMILTON WJ: The giant cells of the pregnant human uterus. J Obstet Gynaecol Br Emp 67:208, 1960

BOYD JD, HAMILTON WJ: The Human Placenta. Cambridge, England, W Heffer and Sons, 1970

EDWARDS RG, HOWE CWS, JOHNSON MH (eds): Immunobiology of Trophoblast. London, Cambridge University Press, 1975

ENDERS AC: Fine structure of anchoring villi of the human placenta. Am J Anat 122:419, 1968

HAMILTON WJ, BOYD JD: Development of the human placenta in the first three months of gestation. J Anat 94:297, 1960

KAUFMANN P, SEN DK, SCHWEIKHART G: Classification of human placental villi I. Histology. Cell Tissue Res 200:409, 1979

KING BF, TIBBITTS FD: The fine structure of the chinchilla placenta. Am J Anat 145:33, 1976

LALA PK, CHATTERJEE–HASROUNI S, KEARNS M ET AL: Immunobiology of the feto-maternal interface. Immunol Rev 75:88, 1983

MCCANN SM: Luteinizing-hormone-releasing-hormone. N Engl J Med 296:797, 1977

MCCANN SM: Present status of LHRH: Its physiology and pharmacology. In McCann SM, Dhindsa DS (eds): Role of Peptides and Proteins in Control of Reproduction, p 3. New York, Elsevier Biomedical Press, 1983

PIERCE GB, Jr, MIDGLEY AR, Jr: The origin and function of human syncytiotrophoblastic giant cells. Am J Pathol 43:153, 1963

PINCUS G: Control of conception by hormonal steroids. Science, 153:493, 1966

SIMMONS RL, CRUSE V, MCKAY DG: The immunologic problem of pregnancy. Am J Obstet Gynecol 97:218, 1967

TERZAKIS JA: The ultrastructure of normal human first trimester placenta. J Ultrastruct Res 9:268, 1963

VILLEE CA: The Placenta and Fetal Membranes. Baltimore, Williams & Wilkins, 1960

VILLEE DB: Development of endocrine function in the human placenta and fetus. N Engl J Med 281:473, 1969

Mammary Glands and Lactation

COWIE AT, FOLLEY SJ: The mammary gland and lactation. In Young WC (ed): Sex and Internal Secretions, 3rd ed, p 590. Baltimore, Williams & Wilkins, 1961

PITELKA DR, HAMAMOTO ST: Ultrastructure of the mammary secretory cell. In Mepham TB (ed): Biochemistry of Lactation. New York, Elsevier Biomedical Press, 1983

VORHERR H: The Breast: Morphology, Physiology, and Lactation. New York, Academic Press, 1974

WAUGH D, VAN DER HOEVEN E: Fine structure of the human adult female breast. Lab Invest 11:220, 1962

WELLINGS SR, GRUNBAUM BW, DEOME KB: Electron microscopy of milk secretion in the mammary gland of the C3H/Crgl mouse. J Natl Cancer Inst 25:423, 1960

24

The Male Reproductive System

The male reproductive system (Fig. 24-1) consists of (1) paired gonads, the *testes,* which produce *spermatozoa* (male germ cells) and *androgens* (male sex hormones); (2) a copulatory organ, the *penis,* by means of which spermatozoa can be introduced into the female reproductive tract; (3) a series of excurrent passageways and ducts of considerable total length that lead from the testes, two of their main functions being to permit the spermatozoa to mature and to store them ready for delivery to the male copulatory organ; and (4) several male *accessory glands.* These glands provide the fluid vehicle for carrying spermatozoa. Also, during ejaculation, contraction of smooth muscle fibers in the walls or stroma of these glands is largely responsible for causing their respective secretions, together with spermatozoa, to be expressed from the penis as a fairly complex mixture called *semen.*

The testes develop in the abdomen and descend into the saclike scrotum (Fig. 24-1) during fetal life. The thin-walled scrotum has a considerable surface area, which under ordinary circumstances enables the testes to be held at a temperature that is slightly below that of the body as a whole. This lower temperature is an important prerequisite for the production of adequate numbers of spermatozoa. The dartos muscle in the wall of the scrotum contracts in response to cold and certain other stimuli; contraction of this muscle makes the scrotum smaller by causing its walls to become corrugated.

The spermatozoa are produced within a mass of tortuous looped *seminiferous tubules* that collectively fill most of the interior of each testis (Figs. 24-2 and 24-3). In the connective tissue stroma between these epithelial tubules, there are small groups of steroid-secreting cells known as *interstitial* or *Leydig* cells. In response to stimulation by luteinizing hormone (LH), these cells produce substantial quantities of androgens, chiefly *testosterone.* Testosterone is the main hormone responsible for (1) promoting formation of spermatozoa (*spermatogenesis*), (2) development and secretory activity of the androgen-responsive accessory glands, and (3) development of the male secondary sexual characteristics.

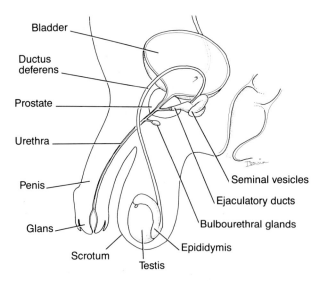

Fig. 24-1. Diagrammatic representation of the parts of the male reproductive system.

A maze of tiny anastomosing passageways called the *rete testis* (L. *rete,* net) connects the straight parts of the seminiferous tubules of each testis (parts referred to as *tubuli recti*) to a number of convoluted *ductuli efferentes* that enter the head of the adjoining crescent-shaped *epididymis* (Fig. 24-2). The ductuli efferentes, in turn, open into a long convoluted *ductus epididymis* (Fig. 24-2). The thick-walled portion of duct that emerges from the tail of the epididymis is called the *ductus (vas) deferens* (Fig. 24-2). This duct ascends in the spermatic cord and enters the pelvis minor by way of the inguinal canal. It then reaches the posterior aspect of the urinary bladder (Fig. 24-1), at which site a tortuous sacculated tubular gland known as a *seminal vesicle* opens into it. On each side of the body, the seminal vesicle lies lateral to the ductus deferens along the posterior aspect of the bladder (Fig. 24-1). A common duct leads from the junction between the relatively wide distal part of the ductus deferens and the associated seminal vesicle; this duct is termed an *ejaculatory duct* (Fig. 24-1). On each side of the body, the ejaculatory duct opens into the *prostatic urethra,* which is the part of the urethra that traverses the prostate gland (Fig. 24-1; see also Fig. 24-21). The *prostate* is a substantial gland that is approximately the size and shape of a horse chestnut and is made up of numerous compound tubuloalveolar glands embedded in a rounded mass of smooth muscle and connective tissue. It is situated around the proximal (prostatic) part of the urethra, close to the neck of the bladder (Fig. 24-1; see also Fig. 24-21). The seminal vesicles produce a thick nutritive fluid, whereas the prostate produces a less viscous but similarly complex secretion; both secretions contribute considerably to the volume of semen. The mixed secretion, containing spermatozoa, passes by way of the *urethra* through the penis,

which, under conditions of sexual arousal, is erect because of engorgement with blood.

Before considering the various parts of the male reproductive system in greater detail, we shall briefly outline the main stages of gametogenesis in males and make some comparisons with the equivalent stages in females. Meiosis has already been considered in some detail in connection with Oogenesis in Chapter 23, so to avoid undue repetition in this chapter, we shall concentrate on those stages of the process that can be recognized microscopically in a testis section.

SYNOPSIS OF SPERMATOGENESIS

Unlike primary oocytes, primary spermatocytes are not produced prior to puberty. An important difference between meiosis in males and the corresponding process in females (described in Chap. 23) is therefore that of *timing.* Hence in males, *meiotic divisions commence at puberty.* A second difference is that whereas only a single ovum results from meiosis I and II in females, all four progeny cells (spermatids) become spermatozoa in males. The entire process of male gametogenesis that results in the formation of spermatozoa is termed *spermatogenesis.*

Male *primordial germ cells* originate from yolk sac endoderm and migrate into the developing testes, whereupon they become incorporated into the epithelial sex cords that will develop into the seminiferous tubules. Here the primordial germ cells give rise to predecessors of male germ cells, sometimes referred to as *primitive spermatogonia* or *prespermatogonia,* that remain quiescent until late adolescence, at which time they begin to undergo mitotic proliferation to form *spermatogonia.* The ordinary epithelial cells of the sex cords, on the other hand, become the constitutive epithelial cells of the seminiferous tubules; these cells are known as *Sertoli cells.*

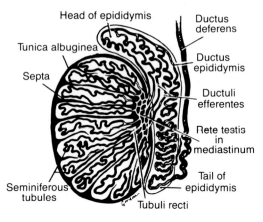

Fig. 24-2. Schematic diagram of the organization of the testis and epididymis.

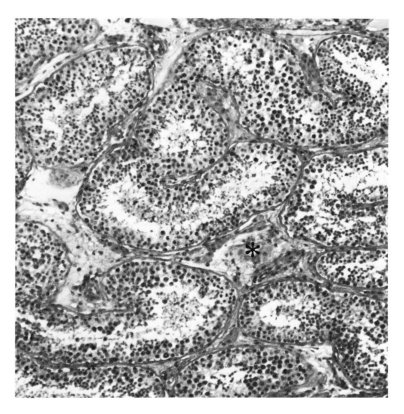

Fig. 24-3. Photomicrograph showing the seminiferous tubules of a testis at low magnification. Asterisk indicates a group of interstitial cells.

By the onset of puberty, many of the spermatogonia have already begun to give rise to *primary spermatocytes*. Other spermatogonia persist throughout reproductive life as unipotential *stem cells* that are capable of giving rise to further spermatogonia. Each new wave of primary spermatocytes that is produced passes through the extended (but in this case, uninterrupted) prophase of meiosis I and then goes on to complete the first maturation division to form two haploid *secondary spermatocytes*. These cells then almost immediately undergo their second maturation division, but *without first going through an S phase*, in other words, without prior replication of their nuclear DNA. Their haploid progeny cells, which are called *spermatids*, transform *with no further division* into *spermatozoa*. Further details will be given in the following section on the Testes.

TESTES

Each *testis* (testicle) is a compact ovoid organ that is 4 cm to 5 cm long and that has an associated more or less crescent-shaped *epididymis* extending along its superior and posterolateral borders. Its mesothelial covering represents the *visceral layer of tunica vaginalis testis*, which is the membranous lining of a serous sac evaginated from the peritoneum. Deep to the mesothelial covering, there is a thick capsule of dense ordinary connective tissue; this layer is known as the *tunica albuginea* because of its white fibrous

appearance (Fig. 24-2). Fibrous septa extend into the testis from the tunica albuginea and subdivide the interior of the organ into incomplete, more or less pyramidal lobules (Fig. 24-2). Where the septa converge on the midline of the posterior border of the testis, there is a ridgelike posterior thickening of the tunica albuginea that is known as the *mediastinum testis*. Along this ridge, both ends of the looped *seminiferous tubules* comprising each lobule (up to four per lobule) open by way of the anastomosing passageways of the *rete testis* into a number of *ductuli efferentes* (Fig. 24-2).

The constitutive columnar supporting cells of the seminiferous tubules are known as *Sertoli cells.* Derived from the epithelial cells of the sex cords in the developing gonads, these tall cells span the entire thickness of the seminiferous epithelium from its surrounding basement membrane to the lumen of the tubule (see Fig. 24-4, stage *I;* see also Fig. 24-16). A proliferating population representing all stages of male germ cell differentiation, with constituent cells that are continually working their way toward the lumen of the tubule, occupies a warren of intercellular cavities between the lateral borders of the Sertoli cells (these cavities are illustrated on the right-hand side of Fig. 24-16).

External to the basement membrane of each seminiferous tubule, there is loose connective tissue containing one or more loose layers of *myoid cells* (shown, but not labeled, at the bottom of each diagram in Fig. 24-4), which resemble smooth muscle cells except that they are squamous. Ex-

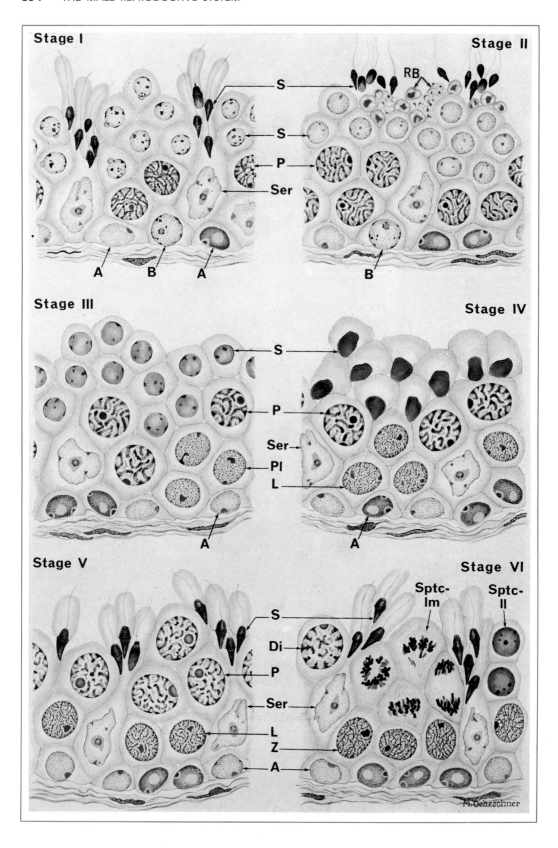

perimental observations in laboratory animals indicate that these cells are contractile and may therefore be capable of generating rhythmic contractions, perhaps even gentle peristaltic waves that pass along the walls of these tubules.

Testicular Changes Occurring During Childhood and Puberty. The small groups of testicular *interstitial cells* that lie between the seminiferous tubules actively secrete androgens during fetal life but later become inconspicuous and manifest less secretory activity during childhood. Then at the onset of puberty, there is a decreasing sensitivity to negative feedback by testosterone, an increasing release of LH in response to GnRH, and a rise in the blood levels of testicular and adrenal androgens that becomes manifested as development of the male secondary sexual characteristics. For the first decade of life, the seminiferous tubules remain inactive and lack a lumen. However, by the time puberty is reached, the testosterone levels attain a concentration that promotes active spermatogenesis, and scattered groups of interstitial cells become more prominent between the tubules (see Fig. 24-14). The tubules themselves acquire a central lumen into which their newly formed spermatozoa are released (Fig. 24-3).

Maldescent of the Testes. Occasionally, however, one or both testes fail to descend into the scrotum during fetal life or immediately after birth. An individual with undescended testes is termed *cryptorchid* (Gr. *kryptos*, concealed; *orchis*, testis). In some instances, undescended testes descend spontaneously during infancy, but in the majority of cases, they do not, and measures must be taken to relocate them in the scrotum. It is important for the testes to descend before the age of 7 years, because this is when the cords become seminiferous tubules if the testes are in their proper environment. Unless the testes gain access to the favorable environment of the scrotum, they *will not produce spermatozoa;* however, the interstitial cells *may still produce androgens.*

Microscopically Recognizable Stages of Spermatogenesis

Spermatogonia. Many different stages of germ cell development can be found in the relatively thick walls of the seminiferous tubules (Fig. 24-4). Nevertheless, in all regions of these tubules, relatively large spherical *spermatogonia* are basally situated adjacent to the surrounding basement membrane (Fig. 24-4). These cells are the diploid predecessors from which spermatocytes arise. Three different subtypes of spermatogonia that have been recognized are

pale type A, dark type A, and *type B spermatogonia.* (Fig. 24-4). The names of the two subtypes of the type A spermatogonia refer to the paler or slightly darker appearance of their nuclear chromatin, much of which is in the extended state (Fig. 24-4). Microscopic identification of the various subtypes of spermatogonia requires some expertise and is less important than understanding the main differences between them. Several lines of evidence indicate that the *pale type A cells* are relatively undifferentiated cells that remain capable of extensive mitotic proliferation.

The respective roles of the pale and the dark type A cells have not yet been clarified in man. However, it seems reasonable to deduce them from the roles of the corresponding cells in other primates. In the monkey, the pale type A cells are believed to be *renewing stem cells* because they yield new pale type A cells and type B cells in approximately equal numbers. Also, the pale type A cells take up tritiated thymidine before their division. In contrast, the dark type A cells remain unlabeled in the adult. It would seem, therefore, that the dark type A cells serve as reserve cells that remain quiescent unless damage to the seminiferous epithelium induces them to give rise to renewing stem cells (Clermont). According to this hypothesis, the pale type A cells are cycling stem cells and the dark type A cells are identical cells that remain out of cycle until the need arises for more of the pale type A cells.

An alternative proposal is that in man it is the pale type A cells that represent the noncycling reserve cells and the dark type A cells that are mitotically active (Schulze). This is an interpretation of results obtained from testicular biopsies of semicastrated patients treated by chemotherapy or radiotherapy for malignant disease of the testis. It is based on the observation that numerous pale type A cells persist whereas the number of dark type A cells is drastically reduced. However, under such compensatory conditions, it could be expected that many dark type A cells would be triggered into cycle to help restore the deficit and that the need for differentiating progeny cells might outweigh the need for self-renewal, making the interpretation of this observation somewhat difficult.

On average, one half the daughter cell population of the dividing type A cells differentiates further to become type B cells, thereby losing their potentiality for producing more type A cells. The other half of this daughter cell population persists as stem cells that maintain the stem cell population. The type B cells undergo mitosis to form *primary spermatocytes.*

Spermatocytes. *Primary spermatocytes* are most readily recognized after they have begun the prophase of meiosis I, the first stage of which is *leptotene.* The double chro-

Fig. 24-4. Drawings of the various stages of spermatogenic differentiation seen in seminiferous tubules. Six cellular associations are found in human seminiferous tubules. The six associations (*stages*) are labeled I to VI. For further details, see caption to Figure 24-8. (*Ser*, nucleus of Sertoli cell; *A*, type A spermatogonia; *B*, type B spermatogonia; *Pl*, preleptotene primary spermatocytes; *L*, leptotene primary spermatocytes; *Z*, zygotene primary spermatocytes; *P*, pachytene primary spermatocytes; *Di*, diplotene primary spermatocytes; *Sptc-Im*, primary spermatocytes in division; *Sptc-II*, secondary spermatocytes in interphase; *S*, spermatids at various steps of spermiogenesis; *RB*, residual bodies) (Clermont Y: Am J Anat 112:35, 1963)

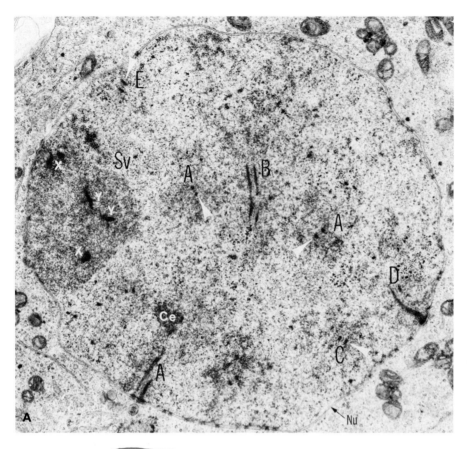

A

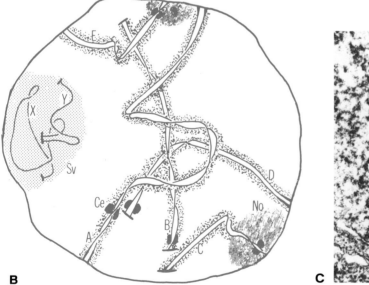

B

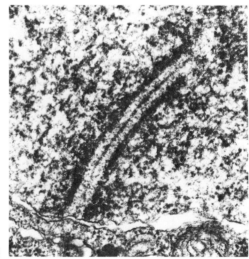

C

Fig. 24-5. (*A*) Electron micrograph of the nucleus of a spermatocyte at the pachytene stage of prophase I (rat). Synaptonemal complexes are labeled A, B, C, D, and E. These complexes are attached to the nuclear envelope (*Nu*). Inside the sex vesicle (*Sv*) are much of the X and the Y chromosomes. (*B*) Interpretive drawing of *A*. In the rat, there are 20 synaptonemal complexes but only the five visible in part *A* are shown. These are identified as A, B, C, D, and E. Each complex represents a set of paired d-chromosomes, has a centromere (*Ce*), and is attached at both ends to the nuclear envelope. A is the longest pair of chromosomes, and C and E are nucleolus-bearing (*No*) chromosomes. The sex vesicle (*Sv*) contains the unpaired region of the X and the Y chromosomes, which have only a small paired region. (*C*) Electron micrograph (×52,000) of part of a synaptonemal complex, showing its medial electron-dense line and its attachment to the nuclear envelope. The nuclear envelope extends across the bottom of the micrograph. (*A*, courtesy of A. Hugenholtz; *B*, courtesy of P. Moens; *C*, courtesy of L. Arsenault)

mosomes (d-chromosomes) that become visible at this stage are very fine and delicate. (*L* in Fig. 24-4, stages IV and V). In *zygotene* (Z in Fig. 24-4, stage VI; see also Fig. 23-2, stage 1), the homologous d-chromosomes pair up as *bivalents*.

Toward the end of this stage, in either primary spermatocytes or primary oocytes, paired electron-dense and parallel ribbons approximately 60 nm wide, separated by a clear space that is roughly 100 nm across, appear along the interface between the members of each bivalent (Fig. 24-5). These ribbonlike structures are known as *synaptonemal complexes* (Gr. *synapsis*, a coming together; *nema*, thread) because they hold the paired chromosomes together

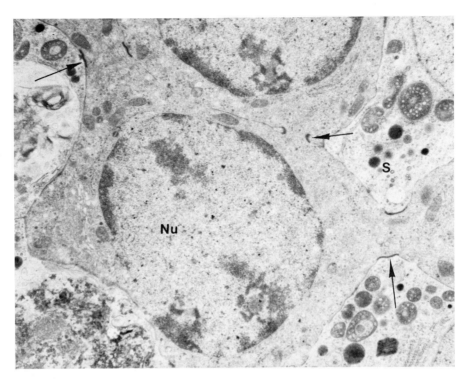

Fig. 24-6. Electron micrograph of a preleptotene spermatocyte showing three of its intercellular bridges in the plane of section. The bridges are marked by arrows. (*Nu,* nucleus; *S,* Sertoli cells). (Courtesy of A. Hugenholtz)

in a structural complex. Formation of these complexes is initiated at several sites along the length of the paired chromosomes. A narrow medial electron-dense line (Fig. 24-5*C*) and fine filaments traversing the central space have also been described. Several synaptonemal complexes can be seen in the nucleus of a pachytene primary spermatocyte in Figure 24-5. Each synaptonemal complex is attached at both ends to the nuclear envelope. (Fig. 24-5*B*).

In man there are 23 synaptonemal complexes. The X and the Y chromosomes become paired only over a short distance; they remain almost entirely single within a region of the nucleus termed the *XY body (sex vesicle)* (which is seen at *left* in Fig. 24-5*A* and *B*). These two chromosomes, too, are attached by both ends to the nuclear envelope.

During *pachytene,* the d-chromosomes become more condensed, appearing thicker and shorter (*P* in Fig. 24-4). In *diplotene,* the two d-chromosomes of each bivalent separate sufficiently for them both to be visible and chiasmata can be seen (*Di* in Fig. 24-4, stage VI; see also Fig. 23-2, stage 4). In *diakinesis,* the final stage of prophase I, the chromosomes thicken further. The primary spermatocyte then enters metaphase I, and the chromosomes become arranged in the equatorial plane. In anaphase I, the two d-chromosomes of each bivalent move toward opposite poles of the cell (Figs. 24-4, stage VI, *Sptc-Im;* see also Fig. 23-2, stage 5). Throughout meiosis I, the two s-chromosomes (single chromosomes) of each d-chromosome remain joined at their centromeres. As a consequence, each secondary spermatocyte receives the haploid number of d-chromosomes instead of the diploid number of s-chromosomes.

Secondary spermatocytes (Fig. 24-4, stage VI, *Sptc-II*) are smaller than primary spermatocytes and are situated in the middle layers and the more superficial layers of the seminiferous epithelium (Fig. 24-4, stage VI). These cells miss the S phase and almost immediately undergo the second maturation division, and for this reason they are seldom found in interphase. In anaphase II, one s-chromosome (chromatid) of each d-chromosome segregates to each daugher cell (see Fig. 23-2, stage 8). The daughter cells of a secondary spermatocyte are called *spermatids* (S in Fig. 24-4). At first, spermatids are rather small round cells with a spherical nucleus (S in Fig. 24-4, stages III and IV). They then elongate and their nucleus takes up a peripheral position relative to the lumen of the tubule (S in Fig. 24-4, stages IV, V, and VI). The series of changes whereby spermatids transform into spermatozoa, a transformation that is referred to as *spermiogenesis,* will be described later in this chapter.

A distinctive feature of spermatogenesis is that with each successive nuclear division, the progeny cells of the individual spermatogonia remain attached to one another by narrow but definite *intercellular bridges* (Figs. 24-6 and 24-7). Because tenuous cytoplasmic continuity is maintained between the members of the entire clone of differentiating progeny cells, they proliferate and differentiate in a synchronized manner and only the spermatozoon stage becomes a completely independent cell. However, a few of the intercellular bridges break down during the first maturation division, and a few of the cells in the clone fail to divide at all (Moens and Go).

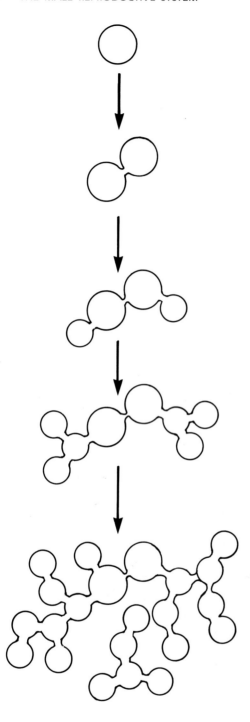

Fig. 24-7. Schematic diagram representing the division of a spermatogonium and subsequent divisions of its progeny cells, which are producing an expanding clone of interconnected spermatocytes. Following each division, the cells remain interconnected by narrow intercellular bridges; this ensures that they will continue to develop in synchrony. (After Moens)

Cycle of Seminiferous Epithelium

Seminiferous epithelium undergoes cyclic changes in its cellular composition. However, in this instance, the turnover time of the whole epithelium is considerably longer than the length of the cycle because only a small proportion of the cells become spermatozoa and leave the epithelium in each cycle.

The *cycle of seminiferous epithelium* is a description of what happens during the course of time at each individual site in a seminiferous tubule. A succession of changes in the cellular composition of each patch of seminiferous epithelium is followed by return of this patch of epithelium to its original cellular composition. The time taken for the entire sequence of changes to occur represents the length of the cycle of the seminiferous epithelium. However, it is not possible to observe the cellular composition of the same patch of seminiferous epithelium for any length of time, so knowledge of this cycle has been gained through indirect means as will be described in the following section.

Cyclically Changing Cell Associations Can Be Recognized Within Seminiferous Epithelium. If a testis obtained from a laboratory animal is cut in cross section at several representative levels along the course of a given seminiferous tubule, the various cross sections of the same tubule will exhibit a number of different microscopic appearances. Indeed, as many as 14 distinctive appearances, described as *cell associations,* have been identified in the seminiferous tubules of the rat (Leblond and Clermont). The cell association that is present at each level of the tubule undergoes a series of changes and then returns to its original cellular composition; the time taken for the original association to reappear at the same level is the cycle time of the seminiferous epithelium. However, in man, the various cell associations that occur in the seminiferous epithelium are not distributed at various levels along the course of a given seminiferous tubule as they are in laboratory animals. Instead, they are present with other patch-shaped cell associations in the same cross section of a tubule, with each of these cell associations occupying a fairly well-defined sector of the section. Furthermore, only six such groupings are seen in seminiferous tubules of the human testis (Clermont). These associations are labeled I to VI in Figure 24-4, which depicts the various cell types found in each association. The general light microscope (LM) appearance of seminiferous epithelium during these six stages is also illustrated and described in Figure 24-8.

Estimating the Total Duration of Spermatogenesis and the Length of the Cycle of Seminiferous Epithelium. In estimating the duration of spermatogenesis or the length of the cycle of seminiferous epithelium, advantage can be taken of the fact that the only cells in this epithelium that undergo replication of their nuclear DNA are spermatogonia and preleptotene primary spermatocytes (Clermont, and Clermont et al). Hence a short pulse of tritiated thy-

Fig. 24-8. Photomicrographs of seminiferous tubules cut transversely (*A*) and longitudinally (*B*) to show the distribution of cell associations (*stages*) of the cycle of the seminiferous epithelium. The six stages illustrated in Figure 24-4 can be identified. The details are as follows.

Stage I (seen in *A*): spermatogonia, pachytene spermatocytes, and two generations of spermatids (one with spherical nuclei, and one with elongated condensed nuclei).

Stage II (seen in *B*); spermatogonia, pachytene spermatocytes, young spermatids with spherical nuclei, and maturing spermatids discarding their residual cytoplasm.

Stage III (*A* and *B*): spermatogonia, preleptotene spermatocytes, pachytene spermatocytes, and spermatids with spherical nuclei.

Stage IV (*A* and *B*): spermatogonia, leptotene and pachytene spermatocytes, and spermatids with slightly elongated nuclei.

Stage V (*B*): spermatogonia, leptotene or zygotene spermatocytes, pachytene spermatocytes, and spermatids with elongated nuclei.

Stage VI (*A*): spermatogonia, early pachytene spermatocytes, maturation divisions of primary spermatocytes, and spermatids with elongated nuclei. The order of stages of the cycle seen around the lumen is variable (not consecutive). (Clermont Y: Am J Anat 112:35, 1963)

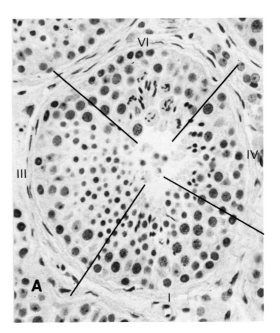

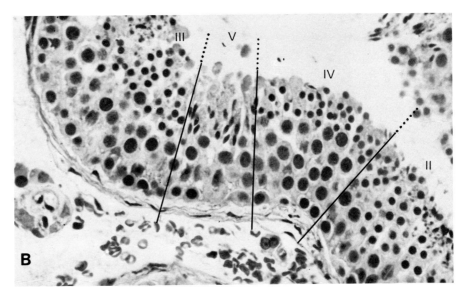

midine becomes incorporated only by spermatogonia and preleptotene primary spermatocytes that are in S phase at the time of labeling. Accordingly, if after an injection of labeled thymidine the label is seen in any cell of the sperm cell series, it will have been incorporated at one of these two stages.

To estimate the total duration of spermatogenesis, all that is necessary is to determine the time that elapses between the administration of labeled thymidine and the time at which label appears in mature testicular spermatozoa. However, in arriving at the duration of spermatogenesis, it is necessary to take into account the fact that the first labeled spermatozoa to appear arise from labeled prelep-

totene primary spermatocytes and not spermatogonia. This is because it takes longer for labeled spermatogonia to give rise to spermatozoa than it takes for labeled preleptotene primary spermatocytes to achieve the same end. From such radioautographic studies, it has been estimated that in man the *total duration of spermatogenesis* is 64 ± 4 to 5 days. The total production time for mature human spermatozoa is commonly estimated to be 74 days.

Estimating the length of the cycle of the seminiferous epithelium by radioautography is more complex. In general, it depends on finding, immediately after labeling, some preleptotene primary spermatocytes that have not only become labeled but are also present in a recognizable cell association. In radioautographs pre-

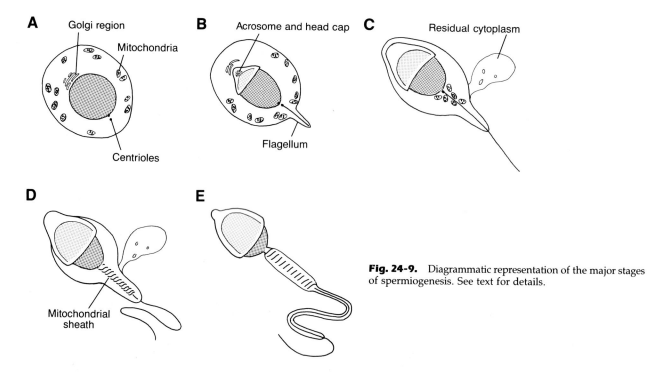

Fig. 24-9. Diagrammatic representation of the major stages of spermiogenesis. See text for details.

pared from successive specimens, it can be reasoned that when labeled cells reappear in an identical cell association, one complete *cycle* will have occurred. However, accurate measurement of the length of a cycle must take into account the fact that the stages of the cycle are not all of equal duration, so that these also have to be determined. Otherwise, it might happen that one labeled cell could be commencing a particular stage when it is seen, while another might be in a late part of that stage. As matters turned out, the stage (Stage III) when preleptotene spermatocytes are in S phase is of short duration.

Radioautographic studies have established that the process of spermatogenesis lasts for 4 cycles and that the length of each cycle is 16 ± 1 day. Thus to proceed from the spermatogonium to the spermatozoon stage, it takes approximately 4 × 16 = 64 days (*i.e.,* just over 2 months) which is the duration of spermatogenesis.

Spermiogenesis

In the last phase of spermatogenesis, the rounded spermatids *transform* directly (*i.e.,* without dividing) into elongated spermatozoa that are still retained in pockets in the surface of the Sertoli cells. The main stages of this transformation process, which is known as *spermiogenesis,* involve the Golgi region and nucleus and the relative positions of the centrioles and mitochondria of the spermatid (Fig. 24-9*A*). The Golgi region becomes closely associated with the nucleus and gives rise to a membranous organelle called the *acrosome vesicle* (Gr. *akron,* extremity). A prominent rounded electron-dense granule termed the *acrosome* then forms inside the acrosome vesicle, and the vesicle

itself flattens and begins to enclose the future anterior pole of the nucleus. The resulting cup-shaped flattened saccule is known as the *head cap* (Fig. 24-9*B*). The acrosome and the head cap comprise the so-called *acrosomic system* of the spermatozoon. The acrosome contains hyaluronidase and several other enzymes (lysosomal hydrolases and a trypsinlike protease), the role of which is to facilitate penetration of the investments surrounding the secondary oocyte (its corona radiata and zona pellucida) by spermatozoa at fertilization.

Concurrently with development of the head cap, the two centrioles migrate to the caudal pole of the nucleus (Fig. 24-9*A*). At this site, the axoneme of the *flagellum (tail)* begins to develop in association with the distal centriole, which at first is aligned with the longitudinal axis of the developing tail (Fig. 24-9*B*) but then disappears (Fig. 24-9*C*). An electron-dense ring-shaped structure called an *annulus* forms around the distal centriole (see Fig. 24-11) but later disappears. However, a second annulus forms externally to the one that disappears. This second annulus, which is less prominent than the first, moves in a caudal direction. Also, a transient structure of uncertain significance and described as a *spindle-shaped body* develops in this region and subsequently disappears (Wartenberg and Holstein).

The nucleus proceeds to condense, flatten, and elongate, and the head cap lengthens so as to cover slightly more than the anterior half of the nucleus (Figs. 24-9*C*, 24-10, and 24-11). Also, the contents of the acrosome become dispersed within the head cap (parts *C* and *D* of Fig. 24-9; also Fig. 24-11). The mitochondria become associated with

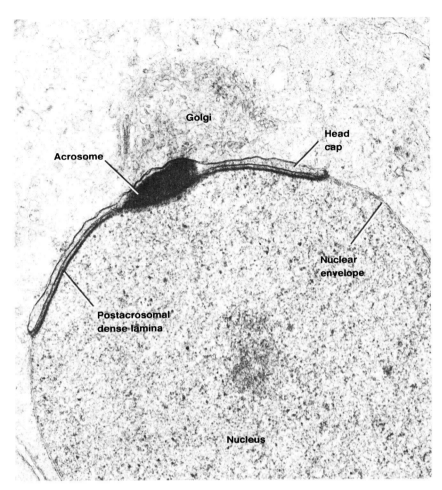

Fig. 24-10. Electron micrograph of the head-cap region of a transforming human spermatid at the stage depicted in Figure 24-9*B* (biopsy of human testis). The Golgi-derived acrosome lies within the lumen of the head cap. (Courtesy of K. Kovacs, E. Horvath, and D. McComb)

the proximal portion of the developing axoneme (Fig. 24-9*C*). Eventually, they become arranged end to end in the form of a tight helix, constituting a collarlike *mitochondrial sheath* (Fig. 24-9*D*) that forms between the nucleus and the annulus. This sheath delineates the future *middle piece* (midpiece) of the developing spermatozoon. Some cytoplasm is left over at the end of this complex metamorphosis and is shed as a residual body between stages D and E in Figure 24-9. It is promptly phagocytosed by Sertoli cells.

Spermatozoa

Each *spermatozoon* is made up of a *head*, a *midpiece* that represents the proximal part of the *tail*, and the main part of the *tail* (Figs. 24-12 and 24-13). The somewhat flattened ellipsoidal head contains the *nucleus*, which is relatively rigid and is packed with highly condensed chromatin. The anterior end of the nucleus is invested by the acrosomal *head cap* (Figs. 24-12 and 24-13). The midpiece and the remainder of the tail comprise the *flagellum*. The midpiece of the spermatozoon also incorporates the *mitochondrial*

sheath and a small quantity of cytoplasmic matrix (Figs. 24-12 and 24-13). The rest of the tail consists of a *principal piece* and an *end piece* (Fig. 24-13).

The microtubular arrangement (nine peripheral doublets and two central single microtubules) in the *axoneme* of the flagellum (Fig. 24-12) is the same as that seen in cilia (as described in Chap. 4 and illustrated in Fig. 4-34). Of particular importance with regard to flagellar motility are the club-shaped dynein arms on the peripheral doublet microtubules (see Fig. 4-34); a congenital absence of these arms leads to spermatozoal immotility and hence infertility. Other incapacitating microtubular defects have also been described (Sturgess and Turner). External to the basic arrangement of microtubules, there is an outer ring of more substantial longitudinal *coarse fibers*, known also as *outer dense fibers*, the arrangement of which depends on which level of the tail is sectioned. Proximally, nine of these accessory longitudinal fibers are interconnected both with the head of the spermatozoon and with each other. In the principal piece, two of the coarse fibers (outer dense fibers) are replaced by substantial supporting structures known as the *dorsal* and *ventral columns*. Furthermore, these two

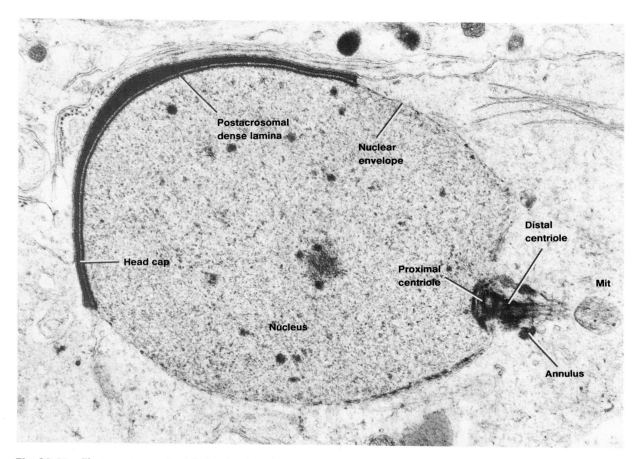

Fig. 24-11. Electron micrograph of the head region of a transforming human spermatid at the stage depicted in Figure 24-9C (biopsy of human testis). The label Mit indicates a mitochondrion in the middle piece. For details, see text. (Courtesy of K. Kovacs, E. Horvath, and D. McComb)

columns are interconnected at intervals by a series of circumferential *fibrous ribs* (Fig. 24-12). The end piece does not have such a complex structure and consists only of the flagellar axoneme and its covering cell membrane (Fig. 24-13). The distal end of the coarse fibers is attached to the peripheral doublet microtubules of the axoneme. For further information, see Fawcett and Bedford.

The function of the *mitochondrial sheath* is to provide the necessary adenosine triphosphate (ATP) for flagellar motility. The *fibrous sheath,* which is the term used for the complex supporting arrangement that is made up of the coarse fibers (outer dense fibers) and their associated fibrous ribs, is believed to harness the forces that result from the sliding of microtubules and to apply these forces to the generation of propulsive lashing movements of the tail.

Male Fertility Levels Depend on the Total Sperm Count and on an Adequate Proportion of Morphologically Normal Spermatozoa in the Ejaculate. As much as 80% of the fluid volume of an ejaculate is made up of the collective fluid secretions of the seminal vesicles and the prostate. The *sperm count* of the ejaculate is normally more than 100

million spermatozoa per ml of semen, with an average volume of 3 ml of ejaculate. The lower the sperm count, the smaller are the chances of being fertile, and men with sperm counts below 20 million per ml are generally sterile. Nevertheless, even in reproductively normal men, up to 20% of the spermatozoa in the ejaculate can have abnormal shapes without this affecting their fertility level. Factors that are known to increase the proportion of abnormally shaped spermatozoa in the mouse include ionizing radiation, heat, pesticides, certain cancer chemotherapy drugs, other pharmaceutical agents, carcinogens, and mutagens. In addition, it is known that x-rays, severe allergic reactions, and certain antispermatogenic agents have similar effects on human spermatozoa. Elevated levels of morphological abnormalities in human spermatozoa are associated with reduced fertility.

As old age advances, there is a steady decline in spermatogenic activity. However, spermatogenesis does not terminate suddenly as does the maturation of ovarian follicles at menopause, and there are many authenticated cases of men becoming fathers at a very advanced age.

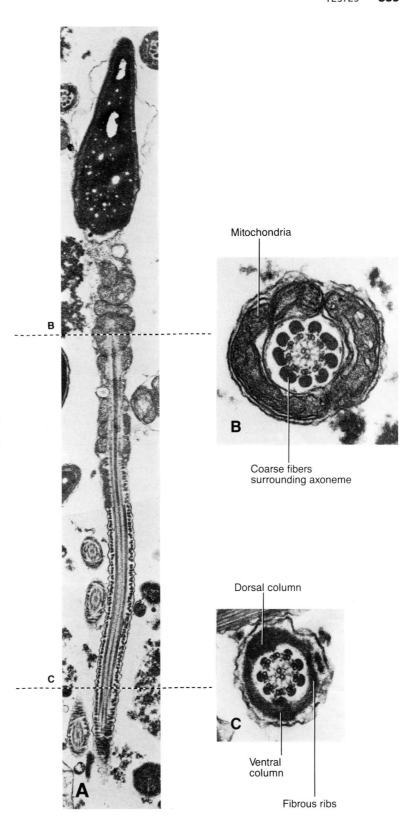

Fig. 24-12. Electron micrographs of spermatozoa (human). (*A*) Longitudinal section. (*B*) Cross section cut at level B (in *A*), showing mitochondrial sheath in middle piece. (C) Cross section cut at level C (in *A*), showing fibrous sheath in principal piece. For interpretive drawing, see Figure 24-13. (Courtesy of J. Sturgess)

Mitochondria

Coarse fibers
surrounding axoneme

Dorsal column

Ventral
column

Fibrous ribs

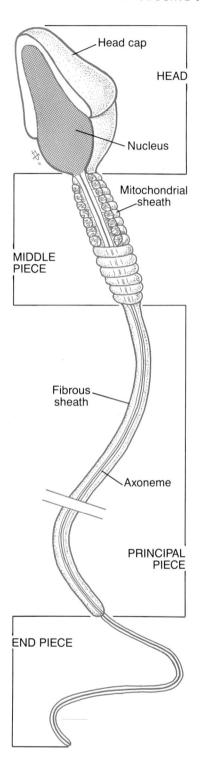

Fig. 24-13. Diagrammatic representation of the main parts of a spermatozoon. (See text for details.) Compare this illustration with Figure 24-12.

Interstitial (Leydig) Cells

For a man to be fertile he must be able to deliver, on some occasions at least, sufficient numbers of normal spermatozoa to bring about fertilization. A *sterile* male cannot accomplish this. *Potency* refers to another matter—the ability of a male to engage in intercourse. This depends on erection of the penis. A potent but sterile male may be able to ejaculate during intercourse, but the semen expressed will not contain a sufficient number of normal spermatozoa to bring about fertilization.

A male may be sterilized either by removing the testes (*castration*) or by tying off the ducti deferentes (*vasectomy*). The latter procedure prevents egress of spermatozoa from the testes, but the interstitial cells continue to produce testosterone, which leaves the testes by way of the bloodstream. The testes of the *cryptorchid* produce testosterone, although in less than normal amounts, and usually do not produce spermatozoa. It is possible for a male to be potent but sterile, and it is also possible for an otherwise fertile male to be impotent. In such males, impotency is usually due to emotional factors that interfere with the functioning of the autonomic nervous system in such a way that the blood flow into the cavernous bodies of the penis is insufficient to cause an erection.

The mesenchyme-derived testicular cells that produce testosterone are diffusely distributed as scattered islands in the loose connective tissue that lies *between* the seminiferous tubules (Fig. 24-14) and are accordingly referred to as *interstitial cells*. An alternative name for them is *Leydig cells*. Approximately 20 μm in diameter, they are fairly large cells with a typically spherical nucleus, and for the most part, they lie near nonfenestrated blood capillaries or lymphatic capillaries (Fig. 24-14). The peripheral region of their cytoplasm is generally pale staining due to accumulation of lipid droplets, and lipochrome pigment may also be present. An extensive smooth-surfaced endoplasmic reticulum (sER), which is a characteristic feature of all steroid-secreting cells, is evident at the electron microscope (EM) level (Fig. 24-15). Also, distinctive crystalloid inclusions called *crystals of Reinke*, the functional significance of which is unknown, are present in these cells (Fig. 24-15, *inset*).

Hormonal Basis of Testicular Function

Adequate amounts of *luteinizing hormone* (LH) and *follicle-stimulating hormone* (FSH) are both necessary to maintain normal levels of spermatogenic activity. There is evidence to suggest that the FSH requirement is greatest during spermatid maturation; *testosterone* secreted in response to LH is a more critical requirement during the earlier stages of spermatogenesis.

LH produced by gonadotrophs of the anterior pituitary stimulates testosterone production by the interstitial cells of the testes. Due to negative feedback that operates pri-

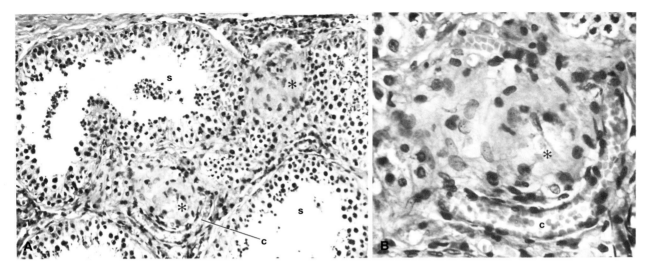

Fig. 24-14. (A) Photomicrograph of two groups of interstitial cells (*asterisks*) lying between seminiferous tubules (*s*) of the testis (medium power). (B) Photomicrograph showing the relation of a group of interstitial cells (*asterisk*) to a wide capillary loop (*c*) in the interstitial connective tissue (high power).

marily at the pituitary level (but conceivably at the hypothalamic level as well), rising testosterone levels then suppress the further release of LH.

FSH produced by gonadotrophs of the anterior pituitary stimulates the Sertoli cells in the seminiferous tubules to secrete an *androgen-binding protein* (ABP) that probably binds estrogen as well. This important protein continually passes into the lumen and the lumen-associated intercellular spaces of the seminiferous tubules, where it binds testosterone and maintains it in the high concentration required for active spermatogenesis. FSH is also believed to augment testosterone production by increasing the number of LH receptors on interstitial cells.

Negative feedback regulation of FSH release appears to be mediated by a polypeptide called *inhibin*, which is also thought to be produced by Sertoli cells of the testes in response to FSH. The further release of FSH is believed to be suppressed by rising levels of inhibin, but the level of the pituitary–hypothalamic axis at which inhibin acts has not yet been established. Inhibin is also present in relatively high concentration in ovarian follicular fluid and appears to be produced by the granulosa cells of ovarian follicles as well as Sertoli cells of the testes. The inhibin activity obtained from bovine follicular fluid, however, is closely associated with a glycoprotein.

Sertoli Cells

The seminiferous tubules, as noted, are lined by a constitutive simple columnar epithelium that is made up of nonproliferating *Sertoli cells*. However, the fact that these cells are actually all contiguous is not evident from LM sections,

in which large gaps appear to be present between some of the adjacent cells (Fig. 24-4). Furthermore, the lateral and luminal borders of Sertoli cells are sufficiently irregular for them to be difficult to discern in the LM. The apparent gaps between these cells, and also their uneven borders, are a consequence of the fact that consecutive generations of differentiating germ cell progenitors are repeatedly passing between Sertoli cells on their way toward the lumen. Throughout the process of their formation, the proliferating and differentiating germ cell progenitors occupy individual pockets in the peripheral cytoplasm of Sertoli cells (Fig. 24-16).

Sertoli cells have a rather large pale-staining nucleus that is commonly located in the basal region of the cell; it is elongated-to-ovoid, with irregular indentations (Fig. 24-4). Seen in the EM, these cells exhibit a very extensive interconnected Golgi complex, patches of rough-surfaced endoplasmic reticulum (rER), and a prominent sER (Fig. 24-17). Lipid droplets, lipochrome pigment, lysosomes, residual bodies, and crystalloid inclusions of unknown function are also present.

Sertoli cells produce a secretion called *testicular fluid* that passes into the lumen of the seminiferous tubules. In response to FSH, for which hormone they possess cell-surface receptors, they also secrete ABP and this enables them to concentrate spermatogenesis-promoting testosterone in their own immediate environment. Other functions ascribed to Sertoli cells include (1) provision of a suitable microenvironment for fostering differentiating germ cell progenitors, (2) active translocation of interconnected differentiating germ cell progenitors toward the lumen, (3) active release of mature spermatozoa into the lumen, and

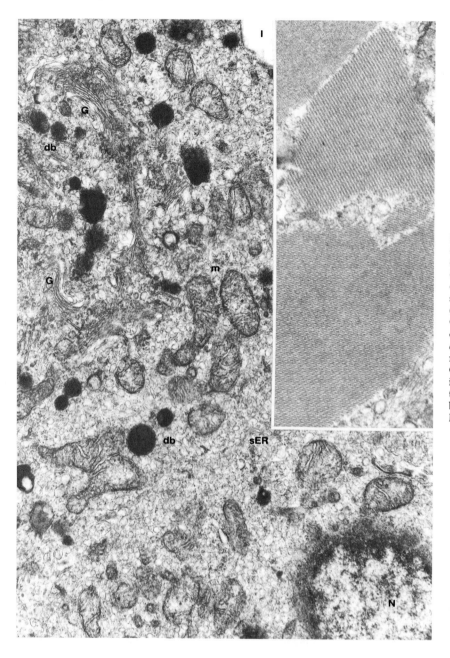

Fig. 24-15. Electron micrograph of part of an interstitial cell of the testis (biopsy of human testis). A portion of the nucleus (*N*) is included at bottom right. The cytoplasm contains an abundance of smooth-surfaced endoplasmic reticulum (*sER*) and mitochondria (*m*), a prominent Golgi complex (*G*), lipid droplets (a part of a lipid droplet, labeled *l*, is seen at *top center*), and some dense bodies (*db*) representing lipochrome pigment. (*Inset*) Crystals of Reinke in the cytoplasm of an interstitial cell from the same source. Between these crystals, tubules of sER can be seen cut in cross section. (Courtesy of K. Kovacs, E. Horvath, and D. McComb)

(4) phagocytic disposal of degenerating germ cells and redundant cytoplasm left over following the formation of spermatozoa.

Sertoli Cells Maintain a Blood–Testis Permeability Barrier. Another functionally important feature of these cells is that the lateral borders of contiguous cells are joined near the base of the cells by well-developed continuous tight junctions of the *zonula occludens* type (Fig. 24-16). As in other zonular junctions of this type, a belt-shaped zone of anastomosing sealing strands occludes the intercellular space (see Figs. 6-10 and 6-11).

Because of their position relative to the lumen, these occluding junctions between the Sertoli cells create two separate compartments in each seminiferous tubule. One compartment, which is known as the *basal compartment* (*light gray* in Fig. 24-16), is situated at the periphery of the tubule and extends inward to the level of the tight junctions. The other compartment, termed the *adluminal compartment* (*dark gray* in Fig. 24-16), extends inward from the level of the tight junctions and includes the lumen. Because of the presence of continuous tight junctions between the Sertoli cells, large molecules with unrestricted access to the inter-

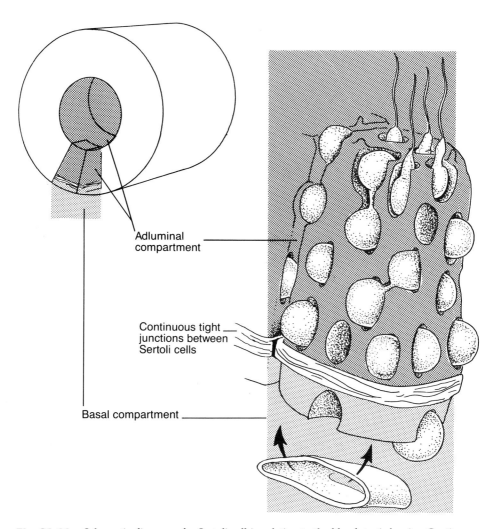

Fig. 24-16. Schematic diagram of a Sertoli cell in relation to the blood–testis barrier. Continuous tight junctions between the lateral walls at the base of Sertoli cells separate an adluminal compartment (*dark gray*) from a basal compartment (*light gray*). These two compartments of the seminiferous tubule are characterized by different populations of spermatogenic cells.

cellular spaces of the basal compartment are restricted from entering the adluminal compartment, and vice versa. One consequence of this arrangement is that certain non–lipid soluble molecules do not readily enter the adluminal compartment from the bloodstream. This permeability barrier is termed the *blood–testis barrier.*

Spermatogonia occupy a basal position in the epithelium, lying next to its basement membrane (Fig. 24-4). Hence mitotic division of spermatogonia occurs in an environment (the basal compartment) with a composition that is similar to the intercellular environment in the remainder of the body (Fig. 24-16). By the time the progeny of these cells reach the leptotene stage of prophase I, however, they enter the adluminal compartment by coming to lie in pockets that are higher up along the lateral borders of the Sertoli cells (Fig. 24-16). These primary spermatocytes and their

progeny thereupon become dependent on the special environment and indirect supply of nutrients provided by the Sertoli cells. Hence the main importance of Sertoli cells is that they (1) provide and maintain the special microenvironment required for spermatogenic differentiation, and (2) secrete ABP and thereby maintain the necessary androgen concentration for adequate levels of spermatogenesis.

New continuous tight junctions form between the Sertoli cells at a level that is below the type B spermatogonia and primary spermatocytes but above the type A spermatogonia. The overlying tight junctions then dissociate, and this allows a wave of type B spermatogonia, along with preleptotene and leptotene primary spermatocytes, to pass from the basal compartment into the adluminal compartment. In this manner, successive waves of germ cell pro-

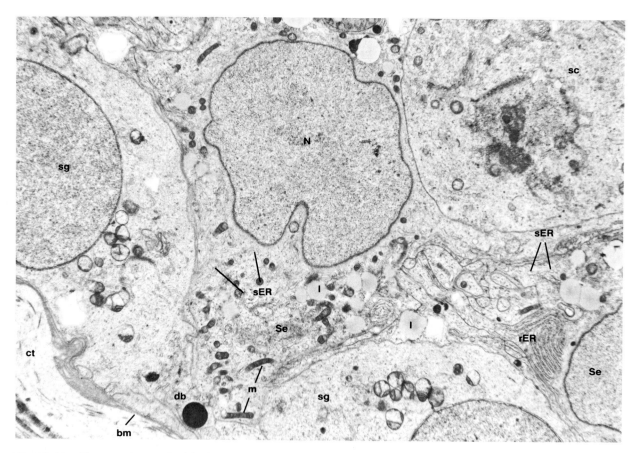

Fig. 24-17. Electron micrograph of the basal region of a Sertoli cell of the testis, with adjacent spermatogonia and a spermatocyte (biopsy of human testis). Bordering on the basement membrane (*bm*) that lies between the connective tissue (*ct*) at bottom left and the seminiferous epithelium are two spermatogonia (*sg*) that are separated by a Sertoli cell (*Se*). Also included in this micrograph are part of a spermatocyte (*sc*), seen at upper right, and part of another Sertoli cell, present at bottom right. In contrast to the spherical or ovoid nuclei of spermatogonia and spermatocytes, Sertoli cell nuclei (*N*) commonly appear irregular in shape in EM sections. This Sertoli cell exhibits fairly numerous lipid droplets (*l*), rod-shaped mitochondria (*m*), patches of rER, an extensive sER, and a few dense bodies (*db*) of lysosomal origin. (Courtesy of K. Kovacs, E. Horvath, and D. McComb)

genitors make their way toward the lumen without disturbing the functional compartmentalization of the tubule. Given the fragile nature of the intercellular bridges between the developing germ cells, this progressive displacement must be a result of coordinated activity of large numbers of Sertoli cells.

This confinement of the developing male germ cells to their own special compartment has several functional implications. First, as a consequence of genetic recombination at the diplotene stage of prophase I, newly expressed antigens can appear on the surface of the developing germ cells. In males, such antigens are expressed only after puberty; hence they can seem foreign to the body's immune system and have the potential to elicit a self-directed (autoimmune) immune response. Keeping these cells in their own adluminal compartment restricts access of their "for-

eign" antigens to the body's lymphatic tissue. Second, in the event that such an immune response does occur, for example in men who have undergone vasectomy (bilateral ligation of the ducti deferentes), the blood–testis barrier restricts the entry of antisperm immunoglobulin molecules into the seminiferous adluminal compartment in which the developing germ cells are being produced. However, such protection is afforded only where these cells are being formed because a similar barrier is lacking along the various ducts that lead from the testis. Also functionally significant is the fact that the permeability barrier in the seminiferous tubules helps to protect their developing germ cells from many drugs, toxic chemicals, and mutagens that can enter the bloodstream. Finally, such an arrangement maintains the appropriate environment for germ cell differentiation. In this connection, we should add that the adluminal com-

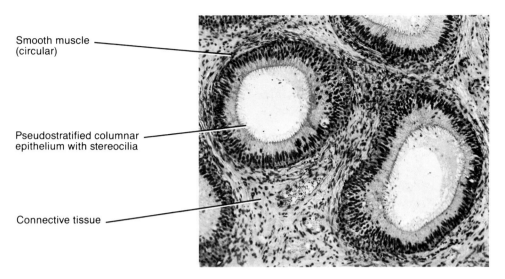

Smooth muscle
(circular)

Pseudostratified columnar
epithelium with stereocilia

Connective tissue

Fig. 24-18.   Photomicrograph of epididymis (medium power), showing the appearance of the ductus epididymis.

partment contains an extracellular fluid of special molecular and ionic composition, rich for example in potassium and ABP and low in sodium.

EPIDIDYMIDES

The *tubuli recti* of each testis, which are lined by tall columnar epithelial cells resembling Sertoli cells, open through its *rete testis* into the *ductuli efferentes* (Fig. 24-2) of its associated *epididymis.* The rete testis is lined by a simple columnar epithelium. The epididymis consists primarily of a long convoluted tube called the *ductus epididymis.* The various windings and convolutions of this tube are covered by a thin fibrous investment, which represents the counterpart of the tunica albuginea, and a superficial visceral layer of tunica vaginalis testis.

Emerging through the tunica albuginea from the upper pole of the testis are a number of *ductuli efferentes* (Fig. 24-2), each of which is irregularly coiled and wound upon itself, constituting a small conical mass. The ductuli efferentes are lined by a simple epithelium made up of groups of tall ciliated columnar cells that alternate with groups of shorter nonciliated columnar resorptive cells, which gives the epithelium a characteristic festooned (garlandlike) appearance. The ciliated cells are provided with typical motile cilia, and the shorter cells resorb some of the testicular fluid. External to the basement membrane of the epithelial lining, there is a thin circular layer of smooth muscle with associated elastic fibers, and this is surrounded by a delicate and fairly vascular loose connective tissue.

Spermatozoa, which at this stage still have not become effectively motile, are carried along by ciliary activity to the *ductus epididymis,* which is a highly convoluted duct that along with its supporting connective tissue comprises the body and the tail of the epididymis. Neither the ductus epididymis nor the series of ducts leading to the exterior of the body possesses motile cilia. Instead of having cilia, the ductus epididymis is provided with prominent groups of extra-long and more or less immotile microvilli that have become known as *stereocilia* (Gr. *stereos,* solid) even though they lack the characteristic internal microtubular arrangement of cilia. The ductus epididymis is lined by pseudostratified columnar epithelium with stereocilia (Fig. 24-18). The tall cells in this epithelium exhibit coated vesicles and other signs of active endocytosis at their apical surface. The basement membrane of the epithelium is again surrounded by a circular layer of smooth muscle that becomes increasingly thick as the distal end of the duct is approached.

Excess fluid is resorbed from the suspension of spermatozoa as it passes along the ductus epididymis. Through both absorption and secretion, the lining cells of this duct also modify the composition of the luminal fluid coming from the rete testis. ABP reaches the epididymis from the testis by way of the rete testis and the ductuli efferentes and is thought to be necessary for maintaining an adequate intraluminal concentration of testosterone.

The spermatozoa that emerge from the testis are still not effectively motile, nor are they capable of fertilization. The epididymis is the site where they are stored, and here they begin maturing and acquiring the capacity for fertilization. However, even the spermatozoa emerging from the epididymis have yet to attain their full capacity for fertilization, as will be explained in the following section.

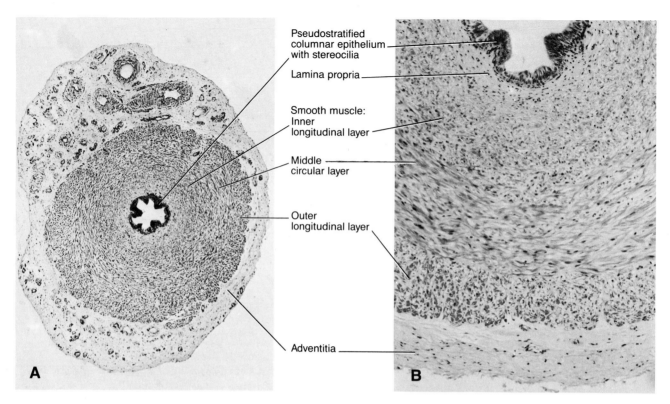

Pseudostratified
columnar epithelium
with stereocilia

Lamina propria

Smooth muscle:
Inner
longitudinal layer

Middle
circular layer

Outer
longitudinal layer

Adventitia

A   **B**

Fig. 24-19.   Photomicrograph of ductus deferens. (*A*) Very low power. (*B*) Medium power, showing the arrangement of smooth muscle in its walls.

Spermatozoa Cannot Fertilize Until They Become Capacitated.   The spermatozoa that are being stored in the epididymis are not effectively motile, yet they will become so the moment they are diluted with an appropriate buffer *in vitro. In vivo,* spermatozoa exhibit forward motility when they become diluted with the secretions of the male accessory glands, indicating that they acquire the potential for such motility in passing along the ductus epididymis. Indeed, it has now been demonstrated in primates that a protein secreted by epithelial lining cells of the ductus epididymis has the capacity to activate forward motility (Hoskins et al).

Capacitation is the term used for a series of biochemical changes in spermatozoa through which they attain their full capacity for fertilization. Representing completion of the maturation process that begins in the ductus epididymis, capacitation involves cell-surface changes and other changes in the periacrosomal region that occur in response to the different environment of the female reproductive tract. Metabolic activity of spermatozoa and effectiveness of their forward motility are also enhanced. Capacitation takes a number of hours and reaches completion only in the uterine or uterine tubal environment. For further information, see Zaneveld; also O'Rand.

DUCTI DEFERENTES

Each *ductus deferens*, alternatively known as a *vas deferens*, is a muscular-walled tube that has three substantial layers of smooth muscle in its walls and a relatively narrow lumen. The thick middle layer of this muscle coat is circularly arranged whereas the inner and outer layers are longitudinal in orientation (Fig. 24-19). The ductus deferens is substantial enough for it to be palpated through the skin and subcutaneous tissue. During *emission*, peristaltic contractions of the thick muscular coat of each ductus deferens result in the transference of spermatozoa from each ductus epididymis to the urethra. The pseudostratified columnar epithelium of this duct is provided with stereocilia except in the ampulla, which is the dilated distal portion of the duct. Its supporting fibroelastic lamina propria raises it into low longitudinal folds and the central lumen appears rather small (Fig. 24-19). Where the ductus deferens becomes part of a spermatic cord, it is attached by its loose and fairly elastic adventitia to the accompanying skeletal muscle (*cremaster* muscle), arteries, lymphatics, nerves, and the associated *pampaniform plexus*, which consists of anastomosing veins that wind around the duct like tendrils (L.

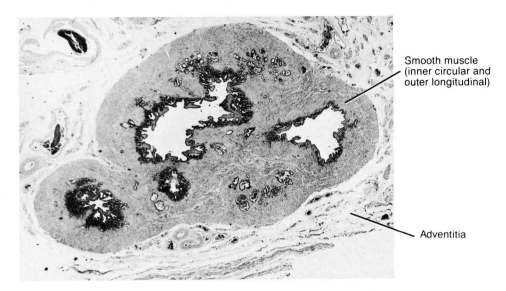

Smooth muscle
(inner circular and
outer longitudinal)

Adventitia

Fig. 24-20. Photomicrograph of seminal vesicle (very low power). See text for details.

pampinus, tendril). This is a site where the veins commonly become varicosed.

Vasectomy. Bilateral ligation of the ducti deferentes (vasa deferentia) can be employed as a means of birth control. Termed a *vasectomy,* this procedure prevents egress of spermatozoa through the urethra. Following a vasectomy, the ejaculate consists only of the secretions made by the male accessory glands (*i.e.,* the seminal vesicles and the prostate). The spermatozoa trapped in the testes and the epididymides become resorbed without discomfort. The only major complication is that in approximately 50% of cases, fertility cannot be restored. Part of the problem is that it is sometimes difficult to restore patency to the ligated ducts, but a more profound problem is that autoimmunity can develop against newly expressed spermatozoal antigens. If sperm-immobilizing or sperm-agglutinating immunoglobulins are formed, this can bring about a permanent reduction in fertility.

SEMINAL VESICLES

Each seminal vesicle is an elongated body, 5 cm to 7 cm or more in length, that opens into the distal end of a ductus deferens. It is essentially an unbranched tubular diverticulum of the duct, that is somewhat longer and narrower than appears to be the case on gross dissection, and that is made up of coils and convolutions held together by connective tissue. When unraveled, this tube has a length of approximately 15 cm. Hence in a transverse section of an undissected seminal vesicle, the same tube is sectioned at several different levels along its course (Fig. 24-20).

The wall of the tube is made up of three coats: an outer coat composed of fibrous connective tissue with a considerable content of elastic fibers, a middle coat composed of smooth muscle, and a mucosal lining. The *muscular coat* is substantial but not quite as thick as that of the ductus deferens. It consists of an inner circular layer and an outer longitudinal layer of smooth muscle fibers. The mucosal epithelium is raised into elaborate folds (Fig. 24-20) that provide a large area of secretory epithelium and that facilitate distension of the vesicle with stored secretion. The *epithelial lining* consists of tall columnar cells, generally with some smaller cells scattered between them and the lamina propria. In some instances, these smaller cells constitute a fairly distinct basal layer under the tall cells. The glandular appearance of the seminal vesicles is entirely due to extensive infolding of the mucosa.

The thick and slightly yellowish secretion produced by the seminal vesicles contains nutrients for the spermatozoa; it is particularly rich in fructose, ascorbic acid, and prostaglandins. During ejaculation it is delivered by way of the ejaculatory ducts and contributes over half the fluid volume of semen.

Finally, it should be noted that full development and normal secretory activity of the seminal vesicles is dependent on adequate levels of testosterone in the circulation.

PROSTATE

Approximately the size and shape of a horse chestnut, the prostate surrounds the urethra where this emerges from the bladder (Fig. 24-1). Hence prostatic enlargement can obstruct the outlet of the bladder, a problem that is fairly common in men past middle age. The cause is obviously hormonal because the prostate atrophies following castra-

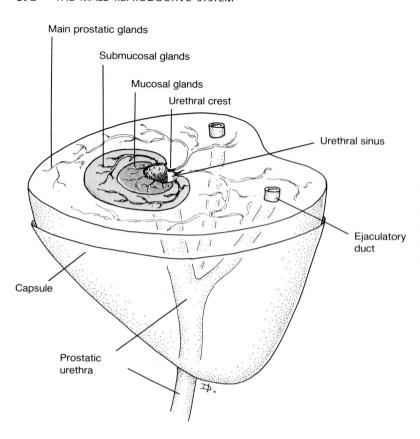

Fig. 24-21. Schematic drawing of the inferior part of the prostate, showing the relation of its mucosal, submucosal, and main prostatic glands to the prostatic urethra. The anterior aspect of the gland is shown on the left. The periurethral zone that contains the greatest number of mucosal glands is indicated in blue.

tion. Partial prostatectomy to free the urethra of obstruction is accordingly a fairly common operation in older men.

The prostate is of a firm consistency. It is surrounded by a thin *capsule* that contains both connective tissue and smooth muscle fibers. The substance of the prostate is made up of a *large number of individual glands;* these open by separate *ducts* into the prostatic urethra and are embedded in a *stroma* that is a mixture of smooth muscle and fibrous connective tissue.

A cross section of the prostate shows that the lumen of the prostatic urethra is V-shaped, with the apex of the V lying anteriorly (Fig. 24-21). The part of the posterior wall of the urethra that bulges forward to make the cross-sectional appearance of its lumen V-shaped is termed the *urethral crest* (Fig. 24-21). The two posterolateral arms of the V constitute the *urethral sinuses* (Fig. 24-21).

Compound tubuloalveolar prostatic glands of three different orders are distributed in three different concentric regions around the urethra. The smallest of these glands are the *mucosal glands,* which are located in the periurethral tissue (Fig. 24-21). These glands are important in connection with *benign prostatic hyperplasia* in older men, because it is these glands that commonly overgrow to form *adenomatous* (Gr. *aden,* gland; *oma,* tumor) *nodules.* The *submucosal glands* are arranged in the ring of tissue surrounding the periurethral tissue (Fig. 24-21). The *main prostatic glands,*

which provide most of the secretion, are situated in the outer and largest portion of the gland (Fig. 24-21). The mucosal glands open at various points around the lumen of the urethra, but the ducts of the submucosal and main prostatic glands open into the posterior margins of the urethral sinuses (Fig. 24-21).

The ejaculatory ducts imperfectly subdivide the prostate into three lobes (Fig. 24-21). Also, each lobe is imperfectly subdivided into lobules that are made up of tubuloalveolar secretory units. These secretory units produce the prostatic secretion and are also adapted for storing it; hence they can have a dilated appearance. Because the secretory epithelium of the prostate is extensively folded (Fig. 24-22), its secretory units are able to fill up with a substantial volume of stored secretion. This arrangement, together with the presence of a *fibromuscular stroma* (*i.e.,* dense ordinary connective tissue intermixed with smooth muscle) between the lobules (Fig. 24-22), gives the prostate a distinctive microscopic appearance.

The *epithelium* of the secretory units and their ducts is usually tall columnar. Smaller flattened or rounded cells may be irregularly distributed between these tall cells. The tall columnar cells have a prominent Golgi complex between their nucleus and their luminal border. Calcified *concretions* are sometimes encountered within the lumina of the prostatic secretory units, particularly in prostate sec-

Fibromuscular stroma   Secretory units with
                              folded epithelium

Secretory epithelium
(tall columnar)

Calcified concretion

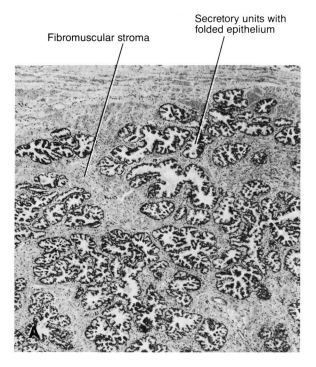

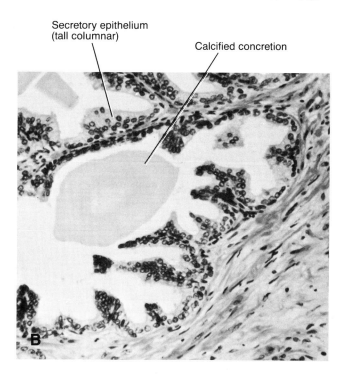

Fig. 24-22. Photomicrograph of prostate. (*A*) Low power. (*B*) High power, showing concretion in a secretory unit.

tions obtained from older men (Fig. 24-22). Beneath the lining epithelium, there is a fibrous lamina propria that is richly supplied with capillaries.

The prostatic secretion is thin in consistency and has a somewhat milky appearance. It contains, among other constituents, the enzyme *acid phosphatase*. Although it is unclear why this particular enzyme is present in the prostatic secretion, detection of elevated levels of acid phosphatase in the bloodstream aids in the diagnosis of malignant tumors of the prostate (carcinoma of the prostate), especially if these have metastasized to bones.

As is the case with the seminal vesicles, normal testosterone levels are necessary to bring about full development and secretory activity of the prostate. Castration after these structures have attained their full size causes them to atrophy, and their tall secretory epithelial cells become low cuboidal and nonsecretory. Furthermore, the growth of some prostatic carcinomas is retarded under conditions of androgen deprivation, which can be achieved by bilateral orchiectomy (castration) or through the administration of estrogen. The rationale for employing estrogen for this purpose is that it inhibits the release of LH and thereby reduces the blood testosterone levels.

PENIS

The body of the penis contains *erectile tissue* that is arranged in the form of three long cylindrical bodies called *cavernous bodies* (*corpora*). These three structures are bound together, and also surrounded, by a *fascia penis* consisting of fairly

elastic loose connective tissue; externally, there is a covering of thin skin (Fig. 24-23). The erectile structures consist of two *corpora cavernosa,* which are fused together along their medial borders, and a somewhat longer *corpus spongiosum,* which lies ventral to them and surrounds the *urethra* (Fig. 24-23). The corpus spongiosum terminates as a short conical structure known as the *glans penis* (Fig. 24-1). The skin of the body of the penis can move relatively freely over the underlying tissues because of the elastic nature of the superficial fascia.

Except in circumcised males, penile skin overlaps the glans (Fig. 24-1) to form the *prepuce* (foreskin), which is a protective fold of extra skin that is normally elastic enough to permit its retraction. In some instances, however, it fits too tightly over the glans, a condition called *phimosis*. When the prepuce cannot be retracted without discomfort, there is a tendency for the secretion from modified sebaceous glands present on the inner surface of the prepuce to accumulate, whereupon it becomes an irritant. *Circumcision* is the common operation by which the prepuce is removed.

A strong fibrous sheath called a *tunica albuginea* encloses each cavernous body (Fig. 24-23). Within each of these bodies, there is a network of characteristic irregular vascular spaces that are lined with endothelium and that are separated from one another by partitions (*trabeculae*) composed of dense fibroelastic tissue with numerous bundles of smooth muscle, many of which are inserted into the tunica albuginea (Fig. 24-23). The fibrous sheath that encloses the

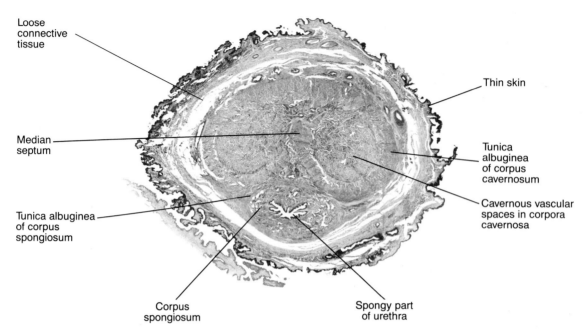

Loose
connective
tissue

Thin skin

Median
septum

Tunica
albuginea
of corpus
cavernosum

Tunica albuginea
of corpus
spongiosum

Cavernous vascular
spaces in corpora
cavernosa

Corpus
spongiosum

Spongy part
of urethra

Fig. 24-23. Photomicrograph of a transverse section of body of penis.

corpus spongiosum is more elastic than those covering the other two cavernous bodies, and the glans penis lacks such a sheath. The penis, especially the glans penis, is richly supplied with various types of sensory receptors.

Mechanism of Erection. In the absence of sexual arousal, the penis maintains a flaccid state because its cavernous bodies do not receive much blood and are therefore mostly collapsed. *Erection* of the penis is an *involuntary parasympathetic response*. It is brought about primarily through relaxation of the smooth muscle in the walls of the relatively large arteries that supply the vascular spaces of the cavernous bodies. The branches of these arteries are provided with unusually thick muscular walls, and many of them have intima-covered longitudinal bundles of smooth muscle encroaching on their lumen. Furthermore, some of the arterial branches extending along the trabeculae are coiled and convoluted when the penis is flaccid; these vessels are called *helicine arteries*. In many cases, the terminal branches of these arteries open directly into vascular spaces of the cavernous bodies. Relaxation of the arterial smooth muscle allows the arteries supplying the cavernous bodies to dilate, whereupon more blood enters the vascular spaces. Relaxation of the smooth muscle in the trabeculae is another factor that contributes to distension of the vascular spaces in the cavernous bodies. The resulting distension of each of these bodies is limited by the strong tunica albuginea that encloses it. Distension of the corpora cavernosa causes compression of the veins that drain their vascular spaces, and this leads to their engorgement with blood, resulting in erection of the penis. However, the corpus spongiosum

does not become as turgid as the outer two cavernous bodies because its surrounding sheath is more elastic, and this avoids undue compression of the part of the urethra that courses through it. After *emission,* which is an *involuntary sympathetic response,* the penis regains its flaccid state because the smooth muscle in the arterial walls regains its former tonus.

MALE URETHRA

There are three parts to the male *urethra.* Traversing the prostate is the *prostatic urethra* (Fig. 24-21). This part of the urethra is lined by a transitional epithelium that becomes pseudostratified or stratified columnar epithelium distally. The short part of the urethra that traverses the urogenital diaphragm is called the *membranous urethra;* this part, too, is lined with stratified columnar epithelium. The last and longest part of the urethra is called its *spongy part* or the *penile urethra.* It begins where the urethra enters the corpus spongiosum, and it extends as far as the external urethral orifice. Its lining is chiefly stratified columnar epithelium, but this is replaced by stratified squamous epithelium in the distal region of the navicular fossa, which is the terminal widening of the urethra within the glans penis. Paired *bulbourethral glands* open into the proximal end of the spongy urethra. These relatively minor compound tubuloalveolar glands secrete a viscid, clear lubricating secretion into the urethra under conditions of sexual excitement. Also associated with the distal part of the spongy urethra are some minor mucus-secreting *urethral glands.*

In some sites, the fibroelastic lamina propria of the urethra also contains smooth muscle fibers. Furthermore, the fibroelastic lamina propria of the prostatic urethra, notably the part of it covering the urethral crest (Fig. 24-21), is highly vascular. In addition, smooth muscle fibers are associated with the mucosa of the prostatic urethra. These are arranged as an inner longitudinal layer and an outer circular layer. The circular layer is most highly developed at the internal urethral orifice, where it contributes to the internal sphincter of the bladder. Skeletal muscle fibers of the urogenital diaphragm surround the membranous urethra and comprise the urethral sphincter.

Finally, three characteristics of the male urethra that medical students will be able to verify in their clinical years when they learn how to pass a urethral catheter are that it is approximately 20 cm long, that its course is not straight but exhibits a reverse curve, and that there are many small diverticula in its lining, which becomes noticeable if the catheter employed is of insufficient caliber.

SELECTED REFERENCES

Comprehensive

AUSTIN CR, SHORT RV (eds): Reproduction in Mammals. Books 1 to 6. London, Cambridge University Press, 1972 to 1976

BEATTY RA: The genetics of the mammalian gamete. Biol Rev 45: 73, 1970

FAWCETT DW: The male reproductive system. In Greep RO, Koblinsky MA, Jaffe FS (eds): Reproduction and Human Welfare: A Challenge to Research, p 165. Cambridge, MA, MIT Press, 1976

HAMILTON DW, GREEP RO (eds): Handbook of Physiology. Vol 5, Sect 7. Male Reproductive System. Washington, DC, American Physiological Society, 1975

JOHNSON MH, EVERITT BJ: Essential Reproduction. Oxford, Blackwell Scientific Publications, 1980

ODELL WD, MOYER DL: Physiology of Reproduction. St. Louis, CV Mosby, 1971

VAN BLERKOM J, MOTTA P: The Cellular Basis of Mammalian Reproduction. Baltimore, Urban & Schwarzenberg, 1979

Testis, Seminiferous Epithelium, Spermatogenesis, Spermiogenesis, and Spermatozoa

AMANN RP: Sperm production rates. In Johnson AD, Gomes WR, Vandemark NL (eds): The Testis. Vol 1. New York, Academic Press, 1970

BRUCE WR: Studies of the genetic implications of abnormal spermatozoa. In Cairnie AB, Lala PK, Osmond DG (eds): Stem Cells of Renewing Cell Populations. New York, Academic Press, 1976

BRUCE WR, FURRER R, WYROBEK AJ: Abnormalities in the shape of murine sperm after acute testicular X-irradiation. Mutat Res 23: 381, 1974

BRUCE WR, MEISTRICH ML: Spermatogenesis in the Mouse. Proc 1st Internat Conf on Cell Differentiation, p 295. Copenhagen, Munksgaard, 1972

BURGOS MH, VITALE–CALPE R, AOKI A: Fine structure of the testis and its functional significance. In Johnson AD, Gomes WR, Vandemark NL (eds): The Testis. Vol 1. New York, Academic Press, 1970

CLERMONT Y: The cycle of the seminiferous epithelium in man. Am J Anat 112:35, 1963

CLERMONT Y: Kinetics of spermatogenesis in mammals: Seminiferous epithelium cycle and spermatogonial renewal. Physiol Rev 52:198, 1972

CLERMONT Y: Spermatogenesis in man. A study of the spermatogonial population. Fertil Steril 17:705, 1966

CLERMONT Y, HERMO L: Spermatogonial stem cells and their behaviour in the seminiferous epithelium of rats and monkeys. In Cairnie AB, Lala PK, Osmond DG (eds): Stem Cells of Renewing Cell Populations. New York, Academic Press, 1976

CLERMONT Y, TROTT M: Duration of the cycle of the seminiferous epithelium in the mouse and hamster determined by means of radioautography. Fertil Steril 20:805, 1969

COUROT M, HOCHEREAU–DE REVIERS M, ORTAVANT R: Spermatogenesis. In Johnson AD, Gomes WR, Vandemark NL (eds): The Testis. Vol 1. New York, Academic Press, 1970

DYM M: The mammalian rete testis—a morphological examination. Anat Rec 186:493, 1976

DYM M, CLERMONT Y: Role of spermatogonia in the repair of the seminiferous epithelium following x-irradiation of the rat testis. Am J Anat 128:265, 1970

DYM M, FAWCETT DW: Further observations on the number of spermatogonia, spermatocytes, and spermatids connected by intercellular bridges in the mammalian testis. Biol Reprod 4:195, 1971

FAWCETT DW: The cell biology of gametogenesis in the male. Perspectives in Biology and Medicine 2, Part 2:S56, 1979

FAWCETT DW: A comparative view of sperm ultrastructure. Biol Reprod (Suppl 2) 2:90, 1970

FAWCETT DW: The mammalian spermatozoon. Dev Biol 44:395, 1975

FAWCETT DW, BEDFORD JM (eds): The Spermatozoon: Maturation, Motility and Surface Properties. Baltimore, Urban & Schwarzenberg, 1979

FAWCETT DW, EDDY E, PHILLIPS DM: Observations on the fine structure and relationships of the chromatoid body in mammalian spermatogenesis. Biol Reprod 2:129, 1970

GIER HT, MARION GB: Development of the mammalian testis. In Johnson AD, Gomes WR, Vandemark NL (eds): The Testis. Vol 1. New York, Academic Press, 1970

HELLER CG, CLERMONT Y: Kinetics of the germinal epithelium in man. Recent Prog Horm Res 20:545, 1964

HOLSTEIN AF: Ultrastructural observations on the differentiation of spermatids in man. Andrologia 8:157, 1975

HOLSTEIN AF, ROOSEN–RUNGE EC: Atlas of Human Spermatogenesis. Berlin, Grosse Verlag, 1981

HOSKINS DD, JOHNSON D, BRANDT H, ASCOTT TS: Evidence for a role for a forward motility protein in the epididymal development of sperm motility. In Fawcett DW, Bedford JM (eds): The Spermatozoon: Maturation, Motility, Surface Properties and Comparative Aspects, p 43. Baltimore, Urban & Schwarzenberg, 1979

HUCKINS C: The spermatogonial stem cell population in adult rats. I. Their morphology, proliferation and maturation. Anat Rec 169:533, 1971

JOHNSON AD, GOMES WR, VANDEMARK NL (eds): The Testis. Vol 1, Development, Anatomy and Physiology; Vol 2, Biochemistry; Vol 3, Influencing Factors. New York, Academic Press, 1970

KOEHLER JK: Human sperm head ultrastructure: A freeze-etching study. J Ultrastruct Res 39:520, 1972

LAM DMK, FURRER R, BRUCE WR: The separation, physical characterization and differential kinetics of spermatogonial cells of the mouse. Proc Natl Acad Sci USA, 65:192, 1970

LEBLOND CP, CLERMONT Y: Definition of the stages of the cycle of the seminiferous epithelium in the rat. Ann NY Acad Sci 55: 548, 1952

MACLEOD J: The significance of deviations in human sperm morphology. In Rosemberg, ER, Paulsen CA (eds): The Human Testis, p 481. New York, Plenum, 1970

MEISTRICH ML, ENG VWS, LOIR M: Temperature effects on the kinetics of spermatogenesis in the mouse. Cell Tissue Kinet 6:379, 1973

MOENS PB: Mechanisms of chromosome synapsis at meiotic prophase. Internat Rev Cytol 35:117, 1973

MOENS PB, GO VLW: Intercellular bridges and division patterns of rat spermatogonia. Z Zellforsch 127:201, 1971

MOENS PB, HUGENHOLTZ AD: The arrangement of germ cells in the rat seminiferous tubule: An electron microscopic study. J Cell Sci 19:487, 1975

MOENS PB, HUGENHOLTZ AD: A new approach to stem cell research in spermatogenesis. In Cairnie AB, Lala PK, Osmond DG (eds): Stem Cells of Renewing Cell Populations. New York, Academic Press, 1976

MORESI V: Chromosome activities during meiosis and spermatogenesis. J Reprod Fertil (Suppl) 13:1, 1971

NAGANO T, SUZUKI F: Cell junctions in the seminiferous tubule and the excurrent ducts of the testis. Int Rev Cytol 81:163, 1983

ODELL WD, MOYER DL: The testis and the male sex accessories. In Physiology of Reproduction. St. Louis, CV Mosby, 1971

OHNO S: Morphological aspects of meiosis and their genetical significance. In Rosemberg E, Paulsen CA (eds): Advances in Experimental Medicine and Biology. The Human Testis. New York, Plenum, 1970

O'RAND MG: Changes in sperm surface properties correlated with capacitation. In Fawcett DW, Bedford JM (eds): The Spermatozoon: Maturation, Motility, Surface Properties and Comparative Aspects, p 195. Baltimore, Urban & Schwarzenberg, 1979

PERCY B, CLERMONT Y, LEBLOND CP: The wave of the seminiferous epithelium in the rat. Am J Anat 108:47, 1961

PHILLIPS DM: Comparative analysis of mammalian sperm motility. J Cell Biol 53:561, 1972

PHILLIPS DM: Substructure of the mammalian acrosome. J Ultrastruct Res 38:591, 1972

DE ROOIJ DG: Proliferation and differentiation of undifferentiated spermatogonia in the mammalian testis. In Potten CS (ed): Stem Cells: Their Identification and Characterization, p 89. Edinburgh, Churchill Livingstone, 1983

ROOSEN-RUNGE EC: The process of spermatogenesis in mammals. Biol Rev 37:343, 1962

ROSEMBERG E, PAULSEN CA (eds): Advances in Experimental Medicine and Biology. The Human Testis. New York, Plenum, 1970

ROWLEY MJ, BERLIN JD, HELLER CG: The ultrastructure of four types of human spermatogonia. Z Zellforsch 112:139, 1971

SATIR P: The basis of flagellar motility in spermatozoa: Current status. In Fawcett DW, Bedford JM (eds): The Spermatozoon: Maturation, Motility, Surface Properties and Comparative Aspects, p 81. Baltimore, Urban & Schwarzenberg, 1979

SCHNEDL W: End to end association of X and Y chromosomes in mouse meiosis. Nature [New Biol] 236:29, 1972

SCHULZE C: Morphological characteristics of the spermatogonial stem cells in man. Cell Tissue Res 198:191, 1979

SETCHELL BP: Characteristics of testicular spermatozoa and the fluid which transports them into the epididymis. Biol Reprod (Suppl 1) 1:40, 1969

SETCHELL BP: Testicular blood supply, lymphatic drainage and secretion of fluid. In Johnson AD, Gomes WR, Vandemark NL (eds): The Testis. Vol 1. New York, Academic Press, 1970

SOLARI AJ, TRES LL: Ultrastructure and histochemistry of the nucleus during male meiotic prophase. In Rosemberg E, Paulsen CA (eds): Advances in Experimental Medicine and Biology. The Human Testis. New Hork, Plenum, 1970

STURGESS JM, TURNER JAP: Transposition of ciliary microtubules: Another cause of impaired ciliary motility. N Engl J Med 303: 318, 1980

STURGESS JM, TURNER JAP: Ultrastructural pathology of cilia in the immotile cilia syndrome. Perspect Pediatr Pathol 8:133, 1984

VILAR O: Histology of the human testis from neonatal period to adolescence. In Rosemberg E, Paulsen CA (eds): Advances in Experimental Medicine and Biology. The Human Testis. New York, Plenum, 1970

WARTENBERG H, HOLSTEIN AF: Morphology of the "spindle-shaped body" in the developing tail of human spermatids. Cell Tissue Res 159:435, 1975

WYROBEK AJ, BRUCE WR: Chemical induction of sperm abnormalities in mice. Proc Natl Acad Sci USA 72:4425, 1975

ZANEVELD LJD: Capacitation of spermatozoa. In Ludwig H, Tauber PT (eds): Human Fertilization, p 128. Stuttgart, Georg Thieme Verlag KG, 1978

Interstitial Cells, Sertoli Cells, Blood–Testis Barrier, Hormonal Basis of Testicular Function, and Male Reproductive Ducts

CHRISTENSEN AK: Fine structure of testicular interstitial cells in humans. In Rosemberg E, Paulsen CA (eds): Advances in Experimental Medicine and Biology. The Human Testis. New York, Plenum, 1970

DORRINGTON JH, ARMSTRONG DT: Effects of FSH on gonadal functions. Recent Prog Horm Res 35:301, 1979

DYM M, CAVICCHIA JC: Functional morphology of the testis. Biol Reprod 18:1, 1978

DYM M, FAWCETT DW: The blood–testis barrier in the rat and the physiological compartmentation of the seminiferous epithelium. Biol Reprod 3:308, 1970

FAWCETT DW: Ultrastructure and function of the Sertoli cell. In Hamilton DW, Greep RO (eds): Handbook of Physiology. Endocrinology. Vol 5, Sect 7. Male Reproductive System. Washington DC, American Physiological Society, 1975

FAWCETT DW, LEAK LV, HEIDGER PM: Electron microscopic observations on the structural components of the blood–testis barrier. J Reprod Fertil (Suppl) 10:105, 1970

FAWCETT DW, NEAVES WB, FLORES MN: Comparative observations on intertubular lymphatics and the organization of the interstitial tissue of the mammalian testis. Biol Reprod 9:500, 1973

FRITZ IB: Sites of action of androgens and follicle stimulating hormone on cells of the seminiferous tubule. In Litwack E (ed): Biochemical Actions of Hormones, Vol 5, p 249. New York, Academic Press, 1979

GILULA NB, FAWCETT DW, AOKI A: Ultrastructural and experimental observations on the Sertoli cell junctions of the mammalian testis. Dev Biol 50:142, 1976

GOMES WR: Metabolic and regulatory hormones influencing testis function. In Johnson AD, Gomes WR, Vandemark NL (eds): The Testis. Vol 3. New York, Academic Press, 1970

HALL PF: Endocrinology of the testis. In Johnson AD, Gomes WR, Vandemark NL (eds): The Testis. Vol 2. New York, Academic Press, 1970

HOOKER CW: The intertubular tissue of the testis. In Johnson AD, Gomes WR, Vandemark NL (eds): The Testis. Vol 1. New York, Academic Press, 1970

LIPSETT MB, SAVARD K: Subcellular structure and synthesis of steroids in the testis. In Rosemberg E, Paulsen CA (eds): Advances in Experimental Medicine and Biology. The Human Testis. New York, Plenum, 1970

LORDING DW, DE KRETSER DM: Comparative ultrastructural and histochemical studies of interstitial cells of rat testis during fetal and postnatal development. J Reprod Fertil 29:261, 1972

ODELL WD, MOYER DL: Dynamic relationship of the testis to the whole man. In Physiology of Reproduction. St. Louis, CV Mosby, 1971

ROSEMBERG E, PAULSEN CA (eds): Regulation of Testicular Function. Role of the hypothalamus. Testicular–pituitary interrelationship. Metabolic effects of gonadotropins. Influence of gonadotropins on testicular function. In Advances in Experimental Medicine and Biology. The Human Testis. New York, Plenum, 1970

ROWLEY MJ, TESHIMA F, HELLER CG: Duration of transit of spermatozoa through the human male ductular system. Fertil Steril 21:390, 1970

SETCHELL BP: The functional significance of the blood–testis barrier. J Androl 1:3, 1980

SETCHELL BP, WAITES GMH: The blood–testis barrier. In Hamilton DW, Greep RO (eds): Handbook of Physiology. Endocrinology. Vol 5, Sect 7. Male Reproductive System. Washington DC, American Physiological Society, 1975

STEINBERGER E: Hormonal control of mammalian spermatogenesis. Physiol Rev 51:1, 1971

TSANG WN, LACY D, COLLINS PM: Leydig cell differentiation, steroid metabolism by interstitium in-vitro and growth of accessory sex organs in rat. J Reprod Fertil 34:351, 1973

25

The Eye and the Ear

THE EYE

The paired *eyes* are the unique and irreplaceable organs of special sense that encode visual information and provide us with the sense of sight. To some extent, they are designed along the same principles as an old-fashioned camera; the excellent image-producing and focusing capabilities of the eye's lens–iris combination and the functional correspondence between retinal photoreceptors and the constituents of an unexposed photographic emulsion will be appreciated by all who are familiar with a camera or a microscope (see Fig. 1-15, *left*). Yet the complexities of the eye still far exceed those of the most sophisticated modern camera, and the unique mechanism by which the

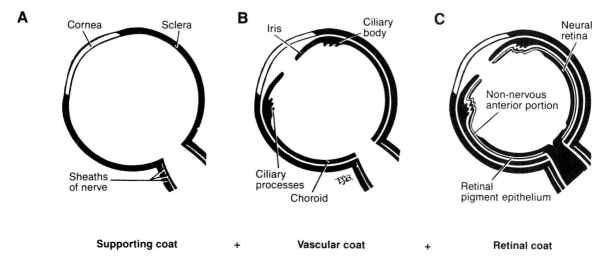

Fig. 25-1. Schematic diagram of the three layers (coats) that make up the wall of the eye.

eye can bring the image of a near object into focus has never been emulated because it depends on the special physical properties of the lens tissue itself.

Our first consideration will be the general wall structure of the eye.

The Wall of the Eye. Three layers (coats) constitute the wall of the eye: (1) an external *supporting layer*, (2) a *middle layer*, and (3) the *retinal layer* (Fig. 25-1). However, these three layers are not all present in every part of the eye wall.

The outermost layer is a *supporting layer* that is made of dense fibrous connective tissue. Over most of the eye surface, this layer is represented by the *sclera* (Gr. *scleros*, hard), which is hard and white compared with the rest of the eye and constitutes the "white" of the eye (Fig. 25-1A). However, where the supporting layer covers the central part of the anterior surface of the eye, it bulges forward slightly and is transparent. This windowlike area in the outermost layer is called the *cornea* (Fig. 25-1A). The supporting layer completely encloses the other two layers of the eye wall, but not where the outermost layer is penetrated posteriorly by the optic nerve (Fig. 25-1C).

The *middle layer* of the eye wall is known as the *uveal layer* or *tract* (L. *uva*, grape) because it is pigmented and surrounds the jellylike contents of the eye like the skin of a dark grape. Because this middle layer is also very vascular, it is sometimes referred to as the *vascular layer* of the eye wall. Anteriorly, this middle layer is represented by the iris and the ciliary body (Fig. 25-1B). The *iris* is an adjustable diaphragm with smooth muscle that regulates the aperture size of the pupil and with melanin-containing cells that, by virtue of their numbers and distribution, confer a variety of different eye colors. The *ciliary body* is a ringlike thickening of the perimeter of the circular corneoscleral junction that projects inward and houses the *ciliary muscle*, the im-

portant smooth muscle that is responsible for bringing images of near objects into focus (Figs. 25-1B and 25-2).

In the part of the eye that lies posterior to the ciliary body, the middle layer is represented by a thin but highly vascular nutritive layer called the *choroid* (Figs. 25-1B and 25-2). The intense dark brown (almost black) color of this layer is due to its substantial content of the pigment melanin, which keeps glare within the eye to a minimum because it absorbs scattered or reflected light.

The innermost layer of the eye wall is termed the *retinal layer* (Fig. 25-1C). This is a complex layer that is made up of the *neural retina*, which is a fairly thick inner layer of highly specialized brain-derived nervous tissue, with an associated outer layer of simple cuboidal pigmented epithelium that is known as the *retinal pigment epithelium* (RPE) because of its substantial melanin content. The neural retina is the light-sensitive layer of the eye wall; it consists largely of two kinds of *photoreceptors* known as retinal *rods* and *cones* together with various orders of interneurons. The RPE absorbs the light that has just passed through the neural retina, preventing its reflection back into the interior of the eye where it would otherwise result in glare. Three other important functional features of the RPE cells are (1) that their lateral borders are interconnected by well-developed continuous tight junctions that form part of a *blood–retina barrier*, (2) that they play a key role in the restoration of photosensitivity to visual pigments that have dissociated in response to light, and (3) that they phagocytose and dispose of membranous disks that have been discarded by the retinal photoreceptors.

There Are Four Refractile Media in the Eye. The eye has four transparent components that are often described as the *refractile media* of the eye. First, there is the *cornea* itself. Posterior to the cornea lies the second refractile medium, a watery fluid called the *aqueous humor*. This fluid is believed to originate from the fenestrated capillaries that

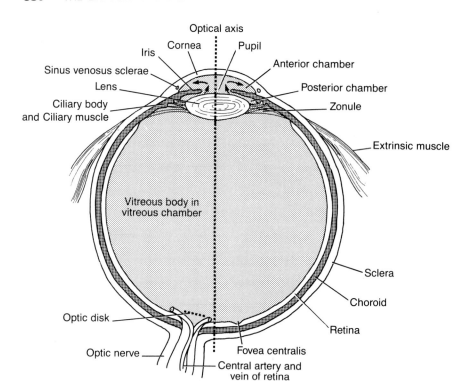

Fig. 25-2. Diagrammatic representation of the right eye, cut in horizontal section so as to disclose its basic structure.

lie under the *ciliary epithelium* covering the ciliary processes, which are folds of vascular loose connective tissue extending from the ciliary body. As in the case of cerebrospinal fluid production by the choroid plexuses, the surface epithelium modifies the composition of the capillary filtrate as this passes through them. As a result, the aqueous humor contains increased concentrations of bicarbonate, sodium, and chloride ions and also of free amino acids and ascorbic acid. The secreted aqueous humor first passes into the *posterior chamber* of the eye, which is the small intraocular cavity that lies posterior to the iris and anterior to the vitreous body (Fig. 25-2). From the posterior chamber, it is able to pass through a valvelike arrangement around the pupillary margin of the iris. Here the posterior border of the pupillary margin of the iris comes into contact with the anterior surface of the lens without being attached to it. Because the iris can be displaced anteriorly by even a slight relative increase in the hydrostatic pressure within the posterior chamber, this arrangement acts as a one-way valve that admits aqueous humor to the *anterior chamber*, which lies between the anterior surface of the iris and the cornea (Fig. 25-2). This pathway taken by the aqueous humor around the pupillary margin is indicated by the arrows in Figure 25-2. From the anterior chamber, excess aqueous humor drains by way of a circumferential venous canal called the *sinus venosus sclerae* (Fig. 25-2), which is also known as the *canal of Schlemm.*

An important role of the aqueous humor is to provide the necessary nutrients for the inner region of the cornea,

which is avascular, and also for the third refractile component, the *lens,* which is also avascular. The fourth refractile medium is the *vitreous body,* which occupies the relatively large *vitreous chamber* of the eye (Fig. 25-2). This structure is a globular mass of very hydrated, transparent jellylike material containing hyaluronic acid, widely dispersed collagen fibrils, and other proteins. Traversing the vitreous body is the *hyaloid canal (Cloquet's canal),* which is an indistinct channel that extends from the optic nerve to the lens and that contains a vestige of the embryonic hyaloid artery. This transparent viscoelastic mass lies in contact with the inner surface of the retina and gently holds the neural retina in place against the rest of the wall. It similarly supports the posterior borders of the lens and the iris (Fig. 25-2).

The convex anterior surface of the cornea, not that of the lens, is the main site of light refraction (bending of light rays). The unique importance of the lens is that it is elastic and that its focal length can therefore be adjusted through contraction of the ciliary muscle that is attached to it. Such contraction releases the tension that is being applied to the margin of the lens and allows it to assume a more globular form. Finally, it should be noted that when light passes through the vitreous body, it does not immediately reach the photoreceptors because these lie deep in the neural retina, next to the RPE (see Fig. 25-8). Light must first penetrate the transparent nerve fibers and nerve cells that are present in the inner layers of the neural retina (*i.e.,* the layers bordering on the vitreous body).

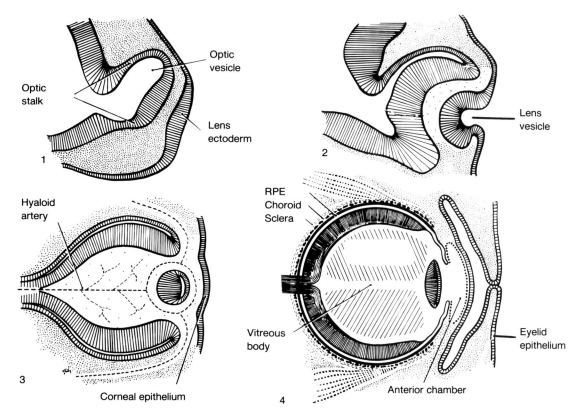

Fig. 25-3. Schematic diagram of four representative stages in the development of the eye. For details, see text.

To understand the detailed structure of the eye, it is necessary to know something about the way it develops, which is briefly outlined in the following section.

Synopsis of Eye Development. The *retina* of each eye develops as an outgrowth of the forebrain, which early in development is hollow. The anterior wall of this outgrowth bulges forward to form a *primary optic vesicle* that remains attached to the forebrain by an *optic stalk* (Fig. 25-3, stage 1). The associated ectoderm thickens and becomes the *lens ectoderm* (Fig. 25-3, stage 1). The anterior wall of the optic vesicle then invaginates, with the result that the optic vesicle becomes cup-shaped and the wall of the *optic cup* thus formed has two layers (Fig. 25-3, stage 2). Also, the lens ectoderm bulges inward to form the *lens vesicle* (Fig. 25-3, stage 2), which later separates from the *corneal epithelium* (Fig. 25-3, stage 3). The lining layer of the optic cup becomes the *neural retina,* and the outer layer becomes the *RPE* (Fig. 25-3, stage 4).

During development of the retina from neuroectoderm, the layer that gives rise to the photoreceptor cells of the neural retina undergoes a series of invaginations and eversions that leads to their appearing to be "upside down" in the retina, with their apical end deep to their basal end. Topologically, however, the polarity of these cells within the membrane does not change. Their apparent inversion is essentially due to invagination of the neural plate during formation of the neural tube (see Fig. 5-3). The photosensitive part of the photoreceptor cells is derived from a single cilium that develops on their apical surface, which now faces the lumen of the neural tube. This apparent inversion persists when the primary

optic vesicle forms as an outgrowth of the forebrain and then invaginates to form the optic cup, the residual slitlike lumen of which constitutes a cup-shaped extension of the lumen of the neural tube. Thus the apical end of the neuroectoderm-derived photoreceptors ends up facing a narrow cup-shaped potential space, which is all that remains of the original cavity of the optic vesicle, in direct apposition to the RPE that constitutes the outer layer of the cup (Fig. 25-3, stage 4; see also Fig. 25-14).

During development, the eye receives blood by way of an artery called the *hyaloid artery* that enters the eye by way of the optic stalk (Fig. 25-3, stage 3). When additional arterial vessels later develop, this artery atrophies, leaving the hyaloid canal in its place.

Both the *middle layer* and the *supporting layer* of the eye wall are derivatives of the mesoderm that surrounds the developing eye. The substance of the *cornea* also forms from mesoderm, but ectoderm persists over its anterior surface as an epithelial covering (Fig. 25-3, stage 4). The *anterior chamber* develops as a space within the mesoderm (Fig. 25-3, stage 4). The *ciliary body* and the *iris* also arise from mesoderm.

We shall now describe the microscopic structure and functions of the various parts of the eye in greater detail.

CORNEA

The *cornea* represents the anterior part of the supporting layer of the eye wall (Fig. 25-1*A*). It is both *transparent* and

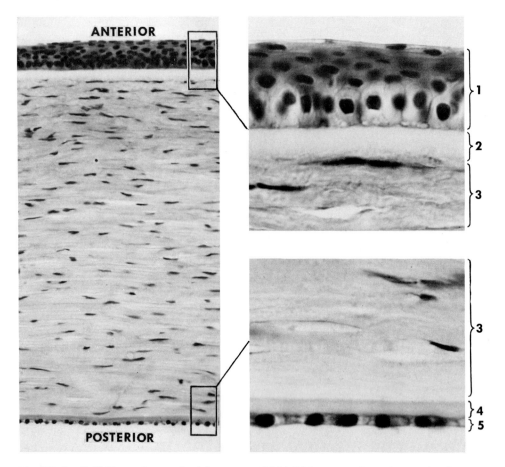

ANTERIOR

POSTERIOR

Fig. 25-4.   (*Left*) Photomicrograph of the cornea. (*Right*) High-power photomicrographs showing representative parts of the cornea: (*1*) stratified squamous epithelium; (*2*) Bowman's layer; (*3*) substantia propria; (*4*) Descemet's membrane; (*5*) endothelium.

avascular, and its radius of curvature is smaller than that of the eye as a whole. Because the cornea is exposed, it is vulnerable to abrasion and other kinds of trauma. In treating injuries of the cornea, it is helpful to know that its thickness is approximately 0.5 mm centrally and approximately double this at its periphery.

The cornea consists chiefly of a dense ordinary connective tissue called its *substantia propria*. This tissue is transparent even though it is made up of a substantial quantity of intercellular substances and cells (Fig. 25-4). Anteriorly, the cornea is covered with *stratified squamous nonkeratinizing epithelium*, and posteriorly it is lined by a single layer of *endothelial cells* (Fig. 25-4).

The anterior epithelium of the cornea is provided with afferent nerve endings that are sensitive to pain. Stimulation of these endings elicits blinking of the eyelids and the flowing of tears. The anterior surface of the cornea must always be kept wet with tears, and microvilli on the free surface of the epithelium retain a film of tears over the entire corneal surface. If the external surface of the cornea is allowed to become dry, the cornea may ulcerate.

The cornea receives its nutrients by diffusion from the aqueous humor and from the scleral capillaries near the corneoscleral junction. In addition to these nutritional requirements, the cornea has to obtain its oxygen directly from the air, and its requirement for sufficient gas exchange has to be taken into account in selecting suitable plastics for the permanent type of soft contact lenses, which are worn for extended periods of time.

The underlying basement membrane of the anterior corneal epithelium attaches this epithelium to an acellular anterior layer of stromal intercellular substances known as *Bowman's layer* (Fig. 25-4). This is a transparent homogeneous layer that in the electron microscope (EM) is seen to contain collagen fibrils in random array. It is regarded as constituting a protective barrier that is resistant to trauma and bacterial invasion; once destroyed, it is not regenerated. Bowman's layer does not extend from the cornea into the sclera; the site where it ends (which is also where the cornea undergoes transition into sclera) is called the *limbus* (L. for border).

The bulk of the corneal stroma, the *substantia propria*, comprises approximately 90% of the thickness of the cornea. It contains layers of flattened fibroblasts sandwiched

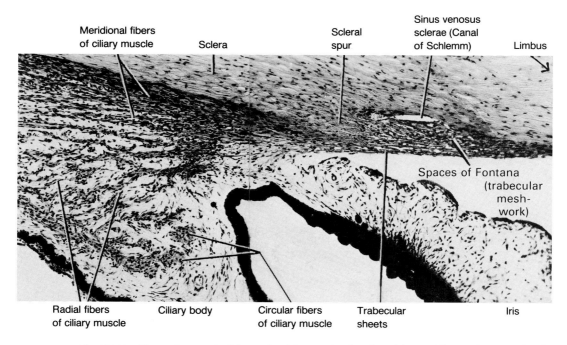

Meridional fibers of ciliary muscle · Sclera · Scleral spur · Sinus venosus sclerae (Canal of Schlemm) · Limbus

Spaces of Fontana (trabecular mesh-work)

Radial fibers of ciliary muscle · Ciliary body · Circular fibers of ciliary muscle · Trabecular sheets · Iris

Fig. 25-5. Photomicrograph of the angle of the anterior chamber of the eye. This site lies immediately posterior to the limbus. In the iridocorneal angle (the acute angle between the iris and the limbus, seen on the *right*) lies a circular canal called the sinus venosus sclerae (the canal of Schlemm). This canal represents the main route by which aqueous humor leaves the anterior chamber.

between approximately 200 to 250 lamellae of type I collagen fibrils. Some of the lamellae can be discerned in the left panel of Figure 25-4. The collagen fibrils are arranged parallel to the corneal surface, and the fibrils of each lamella lie at right angles to those of the next. Also, some of the fibrils extend between adjacent lamellae and hold them together. The collagen fibrils are embedded in an amorphous matrix that contains sulfated gycosaminoglycans (chiefly keratan sulfate with some chondroitin-4-sulfate and chondroitin-6-sulfate) covalently bound to protein as corneal proteoglycan.

Transparency of the cornea depends on limitation of its degree of hydration. For the cornea to stay perfectly transparent, water has to be withdrawn from it (as tissue fluid) on a continuing basis. In this connection, integrity of the single layer of endothelial cells covering its posterior surface seems to be particularly important. In the EM, these cells manifest signs of active transcellular endocytosis, and there is additional evidence that they are able to transfer water from the corneal stroma to the aqueous humor. Consistent with such a role is the clinical finding that corneal edema commonly results from a tear or a break in this thin layer. Furthermore, defects in the corneal endothelium can lead to local clouding of the cornea, and if severe enough, such defects can result in corneal opacity.

Another homogenous acellular layer, termed *Descemet's membrane* (Fig. 25-4), lies posterior to the substantia propria. This layer represents a highly developed basement membrane and contains collagen in a characteristic array (Jakus).

It is produced by the single layer of squamous endothelial cells that covers the posterior surface of the cornea (Fig. 25-4).

Corneal Grafting (Keratoplasty). Corneal transplants made from one person to another (*i.e.*, *allografts*) meet with considerable success. The main reason why they are so successful is that the cornea consists chiefly of intercellular substances and does not contain any blood vessels or recognizable lymphatics. Its substantial content of intercellular substances probably helps to shield the recipient's immune system from detecting the foreign histocompatibility antigens on the engrafted cells, but their main effect is probably that they impede direct contact between any cytotoxic T-cells that are formed and the donor target cells that these cells might otherwise lyse. The original donor-derived stromal cells persist in the allograft and are not replaced by cells from the recipient (Basu). However, it is fairly common for the epithelium of the allograft to become replaced by a layer of epithelial cells from the recipient.

SCLERA

The *sclera* is a tough layer of white fibrous tissue that contains collagen fiber bundles with flattened fibrocytes between them (Fig. 25-5). Some elastic fibers are intermixed with this collagen. The fibers are less regularly arranged than in the substantia propria of the cornea, and the matrix in which they are embedded is of a somewhat different composition. The sclera is sufficiently thick for it to be possible to suture it from the outside without the needle penetrating the vascular middle layer of the eye wall. Moreover, in adults, it is strong enough to withstand increased intraocular pressure if this condition develops. The relative opacity of the sclera in comparison to the cornea is primarily due to its higher water content.

Posteriorly, the sclera is continuous with the dural sheath of the optic nerve (and usually the arachnoid sheath as well). The perforated posterior part of the sclera that is traversed by the optic nerve fibers is called the *lamina cribrosa* (L. *cribrum*, sieve). The sclera is poorly supplied with blood capillaries, but larger vessels penetrate it obliquely in gaining access to the vascular (middle) layer of the eye wall.

CHOROID

The *choroid* is the part of the vascular (middle) layer of the wall of the eye that lies in the posterior part of the eye (*i.e.,* posterior to the ciliary body). Only 0.1 to 0.2 mm thick, the choroid is generally regarded as being made up of four components called the *suprachoroid,* the *vessel layer,* the *choriocapillaris,* and *Bruch's membrane.*

The *suprachoroid,* which is its outermost layer (see Fig. 25-10), is a transitional zone that consists chiefly of elastic fibers attached to the sclera. The intercellular fibers are arranged as six to ten thin interconnected lamellae in which melanocytes, fibrocytes, and macrophages are embedded. Between the lamellae, there is a potential space filled with a watery ground substance and often referred to as the *suprachoroidal (perichoroidal) space.* Numerous nerve fibers and some ganglion cells are also present in this superficial zone of the choroid.

The *vessel layer* (see Fig. 25-10) contains the tortuous choroidal arteries, the choroidal veins, and the four vortex veins that drain the choroidal veins. The loose connective tissue stroma that supports its numerous vessels contains the same kinds of cells as the suprachoroid but is strengthened with a higher content of collagen.

The *choriocapillaris* (see Fig. 25-10) consists of a single layer of unusually wide fenestrated capillaries; these are the only capillaries in the choroid. Their functional importance is that they nourish the outer third of the retina, which is where the photoreceptors are located. In regions where substantial areas of this capillary circulation have been lost as a result of disease, the overlying areas of the retina become atrophied.

Finally, *Bruch's membrane,* alternatively known as the *lamina vitrea* and representing the innermost component of the choroid, is a complex acellular structure that is itself composed of five layers. Its outermost and innermost layers correspond to the basement membranes of the choriocapillaris and the RPE, respectively. Between these two basement membranes lie two layers of collagen with a layer of elastin sandwiched between them.

Bruch's membrane is believed to play a significant role in limiting access of potentially inappropriate macromolecules from the fenestrated capillaries of the choriocapillaris to the adjacent outer part of the retinal layer of the eye wall.

CILIARY BODY

Anteriorly, the choroid becomes continuous with the *ciliary body.* This structure extends forward to a site where a narrow flange of sclera known as the *scleral spur* projects inward (Figs. 25-2 and 25-5). The ciliary body is a thickening of the middle layer of the eye wall that appears as a ring on the inner aspect of the sclera, posterior to the scleral spur (Figs. 25-2 and 25-5). The ciliary body has fibers of *ciliary muscle* in place of the suprachoroid layer; this is a smooth muscle and it comprises the bulk of the ciliary body (Fig. 25-5).

The ciliary muscle fibers can exert pull in three different directions and are accordingly regarded as belonging to three separate functional groups. The *meridional fibers* (a *meridian* of a globe extends from pole to pole and crosses its equator at right angles) arise in the suprachoroid near the ciliary body and pass forward to end at the scleral spur (Fig. 25-5). The *radial fibers* lie internal to the meridional fibers and fan out posteriorly so as to form a wide attachment to the choroid (Fig. 25-5). The *circular* fibers lie at the inner edge of the ciliary body, close to its base (Fig. 25-5), and encircle the eye at this site.

To explain how contraction of the ciliary muscle can change the shape of the lens and bring the image of a near object into focus, it is necessary to describe the lens and how it is suspended.

LENS

The *lens* resembles the cornea in that it is transparent and avascular. However, unlike the cornea, it is composed entirely of modified epithelial cells and lacks a connective tissue component. This is because of the way it develops. It will be recalled that the lens ectoderm bulges inward to form a *lens vesicle* (Fig. 25-3, stage 2) that later pinches off from the surface ectoderm. As a result, the developing lens becomes a hollow structure with a posterior wall that is made up of tall columnar cells and an anterior wall that is made up of cuboidal epithelium (Fig. 25-3, stage 3). The central cavity of the lens vesicle eventually disappears. The vesicle moves inward and gradually assumes a biconvex shape (Fig. 25-3, stage 4).

Lens Epithelial Cells Differentiate into Lens Fibers. As the lens continues to develop, the tall columnar cells that constitute its posterior wall lengthen, dispense with their nucleus, and differentiate into elongated transparent structures known as *lens fibers.* The first-formed group of lens

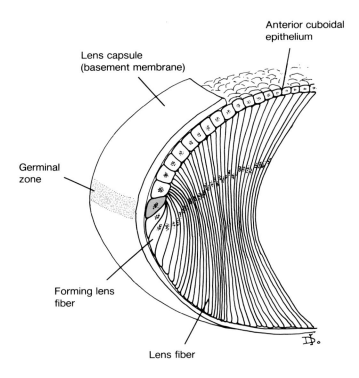

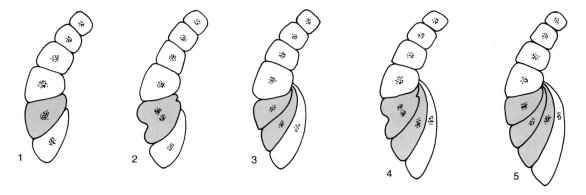

Fig. 25-6. Diagrammatic representation of part of the equatorial region of the lens of the eye, showing its microscopic structure and the mechanism by which it grows (horizontal section oriented with its anterior surface uppermost). The bottom series of diagrams illustrates how the division of anterior epithelial cells in the equatorial germinal zone of the lens produces daughter cells that subsequently elongate and become new lens fibers.

fibers are derived from the posterior wall of the lens vesicle; they are termed the *primary lens fibers.* In contrast, the anterior cuboidal epithelial cells remain less highly differentiated and retain the potential to divide (*e.g.,* in response to injury). Moreover, in the band of anterior cuboidal epithelium that encircles the rim of the lens (*i.e.,* its widest diameter, midway between its anterior and posterior poles), the cells can still divide in adult life and are therefore de-

scribed as constituting the *germinal zone* of the lens. The important contribution made by cells of this zone to growth of the lens will be considered in the following section.

Growth of the Lens. The *germinal zone* of the lens is the marginal band of epithelium that lies around its rim (Fig. 25-6). The rim of the lens is known as its *equatorial region* because it lies midway between the two poles (the anterior and posterior poles) of the lens. In this zone, a mechanism exists for appositional growth of the lens because the most posterior cells of the anterior epithelium, which extends as far as the equator (Fig. 25-6), can elongate and transform into lens fibers. These are called *secondary lens fibers* to distinguish them from the *primary lens fibers* that are derived from the posterior epithelium. Because all lens growth has to occur within the confines of the lens capsule, the only way the elongating lens fibers can fit into the lens is by bending according to the pattern shown in Figure 25-6. Then as each bent lens fiber continues to elongate, it tends to straighten again (Fig. 25-6).

Lens growth occurs because new epithelial cells arise within the germinal zone at the equatorial border of the lens and continue to differentiate into new lens fibers that become added at this border, internal to the capsule and just posterior to the equator (Fig. 25-6). Some of the new anterior epithelial cells generated in this manner continue to serve as progenitor cells for new lens fibers whereas others differentiate into new lens fibers as shown in Figure 25-6. Although the lens continues to increase in diameter in adult life, the original lens fibers still must last a lifetime because they are added to but not replaced.

Before a lens epithelial cell becomes a lens fiber, it possesses a nucleus and all the usual cytoplasmic organelles. During its transformation into a lens fiber, its nucleus degenerates and the nuclear envelope fragments. Lengthening of the cell is believed to involve microfilament assembly and the alignment of its microtubules along its longitudinal axis. The only organelles that persist are a few longitudinal microtubules, a network of filaments, and groups of free ribosomes. The remainder of the cytoplasm appears granular in the EM; it consists primarily of the *crystallins*, a much-studied family of proteins that characterizes lens fibers. Protein synthesis is nevertheless believed to continue for a while in the newly formed lens fibers; because these structures have dispensed with their nucleus, this would require the presence of long-lived mRNA.

Finally, the lateral borders of the lens fibers are extensively interlocked, presumably to prevent sliding of the fibers past each other during focusing of the eye. Scanning EM studies have shown that these borders are provided with surface knobs that fit into corresponding depressions on the adjacent fibers (Hollenberg et al). In addition, desmosomes, tight junctions, and gap junctions between these cells have been described.

The *lens capsule* represents a greatly thickened basement membrane made by both the anterior epithelial cells and the lens fibers. In the EM, it exhibits a lamellar structure suggestive of the deposition of a number of consecutive basement membranes, each discernible as a lamina densa.

The lens is held under tension forces that tend to make it assume a more or less globular shape. However, during the aging process it becomes less elastic, with the result that the range of focus that it can achieve diminishes, most

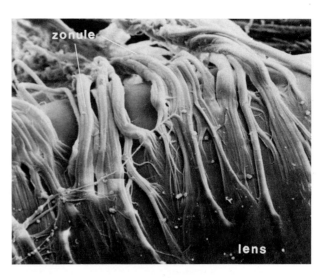

Fig. 25-7. Scanning electron micrograph of a portion of the zonule attached to the periphery of the lens (monkey's eye). The bundles of fibrils are attached to the capsule of the lens. (Courtesy of P. Basu)

commonly around middle age. The wearing of spectacles may then become necessary for focusing on near objects.

ZONULE AND MECHANISM OF ACCOMMODATION

The lens is attached to the ciliary body by means of the *zonule* (Figs. 25-2 and 25-7). Sometimes referred to as the *suspensory ligament* of the lens, the zonule is a rather complex structure that is made up of fibrils and bundles of fibrils (Fig. 25-7), between which there are wide open spaces through which aqueous humor can freely pass. It has a broad zone of attachment both to the equatorial region of the lens (Fig. 25-7) and to the ciliary body. Present evidence indicates that the zonular fibrils are probably made of the same glycoprotein as the microfibrils that are present in elastic fibers.

Accommodation. Contraction of the *ciliary muscle* fibers anchored to the sclera in the region of the scleral spur pulls the part of the ciliary body to which the zonule is attached *forward* and *inward*. Because the zonular attachment to the ciliary body lies posterior to the zonular attachment to the lens, this action *relaxes the tension on the zonule* and permits the lens, which is itself under tension, to assume a more globular shape. This change in the shape of the lens is described as *accommodation* for near objects. Thus muscular contraction is required for viewing near objects, and this is why reading "tires" the eyes. Furthermore, as already noted, accommodation becomes increasingly difficult when the lens loses its elasticity as a result of the aging process.

IRIS AND IRIDOCORNEAL ANGLE

The *iris* is a disk-shaped diaphragm that is situated between the anterior chamber and the posterior chamber of the eye; the *pupil* is its central adjustable aperture (Fig. 25-2). Its *pupillary margin* lies slightly anterior to its periphery (Fig. 25-2). Posteriorly, the iris is lined by two layers of *pigmented epithelial cells* (Fig. 25-5). Anteriorly, it is covered by a discontinuous layer of stromal cells.

The iris is provided with two distinct muscles known as the *sphincter pupillae* and the *dilator pupillae*, respectively. These two muscles are jointly responsible for automatic regulation of the diameter of the pupil so that only the appropriate amount of light enters the eye. The *sphincter pupillae* is a circular band of *smooth muscle fibers* that is situated at the pupillary margin of the iris; increase in its tonus diminishes the size of the pupil and increases the pressure between the posterior aspect of the pupillary margin and the part of the anterior surface of the lens that is in contact with the iris (Fig. 25-2). The *dilator pupillae* is not as distinct as the sphincter muscle and consists of a thin sheet of radial fibers that lie near the posterior border of the iris. Although these fibers have all the structural and functional attributes of smooth muscle fibers, they are actually *myoepithelial cells* that are derived from cells of the anterior layer of the two-layered posterior pigmented epithelium of the iris. Their contraction has the opposite effects to contraction of the sphincter pupillae fibers.

Pupillary size is automatically regulated by pupillary reflexes in which the *retina* acts as the *receptor* and the *iris muscles* act as the *effectors*. When someone looks at a bright object, the pupil is reflexly constricted, thereby decreasing the amount of light that enters the eye, and vice versa. As anyone familiar with photography will know, pupillary size has further significance. A dilated pupil, like a dilated aperture in a camera, results in diminished depth of focus. For this reason, glasses prescribed when the pupil is dilated are likely to be more accurate than those prescribed when the pupil is not dilated.

The *color* of the iris is due to melanin. As mentioned in Chapter 17 in connection with pigmentation of the dermis, melanin seen through a substantial thickness of tissue appears blue. Hence if the melanin in the iris is limited to the epithelial cells that line its posterior surface, the iris (provided that the stroma anterior to the pigment is of usual density) appears blue. If the stroma is somewhat denser than usual, the melanin at the back of the iris gives a gray color to the iris. If sufficient melanin is present in melanocytes in the substance of the stroma as well as in the epithelium at the back of the iris, the iris appears brown. In white races, the ultimate color of the iris is not necessarily evident in newborn infants.

In the so-called *angle of the anterior chamber* (the *iridocorneal angle*) immediately posterior to the *limbus* (the *limbus* is the junctional region between the cornea and the sclera), the *scleral spur* extends forward and inward (Fig. 25-5). Anterior to the scleral spur, a furrow dips down into the inner part of the sclera; this furrow is called the *internal scleral sulcus*. Both the scleral spur and the internal scleral sulcus encircle the eye. At the bottom of the internal scleral sulcus, there is a circular canal called the *sinus venosus sclerae* or the *canal of Schlemm* (Figs. 25-2 and 25-5), which, together with its collector channels, is lined by endothelium. Because the scleral spur and the canal of Schlemm both encircle the eye at the iridocorneal angle, they are both cut in transverse section in a meridional section of the eye (Fig. 25-5).

The bottom of the internal scleral sulcus is occupied by a loose trabecular meshwork of connective tissue, the inner part of which is arranged as a series of *trabecular sheets* (Fig. 25-5). The *trabecular spaces* in the meshwork (which were formerly referred to as the spaces of Fontana, indicated in Fig. 25-5) communicate freely with the anterior chamber. Their endothelial lining is continuous with the posterior endothelial covering of the cornea. The functional and clinical implications of this trabecular arrangement will be considered in the following section.

Outflow Pathway of Aqueous Humor

Aqueous humor that is formed by the ciliary processes passes through the valvelike potential opening between the lens and the iris from the posterior chamber to the anterior chamber of the eye (Fig. 25-2). It then passes to the iridocorneal angle, where most of it enters the trabecular spaces and drains by way of collector channels into the canal of Schlemm (Fig. 25-5). Aqueous humor leaves this canal by way of collector trunks in the sclera. These trunks pass out under the bulbar conjunctiva, where they are known as *aqueous veins* because they contain aqueous humor in place of blood. The aqueous veins communicate with blood-containing veins; hence aqueous humor eventually reaches the venous blood.

Glaucoma Is Due to Impeded Outflow of Aqueous Humor. The contents of the eye remain under constant pressure, the range of normal *intraocular pressure* lying somewhere between 13 and 19 mm Hg. To ensure adequate nourishment of all the tissues in the eye—especially the retina, which has one of the highest oxygen requirements in the body—the blood within the intraocular blood vessels (including capillaries and veins) has to be kept under a hydrostatic pressure that exceeds the intraocular pressure.

Because the supporting layer of the eye wall is unable to stretch, a normal intraocular pressure depends on the proper balance between formation and absorption of aqueous humor. If conditions develop in the eye that cause some impediment to the drainage of aqueous humor, the eye cannot swell; instead, the *intraocular pressure becomes elevated.* Sustained elevation of the intraocular pressure over 25 mm Hg can be sufficient to interfere with normal retinal function and nourishment. This condition is known as *glaucoma*, and it represents a common cause of blindness. In some cases, the impediment to normal outflow of aqueous humor is that the iridocorneal angle is so small that outflow is blocked when the pupil is dilated. In most instances, however, the cause of glaucoma is unknown. Therapeutic management of this condition is directed toward decreasing the rate of production of aqueous humor.

VITREOUS BODY

The *vitreous body* is an avascular mass of transparent gelled intercellular substance; the cells responsible for its formation are not known with certainty. It is bounded by the innermost layer of the retina (the *internal limiting membrane,* which will be described subsequently), the ciliary epithelial covering of the ciliary body and its processes, and the posterior surface of the zonule and lens capsule (Fig. 25-2). In addition to transmitting light, the vitreous body helps to hold the lens in place and also keeps the neural retina in apposition to the RPE. If any of it is lost (*e.g.,* during surgical procedures), these two layers of the retina may separate.

The periphery of the vitreous body is adherent to the internal limiting membrane of the retina, which represents a basement membrane, and is especially adherent at the papilla of the optic nerve (which will be described later in this chapter). It is also strongly adherent to the posterior aspect of the lens capsule and the basement membrane of the ciliary epithelium.

Through the vitreous body runs the *hyaloid (Cloquet's) canal,* which marks the position of the hyaloid artery of the embryonic eye (Fig. 25-3, stage 3). This canal, which extends from the papilla to the posterior surface of the lens, is usually inconspicuous in postnatal life. However, parts of the primitive hyaloid artery occasionally persist and, in some people, may interfere with vision to a minor extent.

The substance of the vitreous body is a highly hydrated viscoelastic colloidal gel containing hyaluronic acid in the form of sodium hyaluronate. This gel is supported by a loose network of randomly dispersed type II collagen fibrils. In addition, it contains the lower molecular weight constituents that are present in aqueous humor. The vitreous body is initially a uniform gel, but it gradually acquires internal pools of sol phase. When denatured by fixation, it exhibits a fibrillar structure in the light microscope (LM).

RETINA

When a *retina* initially develops from an optic vesicle, it consists of two layers because the anterior wall of the optic vesicle invaginates into the posterior half of the vesicle in such a way as to form a two-layered optic cup (Fig. 25-3). The outer layer of the optic cup gives rise to the RPE and the inner layer develops into the *neural retina,* which is responsible for initiating visual impulses (see Fig. 25-8). At this point, it is worthwhile to mention that when applied to the retina, the words *outer* and *inner* continue to be used in the same sense in that they refer to the eye as a whole.

Detached Retina. While the eye is developing, an intraretinal cleft persists between the two layers of the optic cup. Although the RPE and the neural retina later become adherent to each other, the RPE is more strongly attached

to the choroid than to the neural retina. In postnatal life, conditions may develop that lead to the separation of an area of the neural retina from the RPE. This eventuality is referred to as *detachment of the retina* even though it is really a separation between the two parts of the retina. Because the outer third of the neural retina depends on the diffusion of nutrients from the choriocapillaris, a detached neural retina shows degenerative changes unless it is promptly replaced by appropriate surgical procedures. Fortunately, however, a limited supply of nutrients and oxygen can generally reach at least part of the detached tissue from still intact capillaries that are supplied by the central retinal artery, and to some extent this helps the neural retina to survive until a reattachment procedure is performed.

The same kind of separation usually occurs during the preparation of histological sections of the eye because the lack of a strong attachment between the RPE and the neural retina results in these two layers pulling apart during fixation.

Blood–Retina Barrier. Functionally, the presence of continuous tight junctions between the contiguous RPE cells comprising the outermost layer of the retina limits access of substances of high molecular weight from the fenestrated capillaries of the choriocapillaris to the outer part of the retina, which is the part of the retina that contains the photoreceptor cells. These junctions constitute an important part of the *blood–retina barrier,* which represents a functional extension of the blood–brain barrier. Another permeability barrier similarly protects the inner part of the retina; this receives its nutrients from capillaries that are supplied by the central retinal artery, a functionally important artery that enters the eye by way of the papilla (optic disk). This complementary diffusion barrier consists of continuous tight junctions that are present between the endothelial cells of the retinal capillaries that supply the surface layers of the retina.

The Retina Is Made up of Ten Layers. It should be noted that the photoreceptive portion of each rod or cone lies to the *outside* of the other nervous tissue in the neural retina. Light therefore has to penetrate the inner part of the neural retina to reach the photoreceptors (Fig. 25-8). Optic nerve impulses pass through the retina in the reverse direction (*i.e.,* in the opposite direction to light rays; Fig. 25-8).

As a result of LM studies, the retina has come to be regarded as consisting of ten layers. Each of these layers will now be described.

The outermost layer of the retina, as already noted, is the RPE (Fig. 25-8; see also Figs. 25-10 and 25-11). Next to this epithelium lies a layer that contains the photosensitive portions, known as the *outer segments,* of the *rods* and *cones* (Figs. 25-8 and 25-9). The outer segments have a distinctive rodlike or conical shape in the two different types of photoreceptors, and this gives the receptors their

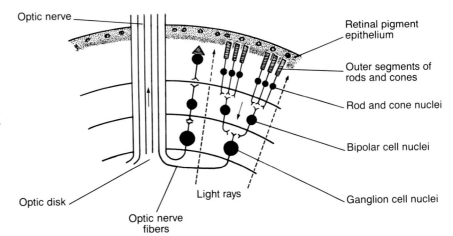

Fig. 25-8. Simplified diagram showing the arrangement of the cells in the retina.

respective names. The inner part of the layer of neural retina next to the RPE contains the *inner segments* of these cells (Fig. 25-9), which will be described later in this chapter. The adjacent layer is termed the *outer nuclear layer* (Fig. 25-9) because it contains the rod and cone nuclei (Figs. 25-8, 25-9, 25-10, and 25-11).

In the next layer, which is called the *outer plexiform layer* (Figs. 25-9, 25-10, and 25-11), the synaptic bodies of the photoreceptors synapse with the dendrites of a second order of neurons. The two types of neurons represented in this layer are (1) *bipolar cells* (Figs. 25-8, 25-9, and 25-11), which relay the photoreceptor impulses inward to a third order of neurons that are called *ganglion cells* because they bear a resemblance to the cells seen in ganglia (Figs. 25-8, 25-9, and 25-11), and (2) *horizontal cells*, which interconnect the photoreceptors laterally (Fig. 25-9).

The next layer of the retina, which is called the *inner nuclear layer* (Figs. 25-9, 25-10, and 25-11), contains the nuclei of the *bipolar cells* (Figs. 25-8 and 25-11) and also the nuclei of horizontally arranged neurons called *amacrine cells* (Fig. 25-9). Amacrine cells (Gr. *a*, without; *makros*, long; *inos*, fiber) are unusual neurons in that they seem to lack an axon; their name denotes this lack of a long fiber. The dendritic processes of amacrine cells constitute the postsynaptic terminal of some synapses and the presynaptic terminal of others. Also present in the inner nuclear layer are the nuclei of *Müller cells*, which are long supporting and nutritive glial cells that span almost the entire thickness of the neural retina.

In the next layer, which is known as the *inner plexiform layer*, (Figs. 25-9, 25-10, and 25-11), the amacrine cells interconnect bipolar cells as well as ganglion cells, and they

Fig. 25-9. Schematic diagram of details of the arrangement of cells in the neural retina. (Compare this illustration with Figure 25-8). The photoreceptor outer segments, which face the retinal pigment epithelium, are shown at the top of this drawing; hence light enters the retina from below. Representative synaptic arrangements between photoreceptors, interneurons, and ganglion cells in the retina are indicated. For a detailed description, see text. (The Human Nervous System, Basic Principles of Neurobiology, 2nd ed, by C. R. Noback and R. J. Demarest. Copyright © 1975, McGraw-Hill Book Company. Adapted from Noback CR, Laemle LK: The Primate Brain. Appleton-Century-Crofts, Inc., 1970. Used with permission of McGraw-Hill Book Company)

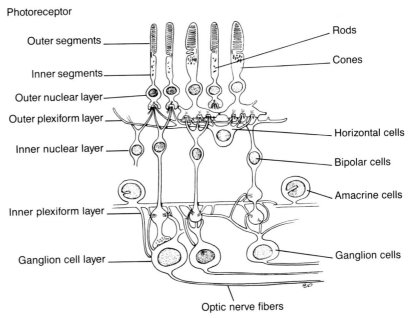

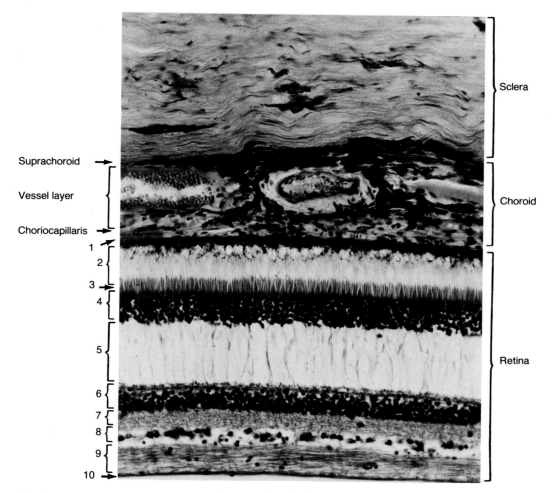

Fig. 25-10.   Low-power photomicrograph of the retina, choroid, and part of the sclera. The numbers refer to the layers of the retina shown diagrammatically in Figure 25-11.

also connect each bipolar cell with several ganglion cells (Fig. 25-9). Bipolar cells can also synapse directly with ganglion cells in this layer (Fig. 25-9). The next layer of the retina, which is termed the *ganglion cell layer* (Figs. 25-9, 25-10, and 25-11), contains the nuclei of the ganglion cells (Figs. 25-8 and 25-11) and retinal blood vessels. For a discussion of the functions of ganglion cells and amacrine cells, see Masland.

The last substantial inner layer of the retina is composed primarily of *retinal (optic) nerve fibers* representing the unmyelinated axons of the ganglion cells, together with processes of Müller cells and retinal blood vessels (Figs. 25-8, 25-9, 25-10, and 25-11). These nerve fibers converge toward the *papilla (optic disk)*, which is the site of exit of the optic nerve (Fig. 25-2). They traverse the sclera at the lamina cribrosa and each acquires a myelin sheath, with the result that the diameter of the optic nerve increases as it leaves the eye (Fig. 25-2). The optic disk is also the site of entry of the central retinal artery and vein (Fig. 25-2; see also

Fig. 25-15). Because the optic disk consists of optic nerve fibers, it is totally devoid of photoreceptors; hence it constitutes a *blind spot*.

The supporting Müller cells are essentially very tall columnar cells. Their long cell body and cytoplasmic processes extend all the way from the retinal *internal limiting membrane* (Figs. 25-10 and 25-11), which is a thin innermost layer of the retina that represents their basement membrane, to the level of the photoreceptor cells. Where the distal ends of the Müller cells abut on these rods and cones, they are joined to them by *zonula adherens* junctions. So much filamentous material is associated with these intercellular junctions that the row of them seen at this level with the LM was erroneously interpreted as being a membrane and was named the *external limiting membrane* of the retina (Fig. 25-11). Its true nature was not established until it could be observed in the EM. Tight (*zonula occludens*) junctions have also been described at this level, but they are present only between adjacent Müller cells and not

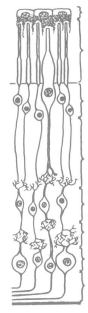

1. Retinal pigment epithelium

2. Outer and inner segments of photoreceptors

3. External limiting membrane
4. Outer nuclear layer

5. Outer plexiform layer

6. Inner nuclear layer (bipolar cells)

7. Inner plexiform layer

8. Ganglion cell layer

9. Retinal (optic) nerve fiber layer

10. Internal limiting membrane

Fig. 25-11. Schematic diagram of the ten layers of the retina. This should be compared with the photomicrograph in Figure 25-10.

between Müller cells and photoreceptors, so the external limiting membrane is a site of strong junctional attachment but not an effective permeability barrier. The distal end of Müller cells is further characterized by having large numbers of long microvillous processes that project into the intercellular spaces between the rods and cones (these processes are just discernible at *lower left* in Fig. 25-13).

Retinal Rods and Cones

The retinae of nocturnal animals are typically provided mainly with rods, whereas those of animals that are active by day have mostly cones. *Rods* are adapted to function in dim light and produce images that are composed of varying shades of black and white; *cones* are adapted to function in bright light and are responsible for the resolution of fine details and for color vision. Thus rats have rather few cones and their color vision is poorly developed compared with man. Birds, on the other hand, have numerous cones and excellent color vision (which is why a certain well-known histologist abandoned attempts at growing his own strawberries).

The basic construction of *rods* and *cones* is essentially similar. However, the rods tend to be taller, and the cones are slightly shorter and somewhat wider, with a conical outer segment instead of a slender cylindrical one (Figs. 25-12 and 25-13). As may be seen in Figure 25-12, both types of photoreceptors are made up of an *outer segment* that is connected by a short narrow region called a *connecting cilium* first to an *inner segment*, then to a *nuclear region*, and finally to a fairly wide *inner fiber* that terminates

as a *synaptic body* (*synaptic process*). In both kinds of cells, the light-sensitive *outer segment* is characterized by the presence of a stack of distinctive *membranous disks*, which are flattened transverse saccules.

The *outer segment* is regarded as a highly modified cilium because the short connecting stalk (*connecting cilium*) that joins it to the inner segment contains nine peripheral doublet microtubules that are arranged as in a cilium, and these are closely associated with a basal body (Fig. 25-12). The other centriole is generally present nearby (Fig. 25-12). The *inner segment* contains the usual organelles seen in a cell that is actively synthesizing cytoplasmic proteins. These include numerous polysomes and mitochondria as well as microtubules, some rough-surfaced endoplasmic reticulum (rER), and a prominent Golgi region (Fig. 25-12). The mitochondria tend to be aggregated in the outer region of the inner segment, which is often referred to as the *ellipsoid*, and the polysomes, rER, and Golgi saccules tend to lie in the inner region of the inner segment, which is known as the *myoid* (Fig. 25-12).

Thin tapering cytoplasmic processes called *calycal processes* extend from the distal end of the inner segment and surround the base of the outer segment (Fig. 25-12). These processes are continuous with longitudinal ridges on the inner segment that are particularly prominent in the case of cones, as may be seen in Figure 25-13*B*.

On the opposite side of the expanded *nuclear region* of the cell lies its club-shaped *synaptic body* or *synaptic process*. Because it has a slightly different shape in rods and cones, this process is often referred to as a *spherule* in the case of rods or as a *pedicle* in the case of cones. It contains synaptic vesicles and mitochondria and represents an expanded presynaptic terminal (Fig. 25-12). This terminal can lie in synaptic contact with synaptic processes of other photoreceptor cells, horizontal cells, or bipolar cells (Figs. 25-9 and 25-12). A distinctive feature of these presynaptic terminals is the presence of a *synaptic ribbon* and associated pre- and postsynaptic densities (Fig. 25-12, *bottom*). The synaptic ribbon of such *ribbon synapses* appears to be anchored to the presynaptic membrane, and it has been proposed that its function may be to guide synaptic vesicles so that impulses are transmitted simultaneously to more than one postsynaptic terminal at synapses where several of these lie in synaptic contact. (For further details about rods and cones, see Borwein, 1981.)

Photoreceptor Disk Membrane Proteins Undergo Active Turnover

The light-sensitive component of the retinal photoreceptors is a visual pigment that, in the case of retinal rods, is called *rhodopsin*. The *visual pigments* are made up of the *cis* form of a vitamin A–derived carotenoid chromophore called *retinal* (*retinene*) that is attached to an integral transmembrane glycosylated disk protein known as an *opsin*. Adequate dietary intake of vitamin A is therefore necessary for normal

(*Text continues on p. 694.*)

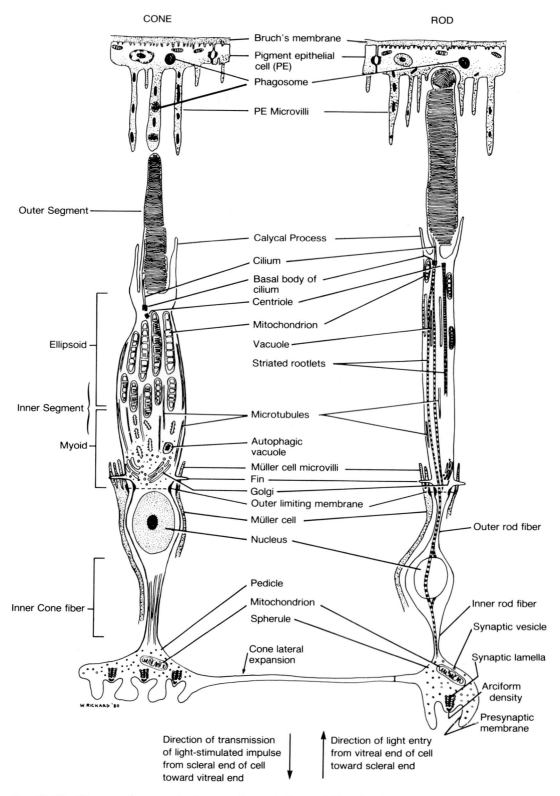

Fig. 25-12.   Diagram of a generalized mammalian retinal cone (*left*) and rod (*right*), showing the detailed structure and specialized parts of both kinds of photoreceptors and their basic pattern of organization in the retina. (Borwein B: The retinal receptor: A description. In Enoch JM, Tobey FL (eds): Springer Series in Optical Sciences, Vol 23: Vertebrate Photoreceptor Optics, p 11. Berlin, Springer-Verlag, 1981)

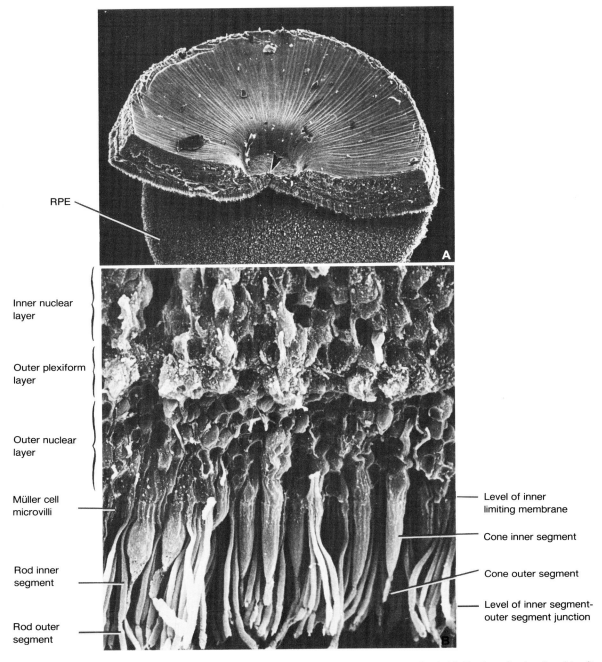

RPE

Inner nuclear
layer

Outer plexiform
layer

Outer nuclear
layer

Müller cell
microvilli

Rod inner
segment

Rod outer
segment

Level of inner
limiting membrane

Cone inner segment

Cone outer segment

Level of inner segment-
outer segment junction

Fig. 25-13.   Scanning electron micrographs of the retina (monkey). (*A*) Portion of retina (trephined) showing the foveal slopes that lead down to the fovea centralis (*arrowhead*), which is the deep pit at center (×70). The associated disk-shaped portion of retinal pigment epithelium (*RPE*) has become detached from the neural retina to which it is attached in life. This epithelium can be seen at the bottom of the micrograph, where it has separated from the outer segments. At the middle of the fovea, the retina is relatively thin. The vitreal surface of the retina has a pattern of radiating ridges that extend as far as the foveal slopes but do not continue across the floor of the pit (the *foveola*). (*B*) Portion of retina obtained from outside the macula lutea, showing the inner nuclear layer, outer plexiform layer, outer nuclear layer (photoreceptor nuclei), and rod and cone inner and outer segments (×1300). The shapes of the rod and cone inner and outer segments, including longitudinal ridging of the cone inner segment, can be seen to advantage at lower left. Many of the outer segments have broken off during tissue preparation. (*A*, Borwein B: Anat Rec 205:363, 1983; *B*, courtesy of B. Borwein)

vision. A prolonged severe deficiency of vitamin A leads to *night blindness,* which is an inability to see properly in dim light. In bright light, however, vision is unimpaired because the rods and cones still contain a sufficient quantity of visual pigment for them to respond adequately.

In rods the opsin is *scotopsin,* whereas in cones there are other opsins called *photopsins.* Light energy converts the *cis* form of the retinal in the visual pigment to the *trans* form, and this brings about a dissociation of the chromophore (retinal) from the protein to which it is attached (opsin). This, in turn, decreases the level of leakage of sodium ions into the cell and brings about its *hyperpolarization,* which is the reverse of the usual effect of a stimulus on a sensory receptor. Both the Müller cells and the pigment epithelial cells of the retina appear to participate in the retinal–retinol interconversions and the isomerization reactions that result in regeneration of the *cis* form of retinal that is necessary for rhodopsin resynthesis. For further information, see Bok.

A pigment called *iodopsin* is the only visual pigment thus far isolated from cones. Yet from a functional point of view, it is known that color vision involves the participation of three different populations of cones with maximal sensitivities to red, green, and blue light, respectively. The basis of wavelength discrimination appears to be the presence of a distinctive photopsin in the visual pigment of each class of cones. *Color blindness* generally results from a lack of functional red- or green-sensitive cones; problems with perception of the color blue are rarer. The various forms of color blindness are X-linked recessive conditions that are more likely to affect males than females.

Retinal rods and cones are terminally differentiated cells with no proliferative capacity that are not renewed in postnatal life. Yet they have to maintain lifelong photosensitivity of the membranous disks in their outer segments. The two different types of photoreceptors achieve this through slightly different means, as will be explained in the following paragraphs.

In both the rods and the cones, the membranous disks form by repetitive transverse infolding of the cell membrane at a level just above the connecting cilium. In the rods, new disks are formed in this manner throughout the entire lifetime of the cell (Young). The radioautographic evidence on which this conclusion is based (see Droz), summarized in Figure 25-14, is described below.

Once radioactively labeled amino acid becomes incorporated into scotopsin and other rod disk proteins, it passes through the Golgi apparatus and migrates from the inner to the outer segment of the rod (Fig. 25-14, stages 1 to 3). It then gradually moves to the tip of the outer segment in the form of a fairly distinct transverse band (Fig. 25-14, stages 4 and 5). This band represents the membranous disks that were being formed at the time, and progressive displacement of the labeled disks toward the tip of the outer segment indicates that new unlabeled disks are repeatedly being formed beneath them.

Cone disks are formed in a manner comparable to that of rod disks, but after cone disks have formed, they are not replaced on a regular basis. Also, soon after rod disks have formed, they lose their continuity with the part of the cell membrane from which they were derived (the part covering the outer segment), and as a consequence, each rod disk becomes a separate membrane-bounded intracellular compartment. Hence away from the region near the connecting cilium, the external membrane of the outer segment of a rod is essentially smooth (Fig. 25-12, *right*). However, this is not the case in cones (Fig. 25-12, *left*) because a considerable proportion of the cone disk membranes retain their original connections with the cell membrane and hence enclose invaginations of the extracellular space instead of constituting the walls of separate compartments within the cell.

The presence of such continuities between the cone disk membranes and the part of the cell membrane covering the outer segment was initially observed in transmission electron micrographs. It was later confirmed by introducing a fluorescent dye (Procion yellow) into the extracellular spaces of the retina. The dye freely enters the cone disks but not the rod disks. This observation indicates that the interior of most (if not all) of the cone disks is continuous with the extracellular space and that direct continuity of cone disk membranes with the cell membrane and with each other is maintained throughout the lifetime of the cell.

To some extent, these findings explain why the visual pigments are renewed by slightly different means in the rods and cones. The details of such renewal are described below.

Radioautographic studies of the rods in monkey retinas indicate that approximately 90 new disks are generated, one at a time, at the base of each rod outer segment per day. Newly synthesized rhodopsin becomes incorporated into the disk membranes during disk formation. From such studies (Fig. 25-14), it is also estimated that in monkeys it takes 9 to 13 days for each disk to be displaced from the base of the outer segment to its apex. In contrast, comparable studies of retinal cones indicate that although labeled proteins are similarly synthesized on a continuous basis in the inner segment of the cell, these proteins can become incorporated into cone disks anywhere in the outer segment, not just at its base. Hence newly synthesized molecules of photopsin are continually being incorporated, along with other membrane proteins, at multiple sites in the cone disk membranes. Thus in contrast to the daily renewal of disks that characterizes the rods, these newly synthesized protein molecules do not seem to be used to generate new disks. As a consequence, there is a steady turnover of cone photopsin but not of the disks into which it is incorporated.

Disk Shedding. Additional evidence that disk turnover occurs in the retinal rods comes from the fact that stacks of shed disks are found within phagosomes in the cytoplasm of RPE cells (Fig. 25-14, stage 6). Such stacks of discarded disks are avidly phagocytosed and degraded by the RPE cells, and a question that is still unanswered is whether the RPE cells play an active role in promoting the shedding process. It is estimated that each RPE cell is capable of phagocytosing and disposing of as many as 7500

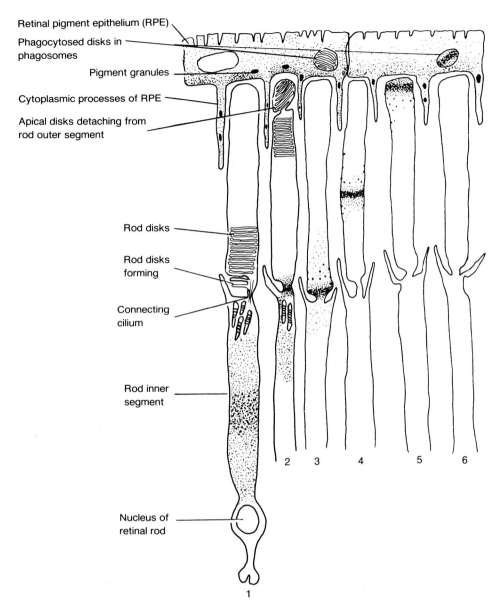

Retinal pigment epithelium (RPE)

Phagocytosed disks in phagosomes

Pigment granules

Cytoplasmic processes of RPE

Apical disks detaching from rod outer segment

Rod disks

Rod disks forming

Connecting cilium

Rod inner segment

Nucleus of retinal rod

1 2 3 4 5 6

Fig. 25-14. Schematic representation of the results of radioautographic EM studies of disk formation and shedding in retinal rods. In stage 1, disks are forming in the basal region of the outer segment. In stage 2, apical disks are about to detach and will be phagocytosed by the retinal pigment epithelium (*RPE*). Stages 1 to 6 illustrate the path taken by labeled amino acid incorporated into rhodopsin. In stage 1, radioactive label (*dark dots*) is seen over the inner segment. By stage 2, the label has reached the connecting cilium. In stage 3, forming basal disks are labeled. Displacement of the labeled disks (stages 4 and 5) culminates in shedding of these disks, which are then found within phagosomes in the RPE (stage 6). Some scattered diffuse labeling of the disks and of the cell membrane is also seen at stages 3 to 5. (Borwein B: The retinal receptor: A description. In Enoch JM, Tobey FL (eds): Springer Series in Optical Sciences, Vol 23: Vertebrate Photoreceptor Optics, p 11. Berlin, Springer-Verlag, 1981)

photoreceptor disks per day. Disk shedding more or less counterbalances new disk production in rods.

There is now evidence that disks are shed by cones as well as by rods and that in both kinds of photoreceptors shedding follows a circadian (daily) rhythm (L. *circa*, about, *dies*, day). This rhythm is based on the light–dark cycle

and is endogenously maintained within each eye. A burst of disk shedding by the rods occurs early in the morning in the first few hours when light would ordinarily enter the eye. Furthermore, studies in albino rats have established that rod disk shedding follows a light–dark–entrained circadian rhythm that continues for up to 2 weeks even in total darkness. However, in monkeys it has also been established that a certain amount of disk shedding occurs during hours of nighttime darkness.

Although disk shedding also occurs in the cones, the time of day at which it occurs is more variable from one mammalian species to another. In Rhesus monkeys, for example, it occurs during hours of darkness as well as during hours of light, whereas in the cat and certain other mammals, it happens along with rod disk shedding soon after early morning light begins to reach the eye. Also, since lifelong production of new basal disks is a feature of rods but not of cones, it could be surmised that disk shedding in cones represents a way of eliminating superfluous and possibly even deteriorating membrane constituents from the system of interconnected disk membranes. Following disk shedding in cones, the next group of disks that move into the apical position become smaller in diameter, and as a consequence, the conical form of the cone outer segment is maintained. For further information regarding disk shedding, see Besharse; also Bok.

Visual Acuity Is Maximal at the Fovea Centralis

Very close to the posterior pole of the eye, there is a slight depression in the retina. Following death, this small circular area has a yellow appearance when compared with the remainder of the retina, so it is known as the *macula lutea* (L. for yellow spot). In the living eye, it appears as described below. Within a shallow central depression of the macula lutea known as the *fovea centralis* (Figs. 25-2 and 25-13*A*), the photoreceptors are less thickly covered by the other components of the neural retina than anywhere else in the retina. This tiny foveal area also lacks overlying retinal blood vessels. Furthermore, the foveal photoreceptors are all *cones,* and more of them are packed into a small area than at other sites in the retina. The fovea centralis therefore provides the greatest degree of visual acuity.

Internal Appearance of the Living Retina. With the aid of an instrument called an *ophthalmoscope,* it is possible to observe the back (*fundus*) of the eye (Fig. 25-15). The living retina appears red because light is reflected back from the blood in the underlying wide capillaries of the choriocapillaris. The general background has a granular appearance because of irregular distribution of the melanin in the RPE and choroid.

The unmyelinated retinal fibers converge to the site of exit of the optic nerve, where they are heaped up as the *papilla,* which is also known as the *optic disk* (Figure 25-15). Here they are loosely arranged. Furthermore, any accumulation of tissue fluid in the neural retina results in obvious *optic disk swelling* (*papilledema*). This condition is a valuable early clinical sign of certain pathological conditions, notably hypertension and elevated intracranial pressure. Because the white lamina cribrosa (fibrous tissue) is penetrated by gray nerve fibers and supplied by capillaries, the papilla normally appears a pale pink in contrast to the red color of the remainder of the retina. Increased intraocular pressure (and certain other conditions) can displace the lamina cribrosa and its nerve fibers posteriorly, causing depression (*cupping*) of the optic disk.

The *central retinal artery* and *vein* enter at the middle of the papilla (Fig. 25-15). The *macula lutea* and its central *fovea centralis*

lie some distance lateral to the margin of the papilla, slightly inferior to its center (Fig. 25-15). The macula appears yellow only if red-free light is used; with ordinary (white) light, it appears somewhat darker and redder than the rest of the retina. The fovea appears as a tiny central bright spot because of reflection from its concave surface.

ACCESSORY STRUCTURES OF THE EYE (ADNEXA)

Several accessory structures called *adnexa* are associated with the eye. The main adnexa are the *conjunctiva, eyelids,* and *tear glands,* which will be described in the following sections.

Conjunctiva

A thin transparent mucous membrane covers the "white" of the eye as the *bulbar conjunctiva* and lines the eyelids as the *palpebral conjunctiva.* Details of this membrane are described below.

The *epithelium* is a characteristically stratified columnar epithelium that is made up of three layers of cells: a basal layer of columnar cells, a middle layer of polygonal cells, and a superficial layer of squamous or low cuboidal cells. The superficial cells are provided with microvilli on their free surface (Fig. 25-16). The middle layer is absent in most of the palpebral conjunctiva. As the epithelium approaches the lid margin, it changes to stratified squamous; this merges with the epidermis of the skin. Scattered through the conjunctival epithelium are mucus-secreting goblet cells. Near the limbus, the epithelium of the bulbar conjunctiva becomes stratified squamous and is provided with deep papillae. It is continuous with the epithelium of the cornea.

The *substantia* (*lamina*) *propria* of the conjunctiva consists of delicate fibrous connective tissue, and it is particularly loose over the sclera. In it are scattered accumulations of lymphocytes. The substantia propria, except in the lid, merges into a more deeply situated and thicker meshwork of collagenous and elastic connective tissue.

The palpebral fissure is the space between the free margins of the two eyelids. At the medial end of the palpebral fissure is a little pool of tears, the *lacus lacrimalis.* A free fold of conjunctiva, the concave border of which faces the pupil, is present at the medial end of the palpebral fissure; this is called the *plica semilunaris.* In the angle of the palpebral fissure at its medial end, a little fleshy mass called the *caruncle* protrudes. Developmentally, this is a detached portion of the marginal part of the lower lid; hence it contains a few skeletal muscle fibers as well as a few hair follicles and sebaceous glands.

Eyelids

The anterior surface of each *eyelid* is covered with a delicate thin skin that is provided with hair follicles, very fine hairs, and some sebaceous glands and sweat glands. Its dermis is of an unusually loose texture, and in white races the subcutaneous tissue deep to it is almost devoid of adipose

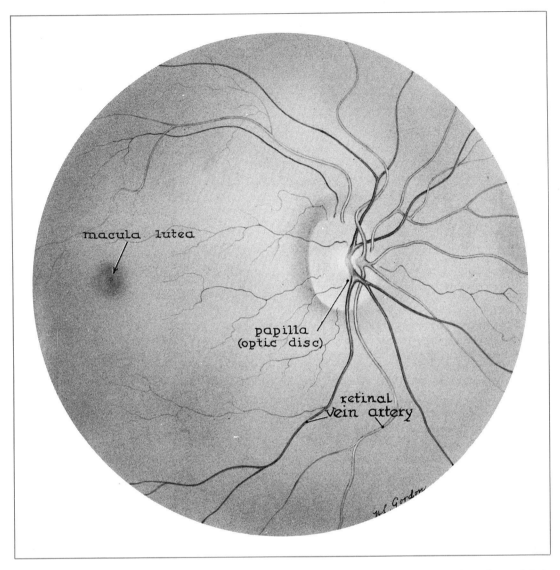

Fig. 25-15. Drawing of the live appearance of the fundus of the right eye, seen through an ophthalmoscope.

tissue. At the free margin of the eyelid, the epidermis becomes continuous with the epithelium of the palpebral conjunctiva that borders the eyelid posteriorly. Deep to the skin covering the anterior surface of the eyelid lies the *orbicularis oculi* muscle.

Each eyelid is reinforced by a plate of fibrous tissue called a *tarsal plate* that lies in its posterior part, immediately anterior to the palpebral conjunctiva. The secretory portions of elongated sebaceous glands termed *meibomian glands* are embedded in the tarsal plate. These glands open onto the posterior part of the free margin of the eyelid. Infection of a meibomian gland can lead to granulomatous inflammation, producing a local painful swelling of the eyelid known as a *chalazion.* The hair follicles of the eyelashes are provided with sebaceous glands known as the *glands of Zeis,* and between these follicles lie the *sweat glands of Moll.* A *sty* is a result of infection of either type of gland.

Tear Glands

Tears are produced by the *lacrimal gland* and *accessory tear glands.* These glands develop from the conjunctiva and are of the compound serous tubuloalveolar type. Their secretory units are provided with myoepithelial cells. The secretion they produce is slightly alkaline and contains *lysozyme,* which is a bactericidal enzyme. Blinking of the eyelids spreads tears evenly over the cornea and conjunctiva, keeping their exposed surfaces moist. Floods of tears

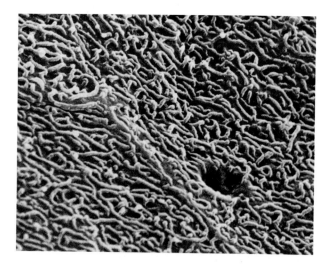

Fig. 25-16. Scanning electron micrograph of the exposed surface of the upper tarsal conjunctiva (hamster). The opening of a tear duct can be seen at lower right. Numerous microvilli cover the free surfaces of these cells and of the corneal epithelial cells; they help to retain a film of tears over these exposed surfaces. (Courtesy of P. Basu and P. Basrur)

can generally be produced for special occasions; those elicited by painful stimuli or irritants serve to wash away extraneous particulate matter or other noxious agents from the corneal and conjunctival surfaces.

Near the medial end of the free margin of each eyelid, there is a small *lacrimal papilla*. A tiny opening termed the *punctum* is just visible on each papilla. From the punctum, tears normally drain by way of the *lacrimal canaliculi, lacrimal sac,* and *nasolacrimal duct* into the nose. The puncta and lacrimal canaliculi are lined by stratified squamous nonkeratinizing epithelium; the lacrimal sac and nasolacrimal duct are lined by two layers of columnar cells with goblet cells.

THE EAR

The *ears* are the paired organs that are responsible for (1) hearing, (2) detecting the position of the head relative to the pull of gravity, and (3) detecting motion of the head. As we shall see, the sensory receptors involved with the maintenance of equilibrium somewhat resemble those involved with hearing.

Each ear is made up of three main parts called the *external ear, middle ear,* and *inner ear* (Fig. 25-17). The *external ear* consists of (1) a substantial appendage known as the *auricle;* (2) the *external acoustic meatus* (L. *meatus,* passage or canal), which is a tube that extends from the auricle to reach the tympanic cavity in the petrous (stonelike) portion of the

temporal bone; and (3) the *tympanic membrane (eardrum),* which is a fibrous partition that extends across the medial end of the external acoustic meatus (Fig. 25-17). The tympanic membrane has the appropriate thickness and tension to vibrate when sound waves reach it by way of the auricle and external acoustic meatus.

Leading to the inner ear is the *middle ear,* which is provided with a chain of *three ossicles* (little bones) that are capable of transmitting the vibrations that occur in the tympanic membrane of the outer ear to the inner ear where they are analyzed.

The *inner ear* possesses special groups of sensory receptors that are selectively stimulated either by sounds or by changes in the relative position or motion of the head. Essentially, this part of the ear consists of a number of membranous ducts that lie in several different planes and a pair of membranous sacs with which they communicate (Fig. 25-17; see also Fig. 25-19). This closed system of interconnected membranous ducts and sacs, which contain a special fluid called *endolymph,* is provided with sensory receptors at strategic sites. The entire system, which is known as the *membranous labyrinth,* is loosely fitted into a system of corresponding channels and cavities in the petrous portion of the temporal bone that constitute the *bony labyrinth* (see Fig. 25-19). At some sites, the membranous labyrinth is anchored to the periosteal lining of the bony labyrinth, but most of it lies suspended in another special fluid called *perilymph* that fills the part of the bony labyrinth that is not occupied by the membranous labyrinth.

Deep to the medial bony wall of the middle ear lies a relatively large chamber of the bony labyrinth called the *vestibule* (see Fig. 25-19). Two closed apertures known as windows, the *fenestra vestibuli (oval window)* and the *fenestra cochleae (round window),* are present in the bony wall that separates the air-filled middle ear from the fluid-filled vestibule (see Fig. 25-19). The free end of the last bone in the chain of ear ossicles fits into the fenestra vestibuli (Fig. 25-17) and is free to rock to and fro into the vestibule. Hence when sound waves cause the tympanic membrane to vibrate, its vibrations are transmitted to the perilymph in the vestibule. Because fluids are incompressible, complementary vibrations have to occur at the fenestra cochleae (see Fig. 25-23), which is closed over by a membrane that has sufficient elasticity to allow this to happen. We shall consider how the vibrations reaching the perilymph affect afferent nerve endings later in this chapter.

Extending from the vestibule are three *semicircular canals,* each of which contains a *semicircular duct,* and the *cochlear canal,* which is a spiral canal that contains the *cochlea,* the structure that houses the organ of hearing. In addition, two interconnected membranous sacs known as the *utricle* and the *saccule* lie within the vestibule (Fig. 25-17).

With this introductory outline of the main parts of the ear as general background, we shall now discuss the microscopic structure of the principal parts in relation to their functions.

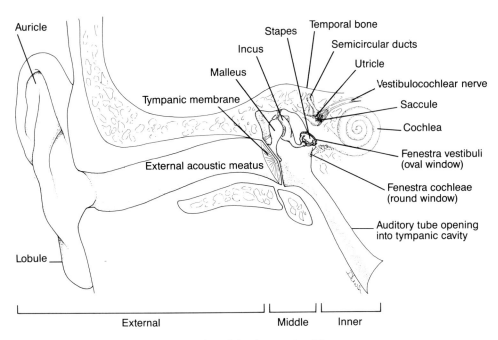

Fig. 25-17. Diagrammatic representation of the three parts of the ear.

EXTERNAL EAR

The central region of the shell-like *auricle* plays a role in the vertical localization of sounds. Its characteristic shape is maintained by an internal supporting plate of *elastic cartilage*. Also, a small quantity of adipose tissue can be found under the thin skin along the posteromedial margin of the auricle and in the ear lobule.

The *external acoustic meatus* is a short canal that is lined with thin skin. Its distal *cartilaginous portion* is prevented from collapsing by the presence of elastic cartilage in its walls. It is also provided with hair follicles, large sebaceous glands, and *ceruminous glands,* which are the glands that produce ear wax (L. *cera,* wax). Ceruminous glands are considered to be modified sweat glands. *Cerumen,* a waxy material that may accumulate in the meatus and interfere with hearing, represents the mixed secretion of the ceruminous glands and the sebaceous glands into which some of the ceruminous glands open. The inner *bony portion* of the external acoustic meatus, which is strongly supported by the tympanic part of the temporal bone (Fig. 25-17), possesses these glands only in its roof.

The thin fibrous *tympanic membrane* that closes over the medial end of the meatus is composed chiefly of two layers of collagen fibers; the outer layer is radial and the inner layer is circular in its arrangement. These two layers, together with a small number of elastic fibers, are covered externally by very thin skin and internally by a very low simple cuboidal or simple squamous epithelium (Fig. 25-18). The upper part of the tympanic membrane is thin and

flaccid because it lacks collagen fibers and is therefore known as its *pars flaccida.*

MIDDLE EAR

The *middle ear* consists primarily of (1) an air-filled cavity called the *tympanic cavity,* which is normally lined by simple cuboidal epithelium and extends posteriorly into the mastoid process of the temporal bone; and (2) a chain of three tiny *auditory ossicles,* known as the *malleus, incus,* and *stapes,* that reaches across the tympanic cavity from its lateral wall to its medial wall (Fig. 25-17; see also Fig. 25-23).

On each side of the body, an *auditory* (Eustachian) *tube* connects the tympanic cavity with the nasopharynx (Fig. 25-17). The role of this tube is to facilitate equilibration of the air pressure in the middle ear with that of the outer ear so that oscillations of the tympanic membrane are not subjected to dampening due to a pressure difference. The tympanic end of the auditory tube is a bony canal, whereas the wider medial portion into which it opens has supporting cartilage in its walls. This cartilaginous portion of the tube is more flexible and, under most circumstances, is partly collapsed. However, it can be opened by yawning or swallowing, a measure frequently resorted to by experienced air travelers that equalizes the air pressures on either side of the tympanic membrane.

Toward the pharynx, the auditory tube becomes lined by ciliated pseudostratified columnar epithelium with goblet cells and associated submucosal mixed glands. Because

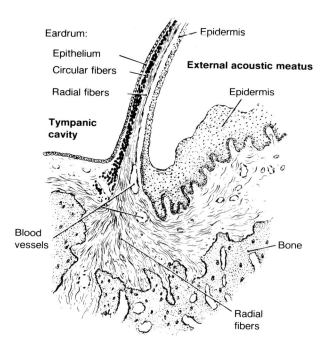

Fig. 25-18. Drawing of part of the tympanic membrane (eardrum) in cross section, showing the relation of this membrane to the external acoustic meatus at right and the tympanic cavity at left.

the middle ear is basically an air-containing cavity, the auditory tube offers a direct route for infections to spread to the middle ear from the nasopharynx. Indeed, middle ear infections sometimes develop as a complication of the common cold, especially in children. Posteriorly, the tympanic cavity is continuous with a variable number of alveolar air spaces within the mastoid and surrounding region of the temporal bone. These spaces are known as the *mastoid air cells*, and they, too, can become involved if infections reach the middle ear by way of the auditory tube.

The three auditory ossicles transmit the vibrations that occur in the tympanic membrane to a tiny oval aperture in the medial wall of the tympanic cavity called the *fenestra vestibuli* or *oval window* (see Fig. 25-23), which is seen in face view in Figure 25-19. This aperture is closed over by the footplate (base) of the stapes, the perimeter of which is flexibly joined to the perimeter of the fenestra vestibuli by the *anular ligament*. The role of the ossicles is to increase the effect of the pressure variations reaching the tympanic membrane. The *fenestra cochleae* (*round window*) in the lower part of the medial wall of the tympanic cavity (Figs. 25-17 and 25-19) is closed over by the *secondary tympanic membrane*, the flexible epithelially covered fibrous membrane that dissipates sound waves when they have stimulated the sensory receptors of the inner ear (see Fig. 25-23).

The *auditory ossicles* are atypical long bones without epiphyses, and their growth is almost entirely prenatal. The malleus and incus

have small medullary cavities whereas the stapes is solid in the adult. The articulating surfaces of these bones are held together by tiny ligaments, and the malleus and incus are suspended by ligaments from the roof of the middle ear. The periosteal surfaces of these bones are covered by the mucous membrane that lines the tympanic cavity.

INNER EAR

The *inner ear* is provided with two important groups of sensory components that are situated in (1) the *cochlea*, which houses the organ of *hearing;* and (2) the *semicircular ducts, utricle,* and *saccule,* which constitute the organ of *vestibular function* (Fig. 25-17). All of these sensory components are housed in the petrous portion of the temporal bone, where they lie within an interconnecting system of bony channels and cavities known as the otic *bony labyrinth.* Each inner ear has four bony channels: the *cochlear canal* and the *anterior, lateral,* and *posterior semicircular canals* (Fig. 25-19). The *vestibule* is the central expanded bony cavity with which all four bony canals communicate. It contains the *utricle* and the *saccule* (Fig. 25-17). These two interconnected membranous sacs and the three *semicircular ducts* lying within the three semicircular canals comprise the *vestibular portion* of the *membranous labyrinth.* The *auditory portion* of the membranous labyrinth is represented by the *cochlear duct,* which lies within the cochlear canal.

The fluid that fills the space between the bony walls of the bony labyrinth and the membranous walls of the membranous labyrinth lying within it is *perilymph,* the composition of which is somewhat similar to that of cerebrospinal fluid. The fluid that fills the lumen of the membranous labyrinth is *endolymph,* a fluid of different composition with a distinctively high potassium ion concentration and a comparatively low concentration of sodium ions. All the sensory receptors of the inner ear are

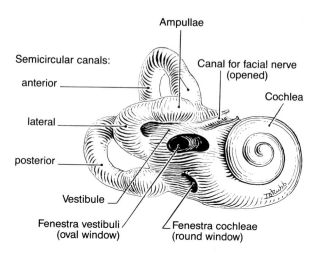

Fig. 25-19. Diagram of the right bony labyrinth (lateral view). See text for details. (After Grant)

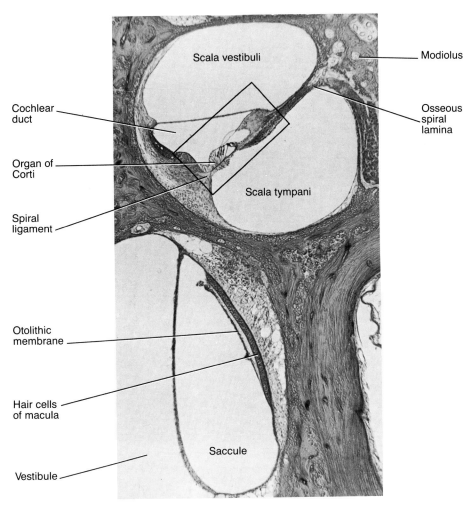

Scala vestibuli

Modiolus

Cochlear
duct

Osseous
spiral
lamina

Organ of
Corti

Scala tympani

Spiral
ligament

Otolithic
membrane

Hair cells
of macula

Saccule

Vestibule

Fig. 25-20.   Photomicrograph of cochlear canal (*top*) and macula of saccule (*lower left*) in horizontal section (low power). Boxed-in area in this figure is depicted in Figure 25-21. (Courtesy of K. Money and J. Laufer)

situated within the endolymph-filled lumen of the membranous labyrinth.

We shall now consider the auditory portion of the membranous labyrinth in further detail.

Cochlea

Situated in the *cochlear canal,* which is a coiled bony canal that opens into the vestibule, lies the *cochlea* (Fig. 25-19). This is a distinctive coiled structure that derives its name from its obvious resemblance to a snail shell (L. *cochlea,* snail shell). The central bony axis of the cochlea, called the *modiolus* (L. for hub), houses the *cochlear* (spiral) *ganglion* and the *cochlear nerve.* Furthermore, a thin bony shelf known as the *osseous spiral lamina* (Fig. 25-20) spirals up the modiolus like the thread on a screw. This spiral lamina provides the necessary support for the nonoscillating parts of the *organ of Corti,* which is described below. As in a snail

shell, the diameter of the spiral turns made by the *cochlear canal* in coiling around the modiolus diminishes as these turns approach the apex of the cochlea.

Extending along the midregion of the cochlear canal is an endolymph-filled compartment of the membranous labyrinth called the *cochlear duct.* This duct is more or less triangular in cross section (Fig. 25-20). The inner side of the duct lying close to the modiolus is fairly sharply pointed, but the outer side remote from the modiolus is taller (Fig. 25-20). A spiral thickening of the periosteal lining of the cochlear canal, known as the *spiral ligament,* secures the outer border of this duct. In addition, a functionally important fibrous partition called the *basilar membrane* extends from the spiral ligament to the osseous spiral lamina. This membrane represents the floor of the cochlear duct (Figs. 25-20 and 25-21). Its lower surface is covered by columnar epithelial cells, and its upper surface supports the spiral organ of Corti (Fig. 25-21). A delicate membrane called

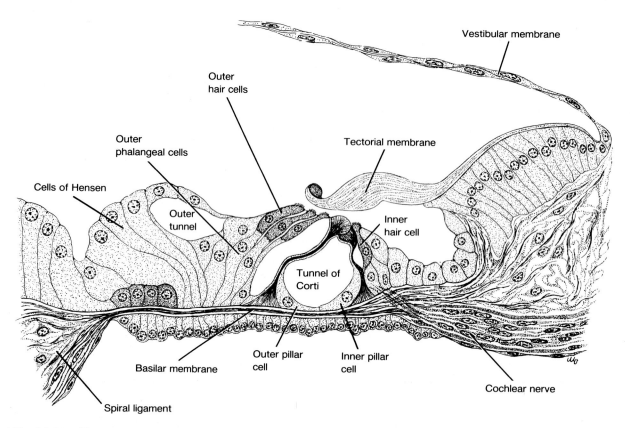

Fig. 25-21. Diagrammatic representation of the organ of Corti, showing the boxed-in area in Figure 25-20, as represented in the guinea pig. See text for details. (Courtesy of C. Leblond and Y. Clermont)

the *vestibular* (Reissner's) *membrane* constitutes the roof of the cochlear duct (Figs. 25-20 and 25-21). This is a very thin membrane consisting only of two apposed layers of simple squamous epithelium separated by a basement membrane (Fig. 25-21).

Substantial chambers filled with perilymph separate the bony walls of the cochlear canal from (1) the roof and (2) the floor of the cochlear duct. The chamber that lies above the roof of the cochlear duct is termed the *scala vestibuli* whereas the chamber that lies below the floor of this duct is termed the *scala tympani* (Fig. 25-20). Because of the intermediate position of the cochlear duct with respect to the scala vestibuli and the scala tympani, the cochlear duct is also known as the *scala media*. Separated by the intervening membranous partitions, these three contiguous spiral compartments extend the entire length of the cochlea. At the apex of the cochlea (which is directed anterolaterally), the scala vestibuli communicates with the scala tympani by way of a tiny aperture known as the *heliocotrema*. We shall consider the functional significance of this parallel arrangement between the three fluid-filled compartments of the cochlea when we discuss the mechanism of hearing later in this chapter.

Organ of Corti

The spiral *organ of Corti* has a very intricate structure. Essentially, it consists of columnar supporting cells and distinctive receptor cells known as *hair cells*. A structure known as the *tectorial membrane* (L. *tectum*, roof) forms a roof over the hair cells (Fig. 25-21). This is a resilient cuticular sheet made of a protein that resembles keratin and produced by the columnar epithelial cells that are supported by the osseous spiral lamina. However, the tectorial membrane is particularly susceptible to fixation artifact, so neither its true shape nor its relation to the underlying hair cells is evident in routine LM sections.

The outermost tall supporting cells of the organ of Corti (known as *cells of Hensen* and shown on the left of the phalangeal cells in Fig. 25-21, next to the spiral ligament lying to the left in this illustration) have no special characteristics. The supporting cells of the remainder of the organ of Corti are known as *phalangeal cells* and *pillar cells*. A distinctive feature of these two types of cells is that they are both strongly reinforced with prominent bundles of microtubules that enable them to provide the necessary rigidity to the bases of the "hairs" on the hair cells (Figs. 25-21 and 25-22).

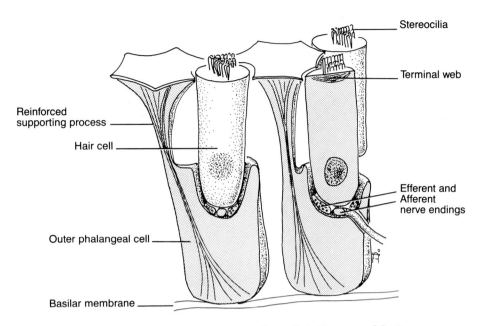

Fig. 25-22. Diagrammatic representation of outer hair cells in the organ of Corti.

Phalangeal Cells and Pillar Cells. The *outer phalangeal cells* (Fig. 25-21) are tall columnar cells that support the outer hair cells of the organ of Corti and also the nerve endings that lie in synaptic contact with the base of these cells (Fig. 25-22). As just mentioned, a noteworthy feature of the outer phalangeal cells is the presence of a prominent bundle of microtubules (which are 27 nm to 28 nm in diameter and therefore unusually wide). Some microfilaments with a parallel orientation are also present in these bundles. The microtubules appear to be firmly anchored to the cell membrane at the base of the cell, and they extend up into a long thin supporting process called a *phalanx* that runs beside the hair cell and terminates as a flat apical platelike expansion (Fig. 25-22). Between the perimeter of this expansion and the apical ends of the adjacent outer hair cells that it supports, there is a well-developed junctional complex. The *inner phalangeal cells,* which support the inner hair cells, are essentially similar except that their phalanx has a different shape.

The *outer* and *inner pillar cells* are regarded as modified phalangeal cells. They, too, extend to the free surface of the organ of Corti. Each of these cells is reinforced with a stout bundle or two of microtubules with associated microfilaments and has a very prominent terminal web. Large adhering junctions attach the apical ends of the outer pillar cells to those of the inner pillar cells.

Cochlear Hair Cells. The specialized auditory and vestibular receptor cells found in the organ of Corti and at strategic sites in the vestibular labyrinth are called *hair cells* because their apical border bears a tuft of long specialized microvilli that, when seen in the LM, somewhat resembles short hairs standing on end.

The columnar hair cells in the organ of Corti are distributed as outer and inner groups (Fig. 25-21). Whereas the hair cells in the outer group are cylindrical, those of the inner group are flask-shaped. Furthermore, the outer group consists basically of three rows of hair cells with an added row or two toward the apex of the cochlea, whereas the inner group consists of only a single row of cells.

Each hair cell lies cradled within the recess of a supporting phalangeal cell and has several afferent and efferent nerve endings synapsing with its base (Fig. 25-22). The apical end of the cell is strongly supported by a prominent terminal web, and at this level, the hair cell is joined by zonula adherens junctions to the adjacent apical plates of the phalangeal cells (Fig. 25-22). Extending from the apical surface of the hair cell is a W-shaped row of tall straight specialized microvilli known as *stereocilia.* A vestigial cilium, represented in adult life solely by its basal body, lies in the notch of the W; this notch faces outward, away from the modiolus. In the outer hair cells, the stereocilia are arranged in several rows that are graded in height, the outermost row also being the tallest. The tips of these outermost stereocilia are embedded in the tectorial membrane. An unusual feature of the stereocilia on hair cells is that their bases are narrower than their tips (Fig. 25-22). However, like microvilli, they contain a bundle of microfilaments that extends down into the terminal web.

The last distinctive feature of each hair cell is that a *synaptic ribbon,* essentially similar to that described earlier in this chapter in the section dealing with retinal rods and

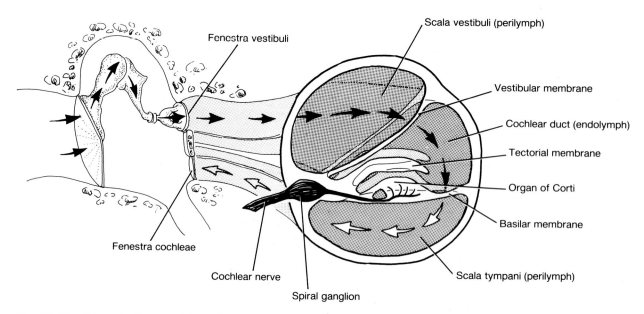

Fig. 25-23. Schematic diagram of the pathway of sound waves entering the ear.

cones, is typically present at each site where the base of the cell is the presynaptic part of an afferent synapse.

Role of the Organ of Corti in Hearing. The perilymph surrounding the membranous labyrinth and the endolymph in its lumen are both incompressible fluids. Furthermore, the vestibular membrane and the basilar membrane of the organ of Corti are both thin flexible membranes that are not kept under much tension. As may be seen in Figure 25-23, vibrations received by the tympanic membrane are transmitted to the fenestra vestibuli by the base of the stapes and then continue on into the scala vestibuli as pressure waves that are transmitted by the perilymph. These pressure waves first pass across the vestibular membrane (the floor of the scala vestibuli) and reach the endolymph that lies in the cochlear duct (the scala media). They then pass across the basilar membrane of the cochlear duct and reach the perilymph in the scala tympani. Finally, they dissipate through the secondary tympanic membrane that extends across the fenestra cochleae.

When these pressure waves pass across the cochlear duct from the scala vestibuli, they *cause its basilar membrane to oscillate.* Different sound frequencies can be discriminated by the cochlea because different zones along the length of the basilar membrane oscillate at different resonant frequencies. The resulting displacement of the basilar membrane is registered by the shearing stresses imposed between (1) the tips of the stereocilia of each hair cell, some of which are known to be firmly embedded in the tectorial membrane; and (2) the bases of these stereocilia, which receive indirect rigid support from the phalangeal cells and the pillar cells of the organ of Corti (Figs. 25-21 and 25-22). Relative movement occurs between the tectorial membrane, which is not known to oscillate at any particular frequency, and the basilar membrane with its rigidly affixed supporting cells and hair cells. Hair cell stereocilia not embedded in the tectorial membrane are thought to be displaced directly by pressure waves passing through the endolymph. Displacement of the hair cell stereocilia due to oscillations of the basilar membrane causes the hair cells to depolarize, and

this contributes to the complex pattern of auditory impulses reaching the auditory cortex by way of the vestibulocochlear nerve.

Vestibular Labyrinth

The part of the inner ear that participates in maintenance of the body's equilibrium consists of the utricle, the three semicircular ducts, and the saccule. The *utricle* is a membranous sac that is filled with endolymph; both ends of each *semicircular duct* open into it. Each of the three semicircular ducts lies in an appropriate plane to detect rotational movement of the head and is provided with an expanded region known as an *ampulla* that lies near one of its ends (Fig. 25-19). The *saccule* is also an endolymph-filled membranous sac, the endolymph of which communicates with that of the utricle, semicircular ducts, and cochlear duct. The thin connective tissue walls of all these membranous structures are lined by simple squamous epithelium. The spot-shaped sensory areas of both the utricle and the saccule are termed *maculae* (L. *macula*, spot), whereas the semicircular ducts are provided with *ampullary cristae (cristae ampullaris)* located within their expanded ampullae. In each instance, the receptor areas are patches of epithelium that are provided with hair cells. The vestibular impulses that these cells generate contribute to the sense of orientation and balance.

Maculae of the Utricle and Saccule. The epithelium of the *maculae* consists of *hair cells* that are interspersed with columnar *supporting cells.* Whereas the cochlear hair cells are covered by the tectorial membrane, the hair cells of the maculae are covered by a layer of protein-containing ex-

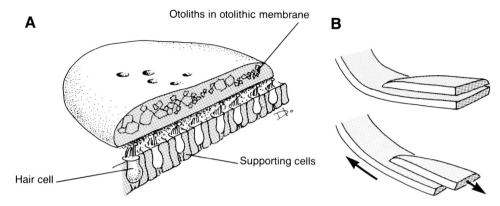

Fig. 25-24. Diagrammatic representations of (*A*) maculae of utricle and saccule and (*B*) relative movement of the otolithic membrane. See text for details.

tracellular material that is studded with crystals of calcium carbonate (Fig. 25-24*A*). Known as *otoliths, otoconia,* or *statoconia,* these crystals are relatively heavy. The layer of extracellular material in which they are embedded is called the *otolithic (otoconial) membrane* (Fig. 25-24*A*). The area of sensory epithelium that is present in the utricle lies in a nearly horizontal plane, whereas that of the saccule is almost vertical. Because of the pull of gravity, the presence of heavy otoliths in the otolithic membrane of each macula causes a shearing force to be exerted on the hair cell stereocilia that are embedded in the underside of this membrane (Fig. 25-24*B*), and this force registers the position of the head. Furthermore, the weight of these crystals provides sufficient inertia to the otolithic membranes for the maculae also to sense linear acceleration or deceleration of the head.

Ampullary Cristae. Each *crista* (L. for crest) is a transverse ridge or crest that projects inward from the membranous walls of the ampulla of a semicircular duct. This ridge has a core of connective tissue, and it is covered by an epithelium that is made up of hair cells with interspersed columnar supporting cells (Fig. 25-25*A*). Here, instead of being covered by a crystal-containing layer, the stereocilia are embedded in a thick flaplike mass of gelatinous extracellular material termed a *cupula* (L. for cup). This flap projects into the lumen of the ampulla like a swing-door (Fig. 25-25*B*). The cupula shrinks to a very marked degree on fixation, but in life it extends for some distance across the ampullary lumen. It hinges freely on the crista and is readily deflected by any movement of the endolymph in which it lies (Fig. 25-25*B*). Rotational acceleration or deceleration of the head in any given plane stimulates the crista in the anterior, lateral, or posterior semicircular duct of the otic labyrinth (Fig. 25-25*B*). This is because the endolymph within each semicircular duct tends to remain stationary because of its own inertia, thereby deflecting the cupula. Thus the three

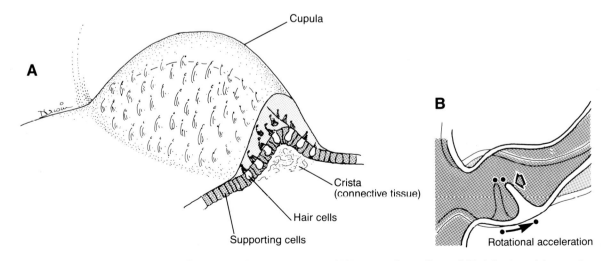

Fig. 25-25. Diagrammatic representations of (*A*) cristae of ampullae and (*B*) deflection of the cupula. See text for details.

ampullary cristae of the vestibular labyrinth register rotational acceleration or deceleration of the head.

Hair Cells of the Vestibular Labyrinth. Both the ampullary cristae and the maculae of the utricle and saccule are provided with *hair cells* of two different kinds. The *type I cells* are flask-shaped and are cradled by challicelike terminal expansions of their basal afferent nerve fibers. These type I cells resemble the inner hair cells of the organ of Corti. The *type II cells* are cylindrical cells that are not cradled by challicelike terminal expansions of the afferent fibers at their basal ends. They resemble the outer hair of the organ of Corti. However, both types of vestibular hair cells differ from those of the organ of Corti in that they retain a single apical cilium. Known as a *kinocilium*, this cilium is not capable of independent motile activity; instead, it forms part of a functional complex with the other apical processes on the cell. Lateral to the kinocilium is a conical bundle of stereocilia that are of graded height; the tallest of them lie next to the kinocilium. Deflection of the kinocilium–stereocilia complex in a direction toward the kinocilium triggers depolarization of the hair cell and leads to the generation of vestibular afferent impulses. Deflection away from the site of the kinocilium hyperpolarizes the cell and decreases the number of vestibular impulses generated.

For further details about the inner ear, see Friedmann and Ballantyne.

SELECTED REFERENCES

The Eye: Comprehensive

AUGUSTEYN RC, ROGERS KM: The Eye, Vol 1. Westmount, Eden Press, 1979

HOGAN MJ, ALVARADO JA, WEDDELL JE: Histology of the Human Eye: An Atlas and Textbook. Philadelphia, WB Saunders, 1971

JAKOBIEC FA (ed): Ocular Anatomy, Embryology, and Teratology. Hagerstown, Harper & Row, 1982

KESSEL RG, KARDON RH: Nervous tissue—eye and ear. In Tissues and Organs: A Text-Atlas of Scanning Electron Microscopy. San Francisco, WH Freeman, 1979

Eye Development, Cornea, Lens, Iris, and Vitreous Body

BASU PK: Immune and nonimmune factors involved in the corneal graft reaction. Indian Med Assoc J 66:229, 1976

BASU PK, CARRÉ F: A study of cells in human corneal grafts. Growth potential in vitro, cellular morphology, and fate of donor cells. Can J Ophthalmol 8:1, 1973

BLOEMENDAL H (ed): Molecular and Cellular Biology of the Eye Lens. New York, John Wiley & Sons, 1981

COULOMBRE AJ: Cytology of the developing eye. Int Rev Cytol 11: 161, 1961

HOLLENBERG MJ, WYSE JPH, LEWIS BJ: Surface morphology of lens fibers

from eyes of normal and microphthalmic (Browman) rats. Cell Tissue Res 167:425, 1976

JAKUS MA: Studies on the cornea: II. The fine structure of Descemet's membrane. J Biophys Biochem Cytol (Suppl) 2:243, 1956

MACDONALD AL, BASU PK, MILLER RG: The systemic production of cytotoxic lymphoid cells in corneal allograft reaction. Transplantation 23:431, 1977

RICHARDSON KC: The fine structure of the albino rabbit iris with special reference to the identification of adrenergic and cholinergic nerves and nerve endings in the intrinsic muscles. Am J Anat 114:173, 1964

SWANN DA: Chemistry and biology of the vitreous body. Int Rev Exp Pathol 22:2, 1980

WILLIS NR, HOLLENBERG MJ, BRACKEVELT CR: The fine structure of the lens of the fetal rat. Can J Ophthalmol 4:307, 1969

Retina and Photoreceptors

ANDERSON DH, FISHER SK, STEINBERG RH: Mammalian cones: Disc shedding, phagocytosis, and renewal. Invest Ophthalmol Vis Sci 17:117, 1978

BESHARSE JC: The daily light-dark cycle and rhythmic metabolism in the photoreceptor-pigment epithelial complex. Progress in Retinal Research 1:81, 1982

BOK D: Retinal photoreceptor-pigment epithelium interactions. Invest Ophthalmol Vis Sci 26:1659, 1985

BORWEIN B: The retinal receptor: A description. In Enoch JM, Tobey FL (eds): Springer Series in Optical Sciences, Vol 23: Vertebrate Photoreceptor Optics, p 11. Berlin, Springer-Verlag, 1981

BORWEIN B: Scanning electron microscopy of monkey foveal photoreceptors. Anat Rec 205:363, 1983

CUNHA-VAZ JG (ed): The Blood–Retinal Barriers. New York, Plenum, 1980

DOWLING JE: Foveal receptors of the monkey retina: Fine structure. Science 147:57, 1965

DROZ B: Dynamic condition of proteins in the visual cells of rats and mice as shown by radioautography with labeled amino acids. Anat Rec 145:157, 1963

HOLLENBERG MJ, BERNSTEIN MH: Fine structure of the photoreceptor cells of the ground squirrel. Am J Anat 118:359, 1966

JACOBS GH: Comparative Color Vision. New York, Academic Press, 1981

KANEKO A: Physiology of the retina. Annu Rev Neurosci 2:169, 1979

MASLAND RH: The functional architecture of the retina. Sci Am 255 No 6:102, 1986

NOBACK CR, LAEMLE LK: Structural and functional aspects of the visual pathways of primates. In The Primate Brain. Advances in Primatology. Vol 1, p 55. New York, Appleton-Century-Crofts, 1970

SCHWARTZ EA: First events in vision: The generation of responses in vertebrate rods. J Cell Biol 90:271, 1982

SJOSTRAND FS: The electron microscopy of the retina. In Smelser GK (ed): The Structure of the Eye. New York, Academic Press, 1961

STEINBERG RH, REID M, LACY PL: The distribution of rods and cones in the retina of the cat (Felix domesticus). J Comp Neurol 148: 229, 1973

WOLKEN JJ: The photoreceptor structures. Int Rev Cytol 11:195, 1961

YOUNG RW: A difference between rods and cones in the renewal of outer segment protein. Invest Ophthalmol 8:222, 1969

YOUNG RW: The organization of vertebrate photoreceptor cells. In Straatsma BR, Hall MO, Allen RA, Crescitelli F (eds): The Retina: Morphology, Function and Clinical Characteristics. UCLA Forum in Medical Sciences, No 8. Berkeley and Los Angeles, University of California Press, 1969

YOUNG RW: The renewal of photoreceptor cell outer segments. J Cell Biol 33:61, 1967

YOUNG RW: The renewal of rod and cone outer segments in the Rhesus monkey. J Cell Biol 49:303, 1971

YOUNG RW: Visual cells. Sci Am 223:80, October, 1970

YOUNG RW: Visual cells and the concept of renewal. Invest Ophthalmol 15:700, 1976

YOUNG RW, BOK D: Autoradiographic studies on the metabolism of the retinal pigment epithelium. Invest Ophthalmol 9:524, 1970

ZINN KM, MARMOR MF (eds): The Retinal Pigment Epithelium. Cambridge, MA, Harvard University Press, 1979

The Ear: General

BATTEAU DW: Role of the pinna in localization: Theoretical and physiological consequences. In Hearing Mechanisms in Vertebrates, A Ciba Foundation Symposium, pp 234. London, J & A Churchill, 1968

FRIEDMANN I, BALLANTYNE J (eds): Ultrastructural Atlas of the Inner Ear. London, Butterworths, 1984

HAWKINS JE, JOHNSSON LG: Light microscopic observations of the inner ear in man and monkey. Ann Otol 77:608, 1968

KESSEL RG, KARDON RH: Nervous tissue—eye and ear. In Tissues and Organs: A Text-Atlas of Scanning Electron Microscopy. San Francisco, WH Freeman, 1979

LIM J, LANE WC: Three-dimensional observations of the inner ear with the scanning electron microscope. Trans Am Acad Ophthalmol Otolaryngol. pp 842, September–October, 1969

LUNDQUIST PG, KIMURA R, WERSÄLL J: Ultrastructural organization of the epithelial lining in the endolymphatic duct and sac in the guinea pig. Acta Otolaryngol 57:65, 1963

SMITH CA: Electron microscopy of the inner ear. Ann Otol 77:629, 1968

WERSÄLL J: Efferent innervation of the inner ear. In Von Euler C, et al (eds): Structure and Function of Inhibitory Neuronal Mechanisms, p 123. Oxford and New York, Pergamon Press, 1968

Cochlea, Hair Cells, Organ of Corti, and Vestibular Labyrinth

ANNIKO M: Development of otoconia. Am J Otolaryngol 1:400, 1980

DUVALL AJ, FLOCK Å, WERSÄLL J: The ultrastructure of the sensory hairs and associated organelles of the cochlear inner hair cell with reference to directional sensitivity. J Cell Biol 29:497, 1966

ENGSTRÖM, H, WERSÄLL J: Structure and innervation of the inner ear sensory epithelia. Int Rev Cytol 7:353, 1958

FERNANDEZ C, GOLDBERG JM, ABEND WR: Response to static tilts of peripheral neurons innervating otolith organs of the squirrel monkey. J Neurophysiol 35:978, 1972

FLOCK Å: The structure of the macula utriculi with special reference to directional interplay of sensory response as revealed by morphological polarization. J Cell Biol 22:413, 1964

GULLEY RL, REESE TS: Freeze fracture studies on the synapses in the organ of Corti. J Comp Neurol 171:517, 1977

HAWKINS JE, Jr: Cytoarchitectural basis of the cochlear transduct. Cold Spring Harbor. Symp Quant Biol 30:147, 1965

HUDSPETH AJ: The hair cells of the inner ear. Sci Am 248 No 1:54, 1983

HUNTER-DUVAR IM: Hearing and hair cells. Canadian Journal of Otolaryngology 4:152, 1975

JOHNSSON LG, HAWKINS JE, Jr: Otolithic membranes of the saccule and utricle in man. Science 157:1454, 1967

KIMURA RS: The ultrastructure of the organ of Corti. Int Rev Cytol 42:173, 1975

KIMURA R, LINDQUIST PG, WERSÄLL J: Secretory epithelial linings in the ampullae of the guinea pig labyrinth. Acta Otolaryngol 57:517, 1963

LAWRENCE M, BURGIO PA: The attachment of the tectorial membrane revealed by scanning electron microscope. Ann Otol Rhinol Laryngol 89:325, 1980

LIM DJ: Formation and fate of the otoconia, scanning and transmission electron microscopy. Ann Otol Rhinol Laryngol 82:23, 1973

MONEY KE, SCOTT JW: Functions of separate sensory receptors of nonauditory labyrinth of the cat. Am J Physiol 202:1211, 1962

PARKER DE: The vestibular apparatus. Sci Am 243 No 5:118, 1980

SOUDIJN ER: Scanning electron microscopy of the organ of Corti. Ann Otol Rhinol Laryngol (Suppl) 86:16, 1976

WERSÄLL J: Studies on the structure and innervation of the sensory epithelium of the cristae ampullares in the guinea pig: A light and electron microscopic investigation. Acta Otolaryngol (Suppl) 126:1, 1956

WERSÄLL J, FLOCK Å, LUNDQUIST PG: Structural basis for directional sensitivity in cochlear and vestibular sensory receptors. Cold Spring Harbor. Symp Quant Biol 30:115, 1965

INDEX

*Page numbers in **boldface** indicate major discussions; t following a page number indicates tabular material.*